Nanotechnologies for the Life Sciences
Volume 10

Nanomaterials for Medical Diagnosis and Therapy

Edited by
Challa S. S. R. Kumar

1807–2007 Knowledge for Generations

Each generation has its unique needs and aspirations. When Charles Wiley first opened his small printing shop in lower Manhattan in 1807, it was a generation of boundless potential searching for an identity. And we were there, helping to define a new American literary tradition. Over half a century later, in the midst of the Second Industrial Revolution, it was a generation focused on building the future. Once again, we were there, supplying the critical scientific, technical, and engineering knowledge that helped frame the world. Throughout the 20th Century, and into the new millennium, nations began to reach out beyond their own borders and a new international community was born. Wiley was there, expanding its operations around the world to enable a global exchange of ideas, opinions, and know-how.

For 200 years, Wiley has been an integral part of each generation's journey, enabling the flow of information and understanding necessary to meet their needs and fulfill their aspirations. Today, bold new technologies are changing the way we live and learn. Wiley will be there, providing you the must-have knowledge you need to imagine new worlds, new possibilities, and new opportunities.

Generations come and go, but you can always count on Wiley to provide you the knowledge you need, when and where you need it!

William J. Pesce
President and Chief Executive Officer

Peter Booth Wiley
Chairman of the Board

Nanotechnologies for the Life Sciences
Volume 10

Nanomaterials for Medical Diagnosis and Therapy

Edited by
Challa S. S. R. Kumar

1st Edition

BICENTENNIAL 1807 WILEY 2007 BICENTENNIAL

WILEY-VCH Verlag GmbH & Co. KGaA

The Editor

Dr. Challa S. S. R. Kumar
The Center for Advanced
Microstructures and Devices
(CAMD)
Louisiana State University
6980 Jefferson Highway
Baton Rouge, LA 70806
USA

Cover
Cover design by G. Schulz based on
Micrograph courtesy of P. Broz,
Medical ICU, University Hospital Basel,
Switzerland

Library of Congress Card No.: applied for

British Library Cataloguing-in-Publication Data
A catalogue record for this book is available from the British Library.

Bibliographic information published by the Deutsche Nationalbibliothek
Die Deutsche Nationalbibliothek lists this publication in the Deutsche Nationalbibliografie; detailed bibliographic data are available in the Internet at ⟨http://dnb.d-nb.de⟩.

Typesetting Asco Typesetters, Hong Kong
Printing betz-druck GmbH, Darmstadt
Binding Litges & Dopf GmbH, Heppenheim
Cover Design Grafik-Design Schulz, Fußgönheim
Wiley Bicentennial Logo Richard J. Pacifico

Printed in the Federal Republic of Germany
Printed on acid-free paper

ISBN 978-3-527-31390-7

Contents of the Series

Kumar, C. S. S. R. (ed.)

Nanotechnologies for the Life Sciences (NtLS)

Book Series

Vol. 1

Biofunctionalization of Nanomaterials

2005, Hardcover
ISBN-10: 3-527-31381-8
ISBN-13: 987-3-527-31381-5

Vol. 2

Biological and Pharmaceutical Nanomaterials

2005, Hardcover
ISBN-10: 3-527-31382-6
ISBN-13: 987-3-527-31382-2

Vol. 3

Nanosystem Characterization Tools in the Life Sciences

2005, Hardcover
ISBN-10: 3-527-31383-4
ISBN-13: 987-3-527-31383-9

Vol. 4

Nanodevices for the Life Sciences

2006, Hardcover
ISBN-10: 3-527-31384-2
ISBN-13: 987-3-527-31384-6

Vol. 5

Nanomaterials – Toxicity, Health and Environmental Issues

2006, Hardcover
ISBN-10: 3-527-31385-0
ISBN-13: 987-3-527-31385-3

Vol. 6

Nanomaterials for Cancer Therapy

2006, Hardcover
ISBN-10: 3-527-31386-9
ISBN-13: 987-3-527-31386-0

Vol. 7

Nanomaterials for Cancer Diagnosis

2006, Hardcover
ISBN-10: 3-527-31387-7
ISBN-13: 987-3-527-31387-7

Vol. 8

Nanomaterials for Biosensors

2006, Hardcover
ISBN-10: 3-527-31388-5
ISBN-13: 987-3-527-31388-4

Vol. 9

Tissue, Cell and Organ Engineering

2006, Hardcover
ISBN-10: 3-527-31389-3
ISBN-13: 987-3-527-31389-1

Vol. 10

Nanomaterials for Medical Diagnosis and Therapy

2006, Hardcover
ISBN-10: 3-527-31390-7
ISBN-13: 987-3-527-31390-7

Foreword

As the traditional compartmentalization of science and engineering into discrete disciplines dissolves, scientists of all backgrounds find that their work is part of a bigger, much more magnificent picture, unrestricted by doctrine, educational plans or other previous, tangible constraints. Hence, nanotechnology and the life sciences enjoy a growing synergy of materials, methods, and mechanisms common or beneficial to both, giving rise to new ideas, novel approaches, understanding of phenomena and a fertile exchange of concepts, strategies and goals.

Although this rapidly growing and evolving field is still in a nascent stage, recent successes are fuelling the vision of "bottom-up" fabrication and assembly processes and man's ability to purposefully control events when nanostructured materials and biological entities encounter each other on the nanoscale.

Some significant functional materials and devices have been realized, especially on the diagnostic front, and an even larger number are waiting to be discovered by pioneering work to come, based upon the foundations laid today.

It is this vision which needs to be transported – between the disciplines, from teachers to pupils, from scientists to policy makers, from experts to the general public, and, especially, from colleague to colleague for fruitful collaboration and success in the search for further pieces of the magnificent puzzle of Everything: Nature, Life, and the Universe.

Nanotechnologies for the Life Sciences (NtLS) aims to fulfill this quest for passing on knowledge to the mutual benefit of its authors and readers by stimulating scientific exchange and disseminating vital knowledge to provide insight into the ongoing exploration of the potent opportunities around the corner.

With over 4600 pages in 124 chapters, these ten volumes are the first major effort to cover the whole breadth and width of this highly dynamic and exciting field, and in leading this effort, Challa S. S. R. Kumar and his numerous authors have brought together an exciting, provocative, and informative source of knowledge and stimulation for all those active in this field or wanting to become so.

Evanston, November 2006 *Chad Mirkin*

Nanotechnologies for the Life Sciences Vol. 10
Nanomaterials for Medical Diagnosis and Therapy. Edited by Challa S. S. R. Kumar

ISBN: 978-3-527-31390-7

Contents

Nanotechnologies for the Life Sciences Vol. 10
Nanomaterials for Medical Diagnosis and Therapy. Edited by Challa S. S. R. Kumar

ISBN: 978-3-527-31390-7

Preface

From the time the human mind emerged, about fifty thousand years ago, our understanding of the human body and of ways and means to protect ourselves better from both natural degradation as well as diseases has been continuously growing. The human mind has been responsible for triggering creative technological breakthroughs at different intervals, significantly improving our quality of life at each of these stages. We are again standing on the threshold of yet another technological mastery with the ability to create nanomaterials akin to natural sub-micron biomolecules for the protection of our body and to prolong its life. The purpose of this book, *Nanomaterials for Medical Diagnosis and Therapy*, is to reveal for the first time how man-made nano-sized materials are being judiciously combined with biological molecules in order to find hitherto unimaginable, superior diagnostic tools and novel therapeutic approaches to alleviate human suffering. Most of what you will read here will provide you with a broader perspective to how nanotechnology is going to revolutionize medicine in the close future. You are unlikely to get such a perspective reading individual articles from the scientific journals. This is the final volume in the ten-volume series on *Nanotechnologies for the Life Sciences (NtLS)* and in a way reflects the ultimate goal of all life scientists, with the other nine volumes as guide posts, to improve our health and quality of living. The book has sixteen chapters, covering all aspects of medical diagnosis and therapy except cancer as this subject is covered in volumes six and seven. With over 700 pages, it is the largest of all the ten volumes. Before I go ahead with giving you details of individual chapters in this final volume, I would like to take this opportunity to provide you glimpses of the information contained in the first nine volumes, which many of you may have already read.

The first volume in the series *Biofunctionalization of Nanomaterials*, with eleven chapters, dealt with various approaches to attach biomolecules to nanomaterials for applications in the life sciences, and the second volume *Biological and Pharmaceutical Nanomaterials*, with twelve chapters, focused on natural nanomaterials that are relevant to the life sciences. The ability to characterize systems in nanoscale is pivotal to the success of nanotechnology, and the third volume *Nanosystem Characterization Tools for the Life Sciences*, with eleven chapters, is a useful source of information both for life scientists interested in nanoscale systems and for characterization specialists interested in applying their tools in biological systems. The

Nanotechnologies for the Life Sciences Vol. 10
Nanomaterials for Medical Diagnosis and Therapy. Edited by Challa S. S. R. Kumar

ISBN: 978-3-527-31390-7

fourth volume of the series, *Nanodevices for the Life Sciences*, contains thirteen chapters and is a compendium of the exciting possibilities that exist in the world of tiny devices. The fifth volume, entitled *Nanomaterials – Toxicity, Health and Environmental Issues*, reviews some of the critical risk assessment issues, which are crucial in life sciences, that are currently being investigated by the health & environmental nano researchers, and has twelve chapters. The sixth and the seventh volumes, *Nanomaterials for Cancer Therapy* and *Nanomaterials for Cancer Diagnosis*, with a total of twenty-two chapters, captured nanotechnological approaches for the treatment of cancer and their utility in developing tools and materials for sensitive and early diagnosis of this serious affliction. While the eighth volume, *Nanomaterials for Biosensors*, containing thirteen chapters, touches upon biomolecular sensing using a variety of Nanomaterials, the ninth volume *Tissue, Cell and Organ Engineering* with its twelve chapters is an encyclopedia on nanotechnological approaches to the engineering of biologically functional matter capable of serving as tissue or organ replacement. The ten volume series on *Nanotechnologies for the Life Sciences* with 122 chapters contributed by about 150 researchers across the globe totaling some 4600 pages comes to conclusion with the publication of the tenth volume.

This tenth volume begins with the chapter entitled *Nanotechnologies for Diagnosis – Present and Future*, which is a contribution by Gareth A. Hughes of Zyvex Corporation in Richardson, Texas, USA. In this chapter, a general discussion on various aspects of diagnostics including *in vitro* diagnostics (IVDs), implantable sensors and imaging techniques is presented in addition to touching upon regulatory and ethical considerations. Moving to a more specific diagnostic tool, authors lead by Jean-Marc Idée from Guerbet, Aulnay-sous-Bois, France, brings out the importance of Superparamagnetic Iron Oxide Nanoparticles (SPIONs) as contrast agents in Magnetic resonance Imaging. The chapter, *Superparamagnetic Nanoparticles of Iron Oxides for Magnetic Resonance Imaging Applications*, is a comprehensive source of information on the unique capability of SPIONs as contrast agents for MRI of the gastrointestinal tract, liver & spleen, lymph node, blood pool, and atheromatous plaque.

The third chapter, *Carbon Nanotube-based Vectors for Delivering Immunotherapeutics and Drugs*, reviews the application of carbon nanotubes in drug delivery and biosensing. Alberto Bianco and co-workers from the Insititute of Molecular and Cellular Biology in Strasbourg, France, have done a commendable job in delineating the pros and cons of utilizing the unique property of CNTs, the penetration ability with capacity for high loading, for innovative medical diagnosis and therapies. The team lead by Soon Hong Yuk from Hannam University in Taejeon, Korea, contributed the fourth chapter, entitled *Core-Shell Nanoparticles for Drug Delivery and Molecular Imaging*. In this chapter, the authors focus on core-shell nanoparticle architecture with a layer of polymeric materials surrounding an organic or inorganic nanoparticle core, and demonstrate that such architectures provide improved stability and a sustained release pattern of protein drug and decreased cytotoxicity. In the fifth chapter, *Nanotechnologies for Targeted Delivery of Drugs*, various aspects of targeted delivery utilizing different types of nanomaterials are highlighted. Authors Pavel Brož and Patrick Hunziker from the Medical Intensive Care unit of Basel University Hospital in Switzerland present successful targeting strategies employed that use both 'natural nanostructures' (such as bacteria and viruses) and 'artificial nanostructures' (lipid-based ones such as liposomes and micelles, protein-based ones such as dendrimers, and polymer-based ones such as nanoparticles, nanospheres and nanocontainers) in areas other than cancer.

The sixth chapter, *Nanoporous and Nanosize Materials for Drug Delivery Systems*, written by Yoshinobu Fukumori, Kanji Takada and Hirofumi Takeuchi from Kyoto Pharmaceutical University, Japan, covers application of a number of inorganic, organic and natural nanoporous materials in general and nanoporous silica-based materials in particular for medical therapy. Continuing on the theme of core-shell nanoparticles as described in a general way in the fourth chapter, Yoko Yamaguchi and Rie Igarashi from the Institute of Medical Science of St Marianna University in Kanagawa, Japan, present their efforts in the seventh chapter towards the development of a specific non-spherical core-shell product, NanoEggTM, for dermatological applications. The chapter, *NanoEggTM Technology for Drug Delivery*, describes the commercialization of these particles for overcoming the limitations of classical ATRA (all-*trans* retinoic acid) treatment through controlled release.

Polymeric nanomaterials have been receiving a lot of attention as materials of choice for both drug delivery as well as diagnostic tools due to their unique physicochemical characteristics that allow for controlling the fate of a drug within the patient. Three chapters, 8, 9 and 10, have been dedicated to bring out comprehensively the information present in the literature on different facets and types of polymeric nanomaterials for application in medical diagnosis and therapy. The eighth chapter, *Polymeric Nanomaterials – Synthesis, Functionalization and Applications in Diagnosis and Therapy*, a contribution from the laboratories of Rachel Auzély-Velty from the Centre de Recherches sur les Macromolécules Végétales (CERMAV) in Grenoble, France, focuses on 'frozen', non-dynamic polymeric nanomaterials, where an exchange between individual polymer chains and polymer chains of the nanoobject cannot take place, unlike the dynamic systems such as micelles and liposomes. On the other hand, the ninth chapter, *Polymeric Nanoparticles for Drug Delivery*, authored by P. Kallinteri and M. C. Garnett from the School of Pharmacy of Nottingham University, UK, brings out the physiology and anatomy underlying the diseases which may be treatable using polymeric nanomaterials and the way these are handled by the body. In the tenth chapter, *Solid Lipid and Polymeric Nanoparticles for Drug Delivery*, the authors José Luis Pedraz and co-workers from the University of Basque Country in Vitoria, Spain, present a comparative analysis of solid lipid nanoparticles (SLNs) and polymeric nanoparticles with reference to their production processes, characterization, and a wide ranging therapeutic applications.

Chapter eleven by Zach Hilt from the University of Kentucky in Lexington, USA, explores the relatively underdeveloped field of hydrogels. In this chapter aptly titled as *Intelligent Hydrogels in Nanoscale Sensing and Drug Delivery Applications*, the author has done a great job in providing an up-to-date review on the application of intelligent hydrogels such as ionic and temperature-responsive, biohybrid and imprinted hydrogels in micro/nanoscale sensing and drug delivery. In the twelfth chapter, *Nanoshells for Drug Delivery*, a layer-by-layer self assembly approach to nanoshell formation is described in addition to the utility of nanoshells in controlled release of pharmaceutical ingredients. Authors Melgardt M. De Villiers and Yuri Lvov from the University of Wisconsin and Louisiana Tech University respectively, compare in a systematic fashion two types of nanoshells – metallic nanoparticles composed of a dielectric core (e.g. silica) coated with an ultra thin metallic layer (e.g. gold) and nanoshells formed by electrostatic layer-by-layer molecular self-assembling (E-LbL) for drug delivery applications. L. Andrew Lee, Hannah N. Barnhill and Qian Wang from University of South Carolina provide an overview on the topic of the programming of the Bionanoparticles (BNPs) and current research on their biomedical applications in the thirteenth chapter entitled *Bionanoparticles and their Biomedical Applications*. This chapter is a must-read for all those interested in BNPs and how they can be exploited for generating novel biotemplates in the nanometer range for a myriad of biomedical applications.

As we reach the end of the book, the last three chapters assume special importance. While chapter fourteen contributed by Hironori Nakagami, Yasuhiko Tabata and Yasufumi Kaneda from Osaka University, Japan, reiterates the importance of nanotechnologies in gene therapy, the fifteenth chapter, written by S. M. Moghimi from the University of Brighton, UK, cautions about the possible toxic effects of a well-known gene transfer vector. The titles of the two chapters are *Nanotechnology for Gene Therapy – HVJ-E Vector* and *Nanotoxicology of Synthetic Gene Transfer Vectors: Poly (ethyleneimine) – and Polyfectin-mediated Membrane Damage and Apoptosis in Human Cell Lines*, respectively. The final chapter by Gang Liu and Ping Men from the University of Utah in Salt Lake City, USA, entitled *Nanoparticles for the Treatment of Alzheimer's Disease: The Theoretical Rationale, Present Status and Future Perspectives* indicates that nanotechnology has potential to treat Alzheimer's disease (AD), the most devastating neurodegenerative disorder with progressive and irreversible damage to thought, memory and language. I am very confident that the information that is presented in these sixteen chapters in this tenth volume will help in furthering the utility of nanotechnological approaches in medical diagnosis and therapy. I am, as always, very grateful to all the authors for their scholarly presentations of their topics, providing timely inputs and corrections in making the final volume in this series a reality.

As I conclude this ten-volume series, I would like to reinforce some of the comments that I made in my preface to the first volume. As I said, nanotechnology's greatest gift to mankind, in my view, is its ability to promote lateral thinking amongst not only scientists, but all those who are associated with this new approach, the so called 'nano thinking' to problem solving. On behalf of all the authors who have made contributions to this exciting series, it is my privilege to play the role of a catalyst in inculcating this new thinking by providing a multi-pronged base of knowledge in nanotechnologies for the life sciences. It is my hope that this book series will help in stretching the limits of thinking in all those who come in contact with it.

It is yet another opportunity for me to convey my thanks to each and every person (unfortunately due to lack of space I am unable to mention all the names) with whom I had the privilege of interacting and who have helped me directly or indirectly during the course of the publication of the whole series. I would like to express my gratitude to the following people for their support and assistance. My employer and colleagues at the Center for Advanced Microstructures and Devices, graduate advisor Prof. N.R. Krishnaswamy who laid the foundation to my career, family and friends, and the Wiley-VCH publishing team, Martin Ottmar, Esther Dörring, Nele Denzau and Eva Wille, with whom I had great pleasure in working.

Finally, my special thanks to you, the readers, for ensuring that the knowledge base provided in this book series will be a building block for further understanding of nanoscience. I do realize that there is a lot of scope for improvement and need to add new topics to this book series. I am hoping that I will be able to, with your comments and suggestions, take this series to a new level in the near future.

October 2006, Baton Rouge *Challa S.S.R. Kumar*

List of Contributors

Maria Angeles Solinis
Department of Pharmacy and Pharmaceutical Technology
University of the Basque Country
P. de la Universidad 7
01006 Vitoria-Gasteiz
Spain

Rachel Auzély-Velty
Centre de Recherches sur les Macromolécules Végétales (CERMAV)
38041 Grenoble Cedex 9
France

Hannah N. Barnhill
Department of Chemistry and Biochemistry and Nanocenter
University of South Carolina
Columbia, SC 29208
USA

Alberto Bianco
Institute of Molecular and Cellular Biology
UPR 9021 CNRS
67084 Strasbourg
France

Bruno Bonnemain
Research Division
Guerbet
93600 Aulnay-sous-Bois
France

Pavel Brož
Medical Intensive Care Unit
University Hospital Basel
4031 Basel
Switzerland

Claire Corot
Research Division
Guerbet
93600 Aulnay-sous-Bois
France

Sun Hang Cho
Nanobiomaterials Laboratories
Korea Research Institute of Chemical Technology
Taejeon
Korea 305-600

Melgardt M. De Villiers
School of Pharmacy
University of Wisconsin-Madison
Madison, WI 53705
USA

Amaia Esquisabel
Department of Pharmacy and Pharmaceutical Technology
University of the Basque Country
P. de la Universidad 7
01006 Vitoria-Gasteiz
Spain

Yoshinobu Fukumori
Department of Pharmacokinetics
Kyoto Pharmaceutical University
Nakauchi-Cho 5, Yamashina-ku
Kyoto 607-8414
Japan

Martin C. Garnett
School of Pharmacy
University of Nottingham
University Park
Nottingham NG7 2RD
UK

Alicia R. Gascón
Department of Pharmacy and Pharmaceutical Technology
University of the Basque Country
P. de la Universidad 7
01006 Vitoria-Gasteiz
Spain

Sung Kyun Han
Department of Polymer Science and Engineering
Hannam University
Daejeon
Korea 306-791

Rosa M. Hernández
Department of Pharmacy and Pharmaceutical Technology
University of the Basque Country
P. de la Universidad 7
01006 Vitoria-Gasteiz
Spain

J. Zach Hilt
Department of Chemical and Materials Engineering
University of Kentucky
Lexington, KY 40506-0046
USA

Gareth A. Hughes
Zyvex Corporation
Richardson, TX 75081
USA

Patrick Hunziker
National Centre of Competence in Research Nanoscale Science
University of Basel
4056 Basel
Switzerland

Jean-Marc Idée
Research Division
Guerbet
93600 Aulnay-sous-Bois
France

Rie Igarashi
Institute of Medical Science
School of Medicine
St Marianna University
Kanagawa-ken 216-8512
Japan

Manoli Igartua
Department of Pharmacy and Pharmaceutical Technology
University of the Basque Country
P. de la Universidad 7
01006 Vitoria-Gasteiz
Spain

Christine Jérôme
Center for Education and Research on Macromolecules (CERM)
University of Liège
4000 Liège
Belgium

Robert Jérôme
Center for Education and Research on Macromolecules (CERM)
University of Liège
4000 Liège
Belgium

Paraskevi Kallinteri
School of Pharmacy
University of Nottingham
University Park
Nottingham NG7 2RD
UK

Yasufumi Kaneda
Division of Gene Therapy Science
Graduate School of Medicine
Osaka University
Osaka 565-0871
Japan

Ree Sun Kim
Department of Polymer Science and Engineering
Hannam University
Daejeon
Korea 306-791

Cédric Klumpp
Institute of Molecular and Cellular Biology
UPR 9021 CNRS
67084 Strasbourg
France

Kostas Kostarelos
Centre for Drug Delivery Research
School of Pharmacy
University of London
London WC1N 1AX
UK

Lara Lacerda
Institute of Molecular and Cellular Biology
UPR 9021 CNRS
67084 Strasbourg
France

Jin Ho Lee
Department of Polymer Science and Engineering
Hannam University
Daejeon
Korea 306-791

L. Andrew Lee
Department of Chemistry and Biochemistry and Nanocenter
University of South Carolina
Columbia, SC 29208
USA

Gang Liu
Radiobiology
University of Utah
729, Arapeen Drive
Suite 2334
Salt Lake City, UT 84102-1218
USA

Yuri Lvov
Institute for Micro-manufacturing and Department of Biomedical Engineering
Louisiana Tech University
Ruston, LA 71272
USA

Ping Men
Radiobiology
University of Utah
729, Arapeen Drive
Suite 2334
Salt Lake City, UT 84102-1218
USA

Seyed M. Moghimi
Molecular Targeting and Polymer Toxicology Group
School of Pharmacy
University of Brighton
Brighton BN2 4GJ
UK

Hironori Nakagami
Division of Gene Therapy Science
Graduate School of Medicine
Osaka University
Osaka 565-0871
Japan

Gorka Orive
Department of Pharmacy and Pharmaceutical Technology
University of the Basque Country
P. de la Universidad 7
01006 Vitoria-Gasteiz
Spain

Marc Port
Research Division
Guerbet
93600 Aulnay-sous-Bois
France

Charalambos D. Partidos
Institute of Molecular and Cellular Biology
UPR 9021 CNRS
67084 Strasbourg
France

Giorgia Pastorin
Institute of Molecular and Cellular Biology
UPR 9021 CNRS
67084 Strasbourg
France

José Luis Pedraz
Department of Pharmacy and Pharmaceutical Technology
University of the Basque Country
P. de la Universidad 7
01006 Vitoria-Gasteiz
Spain

George Perry
Biology Department
University of Texas at San Antonio
San Antonio, TX 78249-1644
USA

Maurizio Prato
Department of Pharmaceutical Sciences
University of Trieste
34127 Trieste
Italy

Philippe Prigent
Research Division
Guerbet
93600 Aulnay-sous-Bois
France

Isabelle Raynal
Research Division
Guerbet
93600 Aulnay-sous-Bois
France

Jutta Rieger
Centre de Recherches sur les Macromolécules Végétales (CERMAV)
38041 Grenoble Cedex 9
France

Philippe Robert
Research Division
Guerbet
93600 Aulnay-sous-Bois
France

Caroline Robic
Research Division
Guerbet
93600 Aulnay-sous-Bois
France

Michel Schaefer
Guerbet
Research Division
93600 Aulnay-sous-Bois
France

Mark A. Smith
Department of Pathology
School of Medicine
Case Western Reserve University
Cleveland, OH 44106-7288
USA

Yasuhiko Tabata
Department of Biomaterials
Fields of Tissue Engineering
Institute for Frontier Medical Sciences
Kyoto University
Kyoto 606
Japan

Giyoong Tae
Department of Material Science and Engineering
Gwangju Institute of Science and Technology
Gwangju
Korea 500-712

Kanji Takada
Department of Pharmacokinetics
Kyoto Pharmaceutical University
Nakauchi-Cho 5, Yamashina-ku
Kyoto 607-8414
Japan

Hirofumi Takeuchi
Department of Pharmacokinetics
Kyoto Pharmaceutical University
Nakauchi-Cho 5, Yamashina-ku
Kyoto 607-8414
Japan

Qian Wang
Department of Chemistry and Biochemistry and Nanocenter
University of South Carolina
Columbia, SC 29208
USA

Wei Wu
Institute of Molecular and Cellular Biology
UPR 9021 CNRS
67084 Strasbourg
France

Yoko Yamaguchi
Institute of Medical Science
School of Medicine
St Marianna University
Kanagawa-ken 216-8512
Japan

Soon Hong Yuk
Department of Polymer Science and Engineering
Hannam University
Daejeon
Korea 306-791

1 Nanotechnologies for Diagnosis – Present and Future

Gareth A. Hughes

1.1 Introduction to Patient Diagnostics

This chapter highlights the capabilities of nanoscale materials and devices for patient diagnostics. Current state-of-the-art diagnostic applications in development are reviewed with an extensive list of references provided for further investigation. The chapter is broken down into four major areas: *in vitro* and *in vivo* diagnostics (optical, electrical, magnetic, mechanical), imaging diagnostics, nanotechnology-enhanced analytical tools and techniques for diagnostics, and the future for patient diagnostics. In comparison to other published chapters on the subject of nanotechnology for diagnostics, this chapter covers the gamut of diagnostics including *in vitro* diagnostics (IVDs), implantable sensors and imaging techniques. Finally, in addition to covering a variety of diagnostic tools and methods where nanotechnology can be implemented, regulatory and ethical considerations are briefly discussed, providing a foundation on which to build scientifically responsible nanotechnology developments for life sciences.

Patient diagnostics involves more than analyzing the symptoms of disease. Diagnostic tools and assays are used to determine tissue type prior to organ transplantation, to determine blood type for patients requiring blood transfusions, and to monitor the progression of disease and the effects of therapy. Diagnosing a patient prior to onset of any symptoms would be ideal. Catching a disease early would allow the patient to take appropriate precautions to slow, halt or possibly reverse the progression of the ailment. The ability to combine diagnostic testing with patient profiling such as a genetic screen could open up the possibility of personalized therapy. Table 1.1 lists examples of applications for patient diagnostics.

A variety of techniques and testing protocols are available for performing patient diagnostics. Many times, a combination of techniques or tests are performed to provide accurate diagnosis. Current diagnostic techniques include immunoassays, genetic-based tests, cell-based assays, tissue or histological tests and medical imaging. Immunoassays are used for numerous diagnostic applications including monitoring levels of endocrine hormones such as estrogen, cortisol and prolactin, detecting biomarkers following myocardial infarction such as troponin and myoglobin, diagnosing hepatitis A–E, and searching for various biomarkers for cancer.

Nanotechnologies for the Life Sciences Vol. 10
Nanomaterials for Medical Diagnosis and Therapy. Edited by Challa S. S. R. Kumar

ISBN: 978-3-527-31390-7

Tab. 1.1. List of diagnostic applications.

Diagnose disease susceptibility, risk assessment
Infectious disease assessment
Tissue typing for organ transplants
Screening for blood transfusions
Monitor therapy activity
Check disease progression
Personalized medicine
Genetic screening

Genetic-based diagnostics involve a variety of analytical techniques and gene expression profiling to determine susceptibility of disease. Cell-based assays involve high-throughput cell sorting along with intracellular imaging techniques. Two of the major focus areas for tissue-based testing are in cancer detection and in tissue typing for transplant patients. A variety of medical imaging tools exist ranging from magnetic resonance imaging to ultrasound. Imaging methods provide noninvasive means to diagnose disease.

There are also numerous specialized diagnostic techniques that are used when symptoms exist that warrant the use of a particular test. Specialized diagnostic techniques include electromyography (EMG) for monitoring nerve and muscle activity, electroencephalograph (EEG) to assess electrical activity of the brain, electrocardiography (ECG or EKG) to monitor electrical activity of the heart, tonometry for measuring internal eye pressure and spirometry to measure lung function. A summary of examples for testing protocols and techniques which are used in diagnostics are listed in Tab. 1.2. A comprehensive resource for diagnostics is the *Merck Manual of Diagnosis and Therapy* [1].

1.2
Nanotechnology and Patient Diagnostics

This chapter will summarize diagnostic applications of nanotechnology currently being development. Life science and medical applications of nanotechnology are numerous, ranging from tissue engineering, drug discovery to drug delivery and diagnostics [2, 3]. Nanotechnology is enabling a variety of diagnostic methods, including optical, electrical, magnetic, electrochemical and mechanical, and is enhancing established methods such as biomedical imaging techniques and spectroscopic methodology [4–22]. Handheld, wearable and implantable diagnostic tools for real-time patient monitoring can be manufactured when comprised of devices and materials precisely fabricated at the nanoscale [23].

Functionalized nanoparticles can enable multiplexed bioassays for simultaneous diagnostic screening of multiple diseases [24, 25]. High-capacity screening and combined molecular and immunological diagnostics will play a role in establishing

Tab. 1.2. Examples of techniques and testing protocols used in patient diagnostics.

Diagnostic type	Tool or technique used	Example applications
Immunoassay	enzyme-linked immunosorbent assay (ELISA)	cancer detection allergy tests, immunoglobulin (IgA, IgE, etc.) levels hormone levels C-reactive protein (CRP) infectious diseases autoimmune diseases diabetes assays prion disease diagnosis pancrease function tests
	bead-based assays	multiplexed assays cytokine levels cystic fibrosis testing blood typing metabolic disorders
	radioimmunoassay (RIA)	hormone levels liver function tests viral detection
	fluorescence polarization immunoassay (FPIA)	kidney function tests homocysteine levels
Genetic	single nucleotide polymorphism (SNP) analysis	sickle-cell cystic fibrosis testing p53 mutation detection metabolic disorders pharmacogenomics drug efficacy
	DNA chips and microarrays	multiplexed assays cancer detection tuberculosis drug efficacy
	polymerase chain reaction (PCR)	DNA amplification infectious diseases inheritable diseases
	Northern blot	mRNA detection gene regulation analysis
	Southern blot	DNA detection inheritable diseases restriction fragment length polymorphisms (RFLP) for prenatal diagnostics

Tab. 1.2 *(continued)*

Diagnostic type	Tool or technique used	Example applications
Cellular	flow cytometry	leukocyte analysis detection of cancer cells in urine and blood monitoring HIV therapies bone marrow transplants
	hematology analyzers	blood cell count
	immunocytochemistry	evaluating intracellular activity
	fluorescent *in situ* hybridization (FISH)	infectious diseases
Tissue	immunohistochemical stains (IHC)	cancer detection organ transplants bone marrow transplants
	laser capture microdissection	cancer detection
	dielectric property analysis	cancer detection
Imaging	magnetic resonance imaging (MRI)	brain disorders spinal cord disorders blood vessel diseases internal organ diseases
	computed tomography (CT)	stroke internal organ diseases soft tissue diagnostics
	X-ray	arthritis osteoporosis congestive heart failure respiratory diseases
	ultrasound	internal organ diseases blood flow analysis
	positron emission tomography (PET)	cancer detection monitoring of cancer therapy coronary heart disease myocardial infarction blood flow analysis memory disorders seizure disorders
	optical coherence tomography (OCT)	high-resolution tissue diagnostics retinal diseases glaucoma

Tab. 1.2 *(continued)*

Diagnostic type	Tool or technique used	Example applications
	optoacoustic tomography (OAT) or photoacoustic tomography (PAT)	cancer detection
Specialty	electromyography (EMG)	muscle activity nerve conduction
	electroencephalography (EEG)	brain electrical activity
	electrocardiography (ECG or EKG)	heart electrical activity
	tonometry	glaucoma
	spirometry	evaluate lung function

a broader range of testing capabilities that will allow diagnostics to be not disease-specific, but patient-specific and support the development of pharmacogenomics [26, 27]. Ultimately, smart nanostructures such as nanoparticles, nanotubes and dendrimers could be fabricated with both targeting capability and therapeutic moieties enabling site-specific delivery of therapy and personalized medicine [28]. Table 1.3 lists diagnostic techniques enhanced or enabled by nanotechnology which will be described in further detail in this chapter.

Nanoscale entities are abundant in biological systems. Viruses, proteins, small molecule drugs and fluorescent dyes are all less than 100 nm, as shown in Fig. 1.1. Through the manipulation of organic and inorganic materials at the atomic level, novel materials, structures and devices can be realized. Thermal, optical, electrical and mechanical properties of materials can be enhanced. Novel properties, not observed in the bulk form of materials, can be harnessed. Chemical activity of substances can be tailored to a desired end use such as improving biocompatibility of implantable materials and developing artificial receptors for targeted analyte binding. Surface properties of materials, such as adhesion, can be modified. Properties of materials at the nanoscale can be quite different than bulk material properties. Due to greater surface area per unit volume, nanomaterials can exhibit higher chemical reactivity, increased mechanical strength, and faster electrical and magnetic responses.

The field of nanotechnology brings about the necessary convergence of technical disciplines such as physics, chemistry, engineering and computer science with the biological disciplines of molecular and cell biology, genetics, neuroscience, biophysics, and biochemistry. Through the convergence of all these disciplines, the field of nanotechnology is poised to create many breakthroughs across all industries. Medical applications show particular promise, including building blocks of

Tab. 1.3. Diagnostic techniques enabled or enhanced by nanotechnology.

Technique	Applications
Optical	enhanced fluorescence quantum dots surface plasmon resonance (SPR) nanoparticles nanoshells bio-barcodes Probes encapsulated by biologically localized embedding (PEBBLEs) fiber optics
Electrical	amperometric conductimetric potentiometric enzymatic
Magnetic	immunoassays magnetofection magnetoresistive
Mechanical	nanocantilevers surface acoustic waves (SAWs) quartz crystal balance
Imaging	contrast agents multifunctional agents
Mass spectrometry	nanoparticle pre-concentrator
Raman spectroscopy	surface enhanced Raman spectroscopy (SERS) tip enhanced Raman spectroscopy (TERS)
Genetics	nanopore sequencing
Immunoassays	luminescent nanoparticles

nucleic acids as structural components as binding agents similar to antibodies rather than typical genetic maps, nanostructured biosensors for implantable patient monitoring and nanoparticles as imaging contrast agents.

Patient diagnostics can be broken down into three major modalities: assays, biosensors and imaging. Nanotechnology plays a role in improving these modalities and also creating novel diagnostic methods. *In vitro* assays are used extensively for diagnostics. Three commonly used assay formats are enzyme-linked immunosorbent assays (ELISAs), polymerase chain reaction (PCR)-based genetic assays, and staining assays such as Giemsa and Gram for viral and bacterial diagnostics. While many diseases and infections can be diagnosed with such assays, most of these assays require laboratory equipment. Point-of-care diagnostics are typically not possible using these assays. Samples are usually shipped to laboratories that

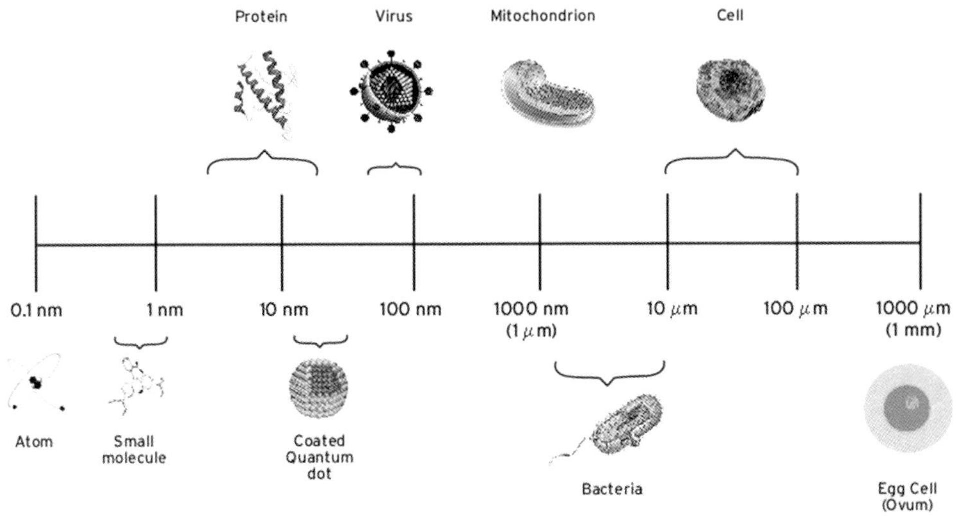

Figure 1.1. Scale of things, from atom to embryo.

specialize in performing these *in vitro* assays. Nanotechnology can improve these assays by increasing throughput for rapid diagnostics or by enhancing sensitivity which could enable catching a disease earlier.

Biosensors provide the ability to perform diagnostics at point-of-care and enable real-time diagnostics in the form of implantable devices. The general format of a biosensor, shown in Fig. 1.2, comprises of a biologically receptive site which binds specifically to the analyte in question and a transducer that translates the binding event into a measurable signal, which can be optical, electrical, magnetic or mechanical. Nanostructures can be used to enhance any of these transduction mechanisms. For example, nanoscale semiconductor materials (quantum dots) can be used in optical biosensors. In comparison to traditional organic fluorophores, quantum dots are much more photostable, have greater quantum efficiency and have much narrower emission. Such advantages could be used to develop highly sensitive optical biosensors and multiplexed assays. Due to high surface area, nanowires and nanotubes can greatly enhance charge transfer in biosensors based on electrical mechanisms. Functionalized magnetic nanoparticles can be targeted to desired analytes and detected with miniature magnetic sensors, creating portable diagnostics. Finally, nanocantilevers, modified with antibodies or other biological receptors, can be sensitive enough to detect a single biomolecule such as an individual viral particle.

Aptamers make up one particular class of biological receptor structures which show increasing potential for use in diagnostics. Aptamers are oligonucleotide sequences that are structured for high affinity and specificity towards a desired ligand, similar to antibodies, but formed from nucleic acids rather than amino acids. Since their discovery in the early 1990s [30] through the use of an *in vitro* technique named systematic evolution of ligands by exponential enrichment (SELEX),

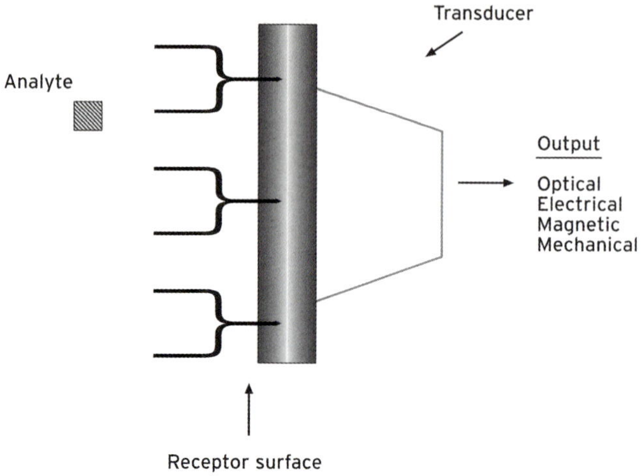

Figure 1.2. Major components of a biosensor.

many aptamers have been developed that bind various targets including thrombin, platelet-derived growth factor (PDGF) and keratinocyte growth factor (KGF). Recently, an anti- vascular endothelial growth factor (VEGF) aptamer was introduced as a new treatment for macular degeneration. Developing therapeutic applications for aptamers is an expanding area of research.

Aptamers have several advantages over monoclonal antibodies which have likewise generated much interest in therapeutics. Aptamers are fully processed *in vitro*. Antibodies require an animal model as a starting point. Therefore, tight process control and scale-up are much more achievable for aptamer production paving the way for lower cost therapeutics. Aptamers, especially DNA aptamers, are much

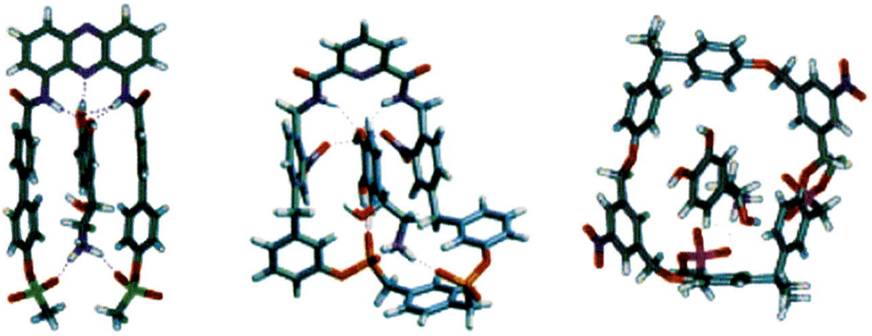

Figure 1.3. Synthetic noradrenaline receptors [42]. Reproduced with permission from J. Am. Chem. Soc., Vol. 127, S. Kolusheva et al., Selective detection of catecholamines by synthetic receptors embedded in chromatic polydiacetylene vesicles, p. 10000–10001. © (2005) American Chemical Society.

more stable than their antibody counterparts, which are large protein molecules that can readily degrade if appropriate storage conditions are not used. Even if the aptamer does denature, the structure can be easily regenerated. Furthermore, aptamers have not shown any appreciable evidence of toxicity or immunogenicity. These same properties show promise for aptamers in the field of diagnostics, both *in vitro* and *in vivo* [30–38].

One strength of aptamer-based diagnostic sensors over antibody- or enzyme-based techniques is the ability to denature and regenerate the aptamer. This ability could enable reusable biosensors that match the affinity and specificity of antibody and enzyme sensors [37, 38]. Combining aptamer recognition with nanoscale sensing capability such as optical, electrochemical or magnetic transduction methods will enable development of highly sensitive, portable and, eventually, implantable diagnostic tools [39–41].

Medical imaging for diagnostics comes in a variety of forms including X-ray imaging such as computed tomography (CT) scans, magnetic resonance imaging (MRI), positron emission tomography (PET) scans, ultrasound and more recent optical techniques such as optical coherence tomography (OCT). The advantage of imaging over assays and biosensors for diagnostics is the elimination of the need for a patient sample, such as blood or tissue. In the case of implantable biosensors, imaging has the advantage of being noninvasive. However, most medical imaging equipment is expensive and requires trained personnel to both operate and interpret. Furthermore, the low resolution of most of these techniques limits sensitivity. Nanoparticles as contrast agents can be used to increase sensitivity which may allow earlier diagnosis of diseases. If sensitivity is greatly increased using contrast agents, then less-powerful imaging components, such as magnets for MRI, may be used reducing size and cost.

1.3 Optical

1.3.1 Fluorescence

Fluorescent tags, such as fluorescein isothiocyanate (FITC) and rhodamine, have been used extensively as optical markers for a variety of biological assays. Traditional fluorophores have a broad user base and are available in many forms such as voltage-sensitivity dyes, membrane-specific chemistries and pH-sensitive structures. However, traditional fluorophores typically have broad emission spectra, exhibit short emission lifetimes and are susceptible to photobleaching. With the desire for greater sensitivity, multiplexed assays, single-molecule detection and *in vivo* diagnostics, enhancement of traditional fluorophores and the development of novel markers are transforming optical detection methods.

Fluorescent tags can be improved by conjugation with receptor molecules, with coatings for improved photostability, and by combining with metals for greater emission. Figure 1.3 shows three synthetic receptors for noradrenaline which

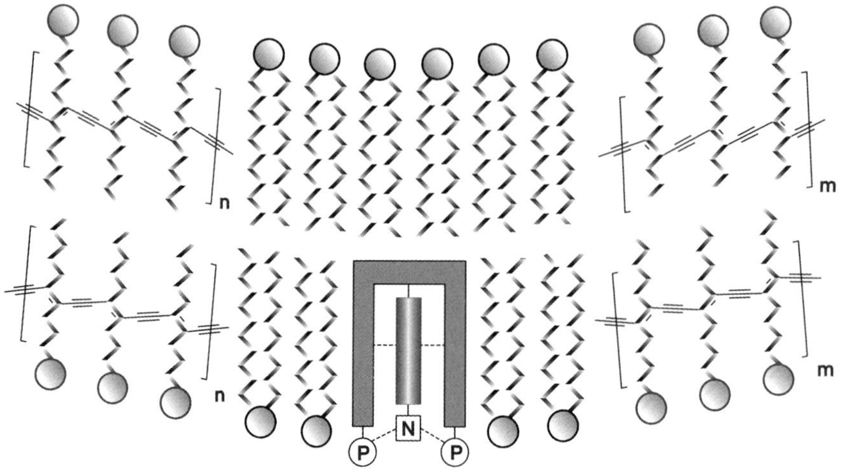

Figure 1.4. Synthetic receptor embedded within a phospholipid/polydiacetylene membrane [42]. Reproduced with permission from J. Am. Chem. Soc., Vol. 127, S. Kolusheva et al., Selective detection of catecholamines by synthetic receptors embedded in chromatic polydiacetylene vesicles, p. 10000–10001. © (2005) American Chemical Society.

provide sensitive fluorescent assays when embedded with phospholipid/polydiacetylene membrane assemblies [42]. By embedding the synthetic receptor within the phospholipid/polydiacetylene membrane (Fig. 1.4), single micromolar detection of catecholamines in urine samples was achieved producing a 1000-fold improvement over existing synthetic receptor-based catecholamine detection systems. Such a sensitive method could provide an earlier diagnostic for Parkinson's disease. Also see Fig. 1.5.

Nanoparticle platforms consisting of surface-functionalized, silica-coated nanophosphors can be used for bioimaging applications [43, 44]. Silica coating enhances aqueous dispersion of nanoparticles, and allows surface functionalization of peptides and nucleic acids for specificity. Fluorescence emission can be tuned by controlling the size of the nanoparticle. A range of nanoparticle sizes can be used simultaneously for multiplexed assays due to each size of nanoparticle emitting a different color. Due to little to no autofluorescence, the signal-to-noise ratio can be quite high, enabling highly sensitive bioimaging techniques for early diagnostics.

Dendrimers are highly branched, monodisperse polymers that have well-defined size and chemical functionality. Voids and channels within the dendritic structure can be carriers for drug molecules. Size, composition and morphology of dendrimer composites can be precisely controlled by pH, temperature and concentration. In addition to drug molecules, metal ions can be entrapped within dendrimer voids creating novel fluorescent nanoparticles [45]. Silver/dendrimer composites absorb in the 300- to 400-nm range with emission from 400 to 500 nm. By using low concentrations of silver/dendrimer composite (below 1 μM) to minimize cytotoxicity, intracellular fluorescent assays can be performed due to cellular uptake of nanoscale dendrimer structures.

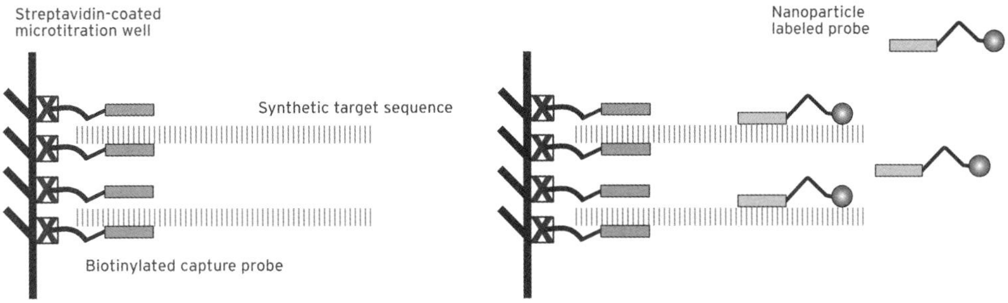

Figure 1.5. Example of assay using nanoparticle tags [48]. Reproduced from Nanotechnology, Vol. 15, P. Huhtinen et al., Europium (III) nanoparticle-label-based assay for the detection of nucleic acids, p. 1708–1715, © (2004), with permission from Institute of Physics and P. Huhtinen.

Fluorescence can also be enhanced using metallic nanostructures such as silver or gold nanorods and nanospheres [46, 47]. Such phenomenon is termed metal-enhanced fluorescence (MEF). When a fluorophore is exposed to a nearby metallic surface, quantum efficiencies can increase due to interactions of the excited-state fluorophore with free electrons in the metal. At short distances between fluorophore and metal (less than 5 nm), quenching can occur. Highly sensitive *in vitro* diagnostic assays may be realized using MEF. Other metals that exhibit enhanced fluorescence are the Lanthanide series of metals or the "rare earth" elements such as europium, samarium and terbium [48, 49].

1.3.2
Quantum Dots

Quantum dots are nanometer-size crystals in which electrons are confined in all three directions. Electron energies are quantized within the nanocrystalline quantum dot enabling an array of emission wavelengths to be produced depending upon the band gap of the crystalline material and quantum dot size as shown in Fig. 1.6. Common quantum dot materials include CdSe which emits blue, InP which emits green and InAs which emits red [50]. Typical quantum dot cores are 3–4 nm in diameter; however, due to water insolubility and possible toxicity of typical cores, polymeric or silica coatings are added to make them water-soluble and biocompatible [51, 52]. ZnS is also a commonly used coating for CdSe core quantum dots for protection against photooxidation [53].

Coatings can increase quantum dot diameter to greater than 30 nm in some cases, creating a tag much larger than standard fluorescent dyes which poses challenges for intracellular delivery and creates potential alterations of the very biological activity that one may be investigating [55]. In addition to water insolubility and large size, quantum dots exhibit thermoquenching where emission decreases as temperature increases. For isothermal bioanalytical applications, thermoquenching poses no problems. However, for *in vitro* assays and, possibly, *in vivo* imaging

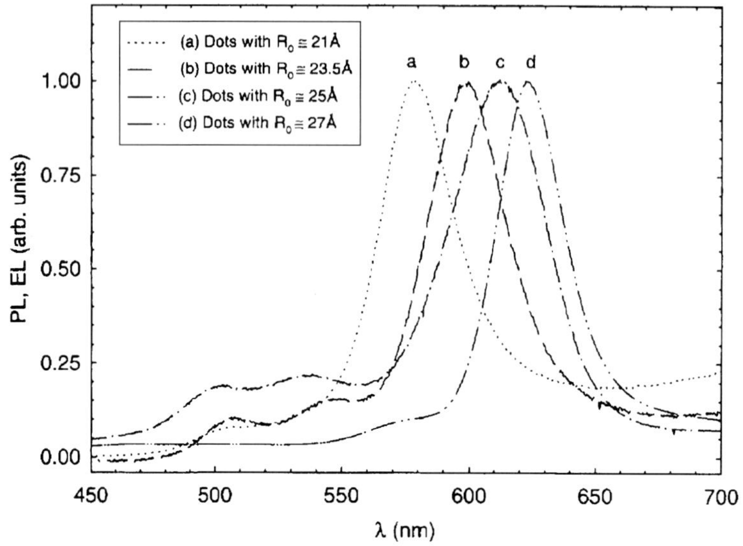

Figure 1.6. Emission wavelength as function of quantum dot size [54]. Reused with permission from H. Mattoussi, J. Appl. Phys., 83, 7965 (1988). Copyright 1998, American Institute of Physics.

applications, where temperatures may fluctuate, thermoquenching effect must be taken into account.

Another limitation of quantum dots is their susceptibility to intermittent emission ("blinking"). Due to their high quantum efficiencies and the use of multiple quantum dots per typical assay, the effects of intermittent emission are negligible. However, where the "blinking" phenomenon becomes a limiting factor is with fluorescence intensity studies, single-molecule spectroscopy and flow cytometry where temporal data is necessary [53, 56, 57].

Despite the larger size, quantum dots are being used for multiplexed *in vitro* assays and *in vivo* imaging applications due to brighter and narrower emission, broader absorption spectra, and high photostability. Quantum dots have much narrower emission spectra (around 30 nm at half maximal emission) in comparison to organic dyes (50–100 nm), such as fluorescein and rhodamine. Due to their narrow emission and the capability of achieving emission over a broad excitation range, multiple quantum dots of different color can be imaged simultaneously using a single excitation source [58–60]. Typical organic dyes limit the ability to perform multiplexed assays because of their overlapping emission spectra and their limited absorption capability, requiring multiple excitation sources to be used when multiple fluorophores are desired.

Through surface functionalization by covalent, noncovalent and chemisorption modifications, quantum dots can be used in protein and DNA immunoassays. Biotinylated, streptavidin-conjugated and antibody-conjugated quantum dots are now readily available, enabling a variety of sandwich-based assays. It is the ability to functionalize quantum dots that make them attractive for diagnostic applications.

By encasing the core quantum dot nanocrystal with a biocompatible, hydrophilic, readily functionalized coating such as silica or polymer and modifying the coating with biologically specific entities such as antibodies, enzymes and nucleic acids, sensitive fluorimetric assays and biosensors can be realized. Assays and biosensors based on quantum dots are being developed for diagnosing breast and prostate cancer, for simultaneously detecting multiple toxins, and for sensing levels of acetylcholine [61].

For *in vivo* applications, it is desirable to have quantum dots that emit in near-infrared (NIR) range of 700–1550 nm, where such energy absorption in tissue is minimal. Example nanocrystalline materials for NIR quantum dots include CdTe, InP and InAs. CdTe-based quantum dots consist of a CdTe core with a CdSe shell which have lower quantum yields and weaker NIR absorption than InP and InAs quantum dots. InP quantum dots are larger (above 6 nm) than most other nanocrystalline structures which, after coating, limits their use for *in vivo* applications. InAs quantum dots are much smaller (below 2 nm), but have limited absorption capability in the NIR due to their small size [62]. Alloys and core–shell structures comprised of nanocrystalline materials improve NIR absorption capability while keeping the quantum dot to a functional size. Figure 1.7 shows the size distributions for InAsP, InP and ZnSe alloys, and core–shell quantum dot structures.

Figure 1.8 shows emission spectra for InP, InAs and InAsP alloy quantum dots. With increasing percentage of arsenic in the alloy, greater NIR luminescence is observed. Figure 1.9 shows the effect of the core–shell structure on emission. As the InAsP alloy core is coated with shell material, first with InP and finishing with ZnSe, the emission of the quantum dot is pushed further into the NIR range.

Another interesting phenomenon of quantum dots is the observation of fluorescent downshift ("blue" shift) when bound to bacterial surfaces [63]. By conjugating antibodies or aptamers to quantum dot surfaces, specific bacteria can be targeted. Upon binding of antibody- or aptamer-conjugated quantum dots to bacterial surfaces, shifts in fluorescent emission peaks ranging from 60 to 140 nm have been

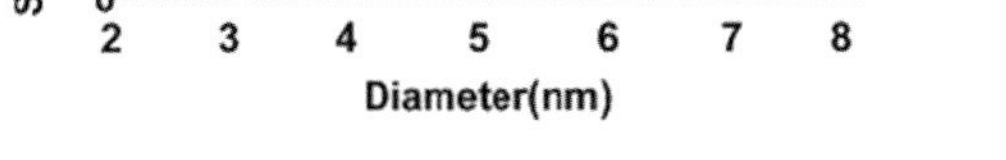

Figure 1.7. Size distribution for quantum dot core and core–shell combinations. $InAs_{0.82}P_{0.18}$ (yellow), $InAs_{0.82}P_{0.18}$ core and InP shell (red), and $InAs_{0.82}P_{0.18}$ core, InP shell and ZnSe outer shell (blue) [62]. Reproduced with permission from J. Am. Chem. Soc., Vol. 127, S.-W. Kim et al., Engineering InAsxP1-x/InP/ZnSe III–V alloyed core/shell quantum dots for the near-infrared, p. 10526–10532. Copyright (2005) American Chemical Society.

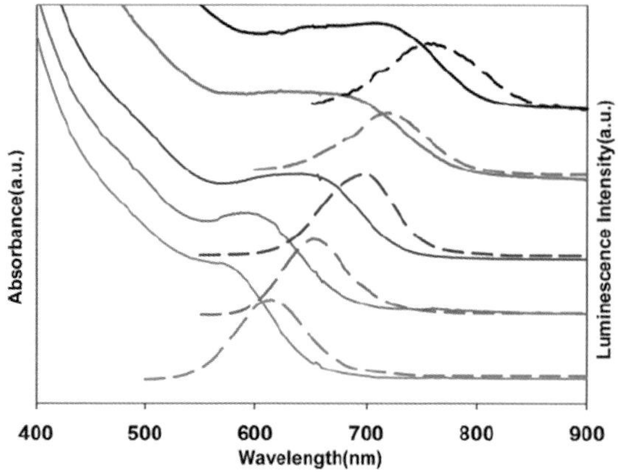

Figure 1.8. Emission of InP (614 nm), $InAs_{0.33}P_{0.66}$ (652 nm), $InAs_{0.66}P_{0.33}$ (699 nm), $InAs_{0.82}P_{0.18}$ (738 nm) and InAs (755 nm) quantum dots. Absorbance shown as solid line [62]. Reproduced with permission from J. Am. Chem. Soc., Vol. 127, S.-W. Kim et al., Engineering InAsxP1-x/InP/ZnSe III–V alloyed core/shell quantum dots for the near-infrared, p. 10526–10532. Copyright (2005) American Chemical Society.

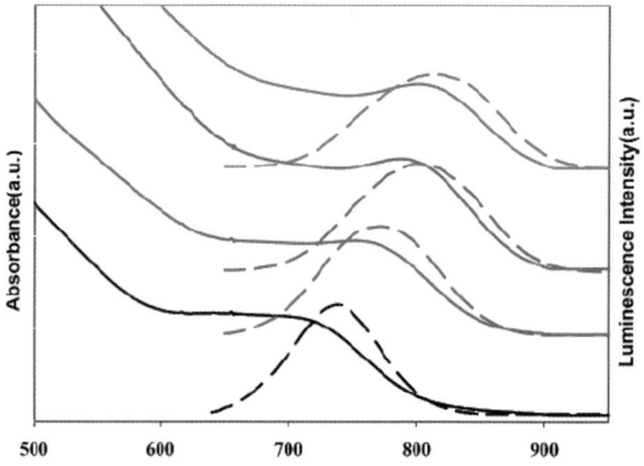

Figure 1.9. Emission of $InAs_{0.82}P_{0.18}$ core (738 nm), with a shell of InP (765 nm), with a second shell of InP (801 nm) and with a final shell of ZnSe (815 nm). Absorbance shown as solid line [62]. Reproduced with permission from J. Am. Chem. Soc., Vol. 127, S.-W. Kim et al., Engineering InAsxP1-x/InP/ZnSe III–V alloyed core/shell quantum dots for the near-infrared, p. 10526–10532. Copyright (2005) American Chemical Society.

observed which can be readily optically detected. This method could be used to determine the presence of bacteria in a sample.

1.3.3
Surface Plasmon Resonance (SPR), Nanoparticles and Nanoshells

Molecular-recognition molecules immobilized using self-assembled monolayers (SAMs) coupled with SPR sensing create sensitive, label-free biosensors [64–74].

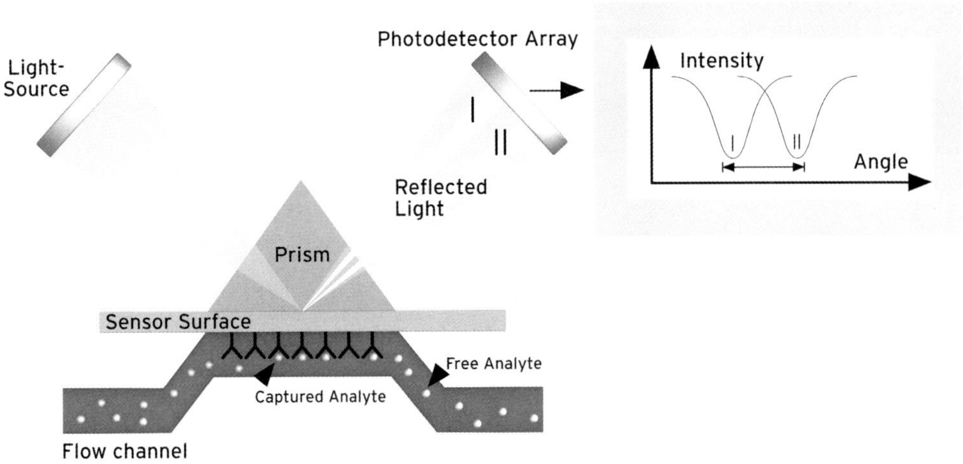

Figure 1.10. Typical set-up for SPR [68].

A typical SPR set-up is depicted in Fig. 1.10, with main components consisting of a sensor substrate (chip) coated with a thin metal film (typically gold or silver), a polarized light source and an optical detection unit. Polarized light is directed toward the sensor chip at an angle such that an evanescent wave is created on the surface of the metal film. Changes in the dielectric constant of the adjacent medium shift the intensity of the evanescent wave, resulting in a change in angle of reflection from the metal surface. The angular shift is detected with a photodetector [70].

By modifying the metal film for biological specificity, the SPR sensor can be tailored to respond to a desired analyte. Upon binding of the analyte to the molecular-recognition site of the modified metal film, the index of refraction changes at the sensor surface, which results in an angular shift of the reflected light. The metal surface is typically first modified with alkane thiol or alkyl siloxane chemistry. Subsequent modification defines the biological specificity of the SPR sensor and can consist of streptavidin for biotinylated analytes, biotin for streptavidin-conjugated analytes or sandwich assays using free streptavidin followed by biotinylated analyte, antibodies for antibody–antigen interactions and enzymes or aptamers for affinity assays.

Using metal nanoparticles and nanoshells with SPR phenomena creates localized SPR (LSPR) which enables field-portable, lower-cost SPR systems with improved capability to detect small molecules, all of which could pave the way for greater use of SPR in patient diagnostics [69, 71–74]. An example of a LSPR set-up using gold-coated silica nanoparticles and a fiber optic probe for excitation and detection is shown in Fig. 1.11.

Optical properties of nanoparticles depend highly on size, shape and local environment. When the nanoparticle diameter is much smaller than the wavelength of light, then the optical interaction of nanoparticles can be described by Mie theory

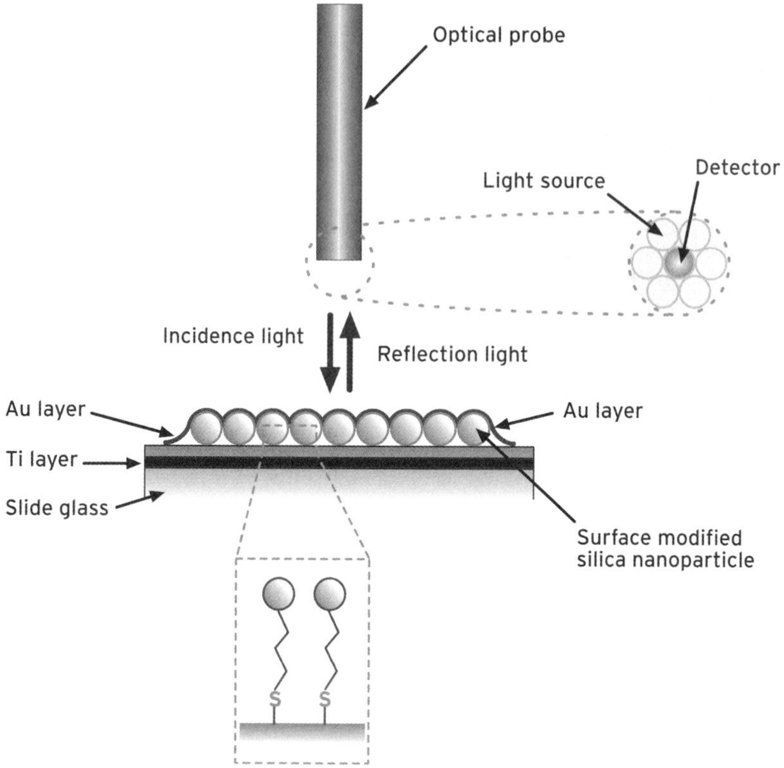

Figure 1.11. LSPR biosensor set-up [71]. Reproduced with permission from Analytical Chemistry, Vol. 77, T. Endo et al., Label-free detection of peptide nucleic acid-DNA hybridization using localized surface plasmon resonance based optical biosensor, p. 6976–6984. Copyright (2005) American Chemical Society.

of electromagnetic radiation scattering stated in Eq. (1) [69, 75, 76]. SPR occurs when $\varepsilon_r = -\chi\varepsilon_m$ and ε_i is small:

$$E(\lambda) = \frac{24\pi N_A a^3 \varepsilon_m{}^{3/2}}{\lambda \ln(10)} \left[\frac{\varepsilon_i}{(\varepsilon_r + \chi\varepsilon_m)^2 + \varepsilon_i{}^2} \right], \tag{1}$$

where $E(\lambda)$ is the optical extinction (sum of absorption and scattering), N_A is the areal density of nanoparticles, a is the radius of nanoparticles, ε_m is the dielectric constant of the medium, λ is the wavelength of the absorbing radiation, ε_i is the imaginary portion of the nanoparticle dielectric constant, ε_r is the real portion of the nanoparticle dielectric constant and χ is the aspect ratio of nanoparticles ($\chi = 2$, for a sphere).

Probes encapsulated by biologically localized embedding (PEBBLEs) are optical nanosensors which can be used to monitor intracellular conditions such as pH and

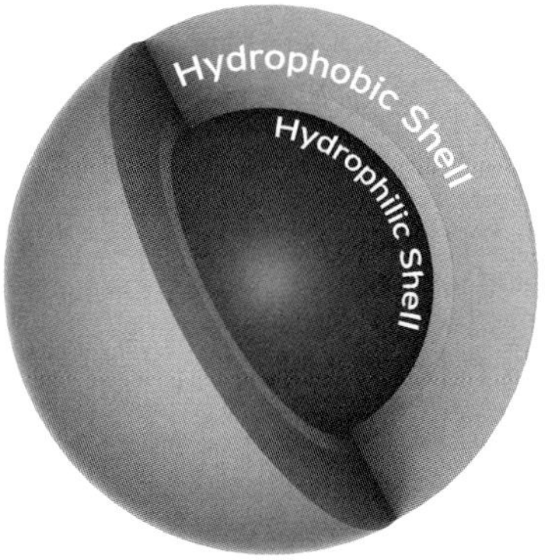

Figure 1.12. Diagram of PEBBLE nanosensor [79]. Reproduced with permission from Analytical Chemistry, Vol. 76, Y.-E. L. Koo et al., Real-time measurements of dissolved oxygen inside living cells by organically modified silicate fluorescent nanosensors, p. 2498–2505. Copyright (2004) American Chemical Society.

calcium ion levels [77–79]. Fluorescent molecules are entrapped within a permeable polymer gel creating PEBBLE nanoparticles typically ranging from 20 to 200 nm, as represented in Fig. 1.12. The polymer gel coating protects the internal fluorophore from nonspecific protein binding and reduces cytotoxicity. Due to the porosity of the polymer coating, small ions such as calcium, oxygen and hydrogen can penetrate the coating, and reach the entrapped fluorophore. Therefore, pH- and calcium-sensitive dyes can be encapsulated while maintaining their desired function.

Single base-pair mismatches in a sequence of DNA can be detected using colorimetric assays comprised of electrostatic absorption of DNA onto colloidal gold nanoparticles [80–83]. Such assays eliminate target labeling and do not require any covalent modifications of DNA or substrate surfaces. Furthermore, sensitivity is high enough to obviate the need for DNA amplification such as PCR. Color detected is dependent upon degree of aggregation of gold nanoparticles. Due to the ability to perform the assay in less than 10 min, RNA degradation is minimized and, therefore, RNA sequences can also be determined.

Another technique which results in high sensitivity without the need for target amplification is the Bio-Barcode Assay (Fig. 1.13), which can be used for both nucleic acid and protein analysis [84–89]. The Bio-Barcode Assay uses both gold nanoparticles and magnetic microparticles functionalized with the same antibody specific for the particular analyte to be detected. Antibody-functionalized gold nanoparticles are further modified with oligonucleotide strands of a known sequence, giving the gold nanoparticles a unique identity or barcode. When exposed to the target analyte, both gold nanoparticles and magnetic microparticles bind to the analyte creating complexes of gold nanoparticle–analyte–magnetic microparticle.

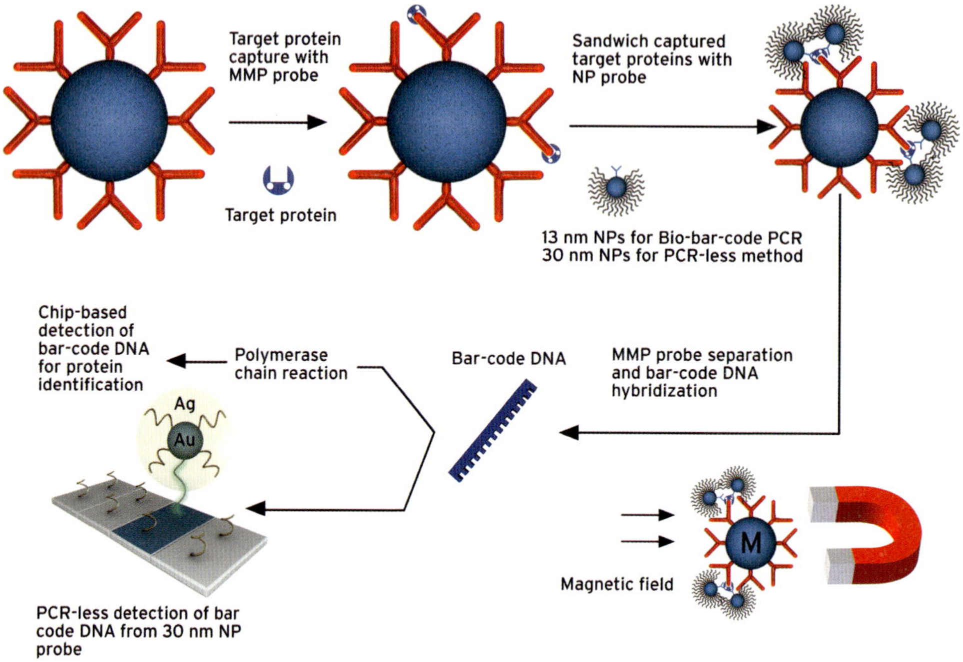

Figure 1.13. Bio-barcode assay [6]. Reproduced from Clinical Chimica Acta, Vol. 358, K. K. Jain, Nanotechnology in clinical laboratory diagnostics, p. 37–54, Copyright (2005), with permission from Elsevier.

After the complexes are magnetically separated and washed, the barcode DNA is dehybridized and released from the gold nanoparticles into solution. The single-stranded barcode DNA is then collected and bound to a microarray containing oligonucleotides complementary to half of the targeted barcode DNA. Gold nanoparticles functionalized with oligonucleotides complementary to the other half of targeted barcode DNA are then hybridized to the microarray-captured DNA. Finally, the gold nanoparticles are coated with silver for amplification and the microarray is read using light scattering intensity measurements. The Bio-Barcode Assay enables detection of molecules down to attomolar sensitivity.

Aptamer-conjugated gold nanoparticles can bind desired protein targets forming gold-tagged proteins for subsequent analysis [90]. The bound gold nanoparticles can be enlarged in catalytic solution of gold chloride resulting in higher absorbance at 540 and 650 nm as the size of gold nanoparticles increases. An example using thrombin as target protein is shown in Fig. 1.14. A greater concentration of protein binds more aptamer–gold nanoparticle conjugates, which provides a greater surface density for catalytic solution to deposit more gold. Observed absorbance then is a function of protein concentration. Sensitivity down to single nanomolar protein concentrations have been achieved with this method.

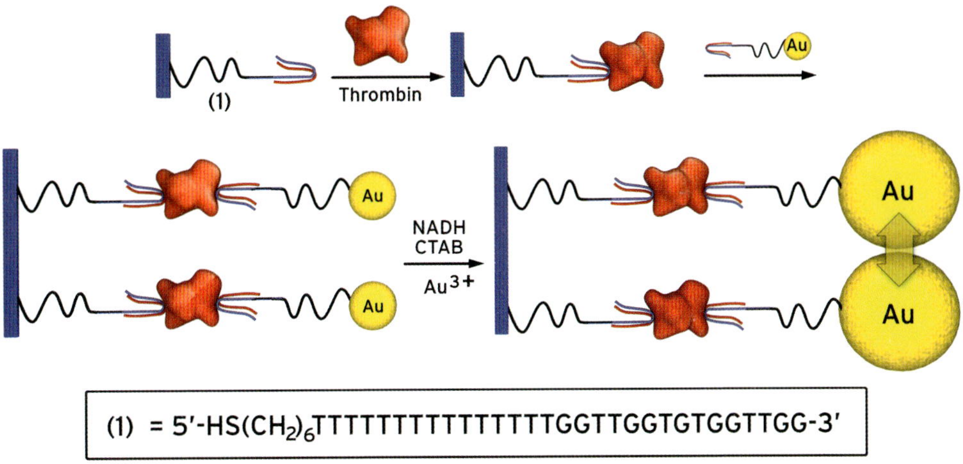

Figure 1.14. Aptamer-functionalized gold nanoparticles for binding assay amplification [90]. Reproduced with permission from J. Am. Chem. Soc., Vol. 126, V. Pavlov et al., Aptamer-functionalized Au nanoparticles for the amplified optical detection of thrombin, p. 11768–11769. Copyright (2004) American Chemical Society.

1.3.4 Fiber Optic Biosensors

Fiber optic biosensors show potential use in intracellular assays and *in vivo* applications [91–95]. Modifying the distal tip of the optical fiber to create a biologically active surface allows for binding events or reactions at the distal tip surface to be monitored optically through fluorescent or spectroscopic (IR and Raman) methods. An example of a modified optical fiber tip is shown in Fig. 1.15. Due to containment of the reactive species to the fiber tip surface, localized detection of the desired analyte can be achieved. Furthermore, highly sensitive diagnostic devices could potentially be developed by combining fiber optic biosensors with nanoparticles or nanoshells for amplification of optical response (i.e. LSPR or surface-enhanced Raman spectroscopy).

1.4 Electrical

Electrical methods to measure analytes include amperometric, conductimetric and potentiometric techniques (Fig. 1.16) [96]. Amperometric techniques utilize a working electrode containing chemistry, typically an enzyme, specific to the analyte being monitored. A voltage potential is set up between the reference electrode and the working electrode. Products from the binding of the analyte to the surface chemistry of the working electrode become oxidized or reduced depending on the voltage potential between the electrodes. Electrical current is measured at the work-

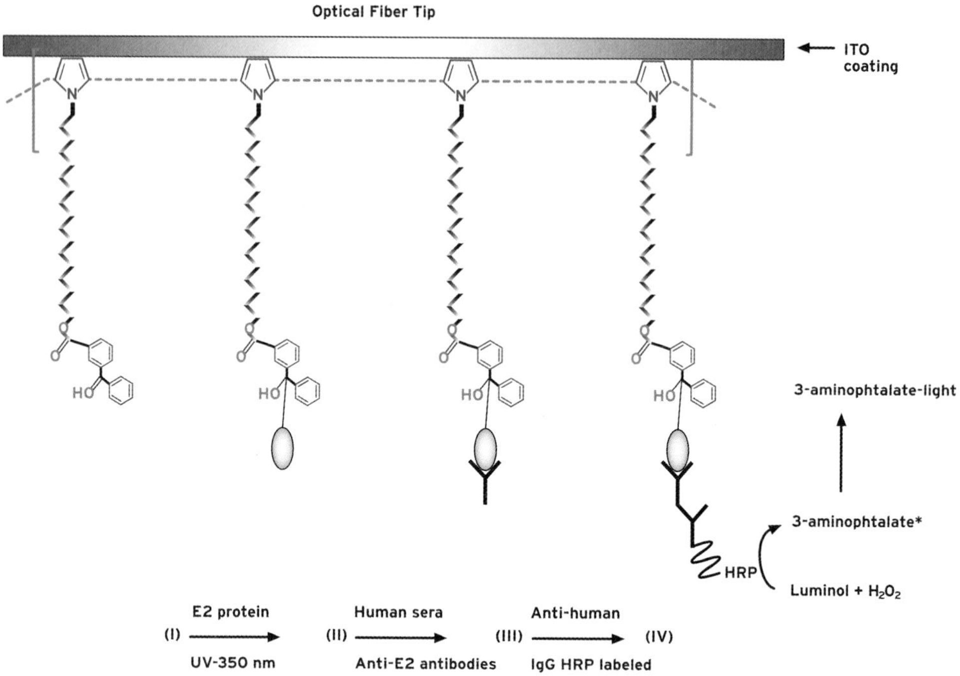

Figure 1.15. Surface modification of optical fiber distal tip [95]. Reproduced with permission from Analytical Chemistry, Vol. 77, T. Konry et al., Optical fiber immunosensor based on a poly(pyrrolebenzophene) film for the detection of antibodies to viral antigen, p. 1771–1779. Copyright (2005) American Chemical Society.

ing electrode providing a method to determine the presence and concentration of the analyte. Conductimetric techniques measure the conductance of the analytical solution as a function of the analyte concentration. Measurement electrodes can be modified with biological receptors concentrating the analyte near the electrode surfaces. Potentiometric techniques are based on field effect transistor devices in which the current flowing between source and drain is affected by analyte concentration. Voltage is monitored as the current is affected providing a method to measure analyte concentration.

1.4.1 Nanomaterials for Enhanced Electron Transfer

Nanomaterials, such as nanotubes and nanoparticles, can enhance electron transfer and can be readily modified for biological specificity [97, 98]. Integrating nanomaterials with microfabricated electrodes and circuits, enable portable, miniature instrumentation. Using electrical methods of detection eliminates the need for enzymatic amplification techniques typically used in optical detection assays. Due to the use of electronics, amplification and signal conditioning can be integrated within the assay substrate.

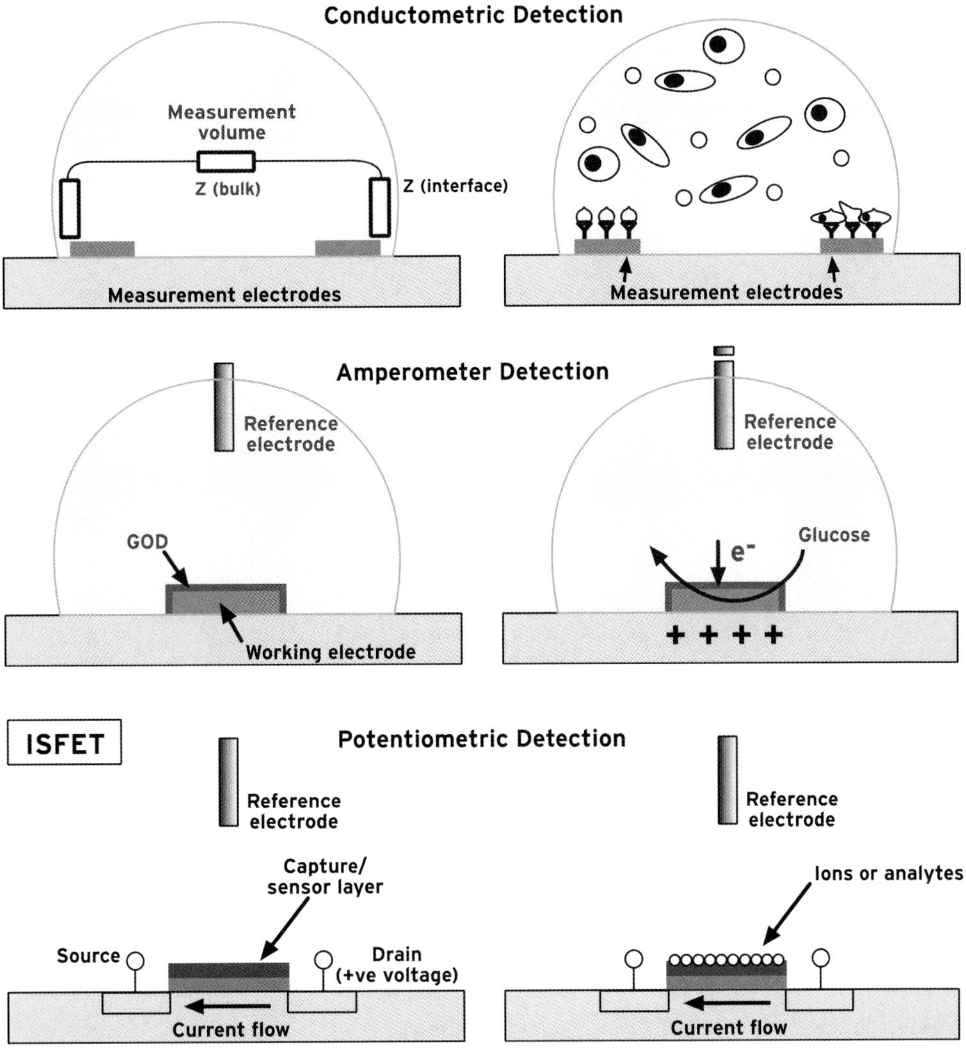

Figure 1.16. Electrical detection methods [96]. Reproduced from Advanced Drug Delivery Reviews, Vol. 56, R. Bashir, BioMEMs: state-of-the-art in detection, opportunities and prospects, p. 1565–1586, Copyright (2004) with permission from Elsevier.

Multiwalled carbon nanotubes (MWNTs) can be functionalized with single-stranded DNA. When exposed to the complementary DNA, after target hybridization, charge conductance through the carbon nanotube changes indicating binding of the cDNA [99]. MWNTs can be selectively grown on electrode surfaces coated with nickel catalyst. A conformal SiO_2 layer passivates the exposed substrate between MWNTs. Ethylene glycol-modified siloxanes can be deposited onto the oxide surface to inhibit nonspecific binding. Finally, siloxanes can be selectively removed

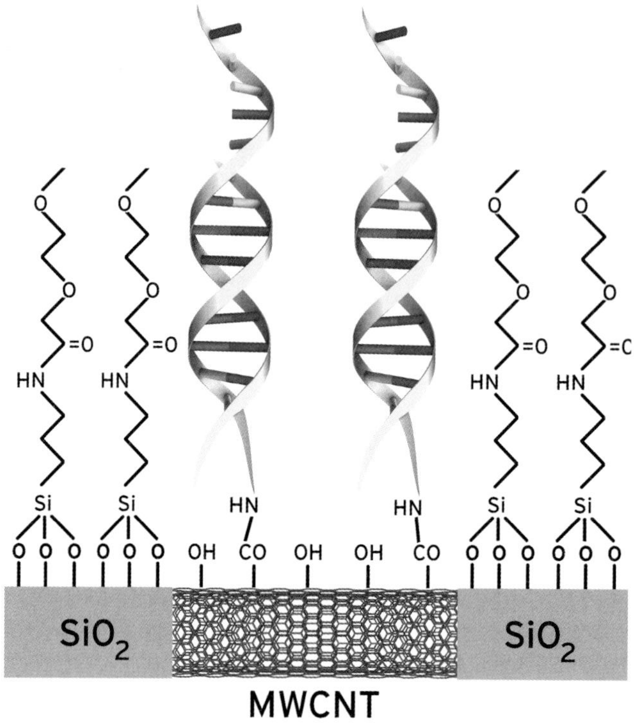

Figure 1.17. MWNT functionalized with DNA [99]. Reproduced from Clinical Chemistry, Vol. 50, J. E. Koehne et al., Miniturized multiplex label-free electronic chip for rapid nucleic acid analysis based on carbon nanotube nanoelectrode arrays, p. 1886–1893, Copyright (2004), with permission from American Association for Clinical Chemistry.

from the MWNTs through electrochemical etching, exposing the MWNT surface for subsequent functionalization with single-stranded DNA (Fig. 1.17). The cycle of siloxane removal from selected MWNTs followed by single-stranded DNA functionalization provides a method to produce dense arrays of different single-stranded DNA probes.

Target DNA, extended with additional guanine bases, is exposed to the MWNT array and allowed to hybridize. The additional guanine produces a small current when electrochemically oxidized. The current generated is transferred to the MWNTs, which transfer the charge to the underlying electronic circuit for eventual signal acquisition. Due to generation of a very small current, electrocatalytic amplification of guanine oxidation current can be achieved using polypyridyl complexes of ruthenium (Fig. 1.18) or osmium.

Nanowires fabricated from semiconducting single-wall carbon nanotubes (SWNTs), silicon and zinc oxide can be integrated into field effect transistors (FETs) [100], and functionalized for biological specificity enabling rapid, label-free, detection of small molecules [61, 65, 101, 102]. The ability of FET devices to sense

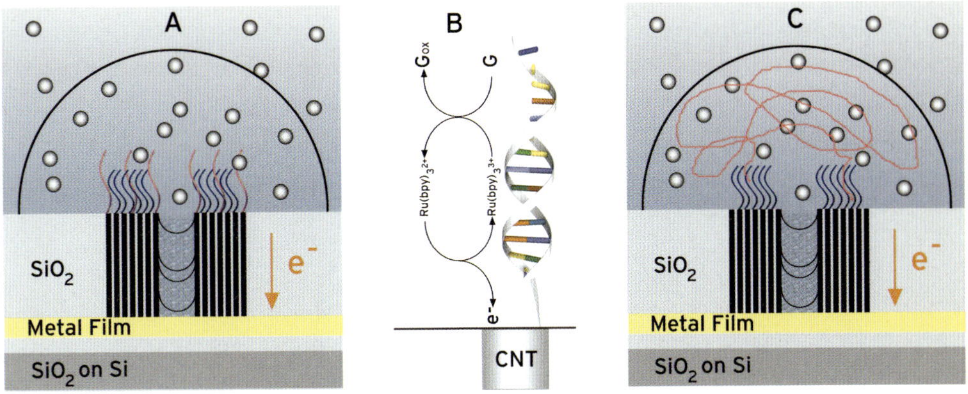

Figure 1.18. Electrochemical detection of nucleic acids with electrocatalytic amplification by ruthenium–polypyridyl complex [99]. Reproduced from Clinical Chemistry, Vol. 50, J. E. Koehne et al., Miniturized multiplex label-free electronic chip for rapid nucleic acid analysis based on carbon nanotube nanoelectrode arrays, p. 1886–1893, Copyright (2004), with permission from American Association for Clinical Chemistry.

small molecules is due to a change in surface charge upon adsorption onto the gate material of target molecules. Nanowire FETs consist of functionalized nanowires as the gate material deposited or placed between transistor source and drain (Fig. 1.19). Such a physical arrangement produces devices highly sensitive to electrical changes. Due to the high surface area to volume of nanowires, extremely minor surface charge changes may be monitored, possibly enabling detection of single molecules.

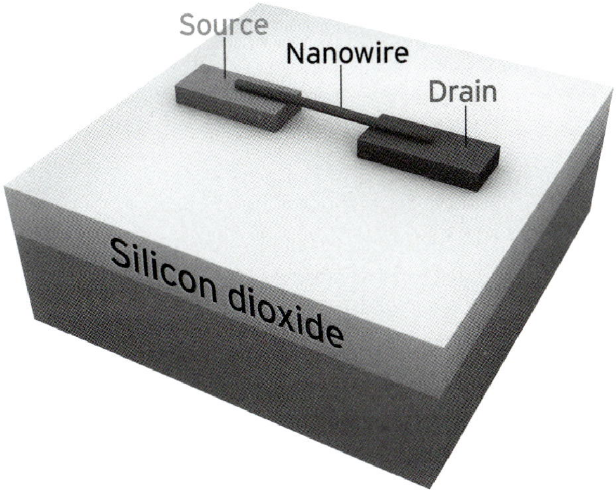

Figure 1.19. Nanowire FET sensor schematic.

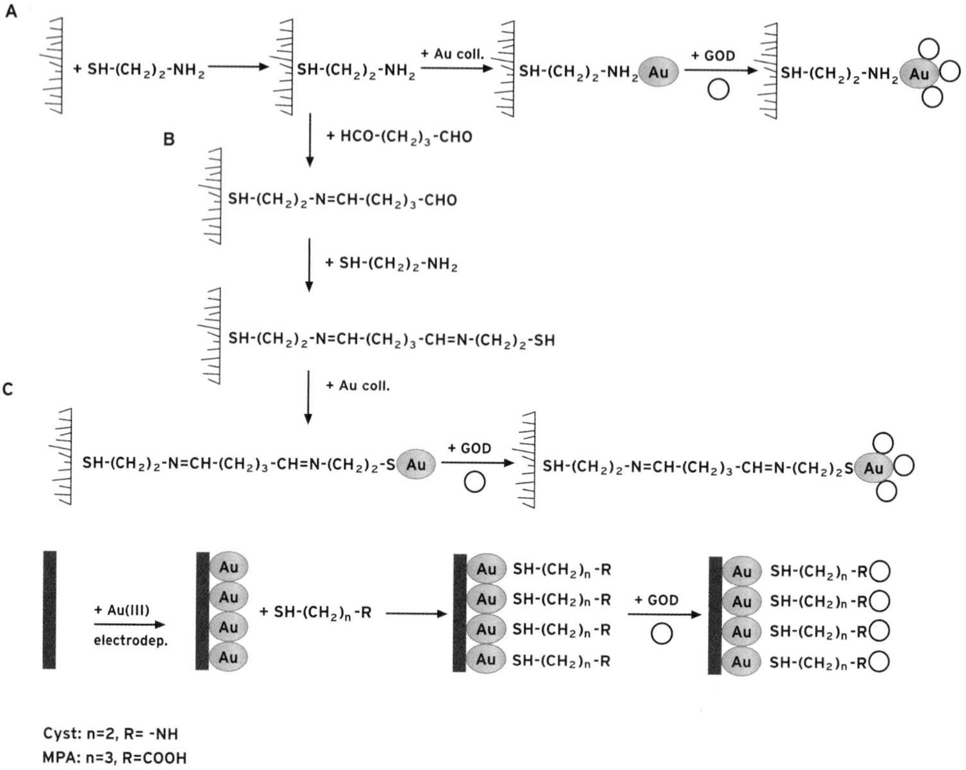

Figure 1.20. Methods to enhance enzyme assays using gold nanoparticles [109]. Reproduced with permission from Anal. Bioanal. Chem., Vol. 382 (2005), p. 884–886, Gold nanoparticle-based electrochemical biosensors, P. Yanez-Sedeno and J. M. Pingarron, Fig. 1. © (2005) with kind permission of Springer Science and Business Media.

1.4.2
Electrochemical Biosensors

Low-cost, portable, fast-response diagnostic systems can be realized with electrochemical biosensors [103]. Glucose biosensors based on glucose oxidase are one of the most common diagnostic tools currently available. Electrochemical DNA analysis has also been widely investigated [104]. Aptamers can also be immobilized onto electrode surfaces and be used in electrochemical sensing systems [105–107]. To enhance charge transfer and to improve immobilization of enzyme or target, nanostructures such as carbon nanotubes and metallic nanoparticles can be used in conjunction with immobilized enzymes to form high specificity and high sensitivity biosensors. Due to their large surface area, nanoparticles provide enhanced adsorption of DNA and enzymes over flat surfaces which are typically used in microarrays and immunoassays [108, 109]. Biosensors can be created by linking silica or gold nanoparticles carrying immobilized DNA or specific enzyme onto gold electrodes. Electrochemical impedance analysis can be used to monitor hybridiza-

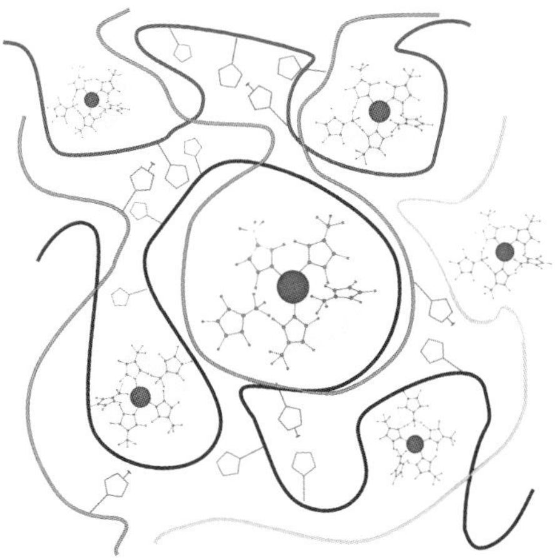

Figure 1.21. PMP complex [110]. Reproduced from Current Applied Physics, Vol. 5, T. Haruyama et al., Bio-, nano-technology for cellular biosensing, p. 108–111, Copyright (2005), with permission from Elsevier.

tion of cDNA or enzyme activity. Several methods for using gold nanoparticles to enhance enzyme-based diagnostic assays are shown in Fig. 1.20.

Through self-assembly of two or more different polymers with metal ions, thin films with nanoscale cavities can be formed (Fig. 1.21). These polymer–metal–polymer (PMP) complexes can be tailored for biochemical specificity and be used as amperometric transducers for electrochemical assays [110]. PMP complexes can be readily spin coated onto metal electrodes for biosensor formation. Another advantage of PMP films is their cellular compatibility. Cells can be cultured directly on the surface of PMP film allowing for cell-based diagnostics to be performed.

Electrochemical detection of DNA hybridization opens up the opportunity for low-cost gene mutation and single nucleotide polymorphism (SNP) analysis. The portability of such genetic sensors (genosensors) provides exciting possibilities for clinical use. Multifunctional gold nanoparticles is one platform that can be used in electrochemical genosensors [111]. First, target single-stranded DNA is immobilized onto the working electrode, such as a pencil graphite electrode (PGE), of the electrochemical cell. Thiol-terminated oligonucleotides, of the sequence to which the target DNA is to be compared, are then added to solution containing gold nanoparticles. The DNA-immobilized working electrode is immersed into the solution which now contains oligonucleotide-functionalized gold nanoparticles and gold oxidation is measured using differential pulse voltammetry which produces an electrical current depending on degree of hybridization (Fig. 1.22). A perfect match produces the highest current. A single point mutation is discernible due to lower current being generated. The absence of hybridization still produces some current, but much less than the single point mutation.

Many electrochemical reactions can be enhanced through electrocatalytic amplification using electron-transfer mediators. These mediators help transfer of

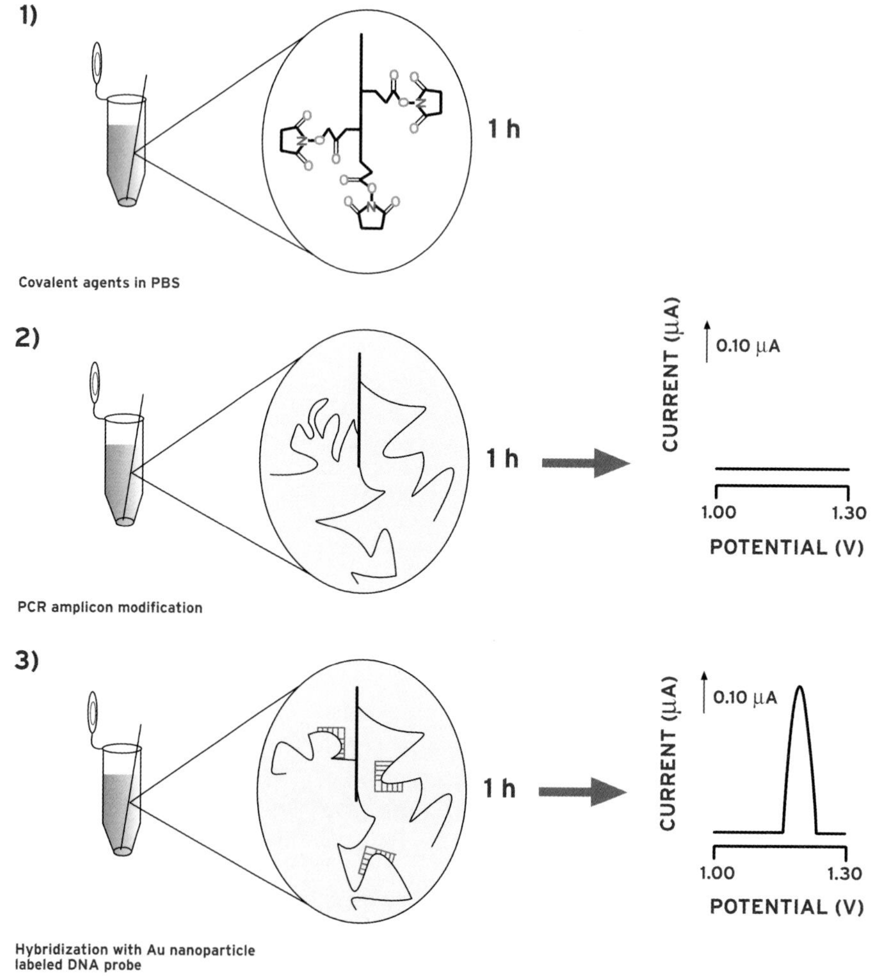

Figure 1.22. DNA hybridization detected electrochemically with gold nanoparticle probes [111]. Reproduced with permission from Analytical Chemistry, Vol. 75, M. Ozsoz et al., Electrochemical genosensor based on colloidal gold nanoparticles for the detection of Factor V Leiden mutation using disposable pencil graphite electrodes, p. 2181–2187. Copyright (2003) American Chemical Society.

electrons between the working electrode and the enzymatic reactants, essentially creating a molecular conduit to shuttle electrons. Without electron-transfer mediators, many of the electrons produced by enzymatic activity may be lost due to diffusion. Methods utilizing electron-transfer mediators involve coimmobilizing them with the enzyme in a conductive polymer matrix, inorganic sol-gel or carbon paste [112–115]. Several frequently used electron-transfer mediators are listed in Tab. 1.4.

Precision assembly of materials is routinely achieved in biological systems through use of proteins. One particular nanostructure formed by bacteria is a monolayer of crystalline proteins called an S-layer. These crystalline proteins can

Tab. 1.4. Examples electron-transfer mediators.

Electron-transfer mediator		
Ferrocene	$C_{10}H_{10}Fe$	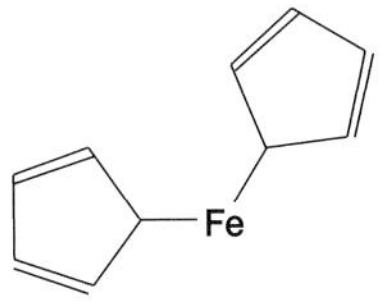
Promazine	$C_{17}H_{20}N_2S$	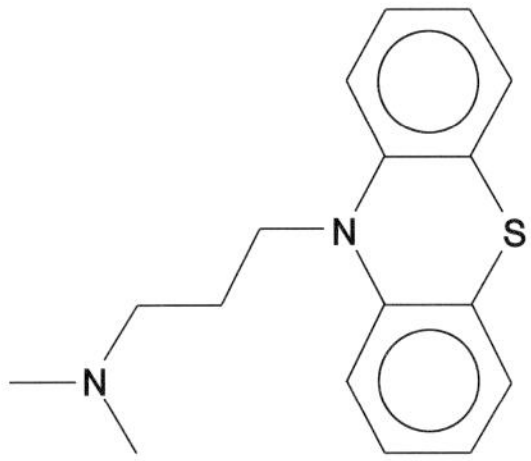
p-Benzoquinone	$C_6H_4O_2$	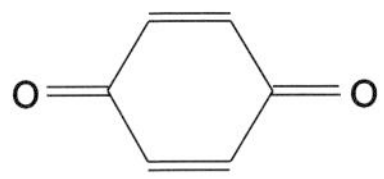
Tetrathiafulvalene	$C_6H_4S_4$	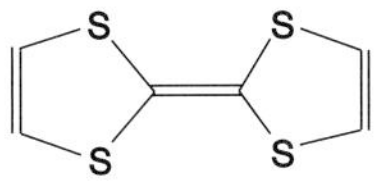
p-Dihydroxydiphenyl	$C_{12}H_{10}O_2$	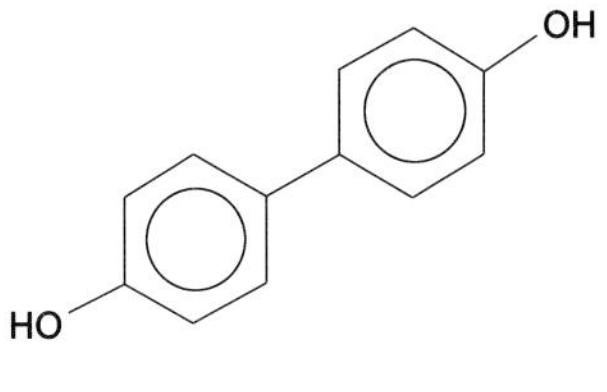
Methylene blue	$C_{16}H_{18}ClN_3S$	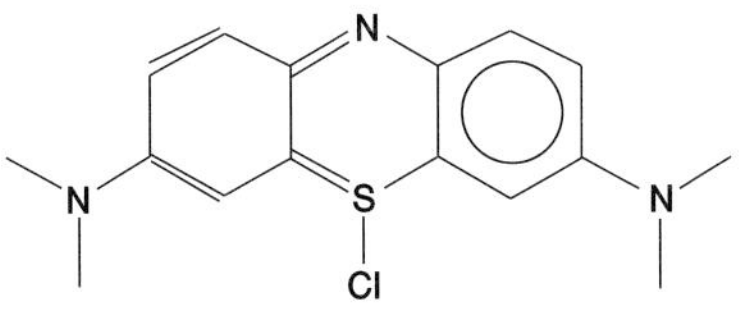

be removed from the exterior of bacteria, resuspended in solution and allowed to self-assemble on solid support surfaces such as silicon, metal or polymer. The self-assembled S-layer monolayer can be modified with enzymes or antibodies for analyte specificity. Optical or electrical measurements can then be used to detect the presence of binding analyte. One such diagnostic tool is an S-layer dipstick shown in Fig. 1.23 [116–118].

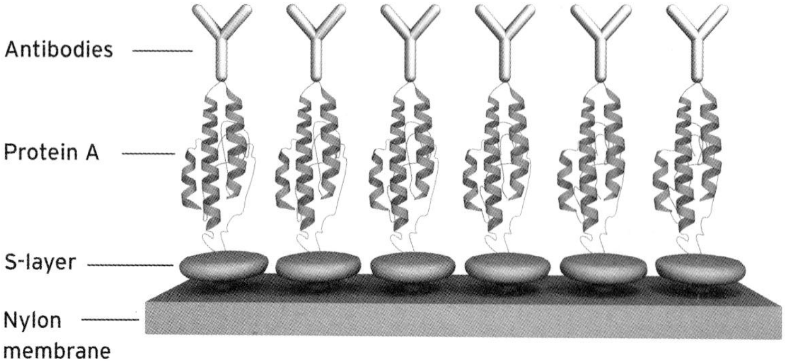

Figure 1.23. Filtration membrane modified with protein A immobilized on S-layer for antibody functionalization.

1.5 Magnetic

Ferrite nanoparticles can be coated with gold (Fig. 1.24) or silica which can then be functionalized with targeting molecules. Antibody-conjugated magnetic nanoparticles can be used to tag proteins for magnetic immunoassays [119]. Using magnetic methods to report binding could enable multiplexed assays to be performance on chip-based substrates.

Genomagnetic nanocapturers are silica-coated, magnetic nanoparticles functionalized to bind with RNA or DNA [121]. Molecular beacons, e.g. loop–stem structures of single-stranded oligonucleotides, can be bound to magnetic nanoparticles to enable capture of single-base mismatched DNA and target mRNAs for intracellular gene expression analysis (Fig. 1.25) [120, 122]. In comparison to linear single-stranded DNA typically used in hybridization assays, the loop–stem structure of molecular beacons provides greater discrimination between perfect match and single-base mismatched DNA [123].

Combining molecular beacons with magnetic nanoparticles, single-base mismatched DNA can be magnetically separated (Fig. 1.26). Genomagnetic nanocapturers (GMNCs) colabeled with molecular beacons perfectly complementary and single-base mismatched to target DNA can be dispersed within a mixture of sample DNA to be analyzed. Both perfectly complementary DNA and single-base mismatched DNA will bind to the molecular beacons on the surface of the GMNCs which can be magnetically separated from solution. Due to the differences in melting temperature for each of the DNA complexes, complementary DNA can be separated from single-base mismatched DNA.

For intracellular applications, magnetic nanoparticles can be coated with cell-penetrating peptides [124]. One class of protein which has been used for efficient cellular internalization is membrane translocating signal (MTS) protein which include HIV-1 tat protein and VP22 herpes virus protein. Other cell-penetrating peptides include penetratin and transportan. These cell-penetrating peptides and proteins show promise as effective carriers to transport impermeable nanoparticles

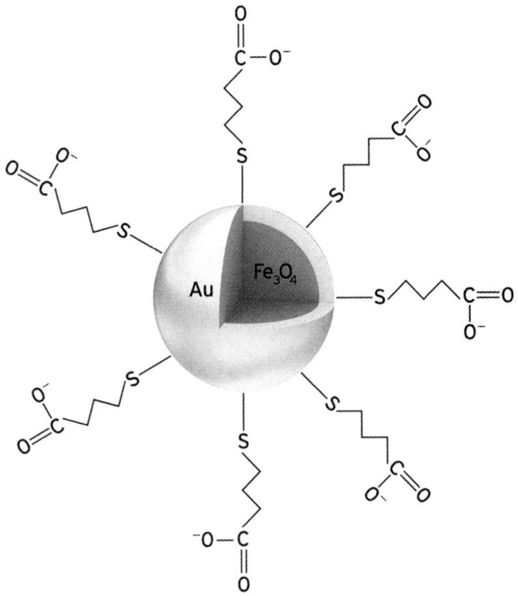

Figure 1.24. Iron oxide nanoparticle with gold coating for surface functionalization [120]. Reproduced from Materials Today, Vol. 7, P. Gould, Nanoparticles probe biosystems, p. 36–43, © (2004), with permission from Elsevier.

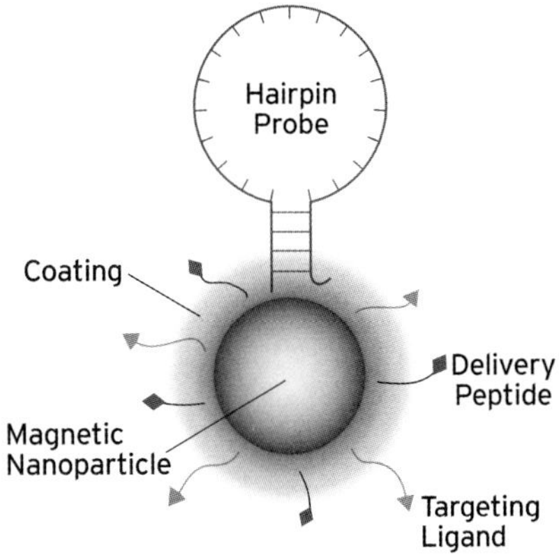

Figure 1.25. Magnetic nanoparticle tagged with molecular beacon oligonucleotide structure [120]. Reproduced from Materials Today, Vol. 7, P. Gould, Nanoparticles probe biosystems, p. 36–43, © (2004), with permission from Elsevier.

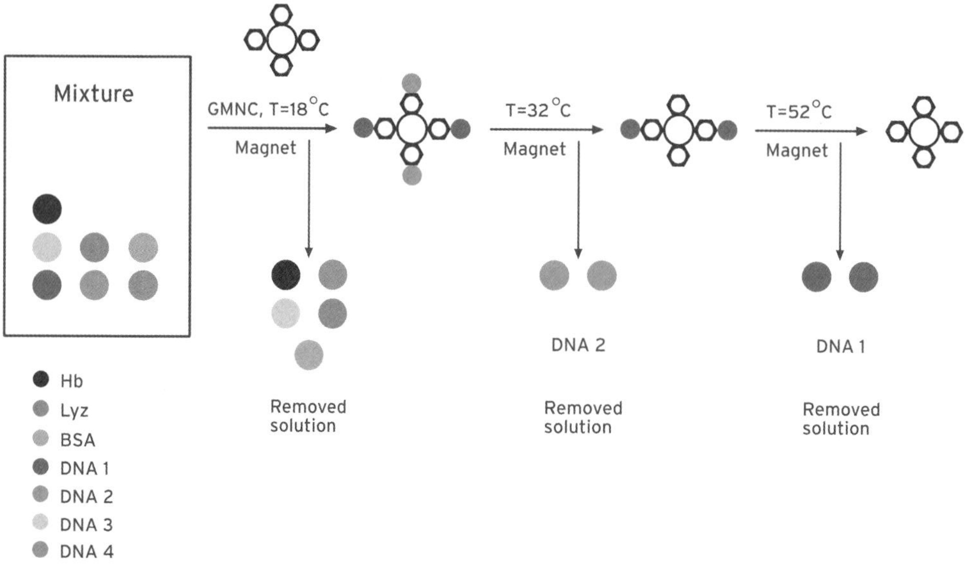

Figure 1.26. Genomagnetic capture separation [121]. Reproduced with permission from Analytical Chemistry, Vol. 75, X. Zhao et al., Collection of trace amounts of DNA/mRNA molecules using genomagnetic nanocapturers, p. 3476–3483. Copyright (2003) American Chemical Society.

across cell membranes. Functionalized magnetic nanoparticles may also be internalized through magnetofection – the application of external magnetic to attract magnetic nanoparticles into the cell (Fig. 1.27) [125–127].

Similar to chip-based electrical methods for biological analysis, sensors based on magnetic nanoparticles could also be used for benchtop and handheld diagnostics. For instance, arrays of DNA probes can be immobilized on surfaces as in DNA chips. Biotinylated complementary target DNA can then be hybridized with the DNA probes on the chip followed by washing of the substrate to remove unbound DNA. Streptavidin-functionalized magnetic nanoparticles can then be exposed to the chip, resulting in the capture of magnetic nanoparticles to target cDNA [120]. The capture sites can be detected with underlying magnetoresistive, spin valve or magnetic tunnel junction sensors which produce signals based on changes in the magnetic field [128]. The magnetic field above the sensor is perturbed due to the presence of bound magnetic nanoparticles. See Fig. 1.28.

1.6 Mechanical

Biosensors based on mechanical transduction methods include cantilevers [129–133], surface acoustic waves (SAWs) [38] and quartz crystal microbalances [134]. These mechanical structures can be mass-produced using combination of photoli-

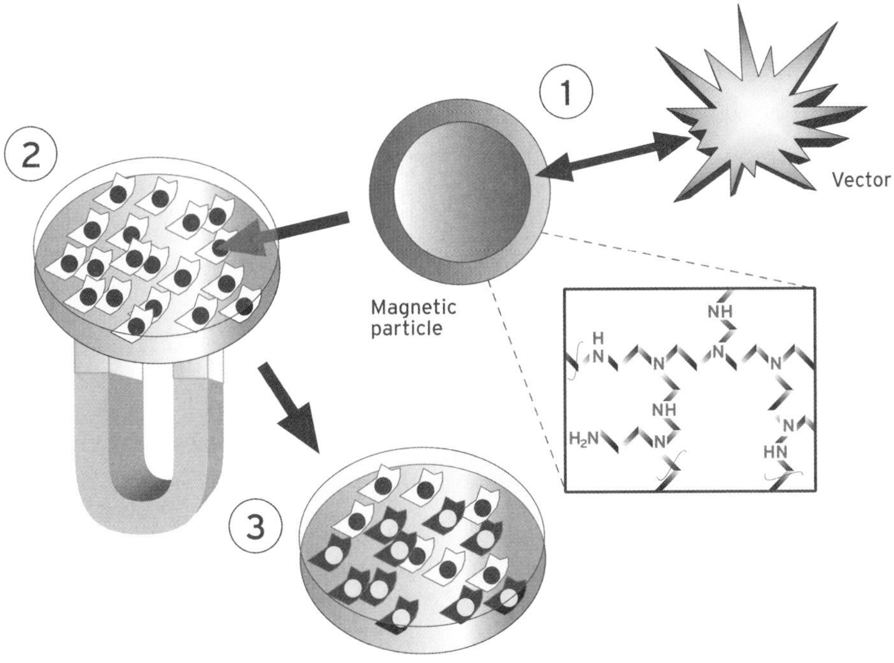

Figure 1.27. Magnetofection [126]. Reproduced from Biological Chemistry, Vol. 384, C. Plank et al., The magnetofection method: using magnetic force to enhance gene delivery, p. 737–747, Copyright (2003), with permission from Walter de Gruyter GmbH & Co. KG and C. Plank.

thographic, micromachining and thin film techniques. As the capabilities of these techniques continue to be improved, nanoscale mechanical structures, such as nanocantilevers, can be fabricated. The advantage of making mechanical structures with nanoscale dimensions is their resulting ability to respond to extremely small mechanical stimuli such as molecular binding. For example, nanocantilevers can be used to detect subfemtograms of material. A single viral particle on a nanocantilever produces a measurable response.

Biosensors based on nanocantilever structures can be fabricated by modifying the cantilever surface with biological receptors such as antibodies, aptamers and complementary DNA. Upon target binding, the cantilever will deflect if operating in static mode or its resonant frequency will shift if operating in dynamic mode. Deflection of the cantilever is typically monitored optically by focusing a laser onto the cantilever and measuring deflection with a photodetector (Fig. 1.29), similar to an atomic force microscope (AFM). Although static mode cantilevers perform better than the dynamic mode due to mechanical damping of the resonating cantilevers, as the cantilevers are reduced to the nanoscale measuring the deflection becomes challenging while resonant cantilevers become much more sensitive to mass loading. Therefore, most nanocantilever biosensors operate in dynamic mode.

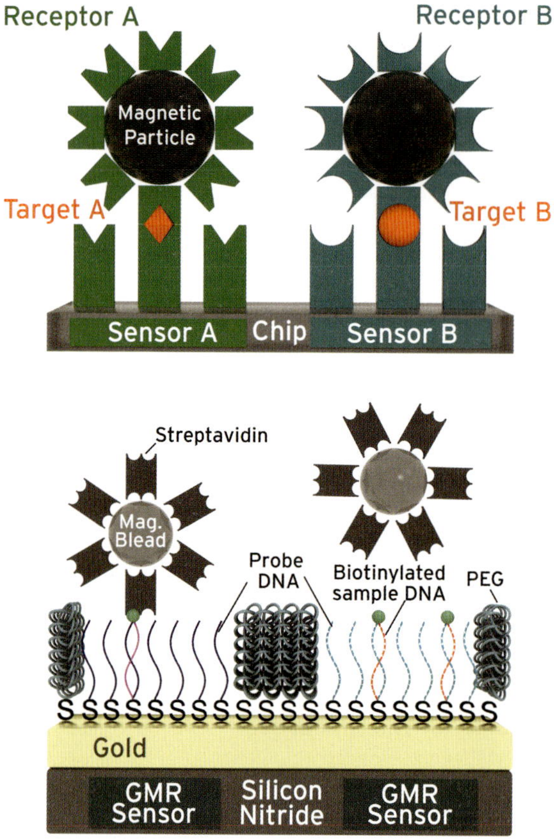

Figure 1.28. Biosensor based on magnetoresistive arrays [120]. Reproduced from Materials Today, Vol. 7, P. Gould, Nanoparticles probe biosystems, p. 36–43, Copyright (2004), with permission from Elsevier.

In dynamic mode, the resonant frequency of the nanocantilever can be monitored with optical methods as described above or with electrical methods such as capacitive or piezoelectric. The binding of additional mass results in a downshift of the resonant frequency as indicated by:

$$\frac{1}{f_1^2} - \frac{1}{f_0^2} = \frac{\Delta m}{4\pi^2 k}, \tag{2}$$

where f_0 is the initial cantilever resonant frequency, f_1 is the resulting cantilever resonant frequency after binding, Δm is the mass of analyte bound to the cantilever and k is the spring constant of the cantilever. The spring constant for a rectangular cantilever is expressed by:

$$k = \frac{Ewt^3}{4L^3}, \tag{3}$$

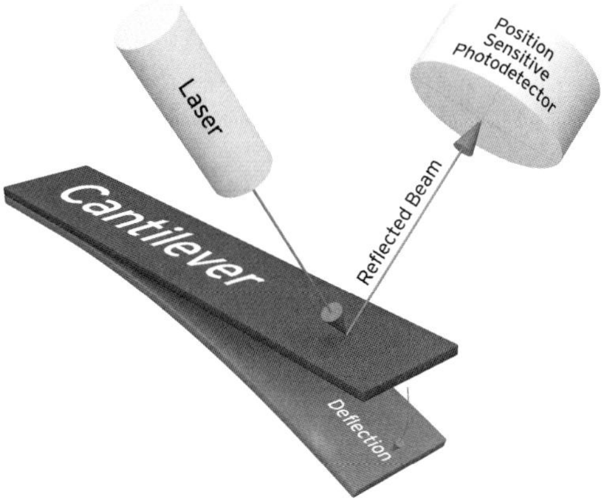

Figure 1.29. Typical optical measurement of cantilever deflection [130]. Reproduced with permission from Nickolay V. Lavrik, Review of Scientific Instruments, 75, 2229 (2004). Copyright 2004, American Institute of Physics.

where E is the Young's modulus of the cantilever, w is the cantilever width, t is the cantilever thickness and L is the cantilever length.

Using techniques based on semiconductor fabrication methods, nanocantilevers can be batch-fabricated in large volumes (hundreds to thousands per substrate) establishing potential for low-cost manufacturing. Nanocantilevers can be individually functionalized such that arrays can be formed providing multiplexing capability. With the use of electrical readout methods instead of optical methods, low-power portable cantilever-based diagnostic systems could be realized.

1.7 Imaging Diagnostics

Medical imaging diagnostics include MRI, PET, CT, OCT, optoacoustic or photoacoustic tomography (OAT or PAT) and NIR imaging. Nanoparticles containing hundreds of contrast agents can greatly enhance the sensitivity of these imaging methods [24, 122, 135, 136]. Examples of MRI contrast agents include gadolinium-diethylene-triamine-pentacetic acid (Gd-DTPA) and superparamagnetic iron oxide particles (SPIOs). Ultrasound contrast agents are designed to affect the propagation of sound waves in the surrounding sample area by altering the acoustic properties. Liquid perfluorocarbon nanoparticles and liposomes are examples of ultrasound contrast agents. Due to the small scale of nanoparticle contrast agents, the body does not quickly clear them, which prolongs the time that can be taken during imaging for a more thorough diagnosis.

Noninvasive detection at the single-cell level may be possible with nanocarriers loaded with contrast agent and functionalized with biological receptors specific to the desired cell. Such sensitivity could greatly improve early disease detection.

Nanocarriers could include liposomes, dendrimers or porous polymeric nanoparticles. Multifunctional nanocarriers combine biological specificity with the ability to use multiple imaging modalities. For instance, crosslinked iron oxide (CLIO) nanoparticles have branched structure which facilitates complexing with targeting entities such as enzymes or aptamers in addition to attachment of fluorophores or quantum dots [137]. Therefore, magnetic nanoparticles which function as MRI contrast agents can be modified to target a specific cell type and can be simultaneously monitored optically due to addition of optical tags.

An advantage of optical imaging methods over MRI, PET and CT is the potential of manufacturing lower cost imaging equipment. Lasers and optical (for OCT and NIR) or acoustic (for OAT/PAT) detectors are relatively inexpensive in comparison to large magnets and X-ray machines. One drawback of optical imaging is tissue absorption and reflection of photonic energy. Nanoparticle contrast agents that possess greater absorption than surrounding tissue or produce enhanced luminescence when irradiated can help alleviate tissue effects. Another advantage of using optics for imaging is the ability to guide the optical path with fiber optics, as in endoscopy, enabling internal imaging of vasculature, deep tissue and possibly the brain.

Optoacoustic or photacoustic tomography uses optical irradiation to induce localized thermal perturbations in the absorbing tissue [138]. Thermal vibrations produce acoustic waves which propagate from the underlying tissue to the skin surface. Acoustic detectors on the surface of the skin pick up the resulting acoustic waves. Optically absorbing gold nanoparticles can be used as contrast agents for optoacoustic imaging [139]. By controlling shape and structure, nanoparticles can be designed to optimally absorb at a desired wavelength. Simultaneously using optically absorbing nanoparticles of various designs that are each targeted to different cell or tissue types could provide a means for multiplexed bioimaging.

Gold nanoparticles as small as organic fluorophores can be irradiated with NIR and produce luminescence from lower excitation intensities than typical bioimaging fluorophores. Gold nanoparticles are also highly photostable (an advantage over organic fluorophores) and do not produce significant blinking (an advantage over semiconductor quantum dots). Furthermore, gold nanoparticles are easier to fabricate than quantum dots, can be readily modified for biological specificity and exhibit very low toxicity. All of these characteristics show promise for gold nanoparticles as an enabling technology to achieve single-molecule *in vivo* imaging for early diagnostics [140].

1.8 Nanotechnology-enhanced Tools

Although nanotechnology promises to develop novel diagnostic methods, current tools and methods can also benefit. Analytical instrumentation such as IR and mass spectrometers are widely used tools which are breaking into patient diagnostics. Enhancements of these instruments and techniques using nanotechnology should further this potential. Genetic-based techniques such as PCR, sequencing and gene chips are being made more affordable and more portable. Even standard immunoassays can be improved upon using multivalent nanoparticles to improve the signal-to-noise ratio.

1.8.1
Analytical Tools

Analytical chemistry techniques such as IR and Raman spectroscopy and mass spectrometry are widely used in life sciences – from pharmaceutical process monitoring to drug discovery. Due to the versatility of these techniques, diagnostic applications are being developed. As discussed earlier, IR spectroscopy, especially in the near IR region, is being used in diagnostic imaging. Raman spectroscopy, with its ability to perform analysis in aqueous samples and less-stringent requirements on sample preparation, is especially promising for diagnostics with the potential for single-molecule detection using Raman enhancement techniques. Finally, mass spectrometry as the gold standard in analytical chemistry and proteomics is already being investigated for use in breath diagnostics and shows potential for diagnosis progression of disease based on protein profiles.

One drawback with using IR, Raman or mass spectroscopy for diagnosis is the need for specialized equipment and trained personnel to operate the equipment. Such equipment is typically situated in separate laboratories, requiring samples to be shipped for analysis. Lower-cost and easier to use equipment may open up the possibility of having analytical spectroscopic techniques at the patient bedside. One advantage of these techniques over biosensor or assay-based diagnostics is their nonspecialization. Biosensors and assays are typically formulated to detect a particular analyte of interest. Enzymes, antibodies, aptamers and complementary DNA strands are all used in biosensors and *in vitro* assays, making the sensors or substrates specific to the target in question. This specificity limits the ability of such diagnostics to detect a multitude of targets unless an array of sensors or substrates are prepared, each with their own specificity. Furthermore, one needs to have an idea of what to target for the biosensor or assay to be useful. Spectroscopic techniques are not target specific, but provide a fingerprint, or spectral signature, based on the chemical profile of the sample. The resulting fingerprint is compared to a database to find matches which delineate the chemicals that exist in the sample. This provides a powerful mechanism to analyze unknown samples and to simultaneously detect a multitude of analytes.

1.8.2
Raman Spectroscopy

One of the challenges using Raman spectroscopy is the weak Raman signal that is generated from the sample being interrogated. The use of more powerful lasers for excitation combined with sensitive detectors has helped Raman spectroscopy become more widespread. For diagnostic use, powerful lasers are not always practical, so another way to improve the Raman signal is to enhance the interaction between the optical excitation and the sample. Two techniques used to enhance

Raman signal are surface-enhanced Raman spectroscopy (SERS) and tip-enhanced Raman spectroscopy (TERS) [141–147].

For SERS, gold or silver nanoparticles are most commonly used to amplify the Raman signal. These nanoparticles can be used within living cells to amplify weak Raman signals from intracellular moieties, enabling the tracking of such entities without the need for fluorescent tags. Nanostructured tips, typically less than 50 nm in tip radius, are used in TERS. These tips can be AFM cantilever tips or scanning tunneling microscope (STM) tips coating with thin gold or silver film. SERS and TERS techniques amplify the Raman signal by establishing resonance between the applied optical field propagating through the sample and the surface plasmon waves propagating through the metallic nanostructures. The potential for single-molecule detection within living cells using SERS or TERS could open up the opportunity for early detection of disease.

1.8.3
Mass Spectrometry

Two of the challenges of using mass spectrometry for diagnostics are sample delivery and sensitivity. For mass spectrometer analysis, samples must be analyzed in an ionized, gaseous form. Therefore, biological samples must be prepared prior to delivery. Two methods are predominantly used for biological sample preparation and delivery with mass spectrometers. The first method involves spotting of the sample onto a substrate. A laser is used to desorb and ionize the sample which is then passed into the mass spectrometer. Matrix-assisted laser desorption and ionization (MALDI) and surface-enhanced laser desorption and ionization (SELDI) are the two commonly used substrate-based techniques. The second method involves use of a fine capillary to deliver the liquid sample towards electrodes situated near the tip of the capillary. The liquid sample aerosolizes upon emission from the capillary and a high field across the electrodes ionizes the aerosol, which travels into the vacuum chamber of the mass spectrometer and transforms to vapor phase.

Nanostructured materials and surfaces can help enhance MALDI and SELDI techniques. By enabling smaller spot sizes, dense arrays could be nanofabricated, helping increase the throughput of MALDI and SELDI systems [148]. Nanoscale surfaces functionalized with an array of biological receptors could be used to bind with desired targets within the protein population of the sample providing a presorting mechanism prior to mass spectrometry analysis. Many proteins of clinical relevance are overshadowed by more abundant proteins and can be difficult to detect. Nanoparticles specific for these lower-abundant proteins could be used as harvesting agents in preparation for mass spectrometry analysis [149].

Finally, protein quantification and binding analysis can be performed in conjunction with fingerprinting and structural elucidation by combining binding-based assay with mass spectrometry. One technique amenable to coupling with mass spectrometry is SPR (Fig. 1.30) [150]. Using immobilized receptors on the SPR substrate, binding of targeted proteins can be detected. Once SPR detection is complete, the substrate can be coated with matrix and used for MALDI mass spectrometry or microfluidics could be used to draw the sample from the SPR sub-

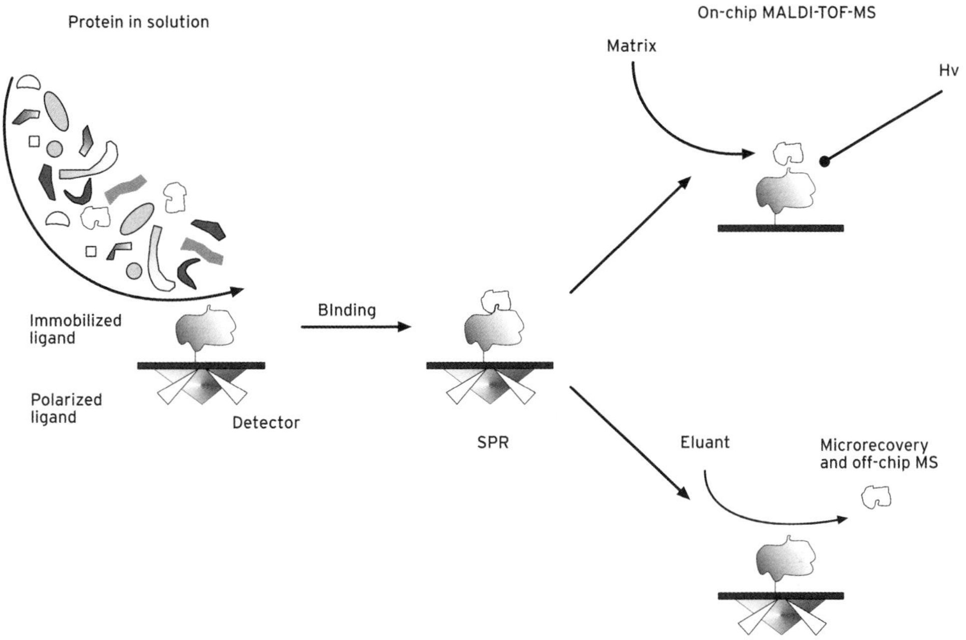

Figure 1.30. SPR mass spectrometry [150]. Reproduced from Trends in Biotechnology, D. Nedelkov and R. W. Nelson, Surface Plasmon resonance mass spectrometry: recent progress and outlooks, p. 301–305. Copyright (2003) with permission from Elsevier.

strate for electrospray ionization (ESI) mass spectrometry. An enhancement of this combination technique would be the use of nanoparticles establishing localized SPR to increase the sensitivity of quantifying low-abundance proteins prior to mass spectrometry.

1.8.4 Genetics

Traditional bacterial diagnostics involve culturing followed by identification and often another confirming step which can take days to weeks for results to be achieved. ELISAs can provide faster results due to higher sensitivity so that fewer cells are required for analysis. However, immunoassays do not necessarily provide information on the particular strain of a pathogen. Here is where strain-specific tests are performed using genetic-based assays. Such assays typically involve amplification of the nucleic acids, such as PCR, to provide enough genetic material to perform the assay. Nanotechnology is enabling even quicker results by speeding up the PCR process or even by obviating the need for amplification altogether.

One nanostructure being investigated is the nanopore for DNA sequencing [151–154]. Nanopores fabricated from organic materials, such as proteins, or inor-

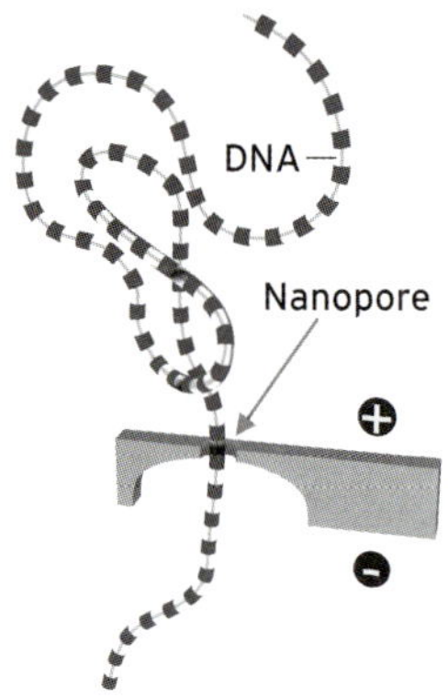

Figure 1.31. DNA nanopore.

ganic materials, such as semiconductors, could be designed to allow only single-stranded DNA to file through (Fig. 1.31). Electrical or optical methods could be used to detect each DNA base as it transcends through the pore, providing a direct readout method for sequencing without the need to amplify the DNA. The resulting sequence can then be analyzed to determine mutations for genetic screening or can be compared to pathogen sequences for diagnosing infections.

Nanopores can be machined within semiconductor materials using focused ion beam (FIB) milling [155]. With FIB milling, a high-energy ion beam is finely focused onto the sample to be machined. Arrays of nanopores can be machined by manipulating the sample stage and alternating the ion beam on and off. Isolated organic structures may also have the capability of nanopore sequencing. One particular biological structure that has an internal pore diameter of 1.5 nm, which will allow only single-stranded DNA to pass through, is the α-hemolysin ion channel shown in Fig. 1.32.

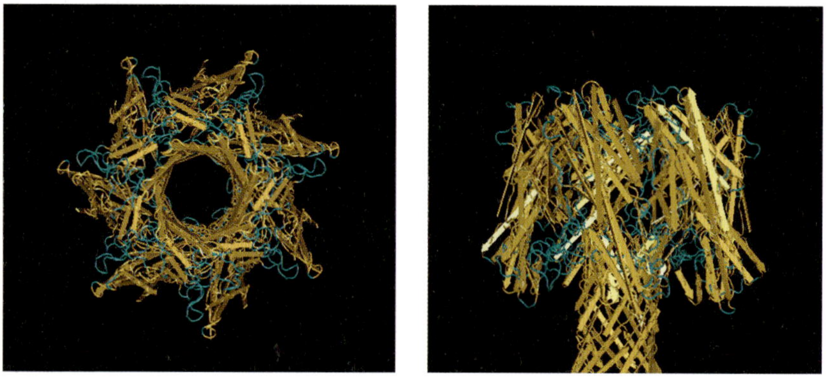

Figure 1.32. α-Hemolysin ion channel, approximately 10 nm long with 1.5 nm internal pore diameter.

1.8.5
Immunoassays

Immunoassays are routinely used for diagnostics due to their high sensitivity and high selectivity. With the growing desire for smaller sample sizes and earlier disease capture, improvements in immunoassays would be welcome. One method to enhance sensitivity of immunoassays is through the use of antibody-conjugated nanoparticles [156]. For instance, lanthanide-based chelate complexes can be attached to antibody-conjugated nanoparticle carriers creating dense luminescent particles with biological specificity. Lanthanide ions, such as Eu(III) and Tb(III), exhibit narrow emission spectra in the visible wavelength range. Therefore, increasing the density of the chelate complexes by nanoparticle immobilization will produce greater emission to enhance sensitivity. A capture probe can be immobilized onto the substrate surface which targets the desired analyte. The detection antibodies conjugated to the nanoparticle carrying the Lanthanide complexes then bind to the captured analyte, if present. Luminescence is then measured to determine the presence of the analyte. Other small molecule dyes could also be used if nanoparticle immobilization of such dyes could be achieved. See Fig. 1.33.

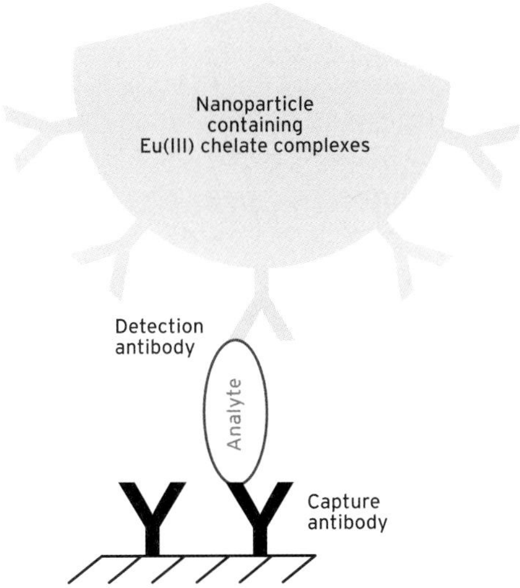

Figure 1.33. Immunoassay enhanced with antibody-conjugated nanoparticle containing luminescent lanthanide complexes [156]. Reproduced with permission from Anal. Bioanal. Chem., Vol. 380 (2004), p. 24–30, Detection strategies for bioassays based on luminescent lanthanide complexes and signal amplification, T. Steinkamp and U. Karst, Fig. 10, Copyright (2004). With kind permission of Springer Science and Business Media.

1.9
Nanotechnology and the Future of Patient Diagnostics

1.9.1
Multifunctional Platforms

An area of future impact of nanotechnology for patient care is the development of *in vivo* modular, multifunctional platforms to target, detect and react [157–160]. Dendrimers, due to their highly branched structure, are potential multifunctional nanostructured platforms. Crosslinking to two or more different types of nanoparticles could also create a multifunctional platform. For targeting, biological receptors such as aptamers or antibodies could be immobilized onto the nanostructured platforms. Reporting moieties such as quantum dots or contrast agents could be attached to a separate branch within the dendrimer or attached to or embedded within the crosslinked, nontargeting nanoparticle. This will allow for tracking of the multifunctional platforms with noninvasive imaging methods. Therapeutics could be harbored within the dendrimer core or coated onto the nontargeting nanoparticle enabling targeted drug delivery in conjunction with imaging for combination diagnosis and therapy.

Figure 1.34 shows a multifunctional dendrimer carrying folic acid as a targeting agent, fluorescein as a reporter and methotrexate as the therapeutic. Folic acid, or folate, has a high affinity for folic acid receptors which many cancer cells overexpress. FITC is a widely used fluorophore. Methotrexate (MTX) is an effective anticancer drug, but with high toxicity. By adding targeting capability to drugs such as MTX, less amounts of drug should be necessary for therapy. Also, systemic side-effects should be minimized. The use of a multifunctional carrier platform not only enables transport of the drug to its desired destination, but also allows for tracking with the addition of reporter entities.

1.9.2
Real-time Monitoring

Implantable sensor technologies that can be remotely monitored enable on-demand and real-time patient monitoring. *In vivo* nanoscale sensors may also provide feedback, based on physiological status, as part of replacement biological systems, such as an artificial kidney or pancreas [161]. Due to the ultraminiature form factor, identical sensors may be implanted for redundancy as a safeguard against sensor failure. Multiple sensors for different targets may also be implanted to simultaneously monitor patient condition.

1.9.3
Multiplexed Diagnostic Assays

Nanoscale sensing platforms combined with microfluidic systems for sample delivery offer the potential to simultaneously perform large numbers of analyses and increase sample throughput [162–164]. Also, biomimetic molecular constructs,

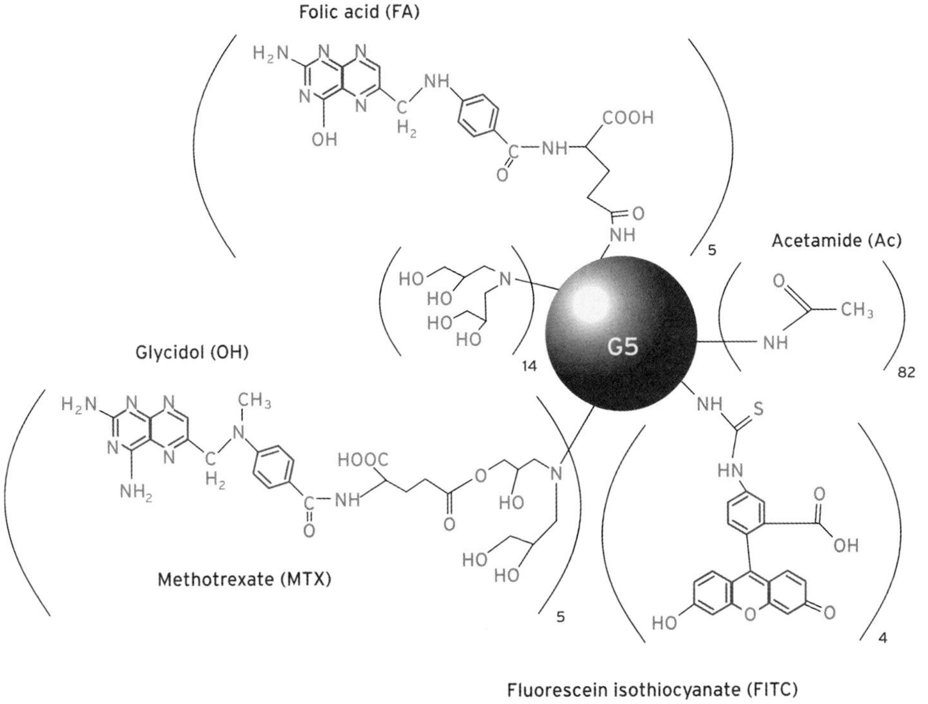

Figure 1.34. Fifth-generation dendrimer simultaneously functionalized with MTX, folic acid and FITC [157]. Reproduced with permission from Molecular Pharmaceutics, Vol. 2, X. Shi et al., Capillary electrophoresis of (poly)amidoamine dendrimers: from simple derivatives to complex multifunctional nanodevices, p. 278–294. Copyright (2005) American Chemical Society.

such as peptide or aptamer structures, have the potential to be derived with high affinity for numerous analytes [165]. Being able to analyze a single sample for a number of disease biomarkers at one time could lower the cost of diagnosis and enable a more accurate assessment of the patient's condition.

1.9.4
Point-of-care Diagnostics

Bringing the diagnostic tool to the patient, i.e. point-of-care, as opposed to sending samples to a laboratory has the potential to benefit everyone in the healthcare chain. The doctor or nurse will be able to perform quicker diagnoses. The healthcare institution may reduce operating costs due to less need to take and process patient samples. The insurance company or other third-party payer may reduce their costs due to fewer reimbursable events that are typically involved in diagnostic procedures, such as drawing patient samples, using laboratory time and purchasing diagnostic reagents. Finally, the patient should also benefit from faster, more accurate and less-costly diagnosis.

Sample handling is one technical hurdle that must be overcome for point-of-care diagnostics to truly reach the clinic. Micro/nanofluidics will likely play a major role in delivering the patient sample to the sensing portion of the diagnostic tool. However, sample delivery is only one of the challenges in getting a sample, such as blood, to the biologically sensitive area of the tool. For instance, in the case of blood analysis, the sample may need to be filtered and desired analytes separated out, all automatically within the portable diagnostic tool. Without filtering and separation, the sensor surface may quickly become saturated with nonspecific proteins.

1.9.5
Regulations, Risks and Ethics

Although a through discussion is beyond the scope of this chapter, the risks and benefits of nanotechnology for patient diagnostics must be carefully addressed. Nanotechnology enables the construction of materials and devices that can intimately interact with biological systems. Such interaction has its benefits, as exhibited by the various opportunities described in this chapter and from numerous other sources. However, we must proceed diligently to understand the effects of artificial nanostructures on biological systems. The benefits of nanotechnology must be understood along with the risks. Early and close interaction with regulatory agencies, such as the Food and Drug Administration (FDA) and the Environmental Protection Agency (EPA), should be part of the technology development process [166, 167].

Currently, additional or special regulatory handling of biomedical nanotechnology products is not being anticipated, although new toxicological testing and standards may need to be developed. For regulatory purposes, the FDA defines nanotechnology as "research and technology or development of products regulated by FDA that involve all of the following:

(1) the existence of materials or products at the atomic, molecular or macromolecular levels, where at least one dimension that affects the functional behavior of the drug/device product is in the length scale range of approximately 1–100 nm;
(2) the creation and use of structures, devices and systems that have novel properties and functions because of their small size; and,
(3) the ability to control or manipulate the product on the atomic scale."

With the potential of multifunctional capability, many biomedical nanotechnology products will likely not fall into a single FDA category, but may be handled as combination products [168]. Examples of existing combination products are listed in Tab. 1.5. To regulate combination products, the FDA established the Office of Combination Products (OCP) in 2002. As defined by the FDA in Section 3.2(e) of 21 CFR (Code of Federal Regulations) Part 3, a combination product includes:

(1) A product comprised of two or more regulated components, i.e. drug/device, biologic/device, drug/biologic or drug/device/biologic, that are physically, chemically or otherwise combined or mixed and produced as a single entity.

Tab. 1.5. Examples of combination products.

Drug-eluting stents
Catheter with antimicrobial coating
Antibody combined with therapeutic
Transdermal drug delivery patches
Orthopedic implant with growth factors

(2) Two or more separate products packaged together in a single package or as a unit and comprised of drug and device products, device and biological products, or biological and drug products.
(3) A drug, device or biological product packaged separately that according to its investigational plan or proposed labeling is intended for use only with an approved individually specified drug, device or biological product where both are required to achieve the intended use, indication or effect and where upon approval of the proposed product the labeling of the approved product would need to be changed, e.g. to reflect a change in intended use, dosage form, strength, route of administration or significant change in dose.
(4) Any investigational drug, device or biological product packaged separately that according to its proposed labeling is for use only with another individually specified investigational drug, device or biological product where both are required to achieve the intended use, indication or effect.

For nanotechnology diagnostic products used *in vitro*, the FDA Office of *In Vitro* Diagnostic Device Evaluation and Safety has regulatory control. As defined by the FDA in 21 CFR 809.3, an *in vitro* diagnostic product includes:

> *In vitro* diagnostic products are those reagents, instruments and systems intended for use in diagnosis of disease or other conditions, including a determination of the state of health, in order to cure, mitigate, treat or prevent disease or its sequelae. Such products are intended for use in the collection, preparation and examination of specimens taken from the human body.

Scientists must not only weigh the health risks, but also the ethical risks. Scientists should be concerned with public perception and ethical issues of nanotechnology [169–175]. With the potential to perform highly sensitive, multiplexed and rapid diagnostics, guidelines and protocols should be established to aid clinicians and patients to make sense of all the data and proceed with the most appropriate course of action. A diagnostic test may be developed and used to which no counter treatment is available. If patients are willing to take such tests, then they should be made well aware of the possible quandaries.

Nanotechnology has the potential to revolutionize medicine as we know it today. Nanostructured materials and devices may make possible the ability for targeted drug delivery, real-time patient monitoring, high-resolution noninvasive imaging, high-throughput screening and multiplexed diagnostics. Such an arsenal of tools and techniques could enable the ability to capture a disease at its earliest onset, specifically target the diseased site and rapidly treat the patient before any physiological damage is done and without any detrimental side-effects.

References

1 Beers, M. H., R. Berkow (Eds.), *The Merck Manual of Diagnosis and Therapy.* 17th edn. Merck, West Point, PA, **1999**.

2 Wilkinson, J. M., Nanotechnology applications in medicine. *Med. Device Technol.* **2003**, *14*, 29–31.

3 Sprintz, M., C. Benedetti, M. Ferrari, Applied nanotechnology for the management of breakthrough cancer pain. *Minerva Anestesiol.* **2005**, *71*, 419–423.

4 Heath, J. R., M. E. Phelps, L. Hood, NanoSystems biology. *Mol. Imaging Biol.* **2003**, *5*, 312–325.

5 Jain, K. K., Nanodiagnostics: application of nanotechnology in molecular diagnostics. *Expert Rev. Mol. Diagn.* **2003**, *3*, 153–161.

6 Jain, K. K., Nanotechnology in clinical laboratory diagnostics. *Clin. Chim. Acta* **2005**, *358*, 37–54.

7 Kubik, T., K. Bogunia-Kubik, M. Sugisaka, Nanotechnology on duty in medical applications. *Curr. Pharm. Biotechnol.* **2005**, *6*, 17–33.

8 Walt, D. R., Chemistry. Miniature analytical methods for medical diagnostics. *Science* **2005**, *308*, 217–219.

9 Emerich, D. F., C. G. Thanos, Nanotechnology and medicine. *Expert Opin. Biol. Ther.* **2003**, *3*, 655–663.

10 Roco, M. C., Nanotechnology: convergence with modern biology and medicine. *Curr. Opin. Biotechnol.* **2003**, *14*, 337–346.

11 Jianrong, C., et al., Nanotechnology and biosensors. *Biotechnol. Adv.* **2004**, *22*, 505–518.

12 Emerich, D. F., Nanomedicine – prospective therapeutic and diagnostic applications. *Expert Opin. Biol. Ther.* **2005**, *5*, 1–5.

13 McNeil, S. E., Nanotechnology for the biologist. *J. Leukocyte Biol.* **2005**, *78*, 585–594.

14 Wiley, C., Nanotechnology and molecular homeostasis. *J. Am. Geriatr. Soc.* **2005**, *53 (9 Suppl.)*, S295–S98.

15 Guetens, G., et al., Nanotechnology in bio/clinical analysis. *J. Chromatogr.* **2000**, *739*, 139–150.

16 Ferrari, M., Cancer nanotechnology: opportunities and challenges. *Nat. Rev.* **2005**, *5*, 161–171.

17 Sahoo, S. K., V. Labhasetwar, Nanotech approaches to drug delivery and imaging. *Drug Discov. Today* **2003**, *8*, 1112–1120.

18 Silva, G. A., Introduction to nanotechnology and its applications to medicine. *Surg. Neurol.* **2004**, *61*, 216–220.

19 Weis, R. P., et al., Calcified nanostructured silicon wafer surfaces for biosensing: effects of surface modification on bioactivity. *Dis. Markers* **2002**, *18*, 159.

20 Bogunia-Kubik, K., M. Sugisaka, From molecular biology to nanotechnology and nanomedicine. *Biosystems* **2002**, *65*, 123–38.

21 Csaki, A., R. Moller, W. Fritzsche, Gold nanoparticles as novel label for DNA diagnostics. *Expert Rev. Mol. Diagn.* **2002**, *2*, 187–93.

22 Leary, S. P., et al., Toward the emergence of nanoneurosurgery: part I – progress in nanoscience, nanotechnology, and the comprehension of events in the mesoscale realm. *Neurosurgery* **2005**, *57*, 606.

23 Hood, E., Nanotechnology: looking as we leap. *Environ. Health Perspect.* **2004**, *112*, A740–A749.

24 Buxton, D. B., et al., Recommendations of the National Heart, Lung, and Blood Institute Nanotechnology Working Group. *Circulation* **2003**, *108*, 2737–2742.

25 Fortina, P., et al., Nanobiotechnology: the promise and reality of new approaches to molecular recognition. *Trends Biotechnol.* **2005**, *23*, 168–173.

26 Barathur, R., et al., New disc-based technologies for diagnostic and research applications. *Psychiatr. Genet.* **2002**, *12*, 193–206.
27 Carella, M., S. Volinia, P. Gasparini, Nanotechnologies and microchips in genetic diseases. *J. Nephrol.* **2003**, *16*, 597–602.
28 Jain, K. K., Applications of biochips: from diagnostics to personalized medicine. *Curr. Opin. Drug Discov. Dev.* **2004**, *7*, 285–289.
29 Wilkinson, J. M., M. H. Kuok, G. Adamson, Biomedical applications of optical imaging. *Med. Device Technol.* **2004**, *15*, 22–24.
30 Proske, D., et al., Aptamers – basic research, drug development, and clinical applications. *Appl. Microbiol. Biotechnol.* **2006**, *69*, 367–374.
31 Achenbach, J. C., R. Nutiu, Y. Li, Structure-switching allosteric deoxyribozymes. *Anal. Chim. Acta* **2005**, *534*, 41–51.
32 Le, X. C., V. Pavski, H. Wang, W. A. E. McBryde, Award Lecture – Affinity recognition, capillary electrophoresis, and laser-induced fluorescence polarization for ultrasensitive bioanalysis. *Can. J. Chem.* **2005**, *83*, 185–194.
33 Shaw, B. R., et al., Reading, writing, and modulating genetic information with boranophosphate mimics of nucleotides, DNA, and RNA. *Ann. NY Acad. Sci.* **2003**, *1002*, 12–29.
34 Vaish, N. K., et al., A Novel, modification-dependent ATP-binding aptamer selected from an RNA library incorporating a cationic functionality. *Biochemistry* **2003**, *42*, 8842.
35 Brody, E. N., L. Gold, Aptamers as therapeutic and diagnostic agents. *J. Biotechnol.* **2000**, *74*, 5–13.
36 Brody, E. N., et al., The use of aptamers in large arrays for molecular diagnostics. *Mol. Diagn.* **1999**, *4*, 381–388.
37 Jayasena, S. D., Aptamers: an emerging class of molecules that rival antibodies in diagnostics. *Clin. Chem.* **1999**, *45*, 1628–1650.
38 Thompson, M., A. K. Deisingh, Biosensors for the detection of bacteria. *Can. J. Microbiol.* **2004**, *50*, 69–77.
39 Danke, X., et al., Label-free electrochemical detection for aptamer-based array electrodes. *Anal. Chem.* **2005**, *77*, 5107–5113.
40 Kawde, A.-N., et al., Label-free bioelectronic detection of aptamer-protein interactions. *Electrochem. Commun.* **2005**, *7*, 537–540.
41 Radi, A.-E., et al., Reusable impedimetric aptasensor. *Anal. Chem.* **2005**, *77*, 6320–6323.
42 Kolusheva, S., et al., Selective detection of catecholamines by synthetic receptors embedded in chromatic polydiacetylene vesicles. *J. Am. Chem. Soc.* **2005**, *127*, 10000–10001.
43 Holm, B. A., et al., Nanotechnology in biomedical applications. *Mol. Crystals Liquid Crystals* **2002**, *374*, 589–598.
44 Prasad, P., Emerging opportunities at the interface of photonics, nanotechnology and biotechnology. *Mol. Crystals Liquid Crystals* **2004**, *415*, 1–7.
45 Lesniak, W., et al., Silver/dendrimer nanocomposites as biomarkers: fabrication, characterization, *in vitro* toxicity, and intracellular detection. *Nano Lett.* **2005**, *5*, 2123–2130.
46 Aslan, K., J. R. Lakowicz, C. D. Geddes, Metal-enhanced fluorescence using anisotropic silver nanostructures: critical progress to date. *Anal. Bioanal. Chem.* **2005**, *382*, 926–933.
47 Aslan, K., et al., Metal-enhanced fluorescence: an emerging tool in biotechnology. *Curr. Opin. Biotechnol.* **2005**, *16*, 55–62.
48 Huhtinen, P., et al., Europium(III) nanoparticle-label-based assay for the detection of nucleic acids. *Nanotechnology* **2004**, *15*, 1708–1715.
49 Valanne, A., et al., A sensitive adenovirus immunoassay as a model for using nanoparticle label technology in virus diagnostics. *J. Clin. Virol.* **2005**, *33*, 217–223.
50 Lakhtakia, A., *Nanometer Structures: Theory, Modeling, and Simulation. The Handbook of Nanotechnology.* ASME Press, New York, **2004**.
51 Ethiraj, A. S., et al., Synthesis and investigation of ZnS nanoparticles adsorbed on functionalised silica particles. *Surf. Eng.* **2004**, *20*, 367–372.

52 Ozkan, M., Quantum dots and other nanoparticles: what can they offer to drug discovery? *Drug Discov. Today* **2004**, *9*, 1065–1071.

53 Riegler, Jr., T. Nann, Application of luminescent nanocrystals as labels for biological molecules. *Anal. Bioanal. Chem.* **2004**, *379*, 913–919.

54 Mattoussi, H., et al., Electroluminescence from heterostructures of poly(phenylene vinylene) and inorganic CdSe. *J. Appl. Phys.* **1998**, *83*, 7965.

55 Cottingham, K., Quantum dots leave the light on. *Anal. Chem.* **2005**, *77*, 354A–357A.

56 Kuno, M., et al., Nonexponential "blinking" kinetics of single CdSe quantum dots: a universal power law behavior. *J. Chem. Phys.* **2000**, *112*, 3117–3120.

57 Kuno, M., et al., "On"/"off" fluorescence intermittency of single semiconductor quantum dots. *J. Chem. Phys.* **2001**, *115*, 1028–1040.

58 Goldman, E. R., et al., Multiplexed toxin analysis using four colors of quantum dot fluororeagents. *Anal. Chem.* **2004**, *76*, 684–688.

59 Gao, X., W. C. Chan, S. Nie, Quantum-dot nanocrystals for ultrasensitive biological labeling and multicolor optical encoding. *J. Biomed. Opt.* **2002**, *7*, 532–7.

60 Gao, X., S. Nie, Quantum dot-encoded beads. *Methods Mol. Biol.* **2005**, *303*: p. 61–71.

61 Wang, Y., Z. Tang, N. A. Kotov, Bioapplication of nanosemiconductors. *Mater. Today* **2005**, *8*, 20–31.

62 Sang-Wook, K., et al., Engineering $InAs_xP_{1-x}/InP/ZnSe$ III–V alloyed core/shell quantum dots for the near-infrared. *J. Am. Chem. Soc.* **2005**, *127*, 10526–10532.

63 Dwarakanath, S., et al., Quantum dot–antibody and aptamer conjugates shift fluorescence upon binding bacteria. *Biochem. Biophys. Res. Commun.* **2004**, *325*, 739–743.

64 Disley, D. M., et al., Covalent coupling of immunoglobulin G to self-assembled monolayers as a method for immobilizing the interfacial-recognition layer of a surface plasmon resonance immunosensor. *Biosensors Bioelectron.* **1998**, *13*, 1213–1225.

65 Jain, K. K., The role of nanobiotechnology in drug discovery. *Drug Discov. Today* **2005**, *10*, 1435–1442.

66 Haes, A. J., R. P. Van Duyne, A unified view of propagating and localized surface plasmon resonance biosensors. *Anal. Bioanal. Chem.* **2004**, *379*, 920–930.

67 Haes, A. J., R. P. V. Duyne, Preliminary studies and potential applications of localized surface plasmon resonance spectroscopy in medical diagnostics. *Expert Rev. Mol. Diagn.* **2004**, *4*, 527–537.

68 Cooper, M. A., Label-free screening of bio-molecular interactions. *Anal. Bioanal. Chem.* **2003**, *377*, 834–842.

69 Haes, A. J., R. P. Van Duyne, A unified view of propagating and localized surface plasmon resonance biosensors. *Anal. Bioanal. Chem.* **2004**, *379*, 920–930.

70 Homola, J., Present and future of surface plasmon resonance biosensors. *Anal. Bioanal. Chem.* **2003**, *377*, 528–539.

71 Endo, T., et al., Label-free detection of peptide nucleic acid–DNA hybridization using localized surface plasmon resonance based optical biosensor. *Anal. Chem.* **2005**, *77*, 6976–6984.

72 Dahlin, A., et al., Localized surface plasmon resonance sensing of lipid-membrane-mediated biorecognition events. *J. Am. Chem. Soc.* **2005**, *127*, 5043–5048.

73 Haes, A. J., et al., Detection of a biomarker for Alzheimer's disease from synthetic and clinical samples using a nanoscale optical biosensor. *J. Am. Chem. Soc.* **2005**, *127*, 2264–2271.

74 Chanda Ranjit, Y., et al., A comparative analysis of localized and propagating surface plasmon resonance sensors: the binding of concanavalin A to a monosaccharide functionalized self-assembled monolayer. *J. Am. Chem. Soc.* **2004**, *126*, 12669–12676.

75 Link, S., M. A. El-Sayed, Optical properties and ultrafast dynamics of metallic nanocrystals. *Annu. Rev. Phys. Chem.* **2003**, *54*, 331.

76 Link, S., M. A. El-Sayed, Shape and size dependence of radiative, non-radiative and photothermal properties of gold nanocrystals. *Int. Rev. Phys. Chem.* **2000**, *19*, 409–453.

77 Clark, H. A., M. Hoyer, Optical nanosensors for chemical analysis inside single living cells. 1. Fabrication. *Anal. Chem.* **1999**, *71*, 4831.

78 Clark, H. A., et al., Optical nanosensors for chemical analysis inside single living cells. 2. Sensors for pH and calcium and the intracellular application of PEBBLE sensors. *Anal. Chem.* **1999**, *71*, 4837–4843.

79 Koo, Y.-E. L., et al., Real-time measurements of dissolved oxygen inside live cells by organically modified silicate fluorescent nanosensors. *Anal. Chem.* **2004**, *76*, 2498–2505.

80 Li, H., L. Rothberg, Detection of specific sequences in RNA using differential adsorption of single-stranded oligonucleotides on gold nanoparticles. *Anal. Chem.* **2005**, *77*, 6229–6233.

81 Li, H., L. Rothberg, Colorimetric detection of DNA sequences based on electrostatic interactions with unmodified gold nanoparticles. *Proc. Natl Acad. Sci. USA* **2004**, *101*, 14036–14039.

82 Li, H., L. J. Rothberg, DNA sequence detection using selective fluorescence quenching of tagged oligonucleotide probes by gold nanoparticles. *Anal. Chem.* **2004**, *76*, 5414–5417.

83 Li, H., L. J. Rothberg, Label-free colorimetric detection of specific sequences in genomic DNA amplified by the polymerase chain reaction. *J. Am. Chem. Soc.* **2004**, *126*, 10958–10961.

84 Nam, J.-M., A. R. Wise, J. T. Groves, colorimetric bio-barcode amplification assay for cytokines. *Anal. Chem.* **2005**, *77*, 6985–6988.

85 Georganopoulou, D. G., et al., Nanoparticle-based detection in cerebral spinal fluid of a soluble pathogenic biomarker for Alzheimer's disease. *Proc. Natl Acad. Sci. USA.* **2005**, *102*, 2273–2276.

86 Nam, J.-M., S.-J. Park, C. A. Mirkin, Bio-barcodes based on oligonucleotide-modified nanoparticles. *J. Am. Chem. Soc.* **2002**, *124*, 3820.

87 Nam, J.-M., C. S. Thaxton, C. A. Mirkin, Nanoparticle-based bio-bar codes for the ultrasensitive detection of proteins. *Science* **2003**, *301*, 1884–1886.

88 Thaxton, C. S., D. G. Georganopoulou, C. A. Mirkin, Gold nanoparticle probes for the detection of nucleic acid targets. *Clin. Chim. Acta* **2006**, *363*, 120–126.

89 Li, Y., Y. T. Cu, D. Luo, Multiplexed detection of pathogen DNA with DNA-based fluorescence nanobarcodes. *Nat. Biotechnol.* **2005**, *23*, 885–889.

90 Pavlov, V., et al., Aptamer-functionalized Au nanoparticles for the amplified optical detection of thrombin. *J. Am. Chem. Soc.* **2004**, *126*, 11768–11769.

91 Monk, D. J., D. R. Walt, Optical fiber-based biosensors. *Anal. Bioanal. Chem.* **2004**, *379*, 931–945.

92 Vo-Dinh, T., Nanobiosensors: probing the sanctuary of individual living cells. *J. Cell Biochem. Suppl.* **2002**, *39*, 154–161.

93 Vo-Dinh, T., Optical nanosensors for detecting proteins and biomarkers in individual living cells. *Methods Mol. Biol.* **2005**, *300*, 383–401.

94 Vo-Dinh, T., P. Kasili, Fiber-optic nanosensors for single-cell monitoring. *Anal. Bioanal. Chem.* **2005**, *382*, 918–25.

95 Konry, T., et al., Optical fiber immunosensor based on a poly(pyrrole-benzophenone) film for the detection of antibodies to viral antigen. *Anal. Chem.* **2005**, *77*, 1771–1779.

96 Bashir, R., BioMEMS: state-of-the-art in detection, opportunities and prospects. *Adv. Drug Deliv. Rev.* **2004**, *56*, 1565–1586.

97 Sotiropoulou, S., N. A. Chaniotakis, Carbon nanotube array-based biosensor. *Anal. Bioanal. Chem.* **2003**, *375*, 103–105.

98 Yemini, M., et al., Peptide nanotube-modified electrodes for enzyme-biosensor applications. *Anal. Chem.* **2005**, *77*, 5155–5159.

99 Koehne, J. E., et al., Miniaturized multiplex label-free electronic chip for rapid nucleic acid analysis based on carbon nanotube nanoelectrode arrays. *Clin. Chem.* **2004**, *50*, 1886–93.

100 Huang, Y., C. M. Lieber, Integrated nanoscale electronics and optoelectronics: exploring nanoscale *science* and technology through semiconductor nanowires. *Pure Appl. Chem.* **2004**, *76*, 2051–2068.

101 Yuqing, M., G. Jianguo, C. Jianrong, Ion sensitive field effect transducer-based biosensors. *Biotechnol. Adv.* **2003**, *21*, 527–534.

102 Friedrich, M. J., Nanoscale biosensors show promise. *J. Am. Med. Ass.* **2005**, *293*, 1965–1965.

103 Castillo, J., et al., Biosensors for life quality: design, development and applications. *Sensors Actuators B* **2004**, *102*, 179–194.

104 Drummond, T. G., M. G. Hill, J. K. Barton, Electrochemical DNA sensors. *Nat. Biotechnol.* **2003**, *21*, 1192–1199.

105 Ikebukuro, K., C. Kiyohara, K. Sode, Electrochemical detection of protein using a double aptamer sandwich. *Anal. Lett.* **2004**, *37*, 2901–2909.

106 Ikebukuro, K., C. Kiyohara, K. Sode, Novel electrochemical sensor system for protein using the aptamers in sandwich manner. *Biosensors Bioelectron.* **2005**, *20*, 2168–2172.

107 Bang, G. S., S. Cho, B.-G. Kim, A novel electrochemical detection method for aptamer biosensors. *Biosensors Bioelectron.* **2005**, *21*, 863–870.

108 Zhang, D., et al., Silica-nanoparticle-based interface for the enhanced immobilization and sequence-specific detection of DNA. *Anal. Bioanal. Chem.* **2004**, *379*, 1025–1030.

109 Yanez-Sedeno, P., J. M. Pingarron, Gold nanoparticle-based electrochemical biosensors. *Anal. Bioanal. Chem.* **2005**, *382*, 884–886.

110 Haruyama, T., et al., Bio-, nanotechnology for cellular biosensing. *Curr. Appl. Phys.* **2005**, *5*, 108–111.

111 Ozsoz, M., et al., Electrochemical genosensor based on colloidal gold nanoparticles for the detection of Factor V Leiden mutation using disposable pencil graphite electrodes. *Anal. Chem.* **2003**, *75*, 2181–2187.

112 Shinkai, S., M. Takeuchi, A.-H. Bae, Rational design and creation of novel polymeric superstructures by oxidative polymerization utilizing anionic templates. *Supramol. Chem.* **2005**, *17*, 181–186.

113 Covington, J. A., et al., Conductive polymer gate FET devices for vapour sensing. *IEE Proc. Circuits Devices Syst.* **2004**, *151*, 326–334.

114 Guang-Ming, Z., et al., Determination of trace chromium(VI) by an inhibition-based enzyme biosensor incorporating an electropolymerized aniline membrane and ferrocene as electron transfer mediator. *Int. J. Environ. Anal. Chem.* **2004**, *84*, 761–774.

115 Jin, L., et al., Amperometric biosensor with HRP immobilized on a sandwiched nano-Au/polymerized *m*-phenylenediamine film and ferrocene mediator. *Anal. Bioanal. Chem.* **2003**, *376*, 902–907.

116 Volkel, D., et al., Immunochemical detection of prion protein on dipsticks prepared with crystalline bacterial cell-surface layers. *Transfusion* **2003**, *43*, 1677–1682.

117 Sleytr, U. B., et al., Applications of S-layers. *FEMS Microbiol. Rev.* **1997**, *20*, 151–175.

118 Sleytr, U. B., M. Sara, Bacterial and archaeal S-layer proteins: structure–function relationships and their biotechnological applications. *Trends Biotechnol.* **1997**, *15*, 20–26.

119 Jain, K. K., Current trends in molecular diagnostics. *Med. Device Technol.* **2002**, *13*, 14–8.

120 Gould, P., Nanoparticles probe biosystems. *Mater. Today* **2004**, *7*, 36.

121 Zhao, X., et al., Collection of trace amounts of DNA/mRNA molecules using genomagnetic nanocapturers. *Anal. Chem.* **2003**, *75*, 3476–3483.

122 LaConte, L., N. Nitin, G. Bao, Magnetic nanoparticle probes. *Mater. Today* **2005**, *8*, 32–38.

123 Wang, Y., et al., Polyacrylamide gel film immobilized molecular beacon array for single nucleotide mismatch

detection. *J. Nanosci. Nanotechnol.* **2005**, *5*, 653–8.

124 Josephson, L., et al., High-efficiency intracellular magnetic labeling with novel superparamagnetic–Tat peptide conjugates. *Bioconjug. Chem.* **1999**, *10*, 186–191.

125 Krotz, F., et al., Magnetofection potentiates gene delivery to cultured endothelial cells. *J. Vasc. Res.* **2003**, *40*, 425–434.

126 Plank, C., et al., The magnetofection method: using magnetic force to enhance gene delivery. *Biol. Chem.* **2003**, *384*, 737–747.

127 Scherer, F., et al., Magnetofection: enhancing and targeting gene delivery by magnetic force *in vitro* and *in vivo*. *Gene Therapy* **2002**, *9*, 102.

128 Wang, S. X., et al., Towards a magnetic microarray for sensitive diagnostics. *J. Magn. Magn. Mater.* **2005**, *293*, 731–736.

129 Sepaniak, M., et al., Microcantilever transducers: a new approach in sensor technology. *Anal. Chem.* **2002**, *74*, 568.

130 Lavrik, N. V., M. J. Sepaniak, P. G. Datsko, Cantilever transducers as a platform for chemical and biological sensors. *Rev. Sci. Instrum.* **2004**, *75*, 2229–2253.

131 Ziegler, C., Cantilever-based biosensors. *Anal. Bioanal. Chem.* **2004**, *379*, 946–959.

132 Majumdar, A., Bioassays based on molecular nanomechanics. *Dis. Markers* **2002**, *18*, 167.

133 Myhra, S., A review of enabling technologies based on scanning probe microscopy relevant to bioanalysis. *Biosensors Bioelectron.* **2004**, *19*, 1345.

134 Hianik, T., et al., Detection of aptamer–protein interactions using QCM and electrochemical indicator methods. *Bioorg. Med. Chem. Lett.* **2005**, *15*, 291–295.

135 Wickline, S. A., G. M. Lanza, Nanotechnology for molecular imaging and targeted therapy. *Circulation* **2003**, *107*, 1092–1095.

136 Morawski, A. M., G. A. Lanza, S. A. Wickline, Targeted contrast agents for magnetic resonance imaging and ultrasound. *Curr. Opin. Biotechnol.* **2005**, *16*, 89–92.

137 Thrall, J. H., Nanotechnology and medicine. *Radiology* **2004**, *230*, 315–318.

138 Wang, X., et al., Photoacoustic tomography of biological tissues with high cross-section resolution: reconstruction and experiment. *Med. Phys.* **2002**, *29*, 2799–2805.

139 Copland, J. A., et al., Bioconjugated gold nanoparticles as a molecular based contrast agent: implications for imaging of deep tumors using optoacoustic tomography. *Mol. Imaging Biol.* **2004**, *6*, 341–349.

140 Farrer, R. A., et al., Highly efficient multiphoton-absorption-induced luminescence from gold nanoparticles. *Nano Lett.* **2005**, *5*, 1139–1142.

141 Zhenjia, W., et al., The structural basis for giant enhancement enabling single-molecule Raman scattering. *Proc. Natl Acad. Sci, USA* **2003**, *100*, 8638.

142 Pettinger, B., et al., Nanoscale probing of adsorbed species by tip-enhanced Raman spectroscopy. *Phys. Rev. Lett.* **2004**, *92*, 096101–096101.

143 Pettinger, B., et al., Surface-enhanced and STM tip-enhanced Raman spectroscopy of CN^- ions at gold surfaces. *J. Electroanal. Chem.* **2003**, *554–555*, 293–299.

144 Dootz, R., et al., Raman and surface enhanced Raman microscopy of microstructured polyethylenimine/DNA multilayers. *Langmuir* **2006**, *22*, 1735–1741.

145 Kneipp, J., et al., Optical probes for biological applications based on surface-enhanced Raman scattering from indocyanine green on gold nanoparticles. *Anal. Chem.* **2005**, *77*, 2381–2385.

146 Kneipp, K., et al., Single molecule Raman detection of enkephalin on silver colloidal particles. *Spectroscopy* **2004**, *18*, 433–440.

147 Kneipp, K., H. Kneipp, Ultrasensitive chemical analysis by Raman spectroscopy. *Chem. Rev.* **1999**, *99*, 2957.

148 Geho, D. H., et al., Opportunities for nanotechnology-based innovation in tissue proteomics. *Biomed. Microdevices* **2004**, *6*, 231–239.

149 Petricoin, E. F., et al., Toxicoproteomics: serum proteomic pattern diagnostics for early detection of drug induced cardiac toxicities and cardioprotection. *Toxicol. Pathol.* **2004**, *32 (s1)*, 122–130.

150 Nedelkov, D., R. W. Nelson, Surface plasmon resonance mass spectrometry: recent progress and outlooks. *Trends Biotechnol.* **2003**, *21*, 301–305.

151 Kasianowicz, J. J., Nanometer-scale pores: potential applications for analyte detection and DNA characterization. *Dis. Markers* **2002**, *18*, 185.

152 LaVan, D. A., D. M. Lynn, R. Langer, Timeline: moving smaller in drug discovery and delivery. *Nat. Rev. Drug Discov.* **2002**, *1*, 77.

153 Fologea, D., et al., Detecting single stranded DNA with a solid state nanopore. *Nano Lett.* **2005**, *5*, 1905–1909.

154 Li, J., et al., DNA molecules and configurations in a solid-state nanopore microscope. *Nat. Mater.* **2003**, *2*, 611–615.

155 Tong, et al., Silicon nitride nanosieve membrane. *Nano Lett.* **2004**, *4*, 283–287.

156 Steinkamp, T., U. Karst, Detection strategies for bioassays based on luminescent lanthanide complexes and signal amplification. *Anal. Bioanal. Chem.* **2004**, *380*, 24–30.

157 Shi, X., I. J. Majoros, J. R. Baker, Jr., Capillary electrophoresis of poly(amidoamine) dendrimers: from simple derivatives to complex multifunctional medical nanodevices. *Mol. Pharmac.* **2005**, *2*, 278–294.

158 Choi, Y., et al., Synthesis and functional evaluation of DNA-assembled polyamidoamine dendrimer clusters for cancer cell-specific targeting. *Chem. Biol.* **2005**, *12*, 35–43.

159 Ferrari, M., G. Downing, Medical nanotechnology: shortening clinical trials and regulatory pathways? *BioDrugs* **2005**, *19*, 203–210.

160 Tkachenko, A. G., et al., Multifunctional gold nanoparticle-peptide complexes for nuclear targeting. *J. Am. Chem. Soc.* **2003**, *125*, 4700–4701.

161 Nissenson, A. R., et al., Continuously functioning artificial nephron system: the promise of nanotechnology. *Hemodial. Int.* **2005**, *9*, 210–217.

162 Lee, S. J., S. Y. Lee, Micro total analysis system (micro-TAS) in biotechnology. *Appl. Microbiol. Biotechnol.* **2004**, *64*, 289–99.

163 Gulliksen, A., et al., Real-time nucleic acid sequence-based amplification in nanoliter volumes. *Anal. Chem.* **2004**, *76*, 9–14.

164 Walter, G., et al., High-throughput protein arrays: prospects for molecular diagnostics. *Trends Mol. Med.* **2002**, *8*, 250–253.

165 Sarikaya, M., et al., Molecular biomimetics: nanotechnology through biology. Nature materials. **2003**, *2*, 577–585.

166 Miller, J., Beyond biotechnology: FDA regulation of nanomedicine. *Columbia Sci. Technol. Law rev.* **2003**, *4*, E5–E5.

167 Rados, C., Nanotechnology: the size of things to come. *FDA Consumer* **2005**, *39*, 40–42.

168 Donawa, M. E., The New FDA Combination Products Programme. *Med. Device Technol.* **2002**, *13*, 25.

169 Bruce, D., The question of ethics. *Mater. Today* **2006**, *1*, 6–7.

170 Mills, K., C. Fleddermann, Getting the best from nanotechnology: approaching social and ethical implications openly and proactively. *IEEE Technol. Soc. Mag.* **2005**, *24*, 18–26.

171 Gordijn, B., Nanoethics: from utopian dreams and apocalyptic nightmares towards a more balanced view. *Sci. Eng. Ethics* **2005**, *11*, 521–533.

172 Grunwald, A., Nanotechnology – a new field of ethical inquiry? *Sci. Eng. Ethics* **2005**, *11*, 187–201.

173 Berne, R. W., Towards the conscientious development of ethical nanotechnology. *Sci. Eng. Ethics* **2004**, *10*, 627–638.

174 Einsiedel, E. F., L. Goldenberg, Dwarfing the social? Nanotechnology lessons from the biotechnology front. *Bull. Sci. Technol. Soc.* **2004**, *24*, 28–33.

175 Lopez, J., Compiling the ethical, legal and social implications of nanotechnology. *Health Law Rev.* **2004**, *12*, 24–27.

2
Superparamagnetic Nanoparticles of Iron Oxides for Magnetic Resonance Imaging Applications

Jean-Marc Idee, Marc Port, Isabelle Raynal, Michel Schaefer, Bruno Bonnemain, Philippe Prigent, Philippe Robert, Caroline Robic, and Claire Corot

2.1
Introduction

Superparamagnetic nanoparticles of iron oxides have become a major tool for medical imaging with a wealth of applications. This chapter will first describe their physicochemical characteristics, which are of paramount importance for their interaction with macrophage-like cells and, more broadly, for their biodistribution. The general pharmacological properties of these nanoparticles (including their interaction with macrophages and pharmacokinetic behavior) will subsequently been reviewed. Nanoparticles of iron oxides are currently marketed or undergoing clinical trials for cancer imaging applications, which will be described, but also for indications related to their blood pool characteristics and their unique potential for interaction with inflammatory cells. Since inflammatory infiltrates are found in a vast number of diseases (from atheromatous plaques to degenerative diseases such as multiple sclerosis), it appeared of clinical interest to numerous researchers to investigate the relevance of nanoparticles in such indications. The results of these studies will be presented for each of these potential new indications. Last, the noninvasive tracking of stem cells with superparamagnetic nanoparticles, which has attracted much attention in both neurological and cardiologic research over recent years, will be detailed.

For nearly 20 years, research in the field of magnetic resonance imaging (MRI) contrast agents has been oriented towards the study and development of superparamagnetic nanoparticles. These are iron oxides – magnetite (Fe_3O_4), maghemite (γ-Fe_2O_3) or other ferrites that are insoluble in water. Unlike ferromagnetic substances and because of their size, superparamagnetic agents have no magnetic properties outside an external magnetic field [1]. These nanoparticles have in common their specific uptake by macrophages, explaining why, even if they are not entirely captured by the liver and spleen, they are widely evaluated as MRI markers for diagnosis of inflammatory and degenerative disorders associated with high macrophage phagocytic activity.

Nanotechnologies for the Life Sciences Vol. 10
Nanomaterials for Medical Diagnosis and Therapy. Edited by Challa S. S. R. Kumar

ISBN: 978-3-527-31390-7

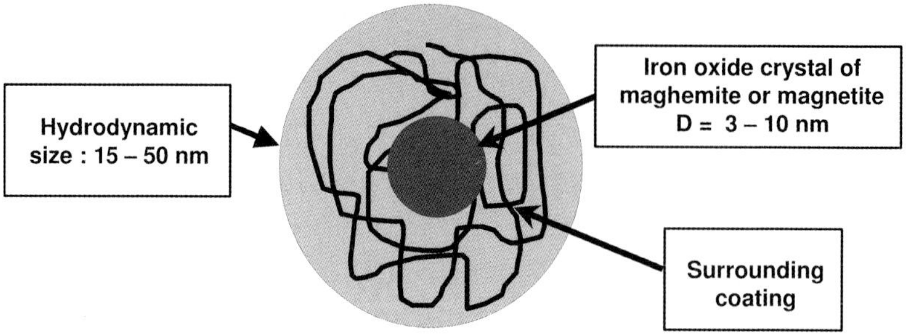

Figure 2.1. General structure of USPIO nanoparticles.

Superparamagnetic agents are highly effective in MRI as they are strong enhancers of proton relaxation.

Superparamagnetic nanoparticles are small coated crystals of iron oxides (Figs. 2.1 and 2.2), characterized by a large magnetic moment in the presence of a static external magnetic field. This large magnetic moment is caused by a crystal ordering (spinels) which induces a cooperativity between the individual paramagnetic ions constituting the crystal. Consequently, the magnetic moment of superparamagnetic particle is greater than the sum of each paramagnetic ions constituting the crystal. These small superparamagnetic crystals are smaller than a magnetic domain (approximately 30 nm) and, consequently, they do not show any magnetic

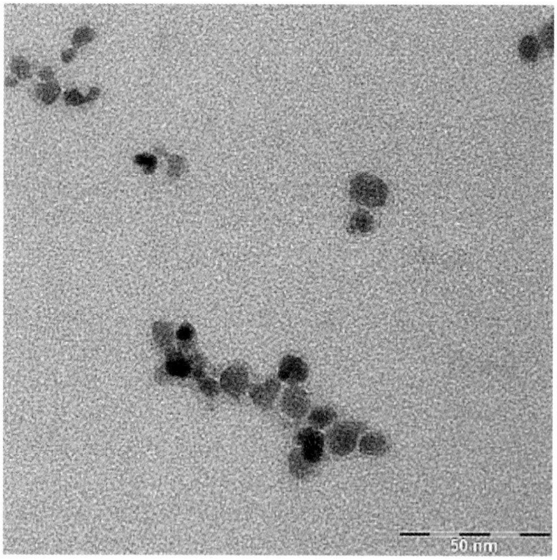

Figure 2.2. Transmission electron microscopy images of USPIOs (iron oxide crystals diameter: 5–7 nm) (Guerbet, unpublished data).

remanence (i.e. restoration of the induced magnetization to zero upon removal of the external magnetic field), unlike ferromagnetic materials. The interaction between surrounding protons of water molecules and the magnetic moment of superparamagnetic particles results in an increase in longitudinal r_1 and transverse r_2 relaxation rates.

The T1 relaxation of superparamagnetic particles has been explained by various models, and Roch and coworkers [2] have proposed a model introducing the anisotropy energy to explain the relaxivity at low magnetic fields while the relaxivity at high fields is mainly related to the outer-sphere Curie relaxation mechanism. The nuclear magnetic relaxation dispersion (NMRD) profile of contrast agents shows the relationship between their relaxivity and the proton Larmor frequency. The NMRD profile of these particles has been obtained, and shows that the magnetic field applied has a considerable and nonlinear influence on the signal [3]. These authors have proposed a new theory which takes account of the magnetic moment of the monodomains and the saturation of the macroscopic magnetization. This fact should be taken into consideration when analyzing the imaging data.

In most situations, it is the significant capacity of superparamagnetic nanoparticles to reduce the spin–spin T2 relaxation time and thus reduce the MRI signal that is used, and such molecules are mostly employed because of their negative enhancement effect on T2-weighted sequences. This drop in signal intensity is related to the field gradients produced by the magnetic particles that dephase nearby diffusing protons and shorten T2/T2*. This effect is rationalized by outer-sphere relaxation (Ayant and Freed's theory).

This predominant effect on the T2 relaxation time does not prevent these agents' properties from being put to use on the T1 relaxation time if the imaging sequences are chosen appropriately [4]. This is why their use in increasing the signal in the myocardium tissue [5] and in magnetic resonance angiography has been proposed [6].

The multiple components which govern the efficacy of these agents require them to be characterized as accurately as possible by information such as the size of the iron oxide crystals, the charge, the nature of the coating, the hydrodynamic size of the coated particle, etc. These physicochemical characteristics not only affect the efficacy of the superparamagnetic particles in MRI, but also their stability, biodistribution, opsonization and metabolism as well as their clearance from the vascular system.

2.2 Physicochemical Characteristics

The synthesis of superparamagnetic nanoparticles is a complex process because of their colloidal nature [7]. Consequently, a full set of analytical methods should be used in order to characterize the efficacy (in terms of magnetization and relaxivity) and purity of nanoparticles and the reproducibility of the synthesis process. Moreover, since the size, the geometry, the composition of the crystals as well as the

Tab. 2.1. Size of iron oxide nuclei (nm) [8].

	X-ray diffraction	Transmission electron microscopy
Ferumoxides	4.96 ± 0.14	4.8 ± 1.9
Ferumoxtran-10	5.85 ± 0.09	4.9 ± 1.5
Ferumoxsil	8.3 ± 1.03	8.4 ± 2.5
Ferumoxytol	6.76 ± 0.41	–

charge of the particles and the nature of the coating strongly influence the physicochemical and biological behavior of the particles, an accurate description of the physicochemical properties of these nanoparticles is crucial in establishing any structure–activity relationship [8, 9].

2.2.1
Physicochemical Properties of the Crystal

The size of the crystals varies from agent to agent, but also depends on the measurement technique. The core size is generally between 4 and 10 nm (Tab. 2.1). The size of the crystal can be appreciated by transmission electronic microscopy (TEM) and needs to be measured on a statistically significant number of crystals. Moreover, the sample preparation can induce aggregation of the colloids and the TEM measurements may consequently not reflect the crystal size in solution. The size of the crystals can also be measured by X-ray diffraction (XRD) by analyzing the X-ray line broadening. Moreover, XRD can provide information concerning the crystal composition and structure. A detailed characterization by TEM and XRD analyses of new nonpolymeric-coated Fe_3O_4 nanoparticles has been recently described by Cheng and coworkers [10].

Composition of the crystal can also be analyzed by Mössbauer spectroscopy. The magnetic properties of the nanoparticles can be studied by the behavior of the magnetization according to the applied magnetic field (magnetometry) which confirms the superparamagnetic property and gives the magnetization at saturation (MS). Of course, the magnetic properties can also be studied by recording the NMRD curve. According to the relaxivity theory developed by Roch and coworkers [2], the fitting of the NMRD curves can provide information on the relaxometric size and the magnetization at saturation.

2.2.2
Hydrodynamic Particle Size and Charge

The hydrodynamic size of the nanoparticles [i.e. the global size of the particle comprising one or several magnetic crystal(s) surrounded by the coating molecules] is usually measured by photon correlation spectroscopy (PCS), which analyses the quasielastic light diffusion of nanoparticles when illuminated by a monochromatic laser beam. The intensity of the diffused light is modulated by the Brownian motion of the particles in solution. Different mathematical analyses of the PCS data can provide an estimation of the hydrodynamic size and the polydispersity of the nanoparticles. However, the values obtained by PCS dramatically depend on the mathematical models and weighting parameters used (unimodal or multimodal distribution, distribution in number, volume or intensity). Consequently, the hydrodynamic size measurements described in the literature for different nanoparticles are very difficult to compare, and any relationship between size and biodistribution should be made with caution.

The size of the particles themselves with their coating varies even more and the measurement method contributes significantly to this variability (Tab. 2.2).

It is currently agreed that two main categories of superparamagnetic agents must be distinguished [9]:

Tab. 2.2. Size and coating agent of the nanoparticles currently marketed or under clinical investigation.

Brand name or common name	Company	Other names	Coating agent	Size (laser light scattering) (nm)
Endorem®/ Feridex®	Guerbet Advanced Magnetics	Ferumoxides AMI-25	dextran	120–180
Sinerem®/ Combidex®	Guerbet Advanced Magnetics	Ferumoxtran-10 AMI-227 BMS-180549	dextran T-10	15–30
–	Advanced Magnetics	Ferumoxytol Code 7228	semisynthetic carbohydrate	30
Lumirem®/ Gastromark®	Guerbet Advanced Magnetics	Ferumoxsil AMI-121	silicon	300
Resovist®	Schering	Ferucarbotran SHU-555A	carboxy-dextran	60
Clariscan®	GE-Healthcare	Feruglose NC100150	pegylated starch	20
Abdoscan®	GE-Healthcare	Ferristene	sulfonated styrene–divinylbenzene copolymer	3500
VSOP-C184	Ferropharm	–	citrate	7.0 ± 0.15

Tab. 2.3. Magnetization and relaxivity measurements [8, 13, 90].

	Magnetization (e.m.u. g Fe^{-1})		Relaxivity ($mM\ s^{-1}$)[a]	
	0.1 T	5.0 T	r_1	r_2
Ferumoxides	37.7 ± 0.6	93.6 ± 1.6	23.7 ± 1.2	107 ± 11
Ferumoxtran-10	53.6 ± 0.4	94.8 ± 0.7	22.7 ± 0.2	53.1 ± 3.3
Ferucarbotran	–	–	25	164
Ferumoxsil	49.4 ± 0.1	91.1 ± 0.2	3.2 ± 0.9	72 ± 12
VSOP	–	–	18.7	30.0
Ferumoxytol	–	–	38	83

[a] At 20 MHz (0.47 T).

- Superparamagnetic iron oxides (SPIOs), the hydrodynamic size of which including coating is greater than 50 nm.
- Ultrasmall superparamagnetic iron oxides (USPIOs) which are less than 50 nm in size.

This difference in size is reflected by significant differences in the ratio of relaxivity constants r_2/r_1 (Tab. 2.3), but also by a significant difference in plasma half-life and biodistribution.

Another fundamental characteristic of these agents is the nature and charge of the particle coating. The charge on the surface of the nanoparticles is usually appreciated by the ζ potential measurement deduced from the measurement of electrophoretic mobility. Unfortunately, the value of ζ potential of superparamagnetic nanoparticles is rarely described in the literature. Although most superparamagnetic particles are covered by dextran or dextran derivatives (e.g. carboxy-dextran), they have occasionally been coated with other molecules such as starch, siloxane, arabinogalactose, amino-functionalized polyvinyl alcohol (PVA), citrate, etc.

Therefore, when referring to superparamagnetic agents, these must be properly characterized and their characteristics compared with the other agents by using the same measurement methods. The relationship between the structure, the composition and the charge of nanoparticles and their potential in terms of efficacy, biodistribution and safety is not yet well understood.

2.3
Pharmacology and Metabolism

Iron oxide nanoparticles are internalized into macrophages (Fig. 2.3) and other phagocytic cells following intravenous administration.

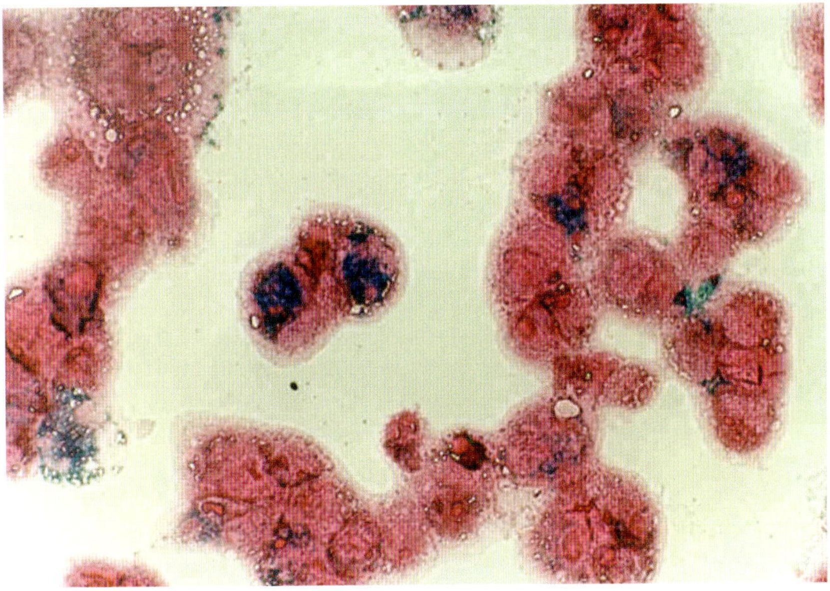

Figure 2.3. Intracellular localization of the USPIO ferumoxtran-10 (7.1 mmol L^{-1}) following a 24-h incubation with activated THP-1 human monocytes. Iron staining with Prussian blue and counter-staining with eosin (Guerbet, unpublished data).

2.3.1
Role of Physicochemical Parameters

The size and physicochemical surface properties of SPIOs and USPIOs strongly interfere with their capacity to be internalized into macrophages or other phagocytic cells following intravenous administration.

Ferumoxtran-10, which has a small hydrodynamic diameter (15–30 nm, see Tab. 2.2), shows a long blood residence time, which allows it to easily access macrophages located in deep and pathologic tissues (such as lymph nodes, kidney, brain, osteoarticular tissues, etc.). Indeed, these tissues are far less accessible than well-vascularized tissues such as the liver or spleen.

Other USPIOs such as ferucarbotran or very small superparamagnetic iron oxide particles (VSOPs) have a higher macrophage uptake. This is associated with a faster blood clearance and, consequently, a more limited access time to the deep compartments [11, 12]. For example, the elimination half-life of VSOP-C184 in healthy volunteers is only 0.5–1.5 h after bolus injection [13]. Conversely, feruglose (Clariscan®), because of the pegylation of the coating starch, can be regarded as "stealth nanoparticles" which are hardly recognized by the macrophage–monocytic system and probably not suitable for macrophage imaging [14].

It has recently been shown that superparamagnetic nanoparticles with an amino-functionalized PVA coating can interact with human melanoma cells without any cytotoxicity. This interaction of the nanoparticles with melanoma cells was found to be active, energy-dependent and saturable [15]. It also depended on the amino-PVA:iron oxide ratio – the increased uptake in the presence of amino groups is consistent with the well-known uptake of cationic liposomes, mainly for transfection purposes.

A recent study compared anionic nanoparticles (AN) (coating: meso-2,3-dimercaptosuccinic acid, hydrodynamic diameter 24 nm) with ferumoxtran-10 [16]. *In vitro* uptake by the human prostatic adenocarcinoma cells PC3 was found to be superior with AN than with ferumoxtran-10. In mice grafted with PC3 cells, the iron concentration inside tumors reached two peaks: first one at 1 h (ferumoxtran-10 > AN) and second one at 12 h (ferumoxytran-10 = AN). Imaging studies showed tumor brightening on T1-weighted images with ferumoxtran-10 and darkening on T2-weighted images with both compounds. With ferumoxtran-10, an early peak at 1 h on T2 imaging and a second peak at 12 h on T1 imaging suggested an initial intravascular distribution and, possibly, a secondary extravasation in the interstitium (or, alternatively, some intracellular uptake) at 12 h [16].

2.3.2
Mechanism and Consequences of Interaction with Macrophages

According to their coating (negative charges and hydrophilicity), nanoparticles display different degrees of uptake by macrophage-like cells, as previously mentioned.

The macrophage is a specialized host defense cell with endocytic properties. Its involvement in the pathogenesis of numerous diseases is well known and makes it a very interesting pharmaceutical target.

It has been shown *in vitro* that ferumoxides endocytosis by mouse peritoneal macrophages was dose-dependently inhibited by polyinosinic acid and fucoidan, suggesting that a scavenger receptor SR-A mediated endocytosis is involved for this contrast agent [17].

On the human activated monocyte THP-1, ferumoxide was shown to undergo a higher macrophage uptake compared with ferumoxtran-10, probably because of its larger size [17]. This result was confirmed in another study [18] which also showed that, apart from particle size, the phagocytic uptake is dependent on the surface properties of the nanoparticles since, both for SPIO or USPIO categories, ionic carboxy-dextran coating leads to a higher uptake than nonionic dextran coating [18].

Another study also found a higher cellular uptake (on hematopoietic progenitor, mesenchymal fibroblast and epithelial HEP-G2 cell lines) with the SPIO ferucarbotran than with the USPIO SHU-555C (hydrodynamic diameter 30 nm) [19].

Rogers and Basu recently showed that the hydroxymethyl glutaryl coenzyme A (HMG-CoA) reductase inhibitor lovastatin dose-dependently reduced the uptake of the SPIO ferumoxides by a murine macrophage-like cell line (J774A) [20]. The mechanism of this effect is unclear, and may be explained by a downregulation of class A types I and II receptors, or, alternatively, by interference of lovastatin in macrophage–receptor binding, reduced receptor recycling or at the level of scavenger receptor mRNA expression. The clinical relevance of such *in vitro* data for the detection and characterization of atheromatous plaques with USPIOs in patients treated with HMG-CoA reductase inhibitors remains unclear.

The same authors also demonstrated that the pro-inflammatory cytokine interferon (IFN)-γ, but also the anti-inflammatory cytokine interleukin (IL)-4 increased SPIO uptake at relatively high concentrations [20].

Another study has investigated the biological consequences of the rat macrophage labeling with the citrate-coated nanoparticles VSOP [21]. Cell growth and viability were minimally affected. However, transient oxidative stress was evidenced by an acute increase in both malonyldialdehyde and protein carbonyls.

In addition to their phagocytic properties, macrophages also possess a high secretory capability leading to the release of growth factors and cytokines. Very low IL-1 release (comparable to negative control) was observed after incubation of macrophages with ferumoxides or ferumoxtran-10, even at a high concentration (500 μg Fe mL^{-1}), thus suggesting a low pro-inflammatory potential for these nanoparticles [17].

2.3.3 Pharmacokinetics

Ferumoxtran-10 is completely degraded in the macrophage lysosomal compartment within 7 days [22]. The plasma elimination half-life is strongly species dependent. It is 2 h in rats (after intravenous injection of a 30 or 45 μmol kg^{-1} dose), approximately 6 h in rabbits whereas it is around 24–36 h in humans following intravenous administration [11, 23]. In both rats and rabbits, increasing the dose caused a longer half-life because of the progressive saturation of uptake by liver and spleen.

Since the access of USPIOs to deep compartments is favored by prolonged blood residence time, animal imaging experiments are generally performed using high doses of USPIO (200–1000 μmol kg^{-1}) compared to the human clinical dose of 45 μmol kg^{-1} [11].

It has been shown that the age of rats significantly influences the half-lives of the signal intensities in vessels and in the liver following injection of VSOP-C43. In the younger animals, the intravascular signal decrease was about 50% of the value seen in older animals [24]. This suggests a higher macrophage uptake in younger animals. Since pharmacokinetic data are classically obtained during phase I clinical studies in young healthy volunteers, caution seems necessary when it comes to extrapolating imaging window to elderly patients.

The iron contained in SPIOs and USPIOs is bioavailable, and is incorporated into the normal body iron pools, such as hemoglobin [25]. This is consistent with the increase in ferritin levels reported in several articles with various USPIOs [13, 26]. Ferritin is the physiologic storage form of iron. Actually, it is believed that Küpffer cells degrade dextran-coated iron oxide nanoparticles by incorporating most of the iron they contain into ferritin and/or hemosiderin (when the intracellular concentration of ferritin becomes relatively high) before exocytosis [27].

The USPIO ferumoxtran-10 (Sinerem®/Combidex®) is currently under clinical trial for the detection of nodal metastases (see Section 2.4.3). After intravenous infusion, USPIO nanoparticles are distributed to the lymph nodes by two distinct pathways: (i) direct transcapillary passage through venules into the medullary sinuses of the lymph node, followed by phagocytosis by macrophages, and (ii) nonselective, endothelial transcytosis into the interstitial space in the body, followed by uptake of the nanoparticles by draining lymphatic vessels and transport to the lymph nodes via afferent lymphatic channels [28, 29].

Several routes of administration have been suggested for SPIOs and USPIOs. The SPIO ferumoxides (Endorem®/Feridex®) is administered using slow intravenous infusion, ferucarbotran (Resovist®) is injected as a bolus. Clinical studies on ferumoxtran-10 have so far used slow intravenous infusion but preclinical studies have shown that this USPIO can also be directed to specific lymph nodes via subcutaneous injections at distinct sites [30]. In human volunteers, it was shown that interstitial administration of ferumoxtran-10 (0.28 mg Fe kg^{-1}) increases the number of lymph nodes that can be adequately detected with MRI.

The site of injection in the pelvis influenced the location of visualized lymph nodes, with the largest number of nodes visualized with periprostatic injection. This interstitial approach may also allow a reduction of the dose when compared with the intravenous route [31].

The optimal temporal window for imaging lymph nodes with ferumoxtran-10 is 24–36 h after intravenous infusion [29].

2.3.4
Nanoparticle Vectorization

Although it has a good temporal and spatial resolution, MRI displays a relatively low sensitivity (about three to six orders of magnitude less than that of isotope techniques). It therefore requires amplification to enable its use in molecular imaging. Molecular imaging includes a large array of applications (study of tissular blood flow changes, spectroscopic quantification of metabolite concentrations, generation of pH maps, studies of vascular volume or permeability, pharmacokinetic studies of chemotherapeutic drugs, denoting of gene expression, specific imaging of molecules that are overexpressed in pathological states, etc.) [32]. A promising option for local signal amplification is vectorization of nanoparticles to enable them to reach their biological target [33]. Several strategies have been selected to vectorize nanoparticles. One example is the oxidative conjugation producing aldehydes on the dextran coating of the particles, at the expense of a substantial loss of the biological activity of the protein. To reduce this effect, the protein that binds the biological target has been linked to the iron oxide nanoparticles through a linker molecule [34].

Nonoxidative strategies have become an interesting alternative method: epichlorhydrin is first coupled to the hydroxyl groups of the dextran coating to provide a terminal halogen derivative which can subsequently be used to link any molecule containing an amine function (peptide, protein, antibodies, etc.) [35]. As an exam-

Tab. 2.4. Functionalized USPIOs: some examples.

Biological target	Type of functionalized USPIO	Experimental model	Reference
Acute inflammation	MION–IgG	rat model of myositis	38
Asialoglycoprotein receptors on hepatocytes	arabinogalactan (AG)–USPIO	blockade of AG–USPIO uptake by hepatocytes with D[+]-galactose	39
Transferrin receptor on tumor cells	dextran-stabilized USPIO covalently labeled with receptor-specific transferrin	SMT/2A tumor-bearing rats	40
$\alpha_{IIb}\beta_3$ integrin	USPIO functionalized with cyclic RGD peptide specific for the $\alpha_{IIb}\beta_3$ integrin	*ex vivo*: clot on a glass tube *in vivo*: clots induced in the jugular veins of domestic pigs	41
Phosphatidylserine	Annexin V-functionalized USPIO	apoptotic Jurkat cells	42
$\alpha_v\beta_3$ integrin	USPIO functionalized with RGD peptide	*in vitro*: PMA-activated Jurkat cells *in vivo*: ApoE$^{-/-}$ atherosclerotic mice	43

ple, vectorizing groups [such as the connecting segment-1 fragment of fibronectin, the peptide GRGD (Gly–Arg–Gly–Asp) or a nonpeptidic small-molecular-weight RGD mimetic] have been grafted with the dextran coating of USPIO previously coated with epichlorhydrin [36].

Another approach uses 2,3-dimercaptosuccinic acid (DMSA) and *N*-succimidyl 3-(2-pyridylthio)propionate (SPDP) [37]. Recent examples of functionalized USPIOs used for experimental molecular imaging are shown in Tab. 2.4 [38–43].

2.4 Current Clinical Uses and Future Developments

2.4.1 Gastrointestinal Tract Imaging

As in computed tomography (CT) scanning, it is clinically necessary to improve the differentiation between the gastrointestinal tract and surrounding organs. Para-

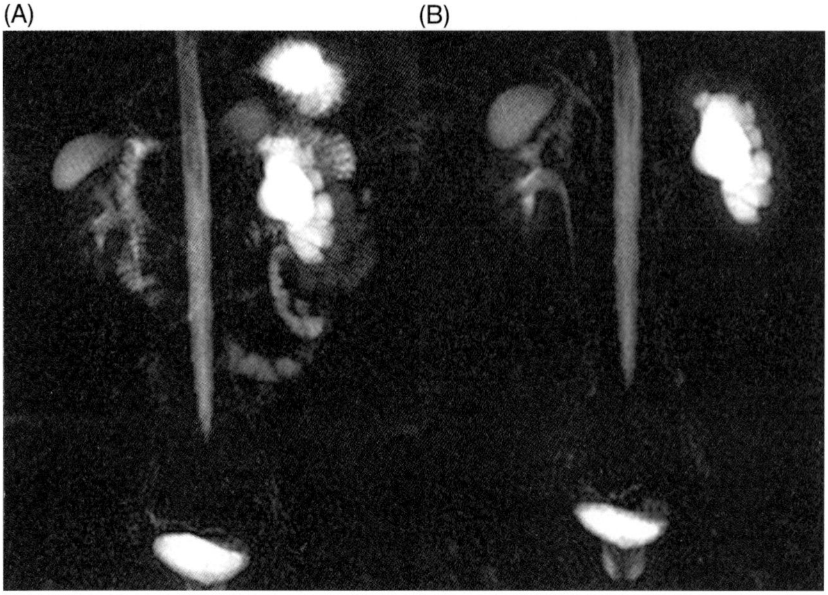

Figure 2.4. Signal suppression of the gastrointestinal structures in pyelography. MRI prior (A) and after (B) oral administration of 500 mL ferumoxsil (courtesy Dr A. Blandino, Policlinico G. Martino, Messina, Italy).

magnetic contrast agents, which increase the gastrointestinal tract signal, may also increase movement artifacts. Specific superparamagnetic contrast agents have been developed for this reason. A first agent, ferumoxsil (AMI-121), has been tested in clinical trials by oral administration at 600–900 mL [44–47] and is licensed in Europe as Lumirem® (or Gastromark® in the USA).

This product is composed of iron oxide particles coated in a layer of inert silicon and its diameter is 300 nm (Tabs. 2.1 and 2.2). After oral administration, it significantly improves the definition of organ boundaries such as the uterus and lymph nodes [47] (Fig. 2.4). Other agents have been developed for the same application: WIN-39996 [48], oral magnetic particles (OMPs), also referred as to ferristene (Abdoscan®) (polystyrene coated) [49–53].

Ferumoxsil has also been used as well in MR enteroclysis in 60 patients with Crohn's disease [54]. Aliquots of 600 mL of ferumoxsil associated with 2.5 L of tide water and methylcellulose were instilled through a transjejunal tube, in order to reduce the signal intensity of the lumen. Additional rectal instillation of water for positive contrast improved the distension and identification of large bowel and terminal ileum.

Similarly, an Italian team [55] used a double-contrast method for evaluating the inflammatory activity in patients with Crohn's disease, after darkening the lumen of the bowel with oral administration of Lumirem®, the gadolinium contrast agent was injected. Parameters such as wall thickness, wall T2-weighted signal, wall contrast enhancement, amount of fibroproliferation and T2-weighted signal of fibrofatty proliferation on fat-suppressed images were evaluated.

These negative contrast agents for gastrointestinal imaging are generally well tolerated, with mild side-effects such as nausea, vomiting (1–5% of patients) or flatulence [56]. Oral SPIO are generally administered over 30–60 min, with a volume of 900 mL for contrast enhancement of the whole abdomen and 400 mL for the upper abdomen [57].

2.4.2 Liver and Spleen Diseases

The first clinical indication for iron oxide nanoparticles was hepatic imaging. Following intravenous injection, SPIOs are rapidly taken up by hepatic Küpffer cells and the spleen (marginal zone and red pulp) macrophages, resulting in a drop in magnetic resonance signal intensity, and therefore in hypointense images, mostly because of a susceptibility effect.

Since Küpffer cells are exclusively located in the healthy hepatic parenchyma [58], SPIOs increase the contrast between healthy and diseased tissue devoid of Küpffer cells. The first agent to be developed (and marketed in Europe more than 10 years ago under the name Endorem®) was ferumoxides (or AMI-25) (Feridex® in the US). These are T10-dextran coated particles and their hydrodynamic size is 120–180 nm (Tabs. 2.1 and 2.2). Many preclinical and clinical trials have demonstrated the efficacy of ferumoxides in the detection of the focal lesions of the liver as well as for their characterization [59–64] (Fig. 2.5).

The same product has been studied in terms of its capacity to detect lesions of the spleen [65, 66]. The most common side-effects reported with ferumoxides are

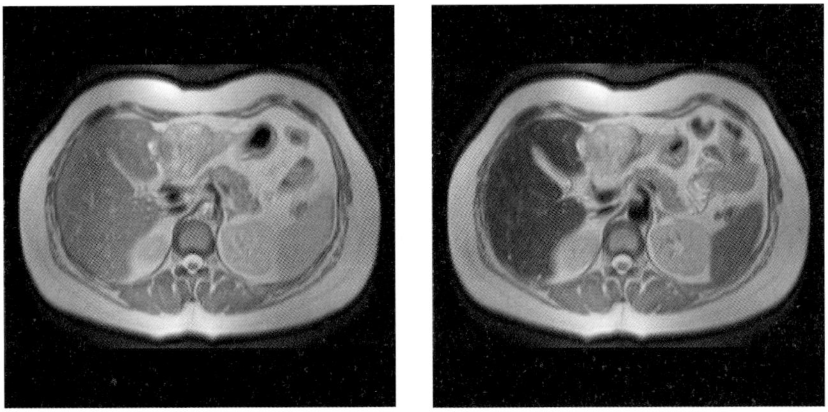

(A) (B)

Figure 2.5. Liver imaging prior (A) and after (B) injection of ferumoxides (HASTE sequence) allowing a better depiction of a cholangiocarcinoma which does not uptake the nanoparticles and appears in isosignal intensity pre/postinjection while the signal of the normal parenchyma becomes dark. (courtesy Dr C. Matos, Erasmus Hospital, Brussels, Belgium) lower back pain (4%), flushing (2%) and various combined gastrointestinal complaints (5.6%) [67].

Another product was subsequently developed for this clinical application in MRI: ferucarbotran (SHU-555A) (Resovist®), the particles of which are coated with carboxy-dextran and are approximately 60 nm in diameter [19, 68]. Safety data obtained during phase I–III trials of this compound revealed a total of 162 side-effects in 1053 patients, of which 75 (7.1%) were possibly, probably or definitely drug related. The majority of events occurred within the first 3 h [69].

Chondroitin sulfate iron colloid (CSIC) has also been put forward [70] as well as MDL (liver-directed nanoparticles) [71], but these particles have not been marketed. Furthermore, other hepatocyte-specific agents were evaluated but not marketed either: asialofetuin-coated USPIO or arabinogalactan-coated USPIO, which are particularly well recognized by the asialoglycoprotein receptor (ASGPR) present on the surface of normal hepatocytes [72]. ASGPR is of interest for hepatocyte targeting in that it is prototypic of the class of receptors that constitutively enters cells and allows delivery of molecules to the intracellular compartments [73]. In addition to their ability to assess focal hepatic lesions, these agents can be used to assess hepatocyte function [57].

In addition to SPIOs, USPIOs such as ferumoxtran-10 can be located in several compartments of the liver (extracellular space, reticuloendothelial cells and possibly hepatocytes). In the rat, ferumoxtran-10 acts mainly as an extracellular agent for at least 1 h (increase in liver signal intensity on T1-weighted images) and is taken up by cells from the reticuloendothelial system at later time points [74]. A subsequent rat study showed that the USPIO feruglose induced an hepatic T2* effect at late (up to 133 days after injection for 5 mg Fe kg^{-1}) time-points when the concentrations of iron oxide nanoparticles in the liver were below method detection limits. This effect is probably a result of nanoparticle breakdown products [27].

In a clinical study comparing the SPIO ferumoxides with the USPIO ferumoxtran-10 in patients with focal hepatic diseases (hepatocellular carcinoma, metastases, hepatocellular adenoma and focal nodular hyperplasia), Mergo and coworkers observed that, although both compounds had similar T2 effects (comparable loss of hepatic signal intensity in their study conditions) and improved the lesion-to-liver contrast when compared with non-contrast-enhanced images, the USPIO allowed more in-depth characterization of the lesions, because of its additional blood pool effect [75].

Further studies are needed to better understand the potential utility of USPIOs for assessment of hepatic vascular structures and clinical benefit in the characterization of focal hepatic lesions, notably by optimizing the USPIO injected dose and the chronology of MRI.

2.4.3
Lymph Node Metastases

Nodal disease is an independent adverse prognostic factor in many types of cancer. The only widely accepted method for assessing nodal involvement by means of imaging so far is measurement of the node size. This preoperative staging will influence the oncologist's decision to use neoadjuvant therapy or the surgeon's decision to perform nodal dissection [76]. Superparamagnetic agents which can be taken up by normal nodes following intravenous or subcutaneous injection have raised great interest. The first agent, and that on which most research has been carried out, is ferumoxtran-10 (or AMI-227). Its iron oxide core is surrounded by a 8- to 12-mm layer of T-10 dextran coating [23], leading to a final size of around 30 nm (Tabs. 2.1 and 2.2). It has similar physicochemical properties to the monocrystalline iron oxide nanocompounds (MION) which have a monocrystalline crystal core with an approximate diameter of 4 nm and a dextran coating resulting in a hydrodynamic diameter of 17 nm [77].

Numerous studies on ferumoxtran-10 have shown its efficacy in metastatic lymph node imaging [78–81] (Fig. 2.6). Schematically, as previously mentioned,

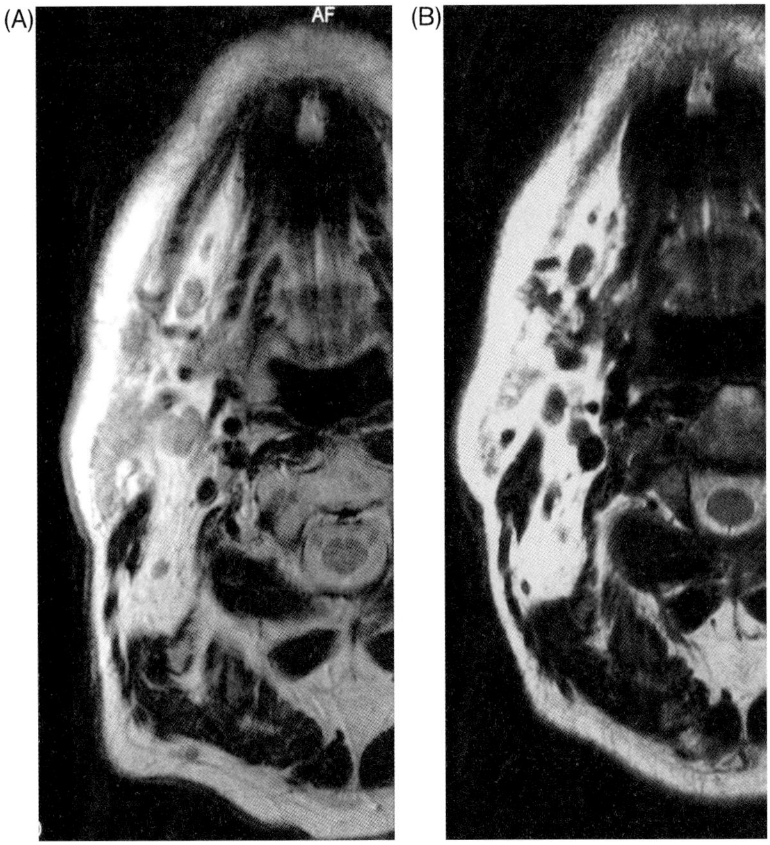

Figure 2.6. MRI (T2* sequence) of lymph node metastases prior (A) and after (B) ferumoxtran-10 injection in a patient with head and neck cancer (courtesy Dr M. Mack, University Hospital, Frankfurt/Main, Germany).

USPIO slowly extravasate from the vessels into the interstitial space, from which they are transported into the lymph nodes through lymphatic vessels [28, 29, 82]. Upon USPIO administration, normal lymph nodes will appear dark on the MR images, while tumor metastases remain isointense with the precontrast image (i.e. before USPIO uptake by lymph node macrophages). In eighty patients with presurgical clinical stage T1, T2 or T3 prostate cancer who underwent lymph-node resection or biopsy, MRI was done before and 24 h after the intravenous injection of 2.6 mg kg^{-1} of ferumoxtran-10. Sixty-three lymph nodes, from 33 patients, had histopathologically detected metastases. Of these, 45 (71.4%) did not fulfill the usual imaging criteria for malignancy. However, the ferumoxtran-10-enhanced MRI correctly identified all patients with nodal metastases. Nodal metastatic infiltration measuring 5–10 mm were identified [81].

Several phase III clinical trials using USPIO ferumoxtran-10 for the detection of lymph node metastases, especially in the head and neck and pelvis regions, are currently in their final stages. Promising results have also been published for rectal cancer [76].

2.4.4
Blood Pool Characteristics

Uptake of ferumoxtran-10 and the MIONs or other USPIOs by the liver and the spleen is quite low because of their physicochemical characteristics. They consequently remain in the blood circulation for a very long time. With their long blood half-life and T1-shortening effect, these agents have been evaluated as blood pool agents for indications such as measurement of cerebral perfusion [83, 84], myocardial or renal perfusion [85], angiography [6], or detection of vascular hepatic lesions [86]. These compounds are classically referred to as slow-clearance blood pool agents. Whereas these agents are confined to the vascular compartment, their molecular volume only allows a slow "sieving" through the glomerular fenestrae. Their renal clearance is consequently much lower than the normal glomerular filtration rate.

These blood pool characteristics provide a much longer time window for data acquisition during radiological procedures, with little loss of intravascular signal intensity.

The potential clinical indications related to these properties are:

- *Cerebral imaging*: measurement of the cerebral blood volume [87] and functional imaging [88]. The MR evaluation of stroke and its functional consequences may benefit from the use of blood pool agents. Even if emergency treatment of cerebral vascular accidents is currently limited, there is reason to believe that a diagnostic aid which precisely defines the cerebral shadow zone would demonstrate the value of better managed care, as was the case in myocardial ischemia.
- *Cardiac imaging*: quantification of the hypoperfused zones and MR coronary angiography.

- *First-pass angiography* [89, 90].
- *Tumor imaging*: detection and characterization of the lesion-associated microvascular environment. These agents would enable prediction of the treatment efficacy by evaluating the endothelial permeability and size of neovessels (calculation of blood volume and vessel size index) [91, 92].
- *Optimization of hyperpolarized ^{3}He gas MRI* [93].

2.4.5
Characterization of the Atheromatous Plaque

The composition and stage of atherosclerotic plaque are clinically more relevant than the severity of stenosis for evaluation of the risk of acute ischemic events. Atherosclerosis is basically an inflammatory disease [94]. Monocytes adhere to the vascular endothelium and accumulate in lesion-prone arterial sites. This adherence is facilitated by the endothelial expression of adhesion molecules. Adherent monocytes are subsequently enticed into the arterial intima where they differentiate into macrophages [95]. Macrophage-rich areas are more frequently found in the atheromatous plaques of patients with unstable angina and non-Q-wave myocardial infarction [96]. This suggests that macrophages are a marker of unstable atherosclerotic plaques and that specific targeting of these cells may lead to the characterization of atheromatous plaques prone to rupture.

Animal studies have clearly shown that USPIO induce focal signal intensity decreases in the aortic wall of atheromatous rabbits [97, 98] or apolipoprotein E (ApoE) knockout mice [99].

Interestingly, the exposure period of atherosclerotic plaque to circulating USPIO seems to be critical for the uptake of nanoparticles: in a comparative study in hyperlipidemic rabbits, the *in vivo* MRI signal intensity was found to be significantly higher with the long half-life agent ferumoxtran-10 than with another USPIO of similar size, ferumoxytol ($T_{1/2} \sim 6$ h), whereas *in vitro* macrophage phagocytosis was greater with the latter compound [100].

Preliminary clinical studies or case reports using ferumoxtran-10 have also shown USPIO-induced signal loss in aorta and pelvic arteries [101] or in carotid atheromatous plaques [102–104]. In one of these clinical trials [102], histological analysis showed USPIO in 27/36 (75%) of the ruptured or rupture-prone plaques and 1/14 (7%) of the stable atheromatous lesions. Postcontrast images should systematically be compared with corresponding precontrast images in order to exclude USPIO-induced signal reduction from other effects such as plaque calcification (which can also lead to strong susceptibility effects).

Given the heterogeneity of plaque formation and progression mechanisms, the macrophages which have endocytosed USPIO could be activated macrophages derived from activated blood-borne monocytes, activated macrophages derived from smooth muscle cells or foam cells which correspond to macrophages at a later stage [11]. Further studies are definitely required to better understand the precise mechanism of USPIO-uptake by atheromatous plaques. Obviously, such preliminary data open very interesting prospects for clinicians.

2.4.6 Other Potential Uses

Given the wide spectrum of inflammatory diseases, it is evident that these nanoparticles have a huge clinical potential. Some clinical applications of high interest are discussed below.

2.4.6.1 Stroke

Ischemic focal lesions are associated with a strong inflammatory local response that involves microglial cell activation as well as infiltration of hematogenous leukocytes, mostly monocytes [105, 106].

Ischemia-associated inflammation plays a major role in the pathogenesis of neurodegeneration associated with stroke. Activated macrophages produce numerous cytokines which exacerbate the ischemic tissue damage [107]. Consequently, noninvasive imaging of inflammation associated with subacute ischemic stroke lesions could be of predictive value and helpful for the development of cytoprotective drugs.

When injected in Fisher rats 5.5 h after permanent occlusion of the middle cerebral artery, the USPIO ferumoxtran-10 was shown to allow MR visualization of macrophage infiltration associated with focal ischemic lesions [108].

However, this technique did not allow determination of the specific contribution of microglia and blood-borne macrophages to USPIO accumulation. These results were confirmed by a subsequent study in rats where cerebral infarction was induced by photothrombosis of cortical microvessels. In this study, ferumoxtran-10 was injected 5 days after the induction of the cerebral ischemic lesions. Magnetic resonance imaging performed 24 h later displayed a rim-like signal loss around the lesion, which was in full spatial agreement with the histological data [109].

In a clinical phase II study, this USPIO was administered at the end of the first week after symptom onset in a series of 10 consecutive patients with ischemic stroke [110]. Two follow-up MR scans were performed 24–36 and 48–72 h after infusion. Vessel-associated changes were noticed (as signal loss on T2/T2*-weighted images) and decreased from the first to second scan. This effect was most likely related to the blood-pool effect of the USPIO. In addition to this effect, a parenchymal enhancement was noticed, mostly on T1-weighted images. This effect increased over time and matched with the expected distribution of macrophages. Larger clinical studies are clearly needed to demonstrate the clinical benefit associated with the use of USPIOs as a MRI surrogate markers for brain inflammation.

2.4.6.2 Cerebral Tumor Characterization

As mentioned above, according to their physicochemical properties, USPIOs can have a long blood half-life and therefore be found into the vascular compartment before being progressively endocytosed by tissue macrophages. Therefore, the nanoparticles can be used both for imaging tumor-associated microvessels during the early vascular equilibrium phase and, later, as a macrophage imaging agent for the characterization of the tumor-associated inflammatory lesion.

Preliminary clinical data [11, 111] have shown that there are distinct contrast enhancement mechanisms between early Gd^{3+} nonspecific contrast agent-based imaging, early USPIO injection, and late (24 h postinfusion) USPIO imaging. This could be of value for brain tumor characterization. USPIO nanoparticles do not cross the ruptured blood–brain barrier at early postinjection stages. This may prove helpful for the assessment of tumoral microvascular heterogeneity. Interestingly, in this preliminary study, the late USPIO-induced tumoral enhancement was found to be higher in high-grade than in low-grade glioblastomas [111].

In a preliminary study comparing the SPIO ferumoxides to the USPIO ferumoxtran-10 in 20 patients with primary and metastatic intracranial tumors, it was found that ferumoxtran-10, in contrast to ferumoxides, can be used as an intravenous contrast agent for MRI of intracranial tumors. Tumor enhancement was found to be comparable to but more variable than that observed with a nonspecific Gd^{3+} chelate. Histological examination showed similar distribution of the USPIO to be similar to that seen on MR images, i.e. primarily at the tumor margin, with less central localization. Most of the staining within the tumor was found in parenchymal cells with fine fibrillar processes, thus suggesting an astrocytic or microglial derivation [112].

2.4.6.3 Multiple Sclerosis

Multiple sclerosis, an idiopathic inflammatory disease of the central nervous system, is characterized pathologically by demyelination and subsequent axonal degeneration. It is currently accepted that MRI with Gd^{3+} nonspecific contrast agent, especially during or following a first attack, can be helpful in providing evidence of lesions in other parts of the brain and spinal cord [113]. Edema formation is detected by T2-weighted MRI, and a second MR scan could be useful at least three months after the initial attack to identify new lesions and provide evidence of dissemination over time [113]. Furthermore, magnetization transfer imaging or T1-weighted imaging can also be used for investigation of the demyelination process.

However, these parameters can only provide information on the consequences of the inflammatory process, but not on inflammation itself.

Some USPIOs (ferumoxtran-10, MION-46L) have been shown to be useful for *in vivo* macrophage activity imaging on experimental autoimmune encephalomyelitis (EAE) – a commonly used animal model that mimics human multiple sclerosis in several aspects [114, 115]. Post-USPIO sensitivity was found to be better than either pre-USPIO or post-nonspecific Gd^{3+} chelate-enhanced images [114].

A phase II pilot study investigated inflammatory lesions in 10 patients with definite relapsing-remitting multiple sclerosis who were included during one relapse episode. MRI with T1-weighted, Gd^{3+}-enhanced, T2- and T2*-weighted images was performed before and 24–48 h post-ferumoxtran-10 infusion. Nine out of the 10 patients studied showed multiple sclerosis lesion enhancement with USPIO. Some lesions enhanced up to 3 days after USPIO infusion. Seven patients showed multiple sclerosis lesion enhancement with the Gd^{3+} chelate.

Several patterns of enhancement were described when comparing USPIO- and Gd^{3+} chelate-induced enhancement: lesions enhancing with both contrast agents

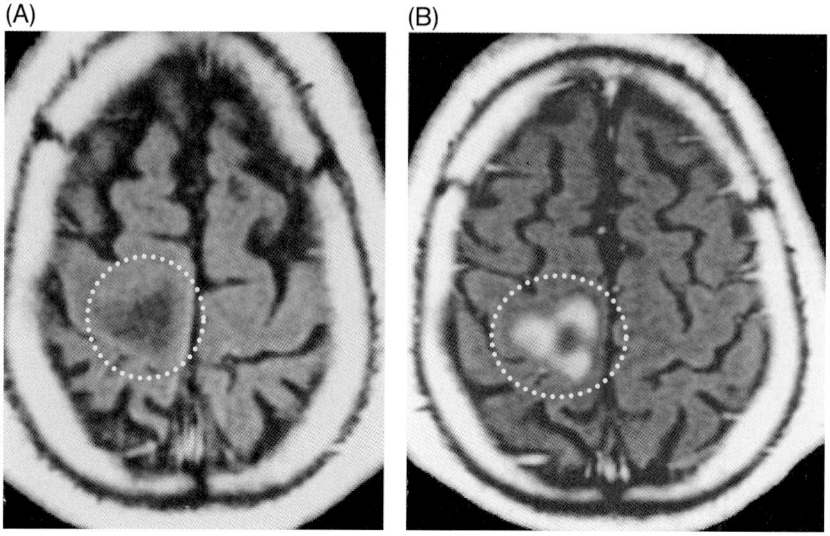

Figure 2.7. Multiple sclerosis: phase II clinical trial – ferumoxtran-10: (A) T1-weighted MRI images before injection and (B) T1-weighted MRI images 24 h postinjection of ferumoxtran-10. (courtesy Professor Vincent Dousset, Pellegrin Hospital, Bordeaux, France)

($n = 31$ lesions), with Gd^{3+} chelate only ($n = 24$) or with USPIO only ($n = 2$). Interestingly, the enhancement with USPIO was not superimposed on that related to the Gd^{3+} chelate [11, 116]. One example of USPIO-enhanced plaque is shown on Fig. 2.7.

2.4.6.4 Arthritis

Arthritis is characterized by infiltration of $CD4^+$ T cells, B cells and macrophages that sometimes organize into discrete lymphoid aggregates with germinal centers [117]. In a rabbit model of unilateral arthritis, MRI at 1.5 T was performed before and 24 h after intravenous injection of the USPIO ferumoxytol. Significant T1 and more predominantly T2* and T2 effects were evidenced in the synovium of all arthritic knees. Conversely, no significant changes in MR signal characteristics were found in the nonarthritic control knees. Histologic examination confirmed iron uptake in the macrophages within the hyperplastic synovium of the arthritic knees [118]. USPIO nanoparticles have also been found in macrophages located in synovial inflammatory infiltrates in a rat model of osteoarthritis (unpublished data) (Fig. 2.8).

2.4.6.5 Infection

Macrophages are activated during infection and migrate to the site of microbiotic invasion, thus providing a theoretical rationale for testing USPIO in such an indi-

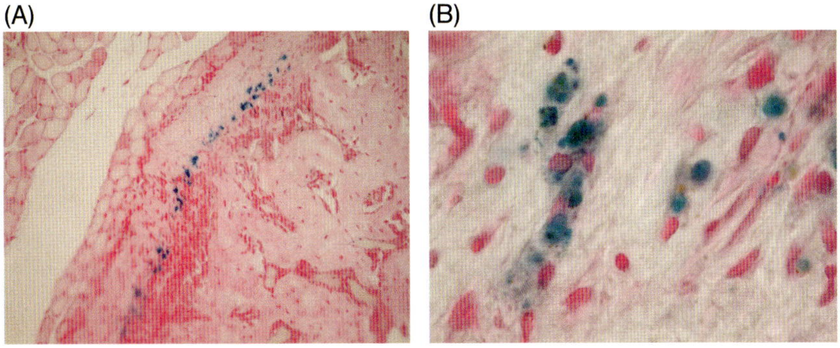

Figure 2.8. Representative photomicrographs of Perl's staining of iron oxide in macrophagic cells located in rat inflammatory synovium: (A) low- and (B) high-power magnification view (unpublished data).

cation. An experimental model of infection was developed in rats (unilateral deep calf muscle abscess following intramuscular injection of a *Staphylococcus aureus* suspension). Animals were imaged before and 3, 24, 48 and 72 h after intravenous injection of the USPIO ferumoxtran-10. Visualization was more sensitive with a T2*-weighted gradient echo sequence. The T2* effect was most prominent 3 h after ferumoxtran injection because of the high amount of intravascular USPIO at this time-point. A significant decrease in T2* relative signal intensity was found at 24 h, reflecting the intracellular iron accumulation within macrophages. Only a slight decrease in T2* signal intensity was found at 48 and 72 h. Local signal intensity changes were correlated with macrophagic uptake of the USPIO [119].

In fact, signal intensity characteristics of abscesses on T1- and T2*-weighted sequences obtained 24 h following USPIO injection strongly depend upon the administered dose. At low dose (50 μmol Fe kg^{-1}), T1 effects were stronger than T2* effects [120].

2.4.6.6 Kidney Imaging

Intravenous injection of puromycin amino-nucleoside (PAN) in the rat is a good model of nephrotic syndrome secondary to glomerular epithelial cell lesions associated with glomerular and tubulointerstitial infiltration by macrophages. In nephrotic rats, the USPIO ferumoxtran-10 injected intravenously (90 μmol kg^{-1}) induced a significant decrease in signal intensity in all compartments of the kidney in the PAN group, whereas the signal from the control group did not vary 24 h postinjection. This effect was correlated with the presence of macrophages with iron oxide nanoparticles at histology [121]. Interestingly, the same USPIO was also found to decrease signal intensity in the cortex in a model of nephrotoxic nephropathy (by injection of sheep anti-rat glomerular basement membrane serum). In this model, equivalent to Goodpasture's syndrome in humans, inflammatory lesions were exclusively located at the level of glomeruli. Conversely, in a rat model of obstructive nephropathy, which is known to induce diffuse interstitial lesions with macrophage infiltration in all kidney compartments, the USPIO induced a decrease in signal intensity in all compartments [122].

Renal allograft rejection is associated with a massive inflammatory infiltration [123]. In a rat renal allograft model, USPIO, when injected on the fourth day following transplantation, induced a decrease in MR signal intensity at 24 h in some rejecting allografts, whereas isografts and allografts with immunosuppressant treatment had no signal reduction [124]. Promising results were obtained in a preliminary clinical study performed in seven patients with suspected proliferative glomerulonephritis and five with suspected renal graft rejection imaged 72 h following injection of ferumoxtran-10. USPIO-enhanced MRI may allow acute tubular necrosis to be distinguished from other acute nephropathies in native and transplanted kidneys and may also allow active proliferative nephropathies to be differentiated from chronic ones [125]. Of course, such preliminary clinical data, obtained in a small number of patients, need to be confirmed by other studies. Dextran-coated USPIOs serving as blood pool agent were also used to evaluate renal perfusion in dynamic MRI in normal and transplanted rat kidneys.

A good agreement between renal graft perfusion and histopathological changes associated with graft rejection suggests that USPIO-enhanced dynamic MRI may be used to evaluate acute allograft rejection [126].

Iodinated contrast agents can be nephrotoxic in at-risk patients by inducing medullary hypoxia [127]. Intravenous injection of USPIO has been used in rat models of contrast nephropathy to assess renal lesions induced by the iodinated contrast agent [128] as well as their reversibility [129].

2.4.6.7 **Acute Cardiac Transplant Rejection**

In addition to kidney graft evaluation, USPIO may be used to noninvasively detect inflammatory changes associated with cardiac graft rejection as elegantly shown in two studies involving intravenous administration of either dextran-coated USPIO (27 nm in diameter) [130] or feruglose (NC100150) [131] in rats with heterotopic heart transplantation. Feruglose was used for its blood pool properties in dynamic T1 MRI whereas the dextran-coated USPIO was used for its ability to be captured by macrophages. However, it is worth mentioning that macrophagic infiltration may be associated with other pathophysiological situations such as reperfusion injury or myocardial infection.

2.4.6.8 ***In Vivo* Monitoring of Cell Therapy**

Recent progress in the field of stem and progenitor cells suggests that their use to correct or replace defective cell populations may soon become a clinical reality. Clinical applications are numerous and promising, both for the central nervous system-related diseases (spinal cord injury, Parkinson's disease, myelin disorders, Huntington's disease, etc) and regeneration of the myocardium. Renal and hepatic pathologies may also benefit from the progress of cell therapies. It is therefore crucial to track the location and *in vivo* distribution of these cells in a noninvasive manner [132].

For this purpose, stem cells must first be magnetically labeled *in vitro* before being administered to a living organism [132].

Several approaches have been described to optimize the internalization process [132], including linking the nanoparticles to the highly cationic HIV *tat* peptide [35] or the use of an anti-transferrin receptor monoclonal antibody covalently linked to nanoparticles (MION-46L) [133].

In fact, it is more convenient to use commercially available and registered nanoparticles. Several studies have shown that ferumoxides or MION-46L can be internalized after mixing with a transfection agent (such as dendrimers, high-molecular-weight poly-L-lysine, lipofectamine, protamine sulfate, etc.) [132, 134] or without such agents [135]. Actually, unmodified SPIOs or USPIOs have been successfully used, at high concentrations, to label cells (fluid phase mediated endocytosis) in the absence of transfection agents [12, 135]. However, it is worth mentioning that SPIO particles, with a diameter of about 100–150 nm were found to be more efficient for cell targeting than were USPIO nanoparticles, which have average hydrodynamic diameters of 20–40 nm [135]. This is probably related to the fact that phagocytic and endocytic uptake increases with increasing particle diameter (at equivalent coating thickness).

Uptake of the nanoparticles increases with time, but cell viability decreases with increasing incubation time. An incubation time of 2–4 h has been considered an acceptable compromise in the case of hematopoietic progenitor cells [135].

There is ample preclinical literature showing that MRI tracking of stem cells is feasible. Some recent examples are shown in Tab. 2.5 [136–139].

Due to the high anatomical spatial resolution of MRI, its potential for quantification, the low cytotoxicity of superparamagnetic nanoparticles and the promising studies currently available, MR monitoring of cell therapy seems to be a technique with a good future.

2.4.6.9 T-staging of Uterine Neoplasms

USPIO ferumoxtran-10, evaluated for MR lymph node staging in uterine carcinoma, was serendipitously found to induce a significant decrease in signal intensity of both myometrum and cervical stroma, thus allowing improved delineation of uterine neoplasms.

A clinical study involving 17 patients subsequently confirmed that the contrast-to-noise ratio between tumor and myometrum and between tumor and cervical stroma was significantly higher on USPIO-enhanced images compared with unenhanced images [140].

2.4.6.10 MRI-detectable Embolotherapy

Embolization is frequently used for the treatment of cancer, but it is so far difficult to locate the injected embolic material and to monitor changes in its structure over time.

SPIOs embedded in polyglucosamine (chitosan) (100–150 μm in diameter) were detected by MRI after selective embolization of a renal artery in rabbits [141]. How-

Tab. 2.5. Animal models of cell tracking: some examples.

Animal model	Stem cells	Nanoparticle used	Result	Reference
Experimental myocardial infarction in pigs	swine mesenchymal stem cells	ferumoxides + poly-L-lysine; intramyocardial injection	successful imaging at 1.5 T and correlation with histology	136
mdx mice (murine model of Duchenne's muscular dystrophy)	multipotent, muscle-derived stem cells	ferumoxides + poly-L-lysine; intramuscular injection	Successful sequential imaging and correlation with histology	137
Healthy rats	mesenchymal stem cells from the bone marrow of a syngenic rat strain	ferumoxides + dendrimer transfection agent (Superfect®); intra-arterial injection into the kidney	Signal intensity loss in the cortex; detection for up to 7 days	138
CCl_4-induced hepatocyte necrosis and inflammation in rats	mesenchymal stem cells from the bone marrow of a syngenic rat strain	ferumoxides + dendrimer transfection agent (Superfect®); intraportal injection	Irregular signal intensity loss, reflecting the lobular structure of the liver; detection for up to 12 days	138
C57Bl/6 mice injected with ovalbumin-transfected B16 melanoma cells (B16-OVA) and B16 F0 melanoma cells	$CD8^+$ cytotoxic T lymphocytes	CLIO-HD (highly-derivatized crosslinked iron oxide) incubated with $CD8^+$ T cells and injected intraperitoneally	*in vivo* detection of CLIO-HD-labeled $CD8^+$ T cells with a threshold of around 3 cells voxel^{-1}	139
Myelin-deficient *md* rats	rat oligodendrocyte progenitor cell line CG-4	MION-46-L targeted to the transferring receptor Tfr and grafted into the spinal cord of neonate *md* rats	Successful *ex vivo* three-dimensional MRI of the migratory capacity of transplanted cells; correlation with histology	133

ever, although they are derived from nanoparticles, such objects can no longer be considered as being nanoparticles.

2.5 Conclusion

The use of superparamagnetic nanoparticulate agents in MRI has been a major development in the range of tools available to clinicians. The efficacy of these agents has led to their being proposed in gastrointestinal tract and hepatic lesion imaging. The prospects for increased use in lymph node and functional imaging look very promising. These nanoparticles are also potential disease-specific agents. This potential depends on improved knowledge of the fundamental mechanisms of the interaction of the superparamagnetic agents with the MR signal and also on the control of the pharmacokinetic behavior of these molecules. In terms of effect on the MR signal, the use of the dose-dependent effect of the nanoparticles on the T1 relaxation time will undoubtedly be an increasingly widely studied research topic in the near future. The importance of the r_2/r_1 ratio as a function of the magnetic field is also emphasized in studies establishing the most appropriate sequences for the molecules under clinical development. In terms of pharmacokinetics, research into preventing the iron oxide particles from being taken up by the liver and spleen reticuloendothelial system by appropriate selection of particle charge, size and coating is of major interest.

The chemical coating of these nanoparticles may also allow them to be linked to molecules ("pharmacophores") capable of specifically targeting a specific area such as an organ, a disease or a particular biological system such as macrophages or stem cells. This opens major research avenues with important potential clinical consequences.

Nanoparticulate molecules can also behave as blood pool contrast agents for MR angiography at both first-pass and equilibrium. Here, again, clinical applications are numerous. Furthermore, the ability for such nanoparticles to target inflammatory lesions offers major and very exciting prospects for the characterization of numerous inflammatory and degenerative diseases.

Last, but not least, nanoparticles used for medical imaging purposes are also at the interface with targeted therapies and can be expected to have the potential to contribute to the follow-up of such treatments.

In addition to the intravenous route, local administration may also be envisaged (aerosol, interstitial, subcutaneous injection, etc). This opens up an important research field into more specific agents adapted to clinicians' needs. Fundamental research is needed to better understand the toxicity issues potentially associated with nanoparticular molecules in general and particularly their interaction with the immune system.

A bright future can be anticipated for nanoparticular contrast agents provided their development is based on a rational design through a thorough understanding of their physicochemistry and biological environment.

References

1 Klaveness J. Particulate agents. In *Enhanced MRI*, Runge VM (Ed.). Mosby, St Louis, MO, **1989**, pp. 117–128.

2 Roch A, Muller RN, Gillis P. Theory of proton relaxation induced by superparamagnetic particles. *J. Chem. Phys.* **1999**, *110*, 5403–5411.

3 Roch A, Muller RN. Longitudinal relaxation of water protons in colloidal suspensions of superparamagnetic crystals. In *11th Annual Scientific Meeting SMRM, Works in Progress*, Berlin, **1992**, p. 1447.

4 Chambon C, Clément O, Le Blanche A, Schouman-Claeys E, Frija G. Superparamagnetic iron oxides as positive MR contrast agents: *in vitro* and *in vivo* evidence. *Magn. Reson. Imaging* **1993**, *11*, 509–519.

5 Canet E, Revel D, Forrat R, Baldy-Porcher C, de Lorgeril M, Sebbag L, Vallée JP, Didier D, Amiel M. Superparamagnetic iron oxide particles and positive enhancement for myocardial perfusion studies assessed by subsecond T1-weighed MRI. *Magn. Reson. Imaging* **1993**, *11*, 1139–1145.

6 Franck H, Weissleder R, Brady TJ. Enhancement of MR angiography with iron oxide: preliminary studies in whole-blood phantom and in animals. *Am. J. Roentgenol.* **1994**, *162*, 209–213.

7 Bomatí-Miguel O, Morales MP, Tartaj P, Ruiz-cabello J, Bonville P, Santos M, Zhao X, Veintemillas-Verdaguer S. Fe-based nanoparticulate metallic alloys as contrast agents for magnetic resonance imaging. *Biomaterials* **2005**, *26*, 5695–5703.

8 Jung CW, Jacobs P. Physical and chemical properties of superparamagnetic iron oxide MR contrast agents: ferumoxides, ferumoxtran, ferumoxsil. *Magn. Reson. Imaging* **1995**, *13*, 661–674.

9 Benderbous S, Corot C, Jacobs P, Bonnemain B. Superparamagnetic agents: physicochemical characteristics and preclinical imaging evaluation. *Acad Radiol.* **1996**, *3 (Suppl. 2)*, S292–S294.

10 Cheng FY, Su CH, Yang YS, Yeh CS, Tsai CY, Wu CY, Wu MT, Shieh DB. Characterization of aqueous dispersions of Fe_3O_4 nanoparticles and their biomedical applications. *Biomaterials* **2005**, *26*, 729–738.

11 Corot C, Petry KG, Trivedi R, Saleh A, Jonkmanns C, Le Bas JF, Blezer E, Rausch M, Brochet B, Foster-Gareau P, Balériaux D, Gaillard S, Dousset V. Macrophage imaging in central nervous system and in carotid atherosclerotic plaque imaging using ultrasmall superparamagnetic iron oxide in magnetic resonance imaging. *Invest. Radiol.* **2004**, *39*, 619–625.

12 Fleige G, Seeberger F, Laux D, Kresse M, Taupitz M, Pilgrimm H, Zimmer C. *In vitro* characterization of two different ultrasmall iron oxide particles for magnetic resonance cell tracking. *Invest. Radiol.* **2002**, *37*, 482–488.

13 Taupitz M, Wagner S, Schnorr J, Kravec I, Pilgrimm H, Bergmann-Fritsch H, Hamm B. Phase I clinical evaluation of citrate-coated monocrystalline very small superparamagnetic iron oxide particles as a new contrast medium for magnetic resonance imaging. *Invest. Radiol.* **2004**, *39*, 394–405.

14 Bjornerud A, Johansson LO, Ahlstrom HK. Pre-clinical results with Clariscan (NC100150 Injection); experience from different disease models. *MAGMA* **2001**, *12*, 99–103.

15 Petri-Fink A, Chastellain M, Juillerat-Jeanneret L, Ferrari A, Hofmann H. Development of functionalized superparamagnetic iron oxide nanoparticles for interaction with human cancer cells. *Biomaterials* **2005**, *26*, 2685–2694.

16 Brillet PY, Gazeau F, Luciani A, Bessoud B, Cuénod CA, Siauve N, Pons JN, Poupon J, Clément O. Evaluation of tumoral enhancement by superparamagnetic iron oxide particles: comparative studies with ferumoxtran and anionic iron oxide

nanoparticles. *Eur. Radiol.* **2005**, *15*, 1369–1377.

17 Raynal I, Prigent P, Peyramaure S, Najid A, Rebuzzi C, Corot C. Macrophage endocytosis of superparamagnetic iron oxide nanoparticles. Mechanisms and comparison of ferumoxides and ferumoxtran-10. *Invest. Radiol.* **2004**, *39*, 56–63.

18 Metz S, Bonaterra G, Rudelius M, Settles M, Rummeny EJ, Daldrup-Link H. Capacity of human monocytes to phagocytose approved iron oxide MR contrast agents *in vitro*. *Eur. Radiol.* **2004**, *14*, 1851–1858.

19 Sun R, Dittrich J, Le-Huu M, Mueller MM, Bedke J, Kartenbeck J, Lehmann WD, Krueger R, Bock M, Huss R, Seliger C, Gröne HJ, Misselwitz B, Semmler W, Kiessling F. Physical and biological characterization of superparamagnetic iron-oxide- and ultrasmall superparamagnetic iron oxide-labeled cells. A comparison. *Invest. Radiol.* **2005**, *40*, 504–513.

20 Rogers WJ, Basu P. Factors regulating macrophage endocytosis of nanoparticles: implications for targeted magnetic resonance plaque imaging. *Atherosclerosis* **2005**, *178*, 67–73

21 Stroh A, Zimmer C, Gutzeit C, Jakstadt M, Marschinke F, Jung T, Pilgrimm H, Grune T. Iron oxide particles for molecular magnetic resonance imaging cause transient oxidative stress in rat macrophages. *Free Radic. Biol. Med.* **2004**, *36*, 976–984.

22 Schulze E, Ferrucci JT Jr, Poss K, Lapointe L, Bogdanova A, Weissleder R. Cellular uptake and trafficking of a prototypical magnetic iron oxide label *in vitro*. *Invest. Radiol.* **1995**, *30*, 604–610.

23 Leenders W. Ferumoxtran-10. *Drugs* **2003**, *6*, 987–993.

24 Schnorr J, Taupitz M, Wagner S, Pilgrimm H, Hansel J, Hamm B. Age-related blood half-life of particulate contrast material: experimental results with a USPIO in rats. *J. Magn. Reson. Imaging.* **2000**, *12*, 740–744.

25 Weissleder R, Stark DD, Engelstad BL, Bacon BR, Compton CC, White DL, Jacobs P, Lewis J. Superparamagnetic iron oxide: pharmacokinetics and toxicity. *Am. J. Roentgenol.* **1989**, *152*, 167–173.

26 Taylor AM, Panting JR, Keegan J, Gatehouse PD, Amin D, Jhooti P, Yang GZ, McGill S, Burman ED, Francis JM, Firmin DN, Pennell DJ. Safety and preliminary findings with the intravascular contrast agent NC100150 injection for MR coronary angiography. *J. Magn. Reson. Imaging* **1999**, *9*, 220–227.

27 Briley-Saebo K, Hustvedt SO, Haldorsen A, Bjornerud A. Long-term imaging effects in rat liver after a single injection of an iron oxide nanoparticles based MR contrast agent. *J. Magn. Reson. Imaging* **2004**, *20*, 622–631.

28 Weissleder R, Elizondo G, Wittenberg J, Rabito CA, Bengele HH, Josephson L. Ultrasmall superparamagnetic iron oxide: characterization of a new class of contrast agents for MR imaging. *Radiology* **1990**, *175*, 489–493.

29 Bellin MF, Beigelman C, Precetti-Morel S. Iron oxide-enhanced MR lymphography: initial experience. *Eur. J. Radiol.* **2000**, *34*, 257–264.

30 Bengele HH, Palmacci S, Rogers J, Jung CW, Crenshaw J, Josephson L. Biodistribution of an ultrasmall superparamagnetic iron oxide colloid, BMS 180549, by different routes of administration. *Magn. Reson. Imaging* **1994**, *12*, 433–442.

31 McCauley TR, Rifkin MD, Ledet CA. Pelvic lymph node visualization with MR imaging using local administration of ultra-small superparamagnetic iron oxide contrast. *J. Magn. Reson. Imaging* **2002**, *15*, 492–497.

32 Pomper MG. Molecular imaging: a review. *Acad. Radiol.* **2001**, *8*, 1141–1153.

33 Morawski AM, Lanza GA, Wickline SA. Targeted contrast agents for magnetic resonance imaging and ultrasound. *Curr. Opin. Biotechnol.* **2005**, *16*, 89–92.

34 Högemann D, Josephson L, Weissleder R, Basilion JP. Improvement of MRI probes to allow efficient detection of gene expression. *Bioconjug. Chem.* **2000**, *11*, 941–946.
35 Josephson L, Tung CH, Moore A, Weissleder R. High efficiency intracellular magnetic labelling with novel superparamagnetic tat–peptide conjugates. *Bioconjug. Chem.* **1999**, *10*, 186–191.
36 Burtea C, Laurent S, Roch A, Vander Elst L, Muller RN. C-MALISA (cellular magnetic-linked immunosorbent assay), a new application of cellular ELISA for MRI. *J. Inorg. Biochem.* **2005**, *99*, 1135–1144.
37 Halbreich A, Roger J, Pons JN, De Fatima da Silva M, Hasmonay E, Roudier M, Boynard M, Sestier C, Amri A, Geldwerth D, Fertil B, Bacri JC, Sabolovic D. Magnetic maghemite nanoparticles: their preparation, properties, and applications in cell sorting and characterization of cellular membrane *in vitro*. In *Scientific and Clinical Applications of Magnetic Carriers (Proceedings of the International Conference on Scientific and Clinical Applications of Magnetic Carriers)*, Haefeli U (Ed.). Plenum Press, New York, **1997**, pp. 399–417.
38 Weissleder R, Lee AS, Fischman AJ, Reimer P, Shen T, Wilkinson R, Callahan RJ, Brady TJ. Polyclonal human immunoglobulin G labeled with polymeric iron oxide: antibody MR imaging. *Radiology* **1991**, *181*, 245–249.
39 Reimer P, Kwong KK, Weisskoff R, Cohen MS, Brady TJ, Weissleder R. Dynamic signal intensity changes in liver with superparamagnetic MR contrast agent. *J. Magn. Reson. Imaging* **1992**, *2*, 177–181.
40 Kresse M, Wagner S, Pfefferer D, Lawaczeck R, Elste V, Semmler W. Targeting of ultrasmall superparamagnetic iron oxide (USPIO) particles to tumor cells *in vivo* by using transferring receptor pathways. *Magn. Reson. Med.* **1998**, *40*, 236–242.
41 Johansson LO, Björnerud A, Ahlström HK, Ladd DL, Fujii DK. A targeted contrast agent for magnetic resonance imaging of thrombus: implications of spatial resolution. *J. Magn. Reson. Imaging* **2001**, *13*, 615–618.
42 van Tilborg GAF, Strijkers GJ, Reutelinsperger CPM, Nicolay K. Annexin V-functionalized USPIO as a contrast agent for apoptotic Jurkat cells. In *Proceedings of the ESMRMB Meeting*, Copenhagen, **2004**, p. 223.
43 Burtea C, Chaabane L, Laurent S, Canet-Soulas E, Vander Elst L, Briguet A, Muller RN. Preclinical evaluation of a new $\alpha_v\beta_3$-targeted nonpeptidic RGD mimetic grafted to USPIO. Preliminary investigations on the molecular imaging of vulnerable atherosclerotic plaques. In *Proceedings of the ESMRMB Meeting*, Copenhagen, **2004**, p. 373.
44 Bonnemain B. Superparamagnetic agents in magnetic resonance imaging: physicochemical characteristics and clinical applications. A review. *J. Drug Target.* **1998**, *6*, 167–174.
45 Hahn PF, Stark DD, Lewis J, Saini S, Elizondo G, Weissleder R, Fretz CJ, Ferrucci JT. First clinical trial of a new superparamagnetic iron oxide for use as an oral gastrointestinal contrast agent in MR imaging. *Radiology* **1990**, *175*, 695–700.
46 Haldemann-Heusler RC, Wight E, Marincek B. Oral superparamagnetic contrast agent (ferumoxsil): tolerance and efficacy in MR Imaging of gynecologic diseases. *J. Magn. Reson. Imaging* **1995**, *4*, 385–391.
47 Johnson WK, Stoupis C, Torres GM, Rosenberg EB, Ros PR. Superparamagnetic iron oxide (SPIO) as an oral contrast agent in gastrointestinal (GI) magnetic resonance imaging (MRI): comparison with state-of-the-art computed tomography (CT). *Magn. Reson. Imaging* **1996**, *14*, 43–49.
48 Rubin DL, Muller HH, Young SW, Hunke WA, Gorman WG, Lee KC. Influence of viscosity of WIN 39996 as

a contrast agent for gastrointestinal resonance magnetic imaging. *Invest. Radiol.* **1995**, *30*, 226–231.

49 MacVicar D, Jacobsen TF, Guy R, Husband JE. Phase III trial of oral magnetic particles in MRI of abdomen and pelvis. *Clin. Radiol.* **1993**, *47*, 183–188.

50 Bach-Gansmo T, Dupas B, Gayet-Delacroix M, Lambrechts M. Abdominal MRI using a negative contrast agent. *Br. J. Radiol.* **1993**, *66*, 420–425.

51 Vlahos L, Gouliamos A, Athanasopoulou G, Kotoulas G, Claus W, Hatziioannou A, Kalovidouris A, Papavasiliou C. A comparative study between Gd-DTPA and oral magnetic particles (OMP) as gastro-intestinal (GI) contrast agents for MRI of the abdomen. *Magn. Reson. Imaging* **1994**, *12*, 719–726.

52 Vlahos L, Gouliamos A, Kalovidouris A, Athanasopoulou A, Kotoulas G, Lygidakis N, Liaou A, Matsaidonis D, Papavasiliou C. Oral magnetic particles as contrast agent for MR imaging of the abdomen. A phase III clinical trial. *Hepatogastroenterology* **1994**, *41*, 82–85.

53 Jacobsen TF, laniado M, Van Beers BE, Dupas B, Boudghene FP, Rummeny E, Falk TH, Rinck PA, MacVicar D, Lundby B. Oral magnetic particles (ferristene) as a contrast medium in abdominal magnetic resonance imaging. *Acad Radiol.* **1996**, *3*, 571–580.

54 Herrmann K, Zech CJ, Michaely HJ, Seiderer J, Ochsenkuehn T, Reiser MF, Schoenberg SO. Comprehensive magnetic resonance imaging of the small and large bowel using intraluminal dual contrast technique with iron oxide solution and water in magnetic resonance enteroclysis. *Invest. Radiol.* **2005**, *40*, 621–629.

55 Maccioni F, Viscido A, Broglia L, Marrollo M, Masciangelo R, Caprilli R, Rossi P. Evaluation of Crohn disease activity with magnetic resonance imaging. *Abdom. Imaging* **2000**, *25*, 219–228.

56 Laghi A, Paolantonio P, Iafrate F, Altomari F, Miglio C, Passariello R. Oral contrast agents for magnetic resonance imaging of the bowel. *Top. Magn. Reson. Imaging* **2002**, *13*, 389–396.

57 Wang YXJ, Hussain SM, Krestin GP. Superparamagnetic iron oxide contrast agents: physicochemical characteristics and applications in MR imaging. *Eur. Radiol.* **2001**, *11*, 2319–2331.

58 Wake K, Decker K, Kirn A, Knook DL, McCuskey RS, Bouwens L, Wisse E. Cell biology and kinetics of Küpffer cells in the liver. *Int. Rev. Cytol.* **1989**, *118*, 173–229.

59 Saini S, Stark DD, Hahn PF, Wittenberg J, Brady TJ, Ferruci JT Jr. Ferrite particles: a superparamagnetic MR contrast agent for the reticuloendothelial system. *Radiology* **1987**, *162*, 211–216.

60 Bellin MF, Zaim S, Auberton E, Sarfati G, Duron JJ, Khayat D, Grellet J. Liver metastases: safety and efficacy of detection with superparamagnetic iron oxide in MR imaging. *Radiology* **1994**, *193*, 657–663.

61 Ros PR, Freeny PC, Harms SE, Seltzer SE, Davis PL, Chan TW, Stillman AE, Muroff LR, Runge VM, Nissenbaum MA, Jacobs P. Hepatic MR imaging with ferumoxides: a multicenter clinical trial of the safety and efficacy in the detection of focal hepatic lesions. *Radiology* **1995**, *195*, 481–488.

62 Séneterre E, Taourel P, Bouvier Y, Pradel J, Van Beers B, Daures JP, Pringot J, Mathieu D, Bruel JM. Detection of hepatic metastases: ferumoxides-enhanced MR imaging versus unenhanced MR imaging and CT during arterial portography. *Radiology* **1996**, *200*, 785–792.

63 Abe Y, Yamashita Y, Namimoto T, Tang Y, Takahashi M. The value of fast and ultrafast T2-weighted MR imaging sequences in hepatic enhancement with ferumoxides: comparison with conventional spin-echo sequences. *Radiat. Med.* **2000**, *18*, 97–105.

64 Kim MJ, Kim JH, Chung JJ, Park MS, Lim JS, Oh YT. Focal hepatic lesions: detection and characterization with combination gadolinium- and superparamagnetic iron oxide-enhanced MR imaging. *Radiology* **2003**, *228*, 719–726.
65 Weissleder R, Hahn PF, Stark DD, Elizondo G, Saini S, Todd LE, Wittenberg J, Ferrucci J Jr. Superparamagnetic iron oxide: enhanced detection of focal splenic tumors with MR imaging. *Radiology* **1988**, *169*, 399–403.
66 Storm BL, Abbitt PL, Allen DA, Ros PR. Splenosis: superparamagnetic iron oxide-enhanced MR imaging. *Am. J. Roentgenol.* **1992**, *159*, 333–335.
67 Schultz JF, Kuhn JA, McCarthy TM. Hepatic imaging with iron oxide magnetic resonance imaging. *Oncology* **2000**, *14 (Suppl. 3)*, 29–36.
68 Weishaupt D, Willmann JK, Lutz AM, Marincek B. Resovist for imaging of hepatocarcinoma in the cirrhotic liver. *Eur. Radiol.* **2004**, *14 (Suppl. 1)*, C5–C6.
69 Reimer P, Balzer T. Ferucarbotran (Resovist): a new clinically-approved RES-specific contrast agent for contrast-enhanced MRI of the liver: properties, clinical development, and applications. *Eur. Radiol.* **2003**, *16*, 1266–1276.
70 Suto Y, Kato T, Matsuo T, Kamba M, Shimatani Y, Ohuchi Y, Nakamura K, Ohta Y. Chondroitin sulfate iron colloid as MR contrast agent in differentiation between hepatocellular carcinoma and adenomatous hyperplasia. *Acta Radiol.* **1993**, *34*, 226–229.
71 Pouliquen D, Lucet I, Chouly C, Perdrisot R, Le Jeune JJ, Jallet P. Liver-directed superparamagnetic iron oxide: quantitation of T2-relaxation effects. *Magn. Res. Imaging* **1993**, *11*, 219–228.
72 Wisner E, Amparo E, Vera D, Brock JM, Barlow TW, Griffey SM, Drake C, Katzberg RW. Arabinogalactan-coated superparamagnetic iron oxide: effect of particle size in liver MRI. *J. Comput. Assist. Tomogr.* **1995**, *19*, 211–215.
73 Stockert RJ. The asialoglycoprotein receptor: relationship between structure, function and expression. *Physiol. Rev.* **1995**, *75*, 591–609.
74 Van Beers BE, Sempoux C, Materne R, Delos M, Smith AM. Biodistribution of ultrasmall iron oxide particles in the rat liver. *J. Magn. Reson. Imaging* **2001**, *13*, 594–599.
75 Mergo PJ, Engelken JD, Helmberger T, Ros PR. MRI in focal liver disease: a comparison of small and ultrasmall superparamagnetic iron oxide as hepatic contrast agents. *J. Magn. Reson. Imaging* **1998**, *8*, 1073–1078.
76 Koh DM, Brown G, Temple L, Raja A, Toomey P, Bett N, Norman AR, Husband JE. Rectal cancer: mesorectal lymph nodes at MR imaging with USPIO versus histopathologic findings. Initial observations. *Radiology* **2004**, *231*, 91–99.
77 Weissleder R, Heautot JF, Schaffer BK, Nossiff N, Papisov MI, Bogdanov A Jr, Brady TJ. MR lymphography: study of a high-efficient lymphotropic agent. *Radiology* **1994**, *191*, 225–230.
78 Rogers JM, Lewis J, Josephson L. Visualization of superior mesenteric lymph nodes by the combined oral and intravenous administration of the ultrasmall superparamagnetic iron oxide, AMI-227. *Magn. Reson. Imaging* **1994**, *12*, 1161–1165.
79 Anzai Y, McLachlan S, Morris M, Saxton R, Lufkin RB. Dextran-coated superparamagnetic iron oxide, an MR contrast agent for assessing lymph nodes in the head and neck. *Am. J. Neuroradiol.* **1994**, *15*, 87–94.
80 Bellin MF, Roy C, Kinkel K, Thoumas D, Zaim S, Vanel D, Tuchmann C, Richard F, Jacqumin D, Delcourt A, Challier E, Lebret T, Cluzel P. Lymph node metastases: safety and effectiveness of MR imaging with ultrasmall superparamagnetic iron oxide particles. Initial clinical experience. *Radiology* **1998**, *207*, 799–808.

81 Harisinghani MG, Barentsz J, Hahn PF, Deserno WM, Tabatabaei S, Hulsbergen van de Kaa C, De la Rosette J, Weissleder R. Noninvasive detection of clinically occult lymph-node metastases in prostate cancer. *New Engl. J. Med.* **2003**, *348*, 2491–2499.

82 Moghimi SM, Hunter AC, Muttay JC. Nanomedicine: current status and future prospects. *FASEB J.* **2005**, *19*, 311–330.

83 Zimmer C, Weissleder R, O'Connor D, LaPointe L, Brady TJ, Enochs WS. Cerebral iron oxide distribution: *in vivo* mapping with MR imaging. *Radiology* **1995**, *196*, 521–527.

84 Reith W, Forsting M, Vogler H, Heiland S, Sartor K. Early MR detection of experimentally induced cerebral ischemia using magnetic susceptibility contrast agents: comparison between gadopentetate dimeglumine and iron oxide particles. *Am. J. Neuroradiol.* **1995**, *16*, 53–60.

85 Trillaud H, Degrèze P, Combe C, Deminière C, Palussière J, Benderbous S, Grenier N. USPIO-enhanced MR Imaging of glycerol-induced acute renal failure in the rabbit. *Magn. Res. Imaging* **1995**, *13*, 233–240.

86 Mergo PJ, Helmberger T, Nicolas AI, Ros PR. Ring enhancement in ultrasmall superparamagnetic iron oxide MR imaging: a potential new sign for characterization of liver tissues. *Am. J. Roentgenol.* **1996**, *166*, 379–384.

87 Berry I, Benderbous S, Ranjeva JP, Gracia-Meavilla D, Manelfe C, Le Bihan D. Contribution of Sinerem used as blood-pool contrast agent: detection of cerebral blood volume changes during apnea in the rabbit. *Magn. Reson. Med.* **1996**, *36*, 415–419.

88 Vanduffel W, Fize D, Mandeville JB, Nelissen K, Van Hecke P, Tootell RB, Orban GA. Visual motion processing investigated using contrast agent-enhanced fMRI in awake behaving monkeys. *Neuron* **2001**, *32*, 565–577.

89 Schnorr J, Wagner S, Abramjuk C, Wojner I, Schink T, Kroencke TJ, Schellenberger E, Hamm B, Pilgrimm H, Taupitz M. Comparison of the iron oxide-based contrast medium VSOP-C184 with gadopentetate dimeglumine for first-pass magnetic resonance angiography of the aorta and renal arteries in pigs. *Invest. Radiol.* **2004**, *39*, 546–553.

90 Li W, Tutton S, Vu AT, Pierchala L, Li BSY, Lewis JM, Prasad PV, Edelman RR. First-pass contrast-enhanced magnetic resonance angiography in humans using ferumoxytol, a novel ultrasmall superparamagnetic iron oxide (USPIO)-based blood pool agent. *J. Magn. Reson. Imaging* **2005**, *21*, 46–52.

91 Troprès I, Grimault S, Vaeth A, Grillon E, Julien C, Payen JF, Lamalle L, Décorps M. Vessel size imaging. *Mag. Reson. Med.* **2001**, *45*, 397–408.

92 Troprès I, Lamalle L, Péoc'h M, Farion R, Usson Y, Décorps M, Rémy C. *In vivo* imaging of tumoral angiogenesis. *Magn. Reson. Med.* **2004**, *51*, 533–541.

93 Vignaud A, Maître X, Guillot G, Durand E, De Rochefort L, Robert P, Vivès V, Santus R, Darrasse L. Magnetic susceptibility matching at the air-tissue interface in rat lung by using a superparamagnetic intravascular contrast agent: influence on transverse relaxation time of hyperpolarized helium-3. *Magn. Reson. Med.* **2005**, *54*, 28–33.

94 Ross R. Atherosclerosis: an inflammatory disease. *N. Engl. J. Med.* **1999**, *340*, 115–126.

95 Keaney JF Jr, Vita JA. The value of inflammation for predicting unstable angina. *N. Engl. J. Med.* **2002**, *347*, 55–57.

96 Moreno PR, Falk E, Palacios IF, Newell JB, Fuster V, Fallon JT. Macrophage infiltration in acute coronary syndromes. Implications for plaque rupture. *Circulation* **1994**, *90*, 775–778.

97 Schmitz SA, Coupland SE, Gust R, Wintherhalter S, Wagner S, Kresse M, Semmler W, Wolf KJ. Superparamagnetic iron-oxide-

enhanced MRI of atherosclerotic plaques in Watanabe hereditable hyperlipidemic rabbits. *Invest. Radiol.* **2000**, *35*, 460–471.

98 Ruehm SG, Corot C, Vogt P, Kolb S, Debatin JF. Magnetic resonance imaging of atherosclerotic plaque with ultrasmall superparamagnetic particles of iron oxide in hyperlipidemic rabbits. *Circulation* **2001**, *103*, 415–422.

99 Litovsky S, Madjid M, Zarrabi A, Casscells SW, Willerson JT, Naghavi M. Superparamagnetic iron oxide-based method for quantifying recruitment of monocytes to mouse atherosclerotic lesions *in vivo*. Enhancement by tissue necrosis factor-α, interleukin-1-β, and interferon-γ. *Circulation* **2003**, *107*, 1545–1549.

100 Yancy AD, Olzinski AR, Hu TCC, Lenhard SC, Aravindhan K, Gruver SM, Jacobs PM, Willette RN, Jucker BM. Differential uptake of ferumoxtran-10 and ferumoxytol, ultrasmall superparamagnetic iron oxide contrast agents in rabbits: critical determinants of atherosclerotic plaque labelling. *J. Magn. Reson. Imaging* **2005**, *21*, 432–442.

101 Schmitz SA, Taupitz M, Wagner S, Wolf KJ, Beyersdorff D, Hamm B. Magnetic resonance imaging of atherosclerotic plaques using superparamagnetic iron oxide particles. *J. Magn. Reson. Imaging* **2001**, *14*, 355–361.

102 Kooi ME, Cappendijk VC, Cleutjens KBJM, Kessels AGH, Kitslaar PJEHM, Borgers M, Frederik PM, Daemen MJAP, Van Engelshoven JMA. Accumulation of ultrasmall superparamagnetic particles of iron oxide in human atherosclerotic plaques can be detected *in vivo* magnetic resonance imaging. *Circulation* **2003**, *107*, 2453–2458.

103 Trivedi RA, U-King-Im JM, Graves MJ, Kirkpatrick PJ, Gillard JH. Noninvasive imaging of carotid plaque inflammation. *Neurology* **2004**, *63*, 187–188.

104 Trivedi RA, U-King-Im JM, Graves MJ, Cross JJ, Horsley J, Goddard MJ, Skepper JN, Quartey G, Warburton E, Joubert I, Wang L, Kirkpatrick PJ, Brown J, Gillard JH. *In vivo* detection of macrophages in human carotid atheroma: temporal dependence of ultrasmall superparamagnetic particles of iron oxide-enhanced MRI. *Stroke* **2004**, *35*, 1631–1635.

105 Arvin B, Neville LF, Barone FC, Feuerstein GZ. The role of inflammation and cytokines in brain injury. *Neurosci. Biobehav. Rev.* **1996**, *20*, 445–452.

106 Stoll G, Jander S, Schroeter M. Inflammation and glial response in ischemic brain lesions. *Prog. Neurobiol.* **1998**, *56*, 149–171.

107 Banati RB, Gehrmann J, Schubert P, Kreutzberg GW. Cytotoxicity of microglia. *Glia* **1993**, *7*, 111–118.

108 Rausch M, Sauter A, Fröhlich J, Neubacher U, Radü EW, Rudin M. Dynamic patterns of USPIO enhancement can be observed in macrophages after ischemic brain damage. *Magn. Reson. Med.* **2001**, *46*, 1018–1022.

109 Saleh A, Wiedermann D, Schroeter M, Jonkmanns C, Jander S, Hoehn M. Central nervous system inflammatory response after cerebral infarction as detected by magnetic resonance imaging. *NMR Biomed.* **2004**, *17*, 163–169.

110 Saleh A, Schroeter M, Jonkmanns C, Hartung HP, Mödder U, Jander S. *In vivo* MRI of brain inflammation in human ischemic stroke. *Brain* **2004**, *127*, 1670–1677.

111 Lamalle L, Kremer S, Troprès I, VSI and BV MRI of human brain. *Proc. Int. Soc. Mag. Reson. Med.* **2003**, *11*, 1271.

112 Varallyay P, Nesbit G, Muldoon LL, Nixon RR, Delashaw J, Cohen JI, Petrillo A, Rink D, Neuwelt EA. Comparison of two superparamagnetic viral-sized iron oxide particles ferumoxides and ferumoxtran-10 with a gadolinium chelate in imaging intracranial tumors. *Am. J. Neuroradiol.* **2002**, *23*, 510–519.

113 Calabresi PA. Diagnosis and management of multiple sclerosis.

Am. Fam. Physician **2004**, *70*, 1935–1944.

114 Dousset V, Ballarino L, Delalande C, Coussemacq M, Canioni P, Petry KG, Caillé JM. Comparison of ultrasmall particles of iron oxide (USPIO)-enhanced T2-weighted, conventional T2-weighted, and gadolinium-enhanced T1-weighted MR images in rats with experimental autoimmune encephalomyelitis. *Am. J. Neuroradiol.* **1999**, *20*, 223–227.

115 Xu S, Jordan E, Brocke S, Bulte JW, Quigley L, Tresser N, Ostuni JL, Yang Y, McFarland HF, Frank JA. Study of relapsing remitting experimental allergic encephalomyelitis SJL mouse model using MION-46L enhanced *in vivo* MRI: early histopathological correlation. *J. Neurosci. Res.* **1998**, *52*, 549–558.

116 Dousset V, Brochet B, Caillé JM, Petry KG. Enhancement of multiple sclerosis lesions with ultrasmall particle iron oxide: phase II study. *Proc. Int. Soc. Magn. Reson. Med.* **2001**, *9*, 261.

117 Firestein GS. Evolving concept of rheumatoid arthritis. *Nature* **2003**, *423*, 356–361.

118 Lutz AM, Seemayer C, Corot C, Gay RE, Goepfert K, Michel K, Marincek B, Gay S, Weishaupt D. Detection of synovial macrophages in an experimental rabbit model of antigen-induced arthritis: ultrasmall superparamagnetic iron oxide-enhanced MR imaging. *Radiology* **2004**, *233*, 149–157.

119 Kaim AH, Wischer T, O'Reilly T, Jundt G, Fröhlich J, von Schulthess GK, Allegrini PR. MR imaging with ultrasmall superparamagnetic iron oxide particles in experimental soft-tissue infection in rats. *Radiology* **2002**, *225*, 808–814.

120 Lutz AM, Weishaupt D, Persohn E, Goepfert K, Froehlich J, Sasse B, Gottschalk J, Marincek B, Kaim AH. Imaging of macrophages in soft-tissue infection in rats: relationship between ultrasmall superparamagnetic iron oxide dose and MR signal characteristics. *Radiology* **2005**, *234*, 765–775.

121 Hauger O, Delalande C, Trillaud H, Deminière C, Quesson B, Kahn H, Cambar J, Combe C, Grenier N. MR imaging of intrarenal macrophage infiltration in an experimental model of nephrotic syndrome. *Magn. Reson. Med.* **1999**, *41*, 156–162.

122 Hauger O, Delalande C, Deminière C, Fouqueray B, Ohayon C, Garcia S, Trillaud H, Combe C, Grenier N. Nephrotoxic nephritis and obstructive nephropathy: evaluation with MR imaging enhanced with ultrasmall superparamagnetic iron oxide. Preliminary findings in a rat model. *Radiology* **2000**, *217*, 819–826.

123 Strom TB, Carpenter CB. Immunobiology of kidney transplantation. In *The Kidney*, 4th edn, Brenner BM, Rector FC (Eds.). Saunders, Philadelphia, PA, **1991**, pp. 2336–2407.

124 Zhang Y, Dodd SJ, Hendrich KS, William M, Ho C. Magnetic resonance imaging detection of rat renal transplant rejection by monitoring macrophage infiltration. *Kidney Int.* **2000**, *58*, 1300–1310.

125 Hauger O, Delmas Y, Deminière C, Merville P, Combe C, Grenier N. Late Sinerem-enhanced MR imaging of renal diseases: a pilot study. *Eur. Radiol.* **2004**, *14 (Suppl. 2)*, 202 (abstr. B-349).

126 Yang D, Ye Q, Williams M, Sun Y, Hu TCC, Williams DS, Moura JMF, Ho C. USPIO-enhanced dynamic MRI: evaluation of normal and transplanted rat kidneys. *Magn. Reson. Med.* **2001**, *46*, 1152–1163.

127 Persson PB, Hansell P, Liss P. Pathophysiology of contrast medium-induced nephropathy. *Kidney Int.* **2005**, *68*, 14–22.

128 Laissy JP, Benderbous S, Idée JM, Chillon S, Beaufils H, Schouman-Claeys E. MR assessment of iodinated contrast medium-induced nephropathy in rats using ultrasmall particles of iron oxide. *J. Magn. Reson. Imaging* **1996**, *7*, 164–170.

129 Laissy JP, Idée JM, Loshkajian A, Benderbous S, Chillon S, Beaufils

H, Schouman-Claeys E. Reversibility of experimental acute renal failure in rats: assessment with USPIO-enhanced MR imaging. *J. Magn. Reson. Imaging* **2000**, *12*, 278–288.

130 Kanno S, Wu YJL, Lee PC, Dodd SJ, Williams M, Griffith BP, Ho C. Macrophage accumulation associated with rat cardiac allograft rejection detected by magnetic resonance imaging with ultrasmall superparamagnetic iron oxides particles. *Circulation* **2001**, *104*, 934–938.

131 Johansson L, Johnsson C, Penno E, Björnerud A, Ahlström H. Acute cardiac transplant rejection: detection and grading with MR imaging with a blood pool contrast agent. Experimental study in the rat. *Radiology* **2002**, *225*, 97–103.

132 Bulte JWM, Kraitchman DL. Monitoring cell therapy using iron oxide MR contrast agents. *Curr. Pharm. Biotechnol.* **2004**, *5*, 567–584.

133 Bulte JWM, Zhang SC, van Gelderen P, Herynek V, Jordan EK, Duncan ID, Frank JA. Neurotransplantation of magnetically-labeled oligodendrocyte progenitors: magnetic resonance tracking of cell migration and myelination. *Proc. Natl Acad. Sci. USA* **1999**, *96*, 15256–15261.

134 Frank JA, Miller BR, Arbab AS, Zywicke HA, Jordan EK, Lewis BK, Bryant LH, Jr, Bulte JWM. Clinically applicable labelling of mammalian and stem cells by combining superparamagnetic iron oxides and transfection agents. *Radiology* **2003**, *228*, 480–487.

135 Daldrup-Link HE, Rudelius M, Oostendorp RAJ, Settles M, Piontek G, Metz S, Rosenbrock H, Keller U, Heinzmann U, Rummeny EJ, Schlegel J, Link TM. Targeting of hematopoietic progenitor cells with MR contrast agents. *Radiology* **2003**, *228*, 760–767.

136 Kraitchmann DL, Heldman AW, Atalar E, Amado LC, Martin BJ, Pittenger MF, Hare JM, Bulte JWM. *In vivo* magnetic resonance imaging of mesenchymal stem cells in myocardial infarction. *Circulation* **2003**, *107*, 2290–2293.

137 Cahill KS, Gaidosh G, Huard J, Silver X, Byrne BJ, Walter GA. Noninvasive monitoring and tracking of muscle stem cell transplant. *Transplantation* **2004**, *78*, 1626–1633.

138 Bos C, Delmas Y, Desmoulière A, Solanilla A, Hauger O, Grosset C, Dubus I, Ivanovic Z, Rosenbaum J, Charbord P, Combe C, Bulte JWM, Moonen CTW, Ripoche J, Grenier N. *In vivo* MR imaging of intravascularly injected magnetically labeled stem cells in rat kidney and liver. *Radiology* **2004**, *233*, 781–789.

139 Kircher MF, Allport JR, Graves EE, Love V, Josephson L, Lichtman AH, Weissleder R. *In vivo* high resolution three-dimensional imaging of antigen-specific cytotoxic T-lymphocyte trafficking to tumors. *Cancer Res.* **2003**, *63*, 6838–6846.

140 Laghi A, Paolantonio P, Panebianco V, Miglio C, Iafrate F, Di Tondo U, Pasariello R. Decrease of signal intensity of myometrum and cervical stroma after ultrasmall superparamagnetic iron oxide (USPIO) particles administration. *Invest. Radiol.* **2004**, *39*, 666–670.

141 Lee HS, Kim EH, Shao H, Kwak BK. Synthesis of SPIO–chitosan microspheres for MRI-detectable embolotherapy. *J. Magn. Magn. Mater.* **2005**, *293*, 102–105.

3
Carbon Nanotube-based Vectors for Delivering Immunotherapeutics and Drugs

Alberto Bianco, Wei Wu, Giorgia Pastorin, Cédric Klumpp, Lara Lacerda, Charalambos D. Partidos, Kostas Kostarelos, and Maurizio Prato

3.1
Introduction

Administration of drugs is very often limited by problems of insolubility, inefficient distribution, lack of selectivity and side-effects raising health concerns. Currently, most of these problems are the subject of very intense studies, aiming to improve efficiency, availability and toxicity profiles. In addition, cell membranes that act as barriers can pose a problem in drug delivery by selectively allowing only certain structures to pass based on hydrophilicity:hydrophobicity ratios. Among the currently available delivery systems, which include liposomes, emulsions, polymers and microparticles [1–3], carbon nanotubes (CNTs) have recently gained high popularity as potential drug carriers, therapeutic agents and for applications in diagnosis [4–10].

CNTs possess a unique and fascinating one-dimensional nanostructure, which imparts intriguing properties to the nanomaterial, such as tremendous strength [11], high thermal conductivity [12] and amazing electronic properties ranging from metallic to semiconducting [13–16]. These all-carbon hollow graphitic tubes with high aspect and nanoscale diameter [17] can be classified by their structure into two main types: single-walled CNTs (SWNTs), which consist of a single layer of graphene sheet seamlessly rolled into a cylindrical tube, and multiwalled CNTs (MWNTs), which comprise multiple layers of concentric cylinders with a space of about 0.34 nm between the adjacent layers (Fig. 3.1) [18].

Several techniques, e.g. arc-discharge [19], laser ablation [20], chemical vapor deposition (CVD) [21] or the gas-phase catalytic process (HiPCO) [22], have been used to synthesize CNTs. However, up to now, the CNTs prepared by all currently known methods are mixtures of different tubes with a broad distribution in diameter and chirality, and often contaminated by impurities (mainly including amorphous carbon and catalyst particles). Various methods have been developed to purify CNTs, such as oxidation of contaminants [23–28], microfiltration [29], chromatographic procedures [30, 31] and microwave irradiation [32–34].

Nanotechnologies for the Life Sciences Vol. 10
Nanomaterials for Medical Diagnosis and Therapy. Edited by Challa S. S. R. Kumar

ISBN: 978-3-527-31390-7

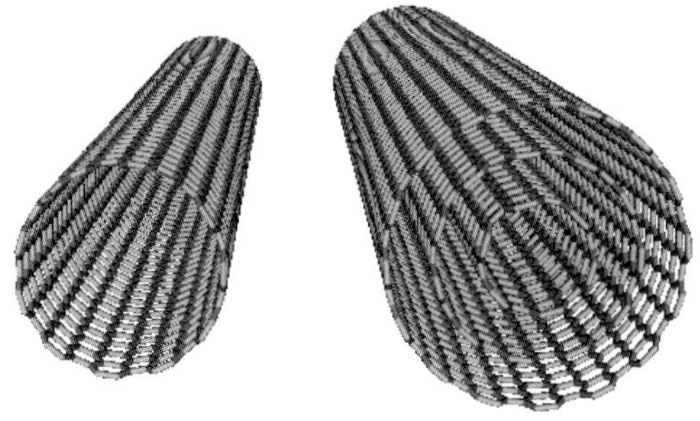

Figure 3.1. Molecular structures of defect-free SWNTs (left) and MWNTs (right) with open ends.

One important feature of CNTs is that this material is practically insoluble in both aqueous and polar/nonpolar organic solvents. Although this characteristic has hindered their chemical manipulation and potential applications in many fields, it has stimulated research in their chemical and physical functionalization.

A great effort has been invested in the search for new ways to chemically derivatize the CNTs. Although their tips are very reactive, similar to fullerenes, their sidewalls are much more inert toward chemical reagents. For this reason, there are not so many methods exhibiting general applicability.

Both covalent and noncovalent functionalization approaches are currently known that are very helpful in disentangling the CNT bundles, but which have different impacts on their electronic properties.

3.2 Chemical Functionalization of CNTs

3.2.1 Noncovalent Functionalization

The methods of functionalization of CNTs based on noncovalent interaction can be performed without destroying the intrinsic sp^2-hybridized structure of the nanotube sidewall, so that the original electronic structure and properties of CNTs can be preserved. Different kinds of noncovalent functionalization have been explored.

3.2.1.1 π–π Stacking Interactions

The noncovalent functionalization of CNTs could be achieved by π–π stacking interactions between conjugated molecules and the graphitic sidewall of CNTs. Compounds with the pyrene moiety, e.g. *N*-succinimidyl-1-pyrenebutanoate (Fig. 3.2), could be adsorbed irreversibly onto the surface of SWNTs through π–π interaction [35]. Furthermore, via the succinimidyl ester group on this bifunctional anchor,

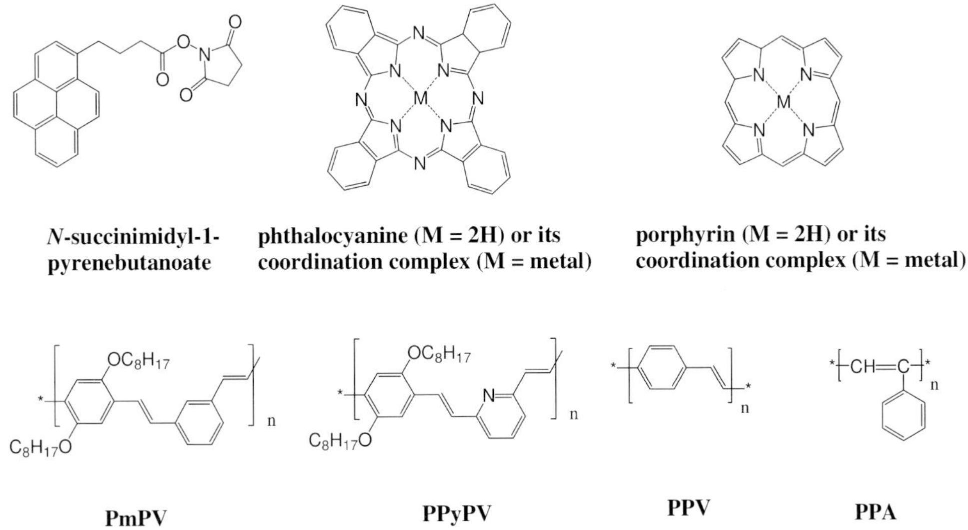

Figure 3.2. Typical molecules that can noncovalently modify CNTs via π–π stacking interaction.

various molecules with primary or secondary amines [such as ferritin, streptavidin (SA) or biotin–polyethyleneoxide-amine] were covalently attached to the activated pyrene by nucleophilic attack of the amino group [35]. Using a similar strategy, some other biomolecules (e.g. protein and DNA) [36–38] and gold nanoparticles [39] were also coupled to CNTs.

Through the π–π stacking interactions, other classes of molecules, including phthalocyanines [40–42], porphyrins [43–53] and their derivatives, have been immobilized onto the surface of CNTs (Fig. 3.2). It was demonstrated that this kind of composite could display photoinduced charge transfer from the dye molecules to CNTs [42, 45]. The selective interaction between the porphyrin derivative and CNTs was also discovered [46]. The use of Raman spectroscopy, near-infrared (NIR) absorption and buck conductivity has shown that porphyrin derivatives could be selectively adsorbed onto semiconducting nanotubes in a solubilized sample. This is a convenient method to separate the semiconductive CNTs from metallic CNTs.

Polymers with conjugated structures could also be coupled to CNTs by π–π forces (Fig. 3.2) [54–75]. The strong interaction between the conjugated polymer and the nanotube remarkably increased CNT dispersibilty [54, 61, 66–68]. Some conjugated polymers have been used to purify CNTs by efficient phase separation from the main impurity, consisting of amorphous graphitic shells [62, 64, 65]. In this way, amorphous carbon impurities tend to sediment out of solution, whereas the nanotubes stay in suspension. In addition, this kind of composite has potential applications in the optoelectronic field because of energy transfer from the excited conjugated polymer to the nanotubes [55–60, 63, 66, 69–75].

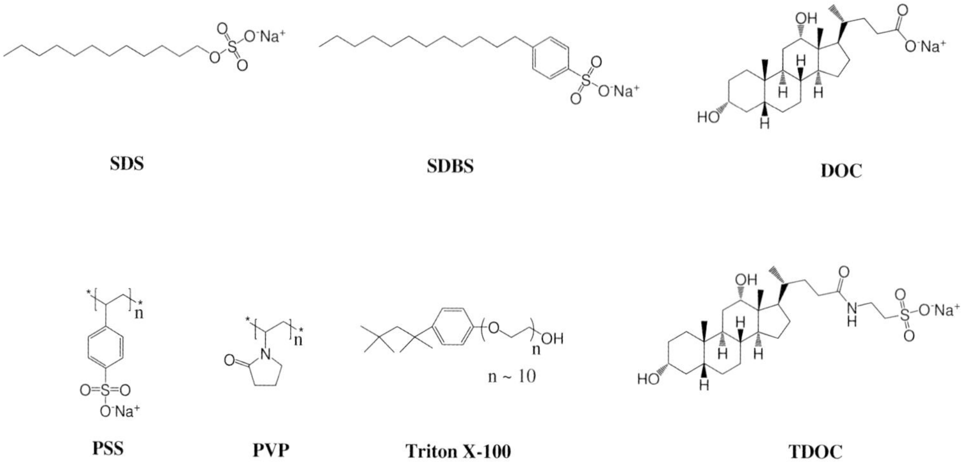

Figure 3.3. Typical molecules that can noncovalently modify CNTs via hydrophobic interactions.

3.2.1.2 **Hydrophobic Interactions**

Another method of noncovalent functionalization of CNTs involves association of CNTs with amphiphilic molecules through hydrophobic interactions in aqueous media. In this system, the amphiphilic molecules interact noncovalently with the aromatic surface of CNTs using their hydrophobic parts, while exposing the hydrophilic parts to the aqueous solution to minimize the hydrophobic interface between the nanotubes and their polar environment.

Through hydrophobic interactions, water-soluble polymers polyvinylpyrrolidone (PVP) and polystyrenesulfonate (PSS) (Fig. 3.3) wrapped helically around the surface of SWNTs helped to dissolve the nanotubes in water [76]. The association between the polymer and SWNTs, which is reversible by changing the solvent system, was very robust, independent of the presence of excess of polymer in solution and uniform along the surface of the nanotubes.

Surfactants were also conjugated to CNTs via hydrophobic interactions. So far, various anionic, nonionic and cationic surfactants have been used to suspend CNTs in aqueous medium (Fig. 3.3) [77–81]. Among them, bile salt surfactants such as deoxycholic acid (DOC) and taurodeoxycholic acid (TDOC) have been found to be very efficient in solubilizing SWNTs. This is because the aggregation was further prevented by the coulombic repulsion between surfactant-coated SWNTs [81]. In addition, if aromatic moieties in the hydrophobic part of the amphiphilic molecule were present, particularly strong interactions between the molecule and the CNTs could be established. This kind of aggregates forms additional π–π stacking between the aromatic part of the molecule and the graphitic sidewalls of CNTs while exposing the hydrophilic groups to the aqueous solution. As an example, sodium dodecylbenzene sulfonate (SDBS) presented an increased ability in suspending CNTs in water [80]. Some of the surfactants including sodium dodecyl sulfate (SDS), SDBS, DOC or TDOC were found to be very effective in dispersing individually SWNTs [79–81]. This provided the possibility to study the properties of individual SWNTs and further manipulate single tubes [82–86].

Hydrophobic interactions were also used to couple biomolecules to CNTs. In particular, an amphiphilic peptide was wrapped around the SWNT surface. The peptide was able to adopt an α-helical structure in aqueous solution, exposing the hydrophobic face of the helix to the nanotube surface [87, 88]. Atomic force microscopy (AFM), transmission electronic microscopy (TEM), and absorption and Raman spectroscopy proved that the SWNTs were debundled by the peptide. The peptide-coated nanotubes were assembled into macromolecular structure through charged peptide–peptide interactions between adjacent peptide-wrapped nanotubes. The size and morphology of the supermolecular structure can be regulated by controlling the factors that affect peptide–peptide interactions. It was also demonstrated that the ability to disperse individual SWNTs increased with increasing the amount of aromatic residues inside the peptide sequence [89]. In a similar manner, different proteins have also been adsorbed onto the surface of SWNTs and uptaken by mammalian cells (see Section 3.4) [90].

Another interesting approach involved the conjugation of single-stranded DNA with SWNTs resulting in helical wrapping around the surface of the tube exposing the hydrophilic sugar-phosphate backbone towards the exterior [91, 92]. Using this strategy, individually dispersed nanotubes in solution were obtained. CNT wrapping by single-stranded DNA was strongly dependent on the DNA sequence. Moreover, the dependence of the electrostatic properties of the DNA–CNT hybrid on the tube diameter and electronic properties enable nanotube separation by anion-exchange chromatography.

In addition to a direct interaction with CNTs, biomolecules have also been attached to SWNTs via amphiphilic molecules as a bifunctional linker. For instance, phospholipid molecules with phospholipid (PL)–poly(ethylene glycol) (PEG) chains and terminal amine (PL–PEG-NH_2) were noncovalently conjugated to SWNTs. PL alkyl chains were adsorbed to the surface of SWNTs via hydrophobic interactions while the PEG chain extended into the aqueous phase for SWNTs dispersion. After incorporation of a heterobifunctional crosslinker sulfosuccinimidyl 6-(3′-[2-pyridyldithio]propionamido)hexanoate (sulfo-LC-SPDP), the functionalized SWNTs (*f*-SWNTs) were coupled with DNA and RNA via disulfide linkage. The complexes were subsequently delivered to cells (see Section 3.7) [93].

3.2.2
Covalent Functionalization

The characteristics of CNTs such as low curvature, low solubility and bundling tendency make these carbon nanomaterials relatively inert to chemical treatment. So far, a number of routes to covalent functionalization of CNTs have been developed. According to the location of the functional groups, the strategies to covalently functionalize CNTs can be classified into two main types: (i) defect functionalization, and (ii) sidewall functionalization. The covalent functionalization of nanotubes is more robust and better controllable compared to functionalization based on non-covalent methods.

3.2.2.1 Defect Functionalization

CNTs synthesized by any available method are not free of defects. The intrinsic defects include five- or seven-membered rings called Stone–Wales defects, sp^3-hybridized defects and vacancies in the sp^2-hybridized six-membered ring carbon structure of the sidewall [94, 95]. A limited number of defects can be tolerated by CNTs without losing their macroscopic electronic and mechanical properties [96–98]. In addition, the tips of the tubes, forming a hemispherical fullerene, have stronger reactivity than the sidewalls because of their higher curvature [99, 100]. When treated with strong oxidizing agents such as nitric acid, $KMnO_4/H_2SO_4$, O_2, $K_2Cr_2O_7/H_2SO_4$ or OsO_4, CNTs could be opened and cut into short tubes. In the meantime defects were introduced around the CNT surface [28, 95, 100, 101]. Moreover, oxygenated functional groups such as carboxylic acid, ketone, alcohol and ester groups were generated by the oxidization process to the ends and the defect sites of the nanotubes [102]. These functional groups were very important to further functionalize CNTs. Sonication could also produce defects on the sidewall of CNTs that were eager for further chemical reactions [103–106].

Using the nanotube-bound carboxylic acid groups introduced by oxidization treatment, further functionalization was performed via amidation, esterification or the zwitterionic $COO^-NH_3^+$ formation. Before covalent modification, the carboxylic acids are often activated by thionyl chloride, carbodiimide [e.g. *N*-(3-dimethylaminopropyl)-*N*′-ethylcarbodiimide (EDC) or *N,N*′-dicyclohexylcarbodiimide (DCC)] or *N*-hydroxysuccinimide (NHS), to get highly reactive intermediate groups (Scheme 3.1). Esterification was achieved by the nucleophilic substitution reaction of nanotube carboxylate salt with alkyl halides [107]. The functionalization of CNTs via nanotube carboxylic acids, located at the ends or pre-existing defects of CNTs, preserved the essential features of the CNT electronic structure as well as the bulk properties of the material [102, 108].

The first shortened soluble SWNTs were obtained through carboxylic amidation using octadecylamine [102]. Since then, various lipophilic and hydrophilic dendrons have been attached to CNTs via amide or ester linkages, which significantly improved the solubility of CNTs in organic or aqueous solvents [109]. These groups could be subsequently removed under basic or acidic hydrolysis conditions [110]. In addition, following this functionalization process, CNT bundles were largely exfoliated into individual nanotubes [96]. This enabled further manipulation and investigation of the spectroscopic properties of individual SWNTs.

Via amidation or esterification, polymers like poly-propionyl-ethylenimine-*co*-ethylenimine (PPEI-EI), poly-*n*-vinylcarbazole (PVK-PS) and PEG were grafted to the surface of CNTs [111]. Another approach called "graft from" was developed to attach polymer to CNTs. The polymerization initiators were first covalently bound to CNTs and then the nanotube-based macroinitiators were exposed to monomers to accomplish the polymerization. In particular, polymer poly-*n*-butyl methacry-

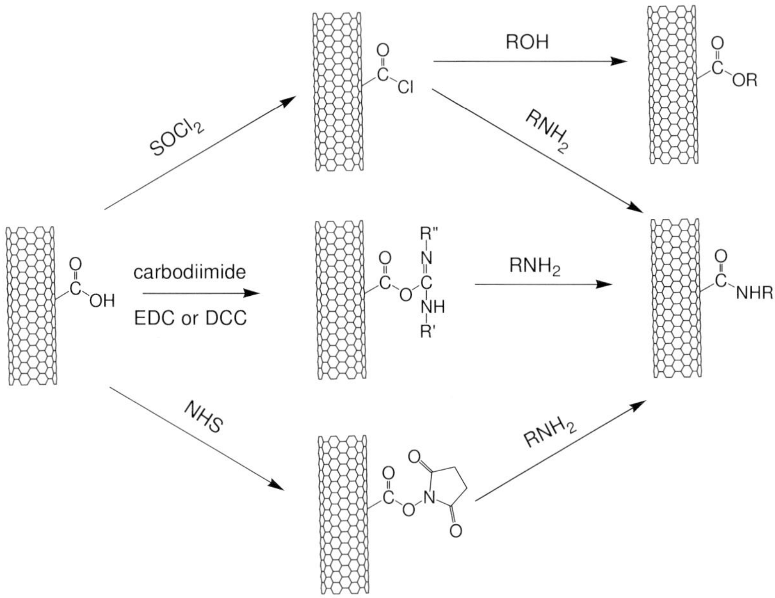

Scheme 3.1. Typical CNT carboxylic acid derivatization routes.

late (PnBMA), poly-methyl methacrylate (PMMA) and copolymer PMMA-*b*-poly-hydroxyethyl methacrylate (PHEMA) have been coupled to CNTs via atom transfer radical polymerization (ATRP) [112, 113].

Defect functionalization was used to link biological molecules to CNTs via stable covalent bonds. For example, *f*-SWNTs and *f*-MWNTs with bovine serum albumin (BSA) were synthesized via diimide-activated amidation at ambient condition. It was found that the protein bound to nanotubes remained active [114]. SA (a protein with potential clinical applications in anticancer therapy) was complexed to SWNTs prefunctionalized with biotin through EDC activated amidation [115]. Similarly, using the biotin–SA interaction, a biotinylated DNAzyme was covalently attached to MWNTs prefunctionalized with SA via amide linkage. The nanotube-bound DNAzymes displayed highly active and classical enzymatic behavior [116].

DNA was also bound to CNTs via amide linkage [117, 118]. DNA–CNT conjugates were hybridized with their complementary sequences and this hybridization was apparently reversible upon a denaturation process. The derived single-strand DNA–CNTs could be reused in a second-round of hybridization. In another case, DNA recognition was achieved by peptide nucleic acid (PNA) *f*-SWNTs, in which PNA was attached to SWNTs via NHS activated SWNTs [119].

3.2.2.2 **Sidewall Functionalization**

The sidewalls of CNTs have an aromatic, six-membered ring structure. So far, various kinds of reactions of the sidewall have been developed such as fluorination, radical addition, nucleophilic addition, electrophilic addition and cycloaddition [120]. There are two principal sources of molecular strain that affect the reactivity in nonplanar conjugated molecules: (i) pyramidalization of the conjugated carbon atom and (ii) π-orbital misalignment between adjacent pairs of conjugate carbon atoms. Unlike fullerene, in which the strain is primarily from pyramidalization, π-orbital misalignment is the main source of the strain for the sidewalls of CNTs. Since π-orbital misalignment, as well as pyramidalization, scales inversely with nanotube diameter, nanotubes with a smaller diameter display a higher chemical reactivity [99]. Differing from defect reactions, sidewall reactions disrupted the conjugated structure of CNTs, as monitored by Raman or absorption spectroscopy. In the Raman spectrum of pristine SWNTs, three main characteristic modes were disclosed: (i) the radial breathing (ω_r) below 350 cm^{-1}, (ii) the tangential (ω_t) mode at 1550–1600 cm^{-1} and (iii) the disorder (sp^3) mode at 1250–1450 cm^{-1}. The radial breathing mode was demonstrated to be in strong relationship with the diameter of the nanotube [121]. The relative intensity of the disorder mode was related to the amount of sp^3-hybridized carbon atoms in the SWNTs and thus provided direct information of the extent of sidewall functionalization, in which the carbons linked to functional groups were converted from sp^2-hybridized into sp^3-hybridized carbon [122]. The absorption spectrum reflected the sidewall covalent modification of SWNTs. The disruption of the conjugated structure caused by the reaction led to the loss of optical transitions between van Hove singularities in the electronic density of state (DOS) of CNTs, which was detected as the loss of the structure of the absorption spectrum [123].

3.2.2.2.1 **Fluorination** The fluorination of SWNTs was accomplished through the reaction of SWNTs with elemental fluorine at temperatures ranging from 150 to 600 °C [124]. By controlling the reaction conditions such as temperature and time, the stoichiometry could be regulated. In some cases, a stoichiometry of C_2F was obtained (see Scheme 3.3). The investigation of absorption and Raman spectra indicated the electronic perturbation of fluorinated SWNTs. The fluorination allowed exfoliation of SWNTs bundles into individual nanotubes and remarkably improved the solubility of SWNTs in tetrahydrofuran (THF), dimethylformamide (DMF) and various alcohols [125]. The C–F bonds were very sensitive to the treatment with hydrazine, which allowed almost complete recovery of the conductivity and the spectroscopic properties of the pristine SWNTs [124]. It was demonstrated that the Fermi energy level of fluorinated SWNTs, as well as the conduction band energy, were significantly shifted to lower values compared to those of the pristine SWNTs. This revealed that fluorinated CNTs were better electron acceptors than pristine nanotubes, and thus displayed higher chemical reactivity to strong nucleophilic reagents like Grignard, alkyllithium reagents and metal alkoxides (Scheme 3.2). The same result was reached by exploiting the eclipsing strain effect that weakened the C–F bonds in fluorinated CNTs relative to the C–F bond in alkyl fluorides [126, 127]. It was proposed that the substitution of fluorine by nucleophilic reagents proceeds via a concerted allylic displacement [126].

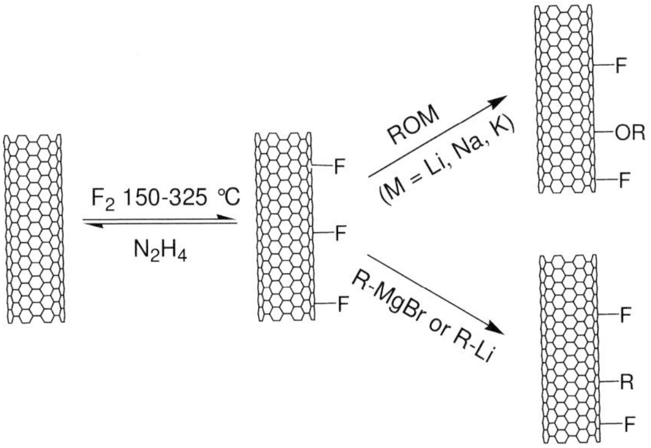

Scheme 3.2. Fluorination of CNTs and further modification routes.

3.2.2.2.2 **Radical Addition** The addition of radicals to SWNTs was carried out using different radical sources including perfluorinated alkyl radicals photoinduced from perfluoroalkyl iodide [128], aryl radicals generated by one-electron reduction of the diazonium salt [129–131], radicals produced by decomposition of benzoyl peroxide in the presence of alkyl iodides [132], or directly produced by decomposition of benzoyl or lauroyl peroxide [133].

The functionalization of SWNTs with diazonium reagents was achieved by three different methods: electrochemical reaction [119], thermochemical reaction in solvent [130] and using a solvent-free system [131] (Scheme 3.3). The resultant SWNTs displayed very high degree of functionalization. It was also demonstrated that metallic SWNTs showed higher reactivity in these types of reactions than semiconductive SWNTs, which would allow CNT separation [134].

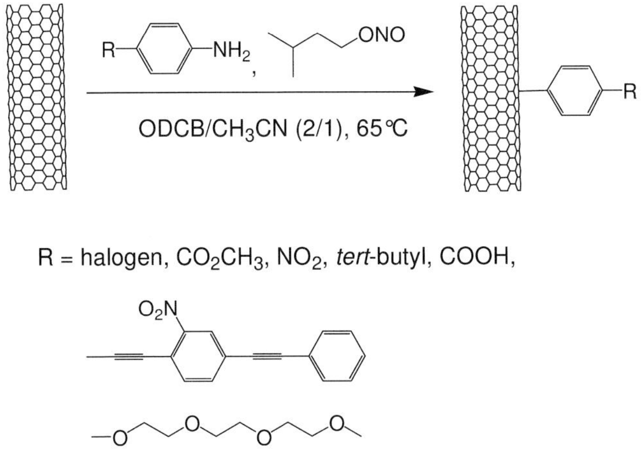

Scheme 3.3. Example of a strategy to functionalize SWNTs with diazonium compounds. ODCB = orthodichlorobenze.

3.2.2.2.3 **Nucleophilic and Electrophilic Addition** Due to the high electron affinity imparted by the curvature of sidewall [135], CNTs were reacted with strong nucleophilic reagents such as nucleophilic carbene [128], *sec*-butyllithium [136], polymeric carbanions [137] and Birch reduction reagents (lithium/1,2-diaminoethane [108] or lithium/ammonia [138]) to form various *f*-CNTs (Scheme 3.4).

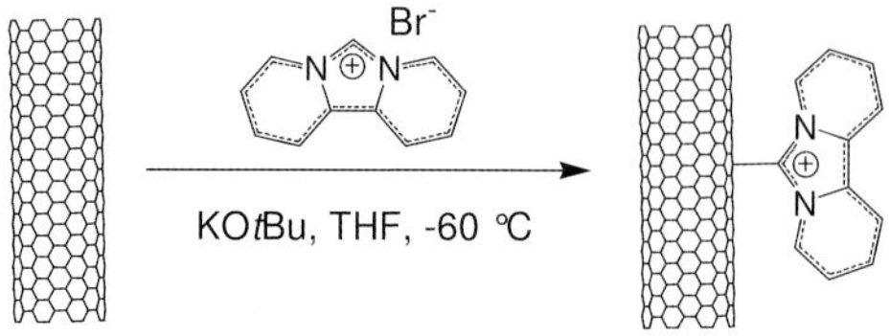

Scheme 3.4. Reaction of SWNTs with nucleophilic carbene.

In addition, the electrophilic addition was also achieved by the reaction of chloroform with the sidewall of CNTs in the presence of Lewis acid [139].

3.2.2.2.4 **Cycloaddition** Various cycloaddition reactions to CNTs have been developed, including [2 + 1] cycloaddition of dichlorocarbene [108], nitrenes [128] and bromomalonates under Bingel reaction conditions [140], [4 + 2] Diels–Alder cycloaddition of *o*-quinodimethane performed under microwave irradiation [141], [3 + 2] cycloaddition of azido groups under ultraviolet (UV) irradiation [142], and azomethine ylides [143]. The 1,3-dipolar addition of azomethine ylides is particularly versatile for the functionalization of CNTs [143–145]. This strategy is suitable for different types of CNTs (e.g. pristine and purified SWNTs or MWNTs), and involves the *in situ* generation of an azomethine ylide through the decarboxylation of an immonium salt derived from condensation of a α-amino acid and an aldehyde in the presence of CNTs. This afforded functionalization of CNTs with the 2-substituted pyrrolidine (Scheme 3.5).

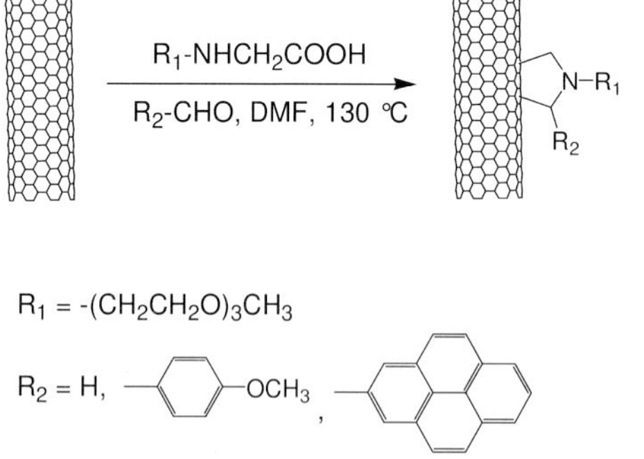

Scheme 3.5. 1,3-Dipolar cycloaddition reaction of azomethine ylides to SWNTs.

The CNTs modified by this method possessed a very high degree of functionalization and improved solubility in organic or aqueous solvents [143, 146]. The disruption of the aromatic structure of the sidewalls of the *f*-SWNTs was proven by absorption spectroscopy [143]. This functionalization technique was also used to purify CNTs [147]. Protected amino groups were introduced onto the surface of CNTs via 1,3-dipolar cycloaddition of azomethine ylides [143, 148]. For instance, *f*-CNTs with N-protected glycine were achieved using N-protected amino acid, which were subsequently used to link biomolecules (e.g. bioactive peptides) by fragment condensation or selective chemical ligation (see Section 3.5) [148, 149].

3.2.2.2.5 **Multifunctionalization of CNTs** The first multifunctionalization of CNTs was achieved using a vertically aligned MWNT membrane. One method involved the protection of the sidewalls of CNTs with polystyrene in the process of plasma oxidation that produced carboxylate derivatization. Under this process, aligned MWNT membranes functionalized with carboxylic acid groups at the terminal parts were obtained. Thereafter, bifunctional CNTs with thiol groups on one end and carboxylic groups on the other end were accomplished by floating on top of a 2-aminoethanethiol reaction solution one side of the oxidized CNTs membrane [150]. Another approach was carried out by floating directly one side of an aligned MWNTs membrane on 3′-azido-3′-deoxythymidine (AZT) solution in ethanol under UV irradiation and, after removal of absorbed AZT molecules by washing with ethanol, laying the unmodified side on the surface of a perfluorooctyl iodide solution in 1,1,2,2-tetrachloroethane (TEC) under UV irradiation. Thus, bifunctionalized MWNTs with AZT molecules and perfluorooctyl chains were obtained [151].

These two methods of CNT bifunctionalization are quite complicated and limited to aligned MWNTs. Using a different method, Wu and coworkers introduced an orthogonal protecting methodology into the chemical modification of nanotube to achieve the multifunctionalization of CNTs [152]. In particular, diaminotriethylene glycol chains mono-protected by phthalimide were linked to the carboxylic acids of oxidized MWNTs. In a second step, a suitable N-substituted glycine with a diaminotriethylene glycol chain mono-protected by *tert*-butyloxycarbonyl (Boc) was introduced via 1,3-dipolar cycloaddition (Scheme 3.6). Since the phthalimide is stable to harsh acidic conditions and orthogonal to the Boc, the selection and control of attachment of different molecules was possible [152]. In this case, CNTs containing both fluorescein and amphotericin B (AmB) were prepared, and bioactivity of the conjugates was studied (see Section 3.6) [152]. This method of bifunctionalization is general and suitable for different types of CNTs.

In summary, the functionalization and consequent applications of CNTs have been dramatically increased in the last few years. The chemical modification of CNTs cannot only endow these intriguing nanomaterials with various functions, but also extend their potential applications to different fields of research.

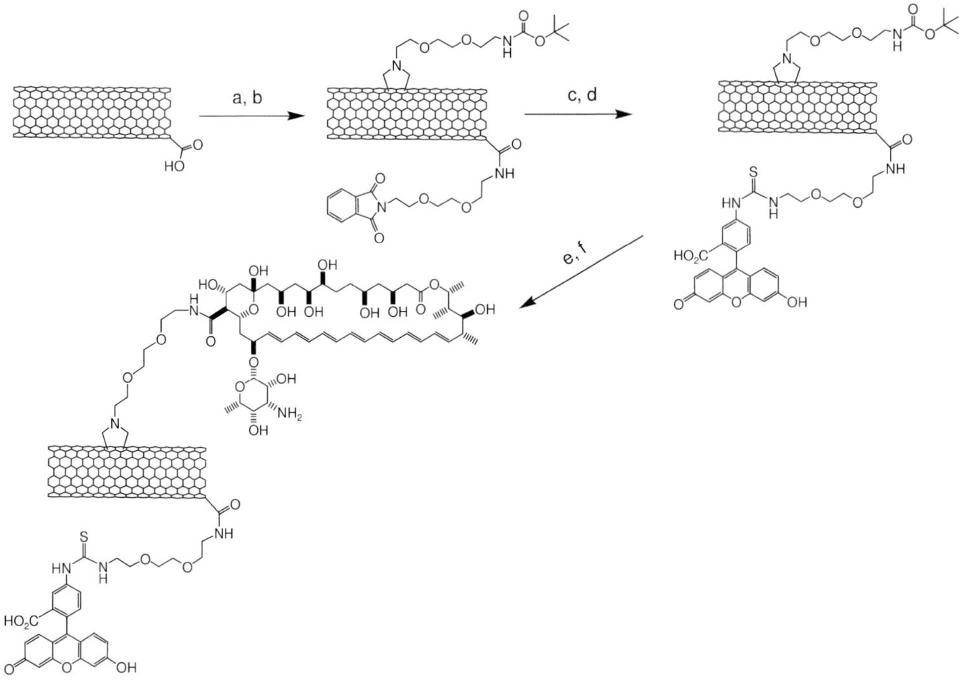

Scheme 3.6. One of the routes to the bifunctionalization of CNTs. (a) Neat $(COCl)_2$; Pht-N$(CH_2CH_2O)_2$-CH_2CH_2-NH_2, dry THF, reflux; (b) Boc-NH-$(CH_2CH_2O)_2$-CH_2CH_2-$NHCH_2COOH/(CH_2O)_n$, DMF, 125 °C; (c) hydrated NH_2-NH_2, EtOH, reflux; (d) FITC, DMF; (e) HCl 4 M in dioxane; (f) Fmoc-AmB, HOBt/EDC × HCl/DIPEA, DMF; 25% piperidine in DMF. Boc = *tert*-butyloxycarbonyl; DIPEA = diisopropylethyl-amine; FMOC = fluorenyl-methyloxycarbonyl; FITC = fluorescein isothiocyanate; HOBt = 1-hydroxybenzo-triazole; Pht = phthalimide.

3.3 CNTs in Diagnosis

A biosensor can be defined as the spatial combination of a biological recognition element and a transduction process into an electrical signal [153]. One of the most used recognition element, due to its high chemical specificity and inherent biocalalytic signal amplification, is an enzyme. Other elements like antibodies, nucleic acid and aptamers are also commonly incorporated into biosensing devices. An important issue in the elaboration of new sensors for application in living systems is to avoid invasive tools, which may cause trauma [154]. In this context, the development of electrical instrumentations has paved the way for miniaturization of noninvasive biosensors. This type of device requires an electronic conductor and a binding agent for recognition [155]. Due to their particular structure [156, 157], CNTs are very promising for the development of new alternative biosensors. The aromatic carbon structure of CNTs is characterized by a (m, n) lattice vector in the graphene plane. The two indices determine the diameter and chirality of the nanotubes. When $n = m$, the rolling process leads to an armchair tube with a metallic behavior. When $n - m = 3i$, where i is an integer, the nanotubes adopt a zigzag conformation and behave as semimetallic species. Finally, when $n - m \neq 3i$, the resulting nanotubes are chiral and semiconductor. Semiconducting nanotubes represent about two-thirds of the SWNTs, whereas metallic tubes represent about one-third. These properties could be exploited for the fabrication of new electronic devices containing CNTs such as field-effect transistors (FETs), nanoelectrode arrays (NEAs), nanoelectrode ensembles (NEEs) or screen-printed electrodes (SPEs) [158–167]. FET devices need semiconductor-type nanotubes. Currently, no method of production permits us to obtain a specific type of nanotubes. Some studies were carried out on the separation or selection of semiconducting and metallic nanotubes [168–171].

This section will describe the utilization of CNTs in FETs and in modified electrodes (NEAs, NEEs and SPEs). Initially, the methods of preparation of the devices will be addressed and then their applications in the field of biosensing will be illustrated.

3.3.1 CNTs in FETs

The FET is a transistor that relies on an electric field to control the shape and hence the conductivity of a channel in a semiconductor material. Basically, two metal electrodes called the source and drain are connected by the channel, and a third component (the gate) is separated from the channel by a thin insulator film. The latter, usually made up of Si, is replaced by semiconducting SWNTs in CNT-based FETs [158, 164]. There are two types of FETs: (i) p-type and (ii) n-type. If a negative charge is placed on the gate and the applied voltage exceeds a certain threshold, then a hole current flows in a p-type system. For a n-type FET, the current flows when a positive charge is present on the gate and the voltage exceeds the threshold [166].

3.3.1.1 Fabrication

As CNTs are still emerging in the field of electronic devices, the protocols for their preparation are not yet optimized. A CNT-based FET was built by positioning a semiconducting SWNT between two metal electrodes. Typically, as-prepared SWNTs were purified by acid treatment to remove metal particles, which can interfere with the electronic properties of the nanotubes. Other, more elaborate techniques to obtain highly pure nanotubes (up to 95% wt) consisted of heating as-grown HiPCO SWNTs in wet air in the presence of H_2O_2, followed by acid treatment, magnetic fractionation and vacuum annealing [168]. Subsequently, the nanotubes were dispersed in an organic (dichloromethane) or aqueous solution with a surfactant like sodium dodecyl benzene sulfonate [164, 168]. The suspension was then deposited on a substrate constituted of a degenerately doped, oxidized silicon

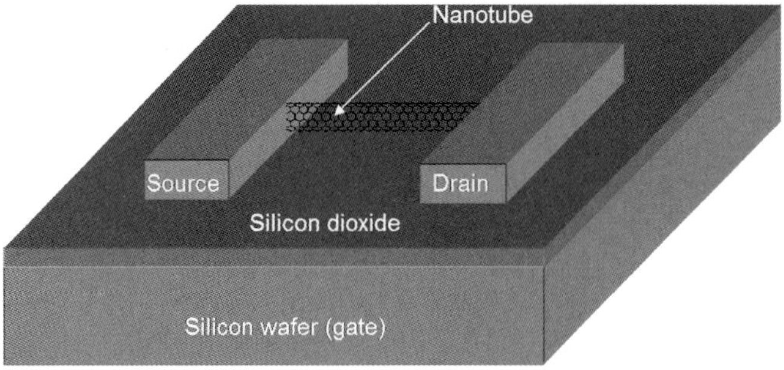

Figure 3.4. A typical CNT-based FET. The nanotube serves as a semiconductor between the source and the drain electrode. The silicon wafer in this case is used as a back gate.

wafer. An alternative technique consisted on the growth of SWNTs directly on the SiO_2/Si water by chemical vapor deposition (CVD) [36, 172–176]. Once the SWNTs were deposited, the electrodes were fabricated with electron beam lithography, followed by thermal evaporation and lift-off. The degenerately doped silicon was used as back gate electrode. At this stage, the channel was composed of a simple SWNTs or a small bundle with properties ranging from semiconducting to metallic behavior (Fig. 3.4). To select only semiconducting SWNTs, a source-drain current I was applied at different bias voltage V_b and gate voltage V_g. Typically, the I–V_g curve at low voltage bias shows a low source–drain resistance and almost no gate response for metallic nanotubes [168]. These types of CNT FET devices behave as p-type FETs with holes as dominant carriers. However, by using a network of SWNTs between the drain and the source, the network exhibited a semiconductor-like conductance as semiconducting SWNTs represented about two-thirds of the tubes [176]. Efforts have been made to improve them, thus now they can be built with a g_m transconductance of 2300 μS μm^{-1} whereas a g_m of 650 μS μm^{-1} was obtained for the same device based on silicon. Moreover, the parasitic contact resistance changed from more than 1 to 100 kΩ or above [166]. In addition, a method to select semiconducting SWNTs by current-induced electrical breakdown was developed. This technique permitted a direct current-induced oxidation only at the metallic SWNT component of the CNT bundle by previously depleting semiconducting SWNTs with the gate [177].

Even at this early stage of development, CNT-based FETs have been shown to outperform the corresponding Si-based devices. Their applications in sensing can therefore offer considerable improvements.

3.3.1.2 FET Biosensors

CNTs have already been successfully employed for sensing chemical species. In fact, molecules were adsorbed onto the surface of nanotubes. The fringing electric field radiating from the CNT surface polarized the molecules, increasing the capacity of the system. Different chemical vapors including NO_2 and NH_3, and a wide range of chemicals were detected [35, 160, 178–181]. A more sophisticated system based on a single-strand DNA-SWNT-FET was designed. The source–drain current was a function of the chemical environment and was modulated by the DNA sequence. In fact, depending on the DNA sequence covering the nanotube, the response for a same gas can be different in both sign and magnitude. Thus, the selection of a DNA sequence can enhance the detection of a specific gas and can serve for the design of "molecular noses" able to detect one molecule in a strong and variable background. The sensor had a rapid response and was also self-regenerating as it could undergo 50 gas exposure cycles [174].

In the field of biosensing, CNT-based FETs appeared as promising devices. Glucose biosensors are particularly requested. In industrialized countries, about 4% of the population is prone to diabetes. Thus, the selective determination of blood glucose is of crucial importance. *In vivo* monitoring requires a biosensor with long-term stability, selectivity and sensitivity in the millimolar range. Usually, the sensor for this type of application requires to couple the enzyme glucose oxidase to the electrochemical transducer. In the case of a CNT-based FET, it was possible to link noncovalently the enzyme via a pyrene moiety [35]. 1-Pyrenebutanoic acid succinimidyl ester was adsorbed onto the nanotube surface by strong van der Waals interactions. The enzyme was subsequently reacted with the active ester, thus forming a covalent linkage. The quantity of enzyme deposited on the CNT support was about one enzyme molecule every 12 nm of nanotube. Such FET allowed the detection of pH changes down to 0.1, by measuring the difference of conductance. Similarly, the CNT sensor could detect the activity of the enzyme in the presence of glucose down to 0.03 mM [36]. This technique was also applied to the recognition of proteins by using biomimetic sensors. One example concerned the sensing of thrombin via an aptamer [172]. An aptamer is an artificial oligonucleotide that can bind any kind of entity (e.g. metal ions, small organic molecules, proteins and/or cells). The affinity, selectivity and specificity are equal or superior to those of antibodies. Practically, the immobilization of thrombin aptamer was achieved by first covering the nanotube in the FET with carbodiimidazole (CDI)-Tween. Tween possess a hydrophobic part, which bound noncovalently to the tube, while the CDI moiety allowed covalent fixation of the aptamer. The measurement of the conductance permitted the detection of thrombin in the millimolar range. The selectivity appeared very high in comparison to elastase. Elastase is another serine protease with an isoelectric point (p*I*) and molecular weight similar to thrombin. However, no changes in the conductance were observed in its presence. Although the specificity and selectivity could be very high, the mechanism of electrical conductance changes is still not well understood. Dai and coworkers fabricated three different types of devices to better comprehend this phenomenon [175]. The first device consisted of a system with unmodified CNTs and Pd/Au electrodes. The second had a methoxy(PEG)thiol covering the metal electrodes to block nonspecific protein adsorption. The third tool was modified at the electrode and the nanotube was coated with Tween 20. The conductance measurements were performed in the presence of different proteins including BSA, human serum albumin (HAS), human chorionic gonadotropin (hCG), α-hCG, human immunoglobulin G (hIgG) and avidin. Unspecific binding led to a decrease of conductance on the first device, a change was detected only for avidin on the second and any change at all was observed on the third. All the proteins used have a p*I* around 5–7, meaning that at physiological pH they are neutral or slightly charged. Avidin was an exception, because its p*I* is between 10 and 11, highlighting the importance of the positive charges. The advanced hypothesis for the mechanism of conductance modifications was that the variation originated from the metal–tube contact. These p-type devices always exhibit a decrease upon protein adsorption. This behavior was similar to a reduction of the work function of a metal. In the case of Pd electrodes, the Schottky barrier to the valence band of the nanotubes is mainly zero. The biomolecular adsorption increased this barrier. However, in the case of avidin, the charges on the CNT surface exerted gating effects or charge transfer causing variations in the electrical conductance.

The CNT-based FETs have also been used in an antibody-based sensor [175]. For example, the hCG–α-hCG antigen–antibody system is currently used for clinical pregnancy tests. The hCG protein could be adsorbed and detected onto the nanotube FET. A signal was observed upon the addition of α-hCG. This biosensor was capable of detecting species in the nanomolar range. The same comparison was done by using antibody-specific binding onto the tubes [176]. CNTs were first covered by Tween. Then U1A RNA splicing factor was linked to the Tween after activation with 1,1-carbonydiimidazole. U1A is a prominent autoantigen target in systemic lupus erythematosus. The measurements revealed the binding of the monoclonal antibody 10E3, which recognizes U1A specifically, at a concentration of 1 nM or below. CNT-based FETs were also functionalized with hemagglutinins (HAs) [173]. Instead of binding the proteins directly to the nanotubes, they were attached on the reverse side of the silicon wafer (Fig. 3.5). The silicon wafer was oxidized with H_2SO_4 for the fixation of a dithiothreitol linker. Next, the introduction of a maleimide linker permitted the coupling of HA. The $I–V_g$ curves measured in the presence of various concentrations of an antibody anti-HA showed a detection limit of approximately of 5×10^{-8} mg mL^{-1}. Comparing these results to the same experiment with an enzyme-linked immunoadsorbent assay (ELISA), the FET increased the limit of detection by three orders of magnitude.

Therefore, the preliminary results on CNT-based FETs displayed an increase in the sensitivity as well as better detection limits. The great advantage of these new FETs stems from their small size, because miniaturization is an important parameter for the development of biosensors able to work at the single-cell level.

3.3.2
CNT-based Electrodes

The construction of nanoelectrodes is a great challenge to create miniaturized sensors. Reducing the size will enable us to detect species in microenvironments with high sensitivity. Thus, the utilization of nanomaterials is highly recommended. CNTs can be considered ideal candidates.

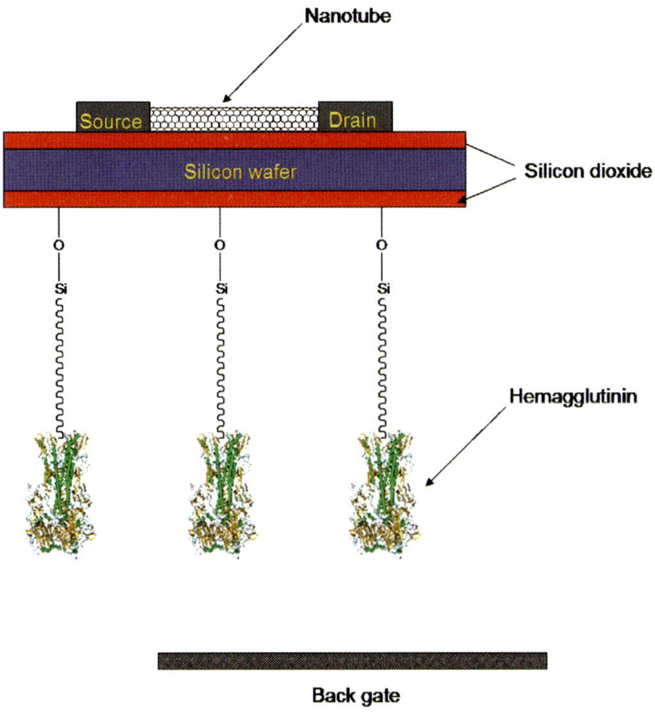

Figure 3.5. CNT-based FET functionalized on its reverse side. The silicon wafer is oxidized on the reverse side to allow the linkage with HA. The current is measured in air by applying a voltage to the back gate facing the reverse side.

3.3.2.1 **Fabrication**

Several techniques were used to prepare CNT-modified electrodes. One approach consisted on the covalent linkage of oxidized nanotubes to a metal electrode (usually Au) [182, 183]. The purification of nanotubes by acid treatment shortened the nanotubes leading to free carboxylic functions mainly at the tips. An Au electrode was functionalized with a mixture of cysteamine and 2-thioethanol. The CNT coupling reaction was performed in the presence of an activator of the carboxylic groups (EDC or DCC). 2-Thioethanol was used to avoid nonspecific adsorption of the nanotubes onto the electrode surface as well as to prevent accumulation of the nanotubes on it. The obtained CNT array was further functionalized with any biological species to finalize the elaboration of the electrode (Fig. 3.6).

Another technique was based on the deposition of a metal film (usually Pt or Cr) on a Si wafer to serve as an electrical contact for the nanotubes. Then, a Ni catalyst was deposited on the top of the metal film and the nanotubes were grown by CVD [165, 184]. The forest-like vertically aligned nanotube array was encapsulated by a dielectric film (SiO_2 or Epon 828 epoxy-based polymer), dramatically increasing the mechanical strength of the nanotube array, so that a chemical mechanical polish-

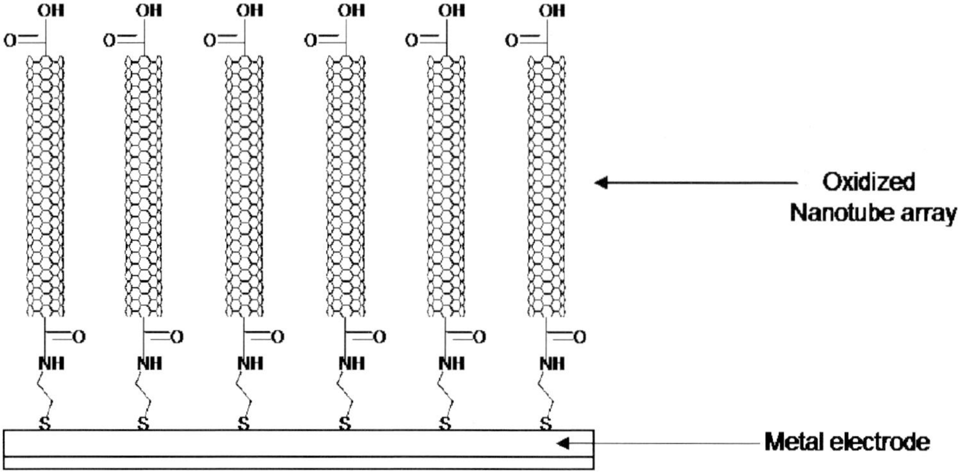

Figure 3.6. Nanoelectrode made of CNT arrays. The CNTs are disposed in a forest-like structure. The carboxylic groups on their tips are not hindered and can be easily functionalized.

ing process could be applied. This treatment oxidized the exposed end of the tubes and allowed control of the quantity of available nanotubes. Again, the nanotubes were ready to be further functionalized to create the nanoelectrode sensor (Fig. 3.7). A third approach to fabricate the electrodes was based on the utilization of the SPE technique [185, 186]. The working and the reference electrodes were made of carbon paste. Three masks were used to form: (i) sliver conducting lead wires, (ii) the carbon film for electrochemical reactions and (iii) the insulating film. In the reaction compartment, the carbon paste film was modified by CNTs. Oxidized CNTs were dropped with a solution of *N*-cyclohexyl-*N′*-(*β*-[*N*-methylmorpholino]ethyl)carbodiimide *p*-toluenesulfonate (CMC) to afford a hydrophilic polymer layer after drying in hot air. Alternatively, oxidized CNTs were dispersed in DMF and then incubated with EDC and NHS to be activated for the coupling of the bioactive molecule.

3.3.2.2 **Nanoelectrode Biosensors**

As mentioned for CNT-based FETs, the environment around the tubes changes their conductance. The measurement of the current will give direct information of the medium. A modified glassy carbon electrode was constructed to detect hydrogen peroxide. Nanotubes were first suspended in Nafion, which possess ion-exchange, discriminative and biocompatibility properties [187]. The suspension was then simply deposited onto the electrode. In this case, cyclic voltammograms displayed oxidation and reduction currents, whereas in comparison no redox activity was observed for a simple glassy carbon electrode. Nevertheless, the preparation of biosensor required the immobilization of a biological entity. This can be done by linking the molecule to the free carboxylic groups of the nanotube tips. To control

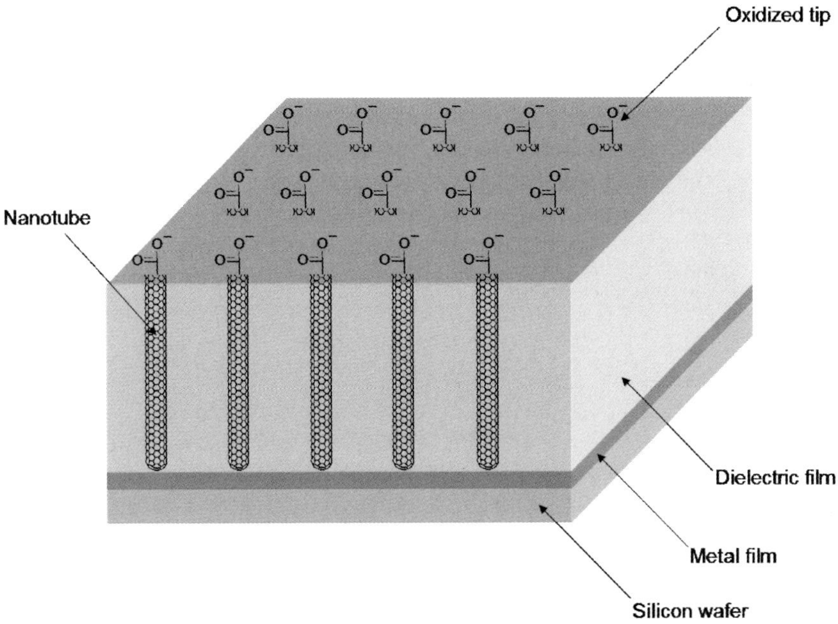

Figure 3.7. A nanoelectrode ensemble. The nanotubes are grown directly on the metal film via a catalyst (usually nickel). After deposition of the dielectric film, the number of nanotubes tips present on the surface can be selected by polishing. A weak polishing lets only the longest tubes appear with a low-density nanoelectrode array.

the specificity of the binding location, it is crucial to avoid any nonspecific absorption. Some reports described the interaction of proteins with nanotubes [188, 189]. For example, SA strongly bound to nanotubes [188]. Hence, the protection of the sidewall of the tube can be performed by wrapping a polymer like Triton X co-adsorbed with PEG [189]. This provided an efficient barrier against protein adsorptions. As a consequence, specific immobilization of glucose oxidase at one tip of the nanotube was achieved via reconstitution of the apo-flavoenzyme glucose oxidase with the flavin adenine dinucleotide (FAD) cofactor [183]. The free amine of the FAD was coupled to the carboxylic end by activation with EDC. After addition of the apo-glucose oxidase, the glucose enzyme was reconstituted at the top of the tubes. The turnover rate of electrons transferred to the electrodes was 6-fold higher than for the active site of the glucose oxidase to its natural O_2 electron acceptor. By controlling the length of the tubes in the array, the measurements of the current revealed that the electrons could be transported along distances greater than 150 nm. Evidently, a shorter length enhances the electrocatalytic current. Another method used the nanoelectrode ensembles where the carboxylic end-groups of the nanotubes were directly coupled to the glucose oxidase [184]. This glucose sensor showed high selectivity towards the substrate. Indeed, a negligible signal was observed for ascorbic, uric acid and acetaminophen. The nanoelectrode gave a linear response up to 30 mM glucose. For practical use, the required linear response is 15 mM. The detection limit of the system was 0.08 mM. These types of sensors could be extended to other enzymes, like microperoxidase MP-11 [182].

The utilization of nanotubes also permitted the development of nucleic acid sensors [165, 185]. The free carboxylic functions on the carbon nanoelectrode were used to covalently link different 5′-amine modified oligonucleotides. In this manner, the oxidation of guanine bases could be monitored to detect DNA hybridization. Several ways were explored to construct this type of sensor. Initially, the sensors exploited the utilization of oligonucleotide probes in which guanines were replaced by nonelectroactive inosines to eliminate the redox background [165]. The complementary DNA sequence was instead modified with a 10-base polyguanine at the 3′ position. However, the background noise remained high because of the low oxidative current resulting from the small number of guanines. To circumvent this problem, a $Ru(bpy)_2{}^{3+}$ mediator was introduced to transfer the electrons from the base to the electrode. Polymerase chain reaction (PCR) amplicons were then detected. An improvement of at least 30 times was obtained in comparison to the use of the same kind of technique with a silane-modified electrode. In a similar approach, hybridization was observed with the single-strand binding (SSB) protein, which plays an important role in DNA replication [185]. The SSB protein binds specifically to the single-strand DNA, while it has almost no affinity toward double-strand DNA. The protein sequence comprises four tyrosines and four tryptophans. The electrochemical oxidation of these residues was measured when the protein was immobilized onto the electrode. Then, specific detection of single-strand DNA in the medium was monitored by signal changes upon binding. At this stage of development, the performances of the biosensor remained constant for 1 week, but decreased 10-fold after 1 month and vanished after 2 months. A third technique of fabrication was applied to carbon nanoelectrodes for monitoring total cholesterol in blood [186]. Cholesterol oxidase, peroxidase, potassium ferrocyanide and threhalose dissolved in a buffer were deposited onto the reaction area of the electrode. Then, a hydrophilic polymer was applied to coat the rest of the electrode. Finally, cholesterol esterase, threhalose and Triton X in a phosphate buffer were deposited. The enzymatic cascade led to the formation of hydrogen peroxide, which was reduced by the ferrocyanide. The resulting current was recorded at various concentrations of cholesterol. While a nonlinear relationship was obtained between the cholesterol concentration and the current response for an unmodified electrode, an almost linear response was observed for a CNT-modified electrode. Moreover, the CNTs provided almost double the sensitivity, an acceptable repeatability over three consecutive assays, no interference effect from ascorbic and uric acids, and a stability at room temperature over 2 months.

In summary, CNTs are endowed with appropriate characteristics for the elaboration of biosensors. They possess high electronic conductivity and nanometric size. Miniaturization is an important parameter in the conception of more efficient sensors, which could be used to control biochemicals at the single-cell level. The current performance of nanotube-based biosensors has already overtaken the other sensors, but optimization still needs to be reached. Glucose biosensors are very

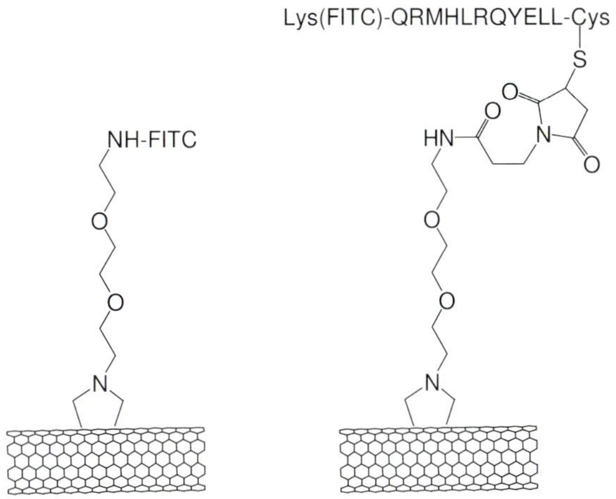

Figure 3.8. Molecular structure of FITC– (left) and fluorescent peptide–CNT (right) conjugates.

promising. However, numerous other oxidases exist and can be employed for the design of novel CNT-based biosensors. A bright future awaits these new sensors for pharmaceutical and clinical use.

3.4 CNT Cell Uptake

CNTs started to develop as new drug delivery systems because of their capacity to penetrate cell membranes and distribute into the cytoplasm and/or the nucleus.

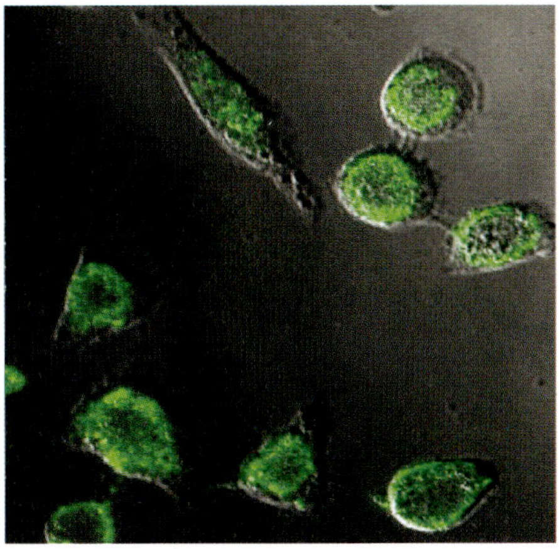

Figure 3.9. Confocal image of HeLa cells incubated with the fluorescent peptide–CNT conjugate.

This behavior was observed for the first time in 2004 by Pantarotto and coworkers [190]. The amino groups of *f*-CNTs were coupled either to fluorescein isothiocyanate (FITC) or to a peptide bearing FITC on the side-chain of a lysine (Fig. 3.8).

Subsequently, fibroblasts were incubated with the fluorescent nanotubes. It was found that these tubes were easily internalized by the cells and could be detected in the cytoplasm and the nucleus using epifluorescence and confocal microscopy [190]. This penetrating capacity was also observed in other types of cells (Fig. 3.9).

The mechanism of uptake of this type of *f*-CNTs was energy independent and nonendocytotic. Indeed, the incubation of the fluorescent tubes with different types of cells in the presence of sodium azide or 2,4-dinitrophenol, well-known endocytosis inhibitors, did not block the penetration capacity of the tubes. The reduction of the temperature of incubation from 37 to 4 °C again did not affect cell uptake to a significant extent.

When the CNTs were devoid of the fluorescent moiety, they could be detected in the cells using transmission electron microscopy (TEM) [191]. Ammonium *f*-CNTs were incubated with HeLa cells. After washing, staining and fixing, the cells were embedded into a polymer that was cut into thin slices of 90 nm thicknesses using a diamond microtome. Each slice was deposited on a TEM grid and observed under the microscope. Functionalized nanotubes were visible in the cytoplasm and the nucleus. The tubes were also identified at the level of the cellular membrane in the process of crossing this barrier [191]. The shape of the tube was elongated, suggesting a behavior as a nanoneedle, capable of piercing the lipid bilayer of the membrane without provoking cell death. This mechanism, which can be defined as nanopenetration, was observed by Cai and coworkers, who developed an efficient molecular delivery technique called nanotube spearing [192]. In this case, CNTs filled with magnetic particles were cultured with MCF-7 cells. Under the action of a magnetic field, the suspended tubes were put in rotation to spear the cells. A second static magnetic field was applied under the plate where the cells were grown to pull the tubes through the cell membrane into the cytoplasm. Scanning electron microscopy showed the nanotubes crossing the cell membrane like tiny needles.

NIR fluorescence microscopy could be also used to detect CNTs in the cells [193]. Macrophages were able to phagocyte pristine CNTs without apparent toxic effects. Subsequently, the tubes were tracked into the cells by irradiation at 1100 nm and recovery of a fluorescence signal. This technique seems very promising since it could be extended to the visualization of CNTs in the tissue and the organs. However, only non-*f*-CNTs were used in this study and concerns are emerging about their toxicity once injected into a body (see Section 3.8).

An alternative pathway of penetration of CNTs into the cells was reported by Dai and coworkers. Oxidized CNTs were initially functionalized with biotin and then complexed to a fluorescent SA [115]. The protein–nanotube conjugates were taken up in an endocytosis-mediated mechanism, as they were localized into the endosomes. This behavior was also confirmed by complexing different proteins or nucleic acids to the nanotubes via noncovalent interactions [90, 194]. HeLa and HL-60 cell lines were treated with fluorescent BSA or SA, and a fluorescent 15-mer oligonucleotide at low temperature and in a adenosine triphosphate (ATP)-depleted environment [194]. Preincubation of the cells with sodium azide or cell culture performed at 4 °C clearly influenced nanotube uptake. In addition, it has been demonstrated that the endocytosis was clathrin dependent. To assess the role of clathrin, experiments were carried out in the presence of sucrose and potassium-depleted medium to disrupt the clathrin-coated vesicles. Under these conditions, the level of nanotube cellular uptake was drastically reduced. In parallel, it has also been demonstrated that the nanotubes were not internalized through the caveolae or lipid-raft pathway. In this case the cells were treated with filipin and nystatin, known to perturb the cholesterol distribution on the cell membrane, which is implicated in the lipid-raft mechanism. The two drugs did not hamper the uptake of the CNTs. Therefore, it could be concluded that *f*-CNTs complexed to proteins and nucleic acids penetrate following a clathrin-dependent endocytotoxic process. Elucidation of the different mechanism of cellular entry is crucial for the development of CNTs as delivery system for therapeutic molecules.

3.5
CNTs as Delivery Devices for Antigens and Adjuvants

The development of new delivery systems for the successful and effective administration of vaccines and immunotherapeutics still remains a great challenge. The listing of "delivery" among the top 10 biotechnologies required for improving global health has recently reinforced this view [195]. Among the novel delivery options, CNTs have emerged as a promising option for biomedical applications. This is because CNTs can enter into the cells and can be functionalized (see Section 3.4) [148, 190]. The later property makes them soluble, nontoxic and permits modification of their surface [7]. Moreover, these molecules in the nanometer size range offer the control that modern drug delivery and targeting demands – control of the chemical nature of the carrier, control of the surface and, important in targeting, control of dimensions. CNTs can serve as vaccine delivery and adjuvant vehicles by virtue of their nanoparticulate nature. The hydrophobic nature of CNTs contributes to vaccine delivery capability by facilitating the interaction of CNTs with antigens or immunostimulatory molecules and uptake of the vaccine particles by immunocompetent cells.

3.5.1
Interaction of *f*-CNTs with CpG Motifs and Potentiation of their Immunostimulatory Activity

Immune responses to vaccine antigens are normally enhanced by immunostimulants called adjuvants. Recently, synthetic oligodeoxynucleotides (ODN) containing immunostimulatory CpG motifs (ODN CpG) have been considered as candidate adjuvants for vaccines or immunomodulators for therapeutic applications against tumors, allergy or to combat bioterrorist threats [196–199]. CpG motifs are unmethylated sequences that derive from bacterial DNA. The activation of the immune system by CpG motifs is a highly evolved defense mechanism, whose actual aim is to detect the microbial nucleic acid [200]. This can be achieved through the Toll-like receptor 9 [201], which belongs to the Toll family of pattern recognition receptors, conserved during the evolution in species from insects to humans [202]. CpG motifs induce B cell proliferation, antibody secretion and activate antigen-presenting cells (APCs) to express costimulatory molecules and secrete cytokines including, interleukin (IL)-12 and tumor necrosis factor (TNF)-α [200, 203]. In particular, the increased production of IL-12 promotes interferon (IFN)-γ production by natural killer (NK) cells and T cells, and enhances the antigen-specific T cell proliferation and differentiation of naive T cells towards the T helper (T_h) 1 phenotype [200, 203]. The triggering of the Toll-like receptor 9 by the ODN CpG is a critical event for the activation of innate immune system [203]. This requires the entry of ODN CpG into the cell for recognition by its receptor, which is expressed in endosomal compartments. Despite the potent immunostimulatory properties of ODN CpGs, their effect is short-lived because of their low uptake by the cells. In order to increase their biological properties, delivery of CpG using CNTs was explored. Therefore, ODN CpGs were first complexed with *f*-CNTs and their interaction analyzed [204], and then the immunostimulatory properties of the complexes were tested *in vitro* [204].

Cationic CNTs lend themselves as vectors for delivery because of their ability to form complexes with ODN CpG. Surface plasmon resonance (SPR) help in the understanding of the interaction that occurred between a *f*-CNT and ODN CpG to form complexes in real time, and gave an insight of how these molecules were bound [204]. Three types of *f*-CNTs were selected in the first series of experiments (Fig. 3.10).

Each *f*-CNT was attached onto the sensor chip by forming a stable amide bond between the amino groups on the tubes and the carboxylic functions on the chip's carboxylated dextran matrix, activated in turn with EDC and NHS. Following attachment, the increase in mass due to the interaction of *f*-CNTs with the ODN CpG 1668 present in the fluid phase was measured using the Biacore 3000 system.

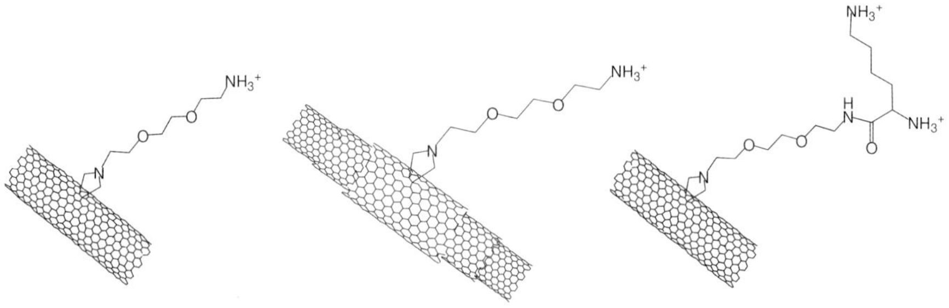

Figure 3.10. Molecular structures of ammonium *f*-CNTs for ODN CpG complexation.

Although there were no significant differences between the affinity of binding between the two SWNT preparations and the ODN CpG 1668, the ODN CpG 1668 bound to the MWNT-NH$_3^+$ formulation with much lower affinity. This difference was probably due to the relative dimensions and charge distributions of the two types of f-CNTs. Both SWNT-Lys-NH$_3^+$ and MWNT-NH$_3^+$ displayed the same amount of positive charges. However, there must be an avidity effect, resulting from a double electrostatic interaction per ODN CpG molecule after their binding to SWNT-Lys-NH$_3^+$ where the two ammonium groups on each lysine residue are in close proximity with respect to the single ammonium on the MWNT-NH$_3^+$.

Following the demonstration of complexation of the ODN CpGs with f-CNTs, their immunopotentiating effect was tested [204]. SWNTs were the CNTs of choice since they bound to ODN CpG 1668 with higher affinity than the MWNTs. After incubating the SWNT-Lys-NH$_3^+$ at various excess ratios with a minimal immunostimulatory dose of the ODN CpG 1668, the complexes were added to a culture of naive mouse splenocytes. Complexes of SWNT-Lys-NH$_3^+$ at 18:1 and 9:1 ratios over the ODN CpG 1668 increased its immunostimulatory properties by 58 and 45%, respectively. There was no significant effect on immunostimulation when lower ratios of SWNT-Lys-NH$_3^+$/ODN CpG were tested. Although the mechanism of this immunopotentiating effect is not quite clear, it could be argued that the high excess of SWNT-Lys-NH$_3^+$ over the ODN CpG 1668 had a neutralizing effect of its negative charge. As a consequence, the repulsion forces by the negatively charged cell membrane were presumably reduced and therefore, the cellular uptake of ODN CpG 1668 was increased.

These preliminary findings pave the way for future *in vivo* experiments using animal models of disease or vaccination protocols to test the therapeutic or adjuvant potential of such complexes. Moreover, further studies will need to address whether serum proteins can alter the surface potential of CNTs, their size, the stability of complexes and the formation of aggregates.

3.5.2
Presentation and Immunogenic Potential of Peptide Antigens Attached onto f-CNTs

Peptides representing selected regions from the amino acid sequence of a protein antigen (epitopes) can be used as immunogens to induce peptide- and pathogen-specific B cell and CD4$^+$ (T$_h$) or cytotoxic CD8$^+$ [cytotoxic T lymphocyte (CTL)] T cell responses. Activated CD4$^+$ T cells help B cells to produce antibodies that neutralize viruses and bacterial toxins [205], enhance the magnitude of cytotoxic T cell responses to clear virus-infected cells [206], and regulate the immune responses to foreign antigens on the basis of the cytokine profile they secrete [207]. CD8$^+$ T cells are the main effector cells responsible for the clearance of viral infections [208]. The development of such peptide vaccines requires a basic knowledge of the role of the various antigens of the pathogen in infection and immunity, the use of a cocktail of epitopes able to induce a broad range of protective antibody and T cell responses, and a delivery system for presentation of these epitopes to immunocompetent cells.

B cell epitopes are mainly located on the surface of a protein antigen. Therefore, the native structure of the antigen is critical for recognition by antibodies. Immunization with flexible peptides normally induces a diverse set of antibody specificities that bind several different conformations of the peptide [209]. However, a subset of these antibodies can cross-react with the native protein, presumably because these peptides adopt a conformation similar to the native epitope [209]. Therefore, for a synthetic peptide vaccine to elicit a protective antibody response it is important the B cell epitope to be presented to the immune system at a conformation mimicking the native structure. The ability of f-CNTs to present a covalently linked synthetic peptide representing a neutralizing and protective B cell epitope from the foot-and-mouth disease virus (FMDV) corresponding to the 141–159 region of the VP1 viral envelope protein was tested [210]. SWNTs-NH$_3^+$ and SWNTs-Lys-NH$_3^+$ modified with a maleimido group were used. This functionality allowed linking the FMDV peptide bearing an additional cysteine at the N-terminus necessary for a selective chemical ligation (Fig. 3.11).

To elucidate the structural and functional relationship between f-CNTs-linked peptide and peptide-specific polyclonal and monoclonal antibodies, the ELISA test and SPR were used. Both methods demonstrated that the SWNTs-linked peptide retained the structural features required for recognition by anti-FMDV peptide monoclonal and polyclonal antibodies [148, 211].

Since the FMDV peptide was not immunogenic (i.e. not capable of eliciting an immune response) in BALB/c mice (T cell help is required) [212] an immunization protocol that has been previously shown to overcome the requirement of coupling nonimmunogenic peptides to carrier proteins or T_h epitopes was employed [213]. To this end, the SWNT-linked FMDV peptide was coimmunized with a protein antigen that provided T cell help, like ovalbumin (OVA) in a Freund's emulsion. After two injections, strong antipeptide antibody responses were induced that had significantly higher virus neutralizing capacity than the antibodies elicited after coimmunizing the free peptide with OVA [211]. This finding highlights the potential of f-CNTs to act as a delivery system capable of presenting critical epitopes at an

Figure 3.11. Molecular structures of FMDV peptide f-CNTs.

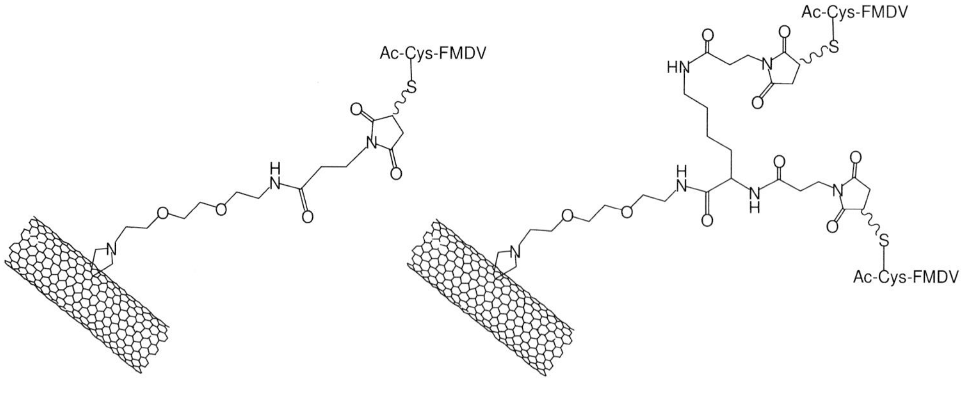

appropriate conformation to elicit antibodies with the right specificity. Moreover, no antibody responses were induced against the f-CNTs, which could potentially hamper the successful outcome of the immunization procedure, particularly when several administrations are required [214].

Although the application of CNTs in the field of vaccine delivery is in its infancy, CNTs offer several attractive features, including the control one has over the primary nature of the system. They provide a platform for the attachment of adjuvants and antigens. Their potential use as vaccine delivery and adjuvant vehicles is likely to have a significant impact on the route that vaccines will be administered in the future and the required dose, conferring a competitive advantage in the market place. Obviously, their immunogenicity, toxicity, biodegradability, stability, biocompatibility, cost and consistent GMP manufacturing with readily scalable production processes has to be studied for each system and each application. These challenging issues should not inhibit research in examining the potential of CNTs to deliver vaccines since the most interesting and valuable delivery systems are yet to come.

3.6
CNTs for Drug Delivery

Drug delivery systems are necessary to improve the pharmacological profile and the therapeutic properties of administered drugs [1]. Among the wide variety of available delivery systems, CNTs may represent a promising alternative [215]. The application of f-CNTs as new nanovectors for drug delivery became possible soon after the demonstration of cellular uptake of this new material. However, only a few examples of delivery of therapeutic agents using CNTs are currently reported in the literature. Dai and coworkers have shown the potential of CNTs to transport proteins into the cells [90]. Single-walled CNTs were shortened to a length between 20 and 100 nm using strong acid conditions. This treatment also allowed the generation of carboxylic groups at the terminal parts of the tubes and at their defect sites. The carboxylated tubes were complexed with different types of proteins including SA, protein A, BSA and cytochrome c (Fig. 3.12).

Mammalian cell lines were incubated with the complexes to study the capacity of CNTs to drive the adsorbed proteins into the cells. The complexes were localized in the endosomes and released into the cytoplasm by addition of chloroquine (a molecule able to destroy the endosomes). In the case of cytochrome c, it was verified that the protein exerted its biological function after liberation from the endosomal trap. Indeed, the cells entered into apoptosis. At the same time, it was shown that CNT–protein complexes were biocompatible by measuring cell proliferation.

In a different approach, Wu and coworkers used f-CNTs with AmB – one of the most effective antimycotic molecules for the treatment of chronic fungal infections (Fig. 3.13) [152].

MWNTs were treated with strong acid conditioned to reduce their length to about 180–940 nm. The carboxylic groups were coupled with a phthalimide

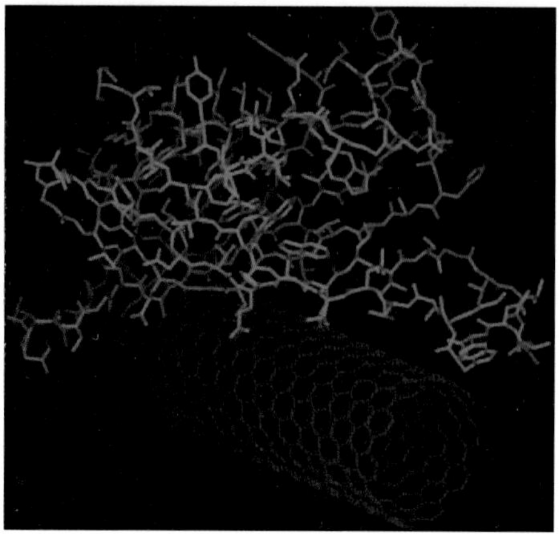

Figure 3.12. Molecular model of the complex between a shortened CNTs and SA.

mono-protected triethylene glycol diamine. Subsequently, the tubes underwent the 1,3-dipolar cycloaddition reaction to introduce a N-functionalized pyrrolidine ring on the external walls of the tubes. A second Boc-protected amino group was therefore introduced on the nanotubes. The two protecting groups are orthogonal and permitted to modify the tubes with a fluorescent probe to follow the cell internalization of the conjugate and the active drug AmB to exert its antifungal activity. It

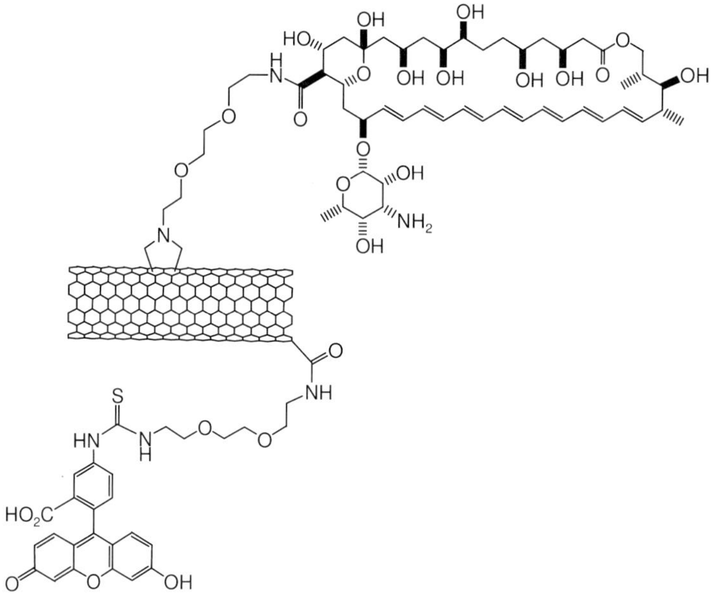

Figure 3.13. Molecular structure of CNTs functionalized with FITC and AmB.

has been shown that AmB–CNTs were rapidly internalized into Jurkat cells in a dose-dependent manner. The process was nonendocytotoxic since the incubation of the cells at 4 °C or in the presence of sodium azide did not completely block the uptake. The drug was internalized into mammalian cells with a remarkable reduction of toxicity. Indeed, AmB is widely used, but it suffers from high toxicity. At the highest dose, more than 40% of cells died by the effect of free AmB, while all cells remained alive following the treatment with AmB covalently conjugated to CNTs. Very interestingly, AmB preserved its high antifungal activity once linked to the nanotubes. Different types of pathogens including *Candida albicans*, *Candida paropsilosis* and *Cryptococcus neoformans* were treated with AmB–CNT conjugates, and the activity was in some cases higher that the drug alone. Although only some hypotheses on the action of the AmB linked to the tubes could be formulated (increase of the solubility of the drug, multipresentation of the drug by CNTs that favor interaction with the fungal membrane), the conjugation of AmB to the tubes modulated its therapeutic effect by decreasing mammalian toxicity and increasing the antifungal activity.

Using another strategy, Hosmane and coworkers prepared SWNTs with a carborane cage for boron neutron capture therapy (BNCT) [216]. CNTs were functionalized with a substituted C_2B_{10} carborane derivative via nitrene cycloaddition. Following treatment with sodium hydroxide, a water-soluble CNT conjugate was obtained (Fig. 3.14).

Then, the biodistribution study on different tissues showed that carborane nanotubes were concentrated more in tumor cells than in blood, liver, lung or spleen when administered intravenously. However, the mechanism for this it is not yet understood. The results are preliminary, although promising for future applications of CNTs on delivery of boron-based agents for effective BNCT treatment of cancer, provided that cytotoxicity and more complete biodistribution studies prove the biocompatibility of this system. Another application of CNTs in cancer therapy was shown by Kam and coworkers [217]. The property of CNTs to adsorb NIR irradiation was exploited to kill cancer cells. Pristine SWNTs were wrapped with PEG modified with a PL moiety on one side and folic acid (FA) on the other side. As

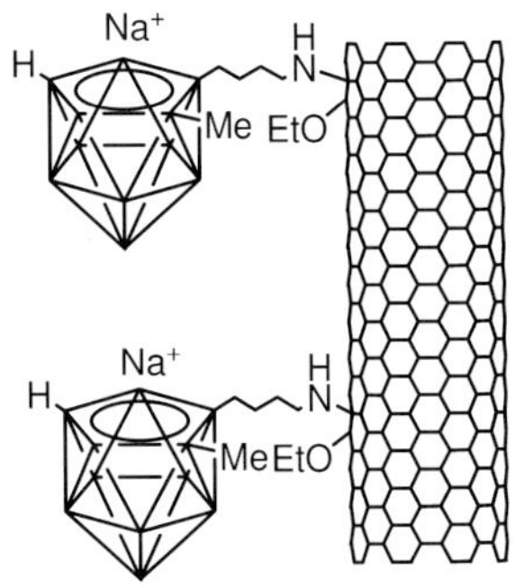

Figure 3.14. Molecular structure of CNTs functionalized with a carborane cage.

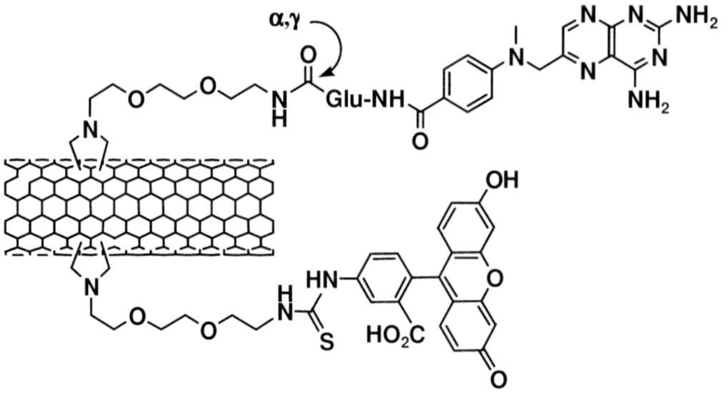

Figure 3.15. Molecular structure of CNTs functionalized with FITC and methotrexate.

tumor cells are known to overexpress folate receptors, the PL–PEG–FA/SWNT construct was mainly taken up by cancer cells, which were then destroyed by using a laser wavelength of 808 nm. Laser pulses induced local heating and consequently death only of those tumor cells that had internalized the CNTs.

Pastorin and coworkers have developed an alternative method to exploit CNTs in cancer [218]. CNTs were doubly functionalized using 1,3-dipolar cycloaddition reaction. Two orthogonally protected amino groups were introduced on the sidewalls and the tips of the tubes. After selective deprotection, an anticancer molecule [methotrexate (MTX)] and a fluorescent probe (FITC) were linked to the tubes (Fig. 3.15).

MTX is a drug widely used against cancer, but it displays a reduced cellular uptake. Therefore, the limited capacity of MTX to cross the cell membrane could be overcome by its conjugation to CNTs, which are able to enhance cell uptake of linked moieties. The presence of fluorescein provided the optical signal for imaging CNT–drug into the cells. Jurkat cells were incubated with different doses of MTX–CNT and the fluorescent tubes were localized around the nuclear membrane in a dose-dependent manner. Preliminary studies have shown that MTX conjugated to the CNTs had the same cytotoxic activity of the drug alone.

Another class of carbon nanomaterials very similar to CNTs called carbon nanohorns were found to be effective systems for delivery of anticancer agents. Single-walled carbon nanohorns (SWCHs) are spherical aggregates of graphitic tubes with dimensions in the nanorange scale. These nanostructures were loaded with dexamethasone [219]. Binding and release of the drug were subsequently evaluated using two types of nanohorns. It was found that oxidized nanohorns were able to adsorb more dexamethasone than as-grown horns. The analysis of activation of glucocorticoid response in mouse bone marrow cells and induction of alkaline phosphatase in mouse osteoblasts confirmed the biological activity of the drug released from the carbon support. Similarly, carbon nanohorns were used to encapsulate cisplatin (another anticancer agent) [220]. Again, the structure of the drug was preserved into the aggregates. Cisplatin was slowly liberated into water and it was effective in blocking the growth of human lung cancer cells. Unloaded oxidized carbon nanohorns were instead not active. Therefore, this type of carbon material is potentially useful as a carrier of anticancer agents.

In view of the overall results, functionalized carbon nanostructures represent an emerging and new class of delivery tools for the transport, encapsulation and release of molecules into mammalian cells. However, it will be important in the near future to assess the metabolism, biodistribution and clearance form the body of nanotubes for further development and complete integration in living systems.

3.7 CNTs for Gene Transfer

3.7.1 Interaction with DNA and RNA

In the quest for a useful nonviral gene transfer system, the interaction between a cationic component (liposome, polymer, nanoparticle) and the negatively charged nucleic acids to be delivered is critical for the eventual effectiveness of the gene transfer construct. CNTs have very recently been explored for the first time as novel materials for the complexation and delivery of gene-encoding nucleic acids [191, 221]. However, the physicochemical interactions between CNTs and DNA have been studied under different contexts for much longer, particularly in attempts to disperse non-f-CNTs, and for the construction of sensors, nanocircuits, nanocomposites and gene delivery vectors.

Theoretical predictions of DNA interactions with CNTs by molecular dynamics simulations have shown that single-stranded DNA spontaneously inserts into non-f-CNTs through a combination of van der Waals and hydrophobic forces [222]. However, a recent molecular modeling simulation has demonstrated that double-stranded DNA can also wrap around non-f-CNTs or, the in case of positively charged CNTs in an aqueous environment, DNA molecules could electrostatically adhere onto the CNTs surface [223].

Experimentally, a range of different techniques has been used to understand the CNT–DNA interactions and the ensuing supramolecular structures between the two components. However, most studies agree that the nature and mechanism of such interactions will be highly dependent on the type of CNTs surface functionalization and the characteristics of the nucleic acids.

UV and IR spectroscopy have both been used to show that non-f-SWNTs and double-stranded DNA interact through hydrogen bonds [224, 225]. Changes in the electronic levels in the nucleotide bases of the DNA molecule were found in these studies and the DNA acquired a chaotic sphere conformation upon interaction with CNTs. π–π interactions between the CNT sidewalls and the nucleic acid bases have been proposed as the mechanistic basis for this wrapping effect. Moreover, the ability of DNA to wrap around the CNT surface has been described for both double-stranded DNA [226, 227] and single-stranded DNA [91], and has been utilized to disperse CNTs in solvents of varying polarity.

As described earlier in this chapter, CNT surface characteristics can be altered through organic and defect functionalization. By strong oxidation, OH and C=O defects are introduced at the tips and sidewalls of CNTs. Several studies describe that these oxidized CNTs (CNT-ox) covalently bond DNA-NH_2 in a controllable assembling process [38, 118, 228, 229] or are helically wrapped (π–π interactions) by double-stranded DNA and single-stranded DNA [230–232]. An alternative functionalization reaction described by Georgakilas and coworkers produces positively charged ammonium-*f*-CNTs (CNT-NH_3^+) [146]. The interaction of CNT-NH_3^+ with plasmid DNA (pDNA) was studied in detail in our laboratories [221, 233]. We have found that these *f*-CNTs interact with pDNA to form complexes primarily through electrostatic forces and that the pDNA was condensed around the CNT-NH_3^+. Moreover, these studies have indicated that the total available surface area and the surface charge density of CNTs were critical parameters in the interaction and complexation of pDNA.

With regard to interactions between RNA and CNTs, to our knowledge there has only been one published report describing the interaction between non-*f*-SWNTs and RNA polymer poly(rU) [234]. In this study the RNA polymer poly(rU) was observed in a blob-like conformation when bound at the surface of CNTs as imaged by scanning electron microscopy, resembling the condensation of pDNA strands. These authors suggested that the binding occurs through π-stacking and hydrophobic interactions; however, no detailed mechanistic study has been published so far describing how the CNT–RNA interactions occur.

3.7.2
Delivery and Expression of Gene-encoding DNA and RNA

The development of water-soluble CNTs automatically renders them compatible with the biological fluids and milieu. The complex formation between CNTs and nucleic acids in combination with the improved CNT biocompatibility recently achieved allowed for exploration of the hypothesis that CNTs can be used as gene-delivery systems. So far, the intracellular translocation and expression of gene-encoding nucleic acids (DNA and RNA) involving CNTs have been shown for mammalian cells to bacteria *in vitro*. The following is a comparative description of the different techniques used to deliver nucleic acids to cells through CNTs.

The first ever study to demonstrate CNT-mediated gene delivery and expression of marker gene-encoding nucleic acids was carried out in our laboratories. Pantarotto and coworkers reported that CNTs covalently functionalized with ammonium groups (CNT-NH_3^+) were able to associate with pDNA through electrostatic interactions [191]. Transmission electron microscopy images of the supramolecular complexes showed the pDNA attaining a condensed globular conformation at the surface of the CNT-NH_3^+. The delivery of pDNA and expression of β-galactosidase (a marker gene) in CHO cells was found to be approximately 10 times higher than naked pDNA. An endosome-independent penetration mechanism was proposed for the complex uptake based on evidence of spontaneous cellular uptake of the *f*-CNTs alone. Similar to other nonviral gene delivery systems based on the electrostatic supramolecular complex formation between a cationic macromolecule or nanoparticle and nucleic acids, the charge ratio (+/−) CNT-NH_3^+:pDNA was found to be a critically important factor determining the level of gene expression.

A similar approach was later followed by Liu and coworkers, which reported a noncovalent association of pDNA onto the surface of CNTs functionalized with polyethylenimine (PEI) – a polymer with high density of terminal amine groups [235]. The complexes were tested at different charge ratios in different cell lines (293, COS7 and HepG2 cells) and the level of gene (pCMV-Luc) expression was found to be much higher than those of DNA alone. This study suggested that the uptake mechanism of the CNT–PEI–pDNA conjugates was took place by endocytosis.

Kam and coworkers later used two distinct methods to deliver nucleic acids via CNTs into HeLa cells. In a first study [217], CNTs functionalized with Cy3-labeled single-stranded DNA through noncovalent adsorption were used. These CNTs were excited with NIR light. The release and nuclear translocation of the single-stranded DNA was reported by confocal microscopy only in the case of NIR treatment. In the absence of cell illumination by NIR, the Cy3-DNA was seen by Kam and coworkers to remain in the cytoplasm. This group also suggested an endosome-mediated cellular uptake.

In a subsequent study by the same group [93], CNTs were functionalized by non-covalent adsorption of PL molecules, which contained a PEG chain terminating in an amine (CNT–PL–PEG-NH_2) or maleimide (CNT–PL–PEG-maleimide) group. Then a thiol-containing SH-DNA–Cy3 was covalently linked to the CNTs via a disulfide bond by a heterobifunctional cross-linker. In this way, a complicated CNT–PL–PEG-single-stranded DNA–Cy3 complex was formed, sensitive to enzymatic cleavage upon endocytosis and translocation to the lysosomal compartments. It was reported in that study that nuclear localization of Cy3–DNA was possible only in the presence of the disulfide linkage. However, in this study gene-encoding nucleic acids were not used therefore no gene expression was reported at all.

A very different strategy to introduce exogenous pDNA into mammalian cells was described recently by Cai and coworkers [192]. The pDNA was immobilized on the CNTs, which contained Ni particles (CNT-Ni) enclosed and suspended with the surfactant Nanosperse AQ. Then, with a magnetic spearing technique (exposure to an external magnetic field followed by centrifugation) the complexes were added to Bal 17 cells, mouse splenic cells and a primary culture of mice cortical neurons. The expression of the enhanced green fluorescent protein (*EGFP*) gene was evaluated by fluorescence microscopy and flow cytometry. Gene delivery through CNT-Ni produced 80–100% fluorescent cells, while CNTs deprived of Ni particles did not produce any fluorescence signal. In this way, another illustration of the possibility to use CNTs to transport intracellularly gene expressing nucleic acids was seen. However, such techniques are only appropriate for *in vitro* or *ex vivo* gene transfer.

The delivery of exogenous genes by CNTs has been shown to be also possible in bacterial cultures. Rojas-Chapana and coworkers have demonstrated that oxidized, water-dispersible CNTs deliver pDNA into *Escherichia coli* through temporary nano-channels across the cell envelope [236]. The pUC19-transformed bacteria were examined by optical microscopy, and an efficient transformation between 9 and 32 transformants was observed. The authors achieved that by an electroporation technique using microwave-activated CNTs, which apparently orient their tips in a conformation perpendicular to the bacterial cell membrane.

CNTs have also been shown to transport RNA into mammalian cells. Lu and coworkers have studied the cellular uptake of CNT–RNA polymer poly(rU) hybrids formed through nonspecific binding. MCF7 cells were examined by confocal microscopy after addition of the hybrids, and their translocation in cellular and nuclear membranes reported [237]. In agreement with these findings, Kam and coworkers, in more a recent report, used a complex CNT–small interfering RNA (siRNA) conjugate linked with disulfide bonds (as described above for single-stranded DNA) and have shown preliminary observations of siRNA-mediated gene silencing [93].

All of these studies have been initiated by our initial observations that it was indeed feasible to use *f*-CNTs to complex, deliver and express gene-encoding nucleic acids. The most recent study in this exploratory exercise has been very recently published using GFP-encoding pDNA condensed with *f*-CNTs carrying positive charges [238]. In this way our initial reports and observations were indeed substantiated and reproduced in an independent study. The development of CNTs as delivery systems for nucleic acids is still in its exploratory stage, and many more studies are needed to determine the advantages and limitations offered by these novel materials.

3.8
Health Impact of CNTs

Nanotechnology has been rapidly developing due to the possibility of engineering at nanometer scales. The resulting nanoproducts display physicochemical characteristics that confer electrochemical, mechanical and thermal properties that are very useful in the medical, scientific, commercial and environmental fields. However, it is too early to say whether the "nanostructures" will wean the world from dirty technologies or if they will definitely backfire, basically because the laws of chemistry or physics are different when particles get down to the nanoscale. Even substances that are normally innocuous can trigger intense chemical reactions and biological anomalies as nanospecies [239].

For this reason, there is a heated debate between the desire of introducing nanomaterials in everyday life and the moralistic tendency of blocking the nanotech factory until the risks will be better understood. Currently, available information concerning the relative environmental and health risks of manufactured nanoparticles or nanomaterials is severely absent and defective. In fact, most of nanomaterials (fullerenes, nanoparticles, nanofibers and nanotubes) are made of carbon atoms, with distinct geometries, different surface areas, and diverse physical and chemical properties. The existence of such variables produced a lot of contrasting evidence. Doses, effects and cell viability of different carbon nanomaterials are summarized in Tab. 3.1. For example, Adelmann and coworkers have studied the *in vitro* effect of fullerenes on alveolar macrophages, prepared in an arc between two graphite electrodes [240]. A 60% reduction in macrophage viability and increased levels of some inflammatory cytokines were found, suggesting that such structures had similar toxicity to quartz particles. Moreover, it was discovered that stable solutions of C_{60} nanoparticles (nano-C_{60}) displayed a high toxicity against bacteria at a concentration of 0.4 μg mL^{-1} [241]. Other highly water-soluble nanofullerenes (13–100 mg mL^{-1}) showed also a remarkable cytotoxicity both in fibroblasts and in liver carcinoma cells at very low concentrations (50 μg mL^{-1}) [242]. It could be deduced that such behavior conveys a common toxicity of all C_{60} materials [243]. On the contrary, it was observed that the lethal doses varied by seven orders of magnitude, strongly depending on the functionalization of the fullerene surface [242]. Therefore, the further modification at the surface deeply influenced the toxicological profile of the nanomaterials [244].

In contrast, some *in vivo* studies on fullerene showed that intraperitoneal injections of amounts of C_{60} up to 2.5 g kg^{-1} in mice and rats had neither lethal effects nor acute toxicity [245, 246]. What was evident was only a hypertrophy of livers and spleens, which could be ascribed to the high amount of compound injected that had exceeded the absorption capacity of the animal. Similarly, mice subcutaneously implanted with Hat-stacked carbon nanofibers did not show severe inflammatory responses such as necrosis or degeneration after 4 weeks of incubation [247]. However, these encouraging results are not exhaustive in representing the reduced harmfulness of all the different nanomaterials.

3.8.1
Parameters of CNTs Related to Health Impact

The data reported above suggest that, in general, carbon nanoparticles can be considered as dangerous as quartz, only on the basis of the common "starting material", i.e. carbon. In particular, CNTs represent a class of substances which are, at the same time, intriguing (for their characteristics) and doubtful. In fact, they revealed unusual toxicological properties, because their shapes can be both fibers and nanoparticles, and they are often characterized by the presence of metallic components even after their purification. CNTs, both single and multiwalled, are classified as "synthetic graphite" by the National Occupational Safety and Health Administration, on the basis of the same hexagonal/honeycomb pattern. However, such extrapolation might not be protective for exposure to CNTs, because they show physicochemical properties that are often influenced by several variables.

3.8.1.1 **Purity**
CNTs generally show different levels of purity, which are strictly dependent on the methods employed for their production. The impurities are essentially made up of

Tab. 3.1. Doses, effects and cell viability of different carbon nanomaterials.

Type of nanomaterial	Amount/ concentration	Cell/animal target	Effect	Possible causes	Ref.
Fullerenes	not specified	alveolar macrophages	60% reduction on cell viability; inflammatory cytokines (IL-6, IL-8)	intrinsic toxicity	240
Nano C_{60}	0.4 μg mL^{-1}	bacteria	growth inhibition		241
Nano C_{60}	50 μg mL^{-1}	fibroblast; liver carcinoma cells	decreasing cytotoxicity with increasing functionalization and solubility	oxidative stress; surface effect	242
Functionalized gold nanoparticles	250 μM	leukemia cells	no remarkable cell death; rapid internalization		244
C_{60}	2.5 g kg^{-1}	mice and rats	no acute toxicity; hypertrophy	too high amount	245, 246
Hat-stacked carbon nanofibers (H-CNF)	not specified	rats	no toxicity		247
SWNTs, MWNTs, fullerenes	≥1.41 μg cm^{-2}	alveolar macrophages	20% reduction on cell viability (SWNTs)	low purity	248
Pristine SWNTs	0.1–10 μg mL^{-1}	HaCaT cells	increased cell death	oxidative stress or solvent (DMF)	249
f-SWNTs	3 μg mL^{-1}– 30 mg mL^{-1}	HDF	cell death 50% or below		252
MWNTs (220 and 825 nm)	50–500 ng mL^{-1} (*in vitro*)	leukemia cells THP-1	inflammation (especially with 825-nm samples)	length	253
	0.1 mg mL^{-1} (*in vivo*)	mice	granulomatous inflammation		253
HiPCO, CVD-SWNTs and CVD-double-walled CNTs	0.62–2.5 mg	red blood cells	complement activation	C1q activation	254
Arc-SWNTs and CVD-H-CNF	10 μg mL^{-1}	leukemia cells THP-1; mouse spleen cells	immune response	Induction of TNF-α	255

Tab. 3.1 *(continued)*

Type of nanomaterial	Amount/ concentration	Cell/animal target	Effect	Possible causes	Ref.
f-SWNTs	<5 μM	fibroblasts	no remarkable cell death (90%); rapid internalization		190
f-SWNTs and *f*-MWNTs + plasmid DNA	1 mg mL^{-1}	HeLa cells	no remarkable cell death; efficient delivery		191
MWNT–PEI + DNA	<5 μg mL^{-1}	HEK293 cells	below 40% reduction on cell viability	increased PEI weight	235
SWNT–CpG ODN	5 ng–5 μg	mouse splenocytes	no remarkable cell death		204
SWNT–RNA	≤1 mg mL^{-1}	breast cancer cells (MCF7)	efficient delivery		237
SWNTs	1–250 μg mL^{-1}	embryo kidney cells (HEK293 cells)	apoptosis; 20/30-kDa protein secretion	downregulation of genes for adhesion; upregulation of genes involved in apoptosis	256
Pristine MWNTs	0.1–0.4 mg mL^{-1}	embryo kidney cells (HEK293)	inflammation	production of IL-8	257
Pristine and oxidized MWNTs	400 μg mL^{-1}	T lymphocytes	40% reduction on cell viability (pristine) 80% reduction on cell viability (oxidation)	better dispersion of oxidized tubes	258
MWNTs	0.5, 2 or 5 mg	rats	upregulation of pro-inflammatory and profibrotic mediators	biopersistence in the lung	259
Raw, HiPCO and arc-SWNTs	0.1 or 0.5 mg per mouse	mice	granulomas	intrinsic toxicity	260
Pristine SWNTs	1 or 5 mg kg^{-1}	rats	pulmonary inflammation, with non-dose-dependent granulomas	blockage of upper airways	261

Tab. 3.1 *(continued)*

Type of nanomaterial	Amount/ concentration	Cell/animal target	Effect	Possible causes	Ref.
Fullerenes and CNTs	0.2 mL (not specified)	four albino rabbits and 40 human volunteers	no remarkable skin irritation or allergen risks		262 263
Carbon fiber particles	not specified	341 workers	contact dermatitis	exposure to organic solvents or to carbonaceous particles	264 265
Pristine HiPCO–SWNTs	0.06, 0.12 or 0.24 mg mL^{-1}	HaCaT cells	alteration of cell morphology and surface integrity	transition metal catalysts	266
Pristine HiPCO or laser ablation SWNTs (aerosol)	15.5 mg	cotton gloves	deposition on individual gloves ranged from 217 to 6020 μg (aerosol below 53 μg m^{-3})	ultrafine powders	267

residual catalysts and amorphous carbon. Their high amount might enhance the toxicity. In this context, Jia and coworkers investigated the cytotoxicity caused by nanostructures such as SWNTs, MWNTs and fullerenes on alveolar macrophages (AM) [248]. The different carbon particles, all with a purity superior than 90%, were suspended in RPMI medium using a Dounce homogenizer and sonicated for 20 min. In this way, a stable suspension was obtained and immediately used to measure the phagocytic ability of AM after a 6-h exposure to carbon materials. The amount of materials used was expressed as μg cm^{-2}, because CNTs are characterized by a wide length distribution. As expected, the tested samples exhibited different cytotoxicity to AM. At low doses (1.41 μg cm^{-2}) SWNTs showed a high cytotoxic effect, corresponding to above 20% inhibition of cell growth with a dose-dependent trend. MWNTs and fullerene were instead much less toxic. One possible reason for such a major difference could be attributed to the purity level of SWNTs that was lower than the other samples. Indeed, residual amorphous carbon and trace amounts of metallic catalysts, such as Fe, Ni and Y, were present in SWNT samples. These impurities, even at a low level, can influence cell viability, so ultrapure material should be employed; in any case, human and environmental heath evaluations of different carbon nanomaterials must be considered individually.

3.8.1.2 Solvents

Any kind of cell evaluation needs a medium to dissolve the sample. Physiological solutions, with the addition of nutritional elements, are the most appropriate, but sometimes the low solubility of the carbon material requires the use of polar, organic solvents. Manna and coworkers investigated the essential mechanism involved in the toxicity of SWNTs [249]. Human keratinocytes (HaCaT cells) were exposed to concentrations between 0.1 and 10 $\mu g\ mL^{-1}$ of nanotubes, displaying increased cell death. This observation was attributed to the excess of oxidative stress within the cells and to the associated activation of transcription factor NF-κB. However, DMF was used to dissolve the samples and might have induced some alterations of the results. In fact, DMF is a solvent known to be toxic and thus it should be avoided in cell manipulation.

3.8.1.3 Surface of CNTs

Until now, the size cut-off below which particles are surely toxic has not been demonstrated. However, there are at least two main reasons that render CNTs potentially harmful: (i) their large surface area and (ii) the reactivity or intrinsic toxicity of the surface [250, 251]. The smaller the particles, the more toxic they become. This is due to the fact that there is more surface area per mass unit. As a consequence, any intrinsic toxicity of the surface will deeply influence the toxicological profile of the samples. For example, Sayes and Ausman investigated the effect on human fibroblasts (HDF) of some water-dispersible SWNTs [252]. It was found that cytotoxicity of compounds decreased significantly with the increased degree of functionalization on the surface. In addition, although a dose–response relationship of toxicity in the considered range of concentrations (0.003–30 $mg\ mL^{-1}$) was observed, cell death did not exceed 50%, apart from in one case in which 1% surfactant was employed. This could be justified by the fact that surfactant was coated on the surface of the nanotubes in a noncovalent, reversible way, whereas the functional groups were covalently bound and were not removed in the conditions of the biological tests.

3.8.1.4 Length

Another parameter that was found to influence the toxicity profile of CNTs is their length. Sato and coworkers separated MWNTs of 220 and 825 nm using controlled strong acid conditions [253]. During a short incubation time, clusters of both samples were shown to be surrounded by macrophages as a consequence of the activation of innate immunity. The shorter tubes displayed a lower inflammatory response. In both cases, no severe effects, such as necrosis or degeneration, were observed around CNTs throughout the experimental period of 4 weeks.

3.8.2 *In Vitro* Effect of CNTs

SWNTs were investigated to verify if they affected the immune system through the activation of complement [254]. For this purpose, SWNTs in concentrations between 0.62 and 2.5 mg were tested in rabbit red blood cells. They displayed a dose-dependent potency in complement activation comparable to that of the known, potent activator zymosan. In particular, it seemed that such activation followed the classical pathway, but with high selectivity. This was confirmed by the demonstration of a direct binding of CNTs to the main complement subunit C1q. On the contrary, chemical modifications at the surface of CNTs reduced or even eliminated the complement activation, but further investigations are necessary to confirm this observation.

In a parallel study, SWNTs were evaluated in terms of their capacity to activate mouse spleen cells [255]. Since different cell types (monocytic leukemia THP-1 and spleen cells) and incubation times were employed, it was difficult to compare the obtained results. It has been confirmed that SWNTs induced an immune response, although the stimulating activity resulted to be lower than that of microbial systems.

The effect of functionalized, water-soluble CNTs on cell viability was also analyzed by Pantarotto and coworkers during the study of translocation of bioactive peptides across the cell membrane [190]. 3T6 and 3T3 fibroblasts were treated with 1–10 μM concentration of fluorescent SWNTs. The cytotoxicity was evaluated by flow cytometry, using the markers Annexin V and propidium iodide as indicators of apoptosis and necrosis, respectively. It was observed that below 5 μM almost 90% of the cell population remained alive, indicating a nontoxic behavior of *f*-CNTs. Low toxicity was not only a characteristic of SWNTs functionalized with peptides. Both *f*-SWNTs and *f*-MWNTs, regardless of cell subtypes, are nontoxic on their own [90, 220]. HeLa cells, incubated for several hours with about 1 mg mL^{-1} of CNTs mixed with plasmid DNA in different charge ratios, did not demonstrate signs of apoptosis [191]. In addition, *f*-CNTs complexed to different types of nucleic acids including plasmid DNA, RNA and oligodeoxynucleotides CpG sequences were not toxic for cells like breast cancer cells (MCF7) or splenocytes [204, 235, 237].

Apart from the investigation of the effect of CNTs on cells, it is also important to understand the mechanism involved in their interaction with biological systems. Cui and coworkers evaluated the activity of human embryo kidney cells (HEK293) during 5 days treatment with SWNTs in concentrations between 1 and 250 μg mL^{-1} [256]. It was found that SWNTs were able to inhibit the proliferation of HEK293, and to induce apoptosis in a dose- and time-dependent way. The most interesting finding was that cells actively responded to SWNTs, secreting a series of 20- to 30-kDa proteins able to aggregate and wrap this unknown material, regardless of the uniformity of the starting samples. The possible mechanism for this phenomenon was attributed to a stimuli induced by SWNTs attached at the cell surface, followed by a downregulation of the genes responsible for adhesion. It was also envisaged that SWNTs could determine an upregulation of the genes associated with apoptosis and secretion of small proteins as protection for cells that were preserved from the contact with the tubes. This phenomenon presents a double advantage, since it allows us to investigate the rules at the basis of this interaction and, at the same time, it offers the possibility to consider these secreted proteins as potential targets in future medical therapy.

The same type of cells was also used to verify if bigger material, like MWNTs, was able to cross the external membrane and to affect the cell functions. It was shown that unmodified MWNTs were able to enter HEK293 cells and to induce the release of the pro-inflammatory cytokine IL-8 [257]. In addition, it was demonstrated that they were less toxic towards T lymphocytes than chemically functionalized tubes [258]. This was attributed to the fact that oxidized MWNTs were better dispersed in aqueous solution, determining higher weight/volume concentrations and, thus, a deeper impact on toxicity. At the dose of 400 $\mu g\ mL^{-1}$, oxidized tubes killed more than 80% of cells in 5 days, while pristine MWNTs decreased the cell viability of less than 40%. However, although it is obvious that CNTs toxicity does not depend only on concentration, the dose used in this study was very high and the same experiments with concentrations below 40 $\mu g\ mL^{-1}$ did not affect the function of T cells [258].

3.8.3 *In Vivo* Effects of CNTs

Apart from *in vitro* experiments, some CNTs were implanted at the subcutaneous level in rats to study their effects *in vivo*. Sato and coworkers demonstrated that coagulated MWNTs of 825 nm determined granulomas, since they were not easily phagocytosed by macrophages in comparison to MWNTs of 220 nm length [253].

MWNTs were also administrated intratracheally to rats to evaluate their respiratory toxicity due to their biopersistence in the lungs [259]. The results clearly showed that, once they reach the lung, MWNTs have the capacity to induce an overexpression of pro-inflammatory and profibrotic mediators. However, there might be some artifacts on the experimental strategy, since the method of administration presents several limitations, such as the formation of big aggregates that could remain entrapped in the airways. A different mode of administration (e.g. inhalation) and the real ability of these materials to translocate from the respiratory system to other organs would give more reliable data.

Other *in vivo* studies were conducted by Lam and coworkers [260] and Warheit and coworkers [261] to investigate the pulmonary toxicity of SWNTs in rodents. In particular, Lam and coworkers evaluated histopathological alterations in mice at 7 and 90 days after exposure to three differently manufactured SWNTs that contained varying amounts of residual catalytic metals: (i) raw nanotubes (RNT) and (ii) purified nanotubes (PNT), both iron-containing HiPCO products from Rice University, and (iii) CarboLex's Ni-containing electric-arc nanotubes (CNTs). Carbon black and quartz were employed as low and high pulmonary toxicity controls, respectively [260]. The experiments indicated that the three types of tubes induced dose-dependent lung lesions characterized by interstitial granulomas, regardless of the amount of metal impurities inside the samples. Even the product containing very low quantities (2% by weight) of iron produced granulomas, suggesting that

CNTs themselves are toxic. However, the methods employed for this study were somehow ambiguous, since the suspension was obtained by briefly shearing and short sonication to avoid any alteration of the nature of SWNTs, but the instillation was performed through a plastic catheter placed in the trachea. Thus, further studies would be needed to elucidate the cause of death. However, it was clear that mice treated with 0.5 mg of nanotubes showed the formation of granulomas, containing macrophages laden with black particles, few lymphocytes, neutrophils, eosinophils and other inflammatory cells. Interestingly, it was encouraging to observe that the lowest dose (0.1 mg per 30 kg) determined no evident clinical signs. The same (5 mg kg^{-1}), or even a lower (1 mg kg^{-1}), amount of SWNTs was employed in the study of Warheit and coworkers, in which histopathological evaluation of lung tissue was conducted after 24 h, 1 week and 3 months postinstillation [261]. In these experiments, SWNTs and graphite particles, together with the corresponding controls (carbonyl iron and quartz particles) were prepared in a volume of 1% Tween 80 surfactant and phosphate saline buffer subjected to polytron dispersion. Rats, intratracheally instilled with carbonyl iron or graphite, did not present adverse effects, while no dose-dependent multifocal granulomas where visible after exposure to SWNTs, even if they did not progress beyond 1 month. In 15% of the rats, the highest dose induced mortality, but the main reason for that was due to mechanical blockage of the upper airways and not to the inner toxicity of SWNTs particulate. The death index was somehow incorrect, because the nanotubes tended to form nanoropes instead of being individually dispersed. A proof was the observation that the surviving animals appeared normal through the whole 3 months. In addition, studies on chemotaxis concerning quartz treatment showed a reduced motility as a consequence of a deficiency in macrophages after 1 week. This phenomenon was not observed in the case of SWNTs, which differed from quartz also in the formation of granulomas in a non-dose-dependent manner.

Additional studies by Huczko and coworkers have contributed to understanding further the impact of nanomaterials on health. They tested the effect of fullerenes and CNTs on skin irritation and allergen risks [262, 263]. There is only some evidence of contact dermatitis caused by exposure to carbon fibers [264, 265]. The authors applied two protocols that are commonly employed for testing skin irritation, i.e. a patch and a Draize rabbit eye test. In the first case, 40 people showing predisposition to irritation and allergy were treated with a patch of Whatman filter paper saturated with a water suspension of CNTs, and then they were examined for 96 h. In the second method, four albino rabbits were administered with 0.2 mL of CNT aqueous suspension, and observed after 24, 48 and 72 h. The absence of adverse effects seemed not to be dependent on the time of exposure nor on the type of material used, since there were no differences in comparison with the reference material (which did not contain CNTs). On the whole, the encouraging results in all experiments on skin irritation suggested that no specific precautions should be adopted while handling such nanomaterial [262, 263].

In general, the manufacturing of carbon nanomaterial is based on the use of transition metal catalysts. Therefore, the eventual health hazards are potentially connected with carbon and metals. In fact, free iron or nickel and transition metal complexes are known to produce reactive radicals, which could induce radical oxidation and enhance oxidative stress. In order to investigate this aspect, Shvedova and coworkers identified and quantified the reactive species that were produced during the manipulation and evaluated the effects of pristine SWNTs on human epidermal keratinocytes (HaCaT) [266]. SEM and TEM allowed us to verify that oxidative stress, caused by treatment with SWNTs, caused a change in the morphology of cells, besides altering surface integrity. These unwanted effects were reduced by the subsequent use of an iron chelator that displayed a protecting role towards HaCaT cells and, thus, confirmed that cytotoxicity of SWNTs was mainly correlated with iron catalytic effects.

A parallel study investigated the adverse effects recorded by aerosol release obtained through mechanical collisions of as-produced SWNTs with bronze beads [267]. The results were somehow ambiguous, since the production of ultrafine powders was not very efficient and it was not possible to discriminate if such particles were made up mainly of nanotubes or of catalyst. Moreover, although nanotubes tended to agglomerate into nanoropes, thus reducing the formation of an appreciable respirable aerosol, it was possible that such nanoparticles remained in the mouth and nasopharyngeal region, causing a potential health risk.

On the whole, CNTs have shown uncommon and interesting physicochemical properties, which increase their possible biomedical applications; however, at the same time, they might persist in biological systems and, consequently, be responsible for adverse health effects and environmental safety. It is imperative that a clear understanding of what really happens to nanoparticles months and years after their release in needed, since some encouraging evidence is not exhaustive in guaranteeing complete innocuous behavior. For all these very important reasons, further studies are required to investigate if CNTs can be widely used for their useful characteristics as well as if they safely represent a promising beginning of the so-called "next industrial revolution".

3.9 General Conclusions

Although still debatable, the use of CNTs in drug delivery and biosensing is acquiring more and more substantiating evidence for efficient development. It is clear that many important issues have to be faced before CNTs can be proposed for clinical trials. However, CNTs show unusual carrier properties, with a very strong tendency to pass cell membranes and seem to perfectly fit into the new discipline of nanobiotechnology. Although the first toxicological reports on pristine CNTs were very discouraging, labeling CNTs as very dangerous species, it is becoming widely accepted that *f*-CNTs are by far less toxic than non-*f*-CNTs. Therefore, the combination of penetration ability with high loading achievable with CNTs makes these new carbon species promising candidates for innovative therapies. Another aspect that should not be disregarded is that other functions can be introduced on CNTs by using different functionalization methods.

In conclusion, we do hope that, in a few years, *f*-CNTs will be considered as valuable building blocks for pharmaceutical uses.

Acknowledgments

The authors are deeply indebted to all their coworkers who have partly contributed to the development of the research described in this chapter and whose names are cited in the references. This work has been supported by the CNRS, MRNT (Gen-Homme 2003), University of Trieste and MIUR (PRIN 2004, prot. 2004035502). G. P. and W. W. are recipients of a fellowship from MNRT. C. K. is grateful to the Università Italo-Francese/Université Franco-Italienne (VINCI Programme 2003) for financing his international PhD.

References

1 Allen, T. M., Cullis, P. R. Drug delivery systems: entering the mainstream, *Science* **2004**, *303*, 1818–1822.
2 Kostarelos, K. Rational design and engineering of delivery systems for therapeutics: biomedical exercises in colloid and surface science, *Adv. Colloid Interface Sci.* **2003**, *106*, 147–168.
3 Merdan, T., Kopecek, J., Kissel, T. Prospects for cationic polymers in gene and oligonucleotide therapy against cancer, *Adv. Drug Deliv. Rev.* **2002**, *54*, 715–758.
4 Bianco, A., Kostarelos, K., Partidos, C. D., Prato, M. Biomedical applications of functionalised carbon nanotubes, *Chem. Commun.* **2005**, 571–577.
5 Lin, Y., Taylor, S., Li, H., Fernando, K. A., Qu, L., Wang, W., Gu, L., Zhou, B., Sun, Y. P. Advances toward bioapplications of carbon nanotubes, *J. Mater. Chem.* **2004**, *14*, 527–541.
6 Kostarelos, K., Lacerda, L., Partidos, C. D., Prato, M., Bianco, A. Carbon nanotube-mediated delivery of peptides and genes to cells: translating nanobiotechnology to therapeutics, *J. Drug Deliv. Sci. Technol.* **2005**, *15*, 41–47.
7 Bianco, A., Hoebeke, J., Kostarelos, K., Prato, M., Partidos, C. D. Carbon nanotubes: on the road to deliver, *Curr. Drug Deliv.* **2005**, *2*, 253–259.
8 Pastorin, G., Kostarelos, K., Prato, M., Bianco, A. Functionalized carbon nanotubes: towards the delivery of therapeutic molecules, *J. Biomed. Nanotechnol.* **2005**, *1*, 133–142.
9 Katz, E., Willner, I. Biomolecule-functionalized carbon nanotubes: applications in nanobioelectronics, *ChemPhysChem* **2004**, *5*, 1084–1104.
10 Fortina, P., Kricka, L. J., Surrey, S., Grodzinski, P. Nanobiotechnology: the promise and reality of new approaches to molecular recognition, *Trends Biotechnol.* **2005**, *23*, 168–173.
11 Yu, M.-F., Files, B. S., Arepalli, S., Ruoff, R. S. Tensile loading of ropes of single wall carbon nanotubes and their mechanical properties, *Phys. Rev. Lett.* **2000**, *84*, 5552–5555.
12 Saito, R., Dresselhaus, G., Dresselhaus, M. S. *Physical Properties of Carbon Nanotubes*. Imperial College Press, London, **1998**.
13 Saito, R., Fujita, M., Dresselhaus, G., Dresselhaus, M. S. Electronic structure of chiral graphene tubules, *Appl. Phys. Lett.* **1992**, *60*, 2204–2206.
14 Saito, R., Fujita, M., Dresselhaus, G., Dresselhaus, M. S. Electronic structure of graphene tubules based on C_{60}, *Phys. Rev. B* **1992**, *46*, 1804–1811.

15 Hamada, N., Sawada, S., Oshiyama, A. New one-dimensional conductors: graphitic microtubules, *Phys. Rev. Lett.* **1992**, *68*, 1579–1581.
16 Kaiser, A. B., Düsberg, G., Roth, S. Heterogeneous model for conduction in carbon nanotubes, *Phys. Rev. B* **1998**, *57*, 1418–1421.
17 Dresselhaus, M. S., Dresselhaus, G., Eklund, P. C. *Science of Fullerenes and Carbon Nanotubes*. Academic Press, New York, **1996**.
18 Iijima, S. Carbon nanotubes: past, present, and future, *Physica B* **2002**, *323*, 1–5.
19 Journet, C., Maser, W. K., Bernier, P., Loiseau, A., Lamy de la Chapelle, M., Lefrant, A., Denard, P., Lee, R., Fischer, J. E. Large-scale production of single-walled carbon nanotubes by the electric-arc technique, *Nature* **1997**, *388*, 756–758.
20 Rinzler, A. G., Liu, J., Dai, H., Nikolaev, P., Huffman, C. B., Rodriguez-Macias, F. J., Boul, P. J., Lu, A. H., Heymann, D., Colbert, D. T., Lee, R. S., Fischer, J. E., Rao, A. M., Eklund, P. C., Smalley, R. E. Large-scale purification of single-wall carbon nanotubes: process, product, and characterization, *Appl. Phys. A* **1998**, *67*, 29–37.
21 Endo, M., Takeuchi, K., Kobori, K., Takahashi, K., Kroto, H. W., Sarkar, A. Pyrolytic carbon nanotubes from vapor-grown carbon fibers, *Carbon* **1995**, *33*, 873–881.
22 Nikolaev, P., Bronikowski, M., Bradley, R. K., Rohmund, F., Colbert, D. T., Smith, K., Smalley, R. E. Gas-phase catalytic growth of single-walled carbon nanotubes from carbon monoxide, *Chem. Phys. Lett.* **1999**, *313*, 91–97.
23 Ajayan, P. M. Nanotubes from carbon, *Chem. Rev.* **1999**, *99*, 1787–1799.
24 Xie, S. S., Chang, B. H., Li, W. Z., Pan, Z. W., Sun, L. F., Mao, J. M., Chen, X. H., Qian, L. X., Zhou, W. Y. Synthesis and characterization of aligned carbon nanotube arrays, *Adv. Mater.* **1999**, *11*, 1135–1138.
25 Dai, L., Mau, A. W. H. Controlled synthesis and modification of carbon nanotubes and C_{60}: carbon nanostructures for advanced polymeric composite materials, *Adv. Mater.* **2001**, *13*, 899–913.
26 Rao, C. N. R., Satishkumar, B. C., Govindaraj, A., Nath, M. Nanotubes, *ChemPhysChem* **2001**, *2*, 78–105.
27 Bahr, J. L., Mickelson, E. T., Bronikowski, M. J., Smalley, R. E., Tour, J. M. Dissolution of small diameter single-wall carbon nanotubes in organic solvents?, *Chem. Commun.* **2001**, 193–194.
28 Liu, J., Rinzler, A. G., Dai, H., Hafner, J. H., Bradley, R. K., Boul, P. J., Lu, A., Iverson, T., Shelimov, K., Huffman, C. B., Rodriguez-Macias, F., Shon, Y.-S., Lee, T. R., Colbert, D. T., Smalley, R. E. Fullerene pipes, *Science* **1998**, *280*, 1253–1256.
29 Bandow, S., Rao, A. M., Williams, K. A., Thess, A., Smalley, R. E., Eklund, P. C. Purification of single-wall carbon nanotubes by microfiltration, *J. Phys. Chem. B* **1997**, *101*, 8839–8842.
30 Duesberg, G. S., Burghard, M., Muster, J., Philipp, G., Roth, S. Separation of carbon nanotubes by size exclusion chromatography, *Chem. Commun.* **1998**, 435–436.
31 Holzinger, M., Hirsch, A., Bernier, P., Duesberg, G. S., Burghard, M. A new purification method for single-wall carbon nanotubes (SWNTs), *Appl. Phys. A* **2000**, *70*, 599–602.
32 Martinez, M., Callejas, M., Benito, A. M., Maser, W. K., Cochet, M., Andres, J. M., Schreiber, J., Chauvet, O., Fierro, J. L. G. Microwave single walled carbon nanotubes purification, *Chem. Commun.* **2002**, 1000–1001.
33 Vazquez, E., Georgakilas, V., Prato, M. Microwave-assisted purification of HIPCO carbon nanotubes, *Chem. Commun.* **2002**, 2308–2309.
34 Harutyunyan, A. R., Pradhan, B. K., Chang, J., Chen, G., Eklund, P. C. Purification of single-wall carbon nanotubes by selective microwave

heating of catalyst particles, *J. Phys. Chem. B* **2002**, *106*, 8671–8675.

35 Chen, R. J., Zhang, Y., Wang, D., Dai, H. Noncovalent sidewall functionalization of single-walled carbon nanotubes for protein immobilization, *J. Am. Chem. Soc.* **2001**, *123*, 3838–3839.

36 Besteman, K., Lee, J.-O., Wiertz, F. G. M., Heering, H. A., Dekker, C. Enzyme-coated carbon nanotubes as single-molecule biosensors, *Nano Lett.* **2003**, *3*, 727–730.

37 Xin, H., Woolley, A. T. DNA-templated nanotube localization, *J. Am. Chem. Soc.* **2003**, *125*, 8710–8711.

38 Taft, B. J., Lazareck, A. D., Withey, G. D., Yin, A., Xu, J. M., Kelley, S. O. Site-specific assembly of DNA and appended cargo on arrayed carbon nanotubes, *J. Am. Chem. Soc.* **2004**, *126*, 12750–12751.

39 Liu, L., Wang, T., Li, J., Guo, Z., Dai, L., Zhang, D., Zhu, D. Self-assembly of gold nanoparticles to carbon nanotubes using a thiol-terminated pyrene as interlinker, *Chem. Phys. Lett.* **2003**, *367*, 747–752.

40 Cao, L., Chen, H., Wang, M., Sun, J., Zhang, X., Kong, F. Photoconductivity study of modified carbon nanotube/oxotitanium phthalocyanine composites, *J. Phys. Chem. B* **2002**, *106*, 8971–8975.

41 Wang, X., Liu, Y., Qiu, W., Zhu, D. Immobilization of tetra-*tert*-butylphthalocyanines on carbon nanotubes: a first step towards the development of new nanomaterials, *J. Mater. Chem.* **2002**, *12*, 1636–1639.

42 Cao, L., Chen, H.-Z., Zhou, H.-B., Zhu, L., Sun, J.-Z., Zhang, X.-B., Xu, J.-M., Wang, M. Carbon-nanotube-templated assembly of rare-earth phthalocyanine nanowires, *Adv. Mater.* **2003**, *15*, 909–913.

43 Guldi, D. M., Rahman, G. N. A., Ramey, J., Marcaccio, M., Paolucci, D., Paolucci, F., Qin, S., Ford, W. T., Balbinot, D., Jux, N., Tagmatarchis, N., Prato, M. Donor–acceptor nanoensembles of soluble carbon nanotubes, *Chem. Commun.* **2004**, 2034–2035.

44 Guldi, D. M., Rahman, G. M. A., Prato, M., Jux, N., Qin, S., Ford, W. Single-wall carbon nanotubes as integrative building blocks for solar-energy conversion, *Angew. Chem. Int. Ed.* **2005**, *44*, 2015–2018.

45 Murakami, H., Nomura, T., Nakashima, N. Noncovalent porphyrin-functionalized single-walled carbon nanotubes in solution and the formation of porphyrin–nanotube nanocomposites, *Chem. Phys. Lett.* **2003**, *378*, 481–485.

46 Li, H., Zhou, B., Lin, Y., Gu, L., Wang, W., Fernando, K. A. S., Kumar, S., Allard, L. F., Sun, Y.-P. Selective interactions of porphyrins with semiconducting single-walled carbon nanotubes, *J. Am. Chem. Soc.* **2004**, *126*, 1014–1015.

47 Chen, J., Collier, C. P. Noncovalent functionalization of single-walled carbon nanotubes with water-soluble porphyrins, *J. Phys. Chem. B* **2005**, *109*, 7605–7609.

48 Satake, A., Miyajima, Y., Kobuke, Y. Porphyrin–carbon nanotube composites formed by noncovalent polymer wrapping, *Chem. Mater.* **2005**, *17*, 716–724.

49 Guldi, D. M., Rahman, G. M. A., Jux, N., Tagmatarchis, N., Prato, M. Integrating single-wall carbon nanotubes into donor–acceptor nanohybrids, *Angew. Chem. Int. Ed.* **2004**, *43*, 5526–5530.

50 Guldi, D. M., Rahman, G. M. A., Jux, N., Balbinot, D., Tagmatarchis, N., Prato, M. Multiwalled carbon nanotubes in donor–acceptor nanohybrids – towards long-lived electron transfer products, *Chem. Commun.* **2005**, 2038–2040.

51 Guldi, D. M., Taieb, H., Rahman, G. M. A., Tagmatarchis, N., Prato, M. Novel photoactive single-walled carbon nanotube–porphyrin polymer wraps: efficient and long-lived intracomplex charge separation, *Adv. Mater.* **2005**, *17*, 871–875.

52 Guldi, D. M., Rahman, G. M. A., Jux, N., Balbinot, D., Hartnagel, U., Tagmatarchis, N., Prato, M. Functional single-wall carbon

nanotube nanohybrids-associating SWNTs with water-soluble enzyme model systems, *J. Am. Chem. Soc.* **2005**, *127*, 9830–9838.

53 Chichak, K. S., Star, A., Altoe, M. V. P., Stoddart, J. F. Single-walled carbon nanotubes under the influence of dynamic coordination and supramolecular chemistry, *Small* **2005**, *1*, 452–461.

54 Tang, B. Z., Xu, H. Preparation, alignment, and optical properties of soluble poly(phenylacetylene)-wrapped carbon nanotubes, *Macromolecules* **1999**, *32*, 2569–2576.

55 Romero, D. B., Carrard, M., de Heer, W., Zuppiroli, L. A carbon nanotube/organic semiconducting polymer heterojunction, *Adv. Mater.* **1996**, *8*, 899–902.

56 Ago, H., Petritsch, K., Shaffer, M. S. P., Windle, A. H., Friend, R. H. Composites of carbon nanotubes and conjugated polymers for photovoltaic devices, *Adv. Mater.* **1999**, *11*, 1281–1285.

57 Ago, H., Shaffer, M. S. P., Ginger, D. S., Windle, A. H., Friend, R. H. Electronic interaction between photoexcited poly(*p*-phenylene vinylene) and carbon nanotubes, *Phys. Rev. B* **2000**, *61*, 2286–2290.

58 Wery, J., Aarab, H., Lefrant, S., Faulques, E., Mulazzi, E., Perego, R. Photoexcitations in composites of poly(paraphenylene vinylene) and single-walled carbon nanotubes, *Phys. Rev. B* **2003**, *67*, 115202 (1–6).

59 Fournet, P., Coleman, J. N., Lahr, B., Drury, A., Blau, W. J., O'Brien, D. F., Horhold, H. H. Enhanced brightness in organic light-emitting diodes using a carbon nanotube composite as an electron-transport layer, *J. Appl. Phys.* **2001**, *90*, 969–975.

60 Fournet, P., O'Brien, D. F., Coleman, J. N., Horhold, H. H., Blau, W. J. A carbon nanotube composite as an electron transport layer for M3EH-PPV based light-emitting diodes, *Synth. Met.* **2001**, *121*, 1683–1684.

61 Dalton, A. B., Stephan, C., Coleman, J. N., McCarthy, B., Ajayan, P. M., Lefrant, S., Bernier, P., Blau, W. J., Byrne, H. J. Selective interaction of a semiconjugated organic polymer with single-wall nanotubes, *J. Phys. Chem. B* **2000**, *104*, 10012–10016.

62 Coleman, J. N., Dalton, A. B., Curran, S., Rubio, A., Davey, A. P., Drury, A., McCarthy, B., Lahr, B., Ajayan, P. M., Roth, S., Barklie, R. C., Blau, W. J. Phase separation of carbon nanotubes and turbostratic graphite using a functional organic polymer, *Adv. Mater.* **2000**, *12*, 213–216.

63 Star, A., Lu, Y., Bradley, K., Gruner, G. Nanotube optoelectronic memory devices, *Nano Lett.* **2004**, *4*, 1587–1591.

64 Murphy, R., Coleman, J. N., Cadek, M., McCarthy, B., Bent, M., Drury, A., Barklie, R. C., Blau, W. J. High-yield, nondestructive purification and quantification method for multiwalled carbon nanotubes, *J. Phys. Chem. B.* **2002**, *106*, 3087–3091.

65 Coleman, J. N., O'Brien, D. F., Dalton, A. B., McCarthy, B., Lahr, B., Barklie, R. C., Blau, W. J. Electron paramagnetic resonance as a quantitative tool for the study of multiwalled carbon nanotubes, *J. Chem. Phys.* **2000**, *113*, 9788–9793.

66 Star, A., Stoddart, J. F., Steuerman, D., Diehl, M., Boukai, A., Wong, E. W., Yang, X., Chung, S. W., Choi, H., Heath, J. R. Preparation and properties of polymer-wrapped single-walled carbon nanotubes, *Angew. Chem. Int. Ed.* **2001**, *40*, 1721–1725.

67 Steuerman, D. W., Star, A., Narizzano, R., Choi, H., Ries, R. S., Nicolini, C., Stoddart, J. F., Heath, J. R. Interactions between conjugated polymers and single-walled carbon nanotubes, *J. Phys. Chem. B* **2002**, *106*, 3124–3130.

68 Star, A., Stoddart, J. F. Dispersion and solubilization of single-walled carbon nanotubes with a hyperbranched polymer, *Macromolecules* **2002**, *35*, 7516–7520.

69 Musa, I., Baxendale, M., Amaratunga, G. A. J., Eccleston, W.

Properties of regioregular poly(3-octylthiophene)/multi-wall carbon nanotube composites, *Synth. Met.* **1999**, *102*, 1250.

70 Alexandrou, I., Kymakis, E., Amaratunga, G. A. J. Polymer–nanotube composites: burying nanotubes improves their field emission properties, *Appl. Phys. Lett.* **2002**, *80*, 1435–1437.

71 Valentini, L., Armentano, I., Biagiotti, J., Frulloni, E., Kenny, J. M., Santucci, S. Frequency dependent electrical transport between conjugated polymer and single-walled carbon nanotubes, *Diam. Rel. Mater.* **2003**, *12*, 1601–1609.

72 Kymakis, E., Amaratunga, G. A. J. Single-wall carbon nanotube/conjugated polymer photovoltaic devices, *Appl. Phys. Lett.* **2002**, *80*, 112–114.

73 Kymakis, E., Alexandrou, I., Amaratunga, G. A. J. High open-circuit voltage photovoltaic devices from carbon-nanotube–polymer composites, *J. Appl. Phys.* **2003**, *93*, 1764–1768.

74 Bhattacharyya, S., Kymakis, E., Amaratunga, G. A. J. Photovoltaic properties of dye functionalized single-wall carbon nanotube/conjugated polymer devices, *Chem. Mater.* **2004**, *16*, 4819–4823.

75 Landi, B. J., Raffaelle, R. P., Castro, S. L., Bailey, S. G. Single-wall carbon nanotube-polymer solar cells, *Prog. Photovolt. Res. Appl.* **2005**, *13*, 165–172.

76 O'Connell, M. J., Boul, P., Ericson, L. M., Huffman, C., Wang, Y., Haroz, E., Kuper, C., Tour, J. M., Ausman, K. D., Smalley, R. E. Reversible water-solubilization of single-walled carbon nanotubes by polymer wrapping, *Chem. Phys. Lett.* **2001**, *342*, 265–271.

77 Islam, M. F., Rojas, E., Bergey, D. M., Johnson, A. T., Yodh, A. G. High weight fraction surfactant solubilization of single-wall carbon nanotubes in water, *Nano Lett.* **2003**, *3*, 269–273.

78 Richard, C., Balavoine, F., Schultz, P., Ebbesen, T. W., Mioskowski, C. Supramolecular self-assembly of lipid derivatives on carbon nanotubes, *Science* **2003**, *300*, 775–778.

79 O'Connell, M. J., Bachilo, S. M., Huffman, C. B., Moore, V. C., Strano, M. S., Haroz, E. H., Rialon, K. L., Boul, P. J., Noon, W. H., Kittrell, C., Ma, J., Hauge, R. H., Weisman, R. B., Smalley, R. E. Band gap fluorescence from individual single-walled carbon nanotubes, *Science* **2002**, *297*, 593–596.

80 Moore, V. C., Strano, M. S., Haroz, E. H., Hauge, R. H., Smalley, R. E. Individually suspended single-walled carbon nanotubes in various surfactants, *Nano Lett.* **2003**, *3*, 1379–1382.

81 Wenseleers, W., Vlasov, I. I., Goovaerts, E., Obraztsova, E. D., Lobach, A. S., Bouwen, A. Efficient isolation and solubilization of pristine single-walled nanotubes in bile salt micelles, *Adv. Funct. Mater.* **2004**, *14*, 1105–1112.

82 Bachilo, S. M., Strano, M. S., Kittrell, C., Hauge, R. H., Smalley, R. E., Weisman, R. B. Structure-assigned optical spectra of single-walled carbon nanotubes, *Science* **2002**, *298*, 2361–2366.

83 Hagen, A., Hertel, T. Quantitative analysis of optical spectra from individual single-wall carbon nanotubes, *Nano Lett.* **2003**, *3*, 383–388.

84 Strano, M. S., Doorn, S. K., Haroz, E. H., Kittrell, C., Hauge, R. H., Smalley, R. E. Assignment of (n, m) Raman and optical features of metallic single-walled carbon nanotubes, *Nano Lett.* **2003**, *3*, 1091–1096.

85 Weisman, R. B., Bachilo, S. M. Dependence of optical transition energies on structure for single-walled carbon nanotubes in aqueous suspension: an empirical Kataura plot, *Nano Lett.* **2003**, *3*, 1235–1238.

86 Dyke, C. A., Tour, J. M. Unbundled and highly functionalized carbon nanotubes from aqueous reactions, *Nano Lett.* **2003**, *3*, 1215–1218.

87 Dieckmann, G. R., Dalton, A. B., Johnson, P. A., Razal, J., Chen, J., Giordano, G. M., Muñoz, E.,

Musselman, I. H., Baughman, R. H., Draper, R. K. Controlled assembly of carbon nanotubes by designed amphiphilic peptide helices, *J. Am. Chem. Soc.* **2003**, *125*, 1770–1777.

88 Zorbas, V., Ortiz-Acevedo, A., Dalton, A. B., Yoshida, M. M., Dieckmann, G. R., Draper, R. K., Baughman, R. H., Jose-Yacaman, M., Musselman, I. H. Preparation and characterization of individual peptide-wrapped single-walled carbon nanotubes, *J. Am. Chem. Soc.* **2004**, *126*, 7222–7227.

89 Zorbas, V., Smith, A. L., Xie, H., Ortiz-Acevedo, A., Dalton, A. B., Dieckmann, G. R., Draper, R. K., Baughman, R. H., Musselman, I. H. Importance of aromatic content for peptide/single-walled carbon nanotube interactions, *J. Am. Chem. Soc.* **2005**, *127*, 12323–12328.

90 Kam, N. W. S., Dai, H. Carbon nanotubes as intracellular protein transporters: generality and biological functionality, *J. Am. Chem. Soc.* **2005**, *127*, 6021–6026.

91 Zheng, M., Jagota, A., Semke, E. D., Diner, B. A., Mclean, R. S., Lustig, S. R., Richardson, R. E., Tassi, N. G. DNA-assisted dispersion and separation of carbon nanotubes, *Nat. Mater.* **2003**, *2*, 338–342.

92 Zheng, M., Jagota, A., Strano, M. S., Santos, A. P., Barone, P., Chou, S. G., Diner, B. A., Dresselhaus, M. S., Mclean, R. S., Onoa, G. B., Samsonidze, G. G., Semke, E. D., Usrey, M., Walls, D. J. Structure-based carbon nanotube sorting by sequence-dependent DNA assembly, *Science* **2003**, *302*, 1545–1548.

93 Kam, N. W. S., Liu, Z., Dai, H. Functionalization of carbon nanotubes via cleavable disulfide bonds for efficient intracellular delivery of siRNA and potent gene silencing, *J. Am. Chem. Soc.* **2005**, *127*, 12492–12493.

94 Hirsch, A. Functionalization of single-walled carbon nanotubes, *Angew. Chem. Int. Ed.* **2002**, *41*, 1853–1859.

95 Banerjee, S., Hemraj-Benny, T., Wong, S. S. Covalent surface chemistry of single-walled carbon nanotubes, *Adv. Mater.* **2005**, *17*, 17–29.

96 Hamon, M. A., Chen, J., Hu, H., Chen, Y., Itkis, M. E., Rao, A. M., Eklund, P. C., Haddon, R. C. Dissolution of single-walled carbon nanotubes, *Adv. Mater.* **1999**, *11*, 834–840.

97 Kukovecz, A., Kramberger, C., Holzinger, M., Kuzmany, H., Schalko, J., Mannsberger, M., Hirsch, A. On the stacking behavior of functionalized single-wall carbon nanotubes, *J. Phys. Chem. B* **2002**, *106*, 6374–6380.

98 Chen, J., Rao, A. M., Lyuksyutov, S., Itkis, M. E., Hamon, M. A., Hu, H., Cohn, R. W., Eklund, P. C., Colbert, D. T., Smalley, R. E., Haddon, R. C. Dissolution of full-length single-walled carbon nanotubes, *J. Phys. Chem. B* **2001**, *105*, 2525–2528.

99 Niyogi, S., Hamon, M. A., Hu, H., Zhao, B., Bhowmik, P., Sen, R., Itkis, M. E., Haddon, R. C. Chemistry of single-walled carbon nanotubes, *Acc. Chem. Res.* **2002**, *35*, 1105–1113.

100 Hiura, H., Ebbesen, T. W., Tanigaki, K. Opening and purification of carbon nanotubes in high yields, *Adv. Mater.* **1995**, *7*, 275–276.

101 Ajayan, P. M., Ebbesen, T. W., Ichihashi, T., Iijima, S., Tanigaki, K., Hiura, H. Capillarity-induced filling of carbon nanotubes, *Nature* **1993**, *361*, 333–334.

102 Chen, J., Hamon, M. A., Hu, H., Chen, Y., Rao, A. M., Eklund, P. C., Haddon, R. C. Solution properties of single-walled carbon nanotubes, *Science* **1998**, *282*, 95–98.

103 Lago, R. M., Tsang, S. C., Lu, K. L., Chen, Y. K., Green, M. L. H. Filling carbon nanotubes with small palladium metal crystallites: the effect of surface acid groups, *Chem. Commun.* **1995**, 1355–1356.

104 Lu, K. L., Lago, R. M., Chen, Y. K., Green, M. L. H., Harris, P. J. F., Tsang, S. C. Mechanical damage of carbon nanotubes by ultrasound, *Carbon* **1996**, *34*, 814–816.

105 Monthioux, M., Smith, B. W., Burteaux, B., Claye, A., Fischer, J. E., Luzzi, D. E. Sensitivity of single-wall carbon nanotubes to chemical processing: an electron microscopy investigation, *Carbon* **2001**, *39*, 1251–1272.

106 Koshio, A., Yudasaka, M., Zhang, M., Iijima, S. A simple way to chemically react single-wall carbon nanotubes with organic materials using ultrasonication, *Nano Lett.* **2001**, *1*, 361–363.

107 Qin, Y., Shi, J., Wu, W., Li, X., Guo, Z., Zhu, D. Concise route to functionalized carbon nanotubes, *J. Phys. Chem. B* **2003**, *107*, 12899–12901.

108 Chen, Y., Haddon, R. C., Fang, S., Rao, A. M., Eklund, P. C., Lee, W. H., Dickey, E. C., Grulke, E. A., Pendergrass, J. C., Chavan, A., Haley, B. E., Smalley, R. E. Chemical attachment of organic functional groups to single-walled carbon nanotube material, *J. Mater. Res.* **1998**, *13*, 2423–2431.

109 Sun, Y.-P., Huang, W., Lin, Y., Fu, K., Kitaygorodskiy, A., Riddle, L. A., Yu, Y. J., Carroll, D. L. Soluble dendron-functionalized carbon nanotubes: preparation, characterization, and properties, *Chem. Mater.* **2001**, *13*, 2864–2869.

110 Fu, K., Huang, W., Lin, Y., Riddle, L. A., Carroll, D. L., Sun, Y.-P. Defunctionalization of functionalized carbon nanotubes, *Nano Lett.* **2001**, *1*, 439–441.

111 Sun, Y.-P., Fu, K., Lin, Y., Huang, W. Functionalized carbon nanotubes: properties and applications, *Acc. Chem. Res.* **2002**, *35*, 1096–1104.

112 Kong, H., Gao, C., Yan, D. Controlled functionalization of multiwalled carbon nanotubes by in situ atom transfer radical polymerization, *J. Am. Chem. Soc.* **2004**, *126*, 412–413.

113 Qin, S., Qin, D., Ford, W. T., Resasco, D. E., Herrera, J. E. Polymer brushes on single-walled carbon nanotubes by atom transfer radical polymerization of *n*-butyl methacrylate, *J. Am. Chem. Soc.* **2004**, *126*, 170–176.

114 Huang, W., Taylor, S., Fu, K., Lin, Y., Zhang, D., Hanks, T. W., Rao, A. M., Sun, Y.-P. Attaching proteins to carbon nanotubes via diimide-activated amidation, *Nano Lett.* **2002**, *2*, 311–314.

115 Kam, N. W. S., Jessop, T. C., Wender, P. A., Dai, H. Nanotube molecular transporters: internalization of carbon nanotube–protein conjugates into mammalian cells, *J. Am. Chem. Soc.* **2004**, *126*, 6850–6851.

116 Yim, T., Liu, J., Lu, Y., Kane, R. S., Dordick, J. S. Highly active and stable DNAzyme–carbon nanotube hybrids, *J. Am. Chem. Soc.* **2005**, *127*, 12200–12201.

117 Baker, S. E., Cai, W., Lasseter, T. L., Weidkamp, K. P., Hamers, R. J. Covalently bonded adducts of deoxyribonucleic acid (DNA) oligonucleotides with single-wall carbon nanotubes: synthesis and hybridization, *Nano Lett.* **2002**, *2*, 1413–1417.

118 Hazani, M., Naaman, R., Hennrich, F., Kappes, M. M. Confocal fluorescence imaging of DNA–functionalized carbon nanotubes, *Nano Lett.* **2003**, *3*, 153–155.

119 Williams, K. A., Veenhuizen, P. T. M., de la Torre, B. G., Eritja, R., Dekker, C. Nanotechnology: carbon nanotubes with DNA recognition, *Nature* **2002**, *420*, 761.

120 Tasis, D., Tagmatarchis, N., Bianco, A., Prato, M. Chemistry of carbon nanotubes, *Chem. Rev.* **2006**, *106*, 1105–1136.

121 Jorio, A., Dresselhaus, G., Dresselhaus, M. S., Souza, M., Dantas, M. S. S., Pimenta, M. A., Rao, A. M., Saito, R., Liu, C., Cheng, H. M. Polarized Raman study of single-wall semiconducting carbon nanotubes, *Phys. Rev. Lett.* **2000**, *85*, 2617–2620.

122 Holden, J. M., Zhou, P., Bi, X., Eklund, P. C., Bandow, S., Jishi, R. A., Chowdhury, K. D., Dresselhaus, G., Dresselhaus, M. S. Raman scattering from nanoscale carbons

generated in a cobalt-catalyzed carbon plasma, *Chem. Phys. Lett.* **1994**, *220*, 186–191.

123 Bahr, J. L., Tour, J. M. Covalent chemistry of single-wall carbon nanotubes, *J. Mater. Chem.* **2002**, *12*, 1952–1958.

124 Mickelson, E. T., Huffman, C. B., Rinzler, A. G., Smalley, R. E., Hauge, R. H., Margrave, J. L. Fluorination of single-wall carbon nanotubes, *Chem. Phys. Lett.* **1998**, *296*, 188–194.

125 Mickelson, E. T., Chiang, I. W., Zimmerman, J. L., Boul, P. J., Lozano, J., Liu, J., Smalley, R. E., Hauge, R. H., Margrave, J. L. Solvation of fluorinated single-wall carbon nanotubes in alcohol solvents, *J. Phys. Chem. B* **1999**, *103*, 4318–4322.

126 Boul, P. J., Liu, J., Mickelson, E. T., Huffman, C. B., Ericson, L. M., Chiang, I. W., Smith, K. A., Colbert, D. T., Hauge, R. H., Margrave, J. L., Smalley, R. E. Reversible sidewall functionalization of buckytubes, *Chem. Phys. Lett.* **1999**, *310*, 367–372.

127 Khabashesku, V. N., Billups, W. E., Margrave, J. L. Fluorination of single-wall carbon nanotubes and subsequent derivatization reactions, *Acc. Chem. Res.* **2002**, *35*, 1087–1095.

128 Holzinger, M., Vostrowsky, O., Hirsch, A., Hennrich, F., Kappes, M., Weiss, R., Jellen, F. Sidewall functionalization of carbon nanotubes, *Angew. Chem. Int. Ed. Engl.* **2001**, *40*, 4002–4005.

129 Bahr, J. L., Yang, J., Kosynkin, D. V., Broniskowski, M. J., Smalley, R. E., Tour, J. M. Functionalization of carbon nanotubes by electrochemical reduction of aryl diazonium salts: a bucky paper electrode, *J. Am. Chem. Soc.* **2001**, *123*, 6536–6542.

130 Bahr, J. L., Tour, J. M. Highly functionalized carbon nanotubes using in situ generated diazonium compounds, *Chem. Mater.* **2001**, *13*, 3823–3824.

131 Dyke, C. A., Tour, J. M. Solvent-free functionalization of carbon nanotubes, *J. Am. Chem. Soc.* **2003**, *125*, 1156–1157.

132 Ying, Y., Saini, R. K., Liang, F., Sadana, A. K., Billups, W. E. Functionalization of carbon nanotubes by free radicals, *Org. Lett.* **2003**, *5*, 1471–1473.

133 Peng, H., Reverdy, P., Khabashesku, V. N., Margrave, J. L. Sidewall functionalization of single-walled carbon nanotubes with organic peroxides, *Chem. Comm.* **2003**, 362–363.

134 Strano, M. S., Dyke, C. A., Usrey, M. L., Barone, P. W., Allen, M. J., Shan, H., Kittrell, C., Hauge, R. H., Tour, J. M., Smalley, R. E. Electronic structure control of single-walled carbon nanotube functionalization, *Science* **2003**, *301*, 1519–1522.

135 Hamon, M. A., Itkis, M. E., Niyogi, S., Alvaraez, T., Kuper, C., Menon, M., Haddon, R. C. Effect of rehybridization on the electronic structure of single-walled carbon nanotubes, *J. Am. Chem. Soc.* **2001**, *123*, 11292–11293.

136 Viswanathan, G., Chakrapani, N., Yang, H., Wei, B., Chung, H., Cho, K., Ryu, C. Y., Ajayan, P. M. Single-step *in situ* synthesis of polymer-grafted single-wall nanotube composites, *J. Am. Chem. Soc.* **2003**, *125*, 9258–9259.

137 Wu, W., Zhang, S., Li, Y., Li, J., Lu, L., Qin, Y., Guo, Z., Dai, L., Ye, C., Zhu, D. PVK-modified single-walled carbon nanotubes with effective photoinduced electron transfer, *Macromolecules* **2003**, *36*, 6286–6288.

138 Pekker, S., Salvetat, J.-P., Jakab, E., Bonard, J.-M., Forro, L. Hydrogenation of carbon nanotubes and graphite in liquid ammonia, *J. Phys. Chem. B* **2001**, *105*, 7938–7943.

139 Tagmatarchis, N., Georgakilas, V., Prato, M., Shinohara, H. Sidewall functionalization of single-walled carbon nanotubes through electrophilic addition, *Chem. Commun.* **2002**, 2010–2011.

140 Coleman, K. S., Bailey, S. R., Fogden, S., Green, M. L. H. Functionalization of single-walled

carbon nanotubes via the Bingel reaction, *J. Am. Chem. Soc.* **2003**, *125*, 8722–8723.

141 Worsley, K. A., Moonoosawmy, K. R., Kruse, P. Long-range periodicity in carbon nanotube sidewall functionalization, *Nano Lett.* **2004**, *4*, 1541–1546.

142 Moghaddam, M. J., Taylor, S., Gao, M., Huang, S., Dai, L., McCall, M. J. Highly efficient binding of DNA on the sidewalls and tips of carbon nanotubes using photochemistry, *Nano Lett.* **2004**, *4*, 89–93.

143 Georgakilas, V., Kordatos, K., Prato, M., Guldi, D. M., Holzinger, M., Hirsch, A. Organic functionalization of carbon nanotubes, *J. Am. Chem. Soc.* **2002**, *124*, 760–761.

144 Lu, X., Tian, F., Xu, X., Wang, N., Zhang, Q. Theoretical exploration of the 1,3-dipolar cycloadditions onto the sidewalls of (n, n) armchair single-wall carbon nanotubes, *J. Am. Chem. Soc.* **2003**, *125*, 10459–10464.

145 Yao, Z., Braidy, N., Botton, G. A., Adronov, A. Polymerization from the surface of single-walled carbon nanotubes – preparation and characterization of nanocomposites, *J. Am. Chem. Soc.* **2003**, *125*, 16015–16024.

146 Georgakilas, V., Tagmatarchis, N., Pantarotto, D., Bianco, A., Briand, J.-P., Prato, M. Amino acid functionalization of water soluble carbon nanotubes, *Chem. Commun.* **2002**, 3050–3051.

147 Georgakilas, V., Voulgaris, D., Vazquez, E., Prato, M., Guldi, D. M., Kukovecz, A., Kuzmany, H. Purification of HiPCO carbon nanotubes via organic functionalization, *J. Am. Chem. Soc.* **2002**, *124*, 14318–14319.

148 Pantorotto, D., Partidos, C. D., Graff, R., Hoebeke, J., Briand, J.-P., Prato, M., Bianco, A. Synthesis, structural characterization, and immunological properties of carbon nanotubes functionalized with peptides, *J. Am. Chem. Soc.* **2003**, *125*, 6160–6164.

149 Bianco, A., Prato, M. Can carbon nanotubes be considered useful tools for biological applications?, *Adv. Mater.* **2003**, *15*, 1765–1768.

150 Chopra, N., Majumder, M., Hinds, B. J. Bifunctional carbon nanotubes by sidewall protection, *Adv. Funct. Mater.* **2005**, *15*, 858–864.

151 Lee, K. M., Li, L., Dai, L. Asymmetric end-functionalization of multi-walled carbon nanotubes, *J. Am. Chem. Soc.* **2005**, *127*, 4122–4123.

152 Wu, W., Wieckowski, S., Pastorin, G., Benincasa, M., Klumpp, C., Briand, J.-P., Gennaro, R., Prato, M., Bianco, A. Targeted delivery of amphotericin B to cells using functionalized carbon nanotubes, *Angew. Chem. Int. Ed.* **2005**, *44*, 6358–6362.

153 Scheller, F. W., Wollenberger, U., Warsinke, A., Lisdat, F. Research and development in biosensors, *Curr. Opin. Biotechnol.* **2001**, *12*, 35–40.

154 Meadows, D. Recent developments with biosensing technology and applications in the pharmaceutical industry, *Adv. Drug. Deliv. Rev.* **1996**, *21*, 179–189.

155 Tess, M. E., Cox, J. A. Chemical and biochemical sensors based on advances in materials chemistry, *J. Pharm. Biomed. Anal.* **1999**, *19*, 55–68.

156 Popov, V. N. Carbon nanotubes: properties and application, *Mater. Sci. Eng.* **2004**, *R43*, 61–102.

157 Special Issue on Carbon Nanotubes, *Acc. Chem. Res.* **2002**, *35*, 997–1113.

158 Tans, S. J., Verschueren, A. R. M., Dekker, C. Room-temperature transistor based on a single carbon nanotube, *Nature* **1998**, *393*, 49–52.

159 Davis, J. J., Green, M. L. H., Hill, H. A. O., Leung, Y. C., Sloan, J., Sadler, P. J., Xavier, A. V., Tsang, S. C. The immobilisation of proteins in carbon nanotubes, *Inorg. Chim. Acta* **1998**, *272*, 261–266.

160 Snow, E. S., Perkins, F. K., Houser, E. J., Badescu, S. C., Reinecke, T. L. Chemical detection with a single-walled carbon nanotube capacitor, *Science* **2005**, *307*, 1942–1945.

161 Qian, K., Yan, B., Lin, Y., Xu, D., Cai, B., Chen, T., Sun, Z. Research

on carbon nanotube array field emission pressure sensors, *Electron. Lett.* **2005**, *41*, 824–825.

162 Postma, H. W. C., Teepen, T., Yao, Z., Grifoni, M., Dekker, C. Carbon nanotube single-electron transistors at room temperature, *Science* **2001**, *293*, 76–79.

163 Merkoçi, A., Pumera, M., Llopis, X., Pérez, B., Del Valle, M., Alegret, S. New materials for electrochemical sensing VI: carbon nanotubes, *Trends Anal. Chem.* **2005**, *24*, 826–838.

164 Martel, R., Schmidt, T., Shea, H. R., Hertel, T., Avouris, P. Single- and multi-wall carbon nanotube field-effect transistors, *Appl. Phys. Lett.* **1998**, *73*, 2447–2449.

165 Li, J., Koehne, J. E., Cassell, A. M., Chen, H., Ng, H. T., Ye, Q., Fan, W., Han, J., Meyyappan, M. Inlaid multi-walled carbon nanotube nanoelectrode arrays for electroanalysis, *Electroanalysis* **2005**, *17*, 15–27.

166 Avouris, P. Molecular electronics with carbon nanotubes, *Acc. Chem. Res.* **2002**, *35*, 1026–1034.

167 Dai, H. Carbon nanotubes: synthesis, integration, and properties, *Acc. Chem. Res.* **2002**, *35*, 1035–1044.

168 Johnston, D. E., Islam, M. F., Yodh, A. G., Johnson, A. T. Electronic devices based on purified carbon nanotubes grown by high-pressure decomposition of carbon monoxide, *Nat. Mater.* **2005**, *4*, 589–592.

169 Niyogi, S., Hu, H., Hamon, M. A., Bhowmik, P., Zhao, B., Rozenzhak, S. M., Chen, J., Itkis, M. E., Meier, M. S., Haddon, R. C. Chromatographic purification of soluble single-walled carbon nanotubes (s-SWNTs), *J. Am. Chem. Soc.* **2001**, *123*, 733–734.

170 Zhao, B., Hu, H., Niyogi, S., Itkis, M. E., Hamon, M. A., Bhowmik, P., Meier, M. S., Haddon, R. C. Chromatographic purification and properties of soluble single-walled carbon nanotubes, *J. Am. Chem. Soc.* **2001**, *123*, 11673–11677.

171 Dyke, C. A., Stewart, M. P., Tour, J. M. Separation of single-walled carbon nanotubes on silica gel. Materials morphology and Raman excitation wavelength affect data interpretation, *J. Am. Chem. Soc.* **2005**, *127*, 4497–4509.

172 So, H.-M., Won, K., Kim, Y. H., Kim, B.-K., Ryu, B. H., Na, P. S., Kim, H., Lee, J.-O. Single-walled carbon nanotube biosensors using aptamers as molecular recognition elements, *J. Am. Chem. Soc.* **2005**, *127*, 11906–11907.

173 Takeda, S., Sbagyo, A., Sakoda, Y., Ishii, A., Sawamura, M., Sueoka, K., Kida, H., Mukasa, K., Matsumoto, K. Application of carbon nanotubes for detecting anti-hemagglutinins based on antigen–antibody interaction, *Biosensors Bioelectron.* **2005**, *21*, 201–205.

174 Staii, C., Johnson Jr., A. T., Chen, M., Gelperin, A. DNA-decorated carbon nanotubes for chemical sensing, *Nano Lett.* **2005**, *5*, 1774–1778.

175 Chen, R. J., Choi, H. C., Bangsaruntip, S., Yenilmez, E., Tang, X., Wang, Q., Chang, Y.-L., Dai, H. An investigation of the mechanisms of electronic sensing of protein adsorption on carbon nanotube devices, *J. Am. Chem. Soc.* **2004**, *126*, 1563–1568.

176 Chen, R. J., Bangsaruntip, S., Drouvalakis, K. A., Kam, N. W. S., Shim, M., Li, Y., Kim, W., Utz, P. J., Dai, H. Noncovalent functionalization of carbon nanotubes for highly specific electronic biosensors, *Proc. Natl Acad. Sci. USA* **2003**, *100*, 4984–4989.

177 Collins, P. G., Arnold, M. S., Avouris, P. Engineering carbon nanotubes and nanotube circuits using electrical breakdown, *Science* **2001**, *292*, 706–709.

178 Kong, J., Franklin, N. R., Zhou, C., Chapline, M. G., Peng, S., Cho, K., Dai, H. Nanotube molecular wires as chemical sensors, *Science* **2000**, *287*, 622–625.

179 Feng, X., Irle, S., Witek, H., Morokuma, K., Vidic, R., Borguet, E. Sensitivity of ammonia interaction with single-walled carbon nanotube bundles to the presence of defect sites

and functionalities, *J. Am. Chem. Soc.* **2005**, *127*, 10533–10538.

180 LUCCI, M., REGOLIOSI, P., REALE, A., DI CARLO, A., ORLANDUCCI, S., TAMBURRI, E., TERRANOVA, M. L., LUGLI, P., DI NATALE, C., D'AMICO, A., PAOLESSE, R. Gas sensing using single wall carbon nanotubes ordered with dielectrophoresis, *Sensors Actuators B* **2005**, *111–112*, 181–186.

181 ZHANG, B., FU, R. W., ZHANG, M. Q., DONG, X. M., LAN, P. L., QIU, J. S. Preparation and characterization of gas-sensitive composites from multi-walled carbon nanotubes/polystyrene, *Sensors Actuators, B* **2005**, *109*, 323–328.

182 GOODING, J. J., WIBOWO, R., LIU, J., YANG, W., LOSIC, D., ORBONS, S., MEARNS, F. J., SHAPTER, J. G., HIBBERT, D. B. Protein electrochemistry using aligned carbon nano-tube arrays, *J. Am. Chem. Soc.* **2003**, *125*, 9006–9007.

183 PATOLSKY, F., WEIZMANN, Y., WILLNER, I. Long-range electrical contacting of redox enzymes by SWCNT connectors, *Angew. Chem. Int. Ed.* **2004**, *43*, 2113–2117.

184 LIN, Y., LU, F., TU, Y., REN, Z. Glucose biosensors based on carbon nanotube nanoelectrode ensembles, *Nano Lett.* **2004**, *4*, 191–195.

185 KERMAN, K., MORITA, Y., TAKAMURA, Y., TAMIYA, E. *Escherichia coli* single-strand binding protein–DNA interactions on carbon nanotube-modified electrodes from a label-free electrochemical hybridization sensor, *Anal. Bioanal. Chem.* **2005**, *381*, 1114–1121.

186 LI, G., LIAO, J. M., HU, G. Q., MA, N. Z., WU, P. J. Study of carbon nanotube modified biosensor for monitoring total cholesterol in blood, *Biosensors Bioelectron.* **2005**, *20*, 2140–2144.

187 WANG, J., MUSAMEH, M., LIN, Y. Solubilization of carbon nanotubes by nafion toward the preparation of amperometric biosensors, *J. Am. Chem. Soc.* **2003**, *125*, 2408–2409.

188 BALAVOINE, F., SCHULTZ, P., RICHARD, C., MALLOUH, V., EBBESEN, T. W., MIOSKOWSKI, C. Helical crystallization of proteins on carbon nanotubes: a first step towards the development of new biosensors, *Angew. Chem. Int. Ed.* **1999**, *38*, 1912–1915.

189 SHIM, M., KAM, N. W. S., CHEN, R. J., LI, Y., DAI, H. Functionalization of carbon nanotubes for biocompatibility and biomolecular recognition, *Nano Lett.* **2002**, *2*, 285–288.

190 PANTAROTTO, D., BRIAND, J.-P., PRATO, M., BIANCO, A. Translocation of bioactive peptides across cell membranes by carbon nanotubes, *Chem. Commun.* **2004**, 16–17.

191 PANTAROTTO, D., SINGH, R., MCCARTHY, D., ERHARDT, M., BRIAND, J.-P., PRATO, M., KOSTARELOS, K., BIANCO, A. Functionalised carbon nanotubes for plasmid DNA gene delivery, *Angew. Chem. Int. Ed.* **2004**, *43*, 5242–5246.

192 CAI, D., MATARAZA, J. M., QIN, Z. H., HUANG, Z., HUANG, J., CHILES, T. C., CARNAHAN, D., KEMPA, K., REN, Z. Highly efficient molecular delivery into mammalian cells using carbon nanotube spearing, *Nat. Methods* **2005**, *2*, 449–454.

193 CHERUKURI, P., BACHILO, S. M., LITOVSKY, S. H., WEISMAN, R. B. Near-infrared fluorescence microscopy of single-walled carbon nanotubes in phagocytic cells, *J. Am. Chem. Soc.* **2005**, *127*, 15638–15639.

194 KAM, N. W. S., LIU, Z., DAI, H. Carbon nanotubes as intracellular transporters for proteins and DNA: an investigation of the uptake mechanism and pathway, *Angew. Chem. Int. Ed.* **2006**, *46*, 577–581.

195 ACHARYA, T., KENNEDY, R., DAAR, A. S., SINGER, P. A. Biotechnology to improve health in developing countries – a review, *Mem. Inst. Oswaldo Cruz* **2004**, *99*, 341–350.

196 MICONNET, I., KOENIG, S., SPEISER, D., KRIEG, A., GUILLAUME, P., CEROTTINI, J. C., ROMERO, P. CpG are efficient adjuvants for specific CTL induction against tumor antigen-derived peptide, *J. Immunol.* **2002**, *168*, 1212–1218.

197 KLINMAN, D. M., CURRIE, D., GURSEL, I., VERTHELYI, D. Use of CpG

oligodeoxynucleotides as immune adjuvants, *Immunol. Rev.* **2004**, *199*, 201–216.
198 KLINMAN, D. M. Immunotherapeutic uses of CpG oligodeoxynucleotides, *Nat. Rev. Immunol.* **2004**, *4*, 249–258.
199 KLINMAN, D. M., VERTHELYI, D., TAKESHITA, F., ISHII, K. J. Immune recognition of foreign DNA: a cure for bioterrorism?, *Immunity* **1999**, *11*, 123–129.
200 KRIEG, A. M. CpG motifs in bacterial DNA and their immune effects, *Annu. Rev. Immunol.* **2002**, *20*, 709–760.
201 HEMMI, H., TAKEUCHI, O., KAWAI, T., KAISHO, T., SATO, S., SANJO, H., MATSUMOTO, M., HOSHINO, K., WAGNER, H., TAKEDA, K., AKIRA, S. A. A Toll-like receptor recognizes bacterial DNA, *Nature* **2000**, *408*, 740–745.
202 HOFFMANN, J. A., KAFATOS, F. C., JANEWAY, C. A., EZEKOWITZ, R. A. B. Phylogenetic perspectives in innate immunity, *Science* **1999**, *284*, 1313–1318.
203 KRIEG, A. M. The role of CpG motifs in innate immunity, *Curr. Opin. Immunol.* **2000**, *12*, 35–43.
204 BIANCO, A., HOEBEKE, J., GODEFROY, S., CHALOIN, O., PANTAROTTO, D., BRIAND, J.-P., MULLER, S., PRATO, M., PARTIDOS, C. D. Cationic carbon nanotubes bind to CpG oligodeoxy-nucleotides and enhance their immunostimulatory properties, *J. Am. Chem. Soc.* **2005**, *127*, 58–59.
205 LEIST, T. P., COBBOLD, S. P., WALDMANN, H., AGUET, M., ZINKERNAGEL, R. M. Functional analysis of T lymphocyte subsets in antiviral host defense, *J. Immunol.* **1987**, *138*, 2278–2281.
206 MATLOUBIAN, M., CONCEPCION, R. J., AHMED, R. CD4$^+$ T cells are required to sustain CD8$^+$ cytotoxic T-cell responses during chronic viral infection, *J. Virol.* **1994**, *68*, 8056–8063.
207 MOSMANN, T. R., COFFMAN, R. L. T$_H$1 and T$_H$2 cells: different patterns of lymphokine secretion lead to different functional properties, *Annu. Rev. Immunol.* **1989**, *7*, 145–173.

208 BARCHET, W., OEHEN, S., KLENERMAN, P., WODARZ, D., BOCHAROV, G., LLOYD, A. L., NOWAK, M. A., HENGARTNER, H., ZINKERNAGEL, R. M., EHL, S. Direct quantitation of rapid elimination of viral antigen-positive lymphocytes by antiviral CD8$^+$ T cells in vivo, *Eur. J. Immunol.* **2000**, *30*, 1356–1363.
209 PARTIDOS, C. D. Peptide mimotopes as candidate vaccines, *Curr. Opin. Mol. Ther.* **2000**, *2*, 74–79.
210 FRANCIS, M. J. Peptide vaccines for viral diseases, *Sci. Prog.* **1990**, *74*, 115–130.
211 PANTAROTTO, D., PARTIDOS, C. D., HOEBEKE, J., BROWN, F., KRAMER, E., BRIAND, J.-P., MULLER, S., PRATO, M., BIANCO, A. Immunization with peptide-functionalized carbon nanotubes enhances virus-specific neutralizing antibody responses, *Chem. Biol.* **2003**, *10*, 991–966.
212 FRANCIS, M. J., HASTINGS, G. Z., SYRED, A. D., MCGINN, B., BROWN, F., ROWLANDS, D. J. Non-responsiveness to a foot-and-mouth disease virus peptide overcome by addition of foreign helper T-cell determinants, *Nature* **1987**, *330*, 168–170.
213 PARTIDOS, C. D., OBEID, O. E., STEWARD, M. W. Antibody responses to non-immunogenic synthetic peptides induced by co-immunization with immunogenic peptides, *Immunology* **1992**, *77*, 262–266.
214 SCHUTZE, M. P., LECLERC, C., JOLIVET, M., AUDIBERT, F., CHEDID, L. Carrier-induced epitopic suppression, a major issue for future synthetic vaccines, *J. Immunol.* **1985**, *135*, 2319–2322.
215 POUTON, C. W., SEYMOUR, L. W. Key issues in non-viral gene delivery, *Adv. Drug. Deliv. Rev.* **2000**, *46*, 187–203.
216 YINGHUAI, Z., PENG, A. T., CARPENTER, K., MAGUIRE, J. A., HOSMANE, N. S., TAKAGAKI, M. Substituted carborane-appended water-soluble single-wall carbon nanotubes: New approach to boron neutron capture therapy drug delivery, *J. Am. Chem. Soc.* **2005**, *127*, 9875–9880.
217 KAM, N. W. S., O'CONNELL, M., WISDOM, J. A., DAI, H. Carbon

nanotubes as multifunctional biological transporters and near-infrared agents for selective cancer cell destruction, *Proc. Natl Acad. Sci. USA* **2005**, *102*, 11600–11605.

218 PASTORIN, G., WU, W., WIECKOWSKI, S., BRIAND, J.-P., KOSTARELOS, K., PRATO, M., BIANCO, A. Double functionalization of carbon nanotubes for multimodal drug delivery, *Chem. Commun.* **2006**, 1182–1184.

219 MURAKAMI, T., AJIMA, K., MIYAWAKI, J., YUDASAKA, M., IIJIMA, S., SHIBE, K. Drug-loaded carbon nanohorns: adsorption and release of dexamethasone in vitro, *Mol. Pharm.* **2004**, *1*, 399–405.

220 AJIMA, K., YUDASAKA, M., MURAKAMI, T., MAIGNÉ, A., SHIBA, K., IIJIMA, S. Carbon nanohorns as anticancer drug carriers, *Mol. Pharm.* **2005**, *2*, 475–480.

221 SINGH, R., PANTAROTTO, D., MCCARTHY, D., CHALOIN, O., HOEBEKE, J., PARTIDOS, C. D., BRIAND, J.-P., PRATO, M., BIANCO, A., KOSTARELOS, K. Binding and condensation of plasmid DNA onto functionalized carbon nanotubes: towards the construction of nanotube-based gene delivery vectors, *J. Am. Chem. Soc.* **2005**, *127*, 4388–4396.

222 GAO, H., KONG, Y., CUI, D. X., OZKAN, C. S. Spontaneous insertion of DNA oligonucleotides into carbon nanotubes, *Nano Lett.* **2003**, *3*, 471–473.

223 LU, G., MARAGAKIS, P., KAXIRAS, E. Carbon nanotube interaction with DNA, *Nano Lett.* **2005**, *5*, 897–900.

224 MATYSHEVSKA, O. P., KARLASH, A. Y., SHTOGUN, Y. V., BENILOV, A., KIRGIZOV, Y., GORCHINSKYY, K. O., BUZANEVA, E. V., PRYLUTSKYY, Y. I., SCHARFF, P. Self-organizing DNA/carbon nanotube molecular films, *Mater. Sci. Eng. C* **2001**, *15*, 249–252.

225 BUZANEVA, E., KARLASH, A., YAKOVKIN, K., SHTOGUN, Y., PUTSELYK, S., ZHEREBETSKIY, D., GORCHINSKIY, A., POPOVA, G., PRILUTSKA, S., MATYSHEVSKA, O., PRILUTSKYY, Y., LYTVYN, P., SCHARFF, P., EKLUND, P. C. DNA nanotechnology of carbon nanotube cells: physico-chemical models of self-organization and properties, *Mater. Sci. Eng. C* **2002**, *19*, 41–45.

226 DOVBESHKO, G. I., REPNYTSKA, O. P., OBRAZTSOVA, E. D., SHTOGUN, Y. V. DNA interaction with single-walled carbon nanotubes: a SEIRA study, *Chem. Phys. Lett.* **2003**, *372*, 432–437.

227 NEPAL, D., SOHN, J. I., AICHER, W. K., LEE, S., GECKELER, K. E. Supramolecular conjugates of carbon nanotubes and DNA by a solid-state reaction, *Biomacromolecules* **2005**, *6*, 2919–2922.

228 DWYER, C., GUTHOLD, M., FALVO, M., WASHBURN, S., SUPERFINE, R., ERIE, D. DNA-functionalized single-walled carbon nanotubes, *Nanotechnology* **2002**, *13*, 601–604.

229 GUO, M. L., CHEN, J. H., LIU, D. Y., NIE, L. H., YAO, S. Z. Electrochemical characteristics of the immobilization of calf thymus DNA molecules on multi-walled carbon nanotubes, *Bioelectrochemistry* **2004**, *62*, 29–35.

230 NAKASHIMA, N., OKUZONO, S., MURAKAMI, H., NAKAI, T., YOSHIKAWA, K. DNA dissolves single-walled carbon nanotubes in water, *Chem. Lett.* **2003**, *32*, 456–457.

231 RAJENDRA, J., BAXENDALE, M., DIT RAP, L. G., RODGER, A. Flow linear dichroism to probe binding of aromatic molecules and DNA to single-walled carbon nanotubes, *J. Am. Chem. Soc.* **2004**, *126*, 11182–11188.

232 RAJENDRA, J., RODGER, A. The binding of single-stranded DNA and PNA to single-walled carbon nanotubes probed by flow linear dichroism, *Chem. Eur. J.* **2005**, *11*, 4841–4847.

233 LACERDA, L., PASTORIN, G., WU, W., PRATO, M., BIANCO, A., KOSTARELOS, K. Luminescence of functionalized carbon nanotubes as a tool to monitor bundle formation and dissociation in water: the effect of plasmid-DNA complexation, *Adv. Funct. Mater.* **2006**, *16*, 1839–1846.

234 RAO, R., LU, Q., KESKAR, G., FREEDMAN, K. O., FLOYD, W. C., RAO, A. M., KE, P. C. Single-molecule

fluorescence microscopy and Raman spectroscopy studies of RNA bound carbon nanotubes, *Appl. Phys. Lett.* **2004**, *85*, 4228–4230.
235 Liu, Y., Wu, D. C., Zhang, W. D., Jiang, X., He, C. B., Chung, T. S., Goh, S. H., Leong, K. W. Polyethylenimine-grafted multiwalled carbon nanotubes for secure noncovalent immobilization and efficient delivery of DNA, *Angew. Chem. Int. Ed.* **2005**, *44*, 4782–4785.
236 Rojas-Chapana, J., Troszczynska, J., Firkowska, I., Morsczeck, C., Giersig, M. Multi-walled carbon nanotubes for plasmid delivery into *Escherichia coli* cells, *Lab on a Chip* **2005**, *5*, 536–539.
237 Lu, Q., Moore, J. M., Huang, G., Mount, A. S., Rao, A. M., Larcom, L. L., Ke, P. C. RNA Polymer translocation with single-walled carbon nanotubes, *Nano Lett.* **2004**, *4*, 2473–2477.
238 Gao, L., Nie, L., Wang, T., Qin, Y., Guo, Z., Yang, D., Yan, X. Carbon nanotube delivery of the GFP gene into mammalian cells, *ChemBioChem.* **2006**, *7*, 239–242.
239 Weiss, R. Nanotech poses big unknowns, *Washington Post*, February **2004**, A01.
240 Adelmann, P., Baierl, T., Drosselmeyer, E., Politis, C., Polzer, G., Seidel, A., Schwegler-Berry, D., Steinleitner, C. Effects of fullerenes on alveolar macrophages *in vitro*, in *Toxic and Carcinogenic Effects of Solid Particles in the Respiratory Tract*. U. Mohr, D. L. Dungworth, J. Mauderly, G. Oberdoerster, (Eds.). ILSI Press, Washington, DC, **1994**, pp. 405–407.
241 Fortner, J. D., Lyon, D. Y., Sayes, C. M., Boyd, A. M., Falkner, J. C., Hotze, M., Alemany, L. B., Tao, Y. J., Guo, W., Ausman, K. D., Colvin, V. L., Huges, J. B. C_{60} in water: nanocrystal formation and microbial response, *Environ. Sci. Technol.* **2005**, *39*, 4307–4316.
242 Sayes, C. M., Fortner, J. D., Guo, W., Lyo, D., Boyd, A. M., Ausman, K. D., Tao, Y. J., Sitharaman, B., Wilson, L. J., Huges, J. B., West, J. L., Colvin, V. L. The differential cytotoxicity of water-soluble fullerenes, *Nano Lett.* **2004**, *4*, 1881–1887.
243 Colvin, V. L. The potential environmental impact of engineered nanomaterials, *Nat. Biotechnol.* **2003**, *21*, 1166–1170.
244 Connor, E. E., Mwamuka, J., Gole, A., Murphy, C. J., Wyatt, M. D. Gold nanoparticles are taken up by human cells but do not cause acute cytotoxicity, *Small* **2005**, *1*, 325–327.
245 Moussa, F., Pressac, M., Hadchouel, M., Arbeille, B., Chrétien, P., Trivin, F., Céolin, R., Szwarc, H. C_{60} fullerene toxicity: preliminary account of an *in vivo* study, Electrochemical Soc. Proc. **1997**, *5*, 332–336.
246 Gharbi, N., Pressac, M., Hadchouel, M., Szwarc, H., Wilson, S. R., Moussa, F. [60]Fullerene is a powerful antioxidant *in vivo* with no acute or subacute toxicity, *Nano Lett.* **2005**, *5*, 2578–2585.
247 Yokoyama, A., Sato, Y., Nodasaka, Y., Yamamoto, S., Kawasaki, T., Shindoh, M., Kohgo, T., Akasaka, T., Uo, M., Watari, F., Tohji, K. Biological behavior of hat-stacked carbon nanofibers in the subcutaneous tissue in rats, *Nano Lett.* **2005**, *5*, 157–161.
248 Jia, G., Wang, H., Yan, L., Wang, X., Pei, R., Yan, T., Zhao, Y., Guo, X. Cytotoxicity of carbon nanomaterials: single-wall nanotube, multi-wall nanotube, and fullerene, *Environ. Sci. Technol.* **2005**, *39*, 1378–1383.
249 Manna, S. K., Sarkar, S., Barr, J., Wise, K., Barrera, E. V., Jejelowo, O., Rice-Ficht, A. C., Ramesh, G. T. Single-walled carbon nanotube induces oxidative stress and activates nuclear transcription factor-κB in human keratinocytes, *Nano Lett.* **2005**, *5*, 1676–1684.
250 Donaldson, K., Stone, V., Tran, C. L., Kreyling, W., Borm, P. J. A. Nanotoxicology, *Occup. Environ. Med.* **2004**, *61*, 727–728.
251 Tran, C. L., Buchanan, D., Cullen, R. T., Searl, A., Jones, A. D., Donaldson, K. Inhalation of poorly

soluble particles. II. Influence of particle surface area on inflammation and clearance, *Inhal. Toxicol.* **2000**, *12*, 113–126.

252 Sayes, C. M., Liang, F., Hudson, J. L., Mendez, J., Guo, W., Beach, J. M., Moore, V. C., Doyle, C. D., West, J. L., Billups, W. E., Ausman, K. D., Colvin, V. L. Functionalization density dependence of single-walled carbon nanotubes cytotoxicity *in vitro*, *Toxicol. Lett.* **2006**, *161*, 135–142.

253 Sato, Y., Yokoyama, A., Shibata, K., Akimoto, Y., Ogino, S., Nodasaka, Y., Kohgo, T., Tamura, K., Akasaka, T., Uo, M., Motomiya, K., Jeyadevan, B., Ishiguro, M., Hatakeyama, R., Watari, F., Tohji, K. Influence of length on cytotoxicity of multi-walled carbon nanotubes against human acute monocytic leukemia cell line THP-1 *in vitro* and subcutaneous tissue of rats *in vivo*, *Mol. BioSyst.* **2005**, *1*, 176–182.

254 Salvador-Morales, C., Flahaut, E., Sim, E., Sloan, J., Green, M. L. H., Sim, R. B. Complement activation and protein adsorption by carbon nanotubes, *Mol. Immunol.* **2006**, *43*, 193–201.

255 Kiura, K., Sato, Y., Yasuda, M., Fugetsu, B., Watari, F., Tohji, K., Shibata, K. Activation of human monocytes and mouse splenocytes by single-walled carbon nanotubes, *J. Biomed. Nanotechnol.* **2005**, *1*, 359–364.

256 Cui, D., Tian, F., Ozkan, S., Wang, M., Gao, H. Effect of single wall carbon nanotubes on human HEK293 cells, *Toxicol. Lett.* **2005**, *155*, 73–85.

257 Monteiro-Riviere, N. A., Nemanich, R. J., Inman, A. O., Wang, Y. Y., Riviere, J. E. Multi-walled carbon nanotube interactions with human epidermal keratinocytes, *Toxicol. Lett.* **2005**, *155*, 377–384.

258 Bottini, M., Bruckner, S., Nika, K., Bottini, N., Bellucci, S., Magrini, A., Bergamaschi, A., Mustelin, T. Multi-walled carbon nanotubes induce T lymphocyte apoptosis, *Toxicol. Lett.* **2005**, *160*, 121–126.

259 Muller, J., Huaux, F., Moreau, N., Misson, P., Heilier, J.-F., Delos, M., Arras, M., Fonseca, A., Nagy, J. B., Lison, D. Respiratory toxicity of multiwall carbon nanotubes, *Toxicol. Appl. Pharmacol.* **2005**, *207*, 221–231.

260 Lam, C. W., James, J. T., McCluskey, R., Hunter, R. L. Pulmonary toxicity of single-wall carbon nanotubes in mice 7 and 90 days after intratracheal instillation, *Toxicol. Sci.* **2004**, *77*, 126–134.

261 Warheit, D. B., Laurence, B. R., Reed, K. L., Roach, D. H., Reynolds, G. A. M., Webb, T. R. Comparative pulmonary toxicity assessment of single-wall carbon nanotubes in rats, *Toxicol. Sci.* **2004**, *77*, 117–125.

262 Huczko, A., Lange, H., Calko, E. Fullerenes: experimental evidence for a null risk of skin irritation and allergy, *Fullerene Sci. Technol.* **1999**, *7*, 935–939.

263 Huczko, A., Lange, H. Carbon nanotubes: experimental evidence for a null risk of skin irritation and allergy, *Fullerene Sci. Technol.* **2001**, *9*, 247–250.

264 Eedy, D. J. Carbon-fibre-induced airbone irritant contact dermatitis, *Contact Derm.* **1996**, *35*, 362–363.

265 Kasparov, A. A., Popova, T. B., Lebedeva, N. V., Gladkova, E. V., Gurvich, E. B. Evaluation of the carcinogenic hazard in the manufacture of graphite articles, *Vopr. Onkol.* **1989**, *35*, 445–450.

266 Shvedova, A. A., Kisin, E. R., Murray, A. R., Gandelsman, V. Z., Maynard, A. D., Baron, P. A., Castranova, V. Exposure to carbon nanotube material: Assessment of nanotube cytotoxicity using human keratinocytes cells, *J. Toxicol. Environ. Health A* **2003**, *66*, 1909–1926.

267 Maynard, A. D., Baron, P. A., Foley, M., Shvedova, A. A., Kisin, E. R., Castranova, V. Exposure to carbon nanotube material: aerosol release during the handling of unrefined single-walled carbon nanotube material, *J. Toxicol. Environ. Health A* **2004**, *67*, 87–107.

4 Core–Shell Nanoparticles for Drug Delivery and Molecular Imaging

Sung Kyun Han, Ree Sun Kim, Jin Ho Lee, Giyoong Tae, Sun Hang Cho, and Soon Hong Yuk

4.1 Introduction

Core–shell nanoparticle structures, in which a layer of polymeric materials surrounds an organic or inorganic nanoparticle core, have been investigated both as a means to improve the stability of the core nanoparticle and as a way of accessing unique physical properties that are not possible from one nanomaterial alone. This chapter describes the preparation method and characterization of a novel protein delivery system and molecular imaging agent composed of core–shell nanoparticles with the variation of core materials such as lipid, polymeric or inorganic nanoparticles.

With rapid advancements in the field of biotechnology/genetic engineering, a growing number of protein drugs have been produced [1, 2]. Although they show potent and specific physiologic actions in small doses, most of them are difficult to administer clinically. Although a wide variety of delivery systems have been designed and characterized, the parenteral route has been most widely selected for the efficient delivery of protein [3–7]. However, the problems still remain in the parenteral delivery of protein because most proteins have a short half-life in the physiological condition. Loss of biological activity and change in immunogenicity as a result of protein aggregation or denaturation are the most important challenges faced in the delivery of protein drugs [8–10]. Hence, they cannot be utilized effectively in conventional dosage forms. For such active agents, new types of drug delivery systems must be developed to deliver the drug more effectively. Among the various approaches investigated, extensive research has been conducted on the ability of colloidal systems such as liposomes and polymeric nanoparticles as an optimal delivery system for protein drugs. A wide variety of drugs such as hydrophilic drugs, hydrophobic drugs, proteins, vaccines and biological macromolecules can be delivered using colloidal systems via a number of routes [11–15]. They can be formulated for targeted delivery to the lymphatic system, brain, arterial walls, lungs, liver or spleen, or made for long-term systemic circulation [16–18]. There-

Nanotechnologies for the Life Sciences Vol. 10
Nanomaterials for Medical Diagnosis and Therapy. Edited by Challa S. S. R. Kumar

ISBN: 978-3-527-31390-7

fore, numerous protocols exist for colloidal systems based on the type of drug used and the desired delivery route.

A number of liposomal formulations have been reported as drug delivery vehicles for sustained release of protein drugs and some have been evaluated for clinical applications [19–21]. Most of the previous studies involved traditional liposomes (unilamellar [22, 23] or multilamellar vesicular systems [24, 25]) and multivesicular liposomes (DepoFoam) [26–29]. However, the liposomal system shows a mechanical instability under physiological conditions, which results in a total release of the internal aqueous content (burst effect). As each multivesicular liposome is composed of discontinuous internal aqueous chambers, bounded by a continuous, nonconcentric network of lipid membranes with a higher aqueous volume:lipid ratio, the multivesicular liposomes have exhibited an improved stability. This enables us to design the sustained release form of encapsulated protein drug since, unlike unilamellar vesicular systems, a single breach in the external membrane of a multivesicular liposome will not result in a total release of internal aqueous content containing protein drug. They have been evaluated with recombinant human insulin [30–32], leuprolide (a 9-amino-acid peptide analog of luteinizing hormone releasing hormone) [33–35], met-enkephalin (an endogenous opioid peptide of 5 amino acids) [36, 37] and octreotide (a cyclic octapeptide analog of somatostatin) [38, 39]. However, the sustained release formulation of protein drugs using multivesicular liposomes still remains a major challenge, achieving high drug loading with high drug recovery and controlling the release pattern over a prolonged period.

Recently, polymersome (polymer vesicle) has be prepared by the molecular assembly of an amphiphilic diblock copolymer composed of poly(ethylene glycol) (PEG) and polyesters or polycarbonates [40, 41]. Biodegradable diblock copolymers based on PEG and poly(lactide) have been used to prepare carriers such as micelles, nano/microparticles and gels for controlled or targeted delivery. However, the formation of polymersomes has been reported and suggests a promising application in drug delivery system for water-soluble drugs and protein drugs; similar advantages and disadvantages founded in the liposomal system are observed in the polymersome.

Polymeric nano/microparticles are the most suitable and preferred systems in the delivery of protein drugs by the parenteral or nonparenteral route. Due to the large amount of toxicological and chemical data available, biocompatibility/histocompatibility, predictable biodegradation kinetics, ease of fabrication, and variety in copolymer ratio and molecular weight, polyesters have been found the most widespread use as a major component of polymeric nano/microparticles and they have been approved in clinical applications [42, 43]. Despite many advantages, polyesters like poly(lactide-*co*-glycolide) (PLGA) also have some inherent shortcomings. Due to the hydrophobic nature of the polymer compared to most of the protein drugs to be encapsulated, the serious problems associated with protein activity were observed during storage or *in vivo* release. Since hydration and degradation of PLGA are prerequisites for the release of protein drugs during the bioerosion phase, this results in an acidic micoenvironment due to the formation of lactic acid and glycolic acid, which leads to denaturation (hydrolytic degradation and aggregation) of protein drugs. Although improvement of protein drug compatibility has been investigated by coencapsulating buffer salts and stabilizer for protein drugs and modification of polyesters, it still remains challenging.

With the significant progress in the treatment of diseases and diagnosis, the importance of molecular imaging as well as that of drug delivery has increased tremendously. The prerequisite for efficient molecular imaging is to prepare the magnetic nanoparticles with a narrow size distribution. Information technology which has been used in data storage devices now enables us to prepare magnetic (metal) nanoparticles with such a narrow size distribution. However, as such particles have a strong tendency to agglomerate due to their large specific surface area, various methods have been studied in order to stabilize the nanoparticles. For this purposes, many attempts have been made to establish the preparation method of magnetic nanoparticles coated with a biocompatible polymer (core–shell nanoparticles with metallic core) to improve the stability and biocompatibility under physiological conditions.

As described previously, there are number of studies on the protein delivery system and molecular imaging agent using a single nanomaterial system. However, these systems showed major drawbacks in terms of the stability, release pattern and cytotoxicity. Recently, a number of investigations have been devoted to understanding the formation of core–shell nanoparticles [44, 45] and much interest has been focused on developing core–shell nanoparticles as an effective means of delivering bioactive materials [46–50]. Due to their distinct geometry, numerous applications have evolved, and core–shell nanoparticles with a variation of core materials have been designed and characterized as drug delivery systems based on the type of drug used. In this chapter, a new type of protein delivery system and molecular imaging agent will be introduced using core–shell nanoparticles, which exhibit the improved stability, a sustained release pattern of protein drug and decreased cytotoxicity.

4.2 Core–shell Nanoparticles with a Lipid Core

As an effective oil-soluble drug carrier, lipid and mixed micelles have been developed. However, lipid-based drug carriers composed of a single lipid phase have several inherent problems, including the burst effect and difficulty in achieving zero-order release. To overcome these difficulties, core–shell nanoparticles with drug-loaded lipid core were prepared (see Fig. 4.1). For the formation of the polymeric shell, drug-loaded lipid cores were usually freeze-dried in the aqueous solution containing polymers used for the shell material. Freeze-drying of vesicular structure and subsequent recovery of the very same structure on the microscale is simple and straightforward [51, 52]. However, with the vesicular structure on the nanoscale, the situation is more complex [51]. A solution to the problem that allows the recovery of vesicular structure on the nanoscale was found to be the inclu-

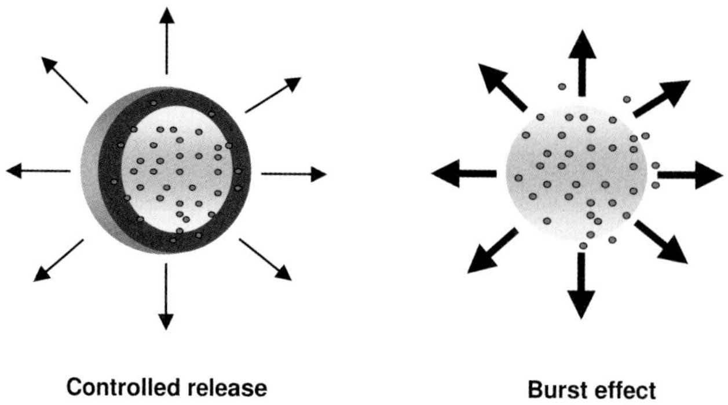

Figure 4.1. Schematic description of the advantages gained with the formation of core–shell nanoparticles.

sion of relatively high concentrations (around 30 wt%) of cryoprotectants such as trehalose, sucrose, mannose or glucose. The role attributed to these cryoprotectants is replacement of structure-stabilizing water-based hydrogen bonds at the liposomal surface, which are lost in the process of drying [53].

Another approach to cryoprotection, which does not require the inclusion of additives such as the sugars listed above, has been made by chemical modification of phospolipid with hydrophilic polymers, surfactants or block copolymers [54].

A novel method for the preparation of core–shell nanoparticles with a lipid core was designed and characterized (see Fig. 4.2). The lipid core is composed of lecithin, which forms a spherical supramolecular structure (multilamellar vesicles) in the concentrated state [55]. The polymeric shell is composed of pluronics [poly(ethylene oxide)–poly(propylene oxide)–poly(ethylene oxide) triblock copolymer, F-127]. In this study, a F-127/trehalose mixture was used to stabilize the drug-loaded lipid core in the form of core–shell nanoparticles. With the combina-

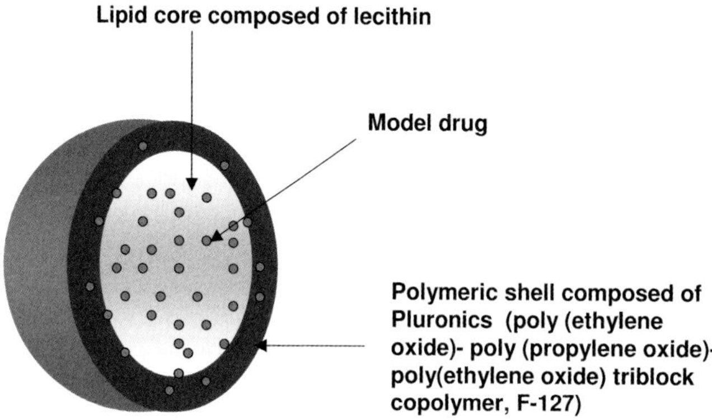

Figure 4.2. Schematic description of core–shell nanoparticles with drug-loaded lipid cores.

tion of F-127 and trehalose, the concentration of cryoprotectant can be reduced into approximately 5 wt% and chemical modification of lipid to improve the stability of vesicular structure on the nanoscale was not required.

First, the core–shell nanoparticles with a drug-loaded lipid core were prepared for a lipophilic drug. A drug suspension composed of 90/10 (w/w) [Tween 80/paclitaxel (model drug)] mixture was prepared in which the oil phase was subsequently dispersed. The oil phase was composed of 40 wt% aqueous solution of lecithin from soy bean oil. The obtained drug dispersion and oil phase were mixed in equal amounts, and were then subjected to sonication in an ice bath for 3 min to prepare the drug-loaded lipid core using a probe-type ultrasonic wave homogenizer (Branson Sonifier Model 185). The solution mixtures composed of 90/10 (w/w) (F-127 aqueous solution/drug-loaded lipid core) were prepared to induce the formation of the polymeric shell on the surface of the drug-loaded lipid core. F-127 aqueous solutions were prepared with or without trehalose to observe the preservation of integrity of the core–shell structure of nanoparticles during the freeze-drying.

Aqueous concentrated lecithin mixtures show typical lamellar liquid crystalline behavior and the individual lamellae tend to form a spherical supramolecular structure [55]. Figure 4.3 shows the particle size distribution of 5 wt% lecithin aqueous solution, which exhibits the formation of a spherical supramolecular structure with a diameter of 45.6 nm. The size, polydispersity and surface charge of nanoparticles were determined using an electrophoretic light-scattering spectrophotometer equipped with a 10 mW He–Ne laser (632.8 nm) (ELS-8000; Otsuka Electronics, Japan). Based on this, paclitaxel solubilized in Tween 80 was added to 40 wt% lecithin aqueous solution and subjected to sonication leading to the complete dissolution of paclitaxel. This is a universal principle for all drugs that are

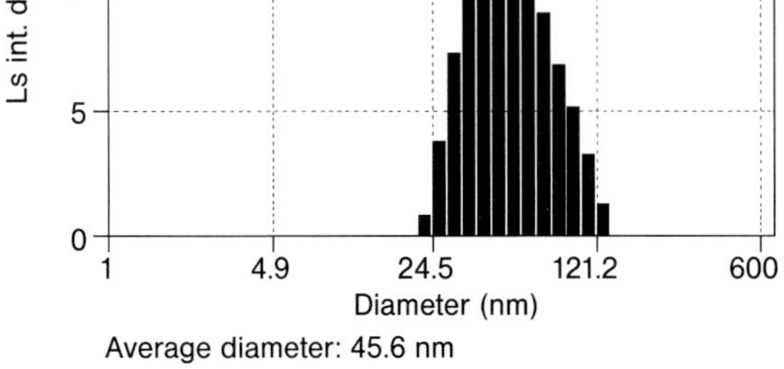

Figure 4.3. Size distribution of 5 wt% lecithin in aqueous medium with 5 wt% Tween 80. (From Ref. [48].)

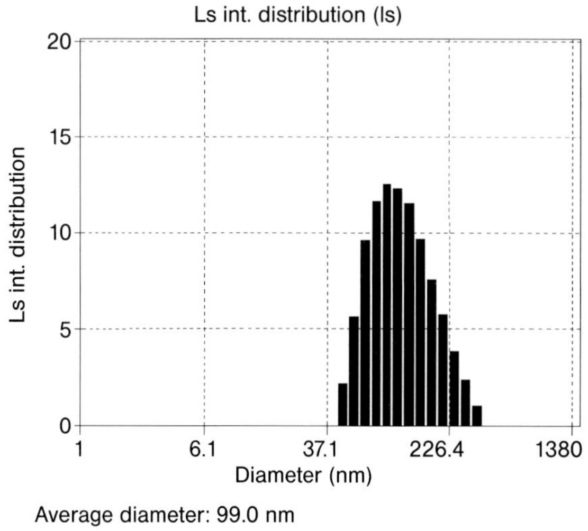

Figure 4.4. Size distribution of paclitaxel-loaded lipid cores in the aqueous medium. (From Ref. [48].)

poorly soluble in the water phase of emulsions and simultaneously in the oil phase, but processing a suitable lipophilicity to interact with the lecithin molecules in the interfacial layer [56]. Of course, the incorporation capacity of an oil-in-water (o/w) emulsion is not unlimited. At a certain stage, the interfacial layer is saturated with paclitaxel, leading to the formation of nondissolved small drug crystals in the dispersion. As shown in Fig. 4.4, paclitaxel-loaded lipid cores dispersed in 10 wt% F-127 aqueous solution exhibit a stable emulsion with diameter of 99 nm.

Freeze-drying was performed for the formation of a polymeric shell composed of F-127. As shown in Fig. 4.5(A), significant aggregation was observed to show that the spherical supramolecular structure was disintegrated during the freeze-drying process. This phenomenon is usually found in the freeze-drying of protein solution. With freeze-drying, the protein activity is significantly decreased due to the disintegration of supramolecular structure. It has been reported that trehalose, a naturally occurring osmolyte, is known to be an efficient stabilizer of proteins and helps the activity of enzymes in solution as well as in the freeze-dried state [57]. This led us to use trehalose as a stabilizer of the spherical supramolecular structure of core–shell nanoparticles. Note that exposure of freshly collected oocytes to a concentration of trehalose between 0.5 and 1.0 M for up to 10 min had no significant effect, indicating that trehalose is not toxic [58]. With adding 5 wt% trehalose in F-127 aqueous solution, freeze-drying was performed to induce the formation of the polymeric shell. As shown in Fig. 4.5(B), nanoparticles with diameter of 267.4 nm were observed, indicating minimal disintegration of spherical supramolecular structure.

A cryogenic transmission electron microscopy (cryo-TEM) image was obtained for the verification of the formation of core–shell nanoparticles. For the measure-

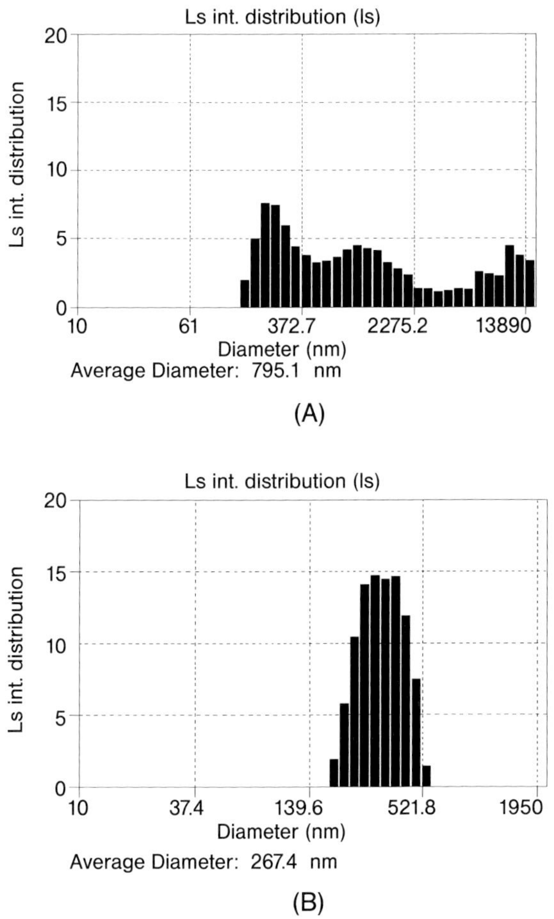

Figure 4.5. (A) Size distribution of nanoparticles formed from 10 wt% F-127 aqueous solution without trehalose. (B) Size distribution of nanoparticles formed from 10 wt% F-127 aqueous solution with 5 wt% trehalose. (From Ref. [48].)

ment, the samples were prepared as a thin liquid film (less than 0.25 μm thick) supported on cryo-grid. These were quenched into liquid ethane at its freezing point and stored under liquid nitrogen. They were later transferred to a Tecnai 12 electron microscope (Philips, The Netherlands). Direct imaging was carried out at a temperature of approximately −170 °C and with a 120 kV acceleration voltage, using the images acquired with a Multiscan 600 W CCD camera (Gatan, USA). With the nanoparticles formed from 10 wt% F-127 aqueous solution, the formation of core–shell nanoparticles was observed as shown in Fig. 4.6.

In this study, lecithin was used as the main component for the preparation of nanoparticles (self-assembled aggregates). The addition of other substances, espe-

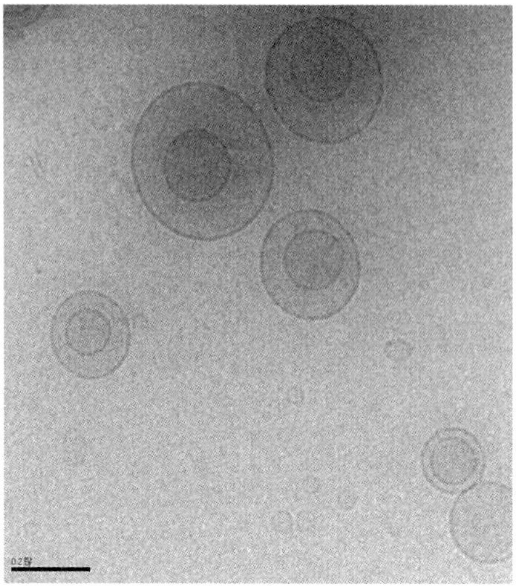

Figure 4.6. Cryo-TEM image of nanoparticles formed from 10 wt% F-127 aqueous solution with 5 wt% trehalose. (From Ref. [48].)

cially surfactants and drug, may result in the alteration of the original structures. Differential scanning calorimetry (DSC) was used to characterize the lipid core with addition of surfactant, F-127 and drug as shown in Fig. 4.7. Although a minimal peak was observed with 15 wt% F-127 aqueous solution, no characteristic peaks

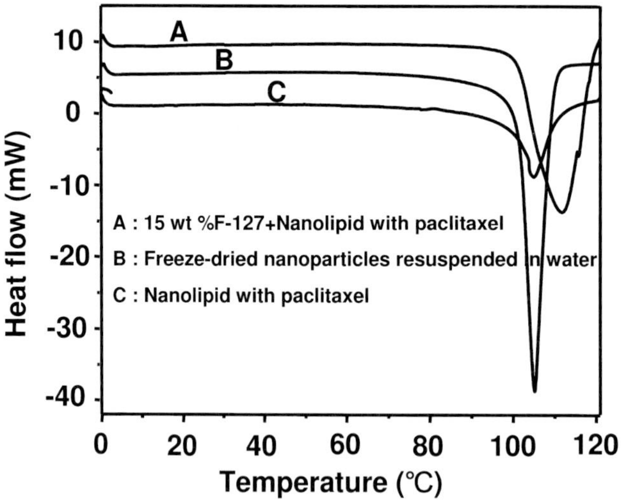

Figure 4.7. DSC thermograms of components used to prepare for the core–shell nanoparticles. (From Ref. [48].)

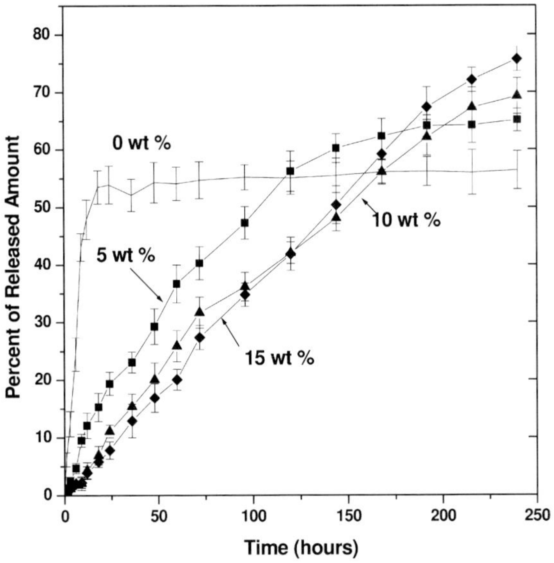

Figure 4.8. The release pattern of paclitaxel from nanoparticles formed as a function of the concentration of F-127 aqueous solution. $N = 3$ experiments. (From Ref. [48].)

were observed with lecithin and Tween 80 mixed with paclitaxel. However, the characteristic peaks were observed at 105.5 and 111.9 °C with paclitaxel-loaded lipid cores (loading amount: 4 wt%) and with paclitaxel-loaded lipid cores in the presence of F-127 and trehalose, respectively. A similar peak was observed at 104.9 °C with the freeze-dried nanoparticles resuspended in water. This indicates that the original structure of the paclitaxel-loaded lipid core was maintained in the presence of F-127 and trehalose during the freeze-drying, resulting in the formation of core–shell nanoparticles with a drug-loaded lipid core.

For application as a drug delivery system for lipophilic drugs, core–shell nanoparticles with paclitaxel-loaded lipid core were prepared and the release behavior of paclitaxel was observed as shown in Fig. 4.8. Without the polymeric shell (0 wt% of F-127 aqueous solution), a significant burst effect was observed, resulting in the precipitation of paclitaxel into the release medium. This is due to the poorly solubilized paclitaxel in the lipid phase and its poor solubility in aqueous media. With the formation of the polymeric shell, released paclitaxel from the lipid phase diffused through the polymeric shell (F-127 phase), resulting in a significant decrease in the burst effect and an almost zero-order release pattern was observed with nanoparticles formed from 10 wt% F-127 aqueous solution.

Based on the formation of core–shell nanoparticles, the application has evolved in the area of protein delivery. Figure 4.9 shows the chemical structure of lecithin used as a core material. Due to its low isoelectric point (below 3.5), zwitterionic lecithin shows anionic characteristics under physiological pH as presented in Fig. 4.9.

Figure 4.9. Chemical structure of lecithin used as a lipid core.

With a proper choice of protein drug with a higher isoelectric point (above 7.4), the ionic interaction between lecithin nanolipid and protein drug can be achieved as presented schematically in Fig. 4.10.

Vascular endothelial growth factor (VEGF) was used as a model protein drug. VEGF is a potent mitogen in embryonic and somatic angiogenesis with a unique specificity for vascular endothelial cells [59, 60]. VEGF has been considered as a potential treatment for stroke due to its angiogenic and direct neuroprotective action [61]. One potential mechanism for the treatment of stroke is the induction of angiogenesis with increasing oxygen availability. The extent of newly formed vessels is probably an important factor in determining the improvement in the blood flow, culminating in the recovery and repair of neurons, and a reduction in the ischemic damage.

Figure 4.10. Schematic description of the formation of protein-loaded core–shell nanoparticles.

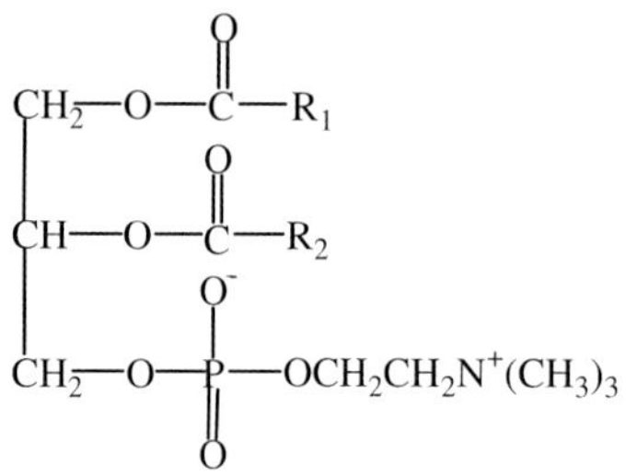

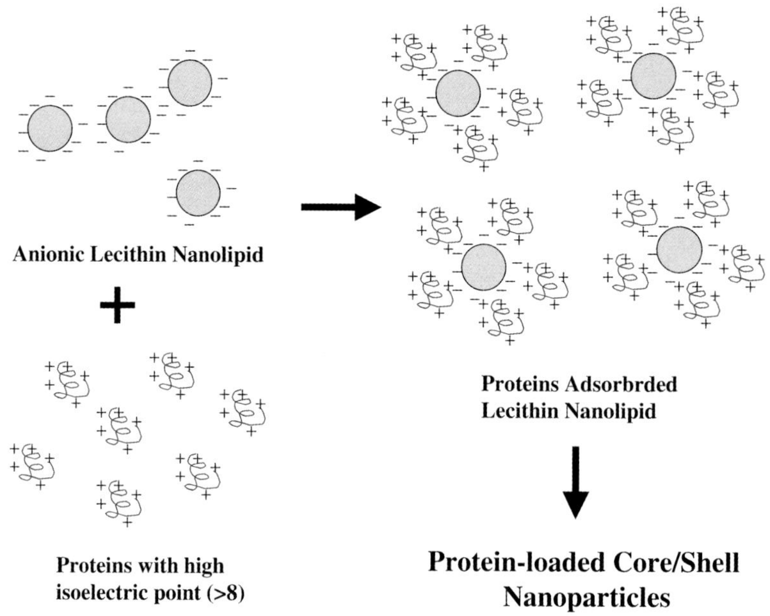

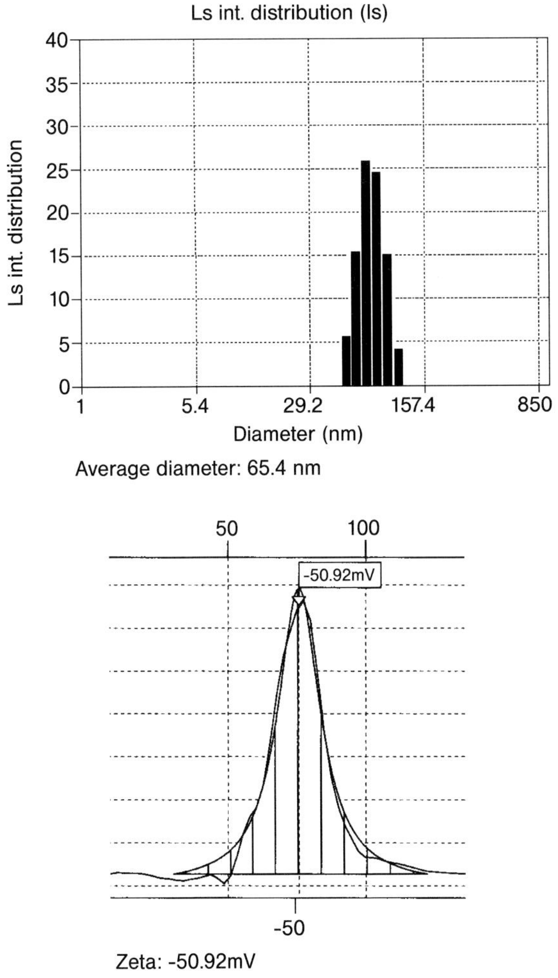

Figure 4.11. The size distribution and ζ potential of lecithin nanoparticles.

The medical product related to VEGF is being developed for the treatment of coronary artery disease [62]. As a result of blocked arteries in the heart, patients with coronary artery disease typically experience severe, often immobilizing, pain from minimum physical activity such as walking. This product is intended to improve blood flow in the heart through the formation of new blood vessels, a process known as angiogenesis, with the delivery the angiogenic protein, VEGF-121. In this approach, the product is directly injected into the heart wall by an endocardial injection catheter and this enables the sustained, controlled production of VEGF-121 protein in the area of the heart with poor blood flow. It was reported that there were no VEGF-related serious adverse events or dose-limiting toxicities.

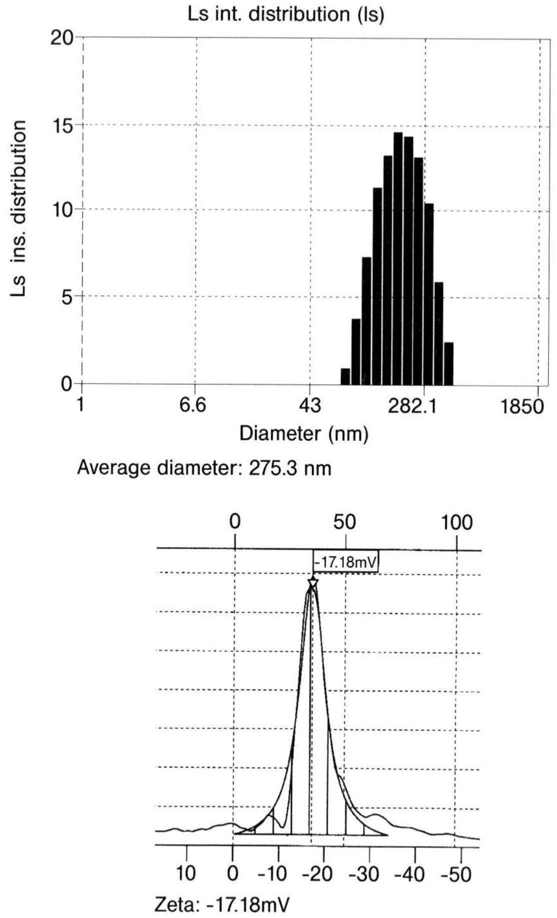

Figure 4.12. The size distribution and ζ potential of core–shell nanoparticles with a VEGF-loaded lecithin core.

The core–shell nanoparticles are utilized as a delivery vehicle of VEGF with a sustained release pattern. For the preparation of the protein-loaded core–shell nanoparticles, a similar process to that described previously was employed. For efficient loading of protein drug, complex formation was induced between lecithin and VEGF, and this complex was mixed with F-127 aqueous solution containing 5 wt% trehalose. Freeze-drying was conducted to form the polymeric shell on the surface of the complex composed of lecithin and VEGF (see Fig. 4.10).

In the freeze-drying process, trehalose used as a cryoprotectant plays two roles. One is to preserve the core–shell structure of nanoparticles, which is very important for the accomplishment of the sustained release pattern of VEGF. The other is to preserve the activity of loaded VEGF. It has been reported that globular proteins invariantly show higher melting (denaturation) temperatures in the presence of sugars (in dilute solution) and concentrated sugar systems confer textural consistency that prevents microbial attack in foods. It is not clear, however, whether these two different types of stabilization have a common physicochemical origin; in particular, whether water–sugar interactions are the only basis of both phenomena. Among all the sugars, trehalose has received the greatest attention, both because of its wide role in nature and its potential use as a highly efficient natural preservative [63].

Figure 4.11 shows the ζ potential and size distribution of lecithin nanolipid. The size of lecithin nanolipid was approximately 65.4 nm and a negative value of the ζ potential was observed, indicating that anionic lecithin nanolipid is suitable for the immobilization of cationic VEGF. After freeze-drying of VEGF/lecithin nanolipid complex in the F-127 aqueous solution containing 5 wt% trehalose, the obtained powder was resuspended in water and characterized with a particle size analyzer. As shown in Fig. 4.12, the diameter was approximately 270 nm and the magnitude of the negative value of the ζ potential was decreased. With the formation of the polymeric shell, the size of the nanoparticles was increased and the negative charge of the lecithin nanolipid was decreased. The cryo-TEM image clearly demonstrates the formation of core–shell nanoparticles as shown in Fig. 4.13.

The release of VEGF from the nanoparticles was measured as shown in Fig. 4.14. A VEGF-loaded nanoparticle suspension (0.2 mL) was subsequently put into a dialysis tube. The dialysis tube was placed into 15 mL PBS containing 2.0 mM sodium azide and 0.1% (w/v) bovine serum albumin (BSA), and kept in reciprocal shaking water bath (Sangwoo Scientific, Korea) at 37 °C and 35 r.p.m. At each timepoint, the whole medium was taken and replaced with the fresh release medium.

Figure 4.13. Cryo-TEM image of core–shell nanoparticles with a VEGF-loaded lecithin core.

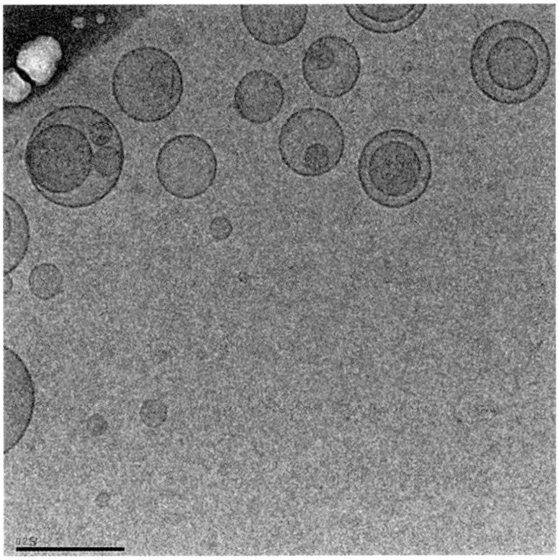

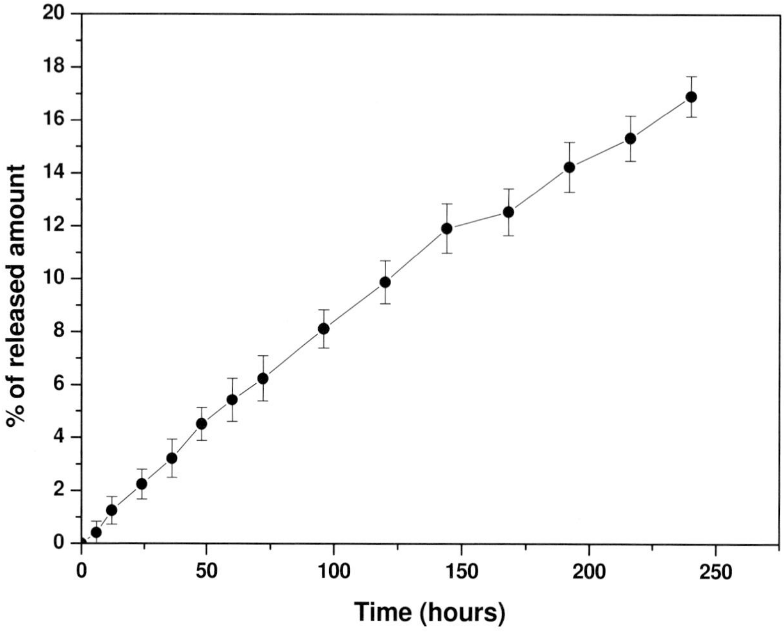

Figure 4.14. The release of VEGF from the core–shell nanoparticles.

The amount of released VEGF into the release medium was determined by ELISA analysis (Neogen, USA). The sustained release pattern was observed up to 10 days, releasing about 16% of the initial loading and this indicates that a 1-month period of VEGF release can be achieved with core–shell nanoparticles.

With the adsorption of F-127 on the surface of lipid core by freeze-drying, the stabilized core–shell nanoparticles were formed in the presence of trehalose. This indicates that trehalose, which is generally used as a protein stabilizer, preserves the integrity of the spherical supramolecular structure of the lecithin core during the freeze-drying. Due to the distinct geometry of core–shell nanoparticles with a lipid core, the lipophilic drug can be loaded in the lipid core and protein drugs can be loaded in the polymeric shell.

4.3 Core–Shell Nanoparticles with a Polymeric Core

PLGA micro/nanoparticles have been designed and characterized for the delivery of a couple of proteins. Biodegradable microspheres containing recombinant human erythropoietin (EPO) were prepared from ABA triblock copolymers, consisting of hydrophobic PLGA A blocks and poly(ethylene oxide) (PEO) B blocks [64]. Using excipients with known protein stabilizing properties, such as BSA, poly(L-histidine), poly(L-arginine) or a combination of poly(L-arginine) and dextran, the EPO aggregate content was significantly reduced to below 5% of the encapsulated

EPO. In particular, the microspheres composed of ABA triblock copolymer (35 mol% PEO; 30 kDa) in combination with 5% BSA yielded both an acceptable level of EPO aggregate and a continuous release profiles under *in vitro* conditions for up to 14 days. Pharmacokinetic characterization of VEGF controlled release microspheres composed of PLGA was performed using a rat model. The microspheres were administered subcutaneously to the rat and the pharmacokinetic parameters were compared with those of VEGF solution [65]. The subcutaneous administration of protein solution resulted in rapid clearance from the tissue, with high plasma concentrations as expressed by rapid absorption and elimination. However, the subcutaneous administration of VEGF microspheres produced low plasma concentrations and high subcutaneous concentrations over a period of 7 weeks.

However, because of the hydrophobic character of PLGA, the loading of protein into PLGA micro/nanoparticles with a minimal decrease of protein activity still remains challenging. In addition, nanoparticles have a further advantage over larger micorparticles because they are better suited for intravenous delivery. The smallest capillaries in the body are 5–6 μm in diameter. The size of particles being distributed into the blood stream must be significantly smaller than 5 μm, without forming aggregates, to ensure that the particles do not form an embolism.

The rapid removal of intravenously administered colloidal drug carrier by the mononuclear phagocytic system, comprising mainly the Kupffer cells of the liver and the macrophages of the spleen, has been identified as the major obstacle to the efficient targeting of colloidal carriers to target sites such as the circulation itself, tumor, sites of inflammation and bone marrow. Various studies have been carried out for the successful avoidance of these difficulties. One of the related studies reported that the *in vitro* interaction with isolated macrophages and the biodistribution of model polystyrene nanospheres after modification of the particle surface using PEO/poly(propylene oxide) (PPO) block copolymers of the poloxamer (Pluronic) poloxamine series and the presence of PEO on the surface of nanospheres decrease the extent of phagocytosis [66]. It was also verified that poloxamer and poloxamine copolymers are bound to the nanosphere surface by hydrophobic interaction of the PPO chains, whereas the hydrophilic PEO chains protrude into the surrounding medium to create a steric barrier and this barrier prevents or decreases the adsorption of plasma proteins onto the particle surface, resulting in the decreased recognition by the liver and spleen macrophages [67–69]. Similar results have been reported with PLGA nanoparticles coated with Pluronic [70]. In particular, the size of nanoparticles and coating layer thickness were measured using photon correlation spectroscopy, indicating the presence of a hydrogel layer on the surface of nanoparticles. These results enable us to design PLGA nanoparticles with a hydrogel layer on the surface, which are utilized as cores in the formation of core–shell nanoparticles with a polymeric core.

4.3.1 Hyaluronic Acid (HA)-functionalized PLGA Nanoparticles

A novel preparation method for core–shell nanoparticles with a hydrophilic polymeric shell was designed and characterized based on the preparation method of hydrophilized PLGA nanoparticles with Pluronics described previously. The core is composed of PLGA and polymeric shell is composed of Pluronics (F-127) and HA. The role of the core is to provide the nucleus for the stable formation of the hydrophilic polymeric shell by physical adsorption and that of the polymeric shell is to provide the hydrophilic network for protein loading. Specifically, HA was used as one of the components for polymeric shell to induce the ionic interaction between protein and HA for the efficient loading and sustained release of ionized and hydrophilic protein. For the characterization of core–shell nanoparticles as a drug carrier, lysozyme, which was used as a model protein drug, was loaded into the nanoparticles, and the loading amount and release pattern was observed with the variation of the composition of the polymeric shell.

In the previous study, PLGA nanoparticles were prepared based on the temperature-induced phase transition in the F-127/PLGA mixture without solvent [71]. This method provides F-127-coated PLGA nanoparticles (hydrophilized nanoparticles) used as a core. Figure 4.15 describes the preparation method of nanoparticles used as a polymeric core schematically. F-127 is in a flaky state and PLGA is in a powdery state at room temperature. The mixtures were prepared individually by weighing 85 mg of polymers with 0.2 weight ratio of (PLGA/F-127) and 3 mg of Tween 80 into 20 mL vials, which were immediately put into a vacuum oven at 60 °C. Within 30 min, both polymers were liquidized completely to form a transparent polymer solution. The melted mixtures were transferred to vacuum oven at 25 °C to induce the phase transition (the solidification of liquidized polymer mixture). With the phase transition, PLGA formed the phase-separated domain with a spherical form and F-127 formed the continuous phase as shown in Fig. 4.16. Following the equilibration period for 3 h, the solidified mixture was withdrawn from the vacuum oven and immersed in distilled/deionized water for 3 days to solubi-

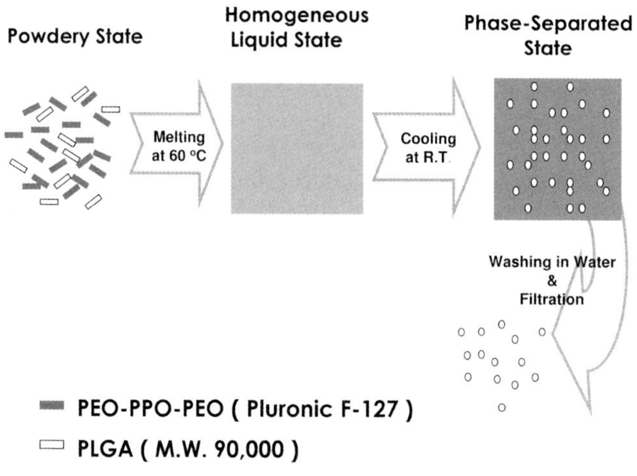

Figure 4.15. Schematic description of the method of preparation of PLGA nanospheres. (From Ref. [71].)

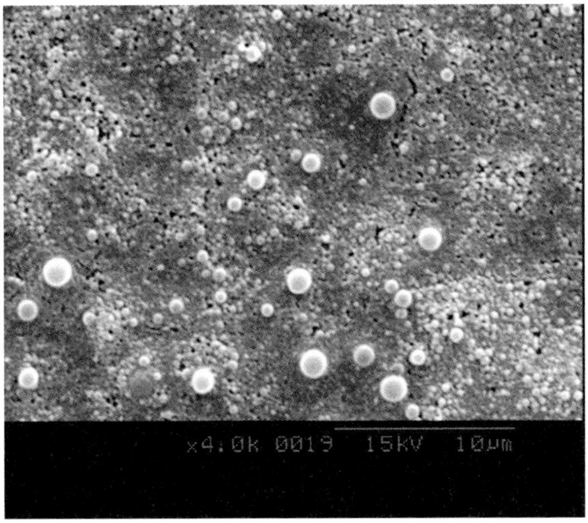

Figure 4.16. SEM image of phase-separated (8:2) (w/w) F-127/PLGA mixture. (From Ref. [71].)

lize F-127 using a dialysis bag (molecular weight cut-off range: 40–50 kDa; Fisher Scientific, USA), replacing the distilled/deionized water every hour. This aqueous solution containing PLGA nanoparticles was centrifuged for 20 min and filtered through the 0.45-µm filter membrane. The obtained PLGA nanoparticles were freeze-dried. In the final stage for preparing PLGA nanoparticles, Pluronics was removed from the phase-separated aggregate. However, the complete removal of Pluronic was impossible due to the hydrophobic interaction between the PLGA and the PPO domain of F-127, resulting in the formation of Pluronic-adhered PLGA nanoparticles. Due to the presence of F-127 on the surface of PLGA nanoparticles, stability in aqueous medium was significantly improved as shown in Fig. 4.17.

For the preparation of core–shell nanoparticles with a hydrophilic polymeric shell, the formation of a gel layer was induced. First, PLGA nanoparticles prepared previously were suspended in HA/F-127 aqueous solution with a variation of the weight ratio of HA/F-127. Subsequently, this aqueous solution mixture was subjected to freeze-drying to induce the formation of the polymeric shell.

Figure 4.18 describes the formation of core–shell nanoparticles with a hydrophilic polymeric shell and the protein-loading process [49]. F-127 forms a spherical micelle at low concentration. In this low micellar concentration regime, micelles are well-separated and the solution is an isotropic fluid. At higher concentrations, the micelles approach close packing and ordered domains, consisting of cubic packing of spherical micelles, are induced resulting in the gelation. With the freeze-drying process in this study, the concentration of F-127 aqueous solution was increased with the evaporation of water and gelation was induced to form a polymeric shell. With the evaporation of water by freeze-drying, F-127 was adsorbed (gelled) into F-127-coated PLGA nanoparticles and HA might be adsorbed

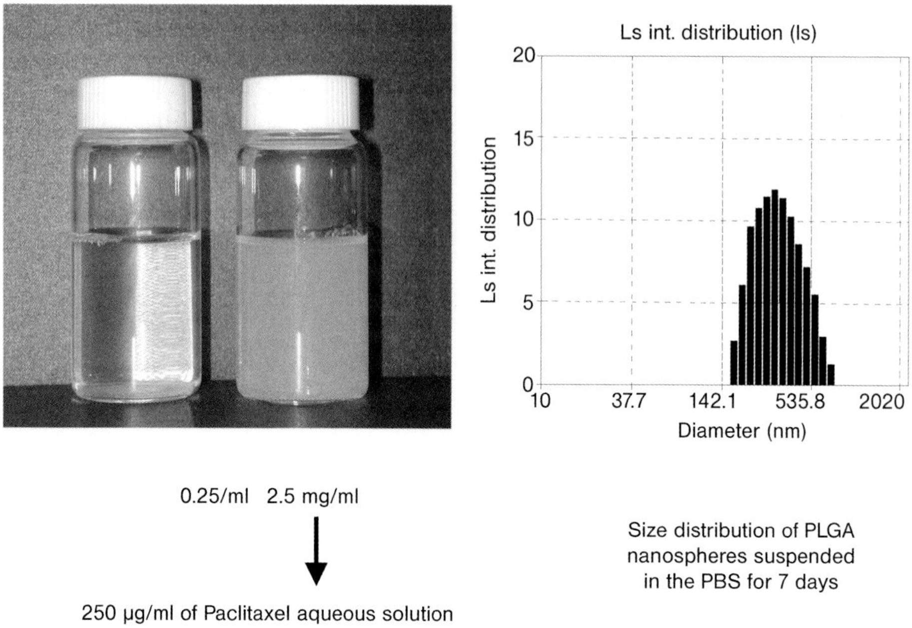

Figure 4.17. The enhanced stability of F-127-coated PLGA nanoparticles in aqueous media.

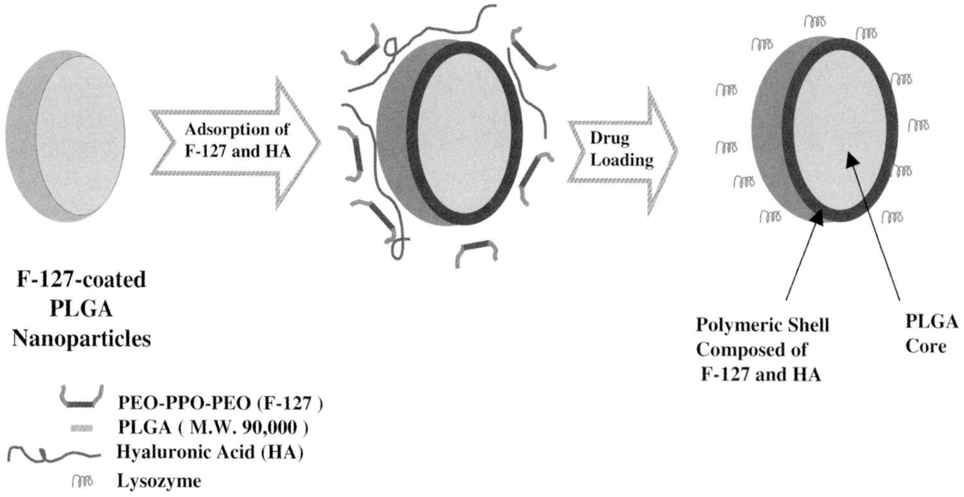

Figure 4.18. The formation of core–shell nanoparticles with a hydrophilic polymeric shell and the protein loading process. (From Ref. [49].)

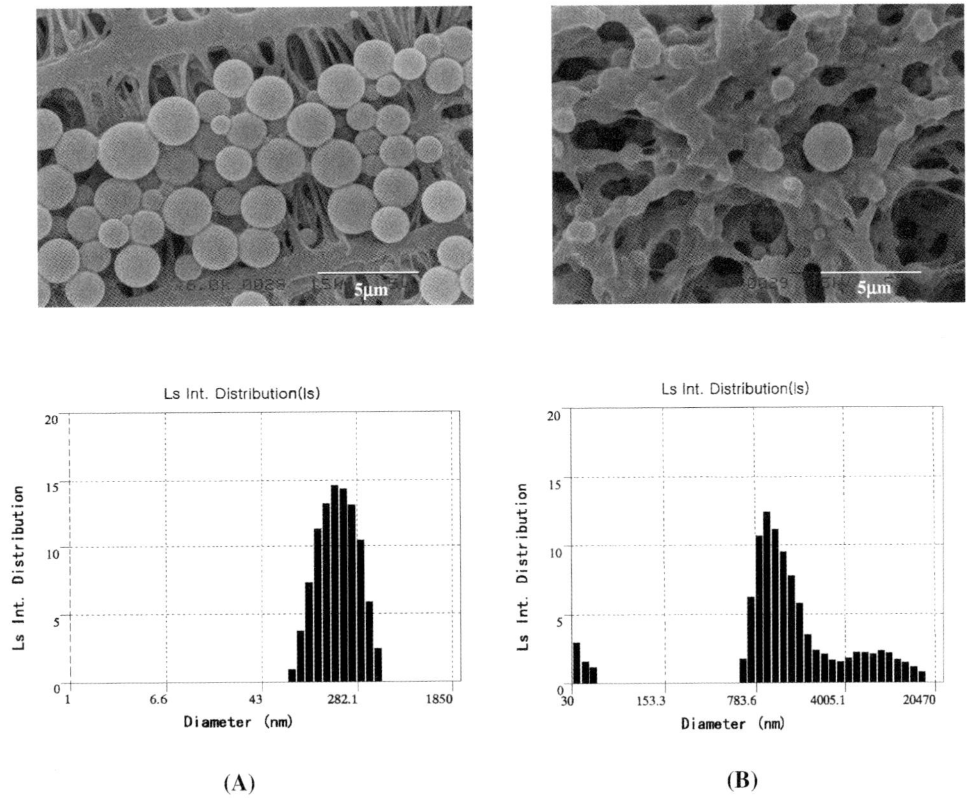

Figure 4.19. (A) SEM image and size distribution of core–shell nanoparticles formed from 5 wt% F-127 aqueous solution.
(B) SEM image and size distribution of core–shell nanoparticles formed from 10 wt% F-127 aqueous solution. (From Ref. [49].)

into F-127-coated PLGA nanoparticles with F-127, resulting in the formation of a polymeric shell composed of F-127/HA composite.

The shape of core–shell nanoparticles formed at different concentrations of F-127 in the absence of HA was examined by scanning electron microscopy (SEM) to observe the optimum concentration of F-127 for the stable formation of the polymeric shell. As shown in Fig. 4.19, the aggregation of nanoparticles was observed at core–shell nanoparticles formed as 10 wt% F-127 aqueous solution. This is due to the formation of a polymer network between free F-127 (which was not adsorbed on the surface of the PLGA nanoparticle). However, aggregation was not observed at the core–shell nanoparticles formed at 5 wt%, indicating that most F-127 in the aqueous media was adsorbed on the surface of PLGA nanoparticles. Therefore, the concentration of polymeric shell material was fixed at 5 wt% throughout the experiment. Note that the fibrous structure in the background of Figs. 4.19(A) and 4.20(A) is from the filter paper.

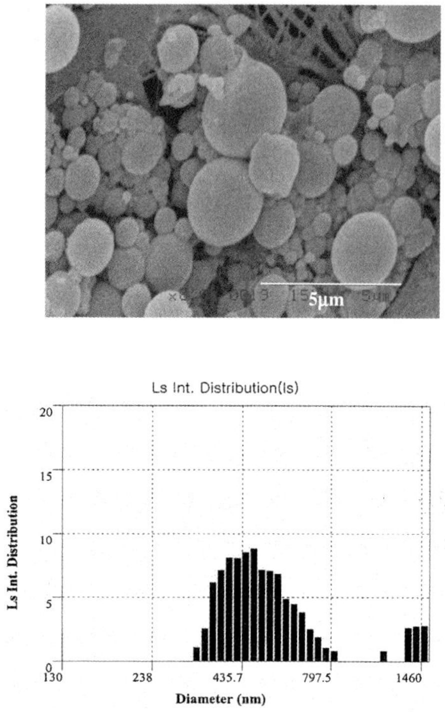

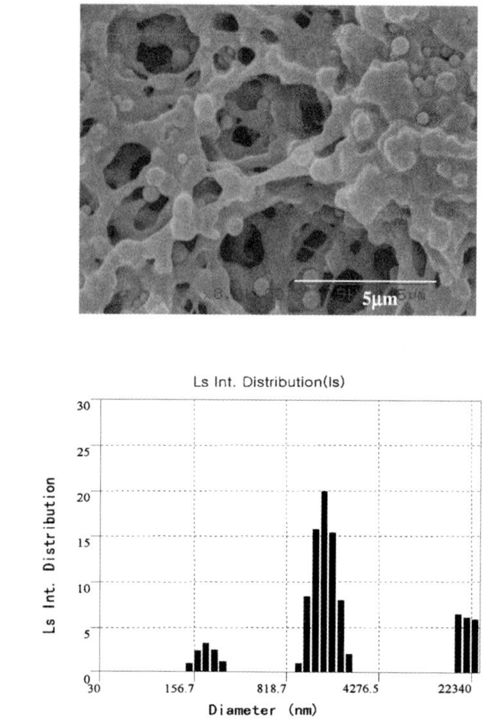

Figure 4.20. (A) SEM image and size distribution of core–shell nanoparticles with 0.2 weight ratio of HA/F-127. (B) SEM image and size distribution of core–shell nanoparticles with 0.4 weight ratio of HA/F-127. (From Ref. [49].)

For the efficient loading of cationic lysozyme (isoelectric point: 11.1) under physiological conditions, anionic HA was incorporated into the polymeric shell by co-adsorption with F-127. Core–shell nanoparticles were prepared with the variation of the HA/F-127 weight ratio. As shown in Fig. 4.20, the aggregation of nanoparticles was observed at 0.4 weight ratio of HA/F-127. This is due to the formation of a polymer network between free HA (which was not incorporated into the polymeric shell). In the adsorption of F-127 and HA on the surface of F-127-coated nanoparticles, the main driving force forming the polymeric shell is the hydrophobic interaction between F-127. As HA does not have intermolecular interactions with F-127 or PLGA nanoparticles, it is embedded physically in the F-127 network within the range of 0–0.3 weight ratio of HA/F-127. However, the formation of the HA/lysozyme complex without the PLGA core could be possible due to unstable embedding of HA in the polymeric shell. This property should be improved for

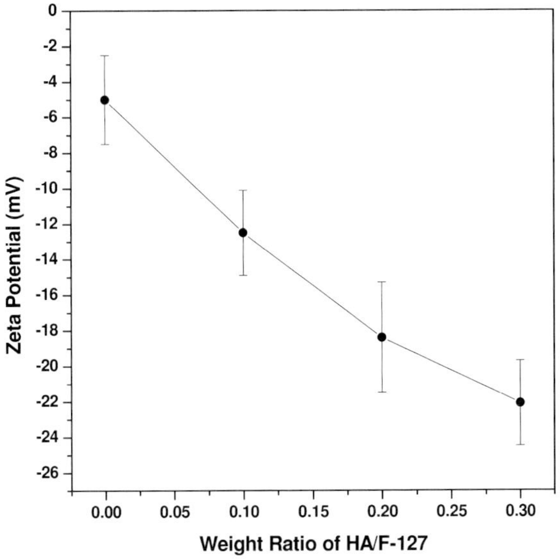

Figure 4.21. The variation of the ζ potential of core–shell nanoparticles as a function of the weight ratio of HA/F-127. (From Ref. [49].)

the exact manipulation of loading lysozyme (or negatively charged proteins under physiological conditions).

Figure 4.21 shows the variation of the ζ potential of core–shell nanoparticles with the variation of weight ratio of HA/F-127. The negative value was observed with the increase of weight ratio of HA/F-127, indicating that anionic HA is embedded in the polymeric shell and that the polymeric shell is suitable for the immobilization of cationic lysozyme.

Figure 4.22 shows the change of loading amount with the variation of weight ratio of HA/F-127. Lysozyme was loaded into core–shell nanoparticles by sorption method. Samples of 100 mg of dried core–shell nanoparticles were suspended in 100 mL of PBS containing 10 mg of lysozyme and stored at 25 °C to induce the ionic interaction between lysozyme and HA in the polymeric shell. After equilibrium for 12 h, this aqueous solution was centrifuged for 20 min and filtered through a 0.45-μm filter membrane. The obtained lysozyme-loaded core–shell nanoparticles were freeze-dried. The amount of unloaded lysozyme in the aqueous media was analyzed by high-performance liquid chromatography (HPLC) to measure the amount of drug loaded. Lysozyme was determined by reversed-phase HPLC using a Shodex RSpak RP 18-415 column and trifluoroacetic acid/acetonitrile (0.1/99.9, v/v%) mobile phase at a flow rate of 1 mL min^{-1}. The elute was monitored by UV absorption at 220 nm. The amount of drug loading is defined as the ratio of the amount of drug in the nanoparticles/total weight of nano-

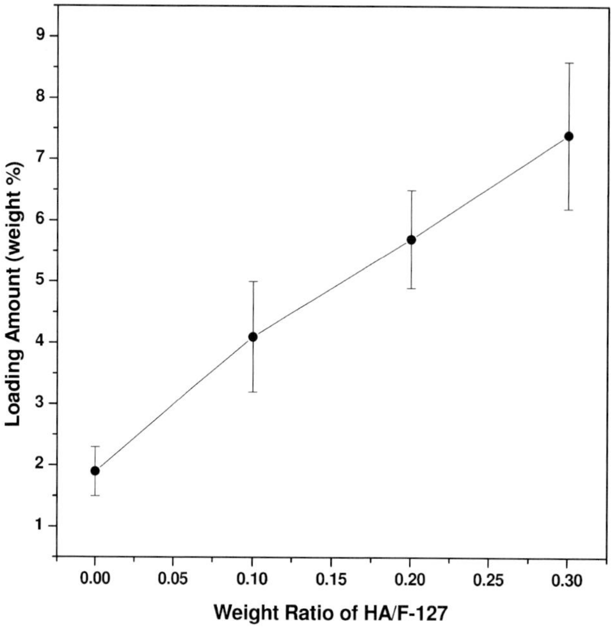

Figure 4.22. The variation of loading amount of core–shell nanoparticles as a function of the weight ratio of HA/F-127. (From Ref. [49].)

particles. The loading amount was increased up to 7 wt% with the increase of HA content in the polymeric shell. Due to the ionic interaction between cationic lysozyme and anionic HA in the PBS (pH 7.4), stable immobilization of lysozyme into the polymeric shell was induced and this led to the increase of the loading amount.

Figure 4.23 shows the release pattern of lysozyme from the core–shell nanoparticles formed as a function of weight ratio of HA/F-127. To measure the release pattern of lysozyme from the nanoparticles, 5 g of freeze-dried core–shell nanoparticles was put into 500 mL of PBS (pH 7.4). Temperature was maintained at 37 °C and stirring was maintained at 600 r.p.m. At given time intervals, 5-mL aliquots were withdrawn from release medium (PBS). HPLC analysis can then be performed as previously described. To maintain the sink condition in the release medium, 5 mL of fresh PBS was added to release medium after sampling. Without HA in the polymeric shell, a significant burst effect was observed. With the formation of the polymeric shell composed of F-127 and HA, the release rate was reduced significantly and an almost zero-order release pattern was observed at nanoparticles with 0.2 weight ratio of HA/F-127. Although HA is embedded in the F-127 network within the range of 0–0.3 weight ratio of HA/F-127 as shown in Fig. 4.21, it does not have intermolecular interactions with F-127 or PLGA nanoparticles and this leads to the release of HA from the polymeric shell. As lysozyme is ionically bound to HA, lysozyme and HA release together with the formation of

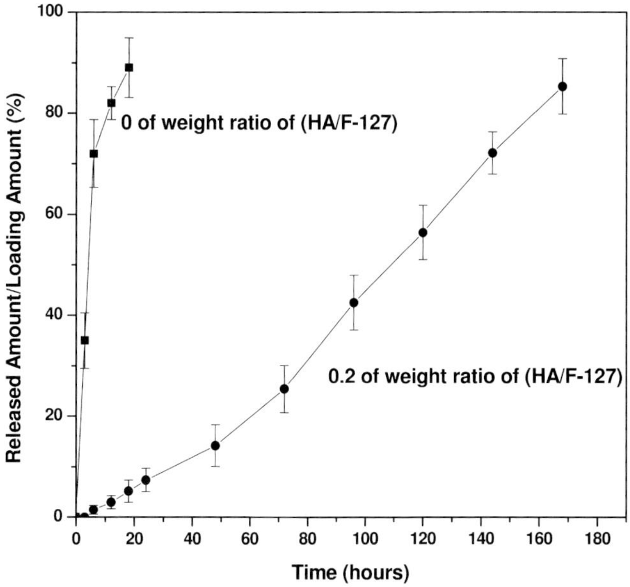

Figure 4.23. The release pattern of lysozyme from the core–shell nanoparticles. (From Ref. [49].)

an ion complex. To verify the release of HA from the polymeric shell, the variation of the ζ potential was measured as a function of time for equilibrium in the release media. Figure 4.24 shows that the ζ potential of core–shell nanoparticles with 0.2 weight ratio of HA/F-127 was increased with the increase of equilibrium time. This indicates that HA is released from the polymeric shell during the release of lysozyme and the sustained release of lysozyme is due to the release of the ionic complex composed of HA and lysozyme, which has a higher molecular weight compared with free lysozyme.

The specific enzyme activity of lysozyme in the release media after the 1-week release experiment was measured. For lysozyme activity assay, a suspension of 0.1 mg mL^{-1} *Micrococcus lysodeikticus* was prepared in PBS (37 °C). To 2.95 mL *M. lysodeikticus* suspension, 0.05 mL lysozyme solution was added and mixed immediately. The turbidity of the suspension was measured at 450 nm by a Shimadzu UV-1601 spectrophotometer. One unit of activity corresponds to a decrease in turbidity of 0.001 min^{-1} at 450 nm [72]. In comparison to the activity of native lysozyme, 81.3% activity was preserved and this indicates that the activity of lysozyme was preserved during the freeze-drying process.

Core–shell nanoparticles with a composite polymeric shell composed of F-127 and HA have been prepared based on the hydrophobic interaction between PLGA and the PPO domain of F-127. Although HA does not have intermolecular interactions in the polymeric shell, the formation of the polymeric shell composed of F-127 and HA within the range of 0.3 weight ratio of HA/F-127 was observed.

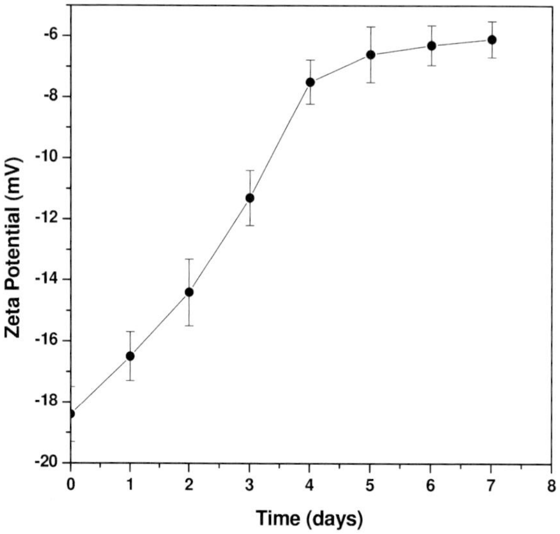

Figure 4.24. The variation of the ζ potential of core–shell nanoparticles as a function of the time for equilibrium in PBS. (From Ref. [49].)

Due to the ionic interaction of cationic lysozyme and anionic HA under physiological conditions, the efficient loading and sustained release of lysozyme were accomplished. This enables us to prepare charged nanoparticles with a core–shell structure for the delivery of protein drug.

4.3.2
Heparin-functionalized PLGA Nanoparticles

A new, facile method to prepare heparin-functionalized PLGA nanoparticles for the controlled release of growth factors has been developed [73]. This system is composed of PLGA as a hydrophobic core, F-127 as a hydrophilic surface layer (polymeric shell) and heparin as the functional moiety. Nanoparticles were prepared by a solvent-diffusion method without chemical modification of the components.

Heparin is a highly sulfated, anionic polysaccharide composed of repeating disaccharides of 1–4-linked glucosamine and uronic acid residues. Heparin is best known for its anticoagulant properties that are mediated through a pentasaccharide sequence that binds antithrombin III (AT-III) and subsequently complexes thrombin [74]. Heparin also interacts with a variety of proteins that have heparin-binding domains, including various growth factors, e.g. fibroblast growth factor (FGF) family [75], VEGF family [76], platelet-derived growth factor (PDGF) family [77], transforming growth factor (TGF)-β family [78] and glial-derived neurotrophic factor (GDNF) [79]. This binding between growth factor and heparin or heparan sulfate proteoglycans enables the growth factors to crosslink their receptors, and the association stabilizes the growth factor and protects it from proteolytic degradation [80, 81].

Based on the high specific binding of heparin for various growth factors, several heparin-containing systems have been developed for the controlled release of the growth factors. Edelman and coworkers encapsulated heparin-conjugated and basic FGF (bFGF)-loaded Sepharose beads in calcium alginate microspheres and demonstrated the controlled release of bFGF [82]. Sakiyama-Elbert and coworkers incorporated heparin-binding peptide 5 domains into a fibrin gel to bind heparin, which was then used to load and release bFGF [75] or β-nerve growth factor (NGF) [83]. Wissink and coworkers grafted collagen matrices with heparin and the sustained release of loaded bFGF was observed [84]. Tanihara and coworkers crosslinked alginate and heparin with diamine using carbodiimide activation to construct a hydrogel which showed sustained release of loaded bFGF [85]. Seal and coworkers covalently attached heparin-binding peptides to multi-arm PEGs, which were then physically crosslinked with heparin [86]. Among the heparin-binding growth factors, VEGF is of particular interest in tissue engineering due to its proangiogenic properties [87, 88]. So far, PLGA microspheres have been generally adapted for the particle-type sustained release system of growth factors [89, 90]. However, the encapsulation of proteins into hydrophobic PLGA cores has easily denatured proteins to aggregate and adsorb on the degrading PLGA surface [91–94], and also the presence of a water/organic solvent interface during protein loading has been identified as a major cause of protein denaturation and aggregation [95–97]. Alginate has also been used to encapsulate growth factors [98–100]. Even though there is no interfacial problem when proteins are encapsulated in alginate beads, rapid release and an initial burst of encapsulated proteins, as well as irreversible complexation with alginate were reported [100, 101]. Growth factor delivery by gelatin microspheres is very similar to the case of the alginate system [102, 103]. The main interaction between protein and gelatin is polyion complexation and the conformational change of the gelatin molecule is also followed. In addition, even though alginate and gelatin are natural polymers, growth factors do not have any binding domains on these polymers, thus limiting the binding events to the proteins with net positive charges [104]. Several heparin-based micelles or nanoparticles have also been developed as drug carriers [105–107]. However, all these systems employed chemical modifications of the functional group sequence of heparin to attach with either hydrophobic polymers or the low-molecular-weight hydrophobic moiety, thus reducing the bioactivity of the heparin, as represented by antithrombic activity [108].

The nanoparticles were prepared by a spontaneous emulsion solvent diffusion method as follows (Fig. 4.25). Samples of 40 mg of PLGA were dissolved in 2 mL DMSO at room temperature. The organic phase was then slowly added to 30 mL of deionized water containing 1.5 g of F-127 and a fixed amount of heparin with vigorous stirring. The amount of heparin was varied to control the entrapped heparin on the nanoparticles. The nanoparticles formed in the aqueous solution were col-

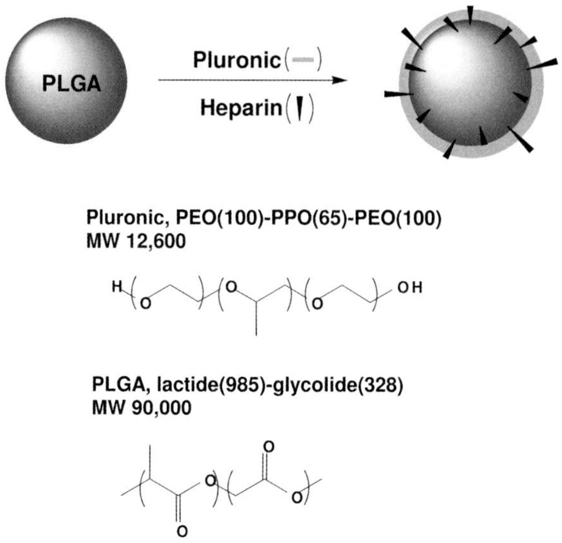

Figure 4.25. Schematic representation of heparin-functionalized PLGA nanoparticle preparation and chemical structures of the components. (From Ref. [73].)

lected by high-speed centrifugation (Hanil Science Industrial, Korea) at 12 000 r.p.m. for 1 h and resuspended in 0.5 mL of PBS solution containing 1.0% (w/v) Tween 80.

The size, polydispersity and surface charge of the nanoparticles were characterized by varying the amount of heparin in the aqueous phase. For the nanoparticles prepared from the aqueous solution containing no heparin, monodispersed nanoparticles with an average diameter of 156 ± 3 nm and polydispersity of 0.09 ± 0.03 were obtained. The surface charge from the ζ potential measurement was -26.0 ± 1.1 mV (Fig. 4.26). By increasing the amount of heparin in the aqueous phase during the preparation of nanoparticles, the ζ potential value decreased significantly, whereas the size and the polydispersity of nanoparticles varied little. However, when the amount of heparin in the aqueous phase was increased to 240 mg, both the size and the polydispersity of the nanoparticles increased noticeably to 188 ± 4 and 0.13 ± 0.04 nm. Thus, it can be concluded that heparin molecules were entrapped in the nanoparticles, maintaining their monodisperse distribution when the amount of heparin in the aqueous phase was less than 240 mg.

To obtain specific information about the amount and distribution of heparin in the nanoparticles, the anti-factor Xa (FXa) assay of the nanoparticles prepared at various conditions was carried out. Anti-FXa assay (Chromogenix Instrumentation Laboratory, Italy) on nanoparticles was carried out to calculate the amount of heparin in nanoparticles. The principle of this assay is that the amount of neutralized FXa binding with a heparin–antithrombin (AT) complex is proportional to the

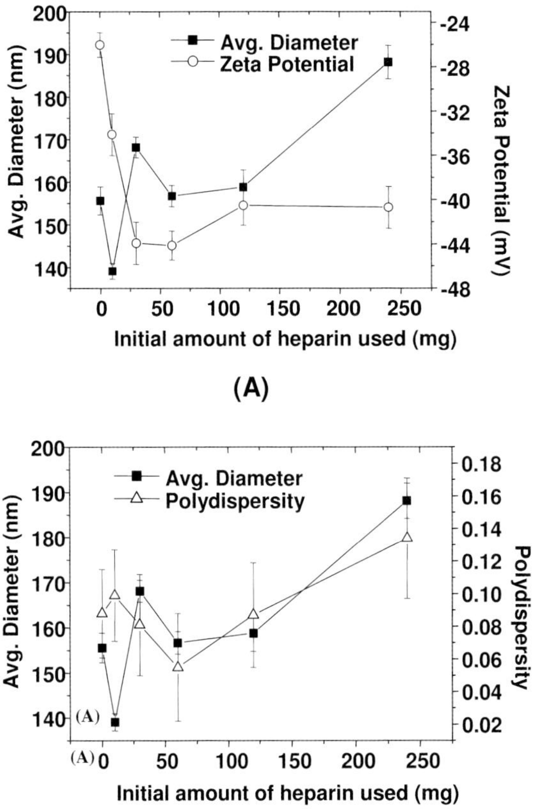

Figure 4.26. The size, surface charge and polydispersity of heparin-functionalized PLGA nanoparticles obtained by varying the amount of heparin in the aqueous phase during preparation. $N = 6$ experiments. (From Ref. [73].)

amount of heparin. In order to measure the total amount of heparin in nanoparticles, the lyophilized nanoparticles were dissolved in methylene chloride to extract PLGA and F-127, and then the precipitated heparin was collected. On the other hand, the amount of heparin available on the nanoparticle surface was directly measured using the nanoparticle–AT complexation. In this assay, the activity of heparin distributed in the nanoparticle surface layer was measured using the diluted nanoparticle suspension and the heparin activity was increased by increasing the amount of heparin in the aqueous phase during the nanoparticle preparation. The activity of total heparin both in the nanoparticle core and surface layer, measured by extracting the entire heparin molecules entrapped in the nanoparticles, was a little higher than the heparin activity in the surface layer. The heparin activity was converted to the amount of heparin by using the anti-FXa activity of the heparin sodium used. The amount of heparin in the surface layer and the core of the nanoparticles, obtained by subtracting the amount in the surface layer from the

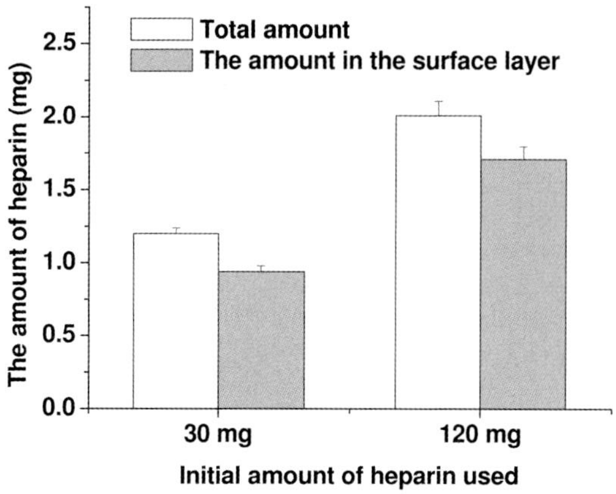

Figure 4.27. The amount of heparin in heparin-functionalized PLGA nanoparticles determined by the anti-FXa assay. $N = 3$ experiments. (From Ref. [73].)

total amount, revealed that heparin molecules were mainly distributed in the nanoparticle surface layer and only a relatively small amount of heparin was in the nanoparticle core (Fig. 4.27).

^{1}H-nuclear magnetic resonance (NMR) analysis of nanoparticles was performed to obtain the mole ratio between F-127 and PLGA in the nanoparticles. The ^{1}H-NMR (JEOL JNM-LA300WB FT-NMR Spectrometer, Japan) analysis was performed to calculate the molar ratio between PLGA and F-127 in the nanoparticles. The suspension of nanoparticles was freeze-dried and then dissolved in $CDCl_3$. The molar ratio was calculated using the integral of separate peaks of CH (5.1 p.p.m.) of PLGA and CH_33 (1.1 p.p.m.) of F-127 (Fig. 4.28).

The weight percentage of the heparin entrapped in the nanoparticles was 0.0, 2.4 and 4.7 for the nanoparticles prepared from an aqueous phase containing 0, 40 and 120 mg of heparin, respectively. Thus, the proposed method can manufacture the monodisperse nanoparticles containing heparin up to 4.7 wt% in total (4.0 wt% at the surface layer) and the amount of heparin can be controlled by adjusting the amount of heparin in the aqueous phase during preparation. The localization of F-127 molecules to the PLGA cores during particle formation is probably due to the hydrophobic interaction between the PPO block of F-127 and PLGA. The interaction between heparin and PEO blocks of F-127 may also contribute to localization of heparin on the nanoparticles, resulting in a high concentration of heparin in the nanoparticles. A similar observation has been reported between alginate and Pluronic F-127; the formation of crosslinks between the carboxyl group of alginate and PEO blocks of PF-127 leads to the formation of a three-dimensional network, resulting in improved shear stress.

Lysozyme was selected as a model protein for the *in vitro* release experiments using the heparin-functionalized PLGA nanoparticles. To load lysozyme into the nanoparticles, the resuspended nanoparticles were mixed with 0.1 mL PBS

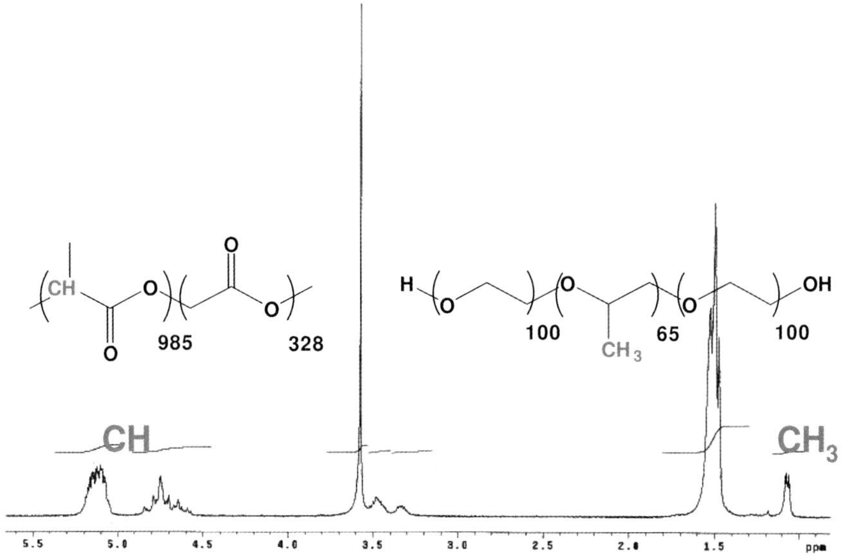

Figure 4.28. ^1H NMR analysis to calculate the molar ratio between PLGA and F-127 constituting the heparin-functionalized PLGA nanoparticles by comparing ^1H from CH of PLGA (5.1 p.p.m.) and ^3H from CH_3 of Pluronic F-127 (1.1 p.p.m.). (From Ref. [73].)

containing 1 mg of lysozyme and then incubated at 4 °C overnight with gentle rotation, which yields the loading of 1 mg of lysozyme into 43.3 mg of heparin-functionalized PLGA nanoparticles. Then, lysozyme-loaded nanoparticle suspension (0.6 mL) was subsequently put into a dialysis tube. The dialysis tube was placed in 100 mL PBS containing 2.0 mM sodium azide and kept under the same conditions as described previously.

Lysozyme can interact electrostatically with the heparin because lysozyme is net positively charged (the isoelectric point of lysozyme is pH 11.1). The average diameter and size distribution of nanoparticles after loading lysozyme were not changed after loading, and there was no aggregated complex among lysozyme-loaded nanoparticles. Figure 4.29 shows release profiles of lysozyme from three kinds of nanoparticles with different heparin contents of 0.0, 2.4 and 4.7%, respectively. In the case of the nanoparticles with no heparin, over two-thirds of the total lysozyme loaded was released within 3 days. In contrast, the nanoparticles with heparin contents of 2.4 and 4.7% showed linear and complete release profiles without any initial burst up to 10 and 19 days, respectively which shows net positively charged lysozyme was well bound in the negatively charged surface layer of the nanoparticles. To characterize the deactivation of lysozyme released from the heparin-functionalized nanoparticles, the concentration of the released lysozyme was analyzed based on the bioactivity of the released lysozyme on *M. lysodeikticus* cell walls using a lysozyme assay kit and compared with the concentration of the total

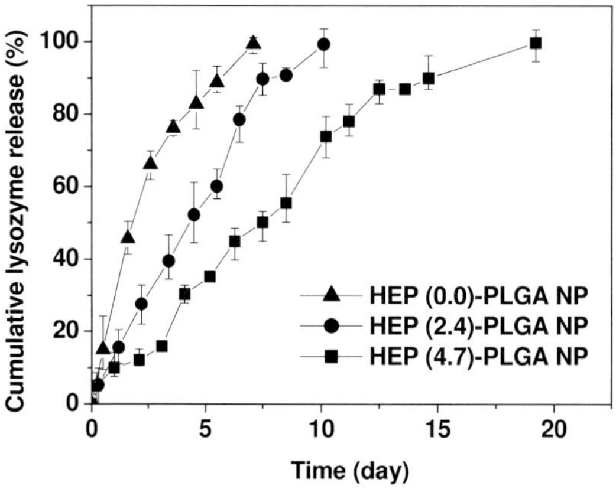

Figure 4.29. Cumulative lysozyme release from three kinds of heparin-functionalized PLGA nanoparticles with different heparin contents. $N = 3$ experiments. (From Ref. [73].)

protein measured using the Micro BCA protein assay (Fig. 4.30). There were no differences between the total protein concentration and the bioactive lysozyme concentration at each time-point, showing that no denaturation of lysozyme occurred during loading into the nanoparticles and release from them.

Nanoparticles with a heparin content of 4.7% were selected as a VEGF release system, based on the result of the lysozyme release experiment. First, the release experiment was performed with loading 250 ng of VEGF into 14.4 mg of the nanoparticles. To load VEGF into the nanoparticles, both one-third and one-tenth of re-

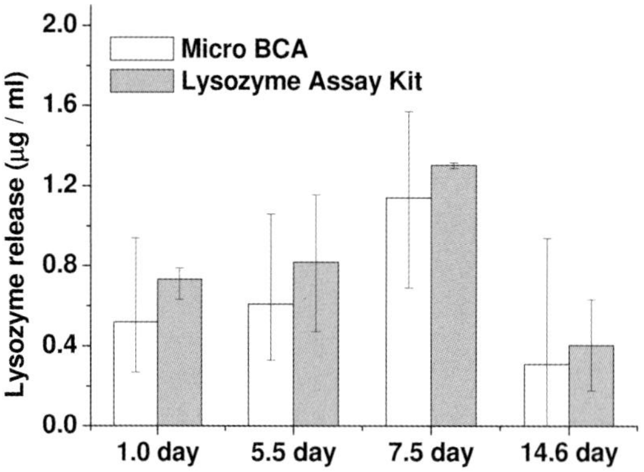

Figure 4.30. Comparison of the concentrations of lysozyme released from heparin-functionalized PLGA nanoparticles measured by the bioactivity on *M. lysodeikticus* cell walls using a lysozyme assay kit and the total protein concentration using a Micro BCA protein assay. $N = 3$ experiments. (From Ref. [73].)

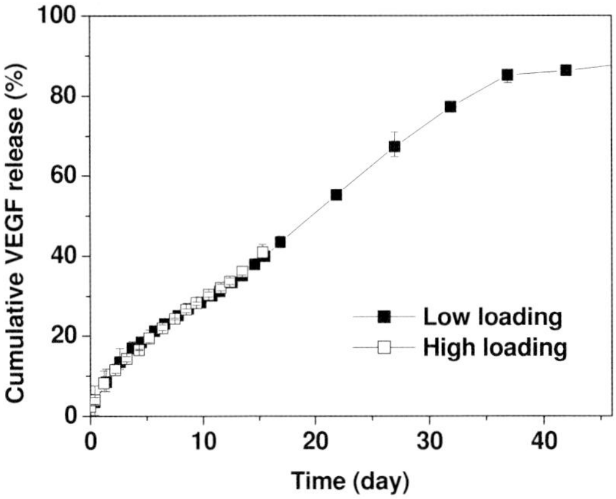

Figure 4.31. Cumulative VEGF release from heparin-functionalized PLGA nanoparticle with 4.7% w/w of heparin for two different loading amounts. $N = 3$ experiments. (From Ref. [73].)

suspended nanoparticles were mixed with 25 μL PBS containing 250 ng of VEGF and 75 μL PBS containing 750 ng of VEGF, respectively, and then incubated at 4 °C overnight with gentle rotation, which yields loading of 250 ng of VEGF into 14.4 mg of nanoparticles and 750 ng of recombinant human VEGF into 4.3 mg of nanoparticles.

After loading, no aggregation among the protein-loaded nanoparticles was observed. The stability of VEGF in the release medium (PBS solution containing 0.1 wt% BSA) was conformed by comparing the concentration of VEGF in the release medium incubated at 37 °C for 24 h. The release of VEGF from the nanoparticles showed a linear profile without any initial burst up to day 37, releasing about 85% of the initial loading amount, and then the release rate was slowed down (Fig. 4.31). This release pattern was similar to the case of lysozyme; however, a much more prolonged release pattern was obtained. To elucidate whether the prolonged release was responsible from the decreased loading amount of the protein or the more specific interaction between VEGF and heparin than that between lysozyme and heparin, the loading amount of VEGF to the nanoparticles was increased 10-fold. The relative release rates (percent of the total amount) were almost same in both cases. Thus, the prolonged release pattern was mainly due to the more strong and specific interaction between VEGF and heparin than that between lysozyme and heparin.

Nanoparticles with heparin molecules on the surface were prepared by solvent diffusion without any chemical reaction. Monodispersed nanoparticles containing heparin up to 4.7 wt% in total (4.0 wt% at the surface layer) were manufactured and the amount of heparin was controlled by adjusting the amount of heparin in the aqueous phase during preparation. The release of lysozyme from the nanoparticles with 4.7 wt% heparin showed a linear and complete release profile without any initial burst over 2 weeks, and the released lysozymes maintained their bioactivity. The release of VEGF from the nanoparticles showed a linear and more prolonged profile without any initial burst over 1 month, mainly due to the stronger and more specific interaction between VEGF and heparin than that between lysozyme and heparin. Thus, the heparin-functionalized PLGA nanoparticles can be employed a growth factor delivery component in tissue engineering scaffolds as well as a sustained release system for various heparin binding growth factors.

4.4 Core–shell Nanoparticles with a Metallic Core

Core–shell nanoparticles with a metallic core have been studied intensively for application in the biomedical areas such as for magnetic resonance contrast agents [109], targeted drug delivery [110], and cancer diagnosis and treatment [111]. With the formation of core–shell nanoparticles with a metallic core (polymer-coated magnetic nanoparticles), a magnetic resonance contrast agent with enhanced stability and biocompatibility under physiological conditions can be achieved. Previously, iron oxide nanoparticles were stabilized with the formation of a polymeric layer on the surface of iron oxide nanoparticles using dextran, starch, albumin, silicones or PEG [112, 113]. The coprecipitation of iron salts in a polymeric coating solution by the microemulsion method [114] or and laser-induced pyrolysis [115] was used to prepare polymer-coated iron oxide nanoparticles. However, the wide size distribution remains still challenging with regard to the formation of a polymer shell on the surface of magnetic nanoparticles.

Recently, PVP-coated iron oxide nanoparticles with a narrow size distribution were prepared [109] based on the thermal decomposition presented previously [117–125]. First, 1 g of PVP was dissolved in 3 mL of DMF and this solution was purged with nitrogen to remove oxygen in a three-neck, round-bottom flask. The resulting mixture was heated to around 160 °C under vigorous mechanical stirring and $Fe(CO)_5$ was injected into the mixture. The reaction mixture was stirred for 2 h at 160 °C. During this process, the initial orange color of the solution gradually became a brownish black colloid solution. The colloid solution was cooled at room temperature and dialyzed for the removal of excess unreacted PVP at 37 °C for 2–3 days whilst being continuously stirred. For the characterization of PVP-coated nanoparticles, the dialyzed colloidal solution was freeze-dried.

Figure 4.32 shows the X-ray diffraction (XRD) data of pure PVP and PVP-coated iron oxide nanoparticles to confirm the crystallinity of the PVP-coated iron oxide nanoparticles. The characteristic patterns of the spinel phases Fe_2O_3 and Fe_3O_4 were observed, and this showed that iron oxide nanoparticles in PVP-coated iron oxide nanoparticles were mixtures of Fe_2O_3 and Fe_3O_4.

The hysteresis loop of PVP-coated iron oxide at in room temperature is shown in Fig. 4.33. The magnetic properties of PVP-coated iron oxide nanoparticles were measured at room temperature with $/H/ \leq 20$ kOe using Quantum Design MPMS 5 superconducting quantum interface device (SQUID) magnetometer. The mass

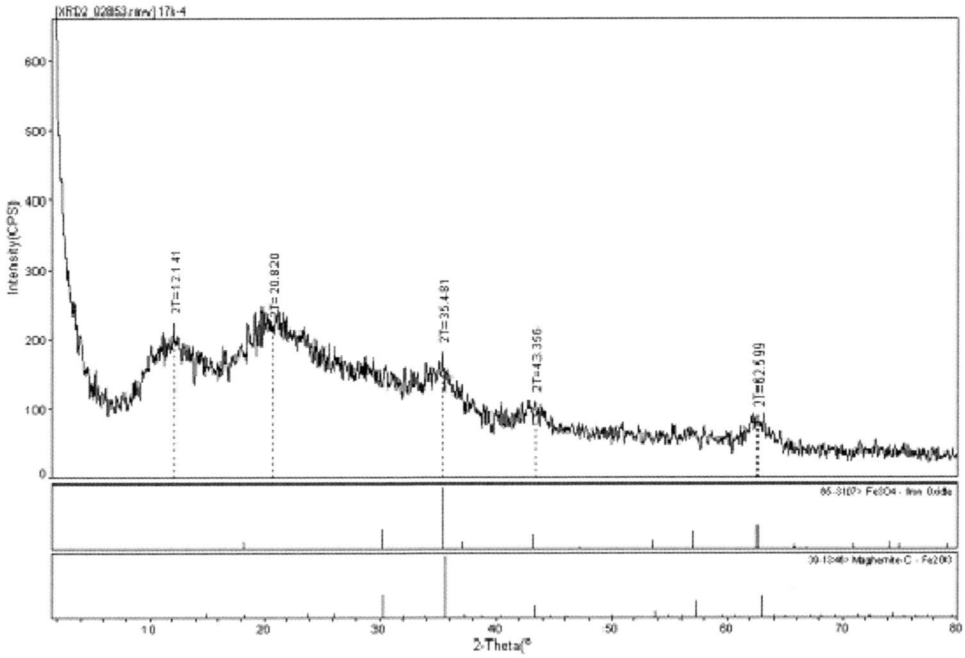

Figure 4.32. XRD pattern of PVP-coated iron oxide. (From Ref. [109].)

magnetization is defined as the magnetic moment per total mass of sample measured. The PVP-coated iron oxide nanoparticles produced were characterized by a high magnetic moment in a high magnetic field (generally, about 5–90 e.m.u. g^{-1} of metal oxide) and a negligible magnetic moment in the absence of an applied field. Such behavior is characteristic of superparamagnetic particles. From the results, 3- and 50- to 100-nm PVP-coated iron oxide nanoparticles exhibited superparamagnetic properties. The saturation magnetization of 3-nm particles was 34 e.m.u. g^{-1} Fe and the saturation magnetization of 50- to 100-nm nanoparticles was 90 e.m.u. g^{-1} Fe. These results showed that bigger iron oxide nanoparticles had larger mass magnetization.

Figure 4.34 shows a TEM image and particle size analysis of PVP-coated iron oxide nanoparticles prepared in DMF. The TEM image shows that the diameter of nanoparticles is 50–100 nm with a spherical shape. Following resuspension of nanoparticles into aqueous media, the size distribution analysis demonstrates that the colloid has the diameter of 200 nm. A similar process was applied to PVP-coated iron oxide nanoparticles prepared in Carbitol as shown in Fig. 4.35. Nanoparticles of 3 nm diameter were observed in the dried state and those of 100 nm diameter were observed in the aqueous media with a narrow size distribution. These size differences are due to the swelling of PVA on the surface of the iron oxide nanoparticles (metallic core); this indicates the formation of PVP-coated iron oxide nanoparticles.

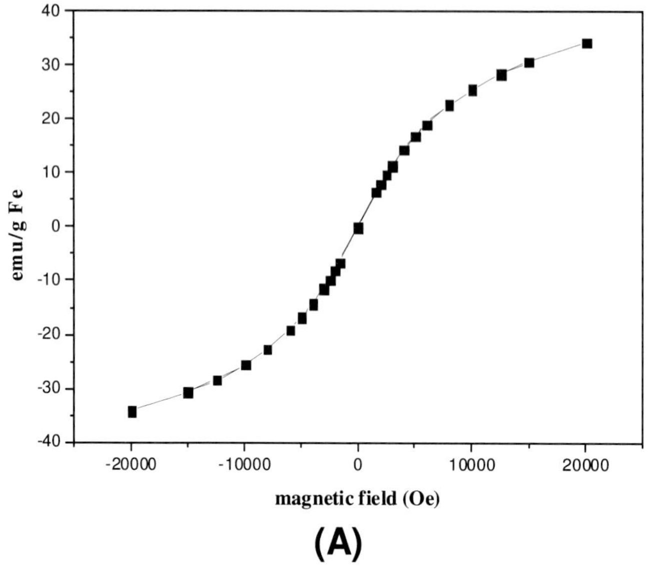

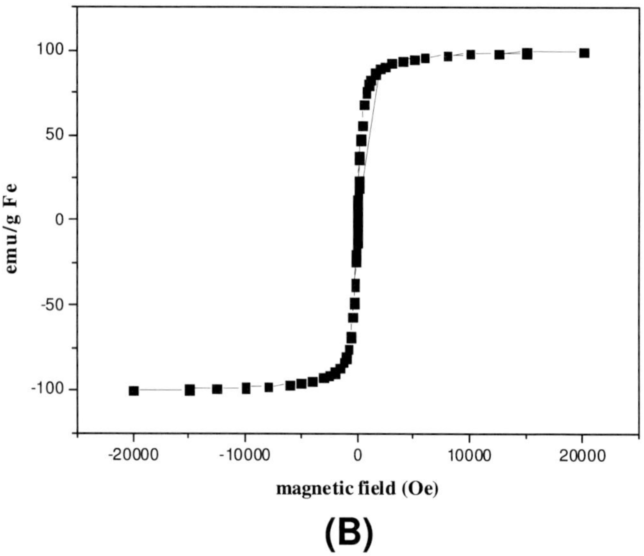

Figure 4.33. Magnetization curve of PVP-coated iron oxide nanoparticles of (A) 3 and (B) 50–100 nm at room temperature. (From Ref. [109].)

Fourier transform IR (FTIR) spectra of pure PVP and PVP-coated iron oxide nanoparticles are presented in Fig. 4.36. With the increase of PVP/$Fe(CO)_5$ molar ratios, the C=O absorption bands were shifted from 1670 to 1653.56 cm^{-1}. The results showed that iron oxide was coordinated through the carbonyl group of PVP,

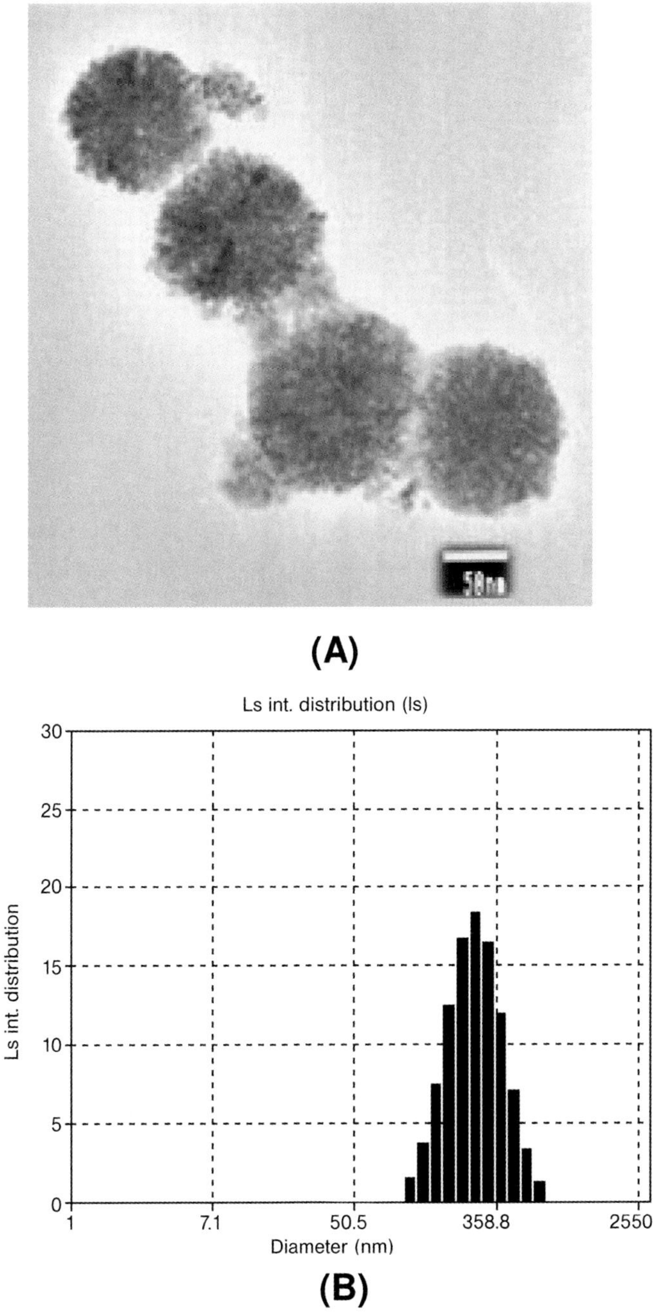

Figure 4.34. (A) TEM image and (B) size distribution of PVP-coated iron oxide nanoparticles prepared with DMF as solvent. (From Ref. [109].)

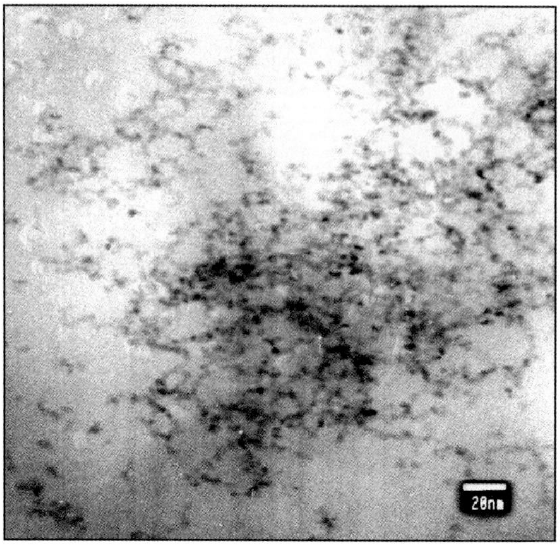

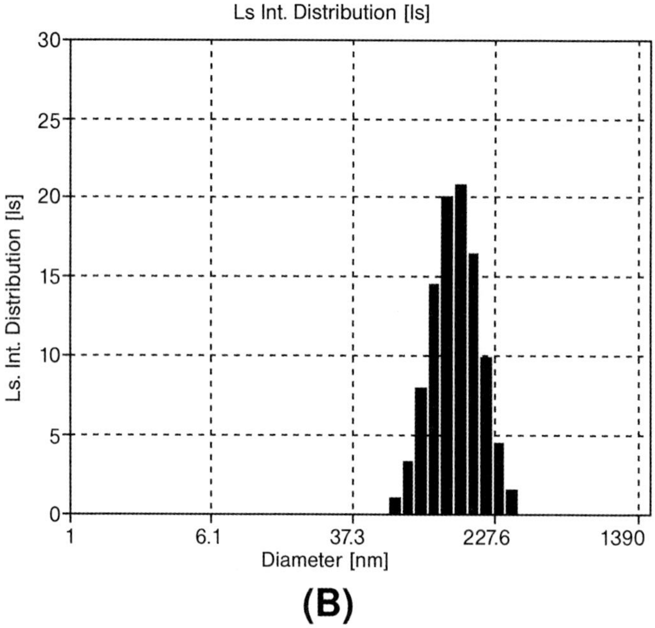

Figure 4.35. (A) TEM image and (B) size distribution of PVP-coated iron oxide nanoparticles prepared with Carbitol as solvent. (From Ref. [109].)

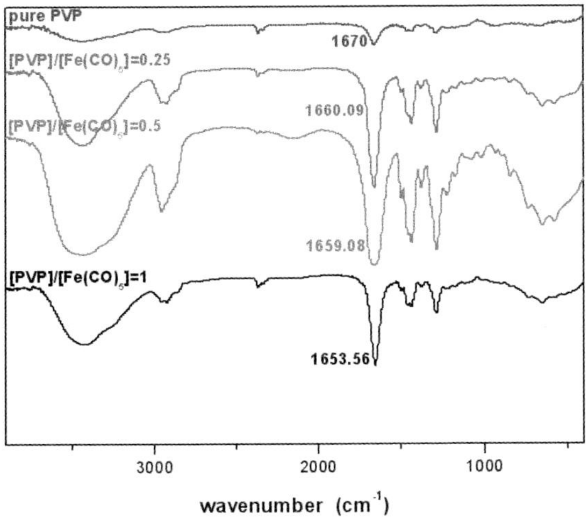

Figure 4.36. FTIR spectra of pure PVP and PVP-coated iron oxide nanoparticles. (From Ref. [109].)

and the interaction between PVP and iron oxide was increased with the increase of the particle size.

For further confirmation of coordination between iron oxide and the carbonyl group of PVP, X-ray photoelectric spectroscopy (XPS) spectra were observed as shown in Fig. 4.37. Correction of the energy shift due to the static charging of the samples was accomplished with the C 1s peak at 284.6 eV as a reference. The accuracy of the reported binding energies was ± 0.1 eV. The photoelectron peaks at 711.3 and 726 eV are the characteristic doublets of Fe 2p from iron oxide. The N

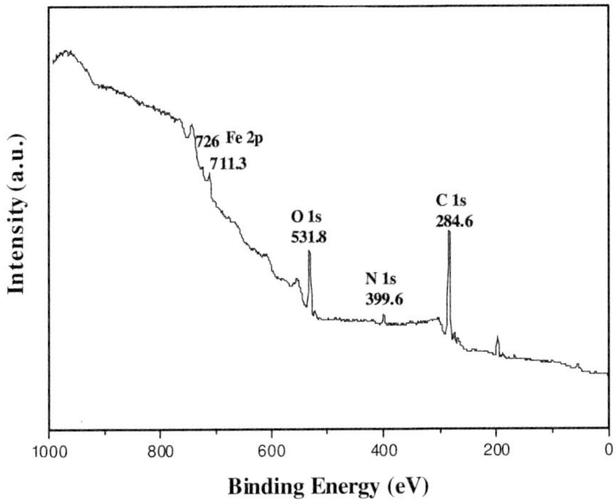

Figure 4.37. XPS spectra of PVP-coated iron oxide nanoparticles. (From Ref. [109].)

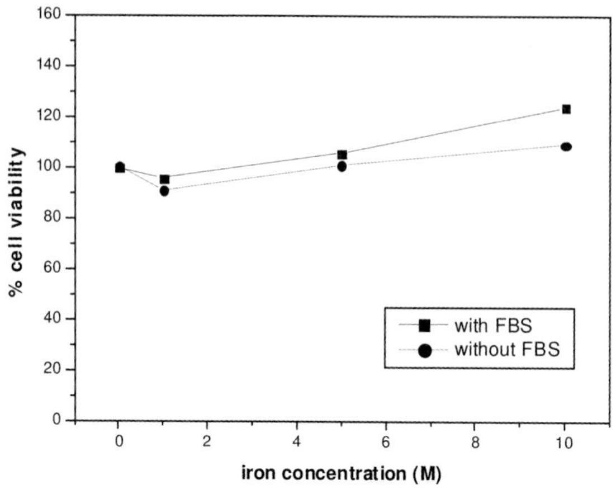

Figure 4.38. Viability of cells exposed to a solution containing PVP-coated iron oxide nanoparticles at various iron concentrations. (From Ref. [109].)

1s peak centered at 399.6 eV indicates that the nitrogen is influenced by the iron oxide. The O 1s peak at 531.8 eV is shifted toward to higher binding energy compared with pure PVP (530.3 eV), implying the decrease of electron density around O atoms in the carbonyl group of PVP, probably due to the interaction between iron oxide and O atoms in PVP [126].

Figure 4.38 shows the viability of cells exposed to the solution containing PVP-coated iron oxide nanoparticles at various iron concentrations for 4 h. To test whether the PVP-coated iron oxide nanoparticles had biocompatibility, a 5-dimethyhlthiazol-2-yl-2,5-diphenyl tetrazolium bromide (MTT) assay was performed. Cell viability is expressed as the mean $\pm$ SE of percentage of absorbance of controls where 100% equals viability of untreated control cells. Although the iron concentration increased, cell viability did not decrease. Following the formation of the PVP layer on the surface of iron oxide nanoparticles, a significant increase in the biocompatibility was observed.

With the administration of 40 μmol PVP-coated iron oxide intravenously into the rabbit, T2-weighted magnetic resonance imaging (MRI) images were observed as shown in Fig. 4.39. Samples 0.24 g of PVP-coated iron oxide nanoparticles were added to 1.4 mL distilled water and this solution was administered to rabbits weighing 4 kg. The concentration was equal to the concentration of commercially available Resovist (40 μmol Fe kg^{-1}). *In vitro* MRI test were performed with a 3.0 T MRI system (Philips, The Netherlands). The T2-weighted MRI images of prepared and commercial samples were observed. The sequence parameter was T2-weighed images; fast gradient echo with repetition time (TR) = 9.6 ms, echo time (TE) = 4.6 ms, flip angle = 8.0°, field of view = 10×5 cm^2. The images are T2-weighted MRI images before injection of contrast agent (left) and after injection

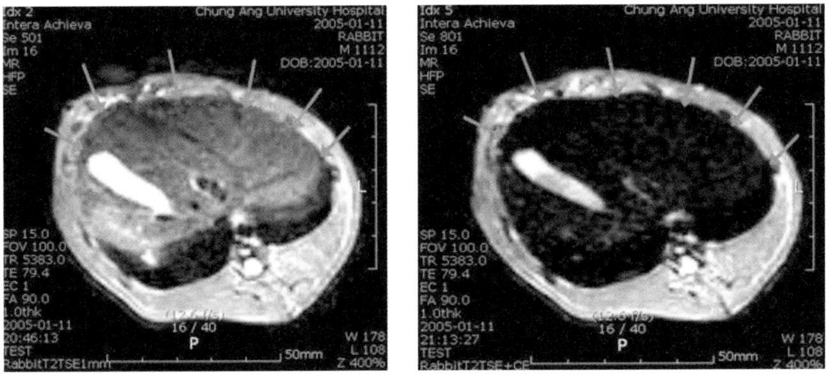

Figure 4.39. T2-weighted MRI images before injection of contrast agent (left) and after injection of PVP-coated iron oxide nanoparticles (right). (From Ref. [109].)

of PVP-coated iron oxide nanoparticles (right). This showed a profound negative enhancement of the liver after injection of PVP-coated iron oxide, indicating that the iron oxide contrast agent improved the detection of the liver lesions significantly.

4.5 Conclusions

With the variation of core materials, various types of core–shell nanoparticles are being introduced Although numerous studies and applications have been made using single-phased nanoparticles mainly composed of lipid, polymer or metal, there remain a number of problems to be solved. With the formation of nanoparticles with a core–shell structure, a significant improvement has been accomplished in the stability of nanoparticles, and the activity and release profile of loaded model drugs. The core–shell nanoparticles discussed in this chapter may be one of the leading examples of biocompatible polymer systems for drug delivery and molecular imaging purposes. Associated considerations may include the characterization in the *in vivo* models and retaining more appropriate physicochemical properties for practical applications in pharmaceutics.

Acknowledgments

This work was financially supported by the Ministry of Science and Technology (M10414030001-05N1403-00130) in Korea.

References

1 Sad, W., Protein drugs: a revolution in therapy?, *Pharm. Res.* **1986**, *3*, 3–6.
2 Lee, V. H., Peptide and protein drug delivery: opportunities and challenges, *Pharm. Int.* **1986**, *7*, 208–212.
3 Pitt, C. G., The controlled parenteral delivery of peptides and protein. *Int. J. Pharm.* **1990**, *59*, 173–196.
4 Leung, S. H. S., Robinson, J. R., Lee, V. H., Parenteral products. In *Controlled Drug Delivery*, Robinson, J. R., Lee, V. H. (Eds.). Marcel Dekker, New York, **1987**, pp. 433–480.
5 Tice, T. R., Mason, D. W., Gilley, R. M., Clinical use and future of parenteral microsphere systems. In *Novel Drug Delivery and its Therapeutic Application*, Prescott, F. and Nimmo, W. S. (Eds.). Wiley, Chichester, **1989**, pp. 223–235.
6 Ogawa, Y., Okada, H., Yamamoto, Y., Shimamoto, T., A new technique to efficiently entrap leuprorelide acetate into microcapsules of poly(lactic acid) or copoly(lactic/glycolic) acid, *Chem. Pharm. Bull.* **1988**, *36*, 1095–1108.
7 Bodmer, D., Kissel, T., Traechslin, E., Factors influencing the release of peptides and proteins from biodegradable parenteral depot systems, *J. Control. Release* **1992**, *21*, 129–138.
8 Manning, M. C., Patel, K., Borchardt, R. T., Stability of protein pharmaceuticals, *Pharm. Res.* **1989**, *6*, 903–918.
9 Lipka, E., Crison, J., Amidon, G. L., Transmembrane transport of peptide type compounds: prospects for oral delivery, *J. Control. Release* **1996**, *39*, 121–129.
10 Cleland, J. L., Powell, S. J., Shire, S. J., The development of stable protein formulation: a close look at protein aggregation, deamidation, and oxidation, *Crit. Rev. Ther. Drug. Carrier Syst.* **1993**, *10*, 307–377.
11 Cowsar, D. R., Tice, T. R., Giley, R. M., English, J. P., Poly(lactide-*co*-glycolide) microcapsules for controlled release of steroids, *Methods Enzymol.* **1985**, *112*, 101–116.
12 Moore, A., McGuirk, P., Adams, S., Jones, W. C., McGee, J. P., O'Hagon, D. T., Mills, K. H., Immunization with a soluble recombinant HIV protein entrapped in biodegradable microparticles induces HIV-specific CD8$^+$ cytoxic T lymphocytes and CD4$^+$ T$_h$1 cells, *Vaccine* **1995**, *13*, 1741–1749.
13 Bittner, B., Morlock, M., Koll, H., Winter, G., Kissel, T., Recombinant human erythropoietin (rHEPO) loaded poly(lactide-*co*-glycolide) microspheres: influence of the en capsulation technique and polymer purity on microspheres characteristics, *Eur. J. Pharm. Biopharm.* **1998**, *45*, 295–305.
14 Ando, S., Putnam, D., Pack, D. W., Langer, R., PLGA microspheres containing plasmid DNA: preservation of super coiled DNA via cryopreparation and carbohydrate stabilization, *J. Pharm. Sci.* **1999**, *88*, 126–130.
15 Wang, D., Robinson, D. R., Kown, G. S., Samuel, J., Encapsulation of plasmid DNA in biodegradable poly(D,L-lactic-*co*-acid) microspheres as a novel approach for immunogene delivery, *J. Control. Release* **1999**, *57*, 9–18.
16 Lewis, K. J., Irwin, W. J., Akhtar, S., Development of a sustained release biodegradable polymer delivery system for site-specific delivery of oligonucleotides: characterization of P(LA–GA) copolymer microspheres *in vitro*, *J. Drug Target.* **1998**, *5*, 291–302.
17 Yamamoto, Y., Nagasaki, Y., Kato, Y., Sugiyama, Y., Kataoka, K., Long–circulating poly(ethylene glycol)–poly(D,L-lactide) block copolymer micelles with modulated surface charge, *J. Control. Release* **2001**, *77*, 27–38.
18 Illum, L., Davis, S. S., Effect of the nonionic surfactant poloxamer 338 on the fate and deposition of polystyrene microspheres following intravenous administration, *J. Pharm. Sci.* **1983**, *72*, 1086–1089.
19 Lasic, D. D., *Liposomes: From Physics To Applications.* Elsevier, Amsterdam, **1993**.

20 Anderson, P. M., Hanson, D. C., Hasz, D. E., Halet, M. R., Blazar, B. R., Ochoa, A. C., Cytokines in liposomes: preliminary studies with IL-1, IL-2, IL-6, GM-CSF and interferon-gamma, *Cytokine* **1994**, *6*, 92–101.

21 Ye, Q., Asherman, J., Stevenson, M., Brownson, E., Katre, N. V., DepoForm^{TM} technology: a vehicle for controlled delivery of protein and peptide drugs, *J. Control. Release* **2000**, *64*, 155–166.

22 Mayer, L. D., Hope, M. J., Cullis, P. R., Vesicles of variable sizes produced by a rapid extrusion procedure, *Biochim. Biophys. Acta* **1986**, *858*, 161–168.

23 Cullis, P. R., Hope, M. J., Bally, M. B., Madden, T. D., Mayer, L. D., Fenske, D. B., Influence of pH gradients on the transbilayer transport of drugs, lipids, peptides and metal ions into large unilamellar vesicles, *Biochim. Biophys. Acta* **1997**, *1331*, 187–211.

24 Huang, C., Studies on phosphatidylcholine vesicles. Formation and physical characteristics, *Biochemistry* **1969**, *8*, 344–352.

25 Bangham, A. D., Standish, N. M., Watkins, J. C., Diffusion of univalent ions across the lamellae of swollen phospholipids, *J. Mol. Biol.* **1965**, *13*, 238–252.

26 Kim, S., Turker, M. S., Chi, E. Y., Sela, S., Martin, G. M., Preparation of multivesicular liposomes, *Biochim. Biophys. Acta* **1983**, *728*, 339–348.

27 Kim, S., DepoFoam-mediated drug delivery into cerebrospinal fluid, *Methods Neurosci.* **1994**, *21*, 118–131.

28 Kim, T., Murdande, S., Gruber, A., Kim, S., Sustained-release morphine for epidural analgesia in rats, *Anesthesiology* **1996**, *85*, 331–338.

29 Katre, N. V., Asherman, J., Schaefer, H., Hora, M., Multivesicular liposome (DepoFoamE) technology for the sustained delivery of insulin-like growth factor-I (IGF-I), *J. Pharm. Sci.* **1998**, *87*, 1341–1346.

30 Heinemann, L., Richter, B., Clinical pharmacology of human insulin, *Diabetes Care* **1993**, *16*, 90–100.

31 Hoffman, A., Ziv, F., Pharmacokinetic considerations of new insulin formulations and routes of administration, *Clin. Pharmacokinet.* **1997**, *33*, 285–301.

32 Spangler, R. S., Insulin administration via liposomes, *Diabetes Care* **1990**, *13*, 911–922.

33 Okada, H., Heya, T., Ogawa, Y., Shimamoto, T., One-month release injectable microcapsules of a luteinizing hormone-releasing hormone agonist (leuprolide acetate) for treating experimental endometriosis in rats, *J. Pharmacol. Exp. Ther.* **1988**, *244*, 744–750.

34 Dlugi, A. M., Miller, J. D., Knittle, J., Lupron depot (leuprolide acetate for depot suspension) in the treatment of endometriosis: a randomized, placebo-controlled, double-blind study, *Fertil. Steril.* **1990**, *54*, 419–427.

35 Okada, H., Doken, Y., Ogawa, Y., Toguchi, H., Preparation of three-month depot injectable microspheres of leuprorelin acetate using biodegradable polymers, *Pharm. Res.* **1994**, *2*, 1143–1147.

36 Hughes, J., Kosterlitz, H. W., Smith, T. W., The distribution of methionine-enkephalin and leucine-enkephalin in the brain and peripheral tissues, *Br. J. Pharmacol.* **1997**, *120*, 428–436.

37 Kuraishi, Y., Hirota, N., Satoh, M., Takagi, H., Antinociceptive effects of intrathecal opioids, noradrenaline and serotonin in rats: mechanical and thermal algesic tests, *Brain Res.* **1985**, *326*, 168–171.

38 Lamberts, S. W., Acromegaly and its treatment, *J. Endocrinol.* **1997**, *155*, S49–S51.

39 Pollak, M. N., Schally, A. V., Mechanisms of antineoplastic action of somatostatin analogs, *Proc. Soc. Exp. Biol. Med.* **1998**, *217*, 143–152.

40 Meng, F., Hiemstra, C., Engbers, G. H. M., Feijen, J., Biodegradable polymersomes, *Macromolecules* **2003**, *36*, 3004–3006.

41 Kukula, H., Schlaad, H., Antonietti, M., Forster, S., The formation of polymer vesicles or

"peptosomes" by polybutadiene-*block*-poly(L-glutamate)s in dilute aqueous solution, *J. Am. Chem. Soc.* **2002**, *124*, 1658–1663.

42 Lewis, D. H., Controlled release of bioactive agents from lactide/glycolide polymers. In *Biodegradable Polymers as Drug Delivery Systems, Drugs and Pharmaceutical Sciences*, Chasin, M., Langer, R. (Eds.). Marcel Dekker, New York, **1990**, pp. 9–41.

43 Jeyanthi, R., Mehta, R. C., Thanoo, B. C., DeLuca, P. P., Effect of processing parameters on the properties of peptide-containing PLGA microspheres, *J. Microencapsul.* **1997**, *14*, 163–174.

44 van Zyl, A. J. P., Sanderson, R. D., Wet-Roos, D., Klumperman, B., Core/shell particles containing liquid cores: morphology prediction, synthesis, and characterization, *Macromolecules* **2003**, *36*, 8621–8629.

45 Pekarek, K. J., Dyrud, M. J., Ferrer, K., Jong, Y. S., Mathiowitz, E., In vitro and in vivo degradation of double-walled polymer microsphere, *J. Control. Release* **1996**, *40*, 169–178.

46 Davis, S. S., Illum, L., Polymeric microspheres as drug carriers, *Biomaterials* **1988**, *9*, 111–115.

47 Pekarek, K. J., Dyrud, M. J., Ferrer, K., Jong, Y. S., Mathiowitz, E., *In vitro* and *in vivo* degradation of double-walled polymer microspheres *J. Control. Release* **1996**, *40*, 169–178.

48 Oh, K. S., Lee, K. E., Han, S. S., Cho, S. H., Kim, D., Yuk, S. H., Formation of core/shell nanoparticles with a lipid core and their application as a drug delivery system, *Biomacromolecules* **2005**, *6*, 1062–1067.

49 Han, S. K., Lee, J. H., Kim, D., Cho, S. H., Yuk, S. H., Hydrophilzed poly(lactide-*co*-glycolide) nanoparticles with core/shell structure for protein delivery, *Sci. Technol. Adv. Mater.* **2005**, *6*, 468–474.

50 Kim, B. K., Kim, D., Cho, S. H., Yuk, S. H., Hydrophilzed poly(lactide-*co*-glycolide) nanospheres with poly(ethylene oxide)–poly(propylene oxide)–poly(ethylene oxide) triblock copolymer, *J. Microencapsul.* **2004**, *21*, 697–707.

51 Liu, S., O'Brien, D. F., Stable polymeric nanoballoons: lyophilization and rehydration of cross-linked liposomes, *J. Am. Chem. Soc.* **2002**, *124*, 6037–6042.

52 Hincha, D. K., Zuther, E., Hellwege, E. M., Heyer, A. G., Specific effects of fructo- and gluco-oligosaccharides in the preservation of liposomes during drying, *Glycobiology* **2002**, *12*, 103–110.

53 Anchordoguy, T., Carpenter, J. F., Loomis, S. H., Crowe, J. H., Mechanisms of interaction of amino acids with phospholipid bilayers during freezing, *Biochim. Biophys. Acta* **1988**, *946*, 299–306.

54 Peer, D., Florentin, A., Margalit, R., Hyaluronan is a key component in cryoprotection and formulation of targeted unilamellar liposome, *Biochim. Biophys. Acta* **2003**, *1612*, 76–82.

55 Robertson, D., Hellweg, T., Tiesch, B., Koetz, J., Polymer-induced structural changes in lecithin/sodium dodecyl sulfate-based multilamellar vesicles, *J. Colloid Interface Sci.* **2004**, *270*, 187–194.

56 Feng, S. S., Gong, K., Chew, J., Molecular interaction between a lipid and an antineoplastic drug paclitaxel (Taxol) within the lipid monolayer at the air/water interface, *Langmuir* **2002**, *18*, 4061–4070.

57 Kaushik, J. K., Bhat, R., Why is threhalose an exceptional protein stabilizer? *J. Biol. Chem.* **2003**, *278*, 26458–26465.

58 Kaleshova, L. L., MacFarlane, D. R., Trounson, A. O., Shaw, J. M., Sugar exert a major influences on the vitrification properties of ethylene glycol-based solutions and have low toxicity to embryos and oocytes, *Cryobiology* **1999**, *38*, 119–130.

59 Muller, Y. A., Li, B., Christinger, H. W., Wells, J. A., Cunningham, B. C., De Vos, A. M., Vascular endothelial growth factor: crystal structure and functional mapping of kinase domain receptor binding site,

Proc. Natl Acad. Sci. USA **1997**, *94*, 7192–7197.
60 Couper, L. L., Shane, R. B., Eldrup-Jorgensen, J., Bredenberg, C. E., Linder, V., Vascular endothelial growth factor increase the mitogenic response to fibroblast growth factor-2 in vascular smooth muscle cells *in vivo* via expression of fms-like tyrosine kinase-1, *Circ. Res.* **1997**, *82*, 932–939.
61 Han, M. K., Kim, M., Bae, S. Y., Kang, L., Han, S. Y., Lee, Y. S., Rha, J. H., Kim, S. U., Roh, J. K., VEGF protects human cerebral hybrid neurons from *in vitro* ischemia, *Neurochemistry* **2004**, *15*, 847–850.
62 GenVec, A randomized, double-blind, placebo-controlled, multicenter, pilot study of the safety and feasibility of Biobypass® (Ad GVVEGF121.10) via an intramyocardial injection catheter in patients with advanced coronary artery disease. Presented at *American College of Cardiology 52nd Annual Scientific Conference* Chicago, IL, **2003**.
63 Sussich, F., Skopec, C., Brady, J., Cesaro, A., Reversible dehydration of trehalose and anhydrobiosis: from solution state to an exotic crystal, *Carbohydrate Res.* **2001**, *334*, 165–176.
64 Morlock, M., Kissel, T., Li, Y. X., Koll, H., Winter, G., Erythropoietin loaded microspheres prepared from biodegradable LPLG–PEP–LPLG triblock copolymers: protein stabilization and *in-vitro* release properties, *J. Control. Release* **1998**, *56*, 105–115.
65 Kim, T. K., Burgess, D. J., Pharmacokinetic characterization of ^{14}C-vascular endothelial growth factor controlled release microspheres using a rat model, *J. Pharm. Pharmacol.* **2002**, *54*, 897–905.
66 Krister, E., Fredrick, T., Equilibrium and kinetics properties of triblock copolymers at hydrophobic surface, *Macromolecules* **1997**, *30*, 6323–6332.
67 Stolnik, S., Daudali, B., Arien, A., Whetstone, J., Heald, C. R., Garnett, M. C., Davis, S. S., Illum, L., The effect of surface coverage and conformation of poly(ethylene oxide) (PEO) chains of poloxamer 407 on the biological fate of model colloidal drug carriers, *Biochim. Biophys. Acta* **2001**, *1514*, 261–279.
68 Prud'homme, R. K., Wu, G., Schneider, D. K., Structure and rheology studies of poly(oxyethylene–oxypropylene–oxyethylene) aqueous solution, *Langmuir* **1996**, *12*, 4651–4659.
69 Coombes, A. G., Scholes, P. D., Davis, M. C., Illum, L. and Davis, S. S., Resorbable polymeric microspheres for drug delivery – production and simultaneous surface modification using PEO–PPO surfactant, *Biomaterials* **1994**, *15*, 673–680.
70 Dunn, S. E., Coombes, A. G. A., Garnett, M. C., Davis, S. S., Davies, M. C., Illum, L. *In vitro* cell interaction and *in vivo* biodistribution of poly(lactide-*co*-glycolide) nanospheres surface modified by poloxamer and poloxamine copolymers. *J. Control. Release* **1997**, *44*, 65–76.
71 Lee, K. E., Kim, B. K., Yuk, S. H., Biodegradable polymeric nanospheres formed by temperature-induced phase transition in a mixture of poly(lactide-*co*-glycolide) and poly(ethylene oxide)–poly(propylene oxide)–poly(ethylene oxide) triblock copolymer, *Biomacromolecules* **2002**, *3*, 1115–1119.
72 Peng, Z. G., Hidajat, K., Uddin, M. S., Adsorption and desorption of lysozyme on nano-sized magnetic particles and its conformational changes, *Colloids Surf. B* **2004**, 35, 169–174.
73 Chung, Y. I., Tae, G. Y., Yuk, S. H., A facile method to prepare heparin-functionalized nanoparticles for controlled release of growth factors, *Biomaterials*, **2006**, *27*, 2621–2626.
74 Sundaram, M., Qi, Y., Shriver, Z., Liu, D., Zhao, G., Venkataraman, G., Langer, R., Sasisekharan, R., Rational design of low-molecular weight heparins with improved *in vivo* activity, *Proc. Natl Acad. Sci. USA* **2003**, *100*, 625–656.
75 Sakiyama-Elbert, S. E., Hubbell, J. A., Development of fibrin derivatives for controlled release of heparin-

binding growth factors, *J. Control. Release* **2000**, *65*, 389–402.

76 Tessler, S., Rockwell, P., Hicklin, D., Cohen, T., Levi, B. Z., Witte, L., Lemischka, I. R., Neufeld, G., Heparin modulates the interaction of VEGF165 with soluble and cell associated flk-1 receptors, *J. Biol. Chem.* **1994**, *269*, 12456–12461.

77 Feyzi, E., Lustig, F., Fager, G., Spillmann, D., Lindahl, U., Salmivirta, M., Characterization of heparin and heparan sulfate domains binding to the long splice variant of platelet-derived growth factor A chain, *J. Biol. Chem.* **1997**, *272*, 5518–5524.

78 Lyon, M., Rushton, G. and Gallagher, J., The interaction of the transforming growth factor-βs with heparin/heparan sulfate is isoform specific, *J. Biol. Chem.* **1997**, *272*, 18000–18006.

79 Hamilton, J. F., Morrison, P. F., Chen, M. Y., Harvey-White, J., Pernaute, R. S., Phillips, H., Oldfield, E., Bankiewicz, K. S., Heparin coinfusion during convection enhanced delivery (CED) increases the distribution of the glial-derived neurotrophic factor (GDNF) ligand family in rat striatum and enhances the pharmacological activity of neurturin, *Exp. Neurol.* **2001**, *168*, 155–161.

80 Saksela, O., Moscatelli, D., Sommer, A., Rifkin, D. B., Endothelial cell-derived heparan sulfate binds basic fibroblast growth factor and protects it from proteolytic degradation, *J. Cell Biol.* **1988**, *107*, 743–751.

81 Sommer, A., Rifkin, D. B., Interaction of heparin with human basic fibroblast growth factor: protection of the angiogenic protein from proteolytic degradation by a glycosaminoglycan, *J. Cell. Physiol.* **1989**, *138*, 215–220.

82 Edelman, E. R., Mathiowitz, E., Langer, R., Klagsbrun, M., Controlled and modulated release of basic fibroblast growth factor, *Biomaterials* **1991**, *12*, 619–626.

83 Sakiyama-Elbert, S. E., Hubbell, J. A., Controlled release of nerve growth factor from a heparin-containing fibrin-based cell in growth matrix, *J. Control. Release* **2000**, *69*, 149–158.

84 Wissink, M. J. B., Beernink, R., Pieper, J. S., Poot, A. A., Engbers, G. H. M., Beugeling, T., van Aken, W. G., Feijen, J., Binding and release of basic fibroblast growth factor from heparinized collagen matrices, *Biomaterials* **2001**, *22*, 2291–2299.

85 Tanihara, M., Suzuki, Y., Yamamoto, E., Noguchi, A., Mizushima, Y., Sustained release of basic fibroblast growth factor and angiogenesis in a novel covalently crosslinked gel of heparin and alginate, *J. Biomed. Mater. Res.* **2001**, *56*, 216–221.

86 Seal, B. L., Panitch, A., Physical polymer matrices based on affinity interactions between peptides and polysaccharides, *Biomacromolecules* **2003**, *4*, 1572–1582.

87 Yancopoulos, G. D., Davis, S., Gale, N. W., Rudge, J. S., Wiegand, S. J., Holash, J., Vascular-specific growth factors and blood vessel formation, *Nature* **2000**, *407*, 242–248.

88 Peters, M. C., Isenberg, B. C., Rowley, J. A. and Mooney, D. J., Release from alginate enhances the biological activity of vascular endothelial growth factors, *J. Biomater. Sci. Polymer Edn* **1998**, *9*, 1267–1278.

89 Murray, J. B., Brown, L., Langer, R., Klagsburn, M., A micro-sustained release system for epidermal growth factor. *In Vitro* **1983**, *10*, 743–748.

90 Mooney, D. J., Kaufmann, P. M., Sano, K., Schwendeman, S. P., Majahod, K., Schloo, B., Vacanti, J. P., Langer, R., Localized delivery of epidermal growth factor improves the survival of transplanted hepatocytes, *Biotechnol. Bioeng.* **1996**, *50*, 422–429.

91 Zhu, G., Mallery, S. R., Schwendeman, S. P., Stabilization of proteins encapsulated in injectable poly(lactide-*co*-glycolide), *Nat. Biotechnol.* **2000**, *18*, 52–57.

92 Li, X., Zhang, Y., Yan, R., Jia, W., Yuan, M., Deng, X., Huang, Z., Influence of process parameters on the protein stability encapsulated in poly-DL-lactide poly(ethylene glycol) microspheres, *J. Control. Release* **2000**, *68*, 41–52.

93 Lu, W., Park, T. G., Protein release from poly(lactic-*co*-glycolic acid) microspheres: protein stability problems, *J. Pharm. Sci. Technol.* **1995**, *49*, 13–19.

94 Crotts, G., Park, T. G., Stability and release of bovine serum albumin encapsulated within poly(D,L-lactide-*co*-glycolide) microparticles, *J. Control. Release* **1997**, *44*, 123–134.

95 Cleland, J. L., Jones, A. J. S., Stable formulations of recombinant human growth hormone and interferon-γ for microencapsulation in biodegradable microspheres, *Pharm. Res.* **1996**, *13*, 1464–1475.

96 Zambaux, M. F., Bonneaux, F., Gref, R., Dellacherie, E., Vigneron, C., Preparation and characterization of protein C-loaded PLA nanoparticles, *J. Control. Release* **1999**, *60*, 179–188.

97 Sah, H., Protein behavior at the water/methylene chloride interface, *J. Pharm. Sci.* **1999**, *88*, 1320–1325.

98 Lee, K. Y., Peters, M. C., Mooney, D. J., Comparison of vascular endothelial growth factor and basic fibroblast growth factor on angiogenesis in SCID mice, *J. Control. Release* **2003**, *87*, 49–56.

99 Elcin, Y. M., Dixit, V., Gitnick, G., Extensive *in vivo* angiogenesis following controlled release of human vascular endothelial cell growth factor: implications for tissue engineering and wound healing, *Artif. Organs* **2001**, *25*, 558–565.

100 Mumper, R. J., Hoffman, A. S., Puolakkainen, P., Bouchard, L. S., Gombotz, W. R., Calcium-alginate beads for the oral delivery of transforming growth factor-β1 (TGF-β1): stabilization of TGF-β1 by the addition of polyacrylic acid within acid-treated beads, *J. Control. Release* **1994**, *30*, 241–251.

101 Lee, K. W., Yoon, J. J., Lee, J. H., Kim, S. Y., Jung, H. J., Kim, S. J., Joh, J. W., Lee, H. H., Lee, D. S., Lee, S. K., Sustained release of vascular endothelial growth factor from calcium-induced alginate hydrogels reinforced by heparin and chitosan, *Transplant. Proc.* **2004**, *36*, 2464–2465.

102 Nakaoka, R., Tabata, Y., Ikada, Y., Potentiality of gelatin microsphere as immunological adjuvant, *Vaccine* **1995**, *13*, 653–661.

103 Mladenovska, K., Kumbaradzi, E. F., Dodov, G. M., Makraduli, L., Goracinova, K., Biodegradation and drug release studies of BSA loaded gelatin microspheres. *Int. J. Pharm.* **2002**, *242*, 247–249.

104 Tabata, Y., Ikada, Y., Protein release from gelatin matrices, *Adv. Drug Delivery Rev.* **1998**, *31*, 287–301.

105 Passirani, C., Barratt, G., Devissaguet, J. P., Labarre, D., Long-circulating nanoparticles bearing heparin or dextran covalently bound to poly(methyl methacrylate), *Pharm Res.* **1998**, *15*, 1046–1050.

106 Chauvierre, C., Marden, M. C., Vauthier, C., Labarre, D., Couvreur, P., Leclerc, L., Heparin coated poly(alkylcyanoacrylate) nanoparticles coupled to hemoglobin: a new oxygen carrier, *Biomaterials* **2004**, *25*, 3081–3086.

107 Park, K., Kim, K., Kwon, I. C., Kim, S. K., Lee, S., Lee, D. Y., Byun, Y., Preparation and characterization of self-assembled nanoparticles of heparin–deoxycholic acid conjugates, *Langmuir* **2004**, *20*, 11726–11731.

108 Lin, H.-R., Sung, K. C., Vong, W.-J., In *situ* gelling of alginate/pluronic solutions for ophthalmic delivery of pilocarpine, *Biomacromolecules* **2004**, *5*, 2358–2365.

109 Lee, H. Y., Lim, N. H., Seo, J. A., Yuk, S. H., Kwak, B. K., Khang, G., Lee, H. B., Cho, S. H., Preparation and magnetic resonance imaging (MRI) effect of polyvinylpyrrolidone (PVP)-coated iron oxide nanoparticles, *J. Biomed. Res. Part B: Appl. Biomater.* **2006**, *79B*, 142–150.

110 Li, Z., Chen, H., Bao, H., Gao, M., One-pot reaction to synthesize water-soluble magnetite nanocrystals, *Chem. Mater.* **2004**, *16*, 1391–1393.

111 Gupta, P. K., Hung, C. T., Lam, F. C., Perrier, D. G., Albumin microspheres. III. Synthesis and characterization of microspheres containing adriamycin and magnetite, *J. Pharm.* **1988**, *43*, 167–177.

112 Jordan, A., Scholz, R., Maier-Hauff, K., Johannsen, M., Wust, P., Nadobny, J., Schirra, H., Schmidt, H., Deger, S., Loening, S., Lanksch, W., Felix, R., Presentation of a new magnetic field therapy system for the treatment of human solid tumors with magnetic fluid hyperthermia, *J. Magn. Magn. Mater.* **2001**, *225*, 118–126.

113 Berry, C. C., Wells, S., Charles, S., Curtis, A. S. G., Dextran and albumin derivatised iron oxide nanoparticles: influence on fibroblasts *in vitro*, *Biomaterials* **2003**, *24*, 4551–4557.

114 Harris, L. A., Goff, J. D., Carmichael, A. Y., Riffle, J. S., Harburn, J. J., St Pierre, T. G., Saunders, M., Magnetite nanoparticle dispersions stabilized with triblock copolymers. *Chem. Mater.* **2003**, *15*, 1367–1377.

115 Liu, Z. L., Ding, Z. H., Yao, K. L., Tao, J., Du, G. H., Lu, Q, H., Wang, X., Gong, F. L., Chen, X., Preparation and characterization of polymer-coated core–shell structured magnetic microbeads. *J. Magn. Magn. Mater.* **2003**, *265*, 98–105.

116 Veintemillas-Verdaguer, S., Bomatí-Miguel, O., Morales, M. P., Effect of the process conditions on the structural and magnetic properties of γ-Fe_2O_3 nanoparticles produced by laser pyrolysis. *Scr. Mater.* **2002**, *47*, 589–593.

117 King, S., Hyunh, K., Tannenbaum, R., Kinetics of nucleation, growth, and stabilization of cobalt oxide nanoclusters, *J. Phys. Chem. B* **2003**, *107*, 12097–12104.

118 Tannenbaum, R., Reich, S., Flenniken, C. L., Goldberg, E. P., Shape control of iron oxide nanoclusters in polymeric media. *Adv. Mater.* **2002**, *14*, 1402–1405.

119 Tannenbaum, R., Flenniken, C. L., Goldberg, E. P., The solid-state decomposition and oxidation of dicobaltoctacarbonyl in a polymer matrix. *J. Polym. Sci. Polym. Phys.* **1987**, *25*, 1341–1358.

120 Tannenbaum, R., Flenniken, C. L., Goldberg, E. P., Magnetic metal–polymer composites: Thermal and oxidative decomposition of $Fe(CO)_5$ and $CO_2(CO)_8$ in a poly(vinylidene fluoride) matrix. *J. Polym. Sci. Polym. Phys.* **1990**, *28*, 2421–2433.

121 Tannenbaum, R., Polymer matrix influence on the kinetics of some fundamental inorganic colloidal reactions, *Langmuir* **1997**, *13*, 5056–5060.

122 He, R., Qian, X., Yin, J., Xi, H., Bian, L., Zhu, Z., Formation of monodispersed PVP-capped ZnS and CdS nanocrystals under microwave irradiation. *Colloid Surf. A* **2003**, *220*, 151–157.

123 Yao, H., Takada, Y., Kitamura, N., Electrolyte effects on CdS nanocrystal formation in chelate polymer particles: optical and distribution properties, *Langmuir* **1998**, *14*, 595–601.

124 Garrec, D. L., Gori, S., Luo, L., Lessard, D., Smith, D. C., Yessine, M. A., Ranger, M., Leroux, J. C., Poly(*N*-vinylpyrrolidone)-block-poly(D,L-lactide) as a new polymeric solubilizer for hydrophobic anticancer drugs: *in vitro* and *in vivo* evaluation. *J. Control. Release* **2004**, *99*, 83–101.

125 Cheng, F.-Y., Su, C.-H., Yang, Y.-S., Yeh, C.-S., Tsai, C.-Y., Wu, C.-L., Wu, M.-T., Shieh, D.-B., Characterization of aqueous dispersions of Fe_3O_4 nanoparticles and their biomedical applications. *Biomaterials* **2005**, *26*, 729–738.

126 Jiang, P., Li, S.-Y., Xie, S.-S., Gao, Y., Song, L., Machinable long PVP-stabilized silver nanowires, *Chem. Eur. J.* **2004**, *10*, 4817–4821.

5
Nanotechnologies for Targeted Delivery of Drugs

Pavel Brož and Patrick Hunziker

5.1
Introduction

Targeting specific tissues, cell types or specific cellular targets such as membrane proteins and intracellular organelles in the body is desirable in modern medicine for improved diagnosis and treatment. Usual therapeutic concepts in somatic medicine involve either targeted mechanical changes of pathological tissues, cells or processes (e.g. cancer surgery, interventional cardiology and orthopedics), or the untargeted application of therapeutic agents (drugs) with an automated function. Both methods have their own limits, which we will highlight to create a common background of understanding that is essential for this chapter.

While modern, minimally invasive (e.g. endoscopic interventions) surgery has increased therapeutic precision and decreased the quantity of negative side-effects to healthy tissues, there still are natural limits to the morphological scale, which direct "human-controlled" (in contrast to automated or self-controlled processes) action can reach. Due to the natural limits of senses, it is most unlikely that we will be able to perform surgical operations at cellular or even subcellular dimensions without the help of nanometer-sized tools with an automated functionality.

On the other hand, medicine knows a huge stockpile of different pharmaceutical agents such as cardiovascular drugs, antibiotics and steroids, which are usually administered on an oral or intravenous route and find their desired therapeutic target (such as cancer cells, bacteria or pathologically altered tissue) on their own or with the help of cellular transport systems. This method allows reaching even subcellular targets such as specific receptors inside or outside the cell for a therapeutic purpose; however, this strategy obviously bears specific problems. Since most of the drugs are transported with the blood flow or bound to plasma proteins, they reach every part of the human body and targets other than just the desired ones. As a result, negative side-effects such as loss of hair, vomiting, diarrhea and destruction of fast growing cells in the bone marrow occur when using cytotoxic anticancer drugs. Some drugs can even lead to fatal complications during the therapeutic process. For further information about adverse drug effects [1], refer to Figs. 5.1 and 5.2.

Nanotechnologies for the Life Sciences Vol. 10
Nanomaterials for Medical Diagnosis and Therapy. Edited by Challa S. S. R. Kumar

ISBN: 978-3-527-31390-7

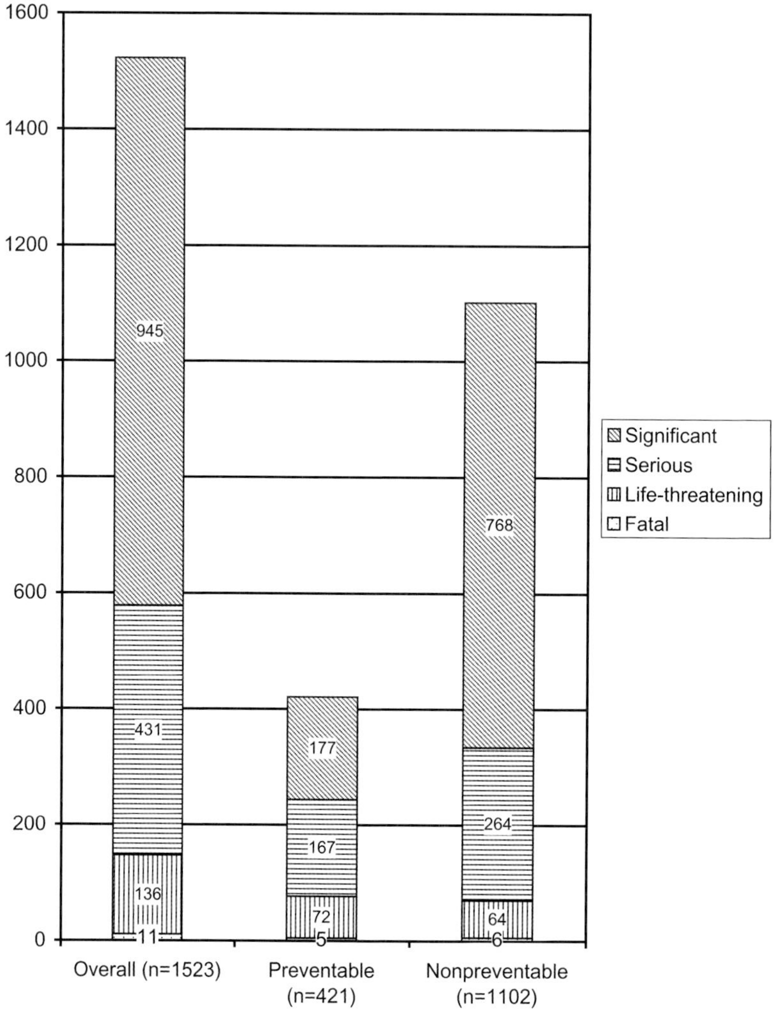

Figure 5.1. Incidence of adverse drug events (data from Ref. [1]). More than 30 000 elderly patients (mean age 74.7 years, 58.7% female, mean prescription drug dispensing over 12 months 21.1!) treated at a Medicare institution were monitored for adverse drug events over a period of 12 months. Observed drug events were rated from significant to fatal. The results show the high impact of adverse drug events on healthcare systems and on patients taking multiple drugs. Even though about one-third of the events may have been prevented by the physician, two-thirds of all adverse drug events are not preventable and have to be explained by unselective drug targeting, which influences physiologic processes other than the expected target process in a negative way.

Modern highly active drugs with strong therapeutic potency that were introduced to medicine in recent years try to overcome these problems of side-effects and unwanted interactions by reaching higher target specificity than older drugs. Examples are therapeutic monoclonal antibodies (e.g. rituximab for non-Hodgkin's

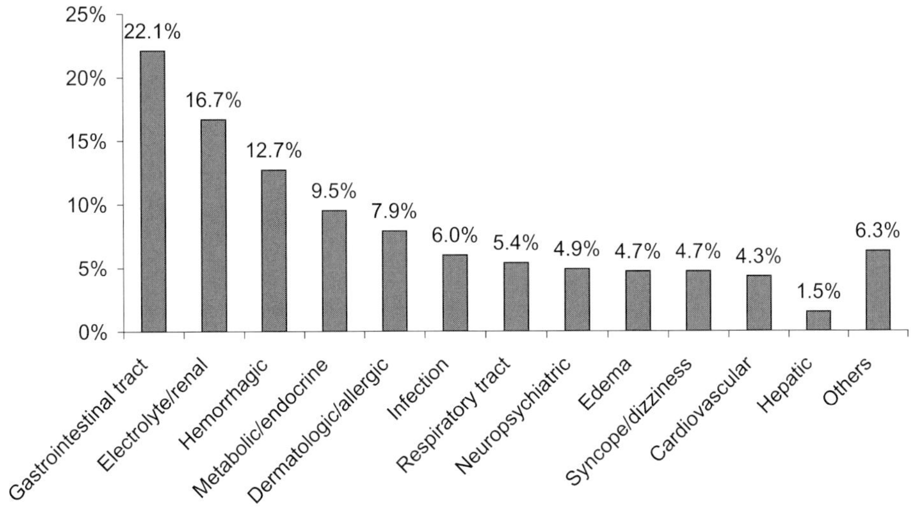

Figure 5.2. Frequency of types of adverse drug events (data from Ref. [1]). In the same study as in Fig. 5.1, adverse drug events were differentiated according to the type of event (organ, physiologic function). One adverse drug event may manifest itself as more than one type; the value gives the probability for an adverse drug event to influence the mentioned organ/physiologic function. Most common events are nausea, vomiting, diarrhea, constipation, electrolyte disorders, renal malfunctioning, bleeding and allergic manifestations.

lymphoma, trastuzumab for breast cancer), which can even bear certain functionality such as (i) a radioactive isotope (e.g. tositumomab, an antibody linked with ^{131}I used for treatment of non-Hodgkin's lymphoma), (ii) monoclonal antibodies for active cancer vaccination (e.g. mitumomab for small cell lung cancer) or (iii) artificially designed agents that can block certain types of intracellular proteins such as kinases (e.g. imatinib inhibits a pathological tyrosine kinase in chronic myeloid leukemia). However, even though these drugs create a much higher therapeutic potency, there are still the known problems with side-effects, even though they tend to be milder than the side-effects of standard anticancer therapy (surgery, chemotherapy and radiotherapy).

Another important area of medicine that will be changed by nanometer-sized tools is diagnostics. Diagnostics can be defined as every method that allows the doctor to assess a certain characteristic or development inside or on the surface of the human body that they cannot assess with their own sensory. This vast area ranges from common techniques such as X-ray imaging, blood cell counting, plasma analysis, drug level measurement, anatomic imagining of certain parts of the body by computed tomography (CT) or magnetic resonance imaging (MRI) and histological inspection of tissue samples to more specialized techniques such as protein assays, gene expression assays and receptor expression studies.

Common to all of these new methods is the trend to miniaturization, small sample measuring, and diagnostics at cellular and subcellular dimensions. Tools such as microchip assays, target-specific contrast agents for imaging and small-sample diagnostics are some of the now commonly used techniques.

Clearly, nanotechnology will be able to introduce even more ground-breaking diagnostic and therapeutic methods to medicine in the years to come, which will contribute to a better detection of pathological processes and to better therapeutic options for sick people. A central problem which nanotechnology has to overcome is the difficulty of targeted delivery as described above. The idea is to increase the diagnostic signal or the therapeutic impact on the desired target with a small range of negative side-effects.

This chapter will highlight some basic problems for targeted delivery of nanometer-sized structures and will present successful targeting strategies employed by both "natural nanostructures" (such as bacteria and viruses) and "artificial nanostructures" (lipid-based such as liposomes and micelles, protein-based such as dendrimers, and polymer-based such as nanoparticles, nanospheres and nanocontainers) in areas other than cancer. The main goal of this chapter is to present different facets of the enormous field of targeted delivery, to present the main literature dealing with targeted delivery and to show the high level of interdisciplinarity. Only by combining parts of scientific disciplines such as pharmacology, microbiology, immunology, chemistry, physics and medicine will it be possible to build nanotechnological devices for targeted delivery.

The chapter is mainly suitable for physicists and chemists working in this research area and showing interest in the biomedical and pharmacological part of targeted delivery to the human body. Nonetheless, it is also written for people with a general interest in "nanomedicine" [2, 3] that share the belief that it will be possible to compose nanostructures with a complex and automated functionality for the benefit of humanity.

Section 2 describes some pharmacological basics and special pharmacological problems concerning targeted delivery of macromolecules and chemically complex carriers. In Section 3, we will discuss strategies for targeted delivery used by microorganisms such as bacteria and viruses, and by the "natural nanoparticle" prion. In Section 4, we will review targeting strategies for site-specific delivery of artificial nanotechnological carriers. In Section 5, we will sum up the main messages of the chapter and try to give an outlook into the future of targeted delivery. The reader is referred to the given references for a deeper insight into a certain topic.

5.2 Basic and Special Pharmacology

5.2.1 Outline

Pharmacology is the scientific discipline that describes and examines the effect of chemical substances on biological systems such as the human body and their use as therapeutic agents. The subspecialty of drug delivery concentrates on the development of new therapeutic systems with high target specificity, low side-effects and controlled release of active substances with complex functionality. The toolbox of nanotechnology has revived this research area and is trying to develop new therapeutic concepts.

In this section, we will first discuss some basic characteristics of drug input and disposition that are essential for a deeper understanding of targeting strategies. In the second part of this section, we will point up specific hurdles for targeted delivery.

For more details about this topic, see Refs. [4–6].

5.2.2 Basic Pharmacology

When giving a drug to the body there exist several steps the chemical substance has to go through before it can unfold its specific effect and other steps before it can be removed from the body. The most important ones are absorption, bioavailability, distribution and elimination. We will discuss these four steps to create a common basis of knowledge. Apart from this, it is obvious that the same physiological pathways and rules apply to both standard drugs and nanotechnological drug formulas, nanospheres, nanocontainers, nanoparticles, "nanobots", etc., making it necessary for all involved researchers to understand these physiological pathways.

5.2.2.1 Absorption

Absorption is the movement the drug has to perform from the administration site direct to the therapeutic site or to the systemic circulation. Absorption is determined by both physicochemical properties of the chemical substance or macromolecule and the biological construction of the administration site. Drugs are administered as solutions, tablets, capsules, aerosols or transdermal permeation systems. Usually the drug builds a complex with other ingredients (e.g. binders, surfactants, dispersants and diluents) that control the stability of the drug and its dissolution speed, and can control the release of the active ingredient. For instance, it is possible to lengthen the absorption time by creating special matrix tablets or tablets with encased granules with substance-specific release characteristics.

The drug complex can be administered by various routes such as oral, intravenous, intra-arterial, intramuscular, sublingual, inhalational, topical (eyes, skin), rectal or vaginal. Administration routes are divided into direct parenteral routes (intravenous, intra-arterial) where the drug does not have to permeate cellular barriers before reaching the circulation (the needle does the permeation) and indirect routes where the drug has to permeate through barriers in organs such as the intestine, the lung or the skin before it can reach the circulation. These barriers are mainly biologic semipermeable cell membranes (triblock hydrophilic–hydrophobic–hydrophilic with a central lipid block containing phospholipids and cholesterol) that selectively block the passage of smaller electrically charged molecules and all macromolecules. Various transmembrane proteins, receptors and transport systems are embedded into this triblock membrane, and are responsible for substance-specific uptake and cellular control. The drug or carrier of complex functionality can cross this cell membrane by passive diffusion, facilitated passive diffusion, active transport or endocytosis according to its physicochemical properties.

Most drugs cross the cell membranes by simple passive diffusion according to the concentration gradient, which is directed from a site with high substance concentration to a site with low substance concentration (e.g. from the intestine to the epithelial cells or the blood vessel near the epithelial cells). Once the drug reaches the systemic circulation, it is washed away and the concentration stays low, thus ensuring a constant substance uptake. Apart from the concentration gradient and the size of the absorption surface, the transmembrane diffusion rate depends on the polarity (the unionized form has a faster permeation rate than the ionized), lipid solubility, drug size and pH of the drug molecule. Small, lipid-soluble substances have the fastest absorption rate.

For facilitated passive diffusion, the molecule (e.g. glucose) binds to substance-specific transmembrane carrier proteins on the cell surface, which speed up the diffusion by building a substance–carrier complex with a higher diffusion rate through the cell membrane without energy consumption. This method relies on a concentration gradient and is characterized by saturability because of the limited amount of carrier complexes.

On the other hand, there exist similar transmembrane proteins responsible for an active, energy-consuming transport. This method is characterized by high specificity (e.g. vitamins, amino acids), saturability and works against a concentration gradient.

Passive diffusion and active transport are limited to small molecules (the size of ions, glucose and amino acids); larger molecules, macromolecules, and micro/nanostructures such as viruses and bacteria can only reach the cell by endocytosis. To perform the endocytosis, the cell (mostly specialized cell types of the immune system such as granulocytes and macrophages) has to engulf the structure, enclose it into a cell membrane-derived vesicle and transport it into the cell interior. There the vesicle is transformed into a so-called lysosome. A major problem of this transport method is the intracellular degradation of the vesicle content by low pH (down to 2–3) and cellular enzymes such as phosphatases, lipases, esterases, proteases, etc., which the cell delivers into the endocytosis vesicle. This method is energy consuming, saturable and needs a ligand–receptor interaction.

Most drugs are administered orally and reach the circulation by crossing the diverse epithelial cell barriers found in the gastrointestinal system, mainly using passive diffusion and scarcely active transport (e.g. L-DOPA – a dopamine-derived drug for Parkinson's disease). Small and lipophilic molecules can use the short contact time inside the mouth to cross the epithelial cells of the buccal or sublingual area and enter the circulation rapidly. An example is nitroglycerin – a drug that dilates the coronary arteries in the case of a myocardial infarction.

Even though the next station in the way of the drug, the stomach, has a larger epithelial surface, almost no drugs enter the circulation here. Reasons are the thick mucous layer protecting the stomach from self-digestion and the usually fast passage time in the stomach. Apart from this, the stomach creates some important problems to drug therapy because of the acidic (pH 1–2) environment and the digestive enzyme pepsin (a protease produced in the stomach wall). Some drugs can be degraded in such an environment (e.g. penicillin), especially when fatty foods or slow stomach emptying slow down the passage time. It is possible to overcome this problem by building gastric acid-resistant capsules and drug formulas when giving an instable drug orally.

Most orally applied drugs are absorbed in the small intestine (especially duodenum and proximal jejunum) over less than 6 h under normal circumstances. Special controlled-release formulations show a slower absorption kinetic and may reach the large intestine, where they can also be absorbed or may be subject to microbial degradation.

When giving a drug in a parenteral way, the substance is directly placed into the circulation (intravenous, intra-arterial) or injected into soft tissues such as the skin or muscles without having to cross the epithelial barriers. These methods are especially suitable for larger and complex molecules such as proteins, and for complex chemical structures such as liposomes or nanoparticles, because here they do not face any problems with degradation and inactivation compared with the intestine. Injections into the fat of the skin (subcutaneous) or into the muscle (intramuscular) are especially suitable for everyday applications of drugs such as insulin for diabetes or low-molecular-weight heparin for perioperative anticoagulation. The patient can perform these injections without facing serious complications such as blood infections and thrombosis when injecting substances into blood vessels. Due to passive diffusion into the porous small capillaries of these soft tissues, proteins up to a molecular weight of 20 kDa face fast and constant absorption, mostly depending on the quantity of capillaries and the perfusion speed. Larger molecules show unstable absorption, since their absorption occurs by the lymphatic system, where they also face contact with degrading enzymes and cells of the immune system such as macrophages that take up all macromolecules and produce an immune reaction (inflammation, allergic reaction) against this substance. On the other hand, parenteral injection of large molecules or rather insoluble drug formulas can be used for controlled release over a large-scale period (e.g. penicillin G benzathine or insulin in crystalline suspensions).

Drugs with a short circulation half-time have to be administered in a controlled-release form to guarantee a stable plasma concentration and persistent therapeutic effect. The best way to achieve this is to apply an intravenous catheter and to infuse the drug constantly. For long-term applications, it is necessary to change the strategy because of complications such as catheter infections, thrombosis and reduced convenience. For oral administration, the drug particles can be coated with wax or other water-soluble material such as biodegradable polymers, or can be embedded into a slow-release matrix. Another administration method is transdermal controlled-release systems consisting of drug-impregnated polymer materials with permeable membranes bonded to an adhesive bandage. These systems provide constant drug release into the skin for 12–24 h, but are restricted to smaller lipophilic molecules that can permeate the skin barrier (e.g. nitroglycerin, opiates).

5.2.2.2 Bioavailability

Bioavailability is the extent and the rate at which the active drug enters the systemic circulation, and is mostly determined by its physicochemical properties and the dosage form (as seen above). Different drug formulations result in different bioavailability and can have clinical significance in the terms of therapeutic effect and toxicity. The bioavailability is also determined by physiologic characteristics of the patient, mainly the gut perfusion rate and the metabolic liver function, or on a smaller scale by sex, genetic phenotype, stress, disease or previous gastrointestinal surgery.

When giving a drug parentally, the bioavailability is, by definition, 1 since all the active formula reaches the systemic circulation. On the other hand, the bioavailability of orally administered drugs is never 1, because the drug has to move down the gastrointestinal tract, has to cross the epithelial barriers of the intestine and has to pass through the metabolically active liver before it can reach the systemic circulation. This primary metabolic degradation and inactivation of the drug is called first-pass metabolism or the first-pass effect. A high first-pass effect results in a low or even zero oral bioavailability (e.g. most protein-based drugs such as insulin and complex molecules such as heparin or testosterone). Some drugs have a high oral bioavailability even though they undergo an extensive chemical change resulting in therapeutically active metabolites – this is called metabolic activation of therapeutically inactive prodrugs (e.g. the antihypertensive drug enalapril, the antiviral drug valaciclovir or heroin).

Physicochemical properties resulting in a low bioavailability are poor water solubility, slow or incomplete absorption during the passage through the gastrointestinal tract (total 1–2 days, but only 2–4 h in the small intestine) and molecule-specific chemical reactivity. Examples for molecule-specific chemical reactivity are (i) complex formation (e.g. the antibiotic tetracycline and polyvalent metal ions), (ii) conjugation in the intestinal epithelium (e.g. sulfoconjugation of the bronchodilatative drug isoproterenol), (ii) hydrolysis by gastric acid (e.g. penicillin), (iv) adsorption to other drugs (e.g. the heart drug digoxin and the bile acid binder cholestyramine) or (v) metabolism by luminal bacterial microflora (normally only in the large intestine, under pathological circumstances even in the small intestine).

To assess the overall bioavailability, one has to take repetitive blood samples, and measure the time (called peak time) and the amount of the peak drug concentration in the plasma (here the drug absorption rate equals the elimination rate), and the so-called area under the plasma concentration–time curve (AUC). A higher absorption rate results in an earlier peak time and higher peak concentration; a slower absorption results in a later peak time. Parentally administered drugs have an early peak time, because the whole dose reaches the systemic circulation in a short time. The AUC is direct proportional to the total amount of drug that reaches the systemic circulation and usually allows the most reliable characterization of the bioavailability.

To increase the overall plasma concentration of the drug, it is possible to give multiple doses of the drug formulation before the entire previous dose is eliminated from the circulation. With fixed-dosing intervals, the drug concentration increases for four to five plasma elimination half-lives (see the following sections for details) before reaching the steady state, where absorption and elimination are equal. Depending on the half-lives of the drug, the dosing interval can vary from some hours to some days.

5.2.2.3 Distribution

After entering the systemic circulation, a drug is delivered to all parts of the body through the bloodstream. Nonetheless the distribution is uneven because of differences in (i) blood flow (e.g. the eye or the kidney have much higher mean perfusion per volume than muscles or the connective tissue), (ii) tissue binding (e.g. lipophilic drugs bind to fatty tissue), (ii) regional pH and (iv) permeability of endothelial membranes of the blood vessels (e.g. very low permeability in the brain and high permeability in liver, spleen and kidney). All of these factors define the organ-specific distribution equilibrium, defined as the time-point when entry rates to the tissue and exit rates from the tissue are the same, and drug concentrations outside and inside the blood vessels are the same (plasma concentration = effective tissue concentration). Richly vascularized areas with high vessel permeability for a specific drug reach the equilibrium more rapidly than poorly vascularized areas with a low permeability, thus making it complex to assess the organ-specific concentrations when researching the borders for therapeutic and toxic effects.

To describe the distribution characteristics of a certain drug, one can use the idea of the apparent volume of distribution, defined as the fluid volume needed to contain the drug in the body at the same concentration as in the plasma. Clearly, a certain quantity of a drug with a high apparent volume of distribution (e.g. the anti-arrythmic drug amiodarone) results in a much lower overall plasma concentration than a drug with a low apparent volume of distribution (e.g. heparin), since the same amount of drug molecules reach a higher fluid volume (e.g. the blood covers roughly 3–4 L and the whole extracellular fluid covers about 17 L). Apart from the fluid volume, other factors such as fat tissue binding, protein binding and pH of the drug influence the apparent volume of distribution, resulting in volumes up to 500 L for fat binding, mostly basic drugs such as digoxin or amiodarone. Acidic drugs such as salicylic acid and warfarin have smaller volumes of distribution than basic drugs such as amphetamine because of their preferential protein binding (the body has much more fat than free proteins for binding).

In the bloodstream, common drugs are transported either or both as unbound, free drug or bound to different blood components such as plasma proteins (mostly albumin for acidic drugs and different glyco/lipoproteins for basic drugs) and blood cells (mostly red blood cells). Differences in blood component concentrations and compositions result in unstable plasma concentrations of the given drugs, possibly decreasing the therapeutic effect or increasing toxicity.

To reach the desired "place of action", the drug has to leave the systemic circulation (similar mechanisms to transcellular passage as described in Section 5.2.2.1) and for most drugs this is only possible for the unbound, free fraction. To assess the possible speed of vessel permeation, it is necessary to know the fraction unbound (defined as the ratio of unbound to total concentration) apart from physicochemical properties of the drug (size, polarity, pH, hydration, chemical functionality) and the endothelial layer of the blood vessel (permeability, transport mechanisms). The fraction unbound usually has a better correlation to the effective pharmacological activity than the overall plasma concentration (both free and bound fraction). At low drug concentrations, not all the available plasma proteins or cells are bound to the drugs; increasing the drug concentration (higher single dose or shorter dosing interval) leaves the fraction unbound unchanged up to a certain upper limit where all the possible binding sites are saturated. By increasing the drug concentration above the saturation limit, the fraction unbound can be raised, thus increasing both possible therapeutic effect in the tissues and possible toxicity and interaction opportunity (e.g. with other drugs or physiological substances in the bloodstream, possibly creating unexpected side-effects).

An important idea when considering the drug effect is the drug reservoir. Clearly, tissues with a fast distribution equilibrium and high drug binding capacity (e.g. bone marrow, fat tissue) can accumulate high amounts of drug molecules before the desired drug target reaches a sufficient drug concentration for the therapeutic effect. Since the plasma and the tissue concentration are at equilibrium, the drug reservoir releases the drug when the plasma concentration decreases because of elimination mechanisms. Therefore, the drug reservoir is both responsible for lower peak concentration and slower concentration decrease, resulting in the same AUC than without a drug reservoir.

Some drugs such as antimalarial drugs, some antibiotics and cytotoxic drugs accumulate inside specific cell types because of substance-specific transport mechanisms, and binding to intracellular components such as proteins, phospholipids or nucleic acids. Thus, the drug concentration is much higher inside the cells (mostly white blood cells such as macrophages, granulocytes and liver cells, but also bacteria) than in the surrounding tissue and in the plasma. Similar to drug reservoirs in the tissue, the intracellular drug is in equilibrium with the plasma and leaves the cell, unless it binds to a certain target or performs a certain chemical reaction.

5.2.2.4 **Elimination**

Elimination is the sum of processes of drug loss from the body, mainly metabolism (chemical alteration) and excretion (elimination without further chemical change).

Metabolism is mostly performed in the hepatocytes (main liver cell type) of the liver – different reaction pathways result in pharmacologically inactive or active metabolites. Drug metabolism pathways usually occur in two apparent phases: phase I and phase II. Phase I reactions involve forming a new or changed functional group or a cleavage (oxidation, reduction, hydrolysis) to ensure a higher rate of reactivity. Phase II reactions involve conjugation with an endogenous compound such as glucuronic acid, glycine or sulfate to ensure higher water solubility. The metabolites of these processes have a higher polarity and are excreted through the kidneys (urine) or the liver (bile) at a much higher rate than the original drug molecule.

The most important enzyme system of phase I metabolism is a microsomal family of isoenzymes called cytochrome P450, which can transfer electrons supplied by certain flavoproteins (NADPH-cytochrome P450 reductase) to catalyze drug oxidation. The cytochrome P450 superfamily is grouped into 14 families with gene sequence identity and 17 subfamilies. The isoenzymes are named by a root symbol CYP, followed by a number/letter combination. The most important CYP isoenzymes for drug metabolism are CYP1A2, CYP2C9, CYP2C19, CYP2D6 and CYP3A4. Every one of these isoenzymes is specific for different drugs and can be upregulated by repetitive drug application of so-called CYP-inductive drugs (e.g. glucocorticoids, rifampicin, carbamazepine, barbiturates, St John's wort, efavirenz, etc.) and downregulated by so-called CYP-inhibiting drugs (e.g. amiodarone, paroxetin, fluconazole, ketoconazole, ciprofloxacin, clarithromycin, ritonavir, grapefruit juice, etc.).

The most important phase II reaction is glucuronidation (conjugation to glucuronic acid), which occurs in the liver microsomal enzyme system (microsomes are intracellular organelles) and results in hydrophilic metabolites suitable for renal or biliary excretion (e.g. morphine, fluoroquinolone or chloramphenicol). Other important reactions are (i) amino acid conjugations with glutamine or glycine (e.g. salicylic acid), (ii) acetylation (e.g. sulfonamides, hydralazine), (iii) methylation (e.g. catecholamines, thiouracil, niacinamide), or (iv) sulfoconjugation of phenolic or alcoholic groups with inorganic sulfate gained from sulfur-containing amino acids such as cysteine (e.g. methyldopa, thyroxin, acetaminophen, estradiol).

All metabolic pathways show different activities according to (i) the genetic background (most important are genetic variations in the CYP2C9 cytochrome P450, resulting in different metabolic activities for certain drugs), (ii) age (newborns and elderly patients show low metabolic activity), (iii) sex, (iv) history of liver diseases, (v) capacity of the enzyme (mostly upper limit of capacity) and (vi) up- or down-regulating endogenous or exogenous substances. Due to these individual variations in drug metabolism, it is difficult to predict the therapeutic effect of a given dose of a drug, especially when the patient is taking other drugs, drinking alcohol or smoking.

The excretion of the now hydrophilic drug metabolite or the original hydrophilic, unmetabolized drug mostly takes place in the kidneys; a smaller degree of the incorporated drug can be excreted through the biliary system (bile is produced in the liver and flows into the small intestine), saliva, sweat, breast milk and lungs (volatile substances such as anesthetics).

Kidney excretion is a complex process that can be separated into glomerular filtration, tubular reabsorption and tubular secretion. The central unit of the kidney is the so-called nephron consisting of a well-perfused capillary congregate called glomerulus and the tubular system that follows the glomerulus. In the glomerulus, plasma is filtered through pores in the glomerular endothelium according to (i) the pressure in the afferent and efferent arterioles, (ii) the perfusion speed, (iii) the filter permeability, (iv) the size and ionization of the molecule (maximum filterable size is 10–15 nm [7]; cationic molecules have higher permeability than anionic molecules because of the anionic charge of the glomerulus), and (v) the pressure in the tubular system. Only unbound drugs up to certain size and ionization can be filtered through the glomerular endothelium, protein-bound drugs cannot be filtered. Most of the filtered ions (such as sodium, chloride, potassium, magnesium, calcium and bicarbonate), all glucose, amino acids, urea and other important substances are reabsorbed by specialized and substance-specific transport systems (active transport systems for glucose, amino acids and some ions; passive diffusion for most ions and water). Filtered drugs can also be reabsorbed if they show molecular closeness with endogenous physiologic substances (e.g. the antidepressant lithium is analogous to sodium). Unionized forms of nonpolar weak acids and weak bases are reabsorbed readily from the tubular filtrate, so acidification of urine increases the reabsorption of filtrated acidic drugs and decreases the reabsorption of basic drugs and *vice versa*.

Another excretion mechanism is the active, energy-dependent tubular secretion process in the proximal part of the tubule, typically used to remove drugs such as penicillin, salicylic acid, procainamide, dopamine, phenylbutazone and trimethoprim. It is possible to distinguish two separate transport mechanisms for anions and cations with a characteristic maximum of secretion. The anion secretory system is more important for drug elimination and transports metabolites conjugated with glycine, sulfate or glucuronic acid (conjugation done by phase II metabolism in the liver) into the tubular system. Due to the saturability of every active transport mechanism, anionic compounds compete with one another for secretion resulting in slower elimination times (e.g. penicillin elimination can be decreased by the therapeutically inactive molecule probenecid to increase therapeutic plasma concentrations of penicillin).

Some drugs can be removed by active biliary excretion (done by hepatocytes) across the biliary epithelium in the liver. This excretion mechanism is especially suitable for larger, lipophilic drugs conjugated with glucuronic acid. Once the excreted drug reaches the small intestine, it is treated in the same way as a drug coming from the stomach, resulting in an absorption by the intestinal epithelium, especially after enzymatic degradation of the "new" functional group (glucuronic acid). This is the enterohepatic cycle.

When assessing the overall rate of elimination, it is necessary to measure the concentrations of both unchanged drugs and possible metabolites in the main excretion routes (urine, bile, milk, saliva, sweat) over a certain time, and to compare these concentrations to the plasma concentrations. The parameter relating total elimination rate to plasma concentration is called total clearance (renal plus extrarenal clearance). The fraction of excreted unchanged drug helps to find out the impact of renal and extrarenal (mainly hepatic) elimination, since the unchanged drug can only be found in the urine and hepatic elimination is only possible for metabolites. A low fraction of unchanged drug shows that hepatic elimination is strongest and that hepatic disease may therefore affect drug elimination. The same applies to drugs with a high fraction of unchanged drug and renal diseases.

Another important assessment value is half-life elimination, defined as the time needed for the plasma drug concentration or the amount of drug in the body to decrease by 50%. This time is usually independent of plasma drug concentration, characterizes both distribution and elimination of the drug, and determines the dosing intervals and time to reach steady state.

5.2.3 Special Pharmacology

Here, we will discuss the key factors found in nature that protect the internal environment from external "macroelements" (bacteria, viruses, proteins, DNA, nanovectors such as liposomes, nanoparticles, nanospheres and nanocontainers). It is important to understand the concept of these defense mechanisms when trying to overcome the challenges and develop a targeting system for site-specific delivery of drugs or diagnostic agents with a minimal negative impact on physiologic pathways. Successful strategies to overcome the defensive obstacles performed by both pathogenic organisms such as bacteria and viruses and therapeutic systems will be presented. For a deeper insight into the immune system and other defense mechanisms, refer to the specialized literature listed in the reference section.

5.2.3.1 Skin Epithelium

The outermost layer of our body consists of multiple layers of squamous epithelial cells, together building the stratum corneum of the epidermis [8]. The stratum corneum can be considered as a two-compartment system consisting of the epithelial cells themselves and the surrounding extracellular matrix. The cells produce and secrete various proteins (e.g. linking proteins for cell–cell adhesion), lipids (e.g. phospholipids, cholesterol, ceramides, sphingomyelin) and enzymes (e.g. lipases, proteases and antiproteases). This two-compartment system of lipid-depleted squamous cells and lipid-enriched, extracellular matrix ensures both physical and chemical protection, preferably against ultraviolet light, chemicals, physical force, temperature, bacteria and viruses, but also against the permeation of macrostructures such as nanovectors.

Nonetheless, the skin can be useful for therapeutic purposes, as transdermal permeation systems for morphine, nitroglycerin or female steroid hormones prove. Factors such as site of application, thickness and integrity of the stratum corneum, size, polarity and pH of the molecule, skin hydration, drug metabolism by bacterial skin flora, and change of blood flow in the skin by additives and body temperature influence the rate of transdermal drug absorption [9, 10].

Small, lipo- or amphiphilic molecules can permeate the complex skin barrier. Permeation is also possible for lipid-based nanostructures such as liposomes up to a diameter of 500 nm [10, 11]; permeation of polymer-based nanostructures is more difficult because of their hydrophilic surface. Once the drug has permeated across the epidermis, it reaches a well-perfused subepidermal layer where it can enter blood vessels through pores in the vessel wall. An intact skin barrier protects the organism from pathogenic microstructures such as bacteria and most viruses; the same applies to nanoparticles bigger than the mentioned 500 nm.

5.2.3.2 Mucosal Epithelium of the Respiratory Tract

The airways can be divided into the upper respiratory tract (nose, mouth, throat and larynx) and the lower respiratory tract (trachea, bronchi and terminal respiratory alveoli). Multilayered squamous epithelium consisting of epithelial cells and special cell types producing mucus and immunoglobulins covers the upper respiratory tract. The physicochemical characteristics of this squamous epithelium are comparable to the skin. Nonetheless, the permeability is much higher because of the absence of a stratum corneum and a strong perfusion with well-permeable blood vessels, making it possible to absorb small, mostly lipophilic drugs such as nitroglycerin, cocaine and steroids at a high rate.

The lower respiratory tract has to be subdivided into the trachea and bronchi with their respiratory epithelium, and the alveoli with their single-layered alveolar epithelium. The respiratory epithelium consists of ciliated epithelial cells and mucus-producing cells, together building a single-layered barrier connected by tight cell–cell adhesion complexes called tight junctions or zonulae occludentes [12].

Drug application to the lower respiratory tract [9] is possible by inhalation of vaporized, nebulized, powdered or aerosolized drugs (e.g. β_2-agonists, corticosteroids, and anticholinergics for asthma and chronic obstructive pulmonary disease therapy, or antibiotics for to treat children with cystic fibrosis). Access to distal airways depends on the particle size, because particles bigger than 4 μm diameter deposit on the epithelium of the upper respiratory tract, and particles smaller than 500 nm diameter fail to deposit on the epithelium and are exhaled. Only particles with a diameter between 0.5 and 4 μm can reach the distal airways and deposit on the epithelium of the bronchi. Once the drug molecule or drug carrier is deposited, it can permeate across the respiratory epithelium (lipophilic drugs better than hydrophilic) and can reach the systemic circulation.

5.2.3.3 Mucosal Epithelium of the Gastrointestinal Tract

The gastrointestinal tract consists of the esophagus, stomach, small intestine and large intestine. Because of the short passage time and the impermeable epithelial barrier in the esophagus and especially in the stomach (low pH, dense mucus layer, and strong intercellular bonds between the epithelial cells), the upper parts of the gastrointestinal tract play no role in absorbing macromolecules and microstructures such as bacteria, viruses or nanoparticles.

The small intestine is the longest section of the gastrointestinal tract, lies between the stomach and the large intestine, and has an overall length of 6 m. The small intestine with its large mucosal surface (250 m^2 because of mucosal folds, mucosal extensions called villi and epithelial cell membrane extensions called microvilli) and epithelial cell (also called enterocytes) lining is responsible for the enzymatic digestion and absorption of small nutritives such as monosaccharides, oligonucleotides, amino acids, fatty acids, vitamins and lipids, and macromolecules such as epidermal growth factor. Dense tight junctions join the enterocytes [13] and build a continuous layer with other cell types that are responsible for other tasks. (i) Enteroendocrine cells sense the luminal environment and can secrete peptide hormones [14] into the blood that influence the digestive process. (ii) Gob-

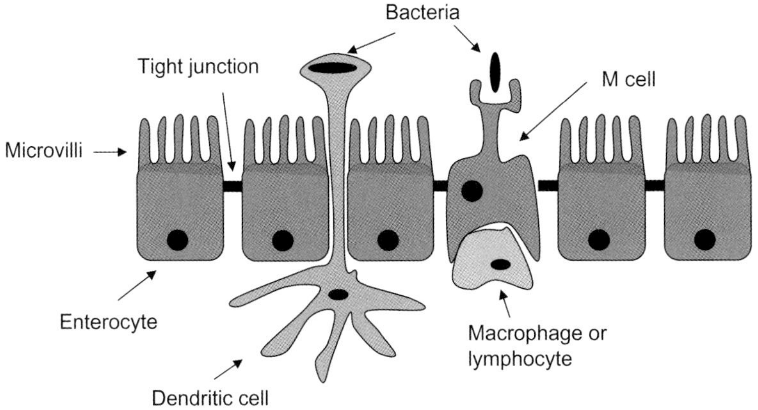

Figure 5.3. Schematic drawing of small intestine epithelium (for details refer to main text).

let cells produce peptides needed for epithelial growth and repair, and lubricating mucus consisting of glycoproteins that covers the mucosal surface, reduces the diffusion of macromolecules, and binds proteins and microorganisms. (iii) Paneth cells secrete antimicrobial digestive enzymes such as cryptidins or defensins. (iv) Finally, the M cells are phagocytic cells that control the luminal microbial environment and can trigger an immune response in the presence of harmful pathogens (see Fig. 5.3).

The epithelium is exposed to a wide variety of potentially harmful bacteria, viruses and other microorganisms that should not be able to permeate the epithelial layer [15]. It is obvious the epithelial cells had to develop sophisticated and specific receptors, transport systems and strong defense systems [16, 17] to cover all necessary functions such as digestion and absorption of all essential nutritives, endocrine functions, and immunologic and mechanical barrier for microorganisms and potentially harmful macromolecules.

The apical surface of the enterocytes is covered by closely placed microvilli (diameter 100 nm, intervillous space is variable and can decrease down to 25 nm) with a filamentous brush border glycocalyx (500 nm thick) consisting of negatively charged mucin-like glycoproteins and enzymes, responsible for terminal digestion of polysaccharides and polypeptides. Apart from this, the glycocalyx is another diffusion barrier that prevents macromolecular particles, bacteria and viruses from direct contact with the enterocyte cell membrane. Microstructures that want to enter the enterocytes have to move into the space between the microvilli or have to produce toxins or inflammatory agents that disrupt the microvilli continuity, thus allowing direct contact with the uncovered enterocytes surface.

Enterocytes take up luminal molecules by different methods. Small nutrient molecules such as glucose, amino acids and ions reach the cell through substance-specific epithelial transporters; larger molecules reach the cell by the receptor-mediated [18, 19], energy-dependent process of pinocytosis (for details, see Section 5.2.3.6). Once the molecules have entered the enterocytes, they can enter different pathways. The first pathways leads to enzymatic degradation in lysosomes, the second pathway leads to transcytotic transport of the intact vesicle content and active release into the subepithelial space, where the molecules can reach the systemic circulation or the lymphatic vessels.

Another pathway for epithelium crossing is the paracellular transport that is only possible under pathological conditions, because normally the intercellular tight junctions block the permeation of large molecules and micro- and nanometer sized structures. Physiologically, the tight junctions can dilate up to a pore radius of 5 nm on activation of certain cellular Na^+-coupled transport systems, enabling a transjunctional osmotic flow for nutrients. Pathological insults such as inflammatory cytokines [e.g. interferon (IFN)-γ, tumor necrosis factor (TNF)-α, interleukin (IL)-1β, IL-4 and IL-13], mechanical damage, infection, bacterial toxins (e.g. cholera toxin) and cell death can open these pores enough to allow the passage of macromolecules or nano/microstructures [15, 20, 21].

5.2.3.4 Mononuclear Phagocyte System (MPS)

Once the drug molecule or drug complex reaches the systemic circulation – be it direct by intravenous or intra-arterial injection or indirect by other application ways – it comes in contact with various metabolic pathways and defensive systems. When discussing the possibility of targeted delivery of nanometer-sized structures (lipid-based such as liposomes and micelles, protein-based such as dendrimers, and polymer-based such as nanospheres, nanoparticles and nanocontainers), the most important hurdle is the MPS [22, 23] [also known as reticuloendothelial system (RES)] – a part of the innate immune system. The MPS consists of bone marrow (pro-) monoblasts, peripheral monocytes and monocyte-derived tissue macrophages in liver (called Kupffer cells), lungs, spleen, lymph nodes, thymus, gut, bone marrow and brain (called microglia). The MPS plays a major role in host defense, and is responsible for clearing unwanted and possibly pathogenic organisms (bacteria, fungi, protozoa, parasites, viruses) and macromolecules such as lipoproteins, polysaccharides, polynucleotides and nanoparticles. Macrophages can also be attracted to an infected focus by various chemotactic substances (bacterial endotoxins, immune complexes, complements factors, collagen fragments), where they phagocyte infectious agents. Apart from this, the cells of the MPS play an important role in the development of pathological conditions such as cancer, atherosclerosis, autoimmune diseases (rheumatoid arthritis, Crohn's disease, systemic lupus erythematosus, multiple sclerosis), diseases of the central nervous system and some infectious diseases (HIV, tuberculosis, leishmaniosis, salmonellosis, schistosomiasis).

When injecting macromolecular formulas such as liposomes, immunoliposomes, polymeric micro/nanospheres and nanoparticles into the circulation, the MPS clears the substances rapidly from the bloodstream, mainly in the well-perfused, macrophage-rich organs liver and spleen. For phagocytosis, the macrophages contact the particles with receptor-equipped pseudopods, attach the particle to the cell membrane and engulf them with lamellipods. After entering the macro-

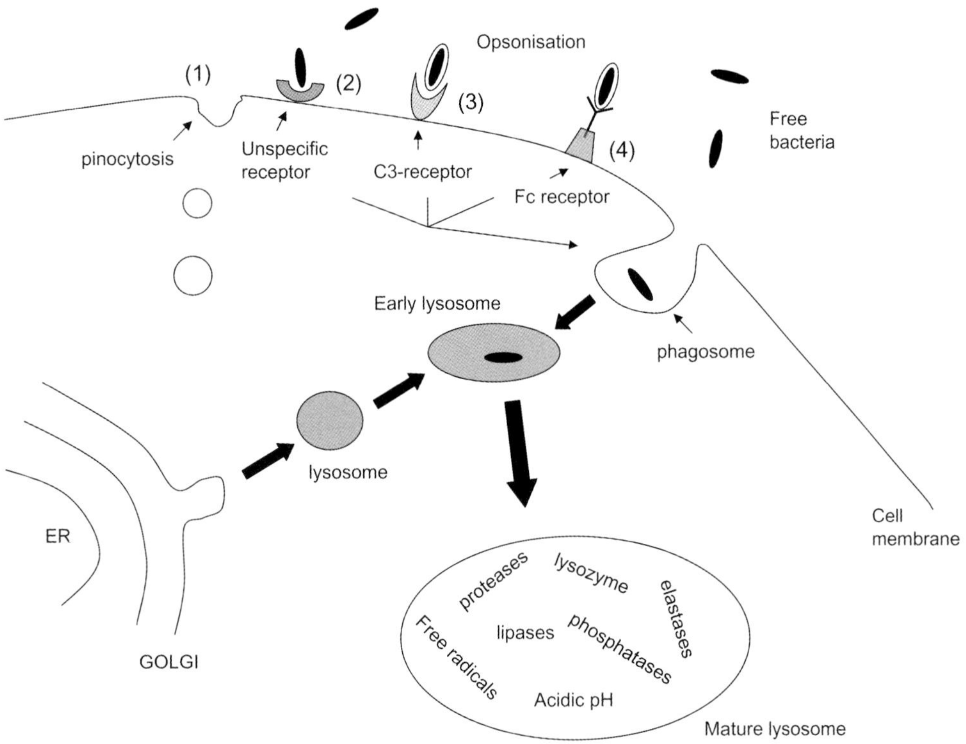

Figure 5.4. Schematic drawing showing the principles of receptor-mediated endocytosis: (1) shows the process of pinocytosis as described in the main text; (2)–(4) show the different pathways that lead to the receptor-mediated endocytosis of various ligands, in this case bacteria. (2) The binding of native, unchanged bacteria to "unspecific" receptors (e.g. scavenger receptors, mannose receptors, TLRs) found on phagocytic cell types (macrophages, dendritic cells). (3) The binding of complement factor-labeled bacteria to the C3 receptor, which binds the activated complement factor 3. (4) The binding of antibody-labeled bacteria to the Fc receptor, which binds a subunit of immunoglobulins. The final steps in the case of receptor-mediated endocytosis consist of the development of the early and mature lysosome with various degrading systems as described in the main text.

phage by membrane–membrane fusion or receptor-mediated endocytosis, the microstructures are subject to aggressive enzymatic (proteases, esterases, glucuronidases, phosphatases, nucleases, lipases, etc.) and nonenzymatic (free radicals, acid) degradation inside specialized, low pH (down to pH 1–2) intracellular vesicles called lysosomes (Fig. 5.4). Most of the macrostructure material gets degraded down to its chemical constituents, but some remaining protein fragments can be used by the cells to create immunogenic antigen fragments for lymphocyte presentation on class I or II major histocompatibility complex (MHC) molecules. (The MHC is a transmembrane multiprotein construct for antigen-presentation to cells of the immune system such as T lymphocytes, which are able to create a specific, antibody-mediated immune response against the presented antigen.) The range of such an immune response reaches from a fast elimination of newly injected micro/nanostructures up to a possibly fatal anaphylactic (allergic) shock. Apart from the obvious loss of material and targeting efficiency, the possible immune response is the main reason why nanostructures for targeted delivery have to be protected from fast uptake into the MPS.

The most important condition for rapid uptake into the MPS [23] is the process of opsonization, defined as the deposition of blood opsonic factors (e.g. fibronectin, immunoglobulins and complement proteins) on the surface of bacteria, viruses, and nanostructures such as liposomes, micelles, nanoparticles, nanocontainers and dendrimers. Once the structures have been labeled by opsonization, the macrophages recognize them with their specialized surface receptors (scavenger receptors, Toll-like receptors (TLRs), Fc receptors, complement receptors, mannose receptors, fibronectin receptors, etc.) and take them up by receptor-mediated endocytosis. Size and surface characteristics of the nanostructures define the opsonization efficiency, the macrostructure–macrophage interaction and thus the clearance kinetics. For instance, smaller polymer-based nanoparticles (below 200 nm diameter) show longer circulation lifetimes than larger ones, but smaller lipid-based nanoparticles show shorter circulation lifetimes than bigger particles [24]. Particles with many available functional groups and stronger polarity also show shorter circulation lifetimes. Lipid-based nanostructures such as liposomes show much shorter circulation life-times than polymer-based nanostructures because of (i) lower physicochemical stability (higher leakage rates in bloodstream turbulences), (ii) better opsonization efficiency, (iii) opsonization-independent receptor interaction of liposome compositions containing phosphatidylserine, phosphatidylglycerol or phosphatidylcholine (all ligands for certain types of macrophage receptors) and (iv) easier uptake into the macrophages because of chemical likeness with the cellular membrane (also based on phospholipids). This allows the macrophages to take up the liposomes by direct membrane-membrane fusion instead of receptor-mediated endocytosis.

Special low-protein absorbing polymeric surfaces such as poly(ethylene glycol) (PEG), poly[*N*-(2-hydroxylpropyl)methacrylamide], distearyl phosphotidyl ethanolamine (DSPE) or poly(2-methyl-oxazoline) (PMOXA) can prolong the circulation lifetime of both liposomes and polymer-based nanoparticles by decreasing the grade of opsonization, making it possible to reach the desired therapeutic target before being removed from the circulation. Nanoparticles with these specialized surfaces are referred to as "stealth" particles [24], since they "hide" themselves from the MPS [25].

5.2.3.5 **Endothelial Barrier**

The endothelial cells cover the interior surface of all blood vessels, and build an important barrier between the blood components and the tissues. The endothelium actively controls the exchange between these two compartments and shows a high grade of impermeability in most tissues. Only a limited number of small molecules such as oxygen, carbon dioxide and water, and small lipophilic molecules diffuse passively across or along the endothelial membrane according to the concentration gradient. For some macromolecules such as glucose and amino acids, the endothelial cells have active transport mechanisms to ensure a sufficient flow of supplies for the underlying organs. Macromolecules can only leave the circulation through so-called endothelial fenestrations, principally holes between the endothelial cells, and across endothelial clefts at the cell–cell junctions. Organs such as the liver, lymph nodes or the spleen show a well-developed endothelial fenestration with an easily permeable endothelial layer. On the other hand, organs such as the testis, the brain or the spinal cord have a dense endothelial barrier with a small permeability for most drugs and all hydrophilic substances. The specialized endothelium of the brain is called the blood–brain barrier and has no fenestrations.

An important characteristic of the endothelial layer is the increase of permeability under certain pathological conditions, known as vascular leakage [26, 27]. For instance, vascular leakage is a complication that can worsen a systemic inflammatory reaction in the case of a severe bacterial infection, and leads to excessive plasma extravasation into the lung, the skin and the abdomen when plasma proteins can leave the blood vessels through enlarged endothelial fenestrations. On the other hand, it allows the white blood cells to leave the circulation in much higher numbers than under physiological conditions, and increases the oxygen and nutrients supply for the tissue. Vascular leakage is also an early step in the development of atherosclerosis, where lipoproteins leave the circulation and gather inside the inner layers of the blood vessels. Some tumors have leaky vessels, making it easier for the tumor cells to reach the systemic circulation.

On the topic of site-specific drug delivery with nanotechnological delivery systems, it is important to consider the physicochemical properties of the endothelial barrier in different tissues and under different states according to the target, size, surface and functionalization of the carrier. For instance, it is almost impossible for "normal" nanoparticles to permeate through the intact blood–brain barrier; on the other hand, the vessels of aggressive brain tumors are leaky, making it possible to reach the tumor cells with nanoparticles. Another interesting target for delivery of nanoparticles is the so-called vulnerable plaque, defined as an inflamed atherosclerotic lesion of the blood vessel wall with a thin fibrous cap covering an amorphous mass of cell detritus, cholesterols, lipoproteins and collagen. A breakup of this instable system [28, 29] leads to the formation of blood clots and may stop the blood flow in the diseased vessel, resulting in potentially fatal diseases such as myocardial infarction, stroke, skin ulcers, etc. The endothelial layer on the vulnerable plaques is known to be leaky, making it possible for nanoparticles to reach the inflamed fibrous cap and influence the diseased state.

5.2.3.6 **Cell Membrane**

The passage across the cell membrane is the last and possibly the most difficult hurdle for targeted delivery of macromolecules because of the complex nature of the membrane, and the variety of different receptors, channel proteins, cell surface functionalizations and transport systems [30, 31]. The membrane consists mainly of phospholipids, cholesterol and proteins building a hydrophilic–hydrophobic–

hydrophilic triblock bilayer membrane stabilized by structure proteins and intercellular connections. Integrated into the bilayer membrane are different transmembrane and nontransmembrane proteins with functions such as ion channels, glucose and amino acid transporters, receptors for ligands, cell communication receptors, cell–cell adhesion, etc.

Small, nonpolar molecules such as oxygen, carbon dioxide or nitrogen dissolve in the lipid bilayer and diffuse passively into the cell according to the concentration gradient. The same applies to small, noncharged molecules such as water or ethanol. Bigger molecules (e.g. glucose, amino acids or urea) and all charged molecules (e.g. sodium, potassium, chlorine or magnesium) have only a limited possibility of passive transmembrane diffusion, making it necessary for the cell to set up transport systems for essential molecules (as described in previous subsections).

When discussing the delivery of macromolecules such as nanoparticles into the cells, one has to be aware that most cells are not intended to take up macromolecules and the nanoparticles have to use transport systems with a different purpose than "nanovehicle transport".

The first step in the transmembrane transport of macromolecules is the binding of a ligand to a specific cell surface receptor. Some receptors answer the ligand binding with a complex process called endocytosis that can be divided into phagocytosis and pinocytosis (Fig. 5.4). Phagocytosis means the uptake of micrometer-sized structures such as bacteria and fungi, which can only be done by specialized phagocytic cell types of the innate immune system such as macrophages, granulocytes, and dendritic cells. These cell types have special cell surface receptors such as (i) Fc receptors (for immunoglobulins bound to bacteria), (ii) complement receptors (for proteins of the complement system, which plays a major role inflammation, immune defense and tumor cell killing), (iii) scavenger receptors [32–36] (for polyanionic molecules such as lipoproteins, polysaccharides and polynucleotides) and (iv) mannose receptors [37] (for mannosylated/*N*-acetylglucosamine-terminal and fucosylated glycoproteins) that stimulate phagocytosis of the mentioned macromolecules. Pinocytosis is possible for all other cell types and is restricted to nanometer-sized structures such as viruses, proteins, lipoproteins, transferrin, cholesterol, etc.

On a molecular level, pinocytosis occurs on different, energy-consuming pathways, e.g. clathrin-mediated, caveolin-mediated, or clathrin- and caveolin-independent. Clathrin-mediated endocytosis is the most important entry pathway for macromolecules in cell types other than phagocytes and is triggered by ligand–receptor binding. It starts with the binding of the protein clathrin to the intracellular part of the transmembrane receptor, followed by the creation of small cell membrane pits. Then the cell membrane pits with the ligand–receptor complexes are dragged into the cell by the cytoskeleton and form enclosed, clathrin-coated vesicles that finally lose the contact with the cell membrane. Once the vesicle is created, it starts to "uncoat" the clathrin coating, allowing the fusion with other intracellular compartments such as lysosomes for degradation and receptor recycling (Fig. 5.5).

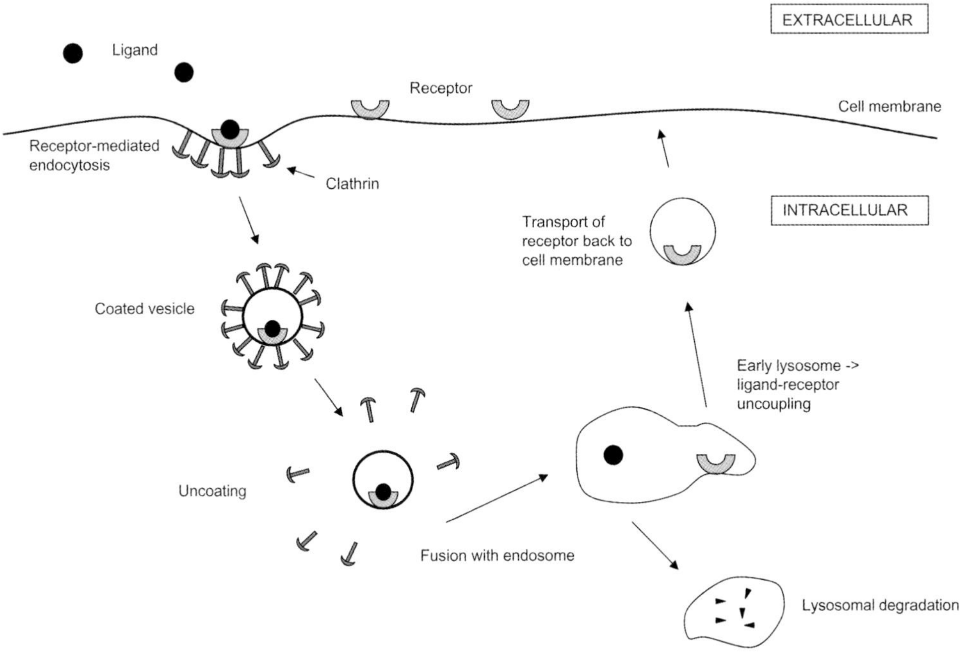

Figure 5.5. Schematic drawing of clathrin-mediated endocytosis (for details refer to main text).

During the process of phagocytosis, the phagocytic cell launches a signaling cascade that results in the formation of cell membrane protrusions that surround the pathogen and engulf it into so-called phagosomes, comparable to giant intracellular vesicles. The content of the phagosomes (bacteria, viruses, nanoparticles) is then attacked by lysosomal enzymes, free acids, and radicals, resulting in a degradation and inactivation of the macrostructure.

For targeted delivery of nanostructures, one has to overcome the inactivating lysosomal pathway when trying to cause a therapeutic impact on intracellular targets in the cytoplasma or nucleus.

5.3 Strategies for Targeted Delivery – Observed in Nature

5.3.1 Outline

When discussing the use of nanotechnologies for targeted delivery, it is essential not to forget the enormous range of "natural micro/nanostructures". Bacteria, viruses, fungi, parasites, prions, etc., have evolved over a long period and have specialized in targeted delivery to targets inside macroorganisms against strong defense mechanisms. To avoid the various defense systems, the microstructures had to develop specialized strategies for adherence, barrier invasion, immune system evasion, targeting and growth.

Obviously, understanding these microorganism strategies is important when trying to develop "artificial micro/nanostructures" for targeted delivery, because it is easier copying an existing targeting strategy than developing a new one. Further, there is no reason why well-tested strategies evolved during the long evolutionary fight between macro- and microorganisms should not work in a similar context like nanostructure delivery. It is also important to show that targeted nano/microstructure delivery is possible through other pathways than parenteral injection. To realize the different possibilities to reach a target inside the body by oral or transbronchial application might perhaps help to break the paradigm that says that nanoparticles can only be delivered by parenteral injection. Apart from this, it allows understanding the defense strategies of the human body from a different perspective and displays the need for a deeper understanding of the complex molecular pathways.

Here, we will discuss major strategies for barrier permeation, immune system evasion, and targeted delivery of bacteria, viruses, and prions. It is not the idea create an outline over all existing pathogenic strategies, but to highlight some of these strategies. Refer to the references section for a deeper insight into certain topics of interest.

5.3.2 Bacteria

To set up an infection of a macroorganism, bacteria have devised a vast range of strategies, also called virulence factors [38, 39]. Here, we will concentrate on two features of bacterial strategies that might become helpful for the design of artificial complex nanostructures for targeted delivery: host invasion and immune system evasion.

5.3.2.1 Host Invasion

The first defense mechanism pathogenic bacteria meet when they try to invade a macroorganism is the native bacterial flora of the skin or the gastrointestinal tract, which consists of normally harmless bacteria that prevent the newly gained pathogenic bacterium from growth and invasion. By successfully erasing or suppressing this protective flora, the bacterium sets up its own nutritive environment on the skin or inside the gut. Iatrogenic (physician-made) elimination of the native flora of the gut by antibiotics also allows the spread of pathogenic bacteria such as *Clostridium difficile.*

The next step of the bacterial attack is bacterial adherence on outer body surfaces such as skin and mucosal epithelium of the respiratory and gastrointestinal tract. As we have discussed above, the outer layer of the body is build of impermeable epithelial barriers that protect the body from the entry of potentially harmful macromolecules and structures of complex functionality. Most bacteria cannot cross the intact epithelial barrier, and can only reach the interior of the body and blood vessels through small mechanical lesions in the epithelial barrier. In particular, the skin is a reliable barrier for bacteria invasion because of the two-compartment, multilayered organization. Permeation across the single-layered epithelium of the mucosa of both the respiratory and gastrointestinal tract is much easier, and can be achieved by specialized bacteria even under physiologic conditions (no mechanical damage to the epithelium). These bacteria have special surface structures for adherence to the epithelial layers, called pili (also called fimbriae) and nonfimbrial adhesins [40]. Pili are rod-shaped protein structures on the cell walls of the bacteria consisting of long cylindrical protein subunits in a helical array. The continuously produced subunits are added from the pili interior and extend the pilus outward. The tip of the pilus adheres and binds to host cell molecules on the surface of the epithelial cells such as glycoproteins and glycolipids. Nonfimbrial adhesins are similar cell-contact structures like pili. The cell adherence structures are specific for certain host cell surface molecules and are one explanation for the tissue tropism of most bacteria (e.g. *Streptococcus mutans* colonizes teeth, but not the epithelium of the tongue). Once the bacteria has fixed the contact with the epithelial cell, it can perform a tighter binding to the cell by other bacterial proteins that can bind to surface structures such as different host cell receptors for cell–cell contact or signal transduction.

The next step is the passage across the intact epithelial layer or the invasion into the epithelial cells. Possible pathways for transepithelial passage without invasion or destruction of the epithelial cells involve paracellular entry, translocation through the M cells and luminal capture by dendritic cells [41].

The easiest method is to profit from temporary disruptions of the dense and normally impermeable cell–cell bonds caused by the paracellular transmigration of polymorphonuclear leucocytes (white blood cells) from the subepithelial tissue into the gut following an inflammatory signal. Leucocytes have the ability to weaken the intercellular connections by enzymatic degradation and cross the epithelial layer actively. Some bacteria such as *Shigella* can use these temporarily created intercellular holes to permeate across the epithelial layer without harming the cells.

The M cells, specialized phagocytic cells, are part of the mucosa-associated immune system and are placed inside the epithelial layer where they constantly take samples of the luminal flora for immunologic controlling. Some bacteria families such as *Shigella*, *Salmonella*, *Yersinia* and *Listeria* have different methods to evade the lysosomal destruction inside the M cells and can leave the M cells without loss of function. While *Listeria* have the ability to escape into the cytoplasma with their pore-forming protein listeriolysin O [42] and *Salmonella* can remodel their phagosomes for intracellular growth with the protein Spi2, *Yersinia* have an antiphagocytic strategy that inactivates the actin cytoskeleton by intracellular injection of the proteins YopE, YopH and YopT. Finally, *Shigella* can synthesize intracellular factors that cause the apoptosis (controlled cell death) of M cells, macrophages and monocytes, leading to the release of the unharmed *Shigella* bacterium after phagocytosis. *Shigella* is even able to synthesize cytokines (substances for cell–cell communication) such as IL-1β and IL-18 that disrupt epithelial impermeability and simplify further bacterial invasion on a paracellular pathway. All of these mechanisms allow the bacteria to cross the epithelial layer without having to kill the epithelial cells [41].

The last pathway for transepithelial passage without epithelial cell invasion is the luminal capture by dendritic cells. Dendritic cells are phagocytic cells of the innate immune system comparable to macrophages. They are not a constant part of the mucosa like the M cells, but have the ability to crawl between two epithelial cells or to send cell extensions called pseudopods through the intercellular compartment into the gut lumen. The pseudopods capture luminal bacteria and phagocyte them for degradation and detection. The bacteria mentioned above have strategies for phagocytosis evasion and can reach the systemic circulation once they leave the dendritic cells. Some bacteria such as the *Salmonella* family can even travel inside the dendritic cells as "blind passengers".

Another method for transepithelial migration is the direct and active (not by phagocytosis [43]) invasion into the epithelial cells; these cell-invasion strategies [41] are more complicated than the methods we have met until now and require sophisticated molecular mechanisms. Bacteria such as *Yersinia pseudotuberculosis* or *Listeria monocytogenes* [44] express proteins such as invasin, internalin or InlB that can bind to surface receptors (mostly receptors for cell-matrix or cell–cell adhesion such as integrin, E-cadherin or Met) of the host cell, leading to a clustering of the bound receptors and a forming of vacuoles that engulf the bacterium through a so-called "zipper" mechanism. The ligand–receptor binding starts a cascade of signals (e.g. protein phosphorylation, recruitment of adaptors and effectors), resulting in an activation of actin cytoskeleton units and finally bacterial internalization through developing membrane extensions that enclose the bacterium.

Other bacteria such as *Shigella* or *Salmonella* can bypass the step of adherence to the host cell and interact direct with the intracellular actin cytoskeleton by injecting effectors through a secretory system that trigger the formation of macropinocytic pits for bacterial entry. A key constituent of this "trigger mechanism" is the type III secretory system [45–48] – a complex multiprotein structure comparable to an injection needle of a syringe. The tip of the secretory system recognizes the surface of the host cell and triggers the insertion of an IpaB/C or SipB/C [49, 50] translocation pore into the cell membrane. This translocation pore allows permeation of the proteins IpaC and SipC that force the cell to form the mentioned macropinocytic pockets by actin cytoskeleton nucleations, and of a protein called VirA that stimulates local destabilization and depolymerization of microtubules, another part of the cytoskeleton. In a next step, more proteins such as SopB/SigD, SopE or IpgD are injected through the type III secretory system and stimulate actin rearrangements and bacterial entry. In the last step, the macropinocytic pocket closed, triggered by the injected proteins SptP and IpaA.

One major effect of these complex mechanisms is the direct invasion into intracellular vesicles or even into the cytoplasma without having to survive the direct contact with the lysosomal compartment. The bacteria can now persist inside the epithelial cell and usually start intracytoplasmic reproduction, finally resulting in host cell killing. The newly created bacteria now can reach the well-perfused subepithelial tissue, where they can enter the blood vessels through the endothelial fenestrations.

Once the bacterium reaches the interior of the body, it has to evade the host defense if it wants to survive. In the tissue or inside the blood vessels, the bacterium meets the cellular and noncellular parts of both unspecific (innate) and specific (adaptive) immune system.

5.3.2.2 Immune System Evasion

One essential requirement for "targeted delivery" of complex structures such as bacteria is the ability to survive in the tissue and in the bloodstream by evading, suppressing or tricking the immune system of the host organism. The immune system [51, 52] consists mainly of the unspecific, innate immune system and the specific, adaptive immune system. The unspecific immune system organizes a first defensive barrier against microorganisms such as bacteria, fungi and parasites. It consists of noncellular (humoral) elements such as the complement system, the acute-phase proteins, the interferons and bactericidal substances such as lysozyme. Then cellular elements such as the epithelial layers, the native microbial flora and the white blood cell granulocytes (neutrophilic, basophilic and eosinophilic), mast cells, monocytes, macrophages, natural killer (NK) cells and dendritic cells. The specific immune system consists of the humoral element antibodies, and the cellular elements B lymphocytes, T lymphocytes and plasma cells. It is responsible for targeted defense against bacteria, viruses, allogenous cells and tumor cells with molecule-specific antibodies and target-specific killer cells.

Bacteria have mainly specialized in manipulating the innate, unspecific immune system with several different strategies [53, 54]. We will discuss some of them to show successful strategies for innate immune system evasion that might be helpful for targeted delivery of artificial micro/nanostructures.

Recognizing microbial molecules by germline-encoded receptors such as the transmembrane TLRs [55, 56] of macrophages and dendritic cells, an important receptor family for the innate recognition of various microorganism, activates the innate immune system. One of the best-characterized of the TLRs is TLR4, which can bind lipopolysaccharides, an essential part of the cell wall of Gram-negative bacteria (e.g. *Escherichia coli, Salmonella*). Binding of a bacterium is a condition for uptake into the phagocyte and for the inflammatory cytokine response. On the other hand, many bacteria have manipulative systems that alter the function of the TLR4 system and enable an infection of the host organism. The *Shigella* bacterium, for instance, synthesizes a surplus of free lipopolysaccharides (also called endotoxins) that bind and block TLR4 of macrophages and stimulate an inflammatory response. As we have seen above, this inflammation can lead to a higher permeability of the intestinal epithelium and to a higher grade of bacterial invasion [57].

Bacteria such as *Yersinia pestis, Helicobacter pylori* and *Chlamydia trachomatis*, on the other hand, synthesize a slightly changed version of the free lipopolysaccharide that also blocks all TLR4, but that does suppress the inflammatory response instead of stimulating it. Thus, the bacterium decreases the efficiency of the immune response and increases its own chance of surviving.

Some pathogenic members of the *Yersinia* family such as *Yersinia enterocolitica* and *Y. pseudotuberculosis* can be considered as specialists for immune system suppression. Not only do they block the TLR4 system with modified free lipopolysaccharides, they can also suppress phagocytosis (see above) and inflammatory response by injecting proteins such as YopM, and by the synthesis and secretion of the immune-suppressive V antigen [47]. The V antigen binds to another TLR, the TLR2, and activates IL-10- and CD14-dependent pathways that lead to immunity downregulation.

The bacterium *L. monocytogenes* produces a membrane-perforating protein to escape the lysosomes as we have seen in the last subsection. Once it reaches the cytoplasma of the macrophages, it can persist there and multiply by forcing the macrophage to produce the cytokine IFN-β that suppresses the ability of the macrophage to fight the infection of its own cytoplasma [42, 58, 59].

Another specialist for innate immune system evasion is the bacterium *Mycobacterium tuberculosis*, responsible for the tuberculosis infection. Similar to *L. monocytogenes*, *M. tuberculosis* has various potent strategies [60] that allow the bacterium to survive and multiply inside macrophages [61]. For instance, it can suppress the response of the innate immune system by (i) downregulating the expression of the cytokine IL-12 [62], (ii) by blocking the response of the macrophage to the cytokine IFN-γ that normally increases the ability and efficiency of the phagocytosis process [63], and (iii) by surrounding its own cell wall with stable and impermeable complex lipids, peptidoglycans and waxes [60] that protect the bacterium from the lysosomal enzymes.

Instead of surviving inside the macrophages or dendritic cells, some bacteria such as Enteropathogenic *E. coli*, *Pseudomonas aeruginosa* and *Yersinia* have strategies that prevent them from being subject to phagocytosis. As we have learned above, these bacteria can inject "antiphagocytic" substances (e.g. ExoS, ExoT, YopH, YopE and YopT) [64–68] into the phagocytic cells with their type III secretion system before the macrophage can bind the bacterium.

Other intracellular bacteria, *Legionella pneumophila* [69] and *Brucella* [70], use a type IV secretion system [71–73] to degrade the function of host lysosomes by intercepting intracellular vesicles from the endoplasmic reticulum that contain the lysosomal enzymes and to stop the presentation of bacterial antigens on class II MHC molecules [74, 75]. *C. trachomatis* [76] and *Chlamydia pneumoniae* [77], also obligate intracellular bacteria, have sophisticated strategies that can block the transition from innate to the adaptive immune system, thus making it hard for the immune system to remove the infected phagocytes. The *Chlamydia* bacteria secrete a proteolytic enzyme called chlamydial protease-like activity factor (CPAF) that degrades the host cell molecules RFX5 and USF-1 – transcription factors essential for activation of class I and class II MHC molecules that would present some *Chlamydia* antigens to lymphocytes for adaptive immune system activation.

The last bacterium we want to discuss here is *Streptococcus pyogenes*, which has evolved complex strategies to evade the inactivation by cells of the innate immune system, in this case by the granulocytes (also called polymorphonuclear leukocytes) [78]. Normally granulocytes can kill invading bacteria and fungi by both phagocytosis and different microbicidal systems such as superoxide, reactive oxygen species, hydrogen peroxide and hypochlorous acid. *S. pyogenes* has the ability to inhibit the recruitment of new granulocytes to the site of infection by producing a serine endoprotease (C5a peptidase) that degrades and inactivates a potent host-derived chemotactic factor of the complement system, C5a [79].

Perhaps the most important defense strategy for our purpose is the ability of *S. pyogenes* to evade the opsonization by plasma proteins that would result in an efficient and fast clearance by phagocytes. To achieve this antiopsonic strategy, the bacterium has a dimeric coiled-coil surface protein called M protein that binds certain nonopsonic factors of the complement system such as C4b-binding protein, factor H, factor H-like protein and the plasma protein fibrinogen. In that way, it impends the binding of the potent opsonic factor C3b to the bacterial surface [80]. Further, the bacterium produces a protein (Streptococcal inhibitor of complement, Sic) that inhibits the formation of the so-called membrane attack complex (MAC) [81, 82], the final cytotoxic formation of the complement factors C5b–C7 that would eventually perforate the bacterial wall (see below). Streptococcal pyrogenic exotoxin B (SpeB), another secretion product of the bacterium, inhibits opsonization and phagocytosis by cleaving opsonic factors such as fibronectin and vitronectin. Further, it blocks the granulocyte function by activating a metalloprotease and the pro-inflammatory and granulocyte-toxic cytokine IL-1β [83]. Finally, *S. pyogenes* produces the enzyme endoglycosidase (EndoS) that inactivates humoral antibodies directed against the bacterial surface for opsonization purposes, thus decreasing the possibilities for antibody-mediated phagocytosis [84].

S. pyogenes has also some interesting physical barriers that protect the bacterium against phagocytosis. A hyaluronic acid capsule composed of *N*-acetylglucosamine and glucuronic acid repeats offering a certain grade of phagocytosis protection covers the cell wall and inhibits the direct interaction of opsonins on the bacterial surface with granulocytes [85]. To increase the physical protection, *S. pyogenes* can cover itself with a matrix of fibronectin and collagen [86], and can even build aggregates with other bacteria, which as a result are difficult to remove for the immune system.

5.3.3
Viruses

When discussing the impact of nanotechnology for targeted delivery in biological systems, viruses are the best example found in nature and can be readily compared to artificial nanometer-sized structures such as nanocontainers. Viruses are nanometer-sized (15–300 nm diameter) complexes with a simple composition of a facultative lipid bilayer envelope with glycoproteins (viruses can be distinguished into viruses with an envelope and viruses without an envelope), a few enzymes such as reverse transcriptase, RNA polymerase or kinases, and a central nucleoprotein complex called a capsid containing the viral DNA or RNA. Viruses themselves have no means of independent locomotion or growth and depend on host cell metabolism. Once they enter the host organism, they have to penetrate the different defense barriers such as mucus layer, epithelial layer, immune system, endothelial layer and finally the cell membrane of their target cell. Here, we will discuss some important virulence factors of different viral species and we will show their enormous ability for target-specific delivery of their content in biological systems. We will also briefly discuss the current state of viral gene therapy and the impact of nanotechnology in gene therapy.

5.3.3.1 Immune System Evasion

Due to the much smaller size compared with bacteria and because of the intracellular reproduction, fighting viral infections is much more difficult for the immune system [87, 88]. To be able to recognize and inactivate the free virus, the immune system has to label the viral surface with opsonins such as unspecific complement factors or specific antibodies. As complement system activation is an important condition for an effective innate and adaptive immune response, most viruses have strategies to evade or manipulate the complement system [89, 90].

The complement system is a defensive method of the humoral innate immune system and consists of an interacting set of plasma enzymes (called C1–C9) synthesized in the liver, and in different cell lines such as monocytes, fibroblasts, endothelial cells and neurons (nerve cell). The complement system can be activated to perform a cascade of reactions leading (i) to the recruitment of antibodies, more complement factors and phagocytic leucocytes to the site of infection by producing potent anaphylatoxins (C3a–C5a), (ii) to the opsonization of viruses and virus-infected cells, and (iii) to the destruction of microorganisms and cells by the final ring-shaped, membrane-perforating MAC (consisting of activated C5–C9) [51]. The complement system activation can be achieved by three different pathways. (i) Classically by binding of the factor C1q to antibody–antigen complexes or certain viruses or virus-infected cells [91–94]. (ii) Lectin-mediated by binding of the mannan-binding lectin protein to oligosaccharides with unprotected repetitive carbohydrates such as mannose on certain viruses or virus-infected cells [95–97]. (iii) Alternatively by spontaneous and indiscriminate breakdown of the factor C3 in the serum or on surfaces of cells or particles when lacking sufficient levels of endogenous complement-regulating proteins such as C1 inhibitor factor 1 (C1-Inh), complement receptor 1 (CR1), decay-accelerating factor (DAF), protectin and Factor H [98–100]. Normally these factors inhibit the complement activation. All three pathways result in the terminal activation of a C3 convertase enzyme that activates C3 by cleavage. Active C3 activates C5, which launches the creation of the MAC. Viruses have a wide variety of complement-evading strategies; we will discuss some of them.

By forcing the virus-infected cell to shed or internalize antibody–antigen complexes on their surface, viruses from the families Herpes and Corona can obstruct the classical complement activation [101]. Further, Herpes and Pox viruses can produce and express proteins such as vaccinia virus complement control protein

(VCP) [102], glycoprotein C1 (gC1) [103, 104], glycoprotein C2 (gC2) [105] and complement control protein homolog (CCPH) [106], with functional likenesses [89] to the complement-regulating proteins that suppress the complement activation (see above). Some viruses of the families Pox [107], Herpes [108], Retro [109–112] and Toga [113] that cannot produce these proteins themselves are able to incorporate some of the complement-regulating proteins produced by the host organism into their envelope or to force the virus-infected cell to synthesize and secrete these proteins.

Another interesting strategy found in some Herpes [114, 115] and Corona [116] viruses enables these viruses to express Fc receptors (receptors for antibody binding) on the viral envelope or on the infected host cell. The Fc receptor binds nonimmune immunoglobulin G (IgG) and protects the virus or the virus-infected cell by sterically blocking the binding of virus-specific IgG [117], and by decreasing the efficiency of an antibody-mediated immune response [118].

5.3.3.2 **Host Cell Invasion**

If a virus wants to multiply, it has to invade a potential host cell [119, 120], has to deliver its capsid and the content of the capsid into the cell, and has to force the infected cell to create new viruses by adding its own genetic information of DNA or RNA to the synthetic machinery of the host cell. One important point is the attachment to the host cell membrane and the invasion into the cell without damaging the cell and without creating an immune response that would finally kill the infected cell.

The first step of cell invasion is the attachment to cell surface proteins, carbohydrates, or lipids that can serve as pure anchors for the virus or can mediate its uptake. The most important cellular receptors for viral attachment are intercellular adhesion molecule (ICAM)-1, integrins, CD4, α-dystroglycan, MHC-I, CXCR4, CCR5, CD46, DAF, CAR, LDLR, PVR, aminopeptidase-N, heparan sulfate glycosaminoglycan, and sialic acids [120].

One well-studied virus, HIV, even binds to multiple attachment factors such as C-type lectin receptors, the ICAM-3-grabbing nonintegrin (DC-SIGN) found on dendritic cells, and the ICAM-3-grabbing nonintegrin (L-SIGN) [121, 122] found in liver and lymph node tissue. Once HIV attaches to its target cell (macrophage, T lymphocyte, dendritic cell), its envelope-bound glycoprotein 120 binds to a surface receptor of the host cell, CD4, and changes its conformation – a condition for the final binding of glycoprotein 120 to the host cell co-receptors CXCR4 or CCR5 [123]. Only by cobinding to both CD4 and CXCR4 or CCR5 can the virus switch its envelope to the fusion-competent conformation [124, 125].

Attachment and binding factors used by other viruses are (i) heparan sulfate proteoglycans (binding site for glycoprotein C of alphaherpes viruses, for Dengue virus, for papilloma virus), (ii) sialic acid groups (for hemagglutinin of influenza virus, for myxo- and paramyxoviruses) [126], (iii) Herpes entry mediator A HVEA (for glycoprotein D of herpes simplex virus 1) [127], (iv) gangliosides GM_1, GD_{1a} and GT_{1b} (for VP1 of polyoma virus) [128, 129], and (v) human lymphocyte antigen (HLA)-DR (for gp43 of Epstein–Barr virus) [130].

For viruses without an envelope, the next step is the endocytosis (clathrin-mediated, caveolin-mediated or clathrin- and caveolin-independent [131]) of the bound capsid that allows the virus to cross the barrier of the cortical cytoskeleton, and to reach deep intracellular structures such as the lysosomes, the endoplasmic reticulum and the Golgi complex [132, 133]. For some viruses the decrease in pH in the endo-lysosome acts as a molecular trigger for membrane penetration mechanisms [134–136]. For most viruses the activation starts at pH 6–6.5, matching early endosomes [137, 138]. Endosome escape is possible by different mechanisms. Adenoviruses become membrane-lytic at low pH and leave the ruptures endosomes intact [139, 140]. Reoviruses can expose a hydrophobic capsid peptide that makes the capsid membrane lytic [141]. Picorna viruses have the ability to sink into the bilayer and to form a protein-lined channel for the viral RNA in the endosomal membrane by exposing a myristic acid end group of the protein VP1 [142].

These methods allow the virus or its genetic information to leave the lysosomal pathway before the enzymatic environment reaches its full degrading power that would inactivate the virus. Further, the lysosomal escape prevents the virus from being subject to an adaptive, MHC-mediated immune response, because the cell does not have any viral antigens to present to lymphocytes on the MHC complex. After leaving the lysosomal compartment, the viral capsid can use the cytoskeleton or intracellular transport motor proteins [143, 144] to reach the cell nucleus or specific cytoplasmic membranes.

Viruses with a protective envelope around the capsid cannot only reach the cell interior by endocytosis as the nonprotected viruses, they can also perform a "simple" membrane fusion to reach the cell. As the protective envelope is a lipid bilayer, membrane fusion is theoretically easy and comparable to the fusion of liposomes and target cells. More complicated is the mechanism that protects the enveloped viruses from fusion with every available cell and allows the membrane fusion only with the desired target cell, thus ensuring a targeted delivery. Membrane fusion is triggered by events such as binding to specific cell surface receptor or a decrease in pH [142, 145], on which the viral envelope changes its conformation and allows the fusion with both host cell membrane and lysosomal membrane.

Viruses have two different fusion factors that can induce the mentioned conformation changes of the lipid bilayer. Type I factors found in the influenza virus consist of homotrimeric spike glycoproteins with coiled-coil subunits and can insert exposed hydrophobic fusion sequences of a lower energy conformation into the target membrane on activation. The released free energy forces both viral and target membranes closer together, resulting in a membrane fusion [124, 126, 146]. Type II factors found in flaviviruses and alpha viruses [147] build a heterodimer with another viral membrane protein and can change their quaternary protein structure after a pH decrease. The fusion subunits of these two proteins dissociate and build a new active homotrimer [148, 149] that forces the membrane fusion. One major advantage of the membrane fusion strategy is the possibility to reach the cytoplasma direct without the complicated way through the receptor-mediated endolysosomal system.

To be able to reach the cellular reproduction machinery, the virus capsid has to cross the membrane of the cell nucleus [150–152], mainly through nuclear pore complexes [153–155] that allow the passage of particles up to a diameter of 39 nm [156]. To activate this transport system, the virus has to bind to cytoplasmic import receptors. For example, HIV and adenovirus bind to importin 7, and papilloma viruses, hepatitis B virus and influenza virus bind to importin α and β [157–161].

Larger viruses and capsids have to deform or disassemble to allow the DNA or RNA to reach the nucleus. Adenovirus disassembles its capsid after binding to a subunit of the nuclear pore and releases its DNA for transmembrane passage [162]. The large capsid (diameter 120 nm) of herpes simplex virus 1 also binds to the nuclear pore and releases its DNA direct into the pore without disassembly of the capsid [163, 164], leaving the empty capsid bound to the nuclear pore.

5.3.3.3 Viral Vectors for Therapeutic Applications

Genetically modified viruses have been used in a wide range of experiments in gene therapy [165, 166] of both hereditary diseases and acquired illnesses such as cancer. The promising idea is to use the sophisticated viral targeting strategies without having to create new lipid-, protein- or polymer-based nanoparticulate carriers for targeted delivery of missing or defective genes to the diseased cells. After replacing the viral DNA with the necessary human sequence vector, the modified virus is applied to the patient and consequently targets its natural host cell according to its surface properties. The genetically modified virus enters the host cell and delivers its genetic content to the cell nucleus, where it can be integrated into the host cell genome.

After first successful results with retrovirus-based gene therapy of patients with different forms of severe combined immune deficiency [167–169] (mostly fatal disorders of the immune system in young children), the field of virus-mediated gene therapy suffered some setbacks such as a lethal complication in a trial of adenovirus-based gene therapy of a metabolic disease and the induction of leukemia in a retrovirus-based gene therapy trial [170–172]. It also became obvious that successful and efficient gene therapy is much more difficult than originally thought because of (i) low *in vivo* targeting efficiency of the used viral vectors, (ii) inadequate targeting specificity resulting in an unwanted gene expression in healthy tissues, (iii) inappropriate integration of the gene vector into the host genome resulting in a long-term decrease in targeted gene expression and (iv) safety problems with insufficiently replication-deficient viral vectors [165]. We will present some widely used targeting systems based on viruses in areas other than cancer therapy.

One well-established virus for gene therapy is the adeno-associated virus [173, 174], popular because of its efficient gene delivery and long-term expression. Disadvantages are its low target specificity with more or less randomized gene delivery, its low gene packing capacity (less than 4000 bases), problems with activation of endogenous genes and problems with pre-existing antibodies in many patients, which lead to inactivation of the viral vector before it can reach the target cell. Adeno-associated virus-based gene therapy has been tried for patients with type IX hemophilia [175] (bleeding disorder), cystic fibrosis [176], α_1-antitrypsin-deficiency [177], peripheral arterial occlusive disease [166] and spinal cord injury [178].

Another popular gene therapy vector is the adenovirus [179–181], known to produce high-titer virus stocks and efficient long-term gene expression. Disadvantages are the strong immunogenicity (especially insufficiently inactivated viral vectors [182]), pre-existing antibodies in most patients (adenovirus is a common virus and makes airway infections) and limited packing capacity of less than 7500 bases. Adenoviral gene vectors have been used for the treatment of brain cancers [183], pulmonary diseases [177] and neurological diseases [184].

The next interesting virus is the herpes simplex virus, popular because of its high packing capacity (above 30 000 bases), good long-term expression, high target specificity for neuronal cell lines, and low toxicity when using gene-deleted non-toxic vectors [185, 186]. Application fields for the use of herpes simplex virus-based gene therapy are various neurological disorders [187] and muscular dystrophy [188].

The last group is the family retrovirus [189], commonly characterized by the enzyme reverse transcriptase that allows the virus to integrate its genetic information precisely into the host genome without the aid of host cells enzymes. Members of the retrovirus family used for gene therapy are HIV [190] and the murine leukemia virus [169] – the pioneer virus for gene therapy. Advantages of the retroviruses are the efficient long-term gene expression, the precise genome integration and the good packing capacity of about 8000 bases. The major disadvantage is the risk of oncogenesis because of an activation of oncogenes after integrating the therapeutic gene into the host genome [166]. Retroviruses are usually restricted to dividing cells; only by modifying the viral envelope (e.g. fusion with other viruses [191]) can the vector also transfect nondividing cells. Retroviruses have been used for gene therapy of hematopoietic disorders [192], immune system deficiencies [167], central nervous system diseases [193] and chronic granulomatous disease [194].

In past years, nanotechnology has enriched the field of virus-based gene delivery with new materials and new ideas, which might help to overcome some of the short- and long-term problems of potentially infectious viruses. In a new approach with adenoviruses, the viral envelope was covered with poly[*N*-(2-hydroxylpropyl) methacrylamide] to protect the virus from inactivating antibodies [195]. Further, fibroblast growth factor (FGF) and vascular endothelial growth factor (VEGF) were incorporated into the polymer to enable a higher grade of target specificity to FGF or VEGF receptor-positive cell lines such as endothelial cells [195].

Other research groups went further and built a chimerical gene carrier consisting of a plasmid DNA encapsulated in liposomes, which themselves were covered with a viral envelope with viral targeting proteins [196] (Fig. 5.6). The construct is called a virosome, and was used for gene delivery to vascular smooth muscle cells [197] and hepatocytes [198]. Disadvantages of the virosome-based delivery system

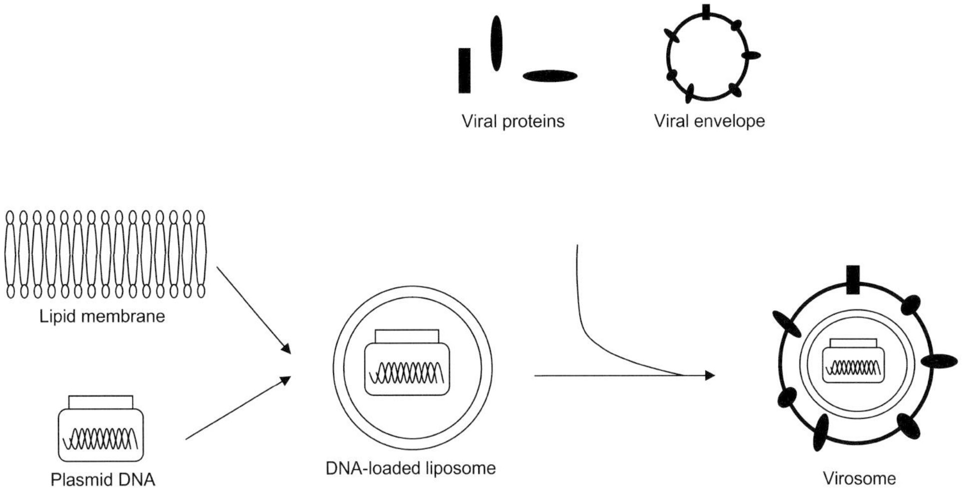

Figure 5.6. Schematic drawing of virosome synthesis. In a first step, a viral-derived and usually genetically modified plasmid DNA in a viral capsid is covered with a liposomal bilayer membrane. In the next step, viral proteins are added to the liposome for targeted delivery or the whole liposomal complex is again covered with a viral envelope, resulting in the formation of the artificial "virosome".

are the antigenicity of the viral proteins [196] and the high uptake into the MPS because of the liposomal constituents.

5.3.4 Prions

Prion is the abbreviation for proteinaceous infectious particle [199–201] and describes the main characteristics of this fascinating infectious agent simply consisting of a badly conformed peptide of 27–30 kDa called prion protein (PrP). It is most surprising that a small peptide with almost no virulence factors, no genetic information, and no protecting envelope, membrane or hull can persist for years or even decades in the host organism and can cause fatal neurodegenerative (spongiform vacuolation and loss of neuronal cells) diseases such as the transmissible spongiform encephalopathies (e.g. bovine spongiform encephalopathy in cows and scrapie in sheep) and Creutzfeldt–Jakob disease in humans [202–204]. Here, we will discuss some important strategies that enable the prion to invade the host organism, to evade the immune system defense, to persist in cells of the innate and adaptive immune system, and to reach its target cells in the central nervous system [205]. It is important to bear in mind that these principles might become helpful for the targeted delivery of artificial protein-based nanoparticles. On the other hand, the prion pathogenesis is a warning example that illustrates the various paths nanoparticles can take in a complex organism, and the huge damage even small particles can cause even after years and decades.

Prions reach the host orally and enter the organism mainly in the small intestine [206, 207] by both M cell-mediated [208] and dendritic cell-mediated luminal capture (as described above for bacteria). After binding or taking up the prions, the infected dendritic cells localized in specialized lymphatic tissue in the gut wall called Peyer's patches can infect other dendritic cells or lymphocytes [209–211]. On the surface or inside the dendritic cells and the lymphocytes, the prions can persist with the help of yet unknown mechanisms and can even "multiply" by passing on their pathological conformation onto normal cellular host-encoded prion protein (PrP^{c}) [212–214]. Further, B-type lymphocytes [215] and complex cytokine functions [203] have been discovered as the main mechanisms responsible for prion spread and for neuroinvasion. One of the few facts is that the prions can spread to various lymphoid organs with a high concentration in the spleen [216].

The next step in the prion pathogenesis is the path from the widely infected lymphoid tissue to the nervous system. It is believed that dendritic cells of spleen and especially Peyer's patches [217, 218] play a major role by setting up a close contact with nervous endings of peripheral nerves. The prions cross the space between the dendritic cell and the nervous ending by passive diffusion or with the help of "mobile elements" such as exosomes (free micellar membrane components with prions) [219], endogenous viruses, B lymphocytes [215, 220] or even special dendritic cells [221, 222]. Once inside the peripheral nerves, the prions enter the neuroretrograde transport system of the nerve that leads to the transport of the prion to structures of the central nervous system, where the destruction of the nervous cells takes place.

One important characteristic of prion pathogenesis important for us is the ability to evade the innate immune system and even use the complement system for simplification of target cell infection. The central role is occupied by the dendritic cells that settle the first contact with the prion in the Peyer's patches and that can store the prions on the surface for lymphocyte presentation. Further, the dendritic cells (and other phagocytes such as macrophages) can also bind complement- or antibody-labeled prions with their Fc and complement receptors [223, 224], usually followed by receptor-mediated endocytosis. Unfortunately, an unknown conformational characteristic allows the prion to "survive" the enzymatic degradation by proteases, making it impossible for the immune system to create an efficient antibody-mediated adaptive immune response by MHC-mediated antigen presentation.

Obviously, an inadequate degradation of the prions in cells of the MPS only leads to widespread spread of the infectious agent when it binds complement factors, because the uptake of complement-labeled prions is much more efficient than the uptake of unlabeled prions to dendritic cells, macrophages and lymphocytes.

Applied to our topic, i.e. targeted delivery of nanostructures, it can be said that unselective uptake of artificial nanometer-sized structures – be it protein-based or polymer-based – can create grave side-effects if the cells of the MPS are not capable of degrading the structure efficiently.

5.4 Strategies for Targeted Delivery – Designed by Man

5.4.1 Outline

In this section, we will discuss strategies for targeted delivery of chemically complex, nanometer-sized structures to a well-defined target site developed by researchers in recent years [225, 226]. We will concentrate on the desired targets and on the targeting strategies and moieties, independent of the nature of the carrier and its content. The section will be divided into the most important targeting pathways and sites other than cancer therapy, i.e. noninvasive and invasive delivery systems, and targeting to the brain, to atherosclerotic plaques and other targets.

5.4.2 Noninvasive Delivery Systems

When discussing the possibilities for targeted drug delivery for pathological conditions other than cancer, we have to be aware that we are dealing with chronic illnesses such as atherosclerosis, arterial hypertension, dyslipidemia, brain disorders (e.g. Parkinson's disease, Alzheimer's disease, psychiatric disorders), chronic inflammatory diseases, diabetes, etc. These diseases normally need a long-term medication. To ensure a good adherence to the therapeutic plan and to limit the possible side-effects, drugs for these chronic disorders have to be ideal from the pharmacological side. Important issues are easy application (oral, inhalatory, transdermal), once-a-day dosage, stable plasma concentrations and no serious adverse side-effects. In particular, the application method is important for the patient's comfort and adherence to the therapeutic procedure.

For diabetes, we have to administer the protein insulin to the systemic circulation, which is right now only possible with parenteral injections (subcutaneous or intravenously). Further, the patient has to inject the insulin up to 5–6 times a day to uphold an acceptable glucose concentration and risks a potentially fatal hypoglycemia when injecting an overdose of insulin. Obviously, such a therapeutic rule decreases the patient's quality of life and is only acceptable if the therapeutic benefit outweighs the negative side-effects to a high degree.

The design of noninvasive (in contrast to invasive methods such as injectable or implantable systems) drug delivery systems for oral, transdermal and transepithelial application and controlled passage of smaller and bigger molecules is therefore an important research area, and has been enriched by nanotechnological tools in recent years [225]. All noninvasive systems we will discuss in this section are a result of a so-called "top-down" manufacturing process, where the final tool is built from larger parts (in contrast to the "bottom-up" process, where atoms and/or molecules come together to build a superstructure). For the details about pharmacology and biology of the barriers, refer to the previous sections of this chapter.

5.4.2.1 Oral Delivery Systems

The most attractive delivery route is oral application – it is convenient, noninvasive and effective because of the large intestinal epithelial surface in the small intestine. In recent years, manufacturers have developed new complex drug formulas for controlled release based on nanotechnology, to ensure a continuous drug release into the systemic circulation over a longer period without toxic initial peak levels [227]. The most important controlled release drug formulation method for tablets is the osmotic oral delivery system (also called osmotic pump technology). It is based on an inner drug reservoir or drug core, a semipermeable membrane with nanometer-sized pores around the drug reservoir and a polymeric push compartment, which triggers the diffusion of the drug through the membrane on activation (e.g. hydration). This method is now commonly used for drugs such as nifedipine (Procardia XL®, Pfizer), oxybutynin chloride (Ditropan XL®, Ortho-McNeil) and methylphenidate (Concerta®, ALZA).

Another important modern drug formulation method is the multilayer matrix tablet, based on a core drug reservoir and one or more surrounding barrier layers such as hydroxypropylmethylcellulose (HPMC) [228, 229]. Various additional ingredients trigger the controlled diffusion process by swelling, gelling or erosion of the barrier layers. This method is being used for drugs such as diltiazem (Dilacor XR®, Watson Labs), paroxetine (Paxil CR®, GlaxoSmithKline) and diclofenac (Voltaren XR®, Novartis).

The last controlled release technology is called spheroidal oral drug absorption system (SODAS), and is based on spherical beads (diameter 1–2 mm) containing drugs and excipients that are coated by controlled-release polymers [225, 230, 231]. In fluids, the polymers start to dissolve at a time-dependent rate and allows the fluid to dissolve the drug core, resulting in an immediate release, a sustained release or a pulsatile delivery. This method is being used for drugs such as diltiazem (Cardizem LA®, Bioavail), methylphenidate (Ritalin LA®, Novartis) and morphine sulfate (Avinza®, Ligand).

5.4.2.2 Transdermal Delivery Systems

Transdermal application of drugs is another elegant method to ensure stable plasma drug concentrations, low maximum–minimum peak concentration differences, low first-pass effect and controlled release of potent, lipophilic drugs.

The most important technology for transdermal drug application is the transdermal delivery patch for drugs such as fentanyl, morphine, nicotine, nitroglycerin and steroid hormones we have already discussed above. Recently, new technologies have been introduced to expand the possibilities for transdermal drug delivery.

First, it is possible to use the so-called iontophoretic delivery by applying an electrical current to the skin, after which the drug molecules move actively trough the epidermis according to the polarity of the electrical field (similar to electrophoresis) [232].

Second, new microtechnological devices called Macroflux® (ALZA) and Microstructured Transdermal System® (3M Drug Delivery) based on microprojection technology [233] allow the skin permeation of macromolecules such as proteins and peptides. The device consists of an array (1–2 cm^2) of drug-coated titanium microprojections (200 μm each) fixed to an adhesive patch backing. The device has to be applied to the skin by using a special applicator, on which the small microprojections pierce the protective stratum corneum of the epidermis mechanically, allowing the coated drug to dissolve and to permeate into the blood vessels of the subepidermal tissue [234].

5.4.2.3 Transmucosal Delivery Systems

Drug application to sites such as the buccal, nasal, rectal, intrauterine, vaginal and ocular mucosa is another interesting alternative to intravenous injection and oral application, especially for special patient groups such as children, elderly or sick people, where the conventional application pathways may be problematic. Further, the absorption is fast in the well-perfused mucosa if the drug molecule is able to cross the epithelial barrier.

Special transmucosal drug delivery systems consist of bioadhesive polymers or hydrogels that increase the contact time and contact intensity to the epithelial layer [235]. For instance, polymers such as polyanhydrides stick physically to the intestinal epithelium and lectins stimulate a ligand–receptor interaction with receptors on the small intestine villi [236], making it possible to couple drug molecules or drug carriers to the lectin molecule [237] for better adhesion and permeation. A similar strategy with drug–polymer conjugates was tested for an oral administration formula for insulin [238].

The drugs in the polymer matrix or hydrogel can be free or attached to special controlled release devices such as microspheres and rings [239, 240], reservoirs [241], or nanoparticles [242].

Further, it is possible to improve the absorption rate across the endothelial layers by disturbing the epithelial barrier with special absorption enhancers [235] such as chitosan, cyclodextrin, poly-L-arginine and various lipids [243]. Formulas enriched with chitosan [244] powder have already been used for nasal administration of insulin and morphine [245].

5.4.3 Invasive Delivery Systems

In this section, we will discuss controlled, "top-down" micro/nanotechnological devices for drug delivery that have to be injected or implanted [246]. The variety of uncontrolled, "bottom-up" liposomes, nanoparticles and other nanometer-sized superstructures will be discussed in the next sections.

One important example of invasive delivery systems are controllable microfabricated devices (based on silicon chips, "off-wafer" techniques or microfluidic devices) with a drug reservoir that can be triggered or programmed to release a certain volume of drugs to the tissue or to the circulation [247]. Older concepts relied on the surgical implantation of the microfabricated device under the skin or into other tissues. Currently, new micro/nanofabrication techniques are being developed that allow the top-down construction of devices down to a size of 10–100 μm. These techniques make it possible to inject the devices into the target tissue with only slight damage or to inhale the macrostructure into the bronchi, where the drug could be released permanently over a certain time. By integrating microfluidic networks with multiple reservoirs, valves and pumps [248], it is possible to program the microfabricated to perform chemical reactions and release several reaction products [249].

One essential requirement for microfabricated device is the possibility for real-time control of the drug release according to changes in chemical and physiological parameters. One approach is the activation of molecular interactions using light radiation, radiofrequency or ultrasound energy. Ferromagnetic seeds [250], rods [251], microparticles [252] or superparamagnetic nanoparticles [253] can be injected or transported to a desired target, where they can be heated using localized radiofrequency or ultrasound for thermal treatment or release activation. Further, it had been shown that high-frequency radiofrequency changes the conformation of nucleic acid conjugates or proteins coupled to nanoparticles.

Another strategy for controlled drug release in microfabricated devices is based on hydrogels, three-dimensional, hydrophilic polymer (e.g. collagen, gelatin, dextrans, chitosans, poly-*N*-vinylpyrrolidone, polyphosphazenes, PLA/polyethylene oxide/PLA copolymers, PEGT–PBT copolymers [254]) networks that swell and change their diffusion properties reversibly when exposed to water. Thus, it is possible to control the drug diffusion out of a drug reservoir or a matrix with a hydrogel covering according to the swelling properties of the hydrogel. Special hydrogels are even sensitive to specific antigens [255], to an enzyme [256], to pH changes (methylacrylates) or to an applied charge and change their swelling properties [257].

Finally, special polymer-based surfaces sensitive to light [258, 259], pH, charge [260] and heat offer further possibilities for triggered controlled release of the content.

Similar to the microfabricated devices are noncontrollable diffusion chambers [261] or diffusion tubes with a central chamber filled with one or more drugs and semipermeable membrane that controls the release rate. Diffusion chambers or tubes have to be implanted into a certain tissue, and have been tested for diseases such as diabetes [262, 263], epilepsy [264] and spinal cord damage [265], and for birth control implants [266]. Diffusion chambers can also be filled with living cells [267] to enable the production of proteins, hormones and other molecules (e.g. erythropoietin [268], insulin [269, 270] or IFN-α [271]), but we are not going to discuss this vast area further in this chapter.

5.4.4 Targeted Delivery to the Brain

The brain is well protected against the diffusion of hydrophilic molecules and macromolecules by the blood–brain barrier, consisting of the dense, unfenestrated endothelial cell layer, the subendothelial space and specialized protecting cells of the brain – the astrocytes. The blood–brain barrier makes it difficult for microorganisms, toxic substances and macromolecules to reach the neurons of the brain, but also complicates therapeutic applications targeting cerebral pathologies such as Parkinson's disease, Alzheimer's disease, multiple sclerosis, meningitis or encephalitis. Only small lipophilic substances are able to cross the blood–brain barrier passively by diffusion; larger or hydrophilic substances need active transport system or a functional disruption of the blood–brain barrier to reach the neurons. Due to these limits, targeted delivery to the brain is one of the most active research areas using nanotechnological devices and researchers have developed a wide range of macromolecular targeting carriers. In recent years, new nanotechnological drug formulas have been tested for transport of bigger molecules such as peptides, proteins, and genes across the blood–brain barrier, both liposomal formulations [272] and polymer-based formulations [273].

Currently used liposomes are typically sterically stabilized for prolonged circulation lifetimes by a protective coating of PEG or other "antiopsonization agents" [24]; some liposomes are further functionalized with targeting moieties such as antibodies (immunoliposomes) [274], proteins, peptides or others [275, 276] for preferred target deposition. For details on the synthesis of nanotechnological carriers, refer to the specialized sections and references.

Well-studied targeting agents for trans-blood–brain barrier delivery are monoclonal antibodies such as OX26 [277] or 8D3 [278] directed against the ubiquitous (especially liver, muscles and brain) transferrin (iron-binding protein in plasma) receptors. The murine antibodies are typically conjugated to PEGylated liposomes that have to been injected intravenously and have shown a certain affectivity to the endothelial cells of the blood–brain barrier [279]. After binding to the transferrin receptor, the antibody with the liposome is transported across the blood–brain barrier by receptor-mediated endocytosis and transcellular transport [280, 281]. The antibody–liposome complex can now diffuse freely and spread into the brain tissue, which shows a clear liposome accumulation compared with native PEGylated liposomes [282].

Other targeting moieties for targeted brain delivery of liposomes are monoclonal antibodies directed against the human insulin receptor such as 83-14 [283], which can be found on endothelial cells and neurons in a high concentration. The functionalized liposomes bind to the cell surface receptor and can be internalized by receptor-mediated endocytosis. To increase the rate of *trans*-blood–brain barrier passage, it is also possible to functionalize the liposomes further with antitransferrin receptor antibodies [284]. In this case, the antitransferrin receptor antibody ensures the passage across the blood–brain barrier, while the anti-insulin receptor ensures the uptake into the neurons.

Due to the well-known limits when using liposomes such as low physicochemical stability, leakage, difficult preparation procedures, low possibility for controlled release, low loading efficiency and short *in vitro* lifetimes, many researchers have turned to polymer-based formulas [273, 285] to overcome these problems.

The first nanoparticles for targeted brain delivery were made using poly(alkylcyanoacrylates) such as polybutylcyanoacrylate (PBCA) [286] coated with the nonionic surfactant polysorbate 80 [287–289], and later using nanoparticles consisting of polylactide homopolymers (PLA) and poly(lactide-*co*-glycolide) heteropolymers (PLGA) coated with PEG [290] to protect the nanoparticles from opsonization and to ensure longer circulation lifetimes [291, 292].

The targeting moiety of PBCA nanoparticles is the polysorbate coating, which ensures a certain nanoparticle accumulation in the brain tissue, probably by a polysorbate-mediated disruption and permeabilization of the blood–brain barrier [293, 294] or by endocytosis by the brain capillary endothelial cells [285]. It has been hypothesized that the endogenous plasma protein apolipoprotein E (ApoE) absorbs to the polysorbate coating and triggers the receptor-mediated endocytosis [285]. On the other hand, a protein-binding nanoparticle surface obviously enables opsonization and leads to a fast uptake into the MPS [288, 295, 296], making it impossible to use these nanoparticles for target-specific delivery. Further, blood–brain barrier permeabilization is a serious adverse drug event [273] that might lead to neuronal damage by exogenous or endogenous toxic substances or microorganisms.

Nanoparticles made of polymers based on glycolic acid and D,L-lactic acid enantiomers have a proven record of good biocompatibility and resorbability [297, 298], and have been used for some years in building biodegradable devices and microspheres [299]. Further, PLA and PLGA are easily degraded by spontaneous hydrolysis of the ester bonds [300] into oligomers and monomers, which are further metabolized and degraded into CO_2 and H_2O [273]. For nanoparticle targeting applications, the PLA/PLGA polymers have to be covered with PEG moieties to ensure a prolonged circulation lifetime [301] of some hours compared with some minutes for native PLA/PLGA nanoparticles [302–306].

Possible targeting moieties for brain-specific delivery of nanoparticles based on PLA/PLGA are the monoclonal antibodies (OX26 and 8D3) against the transferrin or insulin receptors we have already met. The targeting antibodies are bound to the tips of specially functionalized PEG strands (biotinylated [307], amine reactive [308] or thiol reactive [309, 310]) and enable the endocytosis of nanoparticles with a diameter of around 100 nm to the endothelial cells of the brain capillaries and the passage across the blood–brain barrier.

5.4.5
Macrophage Targeting

Macrophages, the main cell type of the innate immune system, play a major role in a wide range of disease states, including infections (e.g. *Leishmania*, *M. tuberculosis*, *L. monocytogenes*), autoimmune diseases (e.g. rheumatoid arthritis, sarcoidosis, type I diabetes), cancer and atherosclerosis [311–318]. Therefore, the macrophage is an interesting pharmaceutical target, despite the fact there exist only a few therapeutic choices until now.

Targeting to macrophages is theoretically easy, because the macrophages of the MPS are the primary target for all nonstealth lipid- or polymer-based nanometer-sized vehicles. Nonetheless, the macrophages of the MPS in liver and spleen are only rarely the desired target when trying to achieve a therapeutic effect; the "desired'' macrophages are those found in vulnerable plaques of the blood vessels, in the peritoneum, the lung and other sites of disease. In contrast to the macrophages in liver (called Kupffer cells) and spleen, the macrophages in these tissues are normally protected from the nanovehicles by a dense endothelial layer (endothelium in liver and spleen has wide fenestrations). To be able to target the ''desired'' macrophages, a nanovehicle has to (i) evade the phagocytic cells of liver and spleen, (ii) uphold long circulation lifetimes, (iii) find a way to leave the circulation intact at a desired therapeutic target, (iv) reach the target cells specifically (v) and enter the macrophages (vi) avoiding the destruction in the endo-lysosomal compartment. All this makes targeting to the ''desired'' macrophages a serious task and calls for innovative solutions based on nanotechnological tools.

Early examples of macrophage-directed drugs are nonstealth liposomes containing the antimicrobial drug amphotericin B (AmBisome®, Gilead Sciences) for the therapy of the intracellular parasite *Leishmania* (which stays in macrophages) and various fungal infections [319–321]. Similar approaches with liposomes and nanoparticles were also used for improved targeting of antimicrobial agents such as β-lactam antibiotics, aminoglycosids and fluoroquinolones to intracellularly infected macrophages (e.g. *Salmonella*, *L. monocytogenes*, *M. tuberculosis*, *Mycobacterium avium*, *Mycobacterium intracellulare*, *Brucella abortus* and *L. pneumophila*) [322]. The liposomal formulas allow reducing the quantity of applied drug molecules and decrease the severity of adverse side-effects [323], because most of the encapsulated drug is rapidly transported to the phagocytic macrophages or the fungi and not to other healthy tissues. Targeting can be further improved using targeting moieties such as tuftsin, a natural macrophage activator tetrapeptide (threonine–lysine–proline–arginine) based on a part of the IgG heavy chain [324].

One interesting application area for nanoparticulate formulations targeting macrophages is the development of new nanotechnological vaccines. The required protein or peptide antigen is coupled physically or covalently to a polymer- or lipid-based nanocarrier adjuvant, which promotes the preferred uptake of the coupled antigen to macrophages of the innate immune system. The antigen is then processed by the endo-lysosomal compartment and presented to T lymphocytes using the MHC class I and especially class II molecules on the surface of antigen-presenting cells (APC), increasing the immunogenic potency of the used vaccination antigen [325–327]. Similar approaches have been tried for new DNA vaccines [328, 329]. Targeting can be further improved using targeting moieties such as various mannose receptor ligands [330].

Much progress has been achieved in the use of nanotechnology-based contrast agents for diagnostic applications. Detection of activated macrophages might help the doctors to find and define a diseased tissue, especially an inflamed tissue such as the vulnerable plaque or autoaggressive immunologic process. In recent years, paramagnetic iron oxide nanoparticles (4–5 nm diameter, usually coated with PEG or dextran) have been used for detecting macrophages using the readily available technique of MRI. Macrophages or other target cells take up the nanoparticles that can be detected by MRI (negative signal in T2), because the iron oxide shortens the spin relaxation compared with surrounding tissues. Paramagnetic iron oxide nanoparticles have been used for detecting lymph nodes metastases [331, 332], arthritis [333], fibrin molecules [334], angiogenesis in atherosclerotic plaques [335] and other constituents of atherosclerotic plaques [253, 336, 337].

The detection of actively inflamed atherosclerotic plaques that are in danger of rupture (leading to heart infarction, stroke and other organ ischemia), called vulnerable plaques [28, 318], is an active and promising research area that has been enriched by nanometer-sized vehicles for targeted delivery [3]. Several characteristics of vulnerable plaques simplify the targeted delivery, i.e. the functional and morphological disruption of the endothelial layer that covers the atherosclerotic plaque and enables the extravasation of larger molecules and superstructures such as lipoproteins, polynucleotides, polypeptides, complex lipids and advanced glycation end-products (AGE). These macromolecules initiate and support the pathological process of atherosclerosis. In the vulnerable plaque, active macrophages take up the plasma proteins and lipids and transform into so-called foam cells, instable macrophages filled with lipids that produce various cytokines and other pro-inflammatory and proliferation-stimulating chemical substances. These substances attract more white blood cells to the plaque, trigger the growth of the plaque and finally cause the breakup of the fibrous cap [338].

Intelligently designed nanovehicles such as polymer nanocontainers [32] have several properties that might enable them to reach the vulnerable plaque and block the central cell type of the pathological process – the macrophage. Covered with the inert antiopsonization polymer PMOXA, the nanocontainers (diameter 100–200 nm) have long circulation lifetimes, allowing them to leave the circulation in sites with a disrupted endothelial layer such as the vulnerable plaque. Functionalized with the polynucleotide tracking ligand polyguanylic acid [339] by multifunctional biotin–avidin–biotin bonds [32], the nanocontainers bind specifically to a highly upregulated receptor subtype of active macrophages called scavenger receptor A1 [340]. It was shown that these innovative, functionalized nanocontainers reach specifically active macrophages that express the scavenger receptor A1 and do not reach macrophage precursor cells and tissue macrophages with a low grade of upregulation [32] (Figs. 5.7–5.9).

5.4.6 Other Targets

PEGylated liposomes coated with plasminogen were designed for fibrin clot targeting. The plasminogen serves as a targeting moiety, because it binds to the fibrin in clots that block the blood flow in a case of heart infarction, lung embolism or stroke. The liposomes were filled with the fibrinolytic substance plasminogen activator, which triggers the degradation of fibrin in the clot and allows the reperfusion of the infarcted area [341].

PEGylated liposomes labeled with the targeting moiety RGD peptide (containing the arginine–glycine–aspartic acid sequence) were designed for targeted delivery to α_V integrin receptors on endothelial cells [342, 343]. The liposomes can be filled with different drugs such as angiogenesis inhibitors, which block this important

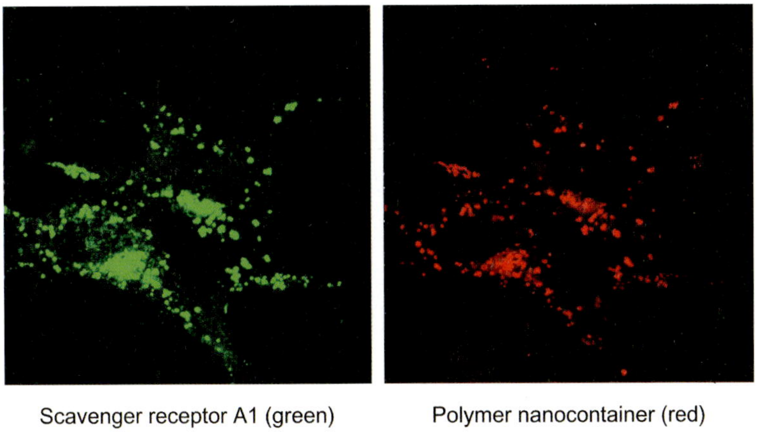

Figure 5.7. Scavenger receptor A1-mediated uptake of polyguanylic acid-functionalized polymer nanocontainers into intracellular vesicles (for details refer to Ref. [32]). PMOXA–PDMS–PMOXA triblock copolymer nanocontainers (diameter 100–200 nm) were functionalized with the oligonucleotide tracking ligand polyguanylic acid for macrophage scavenger receptor A1 targeting via biotin–avidin–biotin bonds. In cell cultures expressing the enhanced green fluorescent protein (EGFP)-labeled scavenger receptor A1, rapid binding to the target receptor was detected by fluorescent microscopy. The nanocontainers were filled with the hydrophilic red fluorescent dye sulforhodamine B and can be detected both on the cell surface and in intracellular vesicles, most probably lysosomes. The colocalization of receptor (green, left) and nanocontainer (red, right) proves the receptor-specific targeting.

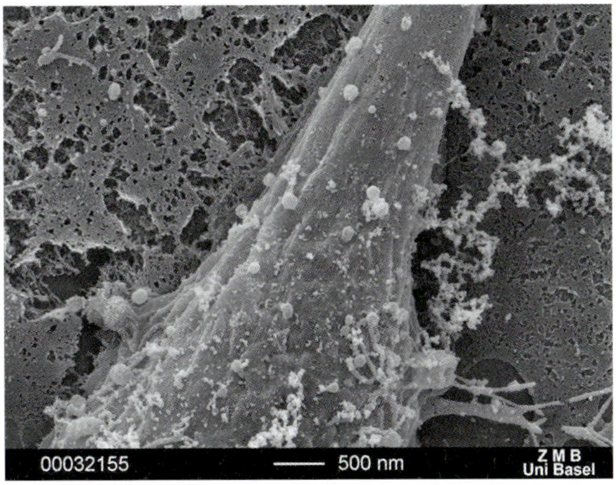

Figure 5.8. Functionalized polymer nanocontainers bound to macrophages (for details refer to Ref. [32]). The same functionalized nanocontainers as in Fig. 5.7 were targeted to endocytosis-inhibited macrophages in culture. Precise analysis of the experimental macrophages by scanning electron microscopy discovered the presence of vesicular formations (diameter 100–200 nm) on the macrophage cell membrane, most probably the intact nanocontainers. Unfunctionalized nanocontainers lacking the tracking ligand polyguanylic acid did not bind to the activated macrophages.

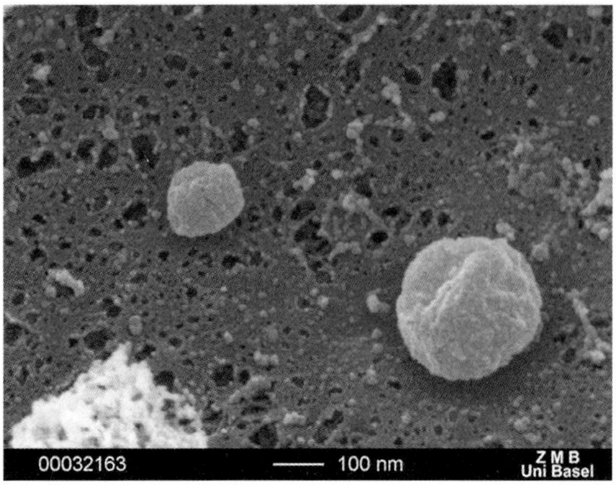

Figure 5.9. Functionalized polymer nanocontainers bound to macrophages – detail (for details refer to Ref. [32]). Same set-up as in Fig. 5.8; the scanning electron microscopy image offers an unique insight into the morphology of polymer nanocontainers bound to the macrophage surface.

step in the development of disease conditions such as atherosclerosis and especially cancer.

Asialoglycoprotein receptor (ASGP-R) ligands such as asialofetuin and galactosylated cholesterol, glycolipids or polymers coupled to PEGylated liposomes or other carriers were used for hepatocyte targeting of both drugs and gene sequences for gene therapy [344–347]. Other strategies for hepatocyte targeting of lipid emulsions involve the use of the lipoprotein protein ApoE as a tracking ligand [348].

The last topic we want to discuss is the field of cell-penetrating peptides, which enable the invasion of nanovehicles into the cytoplasma of the target cell [31]. Cell-penetrating peptides are naturally occurring in viruses such as HIV, herpes virus and hepatitis B virus, and in macroorganisms such as *Drosophila*. They can be divided into two classes: the lysine-rich amphipathic helical peptides (e.g. transportan [349] and model amphipathic peptide [350]) and the arginine-rich peptides (e.g. TAT [351, 352], Antp [353], VP22 [354] and penetratin) [355–359]. We will discuss the principles and applications of the most important cell-penetrating peptide, the TAT (transactivating transcriptional activator) peptide, which is a central protein of HIV [31].

After binding to cell surface receptors such as $\alpha_V\beta_5$ integrin [360], TAT is internalized rapidly and is transported to the nucleus, where it transactivates the HIV promoter [352]. The uptake of TAT peptide and TAT-coupled small molecules is thought to be triggered by strong electrostatic binding of the peptide to the cell membrane, upon which the peptide enters an energy-independent nonlysosomal endocytic pathway [361–363]. On the other hand, TAT-functionalized nanovehicles are taken up by the cell by an energy-dependent macropinocytosis, followed by a facilitated endosome escape into the cytoplasma [356, 364].

TAT-coupling was tested for intracellular and intranuclear delivery of various proteins and peptides [365–368], genes [369–371], oligonucleotides [372], antibodies [373, 374], imaging contrast agents for scintigraphy and MRI [375–377], and finally of various macrostructures. It was shown that TAT-coupling improved the fast and nondegrading internalization of dextran-coated superparamagnetic iron oxide nanoparticles (mean diameter 41 nm) into white blood cells [378, 379], of gold nanoparticles into cell cultures [380] and of various PEGylated liposomes [381–383].

5.5 Conclusion and Outlook

In this chapter, we have defined the major obstacles and barriers that have to be overcome for a targeted delivery of diagnostic or therapeutic agents to a desired cellular or subcellular target. We have discussed microbial targeting and immune system evasion strategies, and tried to give an insight into the vast field of nanotechnology-based delivery tools. We are aware that we rather had to concentrate on general principles than on a precise summary of all available targeted delivery nanovehicles. We apologize to all groups that were not mentioned and we encourage them to send us material about their research activities for future publications from our side. Please refer to other chapters of this book and to the mentioned references for details on some special topics that were not fully covered in this chapter.

As we have seen, the field of targeted delivery using nanotechnological tools is an active and promising research area, and creates new ideas at a very fast pace. Clearly, nanotechnological targeted delivery will split into specialized subtopics in the future according to the desired target. Many medical disciplines such as neurology, cardiology, gastroenterology and surgery will profit from the toolbox of nanoscience that will revolutionize current diagnostic and therapeutic applications, and that will offer possibilities for new concepts.

The final goal of nanomedicine will be to create nanometer-sized, nontoxic and easily built carriers of complex functionality such as (i) undamaging epithelial barrier passage, (ii) long circulation lifetime, (iii) immune system evasion, (iv) controlled bloodstream extravasation, (v) target-specific deposition, (vi) undisruptive target cell invasion, and (vii) precise and (viii) automated diagnostic or therapeutic intervention (Fig. 5.10). Some these criteria have already been developed for certain nanovehicles, others will be developed in future years. Combining all of them will create an exciting and complex nanostructure – some will call it nanorobot or nanobot, others will call it an artificial virus, which is perhaps the best definition.

Obviously, such a nanorobot will create fear and concerns in the public, comparable to the concern we face nowadays with scientific topics such as biotechnology, stem cell research and bioterrorism. Miniaturized defense mechanisms penetrating and probably self-replicating artificial nanorobots that invade our body and have the ability to reach every organ and tissue are much more powerful than cur-

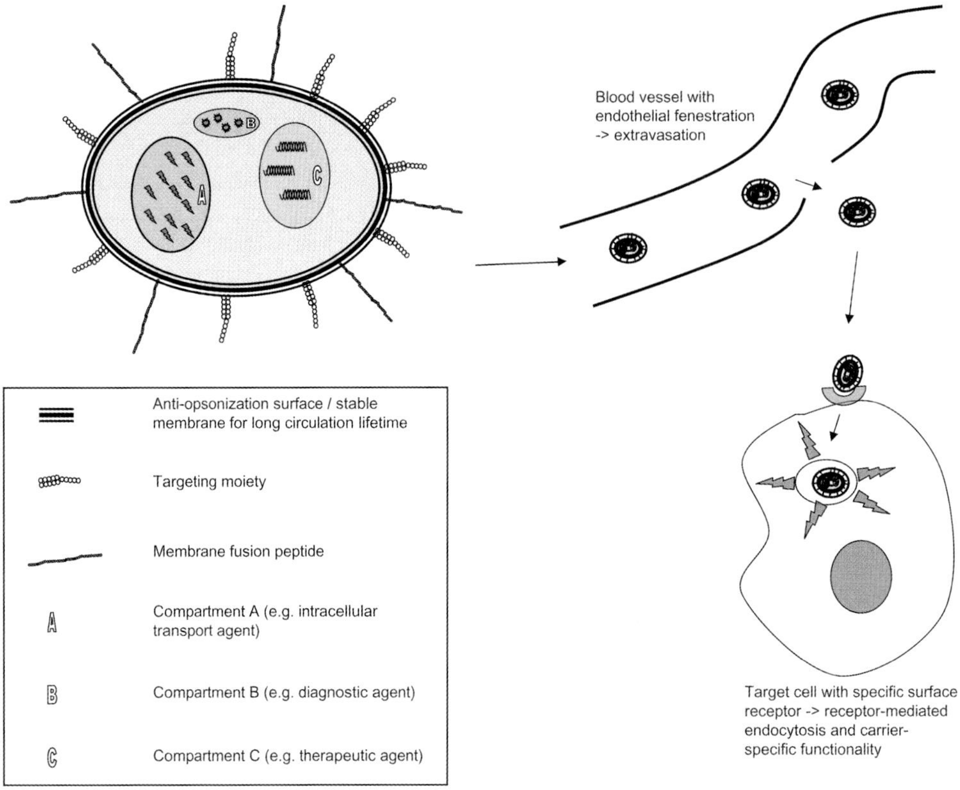

Figure 5.10. Theoretical construction of a long-circulating, receptor-specific nanocarrier with a highly complex functionality (such as cell invasion, intracellular transport, diagnostic and therapeutic agents).

rent scientific tools when it comes to creating worst-case scenarios. Therefore, it is fundamental that nanotechnology researchers understand this problem, and engage themselves actively and without legislative or media pressure in discussions about "nanotoxicity" [384–386] and "nanoethics" [387, 388], which were not covered in this chapter.

Only with careful considerations on the advantages and disadvantages of new technologies will it be possible to create nanoscaled tools that will help us to overcome severe and until now incurable diseases.

References

1 Gurwitz, J. H., Field, T. S., Harrold, L. R., Rothschild, J., Debellis, K., Seger, A. C. et al. Incidence and preventability of adverse drug events among older persons in the ambulatory setting.

J. Am. Med. Ass. **2003**, *289*, 1107–1116.

2 Moghimi, S. M., Hunter, A. C., Murray, J. C. Nanomedicine: current status and future prospects. *FASEB J.* **2005**, *19*, 311–330.

3 Wickline, S. A., Lanza, G. M. Nanotechnology for molecular imaging and targeted therapy. *Circulation* **2003**, *107*, 1092–1095.

4 *The Merck Manual of Diagnosis and Therapy*. 17th edn. Merck, West Point, PA, **1999**.

5 *Pharmacology*. Edinburgh: Churchill Livingstone, **2003**.

6 *Goodman & Gilman's: The Pharmacological Basis of Therapeutics*. McGraw-Hill, New York, **2001**.

7 Tencer, J., Frick, I.-M., Oquist, B. W., Alm, P., Rippe, B. Size-selectivity of the glomerular barrier to high molecular weight proteins: upper size limitations of shunt pathways. *Kidney Int.* **1998**, *53*, 709–715.

8 Elias, P. M. Stratum corneum defensive functions: an integrated view. *J. Invest. Dermatol.* **2005**, *125*, 183–200.

9 Committee on Drugs. Alternative routes of drug administration – advantages and disadvantages (subject review). *Pediatrics* **1997**, *100*, 143–152.

10 Saunders, J., Davis, H., Coetzee, L., Botha, S., Kruger, A., Grobler, A. A novel skin penetration enhancer: evaluation by membrane diffusion and confocal microscopy. *J. Pharm. Pharm. Sci.* **1999**, *2*, 99–107.

11 Pierre, M., Tedesco, A., Marchetti, J., Bentley, M. V. Stratum corneum lipids liposomes for the topical delivery of 5-aminolevulinic acid in photodynamic therapy of skin cancer: preparation and *in vitro* permeation study. *BMC Dermatology* **2001**, *1*, 5.

12 Morita, K., Miyachi, Y. Tight junctions in the skin. *J. Dermatol. Sci.* **2003**, *31*, 81–89.

13 Cheng, H., Leblond, C. P. Origin, differentiation and renewal of the four main epithelial cell types in the mouse small intestine. I. Columnar cell. *Am. J. Anat.* **1974**, *141*, 461–479.

14 Roth, K. A., Hertz, J. M., Gordon, J. I. Mapping enteroendocrine cell populations in transgenic mice reveals an unexpected degree of complexity in cellular differentiation within the gastrointestinal tract. *J. Cell Biol.* **1990**, *110*, 1791–1801.

15 Fasano, A., Shea-Donohue, T. Mechanisms of disease: the role of intestinal barrier function in the pathogenesis of gastrointestinal autoimmune diseases. *Nat. Clin. Pract. Gastroenterol. Hepatol.* **2005**, *2*, 416–422.

16 Snoeck, V., Goddeeris, B., Cox, E. The role of enterocytes in the intestinal barrier function and antigen uptake. *Microb. Infect.* **2005**, *7*, 997–1004.

17 MacDonald, T. T., Monteleone, G. Immunity, inflammation, and allergy in the gut. *Science* **2005**, *307*, 1920–1925.

18 Stern, M., Walker, W. A. Food proteins and gut mucosal barrier I. Binding and uptake of cow's milk proteins by adult rat jejunum *in vitro*. *Am. J. Physiol.* **1984**, *246*, G556–G562.

19 Chu, S. H., Walker, W. A. Development of the gastrointestinal mucosal barrier: changes in phospholipid head groups and fatty acid composition of intestinal microvillus membranes from newborn and adult rats. *Pediatr. Res.* **1988**, *23*, 439–442.

20 McKay, D. M., Baird, A. W. Cytokine regulation of epithelial permeability and ion transport. *Gut* **1999**, *44*, 283–289.

21 Berin, M. C., Yang, P. C., Ciok, L., Waserman, S., Perdue, M. H. Role for IL-4 in macromolecular transport across human intestinal epithelium. *Am. J. Physiol.* **1999**, *276*, C1046–C1052.

22 Brannon-Peppas, L., Blanchette, J. O. Nanoparticle and targeted systems for cancer therapy. *Adv. Drug Deliv. Rev.* **2004**, *56*, 1649–1659.

23 Ahsan, F., Rivas, I. P., Khan, M. A., Torres Suarez, A. I. Targeting to macrophages: role of physicochemical properties of particulate carriers – liposomes and microspheres – on the

phagocytosis by macrophages. *J. Control. Release* **2002**, *79*, 29–40.

24 Moghimi, S. M., Szebeni, J. Stealth liposomes and long circulating nanoparticles: critical issues in pharmacokinetics, opsonization and protein-binding properties. *Prog. Lipid Res.* **2003**, *42*, 463–478.

25 Moghimi, S. M., Hunter, A. C., Murray, J. C. Long-circulating and target-specific nanoparticles: theory to practice. *Pharmacol. Rev.* **2001**, *53*, 283–318.

26 van Nieuw Amerongen, G. P., van Hinsbergh, V. W. M. Targets for pharmacological intervention of endothelial hyperpermeability and barrier function. *Vasc. Pharmacol.* **2002**, *39*, 257–272.

27 Mullin, J. M., Agostino, N., Rendon-Huerta, E., Thornton, J. J. Keynote review: Epithelial and endothelial barriers in human disease. *Drug Discov. Today* **2005**, *10*, 395–408.

28 Boyle, J. J. Macrophage activation in atherosclerosis: pathogenesis and pharmacology of plaque rupture. *Curr. Vasc. Pharmacol.* **2005**, *3*, 63–68.

29 Ohashi, R., Mu, H., Yao, Q., Chen, C. Atherosclerosis: immunopathogenesis and immunotherapy. *Med. Sci. Monit.* **2004**, *10*, RA255–260.

30 Belting, M., Sandgren, S., Wittrup, A. Nuclear delivery of macromolecules: barriers and carriers. *Adv. Drug Deliv. Rev.* **2005**, *57*, 505–527.

31 Gupta, B., Levchenko, T. S., Torchilin, V. P. Intracellular delivery of large molecules and small particles by cell-penetrating proteins and peptides. *Adv. Drug Deliv. Rev.* **2005**, *57*, 637–651.

32 Brož, P., Benito, S. M., Saw, C., Burger, P., Heider, H., Pfisterer, M. et al. Cell targeting by a generic receptor-targeted polymer nanocontainer platform. *J. Control. Release* **2005**, *102*, 475–488.

33 Witztum, J. L. You are right too! *J. Clin. Invest.* **2005**, *115*, 2072–2075.

34 Willekens, F. L., Werre, J. M., Kruijt, J. K., Roerdinkholder-Stoelwinder, B., Groenen-Dopp, Y. A., van den Bos, A. G. et al. Liver Kupffer cells rapidly remove red blood cell-derived vesicles from the circulation by scavenger receptors. *Blood* **2005**, *105*, 2141–2145.

35 Van Eck, M., Bos, I. S., Hildebrand, R. B., Van Rij, B. T., Van Berkel, T. J. Dual role for scavenger receptor class B, type I on bone marrow-derived cells in atherosclerotic lesion development. *Am. J. Pathol.* **2004**, *165*, 785–794.

36 Krieger, M. Scavenger receptor class B type I is a multiligand HDL receptor that influences diverse physiologic systems. *J. Clin. Invest.* **2001**, *108*, 793–797.

37 Linehan, S. A., Martinez-Pomares, L., Stahl, P. D., Gordon, S. Mannose receptor and its putative ligands in normal murine lymphoid and nonlymphoid organs: in situ expression of mannose receptor by selected macrophages, endothelial cells, perivascular microglia, and mesangial cells, but not dendritic cells. *J. Exp. Med.* **1999**, *189*, 1961–1972.

38 Domingue, G. J., Woody, H. B. Bacterial persistence and expression of disease. *Clin. Microbiol. Rev.* **1997**, *10*, 320–344.

39 Finlay, B. B., Falkow, S. Common themes in microbial pathogenicity revisited. *Microbiol. Mol. Biol. Rev.* **1997**, *16*, 136–169.

40 Sauer, F. G., Mulvey, M. A., Schilling, J. D., Martinez, J. J., Hultgren, S. J. Bacterial pili: molecular mechanisms of pathogenesis. *Curr. Opin. Microbiol.* **2000**, *3*, 65–72.

41 Cossart, P., Sansonetti, P. J. Bacterial invasion: the paradigms of enteroinvasive pathogens. *Science* **2004**, *304*, 242–248.

42 Carrero, J. A., Calderon, B., Unanue, E. R. Type I interferon sensitizes lymphocytes to apoptosis and reduces resistance to *Listeria* infection. *J. Exp. Med.* **2004**, *200*, 535–540.

43 Finlay, B. B., Cossart, P. Exploitation of mammalian host cell functions by bacterial pathogens. *Science* **1997**, *276*, 718–725.

44 Cossart, P., Pizarro-Cerda, J., Lecuit, M. Invasion of mammalian cells by *Listeria monocytogenes*: functional mimicry to subvert cellular functions. *Trends Cell Biol.* **2003**, *13*, 23–31.

45 Ghosh, P. Process of protein transport by the type III secretion system. microbiol. *Mol. Biol. Rev.* **2004**, *68*, 771–795.

46 He, S. Y., Nomura, K., Whittam, T. S. Type III protein secretion mechanism in mammalian and plant pathogens. *Biochim. Biophys. Acta Mol. Cell Res.* **2004**, *1694*, 181–206.

47 Mueller, C. A., Brož, P., Muller, S. A., Ringler, P., Erne-Brand, F., Sorg, I. et al. The V-antigen of *Yersinia* forms a distinct structure at the tip of injectisome needles. *Science* **2005**, *310*, 674–676.

48 Goure, J., Brož, P., Attree, O., Cornelis, G. R., Attree, I. Protective anti-V antibodies inhibit and *Yersinia* translocon assembly within host membranes. *J. Infect. Dis.* **2005**, *192*, 218–225.

49 Galan, J. E. *Salmonella* interactions with host cells: type III secretion at work. *Annu. Rev. Cell Dev. Biol.* **2001**, *17*, 53–86.

50 Sansonetti, P. J. Rupture, invasion and inflammatory destruction of the intestinal barrier by *Shigella*, making sense of prokaryote-eukaryote cross-talks. *FEMS Microbiol. Rev.* **2001**, *25*, 3–14.

51 *Immunobiology – The Immune System in Health and Disease*, 5th edn. Garland, New York, **2001**.

52 *Cellular and Molecular Immunology*, 4th edn. Saunders, New York, **2000**.

53 Coombes, B. K., Valdez, Y., Finlay, B. B. Evasive maneuvers by secreted bacterial proteins to avoid innate immune responses. *Curr. Biol.* **2004**, *14*, R856–R867.

54 Portnoy, D. A. Manipulation of innate immunity by bacterial pathogens. *Curr. Opin. Immunol.* **2005**, *17*, 25–28.

55 Takeda, K., Kaisho, T., Akira, S. Toll-like receptors. *Annu. Rev. Immunol.* **2003**, *21*, 335–376.

56 Akira, S. Toll-like receptors and innate immunity. *Adv. Immunol.* **2001**, *78*, 1–56.

57 D'Hauteville, H., Khan, S., Maskell, D. J., Kussak, A., Weintraub, A., Mathison, J. et al. Two *msbB* genes encoding maximal acylation of lipid A are required for invasive *Shigella* flexneri to mediate inflammatory rupture and destruction of the intestinal epithelium. *J. Immunol.* **2002**, *168*, 5240–5251.

58 Auerbuch, V., Brockstedt, D. G., Meyer-Morse, N., O'Riordan, M., Portnoy, D. A. Mice lacking the type I interferon receptor are resistant to *Listeria monocytogenes. J. Exp. Med.* **2004**, *200*, 527–533.

59 O'Connell, R. M., Saha, S. K., Vaidya, S. A., Bruhn, K. W., Miranda, G. A., Zarnegar, B. et al. Type I Interferon production enhances susceptibility to *Listeria monocytogenes* infection. *J. Exp. Med.* **2004**, *200*, 437–445.

60 Nguyen, L., Pieters, J. The Trojan horse: survival tactics of pathogenic mycobacteria in macrophages. *Trends Cell Biol.* **2005**, *15*, 269–276.

61 Sinai, A. P., Joiner, K. A. Safe haven: the cell biology of nonfusogenic pathogen vacuoles. *Annu. Rev. Microbiol.* **1997**, *51*, 415–462.

62 Nau, G. J., Richmond, J. F. L., Schlesinger, A., Jennings, E. G., Lander, E. S., Young, R. A. Human macrophage activation programs induced by bacterial pathogens. *Proc. Natl Acad. Sci. USA* **2002**, *99*, 1503–1508.

63 Fortune, S. M., Solache, A., Jaeger, A., Hill, P. J., Belisle, J. T., Bloom, B. R. et al. *Mycobacterium tuberculosis* inhibits macrophage responses to IFN-gamma through myeloid differentiation factor 88-dependent and -independent mechanisms. *J. Immunol.* **2004**, *172*, 6272–6280.

64 Goehring, U.-M., Schmidt, G., Pederson, K. J., Aktories, K., Barbieri, J. T. The N-terminal domain of *Pseudomonas aeruginosa* exoenzyme S is a GTPase-activating

protein for Rho GTPases. *J. Biol. Chem.* **1999**, *274*, 36369–36372.

65 Cowell, B. A., Chen, D. Y., Frank, D. W., Vallis, A. J., Fleiszig, S. M. ExoT of cytotoxic prevents uptake by corneal epithelial cells. *Infect. Immuni.* **2000**, *68*, 403–406.

66 Garrity-Ryan, L., Kazmierczak, B., Kowal, R., Comolli, J., Hauser, A., Engel, J. N. The arginine finger domain of ExoT contributes to actin cytoskeleton disruption and inhibition of internalization of by epithelial cells and macrophages. *Infect. Immun.* **2000**, *68*, 7100–7113.

67 Hamid, N., Gustavsson, A., Andersson, K., McGee, K., Persson, C., Rudd, C. E. et al. YopH dephosphorylates Cas and Fyn-binding protein in macrophages. *Microbial Pathogenesis* **1999**, *27*, 231–242.

68 Shao, F., Merritt, P. M., Bao, Z., Innes, R. W., Dixon, J. E. A *Yersinia* effector and a avirulence protein define a family of cysteine proteases functioning in bacterial pathogenesis. *Cell* **2002**, *109*, 575–588.

69 Lammertyn, E., Anne, J. Protein secretion in *Legionella pneumophila* and its relation to virulence. *FEMS Microbiol. Lett.* **2004**, *238*, 273–279.

70 Celli, J., Gorvel, J.-P. Organelle robbery: *Brucella* interactions with the endoplasmic reticulum. *Curr. Opin. Microbiol.* **2004**, *7*, 93–97.

71 Ma, Q., Zhai, Y., Schneider, J. C., Ramseier, T. M., Saier, J., Milton, H. Protein secretion systems of *Pseudomonas aeruginosa* and *P. fluorescens*. *Biochim. Biophys. Acta Biomembranes* **2003**, *1611*, 223–233.

72 Yeo, H.-J., Waksman, G. Unveiling molecular scaffolds of the type IV Secretion system. *J. Bacteriol.* **2004**, *186*, 1919–1926.

73 Schroder, G., Dehio, C. Virulence-associated type IV secretion systems of Bartonella. *Trends Microbiol.* **2005**, *13*, 336–342.

74 Kagan, J. C., Roy, C. R. Legionella phagosomes intercept vesicular traffic from endoplasmic reticulum exit sites. *Nat. Cell Biol.* **2002**, *4*, 945–954.

75 Celli, J., de Chastellier, C., Franchini, D.-M., Pizarro-Cerda, J., Moreno, E., Gorvel, J.-P. Brucella evades macrophage killing via VirB-dependent sustained interactions with the endoplasmic reticulum. *J. Exp. Med.* **2003**, *198*, 545–556.

76 Fan, P., Dong, F., Huang, Y., Zhong, G. *Chlamydia pneumoniae* secretion of a protease-like activity factor for degrading host cell transcription factors required for [correction of factors is required for] major histocompatibility complex antigen expression. *Infect. Immun.* **2002**, *70*, 345–349.

77 Zhong, G., Liu, L., Fan, T., Fan, P., Ji, H. Degradation of transcription factor RFX5 during the inhibition of both constitutive and interferon gamma-inducible major histocompatibility complex class I expression in chlamydia-infected cells. *J. Exp. Med.* **2000**, *191*, 1525–1534.

78 Voyich, J. M., Musser, J. M., DeLeo, F. R. *Streptococcus pyogenes* and human neutrophils: a paradigm for evasion of innate host defense by bacterial pathogens. *Microbes Infect.* **2004**, *6*, 1117–1123.

79 Ji, Y., McLandsborough, L., Kondagunta, A., Cleary, P. P. C5a peptidase alters clearance and trafficking of group A streptococci by infected mice. *Infect. Immun.* **1996**, *64*, 503–510.

80 Bisno, A., Brito, M., Collins, C. Molecular basis of group A streptococcal virulence. *Lancet Infect. Dis.* **2003**, *3*, 191–200.

81 Rus, H. G., Niculescu, F. I., Shin, M. L. Role of the C5b–9 complement complex in cell cycle and apoptosis. *Immunol. Rev.* **2001**, *180*, 49–55.

82 Nicholson-Weller, A., Halperin, J. A. Membrane signaling by complement C5b–9, the membrane attack complex. *Immunol. Res.* **1993**, *12*, 244–257.

83 Kapur, V., Majesky, M. W., Li, L. L., Black, R. A., Musser, J. M. Cleavage of interleukin 1 beta (IL-1 beta) precursor to produce active IL-1 beta by a conserved extracellular cysteine

protease from *Streptococcus pyogenes*. *Proc. Natl Acad. Sci. USA* **1993**, *90*, 7676–7680.

84 Collin, M., Svensson, M. D., Sjoholm, A. G., Jensenius, J. C., Sjobring, U., Olsen, A. EndoS and SpeB from *Streptococcus pyogenes* inhibit immunoglobulin-mediated opsonophagocytosis. *Infect. Immun.* **2002**, *70*, 6646–6651.

85 Dale, J. B., Washburn, R. G., Marques, M. B., Wessels, M. R. Hyaluronate capsule and surface M protein in resistance to opsonization of group A streptococci. *Infect. Immun.* **1996**, *64*, 1495–1501.

86 Dinkla, K., Rohde, M., Jansen, W. T. M., Carapetis, J. R., Chhatwal, G. S., Talay, S. R. *Streptococcus pyogenes* recruits collagen via surface-bound fibronectin: a novel colonization and immune evasion mechanism. *Mol. Microbiol.* **2003**, *47*, 861–869.

87 Vossen, M., Westerhout, E., Söderberg-Nauclér, C., Wiertz, E. Viral immune evasion: a masterpiece of evolution. *Immunogenetics* **2002**, *54*, 527–542.

88 Davis, L. A., Rouse, B. T. A skeptical look at viral immune evasion. *Front. Bosci.* **1997**, *2*, 596–605.

89 Favoreel, H. W., Van de Walle, G. R., Nauwynck, H. J., Pensaert, M. B. Virus complement evasion strategies. *J. Gen. Virol.* **2003**, *84*, 1–15.

90 Lee, S.-H., Jung, J. U., Means, R. E. Viral infection: mechanisms for evading innate immunity. *Trends Microbiol.* **2003**, *11*, 449–452.

91 Cooper, N., Jensen, F., Welsh, R., Jr., Oldstone, M. Lysis of RNA tumor viruses by human serum: direct antibody-independent triggering of the classical complement pathway. *J. Exp. Med.* **1976**, *144*, 970–984.

92 Ebenbichler, C., Thielens, N., Vornhagen, R., Marschang, P., Arlaud, G., Dierich, M. Human immunodeficiency virus type 1 activates the classical pathway of complement by direct C1 binding through specific sites in the transmembrane glycoprotein gp41. *J. Exp. Med.* **1991**, *174*, 1417–1424.

93 Ikeda, F., Haraguchi, Y., Jinno, A., Iino, Y., Morishita, Y., Shiraki, H. et al. Human complement component C1q Inhibits the Infectivity of Cell-Free HTLV-I. *J. Immunol.* **1998**, *161*, 5712–5719.

94 Spiller, O. B., Morgan, B. P. Antibody-independent activation of the classical complement pathway by cytomegalovirus-infected fibroblasts. *J. Infect. Dis.* **1998**, *178*, 1597–1603.

95 Reading, P., Morey, L., Crouch, E., Anders, E. Collectin-mediated antiviral host defense of the lung: evidence from influenza virus infection of mice. *J. Virol.* **1997**, *71*, 8204–8212.

96 Sasaki, K., Tsutsumi, A., Wakamiya, N., Ohtani, K., Suzuki, Y., Watanabe, Y. et al. Mannose-binding lectin polymorphisms in patients with hepatitis C virus infection. *Scand. J. Gastroenterol.* **2000**, *35*, 960–965.

97 Hakozaki, Y., Yoshiba, M., Sekiyama, K., Seike, E., Iwamoto, J., Mitani, K. et al. Mannose-binding lectin and the prognosis of fulminant hepatic failure caused by HBV infection. *Liver* **2002**, *22*, 29–34.

98 Meri, S., Pangburn, M. Discrimination between activators and nonactivators of the alternative pathway of complement: regulation via a sialic acid/polyanion binding site on factor H. *Proc. Natl Acad. Sci. USA* **1990**, *87*, 3982–3986.

99 van den Berg, C., Morgan, B. Complement-inhibiting activities of human CD59 and analogues from rat, sheep, and pig are not homologously restricted. *J. Immunol.* **1994**, *152*, 4095–4101.

100 Rushmere, N. K., Tomlinson, S., Morgan, B. P. Expression of rat CD59: functional analysis confirms lack of species selectivity and reveals that glycosylation is not required for function. *Immunology* **1997**, *90*, 640–646.

101 Favoreel, H., Nauwynck, H., Van Oostveldt, P., Mettenleiter, T., Pensaert, M. Antibody-induced and

cytoskeleton-mediated redistribution and shedding of viral glycoproteins, expressed on pseudorabies virus-infected cells. *J. Virol.* **1997**, *71*, 8254–8261.

102 Kotwal, G. J., Miller, C. G., Justus, D. E. The inflammation modulatory protein (IMP) of cowpox virus drastically diminishes the tissue damage by down-regulating cellular infiltration resulting from complement activation. *Mol. Cell. Biochem.* **1998**, *185*, 39–46.

103 Hung, S., Srinivasan, S., Friedman, H., Eisenberg, R., Cohen, G. Structural basis of C3b binding by glycoprotein C of herpes simplex virus. *J. Virol.* **1992**, *66*, 4013–4027.

104 Friedman, H. M., Cohen, G. H., Eisenberg, R. J., Seidel, C. A., Cines, D. B. Glycoprotein C of herpes simplex virus 1 acts as a receptor for the C3b complement component on infected cells. *Nature* **1984**, *309*, 633–635.

105 Rux, A. H., Lou, H., Lambris, J. D., Friedman, H. M., Eisenberg, R. J., Cohen, G. H. Kinetic analysis of glycoprotein C of herpes simplex virus types 1 and 2 binding to heparin, heparan sulfate, and complement component C3b. *Virology* **2002**, *294*, 324–332.

106 Albrecht, J., Fleckenstein, B. New member of the multigene family of complement control proteins in herpesvirus saimiri. *J. Virol.* **1992**, *66*, 3937–3940.

107 Vanderplasschen, A., Mathew, E., Hollinshead, M., Sim, R. B., Smith, G. L. Extracellular enveloped vaccinia virus is resistant to complement because of incorporation of host complement control proteins into its envelope. *Proc. Natl Acad. Sci. USA* **1998**, *95*, 7544–7549.

108 Betts, R. F., Schmidt, S. G. Cytolytic IgM antibody to cytomegalovirus in primary cytomegalovirus infection in humans. *J. Infect. Dis.* **1981**, *143*, 821–826.

109 Stoiber, H., Kacani, L., Speth, C., Wurzner, R., Dierich, M. P. The supportive role of complement in HIV pathogenesis. *Immunol. Rev.* **2001**, *180*, 168–176.

110 Nguyen, D. H., Hildreth, J. E. K. Evidence for budding of human immunodeficiency virus type 1 selectively from glycolipid-enriched membrane lipid rafts. *J. Virol.* **2000**, *74*, 3264–3272.

111 Saifuddin, M., Parker, C., Peeples, M., Gorny, M., Zolla-Pazner, S., Ghassemi, M. et al. Role of virion-associated glycosylphosphatidylinositol-linked proteins CD55 and CD59 in complement resistance of cell line-derived and primary isolates of HIV-1. *J. Exp. Med.* **1995**, *182*, 501–509.

112 Saifuddin, M., Hedayati, T., Atkinson, J., Holguin, M., Parker, C., Spear, G. Human immunodeficiency virus type 1 incorporates both glycosyl phosphatidylinositol-anchored CD55 and CD59 and integral membrane CD46 at levels that protect from complement-mediated destruction. *J. Gen. Virol.* **1997**, *78*, 1907–1911.

113 Hirsch, R. L., Griffin, D. E., Winkelstein, J. A. Natural immunity to sindbis virus is influenced by host tissue sialic acid content. *Proc. Natl Acad. Sci. USA* **1983**, *80*, 548–550.

114 Watkins, J. F. Adsorption of sensitized sheep erythrocytes to HeLa cells infected with herpes simplex virus. *Nature* **1964**, *202*, 1364–1365.

115 Westmoreland, D., Watkins, J. F. The IgG receptor induced by herpes simplex virus: studies using radio-iodinated IgG. *J. Gen. Virol.* **1974**, *24*, 167–178.

116 Oleszak, E. L., Perlman, S., Parr, R., Collisson, E. W., Leibowitz, J. L. Molecular mimicry between S peplomer proteins of coronaviruses (MHV, BCV, TGEV and IBV) and Fc receptor. *Adv. Exp. Med. Biol.* **1993**, *342*, 183–188.

117 Dowler, K. W., Veltri, R. W. *In vitro* neutralization of HSV-2: inhibition by binding of normal IgG and purified Fc to virion Fc receptor (FcR). *J. Med. Virol.* **1984**, *13*, 251–259.

118 Frank, I., Friedman, H. M. A novel function of the herpes simplex virus

type 1 Fc receptor: participation in bipolar bridging of antiviral immunoglobulin G. *J. Virol.* **1989**, *63*, 4479–4488.

119 Smith, A. E., Helenius, A. How viruses enter animal cells. *Science* **2004**, *304*, 237–242.

120 Baranowski, E., Ruiz-Jarabo, C. M., Domingo, E. Evolution of cell recognition by viruses. *Science* **2001**, *292*, 1102–1105.

121 Bashirova, A. A., Geijtenbeek, T. B. H., van Duijnhoven, G. C. F., van Vliet, S. J., Eilering, J. B. G., Martin, M. P. et al. A Dendritic cell-specific intercellular adhesion molecule 3-grabbing nonintegrin (DC-SIGN)-related protein is highly expressed on human liver sinusoidal endothelial cells and promotes HIV-1 infection. *J. Exp. Med.* **2001**, *193*, 671–678.

122 Pohlmann, S., Baribaud, F., Doms, R. W. DC-SIGN and DC-SIGNR: helping hands for HIV. *Trends Immunol.* **2001**, *22*, 643–646.

123 Feng, Y., Broder, C. C., Kennedy, P. E., Berger, E. A. HIV-1 entry cofactor: functional cDNA cloning of a seven-transmembrane, G protein-coupled receptor. *Science* **1996**, *272*, 872–877.

124 Gallo, S. A., Finnegan, C. M., Viard, M., Raviv, Y., Dimitrov, A., Rawat, S. S. et al. The HIV Env-mediated fusion reaction. *Biochim. Biophys. Acta Biomembranes* **2003**, *1614*, 36–50.

125 Carr, C. M., Kim, P. S. A spring-loaded mechanism for the conformational change of influenza hemagglutinin. *Cell* **1993**, *73*, 823–832.

126 Skehel, J. J., Wiley, D. C. Receptor binding and membrane fusion in virus entry: the influenza hemagglutinin. *Annu. Rev. Biochem.* **2000**, *69*, 531–569.

127 Carfi, A., Willis, S. H., Whitbeck, J. C., Krummenacher, C., Cohen, G. H., Eisenberg, R. J. et al. Herpes simplex virus glycoprotein D bound to the human receptor HveA. *Mol. Cell* **2001**, *8*, 169–179.

128 Tsai, B., Gilbert, J. M., Stehle, T., Lencer, W., Benjamin, T. L., Rapoport, T. A. Gangliosides are receptors for murine polyoma virus and SV40. *EMBO J.* **2003**, *22*, 4346–4355.

129 Smith, A. E., Lilie, H., Helenius, A. Ganglioside-dependent cell attachment and endocytosis of murine polyomavirus-like particles. *FEBS Lett.* **2003**, *555*, 199–203.

130 Mullen, M. M., Haan, K. M., Longnecker, R., Jardetzky, T. S. Structure of the Epstein–Barr virus gp42 protein bound to the MHC class II receptor HLA-DR1. *Mol. Cell* **2002**, *9*, 375–385.

131 Conner, S. D., Schmid, S. L. Regulated portals of entry into the cell. *Nature* **2003**, *422*, 37–44.

132 Bantel-Schaal, U., Hub, B., Kartenbeck, J. Endocytosis of adeno-associated virus type 5 leads to accumulation of virus particles in the Golgi compartment. *J. Virol.* **2002**, *76*, 2340–2349.

133 Dales, S. Early events in cell-animal virus interactions. *Bacteriol. Rev.* **1973**, *37*, 103–135.

134 Marsh, M., Helenius, A. Virus entry into animal cells. *Adv. Virus Res.* **1989**, *36*, 107–151.

135 Helenius, A., Kartenbeck, J., Simons, K., Fries, E. On the entry of Semliki forest virus into BHK-21 cells. *J. Cell Biol.* **1980**, *84*, 404–420.

136 Martin, K., Helenius, A. Nuclear transport of influenza virus ribonucleoproteins: the viral matrix protein (M1) promotes export and inhibits import. *Cell* **1991**, *67*, 117–130.

137 Kielian, M., Helenius, A. pH-induced alterations in the fusogenic spike protein of Semliki Forest virus. *J. Cell Biol.* **1985**, *101*, 2284–2291.

138 Schmid, S., Fuchs, R., Kielian, M., Helenius, A., Mellman, I. Acidification of endosome subpopulations in wild-type Chinese hamster ovary cells and temperature-sensitive acidification-defective mutants. *J. Cell Biol.* **1989**, *108*, 1291–1300.

139 Blumenthal, R., Seth, P., Willingham, M. C., Pastan, I. pH-dependent

lysis of liposomes by adenovirus. *Biochemistry* **1986**, *25*, 2231–2237.

140 FitzGerald, D. J., Padmanabhan, R., Pastan, I., Willingham, M. C. Adenovirus-induced release of epidermal growth factor and pseudomonas toxin into the cytosol of KB cells during receptor-mediated endocytosis. *Cell* **1983**, *32*, 607–617.

141 Chandran, K., Farsetta, D. L., Nibert, M. L. Strategy for non-enveloped virus entry: a hydrophobic conformer of the reovirus membrane penetration protein $\mu 1$ mediates membrane disruption. *J. Virol.* **2002**, *76*, 9920–9933.

142 Hogle, J. M. Poliovirus cell entry: common structural themes in viral cell entry pathways. *Annu. Rev. Microbiol.* **2002**, *56*, 677–702.

143 Sodeik, B. Mechanisms of viral transport in the cytoplasm. *Trends Microbiol.* **2000**, *8*, 465–472.

144 Marsh, M., Bron, R. SFV infection in CHO cells: cell-type specific restrictions to productive virus entry at the cell surface. *J. Cell Sci.* **1997**, *110*, 95–103.

145 Poranen, M. M., Daugelavicius, R., Bamford, D. H. Common principles in viral entry. *Annu. Rev. Microbiol.* **2002**, *56*, 521–538.

146 Colman, P. M., Lawrence, M. C. The structural biology of type I viral membrane fusion. *Nat. Rev. Mol. Cell Biol.* **2003**, *4*, 309–319.

147 Gibbons, D. L., Erk, I., Reilly, B., Navaza, J., Kielian, M., Rey, F. A. et al. Visualization of the target-membrane-inserted fusion protein of semliki forest virus by combined electron microscopy and crystallography. *Cell* **2003**, *114*, 573–583.

148 Modis, Y., Ogata, S., Clements, D., Harrison, S. C. Structure of the dengue virus envelope protein after membrane fusion. *Nature* **2004**, *427*, 313–319.

149 Gibbons, D. L., Vaney, M.-C., Roussel, A., Vigouroux, A., Reilly, B., Lepault, J. et al. Conformational change and protein–protein interactions of the fusion protein of Semliki Forest virus. *Nature* **2004**, *427*, 320–325.

150 Kasamatsu, H., Nakanishi, A. How do animal DNA viruses get to the nucleus? *Annu. Rev. Microbiol.* **1998**, *52*, 627–686.

151 Whittaker, G. R., Kann, M., Helenius, A. Viral entry into the nucleus. *Annu. Rev. Cell Dev. Biol.* **2000**, *16*, 627–651.

152 Whittaker, G. R. Virus nuclear import. *Adv. Drug Deliv. Rev.* **2003**, *55*, 733–747.

153 Norkin, L. C. Caveolae in the uptake and targeting of infectious agents and secreted toxins. *Adv. Drug Deliv. Rev.* **2001**, *49*, 301–315.

154 Parton, R. G., Richards, A. A. Lipid rafts and caveolae as portals for endocytosis: new insights and common mechanisms. *Traffic* **2003**, *4*, 724–738.

155 Pelkmans, L., Helenius, A. Insider information: what viruses tell us about endocytosis. *Curr. Opin. Cell Biol.* **2003**, *15*, 414–422.

156 Pante, N., Kann, M. Nuclear pore complex is able to transport macromolecules with diameters of ~39 nm. *Mol. Biol. Cell* **2002**, *13*, 425–434.

157 Merle, E., Rose, R. C., LeRoux, L., Moroianu, J. Nuclear import of HPV11 L1 capsid protein is mediated by karyopherin $\alpha 2\beta 1$ heterodimers. *J. Cell. Biochem.* **1999**, *74*, 628–637.

158 Nelson, L. M., Rose, R. C., LeRoux, L., Lane, C., Bruya, K., Moroianu, J. Nuclear import and DNA binding of human papillomavirus type 45 L1 capsid protein. *J. Cell. Biochem.* **2000**, *79*, 225–238.

159 Kann, M., Sodeik, B., Vlachou, A., Gerlich, W. H., Helenius, A. Phosphorylation-dependent binding of hepatitis B virus core particles to the nuclear pore complex. *J. Cell Biol.* **1999**, *145*, 45–55.

160 O'Neill, R. E., Jaskunas, R., Blobel, G., Palese, P., Moroianu, J. Nuclear import of influenza virus RNA can be mediated by viral nucleoprotein and transport factors required for protein import. *J. Biol. Chem.* **1995**, *270*, 22701–22704.

161 Trotman, L. C., Mosberger, N., Fornerod, M., Stidwill, R. P.,

Greber, U. F. Import of adenovirus DNA involves the nuclear pore complex receptor CAN/Nup214 and histone H1. *Nat. Cell Biol.* **2001**, *3*, 1092–1100.

162 Greber, U. F., Fassati, A. Nuclear import of viral DNA genomes. *Traffic* **2003**, *4*, 136–143.

163 Ojala, P. M., Sodeik, B., Ebersold, M. W., Kutay, U., Helenius, A. Herpes simplex virus type 1 entry into host cells: reconstitution of capsid binding and uncoating at the nuclear pore complex *in vitro*. *Mol. Cell. Biol.* **2000**, *20*, 4922–4931.

164 Newcomb, W. W., Juhas, R. M., Thomsen, D. R., Homa, F. L., Burch, A. D., Weller, S. K. et al. The UL6 gene product forms the portal for entry of DNA into the herpes simplex virus capsid. *J. Virol.* **2001**, *75*, 10923–10932.

165 Lundstrom, K. Latest development in viral vectors for gene therapy. *Trends Biotechnol.* **2003**, *21*, 117–122.

166 Relph, K., Harrington, K., Pandha, H. Recent developments and current status of gene therapy using viral vectors in the United Kingdom. *Br. Med. J.* **2004**, *329*, 839–842.

167 Cavazzana-Calvo, M., Hacein-Bey, S., Basile, G. e. v. d. S., Gross, F., Yvon, E., Nusbaum, P. et al. Gene therapy of human severe combined immunodeficiency (SCID)-X1 disease. *Science* **2000**, *288*, 669–672.

168 Hacein-Bey-Abina, S., Fischer, A., Cavazzana-Calvo, M. Gene therapy of X-linked severe combined immunodeficiency. *Int. J. Hematol.* **2002**, *76*, 295–298.

169 Blaese, R. M., Culver, K. W., Miller, A. D., Carter, C. S., Fleisher, T., Clerici, M. et al. T lymphocyte-directed gene therapy for ADA SCID: initial trial results after 4 years. *Science* **1995**, *270*, 475–480.

170 Raper, S. E., Yudkoff, M., Chirmule, N., Gao, G.-P., Nunes, F., Haskal, Z. J. et al. A pilot study of *in vivo* liver-directed gene transfer with an adenoviral vector in partial ornithine transcarbamylase deficiency. *Hum. Gene Ther.* **2002**, *13*, 163–175.

171 Kimmelman, J. Recent developments in gene transfer: risk and ethics. *Br. Med. J.* **2005**, *330*, 79–82.

172 Raper, S. E. Gene therapy: the good, the bad, and the ugly. *Surgery* **2005**, *137*, 487–492.

173 Rabinowitz, J. E., Samulski, J. Adeno-associated virus expression systems for gene transfer. *Curr. Opin. Biotechnol.* **1998**, *9*, 470–475.

174 Davidson, B. L., Stein, C. S., Heth, J. A., Martins, I., Kotin, R. M., Derksen, T. A. et al. From the cover: recombinant adeno-associated virus type 2, 4, and 5 vectors: transduction of variant cell types and regions in the mammalian central nervous system. *Proc. Natl Acad. Sci. USA* **2000**, *97*, 3428–3432.

175 Russell, D. W., Kay, M. A. Adeno-associated virus vectors and hematology. *Blood* **1999**, *94*, 864–874.

176 Flotte, T. R., Laube, B. L. Gene therapy in cystic fibrosis. *Chest* **2001**, *120*, 124S–131.

177 West, J., Rodman, D. M. Gene therapy for pulmonary diseases. *Chest* **2001**, *119*, 613–617.

178 Hidaka, C., Khan, S. N., Farmer, J. C., Sandhu, H. S. Gene therapy for spinal applications. *Orthop. Clin. North Am.* **2002**, *33*, 439–446.

179 Stecher, H., Shayakhmetov, D. M., Stamatoyannopoulos, G., Lieber, A. A capsid-modified adenovirus vector devoid of all viral genes: assessment of transduction and toxicity in human hematopoietic cells. *Mol. Ther.* **2001**, *4*, 36–44.

180 Haviv, Y. S., Blackwell, J. L., Kanerva, A., Nagi, P., Krasnykh, V., Dmitriev, I. et al. Adenoviral gene therapy for renal cancer requires retargeting to alternative cellular receptors. *Cancer Res.* **2002**, *62*, 4273–4281.

181 Young, L. S., Mautner, V. The promise and potential hazards of adenovirus gene therapy. *Gut* **2001**, *48*, 733–736.

182 Schiedner, G., Morral, N., Parks, R. J., Wu, Y., Koopmans, S. C., Langston, C. et al. Genomic DNA transfer with a high-capacity adeno-

virus vector results in improved *in vivo* gene expression and decreased toxicity. *Nat. Genet.* **1998**, *18*, 180–183.

183 Gomez-Manzano, C., Yung, W. K. A., Alemany, R., Fueyo, J. Genetically modified adenoviruses against gliomas: from bench to bedside. *Neurology* **2004**, *63*, 418–426.

184 Smith, G. M. Adenovirus-mediated gene transfer to treat neurologic disease. *Arch. Neurol.* **1998**, *55*, 1061–1064.

185 Samaniego, L. A., Neiderhiser, L., DeLuca, N. A. Persistence and expression of the herpes simplex virus genome in the absence of immediate-early proteins. *J. Virology* **1998**, *72*, 3307–3320.

186 Krisky, D. M., Wolfe, D., Goins, W. F., Marconi, P. C., Ramakrishnan, R., Mata, M. et al. Deletion of multiple immediate-early genes from herpes simplex virus reduces cytotoxicity and permits long-term gene expression in neurons. *Gene Ther.* **1998**, *5*, 1593–1603.

187 Kennedy, P. Potential use of herpes simplex virus (HSV) vectors for gene therapy of neurological disorders. *Brain* **1997**, *120*, 1245–1259.

188 Akkaraju, G. R., Huard, J., Hoffman, E. P., Goins, W. F., Pruchnic, R., Watkins, S. C., Cohen, J. B., Glorioso, J. C. Herpes simplex virus vector-mediated dystrophin gene transfer and expression in MDX mouse skeletal muscle. *J. Gene Med.* **1999**, *1*, 280–289.

189 Buchschacher, G. L., Jr., Wong-Staal, F. Development of lentiviral vectors for gene therapy for human diseases. *Blood* **2000**, *95*, 2499–2504.

190 Elisa Vigna, L. N. Lentiviral vectors: excellent tools for experimental gene transfer and promising candidates for gene therapy. *J. Gene Med.* **2000**, *2*, 308–316.

191 Burns, J. C., Friedmann, T., Driever, W., Burrascano, M., Yee, J. K. Vesicular stomatitis virus G glycoprotein pseudotyped retroviral vectors: concentration to very high titer and efficient gene transfer into mammalian and nonmammalian cells. *Proc. Natl Acad. Sci. USA* **1993**, *90*, 8033–8037.

192 Baum, C., Dullmann, J., Li, Z., Fehse, B., Meyer, J., Williams, D. A. et al. Side-effects of retroviral gene transfer into hematopoietic stem cells. *Blood* **2003**, *101*, 2099–2113.

193 Suhr, S. T., Gage, F. H. Gene therapy in the central nervous system: the use of recombinant retroviruses. *Arch. Neurol.* **1999**, *56*, 287–292.

194 Malech, H. L., Choi, U., Brenner, S. Progress toward effective gene therapy for chronic granulomatous disease. *Jpn. J. Infect. Dis.* **2004**, *57*, S27–28.

195 Fisher, K. D., Stallwood, Y., Green, N. K., Ulbrich, K., Mautner, V., Seymour, L. W. Polymer-coated adenovirus permits efficient retargeting and evades neutralising antibodies. *Gene Ther.* **2001**, *8*, 341–348.

196 Kaneda, Y. Virosomes: evolution of the liposome as a targeted drug delivery system. *Adv. Drug Deliv. Rev.* **2000**, *43*, 197–205.

197 Morishita, R., Gibbons, G. H., Kaneda, Y., Ogihara, T., Dzau, V. J. Pharmacokinetics of antisense oligodeoxyribonucleotides (cyclin B1 and CDC 2 kinase) in the vessel wall *in vivo*: enhanced therapeutic utility for restenosis by HVJ-liposome delivery. Gene **1994**, *149*, 13–19.

198 Ramani, K., Bora, R. S., Kumar, M., Tyagi, S. K., Sarkar, D. P. Novel gene delivery to liver cells using engineered virosomes. *FEBS Lett.* **1997**, *404*, 164–168.

199 Chatigny, M. A., Prusiner, S. B. Biohazards of investigations on the transmissible spongiform encephalopathies. *Rev. Infect. Dis.* **1980**, *2*, 713–724.

200 Prusiner, S. B. Prions: novel infectious pathogens. *Adv. Virus Res.* **1984**, *29*, 1–56.

201 Prusiner, S. B., Kingsbury, D. T. Prions – infectious pathogens causing the spongiform encephalopathies. *CRC Crit. Rev. Clin. Neurobiol.* **1985**, *1*, 181–200.

202 Mabbott, N. A. The complement system in prion diseases. *Curr. Opin. Immunol.* **2004**, *16*, 587–593.

203 Aguzzi, A., Heikenwalder, M. Prions, Cytokines, and chemokines: a meeting in lymphoid organs. *Immunity* **2005**, *22*, 145–154.

204 Johnson, R. T. Prion diseases. *Lancet Neurol.* **2005**, *4*, 635–642.

205 Aguzzi, A. Prions and the immune system: a journey through gut, spleen, and nerves. *Adv. Immunol.* **2003**, *81*, 123–171.

206 Sigurdson, C. J., Barillas-Mury, C., Miller, M. W., Oesch, B., van Keulen, L. J. M., Langeveld, J. P. M. et al. PrP^{CWD} lymphoid cell targets in early and advanced chronic wasting disease of mule deer. *J. Gen. Virology* **2002**, *83*, 2617–2628.

207 Heggebo, R., Press, C. M., Gunnes, G., Ulvund, M. J., Tranulis, M. A., Lsverk, T. Detection of PrP^{Sc} in lymphoid tissues of lambs experimentally exposed to the scrapie agent. *J. Comp. Pathol.* **2003**, *128*, 172–181.

208 Neutra, M. R., Frey, A., Kraehenbuhl, J.-P. Epithelial M cells: gateways for mucosal infection and immunization. *Cell* **1996**, *86*, 345–348.

209 Aguzzi, A., Heikenwalder, M. Prion diseases: cannibals and garbage piles. *Nature* **2003**, *423*, 127–129.

210 Mabbott, N. A., Young, J., McConnell, I., Bruce, M. E. Follicular dendritic cell dedifferentiation by treatment with an inhibitor of the lymphotoxin pathway dramatically reduces scrapie susceptibility. *J. Virol.* **2003**, *77*, 6845–6854.

211 Prinz, M., Heikenwalder, M., Junt, T., Schwarz, P., Glatzel, M., Heppner, F. L. et al. Positioning of follicular dendritic cells within the spleen controls prion neuroinvasion. *Nature* **2003**, *425*, 957–962.

212 Brandner, S., Isenmann, S., Raeber, A., Fischer, M., Sailer, A., Kobayashi, Y. et al. Normal host prion protein necessary for scrapie-induced neurotoxicity. *Nature* **1996**, *379*, 339–343.

213 Bueler, H., Aguzzi, A., Sailer, A., Greiner, R. A., Autenried, P., Aguet, M. et al. Mice devoid of PrP are resistant to scrapie. *Cell* **1993**, *73*, 1339–1347.

214 Mallucci, G., Dickinson, A., Linehan, J., Klohn, P.-C., Brandner, S., Collinge, J. Depleting neuronal PrP in prion infection prevents disease and reverses spongiosis. *Science* **2003**, *302*, 871–874.

215 Klein, M. A., Frigg, R., Flechsig, E., Raeber, A. J., Kalinke, U., Bluethmann, H. et al. A crucial role for B cells in neuroinvasive scraple. *Nature* **1997**, *390*, 687–690.

216 Kaeser, P. S., Klein, M. A., Schwarz, P., Aguzzi, A. Efficient lymphoreticular prion propagation requires PrPc in stromal and hematopoietic cells. *J. Virol.* **2001**, *75*, 7097–7106.

217 Beekes, M., McBride, P. A. Early accumulation of pathological PrP in the enteric nervous system and gut-associated lymphoid tissue of hamsters orally infected with scrapie. *Neurosci. Lett.* **2000**, *278*, 181–184.

218 Mabbott, N. A., Bruce, M. E. Prion disease: bridging the spleen–nerve gap. *Nat. Med.* **2003**, *9*, 1463–1464.

219 Fevrier, B., Vilette, D., Archer, F., Loew, D., Faigle, W., Vidal, M. et al. Cells release prions in association with exosomes. *Proc. Natl Acad. Sci. USA* **2004**, *101*, 9683–9688.

220 Raeber, A. J., Klein, M. A., Frigg, R., Flechsig, E., Aguzzi, A., Weissmann, C. PrP-dependent association of prions with splenic but not circulating lymphocytes of scrapie-infected mice. *EMBO J.* **1999**, *18*, 2702–2706.

221 Huang, F.-P., Farquhar, C. F., Mabbott, N. A., Bruce, M. E., MacPherson, G. G. Migrating intestinal dendritic cells transport PrP^{Sc} from the gut. *J. Gen. Virology* **2002**, *83*, 267–271.

222 Aucouturier, P., Geissmann, F., Damotte, D., Saborio, G. P., Meeker, H. C., Kascsak, R. et al. Infected splenic dendritic cells are sufficient for prion transmission to the CNS in mouse scrapie. *J. Clin. Invest.* **2001**, *108*, 703–708.

223 Yoshida, K., van den Berg, T. K., Dijkstra, C. D. Two different mechanisms of immune-complex trapping in the mouse spleen during immune responses. *Adv. Exp. Med. Biol.* **1993**, *329*, 377–382.
224 Klein, M. A., Kaeser, P. S., Schwarz, P., Weyd, H., Xenarios, I., Zinkernagel, R. M. et al. Complement facilitates early prion pathogenesis. *Nat. Med.* **2001**, *7*, 488–492.
225 Rosen, H., Abribat, T. The rise and rise of drug delivery. *Nat. Rev. Drug Discov.* **2005**, *4*, 381–385.
226 Duncan, R. The dawning era of polymer therapeutics. *Nat. Rev. Drug Discov.* **2003**, *2*, 347–360.
227 Theeuwes, F., Swanson, D., Wong, P., Bonsen, P., Place, V., Heimlich, K. et al. Elementary osmotic pump for indomethacin. *J. Pharm. Sci.* **1983**, *72*, 253–258.
228 Colombo, P., Conte, U., Gazzaniga, A., Maggi, L., Sangalli, M. E., Peppas, N. A. et al. Drug release modulation by physical restrictions of matrix swelling. *Int. J. Pharm.* **1990**, *63*, 43–48.
229 Conte, U., Maggi, L., Colombo, P., La Manna, A. Multi-layered hydrophilic matrices as constant release devices (Geomatrix™ Systems). *J. Control. Release* **1993**, *26*, 39–47.
230 Versi, E., Appell, R., Mobley, D., Patton, W., Saltzstein, D. Dry mouth with conventional and controlled-release oxybutynin in urinary incontinence. *Obstet. Gynecol.* **2000**, *95*, 718–721.
231 Anderson, R. U., Mobley, D., Blank, B., Saltzstein, D., Susset, J., Brown, J. S. Once daily controlled versus immediate release oxybutynin chloride for urge urinary incontinence. OROS Oxybutynin Study Group. *J. Urol.* **1999**, *161*, 1809–1812.
232 Viscusi, E. R., Reynolds, L., Chung, F., Atkinson, L. E., Khanna, S. Patient-controlled transdermal fentanyl hydrochloride vs intravenous morphine pump for postoperative pain: a randomized controlled Trial. *J. Am. Med. Ass.* **2004**, *291*, 1333–1341.
233 Sebastien Henry, D. V. M., Mark G. Allen, Mark R. Prausnitz. Microfabricated microneedles: a novel approach to transdermal drug delivery. *J. Pharmaceutical Sciences* **1998**, *87*, 922–925.
234 Barry, B. W. Novel mechanisms and devices to enable successful transdermal drug delivery. *Eur. J. Pharm. Sci.* **2001**, *14*, 101–114.
235 Orive, G., Hernandez, R. M., Gascon, A. R., Dominguez-Gil, A., Pedraz, J. L. Drug delivery in biotechnology: present and future. *Curr. Opin. Biotechnol.* **2003**, *14*, 659–664.
236 Kilpatrick, D. C., Pusztai, A., Grant, G., Graham, C., Ewen, S. W. B. Tomato lectin resists digestion in the mammalian alimentary canal and binds to intestinal villi without deleterious effects. *FEBS Lett.* **1985**, *185*, 299–305.
237 Carreno-Gomez, B., Woodley, J. F., Florence, A. T. Studies on the uptake of tomato lectin nanoparticles in everted gut sacs. *Int. J. Pharm.* **1999**, *183*, 7–11.
238 Veronese, F. M., Harris, J. M. Introduction and overview of peptide and protein pegylation. *Adv. Drug Deliv. Rev.* **2002**, *54*, 453–456.
239 Foran, T. M. New contraceptive choices across reproductive life. *Med. J. Aust.* **2003**, *178*, 616–620.
240 Jain, S. K., Chourasia, M. K., Jain, A. K., Jain, R. K., Shrivastava, A. K. Development and characterization of mucoadhesive microspheres bearing salbutamol for nasal delivery. *Drug Deliv.* **2004**, *11*, 113–122.
241 Luukkainen, T., Pakarinen, P., Toivonen, J. Progestin-releasing intrauterine systems. *Semin. Reprod. Med.* **2001**, *19*, 355–363.
242 Eley, J. G., Pujari, V. D., McLane, J. Poly (lactide-*co*-glycolide) nanoparticles containing coumarin-6 for suppository delivery: *in vitro* release profile and *in vivo* tissue distribution. *Drug Deliv.* **2004**, *11*, 255–261.
243 Merkus, F. W. H. M., Verhoef, J. C., Marttin, E., Romeijn, S. G., van der Kuy, P. H. M., Hermens, W. A. J. J.,

et al. Cyclodextrins in nasal drug delivery. *Adv. Drug Deliv. Rev.* **1999**, *36*, 41–57.

244 DODANE, V., AMIN KHAN, M., MERWIN, J. R. Effect of chitosan on epithelial permeability and structure. *Int. J. Pharm.* **1999**, *182*, 21–32.

245 ILLUM, L., JABBAL-GILL, I., HINCHCLIFFE, M., FISHER, A. N., DAVIS, S. S. Chitosan as a novel nasal delivery system for vaccines. *Adv. Drug Deliv. Rev.* **2001**, *51*, 81–96.

246 LAVAN, D. A., MCGUIRE, T., LANGER, R. Small-scale systems for *in vivo* drug delivery. *Nat. Biotechnol.* **2003**, *21*, 1184–1191.

247 SANTINI, J. T., JR., CIMA, M. J., LANGER, R. A controlled-release microchip. *Nature* **1999**, *397*, 335–338.

248 UNGER, M. A., CHOU, H.-P., THORSEN, T., SCHERER, A., QUAKE, S. R. Monolithic microfabricated valves and pumps by multilayer soft lithography. *Science* **2000**, *288*, 113–116.

249 HANSEN, C. L., SKORDALAKES, E., BERGER, J. M., QUAKE, S. R. A robust and scalable microfluidic metering method that allows protein crystal growth by free interface diffusion. *Proc. Natl Acad. Sci. USA* **2002**, *99*, 16531–16536.

250 LILLY, M. B., BREZOVICH, I. A., ATKINSON, W. J. Hyperthermia induction with thermally self-regulated ferromagnetic implants. *Radiology* **1985**, *154*, 243–244.

251 TUCKER, R. D., HUIDOBRO, C., LARSON, T., PLATZ, C. E. Use of permanent interstitial temperature self-regulating rods for ablation of prostate cancer. *J. Endourol.* **2000**, *14*, 511–517.

252 ROTARIU, O., IACOB, G., STRACHAN, N. J. C., CHIRIAC, H. Simulating the embolization of blood vessels using magnetic microparticles and acupuncture needle in a magnetic field. *Biotechnol. Prog.* **2004**, *20*, 299–305.

253 LANZA, G. M., WINTER, P., CARUTHERS, S., SCHMEIDER, A., CROWDER, K., MORAWSKI, A. et al. Novel paramagnetic contrast agents for molecular imaging and targeted drug delivery. *Curr. Pharm. Biotechnol.* **2004**, *5*, 495–507.

254 BOS, G. W., CROMMELIN, D. J. A., HENNINK, W. E., VERRIJK, R., FRANSSEN, O., BEZEMER, J. M. Hydrogels for the controlled release of pharmaceutical proteins. *Pharm. Technol. Eur.* **2001**, *13*, 64+67–68+70+72+74.

255 MIYATA, T., ASAMI, N., URAGAMI, T. A reversibly antigen-responsive hydrogel. *Nature* **1999**, *399*, 766–769.

256 HELLER, J., TRESCONY, P. V. Controlled drug release by polymer dissolution. II: Enzyme-mediated delivery device. *J. Pharm. Sci.* **1979**, *68*, 919–921.

257 KWON, I. C., BAE, Y. H., KIM, S. W. Electrically credible polymer gel for controlled release of drugs. *Nature* **1991**, *354*, 291–293.

258 ICHIMURA, K., OH, S.-K., NAKAGAWA, M. Light-driven motion of liquids on a photoresponsive surface. *Science* **2000**, *288*, 1624–1626.

259 ABBOTT, S., RALSTON, J., REYNOLDS, G., HAYES, R. Reversible wettability of photoresponsive pyrimidine-coated surfaces. *Langmuir* **1999**, *15*, 8923–8928.

260 LAHANN, J., MITRAGOTRI, S., TRAN, T.-N., KAIDO, H., SUNDARAM, J., CHOI, I. S. et al. A reversibly switching surface. *Science* **2003**, *299*, 371–374.

261 DESAI, T. A., CHU, W. H., TU, J. K., BEATTIE, G. M., HAYEK, A., FERRARI, M. Microfabricated immunoisolating biocapsules. *Biotechnol. Bioeng.* **1998**, *57*, 118–120.

262 SEFTON, M. V., HORVATH, V., ZINGG, W. Insulin delivery by a diffusion-controlled micropump in pancreatectomized dogs: phase 1. *J. Control. Release* **1990**, *12*, 1–12.

263 HANAS, R. Selection for and initiation of continuous subcutaneous insulin infusion. *Hormone Res.* **2002**, *57*, 101–104.

264 FISHER, R. S., HO, J. Potential new methods for antiepileptic drug delivery. *CNS Drugs* **2002**, *16*, 579–593.

265 GARDNER, B., JAMOUS, A., TEDDY, P., BERGSTROM, E., WANG, D.,

Ravichandran, G. et al. Intrathecal baclofen – a multicentre clinical comparison of the Medtronics Programmable, Cordis Secor and Constant Infusion Infusaid drug delivery systems. *Paraplegia* **1995**, *33*, 551–554.
266 Diaz, S., Pavez, M., Miranda, P., Robertson, D. N., Sivin, I., Croxatto, H. B. A five-year clinical trial of levonorgestrel silastic implants (Norplant™). *Contraception* **1982**, *25*, 447–456.
267 Chang, T. M. S. Therapeutic applications of polymeric artificial cells. *Nat. Rev. Drug Discov.* **2005**, *4*, 221–235.
268 Regulier, E., Schneider, B. L., Deglon, N., Beuzard, Y., Aebischer, P. Continuous delivery of human and mouse erythropoietin in mice by genetically engineered polymer encapsulated myoblasts. *Gene Ther.* **1998**, *5*, 1014–1022.
269 Jolley, W. B., Hinshaw, D. B., Call, T. W., Alvord, L. S. Xenogeneic pancreatic islet transplantation in proteolytic enzyme-bonded diffusion chambers in diabetic rats. *Transplant. Proc.* **1977**, *9*, 363–365.
270 Desai, T., Chu, W., Rasi, G., Sinibaldi-Vallebona, P., Guarino, E., Ferrari, M. Microfabricated biocapsules provide short-term immunoisolation of insulinoma xenografts. *Biomed. Microdevices* **1998**, *1*, 131–138.
271 Ogura, H., Tani, K., Ozawa, K., Nagata, S., Asano, S., Takaku, F. Implantation of genetically manipulated fibroblasts into mice as antitumor alpha-interferon therapy. *Cancer Res.* **1990**, *50*, 5102–5106.
272 Schnyder, A., Huwyler, J. Drug transport to brain with targeted liposomes. *NeuroRx* **2005**, *2*, 99–107.
273 Olivier, J. C. Drug transport to brain with targeted nanoparticles. *NeuroRx* **2005**, *2*, 108–119.
274 Torchilin, V. P. Immunoliposomes and PEGylated immunoliposomes: possible use for targeted delivery of imaging agents. *Immunomethods* **1994**, *4*, 244–258.
275 Lee, R., Low, P. Delivery of liposomes into cultured KB cells via folate receptor-mediated endocytosis. *J. Biol. Chem.* **1994**, *269*, 3198–3204.
276 Wu, D., Yang, J., Pardridge, W. M. Drug targeting of a peptide radiopharmaceutical through the primate blood–brain barrier *in vivo* with a monoclonal antibody to the human insulin receptor. *J. Clin. Invest.* **1997**, *100*, 1804–1812.
277 Huwyler, J., Wu, D., Pardridge, W. M. Brain drug delivery of small molecules using immunoliposomes. *Proc. Natl Acad. Sci. USA* **1996**, *93*, 14164–14169.
278 Shi, N., Zhang, Y., Zhu, C., Boado, R. J., Pardridge, W. M. Brain-specific expression of an exogenous gene after i.v. administration. *Proc. Natl Acad. Sci. USA* **2001**, *98*, 12754–12759.
279 Bickel, U., Yoshikawa, T., Pardridge, W. M. Delivery of peptides and proteins through the blood–brain barrier. *Adv Drug Deliv. Rev.* **2001**, *46*, 247–279.
280 Friden, P. M., Walus, L. R., Musso, G. F., Taylor, M. A., Malfroy, B., Starzyk, R. M. Anti-transferrin receptor antibody and antibody-drug conjugates cross the blood–brain barrier. *Proc. Natl Acad. Sci. USA* **1991**, *88*, 4771–4775.
281 Pardridge, W. M., Buciak, J. L., Friden, P. M. Selective transport of an anti-transferrin receptor antibody through the blood–brain barrier *in vivo*. *J. Pharmacol. Exp. Ther.* **1991**, *259*, 66–70.
282 Huwyler, J., Yang, J., Pardridge, W. M. Receptor mediated delivery of daunomycin using immunoliposomes: pharmacokinetics and tissue distribution in the rat. *J. Pharmacol. Exp. Ther.* **1997**, *282*, 1541–1546.
283 Zhang, Y., Zhang, Y.-f., Bryant, J., Charles, A., Boado, R. J., Pardridge, W. M. Intravenous RNA interference gene therapy targeting the human epidermal growth factor receptor prolongs survival in intracranial brain cancer. *Clin. Cancer Res.* **2004**, *10*, 3667–3677.

284 Zhang, Y., Zhu, C., Pardridge, W. M. Antisense gene therapy of brain cancer with an artificial virus gene delivery system. *Mol. Ther.* **2002**, *6*, 67–72.

285 Kreuter, J. Nanoparticulate systems for brain delivery of drugs. *Adv. Drug Deliv. Rev.* **2001**, *47*, 65–81.

286 Couvreur, P., Tulkens, P., Roland, M., Trouet, A., Speiser, P. Nanocapsules: a new type of lysosomotropic carrier. *FEBS Lett.* **1977**, *84*, 323–326.

287 Kreuter, J., Alyautdin, R. N., Kharkevich, D. A., Ivanov, A. A. Passage of peptides through the blood–brain barrier with colloidal polymer particles (nanoparticles). *Brain Res.* **1995**, *674*, 171–174.

288 Gulyaev, A. E., Gelperina, S. E., Skidan, I. N., Antropov, A. S., Kivman, G. Y., Kreuter, J. Significant transport of doxorubicin into the brain with polysorbate 80-coated nanoparticles. *Pharm. Res.* **1999**, *16*, 1564–1569.

289 Alyautdin, R. N., Petrov, V. E., Langer, K., Berthold, A., Kharkevich, D. A., Kreuter, J. Delivery of loperamide across the blood–brain barrier with polysorbate 80-coated polybutylcyanoacrylate nanoparticles. *Pharm. Res.* **1997**, *14*, 325–328.

290 Gref, R., Minamitake, Y., Peracchia, M. T., Domb, A., Trubetskoy, V., Torchilin, V. et al. Poly(ethylene glycol)-coated nanospheres: potential carriers for intravenous drug administration. *Pharm. Biotechnol.* **1997**, *10*, 167–198.

291 Douglas, S. J., Davis, S. S., Illum, L. Nanoparticles in drug delivery. *Crit. Rev. Ther. Drug Carrier Syst.* **1987**, *3*, 233–261.

292 Peracchia, M. T., Fattal, E., Desmaele, D., Besnard, M., Noel, J. P., Gomis, J. M. et al. Stealth® PEGylated polycyanoacrylate nanoparticles for intravenous administration and splenic targeting. *J. Control. Release* **1999**, *60*, 121–128.

293 Calvo, P., Gouritin, B., Chacun, H. L. N., Desmaele, D., D'Angelo, J., Noel, J.-P. et al. Long-circulating PEGylated polycyanoacrylate nanoparticles as new drug carrier for brain delivery. *Pharm. Res.* **2001**, *18*, 1157–1166.

294 Azmin, M. N., Stuart, J. F., Florence, A. T. The distribution and elimination of methotrexate in mouse blood and brain after concurrent administration of polysorbate 80. *Cancer Chemother. Pharmacol.* **1985**, *14*, 238–242.

295 Lode, J., Fichtner, I., Kreuter, J., Berndt, A., Diederichs, J. E., Reszka, R. Influence of surface-modifying surfactants on the pharmacokinetic behavior of ^{14}C-poly(methylmethacrylate) nanoparticles in experimental tumor models. *Pharm. Res.* **2001**, *18*, 1613–1619.

296 Darius, J., Meyer, F. P., Sabel, B. A., Schroeder, U. Influence of nanoparticles on the brain-to-serum distribution and the metabolism of valproic acid in mice. *J. Pharm. Pharmacol.* **2000**, *52*, 1043–1047.

297 Anderson, J. M., Shive, M. S. Biodegradation and biocompatibility of PLA and PLGA microspheres. *Adv. Drug Deliv. Rev.* **1997**, *28*, 5–24.

298 Vert, M., Schwach, G., Engel, R., Coudane, J. Something new in the field of PLA/GA bioresorbable polymers? *J. Control. Release* **1998**, *53*, 85–92.

299 Ueda, H., Tabata, Y. Polyhydroxyalkanonate derivatives in current clinical applications and trials. *Adv. Drug Deliv. Rev.* **2003**, *55*, 501–518.

300 Suming Li. Hydrolytic degradation characteristics of aliphatic polyesters derived from lactic and glycolic acids. *J. Biomed. Mater. Res.* **1999**, *48*, 342–353.

301 Riley, T., Stolnik, S., Heald, C. R., Xiong, C. D., Garnett, M. C., Illum, L. et al. Physicochemical evaluation of nanoparticles assembled from poly(lactic acid)–poly(ethylene glycol) (PLA–PEG) block copolymers as drug delivery vehicles. *Langmuir* **2001**, *17*, 3168–3174.

302 Stolnik, S., Dunn, S. E., Garnett, M. C., Davies, M. C., Coombes, A. G. A., Taylor, D. C. et al. Surface modification of poly(lactide-*co*-glycolide) nanospheres by biodegradable poly(lactide)–poly(ethylene glycol) copolymers. *Pharm. Res.* **1994**, *11*, 1800–1808.
303 Li, Y.-P., Pei, Y.-Y., Zhang, X.-Y., Gu, Z.-H., Zhou, Z.-H., Yuan, W.-F. et al. PEGylated PLGA nanoparticles as protein carriers: synthesis, preparation and biodistribution in rats. *J. Control. Release* **2001**, *71*, 203–211.
304 Zambaux, M.-F., Faivre-Fiorina, B., Bonneaux, F., Marchal, S., Merlin, J.-L., Dellacherie, E. et al. Involvement of neutrophilic granulocytes in the uptake of biodegradable non-stealth and stealth nanoparticles in guinea pig. *Biomaterials* **2000**, *21*, 975–980.
305 Verrecchia, T., Spenlehauer, G., Bazile, D. V., Murry-Brelier, A., Archimbaud, Y., Veillard, M. Non-stealth (poly(lactic acid/albumin)) and stealth (poly(lactic acid–polyethylene glycol)) nanoparticles as injectable drug carriers. *J. Control. Release* **1995**, *36*, 49–61.
306 Le Ray, A. M., Vert, M., Gautier, J. C., Benoit, J. P. Fate of [^{14}C]poly-(lactide-*co*-glycolide)nanoparticles after intravenous and oral administration to mice. *Int. J. Pharm.* **1994**, *106*, 201–211.
307 Salem, A. K., Cannizzaro, S. M., Davies, M. C., Tendler, S. J. B., Roberts, C. J., Williams, P. M. et al. Synthesis and characterisation of a degradable poly(lactic acid)–poly(ethylene glycol) copolymer with biotinylated end groups. *Biomacromolecules* **2001**, *2*, 575–580.
308 Tessmar, J. K., Mikos, A. G., Gopferich, A. Amine-reactive biodegradable diblock copolymers. *Biomacromolecules* **2002**, *3*, 194–200.
309 Tessmar, J., Mikos, A., Gopferich, A. The use of poly(ethylene glycol)-block-poly(lactic acid) derived copolymers for the rapid creation of biomimetic surfaces. *Biomaterials* **2003**, *24*, 4475–4486.
310 Olivier, J.-C., Huertas, R., Lee, H. J., Calon, F., Pardridge, W. M. Synthesis of pegylated immuno-nanoparticles. *Pharm. Res.* **2002**, *19*, 1137–1143.
311 Munn, D. H., Mellor, A. L. Macrophages and the regulation of self-reactive T cells. *Curr. Pharm. Des* **2003**, *9*, 257–264.
312 Takahashi, K., Takeya, M., Sakashita, N. Multifunctional roles of macrophages in the development and progression of atherosclerosis in humans and experimental animals. *Med. Electron Microsc.* **2002**, *35*, 179–203.
313 Kamradt, T., Mitchison, N. A. Tolerance and autoimmunity. *N. Engl. J. Med.* **2001**, *344*, 655–664.
314 Tetley, T. D. Macrophages and the pathogenesis of COPD. *Chest* **2002**, *121 (5 Suppl.)*, 156–159.
315 Barnes, P. J. Chronic obstructive pulmonary disease. *N. Engl. J. Med.* **2000**, *343*, 269–280.
316 Davidson, A., Diamond, B. Autoimmune diseases. *N. Engl. J. Med.* **2001**, *345*, 340–350.
317 Geske, F. J., Monks, J., Lehman, L., Fadok, V. A. The role of the macrophage in apoptosis: hunter, gatherer, and regulator. *Int. J. Hematol.* **2002**, *76*, 16–26.
318 Libby, P., Ridker, P. M., Maseri, A. Inflammation and atherosclerosis. *Circulation* **2002**, *105*, 1135–1143.
319 Veerareddy, P. R., Vobalaboina, V. Lipid-based formulations of amphotericin B. *Drugs Today* **2004**, *40*, 133–145.
320 Lavasanifar, A., Samuel, J., Sattari, S., Kwon, G. S. Block Copolymer micelles for the encapsulation and delivery of amphotericin B. *Pharm. Res.* **2002**, *19*, 418–422.
321 Miller, C. B., Waller, E. K., Klingemann, H. G., Dignani, M. C., Anaissie, E. J., Cagnoni, P. J. et al. Lipid formulations of amphotericin B preserve and stabilize renal function in HSCT recipients. *Bone Marrow Transplant.* **2004**, *33*, 543–548.
322 Pinto-Alphandary, H., Andremont, A., Couvreur, P. Targeted delivery of

antibiotics using liposomes and nanoparticles: research and applications. *Int. J. Antimicrob. Agents* **2000**, *13*, 155–168.

323 Shadkchan, Y., Keisari, Y., Segal, E. Cytokines in mice treated with amphotericin B-intralipid. *Med. Mycol.* **2004**, *42*, 123–128.

324 Agrawal, A. K., Gupta, C. M. Tuftsin-bearing liposomes in treatment of macrophage-based infections. *Adv. Drug Deliv. Rev.* **2000**, *41*, 135–146.

325 Singh, M., O'Hagan, D. Advances in vaccine adjuvants. *Nature Biotechnology* **1999**, *17*, 1075–1081.

326 Dileo, J., Banerjee, R., Whitmore, M., Nayak, J. V., Falo, J., Louis, D., Huang, L. Lipid-protamine-DNA-mediated antigen delivery to antigen-presenting cells results in enhanced anti-tumor immune responses. *Mol. Ther.* **2003**, *7*, 640–648.

327 Mischler, R., Metcalfe, I. C. Inflexal®V a trivalent virosome subunit influenza vaccine: production. *Vaccine* **2002**, *20*, B17–B23.

328 Salem, A. K., Searson, P. C., Leong, K. W. Multifunctional nanorods for gene delivery. *Nat. Mater.* **2003**, *2*, 668–671.

329 Cui, Z., Mumper, R. J. Microparticles and nanoparticles as delivery systems for DNA vaccines. *Crit. Rev. Ther. Drug Carrier Syst.* **2003**, *20*, 103–137.

330 Taylor, P. R., Zamze, S., Stillion, R. J., Wong, S. Y. C., Gordon, S., Martinez-Pomares, L. Development of a specific system for targeting protein to metallophilic macrophages. *Proc. Natl Acad. Sci. USA* **2004**, *101*, 1963–1968.

331 Harisinghani, M. G., Barentsz, J., Hahn, P. F., Deserno, W. M., Tabatabaei, S., van de Kaa, C. H. et al. Noninvasive detection of clinically occult lymph-node metastases in prostate cancer. *N. Engl. J. Med.* **2003**, *348*, 2491–2499.

332 Moghimi, S. M., Bonnemain, B. Subcutaneous and intravenous delivery of diagnostic agents to the lymphatic system: applications in lymphoscintigraphy and indirect lymphography. *Adv. Drug Deliv. Rev.* **1999**, *37*, 295–312.

333 Dardzinski, B. J., Schmithorst, V. J., Holland, S. K., Boivin, G. P., Imagawa, T., Watanabe, S. et al. MR imaging of murine arthritis using ultrasmall superparamagnetic iron oxide particles. *Magn. Reson. Imaging* **2001**, *19*, 1209–1216.

334 Flacke, S., Fischer, S., Scott, M. J., Fuhrhop, R. J., Allen, J. S., McLean, M. et al. Novel MRI contrast agent for molecular imaging of fibrin: implications for detecting vulnerable plaques. *Circulation* **2001**, *104*, 1280–1285.

335 Winter, P. M., Morawski, A. M., Caruthers, S. D., Fuhrhop, R. W., Zhang, H., Williams, T. A. et al. Molecular imaging of angiogenesis in early-stage atherosclerosis with $\alpha_v\beta_3$-integrin-targeted nanoparticles. *Circulation* **2003**, *108*, 2270–2274.

336 Ruehm, S. G., Corot, C., Vogt, P., Kolb, S., Debatin, J. F. Magnetic resonance imaging of atherosclerotic plaque with ultrasmall superparamagnetic particles of iron oxide in hyperlipidemic rabbits. *Circulation* **2001**, *103*, 415–422.

337 Kooi, M. E., Cappendijk, V. C., Cleutjens, K. B. J. M., Kessels, A. G. H., Kitslaar, P. J. E. H. M., Borgers, M. et al. Accumulation of ultrasmall superparamagnetic particles of iron oxide in human atherosclerotic plaques can be detected by *in vivo* magnetic resonance imaging. *Circulation* **2003**, *107*, 2453–2458.

338 Lutgens, E., van Suylen, R. J., Faber, B. C., Gijbels, M. J., Eurlings, P. M., Bijnens, A. P. et al. Atherosclerotic plaque rupture: local or systemic process? *Arterioscler. Thromb. Vasc. Biol.* **2003**, *23*, 2123–2130.

339 Pearson, A. M., Rich, M., M., K. Polynucleotide binding to macrophage scavenger receptors depends on the formation of base-quartet-stabilized four-stranded helices. *J. Biol. Chem.* **1993**, *268*, 3546–3554.

340 Matsumoto, A., Naito, M., Itakura, H., Ikemoto, S., Asaoka, H.,

Hayakawa, I. et al. Human macrophage scavenger receptors: primary structure, expression, and localization in atherosclerotic lesions. *Proc. Natl Acad. Sci. USA* **1990**, *87*, 9133–9137.
341 Leach, J. K., Patterson, E., O'Rear, E. A. Improving thrombolysis with encapsulated plasminogen activators and clinical relevance to myocardial infarction and stroke. *Clin. Hemorheol. Microcirc.* **2004**, *30*, 225–228.
342 Holig, P., Bach, M., Volkel, T., Nahde, T., Hoffmann, S., Muller, R. et al. Novel RGD lipopeptides for the targeting of liposomes to integrin-expressing endothelial and melanoma cells. *Protein Eng. Des. Select.* **2004**, *17*, 433–441.
343 Kumar, C. C. Integrin alpha v beta 3 as a therapeutic target for blocking tumor-induced angiogenesis. *Curr. Drug Targets* **2003**, *4*, 123–131.
344 Wu, J., Nantz, M. H., Zern, M. A. Targeting hepatocytes for drug and gene delivery: emerging novel approaches and applications. *Front. Biosci.* **2002**, *7*, d717–725.
345 Wu, G. Y., Wu, C. H. Receptor-mediated gene delivery and expression *in vivo*. *J. Biol. Chem.* **1988**, *263*, 14621–14624.
346 Hashida, M., Kawakami, S., Yamashita, F. Lipid carrier systems for targeted drug and gene delivery. *Chem. Pharm. Bull. (Tokyo)* **2005**, *53*, 871–880.
347 Nishikawa, M. Development of cell-specific targeting systems for drugs and genes. *Biol. Pharm. Bull.* **2005**, *28*, 195–200.
348 Rensen, P. C., Herijgers, N., Netscher, M. H., Meskers, S. C., van Eck, M., van Berkel, T. J. Particle size determines the specificity of apolipoprotein E-containing triglyceride-rich emulsions for the LDL receptor versus hepatic remnant receptor *in vivo*. *J. Lipid Res.* **1997**, *38*, 1070–1084.
349 Pooga, M., Hallbrink, M., Zorko, M., Langel, U. Cell penetration by transportan. *FASEB J.* **1998**, *12*, 67–77.
350 Oehlke, J., Scheller, A., Wiesner, B., Krause, E., Beyermann, M., Klauschenz, E. et al. Cellular uptake of an α-helical amphipathic model peptide with the potential to deliver polar compounds into the cell interior non-endocytically. *Biochim. Biophys. Acta Biomembranes* **1998**, *1414*, 127–139.
351 Green, M., Loewenstein, P. M. Autonomous functional domains of chemically synthesized human immunodeficiency virus tat *trans*-activator protein. *Cell* **1988**, *55*, 1179–1188.
352 Frankel, A. D., Pabo, C. O. Cellular uptake of the tat protein from human immunodeficiency virus. *Cell* **1988**, *55*, 1189–1193.
353 Joliot, A., Pernelle, C., Deagostini-Bazin, H., Prochiantz, A. Antennapedia homeobox peptide regulates neural morphogenesis. *Proc. Natl Acad. Sci. USA* **1991**, *88*, 1864–1868.
354 Elliott, G., O'Hare, P. Intercellular trafficking and protein delivery by a herpesvirus structural protein. *Cell* **1997**, *88*, 223–233.
355 Lundberg, M., Johansson, M. Positively charged DNA-binding proteins cause apparent cell membrane translocation. *Biochem. Biophys. Res. Commun.* **2002**, *291*, 367–371.
356 Snyder, E., Dowdy, S. Cell penetrating peptides in drug delivery. *Pharm. Res.* **2004**, *21*, 389–393.
357 Fawell, S., Seery, J., Daikh, Y., Moore, C., Chen, L. L., Pepinsky, B. et al. Tat-mediated delivery of heterologous proteins into cells. *Proc. Natl Acad. Sci. USA* **1994**, *91*, 664–668.
358 Kim, D. T., Mitchell, D. J., Brockstedt, D. G., Fong, L., Nolan, G. P., Fathman, C. G. et al. Introduction of soluble proteins into the MHC class I pathway by conjugation to an HIV tat peptide. *J. Immunol.* **1997**, *159*, 1666–1668.
359 Schwarze, S. R., Ho, A., Vocero-Akbani, A., Dowdy, S. F. *In vivo* protein transduction: delivery of a

biologically active protein into the mouse. *Science* **1999**, *285*, 1569–1572.

360 Vogel, B., Lee, S., Hildebrand, A., Craig, W., Pierschbacher, M., Wong-Staal, F. et al. A novel integrin specificity exemplified by binding of the alpha v beta 5 integrin to the basic domain of the HIV Tat protein and vitronectin. *J. Cell Biol.* **1993**, *121*, 461–468.

361 Caron, N. J., Quenneville, S. P., Tremblay, J. P. Endosome disruption enhances the functional nuclear delivery of Tat-fusion proteins. *Biochem. Biophys. Res. Commun.* **2004**, *319*, 12–20.

362 Rothbard, J. B., Jessop, T. C., Lewis, R. S., Murray, B. A., Wender, P. A. Role of membrane potential and hydrogen bonding in the mechanism of translocation of guanidinium-rich peptides into cells. *J. Am. Chem. Soc* **2004**, *126*, 9506–9507.

363 Shen, H., Mai, J. C., Qiu, L., Cao, S., Robbins, P. D., Cheng, T. Evaluation of peptide-mediated transduction in human $CD34^+$ cells. *Hum. Gene Ther.* **2004**, *15*, 415–419.

364 Wadia, J. S., Stan, R. V., Dowdy, S. F. Transducible TAT–HA fusogenic peptide enhances escape of TAT-fusion proteins after lipid raft macropinocytosis. *Nature Medicine* **2004**, *10*, 310–315.

365 Becker-Hapak, M., McAllister, S. S., Dowdy, S. F. TAT-mediated protein transduction into mammalian cells. *Methods* **2001**, *24*, 247–256.

366 Embury, J., Klein, D., Pileggi, A., Ribeiro, M., Jayaraman, S., Molano, R. D. et al. Proteins linked to a protein transduction domain efficiently transduce pancreatic islets. *Diabetes* **2001**, *50*, 1706–1713.

367 Nagahara, H., Vocero-Akbani, A. M., Snyder, E. L., Ho, A., Latham, D. G., Lissy, N. A. et al. Transduction of full-length TAT fusion proteins into mammalian cells: TAT-p27Kip1 induces cell migration. *Nature Medicine* **1998**, *4*, 1449–1452.

368 Dolgilevich, S., Zaidi, N., Song, J., Abe, E., Moonga, B. S., Sun, L. Transduction of TAT fusion proteins into osteoclasts and osteoblasts. *Biochem. Biophys. Res. Commun.* **2002**, *299*, 505–509.

369 Eguchi, A., Akuta, T., Okuyama, H., Senda, T., Yokoi, H., Inokuchi, H. et al. Protein transduction domain of HIV-1 Tat protein promotes efficient delivery of DNA into mammalian cells. *J. Biol. Chem.* **2001**, *276*, 26204–26210.

370 Rudolph, C., Plank, C., Lausier, J., Schillinger, U., Muller, R. H., Rosenecker, J. Oligomers of the arginine-rich motif of the HIV-1 TAT protein are capable of transferring plasmid DNA into cells. *J. Biol. Chem.* **2003**, *278*, 11411–11418.

371 Jin, L. H., Bahn, J. H., Eum, W. S., Kwon, H. Y., Jang, S. H., Han, K. H. et al. Transduction of human catalase mediated by an HIV-1 TAT protein basic domain and arginine-rich peptides into mammalian cells. *Free Radic. Biol. Med.* **2001**, *31*, 1509–1519.

372 Astriab-Fisher, A., Sergueev, D., Fisher, M., Shaw, B. R., Juliano, R. L. Conjugates of antisense oligonucleotides with the tat and antennapedia cell-penetrating peptides: effects on cellular uptake, binding to target sequences, and biologic actions. *Pharm. Res.* **2002**, *19*, 744–754.

373 Stein, S., Weiss, A., Adermann, K., Lazarovici, P., Hochman, J., Wellhoner, H. A disulfide conjugate between anti-tetanus antibodies and HIV (37–72)Tat neutralizes tetanus toxin inside chromaffin cells. *FEBS Lett.* **1999**, *458*, 383–386.

374 Mie, M., Takahashi, F., Funabashi, H., Yanagida, Y., Aizawa, M., Kobatake, E. Intracellular delivery of antibodies using TAT fusion protein A. *Biochem. Biophys. Res. Commun.* **2003**, *310*, 730–734.

375 Polyakov, V., Sharma, V., Dahlheimer, J. L., Pica, C. M., Luker, G. D., Piwnica-Worms, D. Novel Tat–peptide chelates for direct transduction of technetium-99m and rhenium into human cells for imaging and radiotherapy. *Bioconjug. Chem.* **2000**, *11*, 762–771.

376 Bhorade, R., Weissleder, R., Nakakoshi, T., Moore, A., Tung, C. H. Macrocyclic chelators with paramagnetic cations are internalized into mammalian cells via a HIV-tat derived membrane translocation peptide. *Bioconjug. Chem. 11*, 301–305.
377 Kaufman, C. L., Williams, M., Ryle, L. M., Smith, T. L., Tanner, M., Ho, C. Superparamagnetic iron oxide particles transactivator protein–fluorescein isothiocyanate particle labeling for *in vivo* magnetic resonance imaging detection of cell migration: uptake and durability. *Transplantation* **2003**, *76*, 1043–1046.
378 Josephson, L., Tung, C. H., Moore, A., Weissleder, R. High-efficiency intracellular magnetic labeling with novel superparamagnetic–Tat peptide conjugates. *Bioconjug. Chem. 10*, 186–191.
379 Dodd, C. H., Hsu, H.-C., Chu, W.-J., Yang, P., Zhang, H.-G., Mountz, J., John, D. et al. Normal T-cell response and *in vivo* magnetic resonance imaging of T cells loaded with HIV transactivator-peptide-derived superparamagnetic nanoparticles. *J. Immunol. Methods* **2001**, *256*, 89–105.
380 Tkachenko, A. G., Xie, H., Liu, Y., Coleman, D., Ryan, J., Glomm, W. R. et al. Cellular trajectories of peptide-modified gold particle complexes: comparison of nuclear localization signals and peptide transduction domains. *Bioconjug. Chem. 15*, 482–490.
381 Torchilin, V. P., Rammohan, R., Weissig, V., Levchenko, T. S. TAT peptide on the surface of liposomes affords their efficient intracellular delivery even at low temperature and in the presence of metabolic inhibitors. *Proc. Natl Acad. Sci. USA* **2001**, *98*, 8786–8791.
382 Levchenko, T. S., Rammohan, R., Volodina, N., Torchilin, V. P. Tat peptide-mediated intracellular delivery of liposomes. *Methods Enzymol.* **2003**, *372*, 339–349.
383 Torchilin, V. P., Levchenko, T. S., Rammohan, R., Volodina, N., Papahadjopoulos-Sternberg, B., D'Souza, G. G. M. Cell transfection *in vitro* and *in vivo* with nontoxic TAT peptide–liposome–DNA complexes. *Proc. Natl Acad. Sci. USA* **2003**, *100*, 1972–1977.
384 Oberdorster, G., Oberdorster, E., Oberdorster, J. Nanotoxicology: an emerging discipline evolving from studies of ultrafine particles. *Environ. Health Perspect.* **2005**, *113*, 823–839.
385 Seaton, A., Donaldson, K. Nanoscience, nanotoxicology, and the need to think small. *Lancet 365*, 923–924.
386 Hampton, T. Researchers size up nanotechnology risks. *J. Am. Med. Ass.* **2005**, *294*, 1881–1883.
387 Gordijn, B. Nanoethics: from utopian dreams and apocalyptic nightmares towards a more balanced view. *Sci. Eng. Ethics* **2005**, *11*, 521–533.
388 Joachim, C. To be nano or not to be nano? *Nat. Mater.* **2005**, *4*, 107–109.

6
Nanoporous and Nanosize Materials for Drug Delivery Systems

Yoshinobu Fukumori, Kanji Takada and Hirofumi Takeuchi

6.1
Introduction

Nanomaterials have attracted much attention recently in the pharmaceutical field as structural components of pharmaceutical dosage forms. Such an application for nanomaterials has been found in coating materials in aqueous latex systems. Their use for granules and tablets has led to the successful development of many types of controlled release dosage forms. These have provided many excellent examples of nanostructure construction in micro- and macro-devices in the field of nanotechnology. In Section 6.2, nanomaterials for particle coating that are still useful and are expected to achieve further developments in pharmaceutical manufacturing, including commercially available polymeric nanoparticles, novel terpolymer nanoparticles, core–shell nanoparticles and biodegradable chitosan nanoparticles, are described.

Further, the recent development of biotechnology and its application to therapy and diagnosis requires nanoparticulate delivery of a variety of agents. The nanomaterials prepared for various purposes are simply analyzed according to their structural characteristics in Section 6.3.

In addition, the development of nanotechnology has produced many compounds that are specially structured to be nanoporous, and the obtained compounds are applied to many fields such electronics, microfabrication technology and biotechnology, including drug delivery systems. Section 6.4 deals with this hot and attractive topic. The purpose of drug delivery systems is to deliver drug molecules to their target sites for a desired period with a desired concentration. To accomplish this, several functions including sensing, targeting and controlled release are required. Nanoporous compounds are generally used to facilitate the controlled release function to drug delivery systems. Many nanoporous materials, mostly organic and some inorganic, have been studied for drug delivery system usage. Among them, calcium compounds like calcium carbonate ($CaCO_3$), calcium phosphate [$Ca(H_2PO_4)_2$], tricalcium phosphate [$Ca_3(PO_4)_2$] hydroxyapatite [$Ca_{10}(PO_4)_6(OH)_2$] and silastic compounds are well-known drug delivery system carriers. In addition, nanofabrication technology has recently prepared new nano-

Nanotechnologies for the Life Sciences Vol. 10
Nanomaterials for Medical Diagnosis and Therapy. Edited by Challa S. S. R. Kumar

ISBN: 978-3-527-31390-7

porous materials like carbon nanotubes (CNTs), fullerene and single-wall carbon nanohorns (SWNHs). These novel nanomaterials have also been used to clarify the possible biocompatibility, potential utilities and applications in biological settings, i.e. a drug delivery system carrier.

Section 6.5 will focus on the pharmaceutical application of porous silica, which includes both conventional and newly developed uses. One of the topics involves a solid dispersion system to improve the dissolution property of poorly water-soluble drugs. It is demonstrated that the well-ordered porous structure of silica particles can control the crystalline form of drugs in the solid dispersion system, which leads to a much improved dissolution rate. Mesoporous silica, having a highly controlled pore size and structure, is an attractive material. Some experimental data shown encourage us to use this novel material as a carrier of peptide drugs as well as poorly water-soluble drugs.

Thus, this chapter is the first challenge to describe the role of nanomaterials in pharmaceutics in an integrated manner.

6.2 Nanomaterials for Coating

The pharmaceutical application of nanomaterials can be found in latex systems that have been used as coating materials for the last 40 years. Several types of latex are commercially used worldwide. Their application in granules and tablets has led to many controlled release dosage forms on the market. Therein, spray-coating processes such as fluidized bed, spouted bed and tumbling fluidized bed processes can easily provide multilayered particle structures with each layer being monolithic, a random multiphase nanostructure or ordered multiphase nanostructure, etc., as shown in Fig. 6.1. In general, the combination of different monolithic

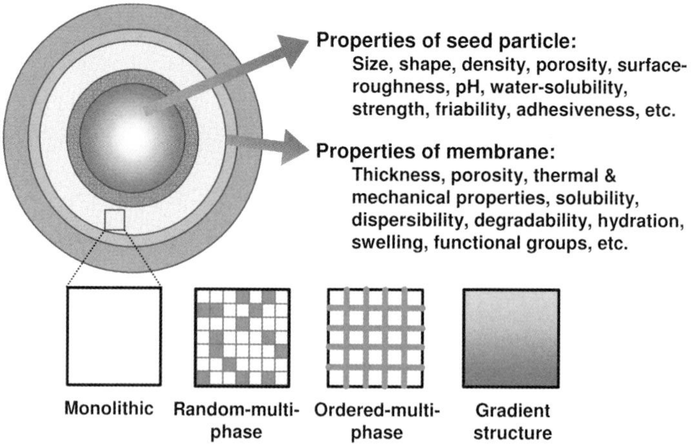

Figure 6.1. Construction of microparticles with nanomaterials.

nanomaterials and, especially, nanostructured nanomaterials can produce an almost infinite array of functional microparticulate products. However, commercially available latexes are formed as monolithic structures from random co- or terpolymers that are designed to be used chiefly for coating such coarse particles as granules and tablets. For further and broader application of this technique, Fukumori and coworkers [1, 2] have been proposing the novel terpolymer and core–shell latexes through their development of fine particle-coating technology and highly functional microcapsules, such as thermosensitive drug-releasing microcapsules using sophisticated latexes with temperature-dependent swelling properties.

6.2.1 Commercially Available Aqueous Polymeric Nanomaterials

Table 6.1 lists commercially available nanomaterials for particle coating [1, 3, 4–16]. They are classified into two types based on the preparation methods [17]: (i) 1atexes synthesized by emulsion polymerization, and (ii) pseudolatexes prepared by emulsion processes such as emulsion-solvent evaporation, phase inversion and solvent change. Cellulose derivatives cannot be synthesized directly in latexes;

Tab. 6.1. Typical manomaterials for coating

Brand	Supplier	Solubility	Main component	References
Aquacoat ECD	FMC	insoluble	ethylcellulose pseudolatex	4, 11, 13
Aquacoat CPD	FMC	enteric	cellulose acetate phthalate pseudolatex	
Surelease	Colorcon	insoluble	ethylcellulose pseudolatex	9
Eudragit RS30D	Röhm	insoluble	1:2:0.1 poly(EA–MMA–TAMC1) pseudolatex	7, 10–13, 16
Eudragit RL30D	Röhm	insoluble	1:2:0.2 poly(EA–MMA–TAMC1) pseudolatex	7, 16
Eudragit NE30D	Röhm	insoluble	2:1 poly(EA–MMA) latex	5, 6, 8, 11
Eudragit L30D	Röhm	enteric	1:1 poly(EA–MAA) latex	8, 12, 14
Eudragit FS30D	Röhm	enteric	7:3:1 poly(MA–MMA–MAA) latex	14–16
Kollicoat MAE30D/DP	BASF	enteric	1:1 poly(EA–MAA) latex	4
Kollicoat EMM30D	BASF	insoluble	2:1 poly(EA–MMA) latex	4
Kollicoat SR30D	BASF	insoluble	polyvinyl acetate latex	4

therefore, they are prepared as pseudolatexes (Aquacoat ECD [18], Aquacoat CPD and Surelease [19] in Tab. 6.1).

Eudragit™ L30D and NE30D are acrylic copolymer latexes synthesized by emulsion polymerization [20]. The particle sizes of these latexes are in the submicron order. L30D is a copolymer of ethyl acrylate (EA) as an ester component with methacrylic acid (MAA) (MAA:EA 1:1). It is used for enteric coating because of the presence of carboxyl groups in the copolymer. NE30D is a copolymer of ester components only, EA and MMA (2:1). The films formed from NE30D have a very low softening temperature (T_s), and hence are flexible and expandable even under normal room conditions.

Eudragit RS and RL are terpolymers of EA and MMA as ester components with trimethylaminoethyl methacrylate chloride (TAMC1) as hydrophilic quaternary ammonium groups; RS and RL are 1:2:0.1 and 1:2:0.2 terpoly(EA–MMA–TAMC1), respectively. As Eudragit RS and RL contain MMA-rich ester components (EA:MMA 1:2), they have T_ss higher than those of NE30D (EA:MMA 2:1) and form hard films under room conditions. Eudragit RS and RL powders are easily transformed into pseudolatexes by emulsifying their powders in hot water without additives [20].

The film formation process from aqueous dispersion is shown schematically in Fig. 6.2. The mechanisms of film formation from aqueous polymeric dispersions have been discussed for a long time and many theories have been proposed. The

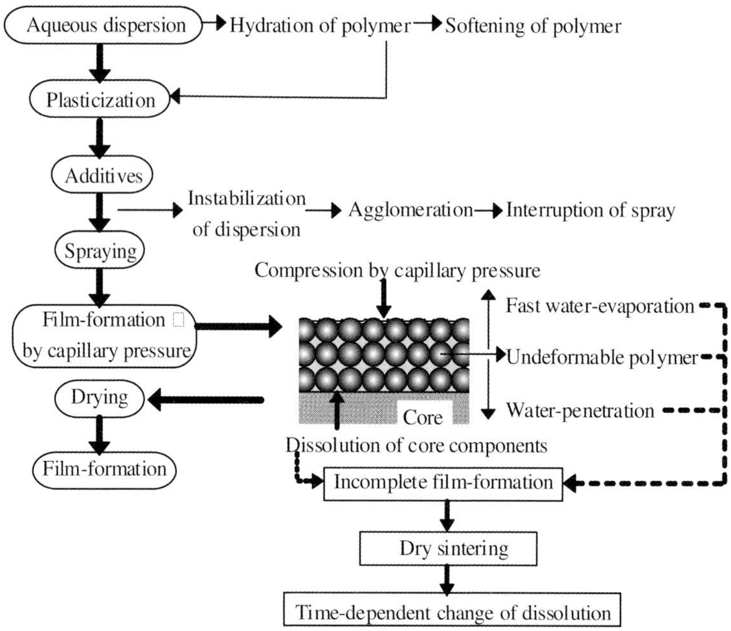

Figure 6.2. Film formation from aqueous dispersions of polymeric nanoparticles.

mechanisms were reviewed by Muroi [21]. Film formation in pharmaceutical applications was discussed by Steuernagel [18], Lehmann [20] and Fukumori [17]. Fusion and film formation of polymeric particles during the coating process can be explained by the wet sintering theory for particles suspended in water, the capillary pressure theory for particle layers containing water in various degrees of saturation and the dry sintering theory for dry particle layers. In all cases, as the particle size becomes smaller, film formation is further enhanced. This is the reason why nanomaterials have been used for aqueous suspension coating.

6.2.2
Novel Terpolymer Nanoparticles for Coating

The most serious problem encountered in fine particle coating using a wet-spraying process is agglomeration. Agglomeration takes place when coating materials supplied among seed particles possess a binding strength stronger than the separation force exerted on core particles. In water- or organic solvent-based solution systems, 10% of 53- to 63-μm lactose particles was unavoidably agglomerated, although various additives to hydroxypropylcellulose (HPC) or ethylcellulose (EC) were sought to reduce the binding strength of sprayed materials [22–25]. In contrast, when aqueous lattices were sprayed, there were some cases where only a minor degree of agglomeration was observed, even for 32- to 44-μm lactose particles [26].

In order to investigate latex as a candidate for spray liquid in fine particle coating, aqueous latexes of terpoly[EA–MMA–2-hydroxyethyl methacrylate (HEMA)] were newly synthesized [27, 28] (Fig. 6.3). When the molar ratio of the monomers used in polymerization was changed, the increase in MMA content raised the T_s of the cast film; HEMA affected T_s far less than MMA, but remarkably enhanced film formation and the release of a water-soluble substance (lactose) in aqueous medium. Further, when T_s was higher than the inlet air temperature, the terpolymer latexes exhibited a very low degree of agglomeration in the coating, due to their poor film-formability and, consequently, their low binding strength. This means

Figure 6.3. Chemical structure of poly(EA–MMA–HEMA).

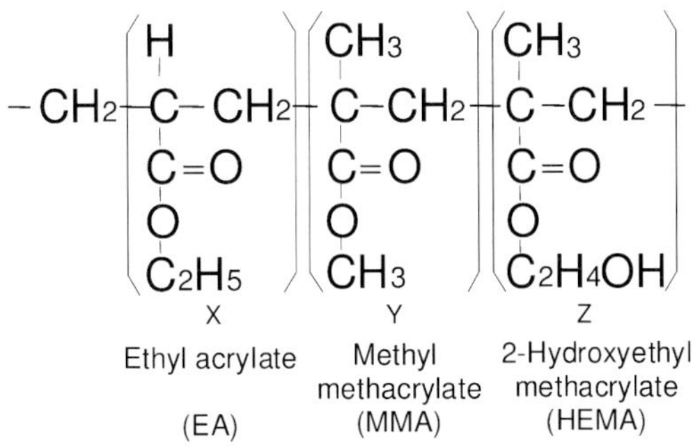

that the drying/layering of latex particles has to be separated from the film-forming process to avoid agglomeration in fine particle coating; when both occur simultaneously, as in the solution systems; agglomeration of particles smaller than 50 µm cannot be avoided. This consequently led to a poor fixing efficiency of cosuspended solid particles, but the coating efficiency of the polymer dispersed as nanoparticles remained high [26]. This low tendency towards agglomeration was confirmed even in the coating of particles as fine as 32–44 µm.

6.2.3
Core–shell Nanoparticles for Fine Particle Coating

An aqueous latex exhibiting a low degree of agglomeration, low membrane permeation and high coating efficiency was developed using poly(EA–MMA–HEMA), whose monomer molar ratio was 6:12:8 or 12:6:4 [29]. Differing from blend latexes, the composite latexes (Fig. 6.4) composed of the low-permeable 12:6:4 polymer core and the nonadhesive 6:12:8 polymer shell with a 6:4 core–shell weight ratio formed a low-permeable membrane by curing. Thus, the 40% coated microcapsules of 53- to 63-µm lactose released only 10% of the lactose at 3 h. Moreover, the composite latexes exhibited a very low degree of agglomeration, with the polymer yield remaining very high, and they did not induce any adhesive behavior during the coating operation. These properties were still effective even in the coating of cornstarch as fine as 12 µm: at a 50% level of coating, the mass median diameter of the product was 16 µm and it contained only 3% agglomerates. These results showed that by using the composite latex, particles of the order of 10 µm could be discretely coated as single-core microcapsules in the spouted bed process assisted with a draft tube.

However, there still remained five serious problems with the coating process of 12-µm particles; (i) particle circulation and fluidization was too unsteady, (ii) the process was too time consuming, (ii) drug loading by spraying was not accom-

Figure 6.4. Composite nanoparticle with a core–shell structure for fine particle coating.

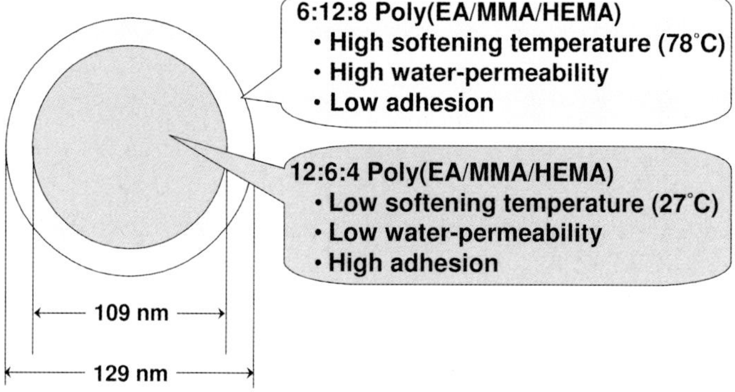

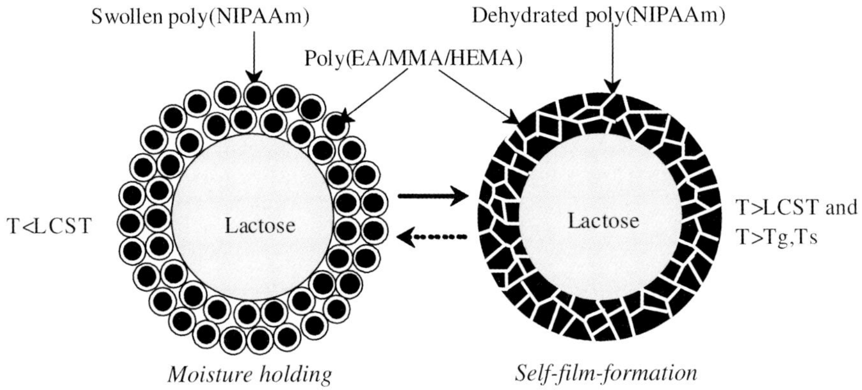

Figure 6.5. Microcapsules coated with composite nanoparticles with a poly(EA–MMA–HEMA) core and a poly(NIPAAm) shell.

plished because the corn starch particles were too small to avoid agglomeration, (iv) surfaces of the coated corn starch were too rough and porous to be cured by heating, and (v) to avoid agglomeration of core particles, spray liquid flow had to be adjusted to a low rate, leading to particle adhesion to the chamber wall due to electrostatic charge. Thus, in order to overcome the last two problems, aqueous composite latex that suppressed the particle adhesion in the coating process and had a self-film-formability in water was developed as a coating material [30]. This composite latex consisted of a poly(EA–MMA–HEMA) core and a thermosensitive poly(*N*-isopropylacrylamide) (NIPAAm) shell (Fig. 6.5). When compared to homogeneous latexes with no poly(NIPAAm) shell, the composite latexes reduced the production of poorly coated particles and the particle size dependence of polymer yield when the coating operation was done at a temperature where poly(NIPAAm) shells were able to swell, i.e. below the lower critical solution temperature (LCST: 32 °C) of poly(NIPAAm). Further, the microcapsules coated with the composite latexes also exhibited a self-film-formability in water at 37 °C, resulting from shrinkage of the poly(NIPAAm) shells in the membrane at temperatures above the LCST.

6.2.4 Core–Shell Nanoparticles for Thermosensitively Drug-releasing Microcapsules

Recently, much attention has been focused on thermosensitive controlled-release systems developed from polymer networks with specific temperature-dependent swelling behaviors [31, 32]. In these systems, temperature variation triggers alteration of polymer configurations, leading to a thermally responsive change in the release rate of therapeutic agents to the systems.

One of the important issues in current thermosensitive release systems is how to facilitate the swelling/shrinking rate of hydrogels involving thermosensitivity. Improving swelling kinetics is an important subject for controlled drug release,

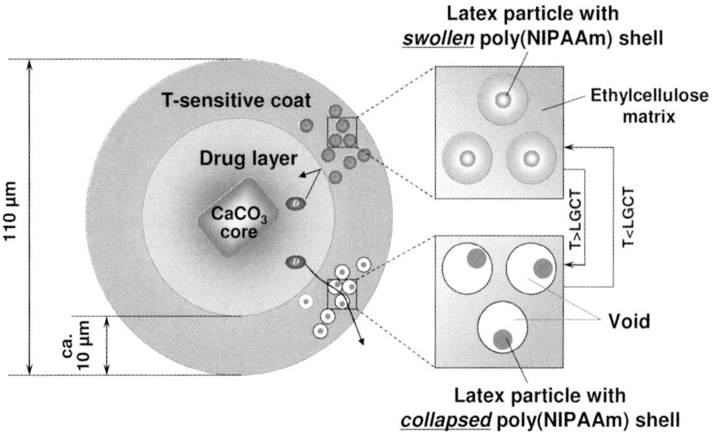

Figure 6.6. Microcapsules exhibiting positive thermosensitive drug release.

particularly pulsatile release with a thermal "on–off" switching response. The gel swelling/shrinking rate can be increased by an appropriate molecular and structural design of the polymer network. These include hydrogels with macroporous [33] and comb-type structures [34]. Incorporating thermosensitive hydrogels into fine particulate systems may be an alternative approach to make systems respond more rapidly to an external temperature change. Additionally, their small dimensions simultaneously offer considerable advantages over disk- or film-shaped macrogels hitherto developed in terms of a wide variety of biomedical applications.

The composite latexes composed of a hydrophobic poly(EA–MMA) core and a thermosensitive poly(NIPAAm) shell (Fig. 6.6) [35] were synthesized by a semicontinuous two-stage emulsion polymerization technique. The poly(NIPAAm) shell was crosslinked with methylene bisacrylamide. The microcapsules with thermosensitive coats were prepared using a Grow Max (140) spouted bed coater assisted with a draft tube and bottom spray (Fuji Paudal, Japan), known as the Wurster process. The microcapsules were cured by heating at 80 °C for 12 h and their dissolution properties were tested by a column method.

The key structure of the microcapsule designed here is its composite coat, consisting of nanosized thermosensitive hydrogels dispersed in a thermo-insensitive polymeric matrix. Ethyl cellulose pseudo latex, Aquacoat ECD (Tab. 6.1), was chosen as the polymeric matrix. As the nanosized thermosensitive hydrogels, a newly synthesized composite latex with a poly(NIPAAm)-rich shell was used. It is well known that poly(NIPAAm) has a phase transition temperature (LCST) of around 32 °C in water. The crosslinked network (hydrogel) constituted from this polymer shows an inverse temperature dependence of swelling: the hydrogel swells by imbibing water below a lower gel collapse temperature (LGCT; temperature for complete deswelling), while it shrinks at temperatures above the LGCT. At high temperatures, therefore, the poly(NIPAAm)-gel domains in the microcapsule membranes shrink, probably leading to the creation of many voids in the membranes. Consequently, the water permeability increases as if a molecular valve has been opened. Due to the voids thus formed, the drug release rate at high temperatures is expected to become higher than that at low temperatures.

In order to confirm the reversibility of thermosensitive changes causing swelling, hydrodynamic size changes of the composite lattices in response to a stepwise shift in temperature were measured by photon correlation. As the temperature was elevated, particle size gradually decreased up to approximately 35 °C, near the volume transition temperature of crosslinked poly(NIPAAm) in water. Above 35 °C, particle size did not remarkably decrease any further. On the other hand, particle size became large again upon cooling. There was no significant difference between the traces of the particle size changes upon heating and cooling, indicating thermally reversible changes in the swelling/shrinking of the poly(NIPAAm) shells on the latex particles. Such a reversible change is a prerequisite to facilitate an "on–off" pulsatile drug release from the microcapsules.

No significant thermosensitivity was found in the release rate of the microcapsules with only Aquacoat film. In contrast, the microcapsules with the composite latex-dispersing coat in an 85:15 blending ratio of Aquacoat and the composite latex exhibited pulsatile thermosensitive release rate changes. Additionally, these microcapsules demonstrated a positive thermosensitivity of drug release, i.e. high release rates at high temperature (50 °C) and low release rates at low temperature (30 °C), except for a less pronounced burst effect in the initial period at 30 °C. It is noteworthy that the sharp release rate changes from the "on" state to the "off" state, and *vise versa*, occurred within a few minutes. Fabrication of composite latex having nanosized thickness poly(NIPAAm) shells and thin microcapsule coats in the order of 10 μm would be responsible for the resulting fast response.

6.2.5
Chitosan Nanoparticles for Microparticle Coating

As is well-known, chitosan (poly[β-(1–4)-2-amino-2-deoxy-D-glucopyranose]) is a hydrophilic and cationic polysaccharide derived from chitin deacetylation, which is the second most abundant polysaccharide in the world after cellulose and a promising resource originating from crustaceans shells and insects [36]. Chitosan has some interesting properties such as acting as a bioadhesive (cationic), with biocompatible (nontoxic) and biodegradable (bioerodible) capabilities. Therefore, it has been investigated in depth, and used in various industrial and medical applications. Furthermore, these interesting properties make it one of the most promising biopolymers for drug delivery [37–46]. Indeed, chitosan has been studied as a drug carrier in various forms, such as tablets, beads, granules, microparticles and nanoparticles. In particular, micro/nanoparticles are the most widely studied as drug carriers for protein, peptide, vaccine and DNA delivery.

A wide variety of preparation methods of chitosan particles such as solvent evaporation techniques, multiple emulsion methods, spray-drying methods, electrostatic complex formation with anionic materials (ionotropic gelation) and block copolymerization have been investigated. These methods often require a crosslinking agent, such as glutaraldehyde. While the use of the crosslinking agent produces hardened particles as well as a drug-release rate possibly controllable in response to the degree of crosslinking, the toxicity of the crosslinking agent would become a major concern. In addition, it leads to a low loading of anionic drugs because amino groups in chitosan responsible for electrostatic interactions with anionic drugs become unavailable due to the crosslinking reaction between the amino groups in chitosan and aldehyde groups in crosslinking agents.

Masui and coworkers [47] reported a study aimed at preparing noncovalently crosslinked chitosan nanoparticles (CNSs) without the use of any organic solvents and additives. For this purpose, an aqueous neutralization–precipitation technique was newly developed. They prepared chitosan nanoparticles in the range of 150–300 nm. Furthermore, spouted-bed spray-coating of protein-layered particles with the noncovalently crosslinked chitosan nanoparticles was carried out and their excellent performance as a biodegradable coating agent was then demonstrated.

6.3
Materials for Nanoparticulate Therapy and Diagnosis

In general, nanoparticles for drug delivery, such as in cancer therapy and diagnosis, are simply constructed, and have a core, shell and surface (Fig. 6.7) [48]. The core determines the particle size and generally consists of an inactive matrix, the active agent itself or an active agent-containing matrix. The shell chemically or physically bound to the core acts as a base to which surface molecules, that sometimes include active agents, are anchored or bound with or without intermediate spacers; in some cases, it acts as an active agent-dispersed matrix. The surface

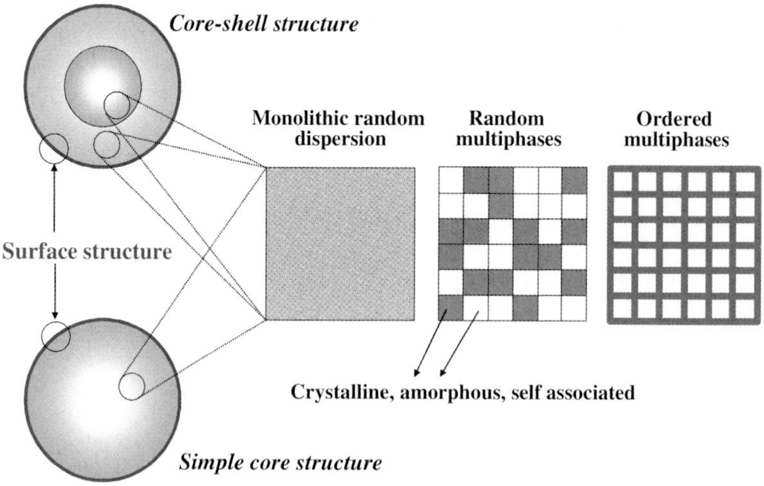

Figure 6.7. Typical structures of composite nanoparticles.

molecules strongly affect the biodistribution of the nanoparticles that usually consist of site-, tissue-, cell- and/or receptor-specific molecules (targeting agents). The poly(ethylene glycol) (PEG) molecules that possibly induce a bound water layer on the particle surface are attached to the shell or surface molecules by physical adsorption or covalent bonding with or without intermediate spacers. The mode of bonding used in particle construction is important from the viewpoint that the rate and timing of release or degradation of the components from the particles have to be controlled in order to achieve their biodistribution and active agent delivery in cancer treatment and diagnosis. The nanoparticles have to be degraded in the body and finally eliminated by globular filtration as molecules with a molecular weight of less than 30 000 or as particles with a size smaller than a few nanometers.

The structures of nanoparticles for cancer therapy and diagnosis are simple, as described above. Tables 6.2 and 6.3 show typical examples of the structures and components of nanoparticles.

6.3.1 Inorganic Nanoparticles

Recently, inorganic nanoparticles that interact with biological systems have attracted widespread interest in biology and medicine (Tab. 6.2). Such nanoparticles are thought to have potential as novel intravascular probes for both diagnostic (e.g. imaging) and therapeutic purposes (e.g. drug delivery). Critical issues for successful nanoparticle delivery include the ability to target specific tissues and cell types, and escape from the biological particulate filter – the reticuloendothelial system (RES).

Among inorganic materials, magnetite has been investigated most widely for cancer therapy and diagnosis [49–56]. Magnetite nanoparticles are used directly or dispersed in the polymeric matrix as cores. They have been used chiefly in hyperthermia treatment of cancer [49, 55] and, in some cases, for magnetic field-assisted targeting of nanoparticles [55]. For diagnostic purposes, they are used in magnetic resonance imaging (MRI) as contrast-enhancing agents for cancer diagnosis [49], hyperfusion region visualization [50], cell labeling in T cell-based therapy [51–53], and for detection of angiogenesis [50], apoptosis [54] and gene expression [56]. PEG [55] or oxidized starch [50] as a hydrophilic surface modifier, antibodies [49], fluorescein isothiocyanate (FITC)-labeled TAT peptide [51–53] or the Annexin V protein [54] as a specific targeting agent, and folic acid [55] or transferrin [56] as a ligand of the receptors overexpressed in tumor cells have been used as surface molecules.

Akerman and coworkers [57] (Tab. 6.2) explored the feasibility of *in vivo* targeting using semiconductor quantum dots. Quantum dots are small (less than 10 nm) inorganic nanocrystals that possess unique luminescent properties; their fluorescence emission is stable and is tuned by varying the particle size or composition. Akerman and coworkers showed that ZnS-capped CdSe quantum dots coated with a lung-targeting peptide accumulated in the lungs of mice after intravenous

Tab. 6.2. Typical examples of inorganic materials for nanoparticulate drug delivery

No.	Therapeutic purpose	Particle size (nm) [structure]	Characterization	Delivery agent	Core–shell component (additive)	Surface component	References
1	Hyperthermia, cancer diagnosis	[agglome rate-liposome]	biodistribution, anti-cancer effect, diagnosis	magnetite	magnetite	phospholipid bilayer, antibody	49
2	MRI, hyperfusion region visualization, angiogenesis		kidney perfusion, tumor capillary leakage	clariscan (superpara-magnetite)	magnetite	oxidized starch	50
3	Cell-based therapy, cell labeling		T cell delivery to tumor, MRI	dextran-coated CLIO	CLIO	Tat peptide–FITC	51–53
4	MRI of apoptosis (phosphatidylserine recognition)		MRI imaging	CLIO	CLIO	Annexin V (protein)	54
5	MRI, hyperthemia, magnetic field-assisted radionuclide therapy	10	tumor and macrophage cell uptake	magnetite	magnetite	PEG, folate	55
6	MRI, detection of gene expression		conjugation number, cell binding, cell uptake, transferrin receptor expression	dextran-coated CLIO, MION	CLIO, MION	transferrin (Tf-S-S-CLIO)	56
7	Disease sensing, drug delivery	<10 (uncoated: 3.5, 5.5) [core–shell]	cell binding, *in vivo* targeting, RES uptake		CdSe (core)–ZnS (shell)	peptide/PEG	57
8	Intracellular diagnostics, therapeutic delivery	20 (gold), 25 (whole) [core–shell]	nuclear targeting		gold (core)–BSA (shell)	five peptides (nuclear localiza-tion signal, etc.)	58

CLIO: crosslinked ion oxide; MION: monocrystalline ion oxide nanoparticle.

injection, whereas two other peptides specifically directed quantum dots to blood vessels or lymphatic vessels in tumors. They also showed that adding PEG to the quantum dot coating prevented quantum dots from nonselective accumulation in reticuloendothelial tissues.

Tkachenko and coworkers [58] (Tab. 6.2) explored the ability of peptide-modified gold nanoparticles to target the nucleus of HepG2 cells. Five peptide/nanoparticle complexes were investigated to modify particles. They used gold nanoparticles because they are easy to identify using video-enhanced color differential interference contrast microscopy. Their studies highlight the challenges associated with nuclear targeting and the potential advantages of designing multifunctional nanostructured materials as tools for intracellular diagnostics and therapeutic delivery.

6.3.2 Polymeric Nanoparticles

The active agents are mostly incorporated in the cores to control or suppress their release. Polymers have been widely used as matrix materials. Table 6.3 shows examples of polymeric nanoparticles [59–78] that have recently been investigated for delivery; as an anticancer drug, doxorubicin, whose liposomes are on the market as Doxil^{TM} (Alza) has often been used [62]. In these nanoparticles, biodegradable polymers, such as poly(lactic acid) (PLA) [59, 62], poly(lactic-*co*-glycolic acid), poly(ε-caprolactone) (PCL) [60, 61], chitosan [64, 69–72], poly(acrylcyanoacrylate) (PACA), poly(lysine) [62] and poly(aspartic acid) [62], are used as the core matrix. Lipid [65, 78] and wax matrixes [63, 73–77] have also been used in nanoparticles, as shown in Tab. 6.2. The particles used in gene therapy are often cationic to enhance association with anionic cell surfaces and/or DNAs [63–66].

Kataoka and coworkers [62] developed block copolymer micelles for drug and gene delivery. They reported the utility of polymeric micelles formed through the multimolecular assembly of block copolymers as novel core–shell-type nanoparticles for drug and gene targeting. The segregated core embedded in the hydrophilic palisade was shown to function as a reservoir for genes, enzymes and a variety of drugs with diverse characteristics. Functionalization of the outer surface of the polymeric micelle to modify its physicochemical and biological properties was carried out for long circulation and receptor-mediated drug delivery.

6.3.3 Other Case Studies

A variety of methodologies of treatment and strategies of delivery have been applied to cancer therapy and diagnosis. In order to achieve an efficient outcome, nanoparticles have been designed using materials that are thought to be optimal for their respective applications. The following typical applications of nanoparticles have been reported: targeting lectin present on the intestinal epithelial cell surface by wheat germ agglutinin on a PCL matrix [67], antileishmania treatment by PCL matrix nanoparticles [68], gadolinium neutron capture therapy (GdNCT) by intra-

Tab. 6.3. Typical examples of organic materials for nanoparticulate drug delivery

No.	Therapeutic purpose	Particle size (nm) [structure]	Characterization	Delivery agent	Core–shell component (additive)	Surface component	References
1	Passive drug targeting	118 [polymeric matrix]	drug content, antitumor effect, plasma concentration	irinotecan	PLA, PEG–PPG–PEG	PEG–PPG–PEG	59
2	Passive and estrogen receptor targeting	250–300 [polymeric matrix]	cell uptake, intracellular distribution, localization	tamoxifen	PCL (MW: 14.8)	Pluronic F-68	60, 61
3	Passive and active targeting	50–100/32 [polymeric matrix]	biodistribution, transfection	doxorubicin, DNA	PEG–poly(aspartic acid)/PEG–PLA/PEG–Poly(lysine)	PEG	62
4	Gene therapy	100–160 [wax matrix]	DNA stability, transfection, biodistribution	plasmid DNA lipophilized with cationic lipid	Wax, Brij 78, Tween 20, Tween 80	Chol-pullulan	63
5	Gene therapy	309 [polymeric matrix]	*in vitro* proliferation, degradation	*Mycobacterium phlei* DNA	Chitosan (MW: 500 000, 84% deacetylated [TPP]		64
6	Anti-angiogenic gene therapy	40 (core) [lipid matrix]	tumor cell apotosis, tumor regression	plasmid DNA (APTmu-Raf)	polymerized cationic lipid	Integrin $\alpha_v\beta_3$	65

7	Gene therapy	100–150 [polymeric matrix]	*in vitro* transfection	nucleic acid	cyclodextrin polycation	transferrin–PEG–adamantane	66
8	Neutron capture therapy	300–500 [polymeric matrix]	tumor retension, growth suppression	gadopentatete dimeglumine	chitosan		69–72
9	Neutron capture therapy	50–80 [wax matrix]	cell uptake, biodistribution, tumor retention	gadolinium hexan edione	wax [Brij 78/Brij 72/ Tween 80]	folate/thiamine–PEG–DSPE, PEG–DSPE	73–77
10	Photodynamic therapy	120 [lipid matrix]	cytotoxicity, receptor binding	hematoporphyrin	triolein [egg PC, Tween 80]	folate, PEG spacer	78

Chol-pullulan: {*N*-[2-(cholesterylcarboxyamino)ethyll]carbamorylmethyl}-pullulan; DSPE: distearoylphosphatidylethanolamine.

tumorally injectable chitosan nanoparticles [69–72] (Tab. 6.2) and wax matrix nanoparticles surface-modified with folic acid or thiamine whose uptake is enhanced in tumor cells [73–77] (Tab. 6.2), photodynamic therapy by solid lipid nanoparticles (SLNs) [78] (Tab. 6.2) or silicate matrix nanoparticles [79], application of dendrimer [80], antiangiogenesis radiotherapy by ^{90}Y chelated on the liposome surfaces using an integrin antagonist [81], drug delivery to the brain by PACA matrix nanoparticles [82] and detection of antigen by immunolabeled europium-holding poly(styrene)nanoparticles [83].

6.4 Nanoporous Materials as Drug Delivery System Carriers

6.4.1 Inorganic Calcium Compounds

Nanoporous materials have been used as a drug delivery system carrier [84–86]. Among them, Higuchi and coworkers used hydroxyapatite as a carrier for delivering drugs to skeletal tissue at high enough local concentrations for desirable therapeutic effects [87]. Using a self-setting hydroxyapatite cement with cephalexin, norfloxacin and indomethacin (IMC), the cement was transformed into hydroxyapatite with affinity for hard bone tissue. Continuous *in vitro* drug release profiles from loaded cement pellets in phosphate buffer, pH 7.4, were obtained. As the cements have good biocompatibility in both periodontal and periapical environments, self-setting cement skeletal drug delivery systems are thought to provide temporary replacement therapy for bone [88].

Porous $CaCO_3$ particles were reported to be useful as an intranasal carrier of insulin and hydrophilic compounds, because of their easy production and slow biodegradability [89–91]. However, the binding of adsorbed drugs to $CaCO_3$ was weak, i.e. drugs and proteins were adsorbed on the surface of solid particles or porous $CaCO_3$ material. Therefore, sufficient sustained release was not obtained. Mizushima and coworkers devised a simple method to incorporate hydrophilic drugs and proteins into nano-$CaCO_3$ and regulate the size of the particles. The mean particle size of the $CaCO_3$ was 44.8–140.7 nm depending on the mixing speed of both particles and the drug. Sustained-release of erythropoietin (EPO), granulocyte colony-stimulating factor (G-CSF) and bethamethasone phosphate (BP) was observed for 1 week both in *in vitro* and *in vivo* experiments [92].

On the other hand, Ogawa and coworkers used porous hydroxyapatite particles, of which the mean inside diameter was 100 nm, as a drug delivery system carrier for long-term sustained release peptide/protein preparation for injection [93]. After protein drug is entrapped into the hydroxyapatite particles, the obtained particles are coated with a biodegradable polymer which has a hydrophilic part, as shown in Fig. 6.8.

Human growth hormone (hGH) was at first entrapped into nanoporous hydroxyapatite particles where an inorganic metal compound was added to prevent the initial release of hGH, i.e. burst phenomenon. The obtained particles were coated

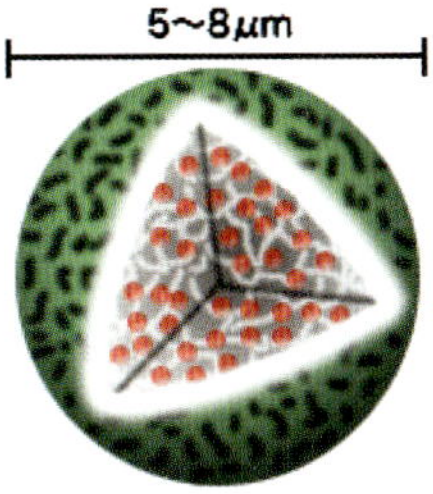

Figure 6.8. Basic concept of a hydroxyapatite drug delivery system for sustained-release protein [10].

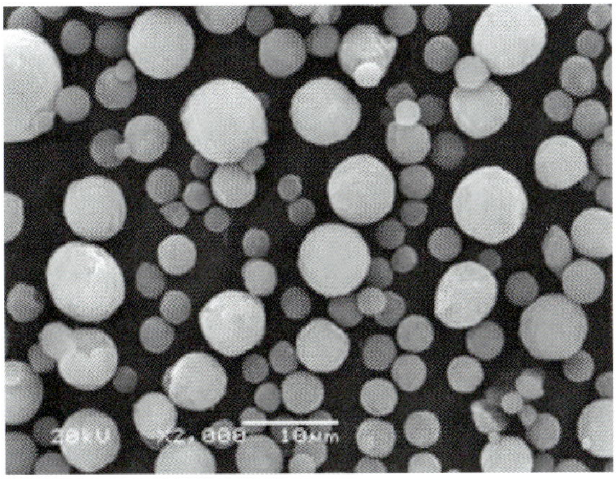

Figure 6.9. SEM images of a hydroxyapatite drug delivery system containing hGH [10].

with a hydrophilic biodegradable polymer like PEG–PLA. The mean particle size of the system is 5–8 μm, as shown in Fig. 6.9. The hGH content of this system is around 15 wt%. About 80 mg of the preparation was injected to patients with dwarfism every 2 weeks with 27 G syringe needle. To evaluate the system, they injected the preparation into rats who received immunosuppressive therapy and it was confirmed that serum hGH levels were maintained over 2 weeks. In addition, the injected particles were not detected at the end of the experiment. They also performed a pharmacodynamic study using hypophysectomized rats. In the sustained-release hGH preparation group, the rat body weights gradually increased over 3 weeks. However, body weights did not increase in the control group rats [94].

6.4.2 Silastic Compounds

6.4.2.1 Nanoporous Silastic Materials for Solidifying Oily Drugs

Porous calcium silicate, Florite™ RE (FLR; Eisai, Japan) has the structure of assembled petal-like flakes, presenting a lot of pores in its surface. Pores show a par-

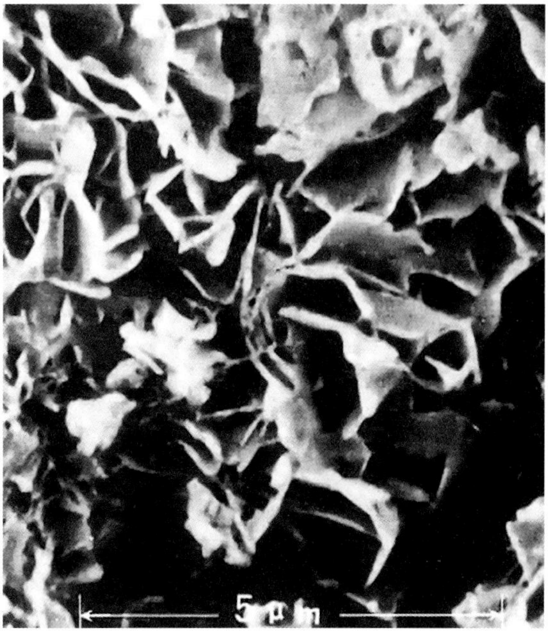

Figure 6.10. SEM image of FLR (www.eisai-fc.co.jp/).

ticular size distribution with two peaks at 12 and 0.15 μm, which are attributed to interparticle and intraparticle pores, respectively. The mean inside diameter is 150 nm. FLR has a porous structure, as shown in Fig. 6.10, and has an excellent liquid-holding ability, about 5.0 mL g^{-1}, through its numerous pores. Both FLR and colloidal silica (Aerosil^{TM} 200, AER; Nippon Aerosil, Japan) have greater adsorption efficiency than other adsorbents, i.e. microcrystalline cellulose, cornstarch and lactose dibasic calcium phosphate. Although AER does not have interparticle pores, FLR has both interparticle and intraparticle pores. AER absorbs liquid into interparticle pores by forming liquid bridges among the particles. On the other hand, FLR adsorbs liquid into the interparticle pores by a capillary phenomenon.

As oily drugs do not dissolve in water, they are usually developed as a soft capsule preparation. As the size of the oily capsule preparation is large, pediatric and elder patients often have trouble swallowing them. In particular, when the oily capsule is taken with a small amount of water, the possibility of capsule adhesion onto the esophageal mucosa increases. In the worst case, esophageal ulcer occurs. To solve these problems, Takeuchi and coworkers formulated vitamin E acetate into a drug emulsion system with colloidal silica [95].

On the other hand, Hanawa and coworkers reported the solidification of ethenzamide (EZA) by a "melt-adsorption" method [96]. When EZA crystals were heated with FLR in a sealed glass ampoule without any solvent, EZA melted and adsorbed on FLR in an amorphous state. The dissolution rate of EZA from the preparation was greatly enhanced as compared with crystal EZA. To enable large-scale manufacturing, Kinoshita and coworkers used a twin-screw extruder, in which both temperature and kneading force can be controlled simultaneously [97]. The extruder allows EZA to melt and adsorb onto FLR. Therefore, the process is also called the "melt-adsorption" method. They prepared melt-adsorbed products of TAS-301 [3-bis(4-methoxyphenyl)methylene-2-indolinone] which were adsorbed on FLR using a twin-screw extruder. TAS-301 is an antirestenosis drug for use after percutaneous transluminal coronary angioplasty (PTCA). The crystallinity, solubility and oral bioavailability (BA) of TAS-301 in the melt-adsorbed products were examined. The particle size distributions of FLR, physical mixture [TAS-301:FLR (1:2)] and the melt-adsorbed product [TAS-301: FLR(1:2)] made by both methods were approximately consistent. The specific surface area decreased in the following order: FLR > physical mixture > melt-adsorbed product > TAS-301 crystal. The specific surface area decreased by mixing due to partial adsorption of TAS-301 on FLR and further decreased by heating due to its penetration into FLR pores. TAS-301 was amorphized by heating with an adsorbent above its melting point. In addition, the decreased crystallinity of TAS-301 was suggested by the endothermic X-ray diffraction (XRD) peaks. Therefore, both the amorphization and decreased crystallinity of TAS-301 might be associated with hydrogen bonding between the C=O group of TAS-301 and the sylanol group of FLR. Although the solubility of the TAS-301 crystal and physical mixture was similar, the melt-adsorbed products prepared by both methods showed temporary super-saturation in water and their initial solubility was approximately 20-fold greater than that of the TAS-301 crystal. The dissolution rates of TAS-301 from the melt-adsorbed products prepared by the two methods were markedly faster than those from the physical mixture and the drug crystal. Figure 6.11 shows the results on the absorption of TAS-30 from the system

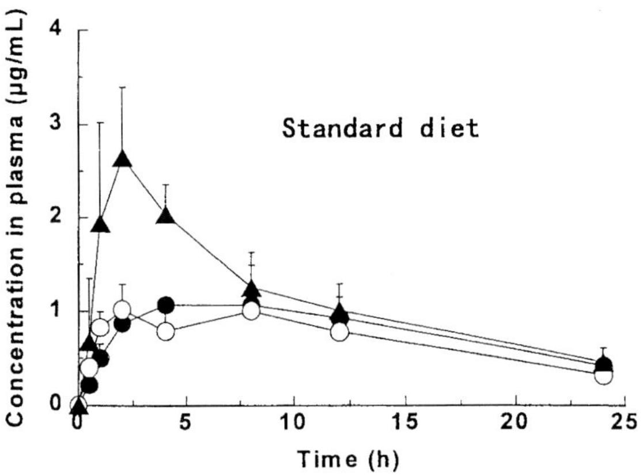

Figure 6.11. Plasma concentration of TAS-301 versus time profiles after oral administration of test preparations at a dose of 300 mg per dog. ▲ = Melt-adsorbed product (capsule). ● = TAS-301 crystal (aqueous suspension). ○ = TAS-301 crystal (capsule). Each point represents the mean ± SD ($n = 3$–6).

after oral administration of three preparations to dogs being fed a standard diet. The AUC (area under the plasma drug concentration–time curve) values of the three test preparations were 1.12 ± 0.03 (crystal suspension), 1.18 ± 0.43 (crystal) and 2.75 ± 0.53 μg h mL^{-1} (melt-adsorbed products), respectively. Thus, melt-adsorption on a porous calcium silicate, FLR, is useful for improving the solubility and BA of hydrophobic drugs like TAS-301.

Yuasa and coworkers applied FLR to granulate a representative oily drug, D,L-tocopheryl nicotinate (TN), by adsorbing TN [98]. They also showed the possibility of tableting TN with FLR as an adsorbent and studied the possibility of the reduction of tablet coloration by TN exudation at compression, because TN was expected to be excluded from TN powder to the surface of the tablet by compression. With mixing, ethanol solution containing TN, 10–60 wt%, was added to FLR. After the adsorbents were dried, TN powder was obtained. In addition, TN powder was used to form granules. When the TN powder in which TN is adsorbed to FLR is compressed, the degree of tablet coloration caused by TN exudation from TN powder becomes larger with a higher TN content and compression pressure. It was clarified that the reduction of tablet coloration at tableting of TN is possible by compressing TN powder added with FLR or AER, both of which have a high liquid holding ability. In particular, when FLR is added at compression, a shorter disintegration time and a higher release property of TN were obtained when AER was added due to the difference of the liquid adsorbing and holding mechanism of FLR and AER. They proposed the models of the existent state of TN in the tablet at compression, which are shown in Fig. 6.12. When TN powder with hydroxypropylstarch (HPS) as a disintegrator is compressed, as shown in Fig. 6.12(A), TN is extruded by compression and readsorbed by forming liquid bridges to the particles of TN powder and HPS. It was considered that the interparticle space decreased as these liquid bridges were formed, with the result that the penetration rate of water into the TN tablet decreased, and therefore the disintegration time was longer and the release rate of TN was slower. When TN powder with FLR and HPS is compressed, as shown in Fig. 6.12(B), TN is extruded by compression and readsorbed to the pores in newly added FLR, with the result that a lot of interparticle spaces without TN are formed. In addition, they confirmed, by determining the pore size distributions in the tablets produced from FLR or AER alone, that the mean interparticle pore diameters among FLR or AER particles in the tablets were about 250 and 150+, respectively. It was considered that, since the interparticle space in the TNF tablet, i.e. the mean pore diameter, was larger than that in the TNA tablet, water easily penetrated into the TNF tablet. As a result, the disintegration time was shorter and the release property of TN was improved in comparison with TN and TN tablets with AER. When TN powder with AER and HPS is compressed, as shown in Fig. 6.12(C), TN is extruded by compression and readsorbed by forming liquid bridges to the particles of TN powder, AER and HPS. When the formulated amount of AER increased, the disintegration time became shorter because the interparticle space without TN bridges increased. Furthermore, because the mean pore diameter of the TN tablet with AER is smaller and the amount of TN forming bridges to the particles in the TN tablet with AER is larger, it may be difficult to

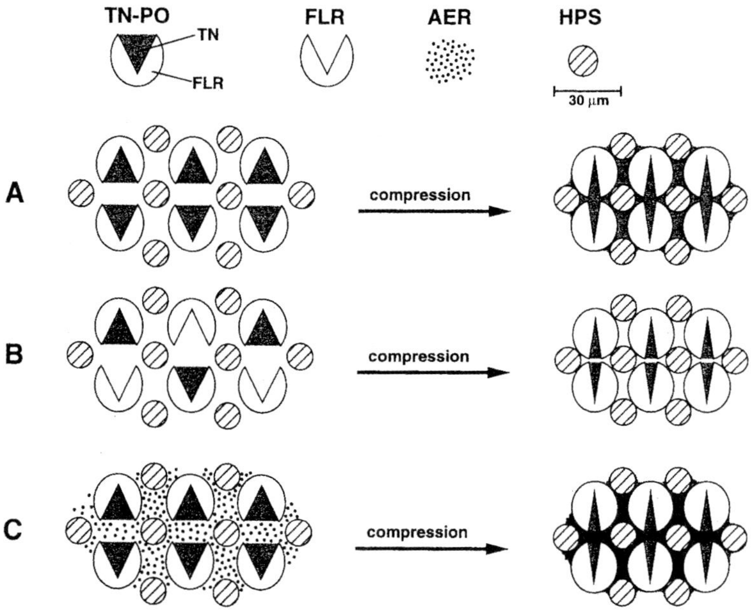

Figure 6.12. Model of the existent state of TN at compression of (A) TN powder, (B) TN tablets with FLR and (C) TN tablets with AER where HPS was used as a disintegrator of tablets.

penetrate into the TN tablet with AER. As a result, the rate of TN from the TN tablet with AER was slower than that from the TN tablet with FLR.

Hwang and coworkers prepared silica particles containing retinal with a fabrication method using an oil/water/oil (o/w/o) emulsion and the sol-gel method [99]. By controlling the formulated amount of surfactants, Span 80 and Tween 20, sustained-release characteristics of retinal were obtained for 100 h.

6.4.2.2 Nanoporous Silastic Materials for Poorly Absorbable Drugs

The BA of hydrophobic drugs after oral administration is very low due to their poor solubility in the gastrointestinal tract. Solid dispersion and microemulsion have been applied to improve the solubility of poorly soluble drugs [100]. These drug delivery system technologies are often used to improve the oral BA of insoluble drugs, e.g. cyclosporin A (microemulsion, Neoral™) and tacrolimus (solid dispersion) [101, 102]. However, solid dispersion technology has limited applicability in improving the oral BA of drugs having both low solubility and low membrane permeability. The principles of the intestinal absorption mechanism of drugs are classified into the following categories: (i) passive diffusion, (ii) facilitated diffusion (endocytosis) and (iii) carrier-mediated active transport [103]. Active transport takes part in the absorption process of a limited number of drugs like vitamin B_{12}, 5-fluorouracil, etc. [104]. Most of the clinically applied drugs are absorbed from the gastrointestinal tract by a passive diffusion mechanism. In this case, the concentration gradient of drug molecules between the intestinal luminal side and the enterocytes is the rate-limiting process for the overall absorption process. In addition, absorption-enhancing technologies have been developed for poorly absorbable drugs, i.e. macromolecular drugs such as protein/peptide drugs, e.g. insulin, low-molecular-weight heparin (LMWH), etc. [105–107]. Emisphere developed nonacylated non-α-amino acid, sodium *N*-[8-(2-hydroxybenzoyl) amino] caprylate (SNAC) as an absorption enhancer for LMWH [108]. After oral administration of LMWH, 30 mg kg^{-1} (4971 IU mL^{-1}), in accordance with SNAC, 150 mg kg^{-1}, the peak plasma LMWH level measured as an anti-Xa activity level of 1.2 IU mL^{-1} was obtained. SNAC thus effectively enhanced the oral absorption of LMWH. However, after the oral administration of LMWH with SNAC, both LMWH and SNAC are diluted in the small intestine. Therefore, the absorption enhancing effect of SNAC is insufficient. Takada and coworkers used nanoporous silastic materials as oral drug carriers [109]. In their system, both the drug and absorption enhancer are held in the carrier at high concentrations. As the result of the high concentration gradients of the drug and absorption enhancer between inside the system and the enterocytes, the formulated drug can be efficiently absorbed. This drug delivery system technology is termed a "liquid formulation holding microparticulate system (LFMPS)", as shown in Fig. 6.13. In the LFMPS system, a hydrophobic drug is solubilized in either an oil or water phase with the help of surfactant(s). Thus, the obtained particles can be formulated either as a capsule or tablet. After the

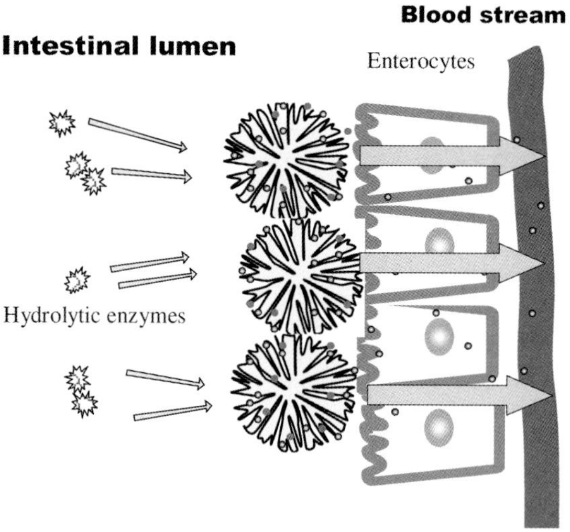

Figure 6.13. Concept of LFMPS. After oral administration of microparticles and adsorbent, holding both absorption enhancer and macromolecular drug-like protein drug in enteric capsules, the microparticles are delivered to the enterocytes where high concentration gradients of enhancer and drug are formed. Consequently, high absorption efficiency of drug is obtained.

oral administration of LFMPS in an enteric capsule, the microparticles are exposed to the enterocytes, and form a high drug concentration gradient between the system and the enterocytes. In addition, when an absorption enhancer is formulated with the drug, good BA can be obtained. LFMPS can be also applied to highly soluble and poorly absorbable drugs that have a high molecular weight (e.g. gentamicin) [110] or high surface charge (e.g. LMWH) [111], resulting in poor membrane permeability. These drugs require the use of an absorption enhancer (e.g. surfactant) to improve their oral BA. The drug and absorption enhancer can be dissolved in water and, thus, the obtained mixture is introduced into the nanoporous material. Takada and coworkers first studied the effect of nanoporous materials on the BA of lansoprazole (LPZ) [109]. LPZ is a representative proton pump inhibitor, and has been clinically used in gastric and duodenal ulcerative disease therapy. LPZ is sparingly soluble in water and is unstable in the stomach, i.e. in gastric acid. According to the classification of drugs with low BA proposed by Amidon and coworkers [112], LPZ is a class II compound (low solubility and high membrane permeability) in the biopharmaceutical classification system (BCS). Clinically, gelatin capsules containing enteric-coated LPZ granules are supplied. Even if LPZ is protected from hydrolysis in the stomach, there is a possibility that LPZ does not dissolve well in the small intestine because of there being less water. Therefore, the oral BA of LPZ is low and shows wide intersubject variation. To solve these problems, nonionic surfactants were used to accelerate dissolution and improve the BA of LPZ. However, a liquid formulation is not as preferable as an oral formulation because no capsule can retain a liquid formulation without dissolution or degradation. LFMPS is composed of a surfactant, nanoporous adsorbent and LPZ. Its function is to improve the dissolution and absorption of LPZ. The BA of LPZ was measured in rats. As surfactants, Tween 80, polyoxyethylated, 60 mol, caster oil derivative (HCO-60^{TM}) and PEG-8 caprylic/capric glycerides (Labrasol^{TM}) were used. As adsorbents, porous silicon dioxide (Sylysia^{TM} 550, 320), magnesium aluminometa silicate (Neusilin^{TM} S_2, NS_2N, US_2) and porous calcium silicate (FLR) were used. Among the used surfactants, HCO-60 showed the highest absorption enhancing effect after the intra-small intestinal administration of LPZ solution. To solidify the LPZ solution with HCO-60, adsorbents were used and the obtained solid preparations were first used in an *in vitro* release experiment. Sylysia 320, Neusilin S_2 and Neusilin NS_2 showed a $T_{50\%}$, the time when half of the formulated amount of drug is released from the test preparation, of about 1 h. To evaluate the BA of LPZ from these solid preparations, an absorption study was performed in rats. The Sylysia 550 system showed a higher AUC than other systems, showing a BA of 28.1%. The Sylysia 550 system was placed in an enteric capsule and orally administered to dogs, and the BA was compared with an enteric tablet. The Sylysia 550 system had a BA of 71.7%, which was significantly greater than the enteric tablet. Thus, the solid system composed of LPZ, surfactant and nanoporous adsorbent, Sylysia 550, was shown to be a good system to improve the BA of LPZ.

Takada and coworkers also applied this system to gentamicin (GM), of which an oral preparation is not available because of a poor BA from the gastrointestinal tract [110]. As GM is a polar water-soluble compound, it is commonly recognized that the intestinal membrane permeability of GM is poor. GM is a class III compound (high solubility and low membrane permeability) of BCS. They previously showed that the BA of GM was greatly increased by formulating GM in a self-microemulsifying drug delivery system (SMEDDS) using PEG-8 caprylic/capric glycerides (Labrasol™) as an absorption enhancer. Labrasol contains saturated polyglycolysed C_6–C_{14} glycerides, where C_8 is 58.1% and C_{10} is 39.8%. Labrasol is a safe pharmaceutical additive, showing a high tolerance and low toxicity in animals; the LD_{50} is 22.0 g kg^{-1} for rats and is a surfactant listed in the European Pharmacopoeia. A SMEDDS is expected to self-emulsify rapidly in the aqueous environment of the small intestine, thereby presenting the drug in solution in small droplets of oil. The gentle agitation required for emulsification is provided by the digestive motility of the small intestine. By formulating GM in a Labrasol SMEDDS, a high BA value of GM, approximately 55%, was obtained after administration to the rat small intestine [113]. The dosage form that results from a SMEDDS is usually either a liquid or liquid-filled soft gelatin capsules. However, from the standpoint of pharmaceutics, the solid dosage form is preferable to the liquid preparation in terms of cost-performance and the convenience of the manufacturing process. After GM was dissolved with Labrasol, the mixture was solidified with several kinds of adsorbents. The adsorbents were microporous calcium silicate (FLR), magnesium alminometa silicate (Neusilin US_2) and silicon dioxide (Sylysia 320). An *in vitro* release study showed no significant difference between the three adsorbents. The *in vivo* rat absorption study showed that the preparation containing 10 mg of FLR had the highest C_{max}, 2.14 ± 0.67 μg mL^{-1} of GM. Other preparations had a C_{max} of 0.69 ± 0.10 μg mL^{-1} for FLR 20 mg, 1.07 ± 0.31 μg mL^{-1} for Neusilin US_2 and 0.99 ± 0.21 μg mL^{-1} for Sylysia 320, respectively. The BA of GM from the FLR 10 mg system was 14.1%. The system was also evaluated in dogs after oral administration in an enteric capsule made of Eudragit S100. High plasma GM levels with a C_{max} of 1.26 ± 0.20 μg mL^{-1} were obtained. These results suggest that the FLR system is useful as an oral solid delivery system of poorly absorbable drugs such as GM [110]. LFMPS can also be applied to highly soluble and poorly absorbable drugs that have a high surface charge (e.g. LMWH) resulting in poor membrane permeability. Thus, LFMPS is a useful system for solving the low BA problem of both hydrophilic and hydrophobic drugs.

6.4.2.3 **Nanoporous Silica Materials for Controlled Release of Drugs**

Calcium silicate was used as a porous carrier for repaglinide, an oral hypoglycemic agent, to prepare microspheres, and a gastroretentive floating drug delivery systems was challenged, as shown in Fig. 6.14 [114]. An *in vitro* release study showed the sustained-release characteristics of repaglinide for 8 h.

On the other hand, porous particle technology was applied to obtain an immediately dissolving intravenous preparation. Straub and coworkers prepared drug powder particles of paclitaxel, a water-insoluble hydrophobic anticancer drug. Ethanol solution containing paclitaxel, Tween 80 and polyvinylpyrrolidone (PVP) C15 was mixed with an aqueous solution containing the pore-forming agent, ammonium bicarbonate and mannitol. The mixture was spray-dried and porous dry

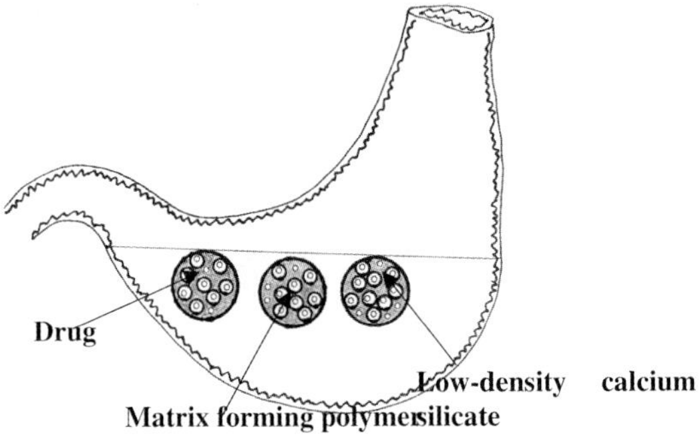

Figure 6.14. Gastroretentive floating drug delivery system made of calcium silicate-based microspheres.

powder particles (shown in Fig. 6.15) were obtained. The mean particle size was about 1 μm and nanosize pores were formed. An *in vitro* dissolution experiment showed that more than 90% of paclitaxel was dissolved from the dry powder within 10 min, although about 80% of the authentic paclitaxel bulk was dissolved at 2 h after the start of the dissolution experiment [115].

Foraker and coworkers applied porous silicon (pSi) as a platform technology for a new generation of drug delivery systems. Macropores (above 50 nm), mesopores (2–50 nm) and nanopores (below 2 nm), occupying 1–95% of the Si volume, were used as a scaffold suitable for loading of drugs. As a model hydrophilic macromolecular drug, insulin was loaded into pSi particles by freeze drying, where sodium laurate was used as an absorption enhancer. Using an *in vitro* permeation system using Caco-2 monolayer, a 10- to 50-fold increase in insulin transport efficiency was obtained by the pSi particle system [116].

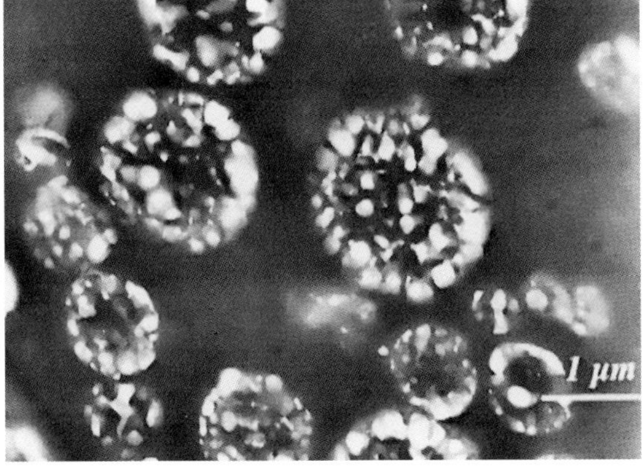

Figure 6.15. TEM image of a cross-section of paclitaxel porous particles.

6.4.3 Carbon Nanotubes (CNTs)

6.4.3.1 CNTs for Oral Delivery of Protein Drug

CNTs are produced by deposition of carbon atoms vaporized from graphite by an electric arc or by a laser onto metal particles. Recently, CNTs have been produced by the chemical vapor deposition (CVD) method. The obtained CNTs often aggregate into bundles or ropes. An individual CNT molecule is about 1 nm in diameter and several microns long [117]. The specific gravity of CNTs is very light because of their large outer and inner surface areas. The adsorption efficiency of CNTs is larger than the conventional adsorbents like silastic compounds. Takada and co-workers used CNTs as an adsorbent of both the absorption enhancer and drug, and the resulting system was evaluated as an oral drug delivery system for poorly-absorbable drugs like peptide/protein drugs [118]. Surfactants such as a saturated polyglycolysed C_8–C_{18} glyceride (Gelucire™ 44/14), Labrasol and HCO-60 were used as absorption enhancers at 50 mg kg^{-1} and EPO was used as a model protein drug. As adsorbents, solid particles such as Sylysia 550, CNTs, carbon nanohorns (CNHs), fullerene, charcoal and bamboo charcoal were used. After either surfactant was loaded into the adsorbent by mixing well, disintegrator (Explotab™) was added and mixed thoroughly. Finally, EPO solution was added to this mixture and mixed well. The test preparations were directly administered into the rat small intestine at the EPO dose level of 100 IU kg^{-1} and EPO absorption was studied by measuring serum EPO levels by ELISA. Labrasol showed the highest absorption

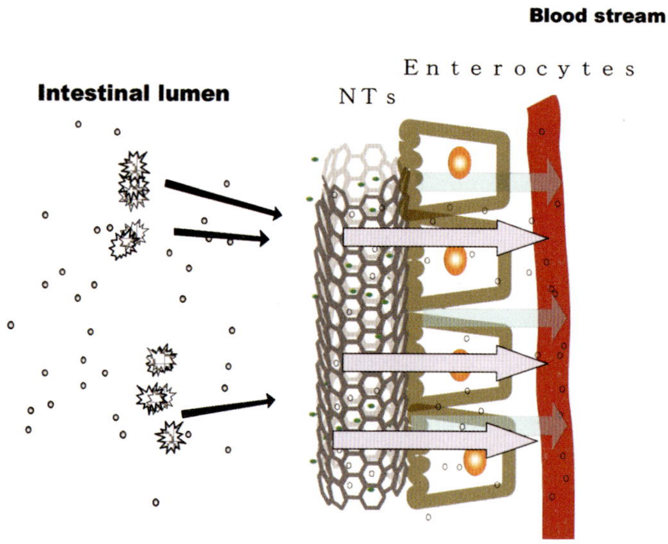

Figure 6.16. CNTs as carriers for oral delivery of macromolecular drug. After the oral administration of CNTs holding both absorption enhancer (Labrasol) and EPO in enteric capsules, CNTs are delivered to the enterocytes where high concentration gradients of Labrasol and EPO are formed. Consequently, high absorption efficiency of EPO is obtained.

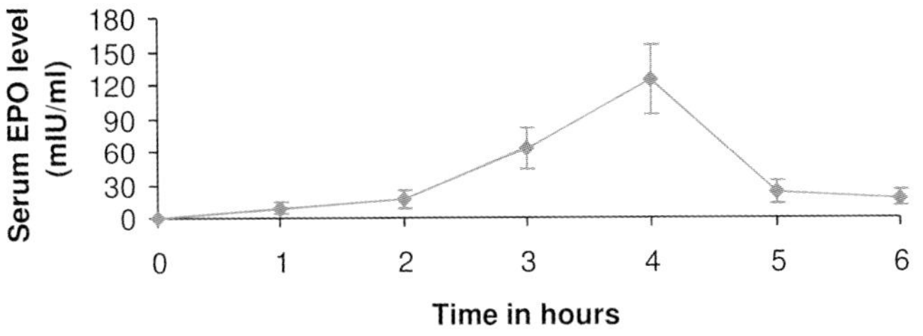

Figure 6.17. Serum EPO concentration versus time curve after small intestinal administration of CNTs holding both absorption enhancer (Labrasol) and EPO (100 IU kg^{-1}).

enhancing effect after intra-jejunum administration than Gelucire 44/14 and HCO-60. Therefore, Labrasol was used as an absorption enhancer for EPO and the systems were evaluated by an *in vivo* absorption model using rats. As in the case of LFMPS, CNTs can deliver both absorption enhancer and EPO by holding onto the enterocytes, and a high concentration gradient between the intestinal mucosal site and enterocytes is formed (Fig. 6.16). Scanning electron microscopy (SEM) image of CNTs used in this system is shown in Fig. 6.18. As a result, a high peak serum EPO level (C_{max}), 62.7 ± 11.6 mIU mL^{-1}, was obtained. Other adsorbents showed lower C_{max}s, 25.9 ± 3.7 mIU mL^{-1} for Sylysia 550, 18.7 ± 5.3 mIU mL^{-1} for CNH, 50.0 ± 11.4 mIU mL^{-1} for fullerene, 40.4 ± 13.1 mIU mL^{-1} for charcoal and 34.1 ± 7.5 mIU mL^{-1} for bamboo charcoal, respectively. The other BA parameter, AUC, also showed the same absorption enhancing order. Among the used adsorbents, the BA values were in the order of CNT > fullerene > Sylysia 550 > CNH > bamboo charcoal > charcoal, where the BA of EPO from the CNT system was 6.7%. By formulating an enzyme inhibitor, casein, into the adsorbent system, the BA of EPO was increased, as shown in Fig. 6.17, where

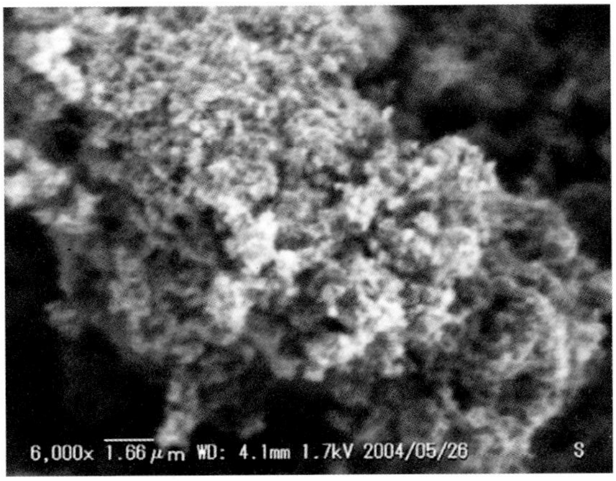

Figure 6.18. TEM image of CNTs used for the oral delivery of EPO.

C_{max} was 143.1 ± 15.2 mIU mL^{-1}, resulting in the highest BA of EPO, i.e. 11.5%. Labrasol also showed good absorption enhancing effects on other poorly absorbable drugs like insulin, vancomicin and gentamicin [119, 120]. CNT is a good adsorbent of Labrasol for the oral delivery of these poorly absorbable drugs.

6.4.3.2 CNTs for Intracellular Delivery of Protein

CNTs were applied to the intracellular delivery of drugs, genes and proteins. Kam and coworkers suggested the ability of single-walled CNTs (SWNTs) to penetrate mammalian cells and deliver various drugs i.e. peptides, the protein streptavidin (SA) and nucleic acids inside living cells, as shown in Fig. 6.19 [121]. The investi-

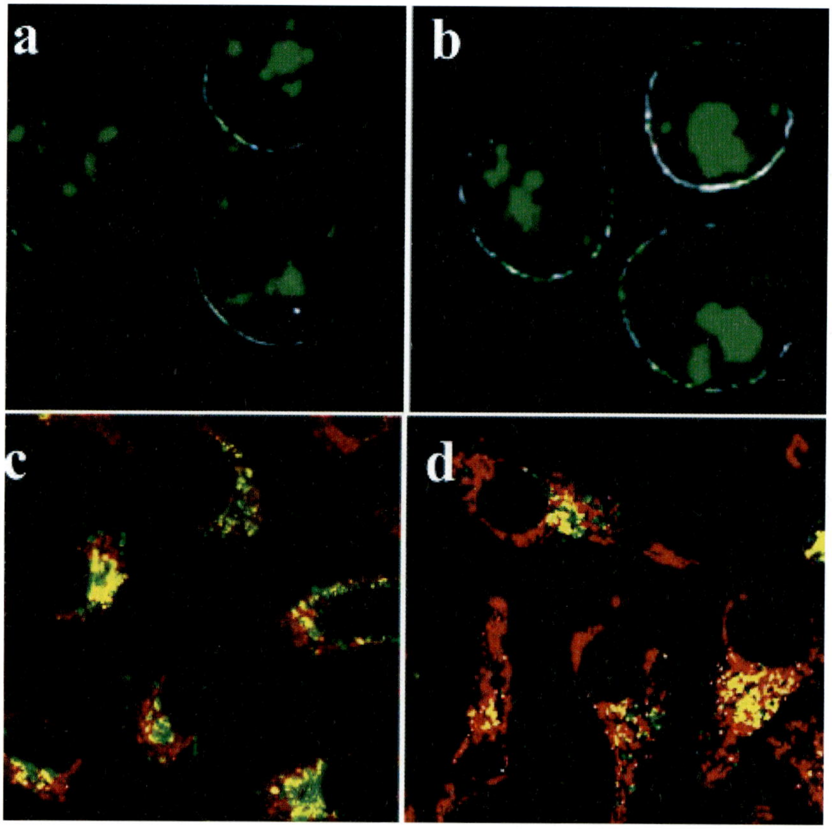

Figure 6.19. Confocal microscopy of cells after incubation in protein–SWNT (proteins labeled to be green fluorescent) solutions for 2 h. (a) HL60 cells after incubation in SA–SWNTs. (b) HL60 cells after incubation in BSA–SWNTs. (c) HeLa cells after incubation in SA–SWNTs in the presence of the FM 4-64, a red membrane and endocytotoxic vesicle marker. Yellow color in the image is due to colocalization of fluorescently labeled green proteins and red FM 4-64. (d) HeLa cells alter incubation in cytochrome *c*–SWNTs in the presence of FM 4-64.

gated proteins were SA, protein A (SpA), bovine serum albumin (BSA) and cytochrome *c*. Intracellular protein transport and uptake by SWNT were also generic for various adherent and nonadherent mammalian cell lines, including HeLa, NIH-3T3 fibroblasts, HL60 and Jurkat cells. Energy-dependent endocytosis was confirmed to be the internalization mechanism. Furthermore, with cytochrome *c* as the cargo protein, they explored the fate of internalized protein–SWNT conjugates, attempted to release the conjugates from the endosome vesicles into the cell cytoplasm using chloroquine and investigated the biological functions of the released proteins. Once released into the cytoplasm of cells, the proteins can perform biological functions, i.e. apoptosis, or programmed cell death, induced by cytochrome *c* transported inside cells by SWNTs after their release from the endosomes. On the other hand, Pantarotto and coworkers and Bianco and coworkers showed that SWNTs were generic intracellular transporters for various types of proteins (below 80 kDa) noncovalently and nonspecifically [122, 123]. The SWNT uptake mechanism was suggested to be via insertion and diffusion through the lipid bilayer of the cell membrane. Therefore, a precise study must be performed to clarify the uptake mechanism of SWNTs. Thus, SWNTs may constitute a new class of molecular transporters for various *in vitro* and *in vivo* delivery applications.

Electroporation has been used to transfer molecules, like DNA or drugs, into living cells, where pulsed electric fields of several kV cm^{-1} in amplitude and submicrosecond duration are required. Thereby, membrane pores are formed temporarily and DNA or drugs penetrate. However, existing electroporation technology has limitations, i.e. a low efficiency. In addition, high electric field pulses lead to cell lysis. Chapana and coworkers applied CNTs to increase the efficiency of electroporation [124]. Their technology reduces to the nanoscale the large-scale process of electroporation by the use of CNTs as physical "electroporation vectors". Their technique differs fundamentally from other methods used today, because electrodes are not needed. Water dispersible CNTs have an anionic surface charge attached to the surface of Gram-negative bacteria. This arises mainly due to an electrostatic interaction between the CNTs and the likewise charged bacterial surface. On the other hand, the effect of a microwave electromagnetic field pulse on the interaction of CNTs with the cells leads to electropermeabilization through individual CNTs. At first, they prepared water dispersible CNTs by treating them with acid solution for 1 h in a nitric:sulfuric (1:3) acid solution, which generates carboxylic groups at the ends as well as in the defects on the sidewalls of the CNTs. After purification, they obtained a stable CNT suspension with no precipitation after several months. Transmission electron microscopy (TEM) examination of the sample shows the presence of individual CNTs approximately 40 nm in diameter and less than 0.6 μm in length. Plasmid DNA pUC19 was successfully introduced into *Escherichia coli* cells. TEM examination showed that the electroporation process proceeded through the intact cell wall of the suspended cells without inducing changes in their morphology. They could isolate pUC19 DNA from cultures made from blue colonies, because β-galactosidase activity was visualized by feeding the transformed cells a lactose analog called X-Gal that turns blue when hydrolyzed by β-galactosidase. Therefore, the transformation of *E. coli* was successfully facilitated by CNTs. CNTs having hollow structures were used to fulfill both requirements, i.e. electroporation and injection (nanopipette). If CNTs recognizing cell surfaces can be designed, it will be possible to deliver DNA molecules and colloidal particles confined in their interstitial channels to a particular cell type through the cell envelope and into compartments. These applications are new challenges in cell biology and biomedicine.

6.4.3.3 Toxicity of CNTs

In the study of Takada and coworkers, CNTs were used as carriers of oral drug delivery systems. However, no toxicity information about CNTs after oral or systemic administration is available. On the other hand, when fine particles of CNTs are aspirated by humans, a health risk occurs. The Occupational Safety and Health Administration (OSHA) set the permissible inhalation exposure limit (PEL) for synthetic graphite at 15 mg m^{-3} of total dust and 5 mg m^{-3} for the respirable fraction [125]. Lam and coworkers performed a pulmonary toxicity study on SWNTs in mice 7 and 90 days after intratracheal instillation [126]. Three CNT products made by different methods and containing different types or amounts of residual metals, i.e. raw CNTs (RNTs) and purified CNTs (PNTs), iron-containing HiPco products of Rice and CarboLex's nickel-containing electric-arc product (CNT), were used for the toxicity study. For their study, mice were intratracheally administered 0, 0.1 or 0.5 mg of CNTs, a carbon black negative control or a quartz positive control and euthanized 7 days or 90 days after treatment for histopathological study of the lungs. All CNT products induced dose-dependent epithelioid granulomas and, in some cases, interstitial inflammation in the animals of the 7-day groups. The lesions persisted and were more pronounced in the 90-day groups; the lungs of some animals were also revealed to have peribronchial inflammation and necrosis that had extended into the alveolar septa. The lungs of mice treated with carbon black were normal, whereas those treated with high-dose quartz had mild to moderate inflammation. Their results showed that if CNTs reach the lungs, they are more toxic than carbon black and can be more toxic than quartz, which was considered a serious occupational health hazard in chronic exposures. Lung toxicity of intratracheally instilled SWNT was also studied in rats [127]. The lungs of rats were instilled either with 1 or 5 mg kg^{-1} of the following control or particle types: (i) SWNT, (ii) quartz particles (positive control), (iii) carbonyl iron particles (negative control), (iv) phosphate buffered saline (PBS) + 1% Tween 80 or (v) graphite particles. Exposures to high-dose (5 mg kg^{-1}) SWNT resulted in about 15% mortality in the SWNT-instilled rats within 24 h postinstillation. This mortality resulted from mechanical blockage of the upper airways by the instillation and was not due to inherent pulmonary toxicity of the instilled SWNT particulate. Exposures to quartz particles produced significant increases versus controls in pulmonary inflammation, cytotoxicity and lung cell parenchymal cell proliferation indices. Exposures to SWNT produced transient inflammatory and cell injury effects. Histopathological study indicated that pulmonary exposures to SWNT in rats produced a non-dose-dependent series of multifocal granulomas, which were evidence of a foreign tis-

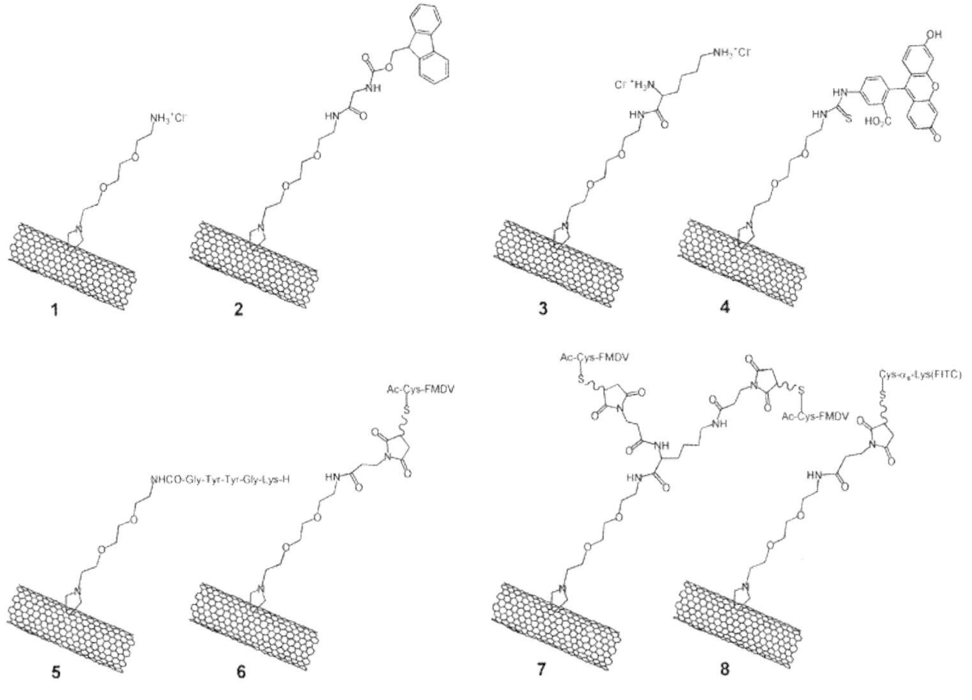

Figure 6.20. Structure of *f*-CNTs.

sue body reaction and were nonuniform in distribution and not progressive beyond 1-month postexposure.

6.4.3.4 Functionalized CNTs (*f*-CNTs) for Drug Delivery

As shown in Fig. 6.20, Bianko and coworkers synthesized several hydrophilic CNT derivatives called *f*-CNTs), *f*-CNT **1–8** [128]. The aqueous solubility and cationic surface character of *f*-CNTs **1** render them potentially novel delivery vehicles. They initially showed the efficiency of *f*-CNTs to transport across the plasma membrane and penetrate into the cytoplasm of cells. To obtain the proof of the concept experiment, they prepared two different FITC-labeled *f*-CNTs, by introducing either FITC directly to the amino functions of the soluble CNTs or a fluorescent peptide. Their molecular structures are shown as conjugate **4** and **8** in Fig. 6.20. This peptide mimics the effect of G_S-protein by increasing the agonist affinity for the P-adrenergic receptor. The free peptide did not penetrate the cell membrane. To evaluate the ability of the *f*-CNTs to penetrate HeLa cells, both conjugates were incubated with the cells and analyzed. The intracellular distribution of the fluorescence was studied by fluorescence microscopy. While *f*-CNT conjugate **4** with the FITC alone mainly distributed into the cytoplasm, slowly moving towards the nucleus, peptide–CNTs **8** rapidly translocated into the cell nucleus. The same results were obtained using other types of cells including human and murine fibroblasts and keratinocytes.

6.4.3.5 *f*-CNTs for Gene Delivery

f-CNTs were also used for gene delivery. Gene therapy is one of the possible methods for cancer and genetic disorder therapy. For gene targeting, viral and nonviral vector systems must be developed. However, these vectors have several pitfalls, i.e. induction of undesirable immune responses, inflammations and oncogenic side-effects. Therefore, nonviral vectors have been studied because of their higher level of safety. However, they have several limitations: (i) poor membrane permeability of the administered oligonucleotide and plasmid DNA conjugates, and (ii) low levels of gene expression. As a vector system, Bianko and coworkers also examined the potential of *f*-CNTs [128]. The observation of the ensuing supramolecular assemblies using TEM indicated that nanotube–DNA complexes were formed. In addition, they obtained a clear effect using the DNA complexes with *f*-CNTs **1** to carry the P-gal gene inside the cells, by monitoring the expression of P-galactosidase. Improved levels of gene expression were also obtained for the *f*-CNT **1**–DNA complex in the range of positive:negative charge ratios between 2:1 to 6:1. Gene expression offered by the complexes between plasmid DNA with *f*-CNTs was 5–10 times higher than that of DNA alone. These promising results suggest the possibility of exploiting *f*-CNTs in gene therapy and genetic vaccination.

6.4.4 CNHs for Drug Delivery

Single-wall CNHs (SWNHs) are aggregates of graphitic tubes that have closed ends with cone-shaped caps (horns). Each tube has a diameter of 2–3 nm, which is larger than the 1.4 nm of typical SWNTs, while the aggregates are 80–100 nm in diameter and have "dahlia-1ike" or "bud-like" spherical structures [129]. SWNHs have extensive surface areas and multitudes of horn interstices, which enable large amounts of guest molecules to be adsorbed on SWNHs [130]. Moreover, the surface area can be further enlarged by oxidization, which causes the formation of nanowindows in the SWNH walls [131]. Through these nanowindows, a variety of small molecules [e.g. N_2, Ar and fullerene (C_{60})] infiltrate into their inner space and quadruple the adsorptive surface areas. In addition, the sizes of the pores can be controlled by changing the oxidization conditions. Murakami and coworkers prepared a series of oxidized SWNHs (oxSWNHs) having distinct molecular sieving effects and their utility as a drug delivery system carrier was studied using dexamethasone (DEX), an anti-inflammatory drug, as a model drug [132]. DEX was adsorbed on oxSWNHs. oxSWNHs (100 μg mL^{-1}) were dispersed by sonication in 0.1–20 mL of a 1:1 mixture of ethanol and water and was filtrated with a 0.22-μm filter, after which DEX (1000 μg mL^{-1}) in ethanol:H_2O (1:1) solution was added at a volume ratio of 1:1. The resultant mixture was incubated at room temperature overnight and then centrifuged at 18 000 g for 5 min to collect DEX–oxSWNH complexes, which were then dried in the vacuum overnight for experiments. At first, they studied the release characteristics of DEX from the DEX–oxSWNHs complex. In the case of *in vitro* release experiments in PBS (pH 7.4) at 37 °C, the amount of DEX released was nearly proportional to the incubation time, i.e. 7–10% per day during the first few days. The release rate then gradually declined and about 50% of the total bound DEX was released from the complex within a period of 2 weeks. When cell culture medium was used instead of PBS, distinctly different release profiles were obtained. Almost half of the DEX was released within the first 8 h, after which the release rates sharply declined, so that by 24 h about 50% of the total bound DEX had been released into the RPMI 1640 medium. As mentioned above, only about 10% was released into PBS during the same time period. One possible explanation for this difference in the release profiles is that hydrophobic organic compounds present in the culture medium are competitively absorbed onto the surface of oxSWNHs or they may increase the apparent solubility of DEX in medium. They also performed the biological assay of the DEX–oxSWNH complex and showed that the DEX released from DEX–oxSWNHs had biological activity.

Murakami and coworkers also applied oxSWNHs for the delivery of the anticancer drug, doxorubicin (DXR) [133]. At first, they prepared the complex, PEG–DXR, of PEG and DXR by introducing PEG into the amino groups of DXR. With PEG–DXR, oxSWNHs were well dispersed in water and the mean diameter was about 200 nm. The obtained PEG–DXR–oxSWNH had a strong antitumor activity in the *in vitro* assay system.

6.5 Physicochemical Aspects of Porous Silastic Materials for Drug Delivery

In the pharmaceutical field, several porous materials, such as silica, calcium silicate [97, 98], controlled pore glass [134, 135] and porous cellulose [136], are used to formulate solid dosage forms. Among them, silica particles are characteristic in having many sylanol groups on their surfaces, which may be able to form hydrogen bonds with drug molecules [137]. There are several grades of silica particles with different properties, such as particle size, degree of hydrophilicity and pore structure. Recently, a new grade of porous silica, mesoporous silica, has also been developed. It has been pointed out that the porous structure itself confers special characteristics, such as a decrease of melting point and a decrease in the crystallinity of drugs entrapped in the pores [134–136, 138]. Using these characteristics of porous silica particles, several applications have been reported in the field of pharmaceutical preparations.

In this section, two different types of applications with porous silastic materials, i.e. improvement in the drug dissolution properties and entrapment of peptide drugs for their sustained release, will be introduced.

6.5.1
Solid Dispersion Particles with Porous Silica

Improvement of the dissolution property of pharmaceuticals is extremely important, especially since the percentage of drugs with poor water solubility has increased in recent years. According to the Noyes–Whitney equation [139], the dissolution rate of a drug depends on its surface area and solubility. It is easier to increase the surface area by reducing the particle size of drug crystals than to increase the drug solubility. The particle size may be easily reduced by simple grinding. However, the ground crystals tend to agglomerate, thereby creating a surface with higher energy than that of the original crystals and reducing the effective surface area for dissolution.

To improve the dissolution properties of drugs, several methods have been studied as pharmaceutical engineering techniques such as grinding with additive [140], formation of salt [141] and preparation of an inclusion compound with cyclodextrin [142], as well as simple grinding [143]. Solid dispersion is a useful method to disperse drugs in the molecular state in a carrier matrix [144, 145]. The interaction between the drug molecule and carrier is responsible for drug dispersion, and may depress the crystallization of the drug in the prepared system. The most popular carrier materials are water-soluble polymers such as PEG [146] or PVP [147]. However, it is often reported that drugs prepared by solid dispersion with a water-soluble polymer carrier tend to be sticky or tacky. This property leads to a decrease in the recovery of solid dispersion in the preparation and also a difficulty in handling in the subsequent processes. Milling or mixing with other excipients is required before preparing the final dosage forms by plugging into capsules or tabletting. These processes sometimes facilitate crystallization of the drug in an amorphous state in the solid dispersion. The change in the crystalline forms of the drug in the dosage form affects its BA after administration.

Takeuchi and coworkers [148] demonstrated that solid dispersion particles of a poorly water soluble drug, tolbutamide (TBM), could be prepared by spray-drying the diluted ammonium solution of the drug with nonporous silica, AER 200. The spray-drying technique is a useful method to obtain spherical particles with a small size and narrow distribution. This method also has the advantage that granulation and drying are completed in one step. It was also confirmed that the drug was molecularly dispersed in the matrix formed with silica particles. The resultant solid dispersion particles were free-flowing and remarkably improved the dissolution property of the drug.

In preparing the solid dispersion particles of TBM using porous silica (Sylysia 350; Fuji Silisia, Japan) as a carrier from ethanol solution, the metastable crystalline form (type II) was observed in the resultant particles [149]. It is well known that the drug crystalline form can be controlled by controlling the crystallization conditions, such as the type of solvent and crystallization rate. In the case of TBM, four types of crystalline forms including the stable form of type I and three types of metastable crystalline forms (types II, III and IV) were characterized based on their physicochemical properties, and the dissolution, BA and stability of these polymorphs have been investigated [150–152].

To confirm the factors controlling the crystalline forms of drug in the silica solid dispersion particles, solid dispersion particles of TBM were prepared by formulating various types of silica such as nonporous [AER 200 (hydrophilic), AER R972 (hydrophobic)] or porous [Sylysia 350 (hydrophilic), Sylophobic 200 (hydrophobic)] silica as carriers and applying the spray-drying or evaporation method. In the solid dispersion particles prepared by the spray-drying method, TBM existed in a metastable form (form II) irrespective of the type of silica. On the other hand, when the evaporation method was used, various crystalline forms of TBM were observed in the solid dispersion particles depending on the type of silica. Polymorphs of forms III and IV were prepared with AER 200 and AER R972, respectively, while crystalline form II was obtained when either of the forms of porous silica, Sylysia 350 or Sylophobic 200, was formulated [149].

There may be two main factors affecting the final crystalline form of the drug in this process – the removal rate of solvent from the drug solution and the type of carrier formulated with the solid dispersion. The rapid solvent evaporation from the drug solution in the spray-drying method facilitated formation of the metastable form II of TBM in the resultant particles irrespective of the type of silica. Formation of this crystalline form was also observed for evaporation solid dispersion with porous silica (Sylysia 350 or Sylophobic 200), although the solvent evaporation speed was not rapid. In this case, formation of the metastable crystalline form (form II) may have been due to restriction of the crystallization of drug molecules in the pores of carrier particles during evaporation.

To examine the pore size effect on the resultant crystalline form of TBM in evaporation solid dispersion particles, several types of porous silica with different average pore sizes (Tab. 6.4) were used. The solid dispersion with Sylysia 740, having an extremely small pore size, showed metastable form III, while form II was detected in other types of silica solid dispersion. This result suggested that pores of this type of silica were not effectively utilized in this solid dispersion formulation. In the case of other porous materials, a similar tendency was observed. Porous cel-

Tab. 6.4. Properties of porous silica and other materials

Commercial name	Average particle size (μm)	Specific surface area ($m^2\ g^{-1}$)	Pore size (nm)	Pore volume ($mL\ g^{-1}$)
Sylysia 350	3.9	300	21.0	1.60
Sylysia 470	14.1	300	17.0	1.25
Sylysia 440	6.2	300	17.0	1.25
Sylysia 740	5.0	700	2.5	0.44
FLR	26.1	120	no data	150.0

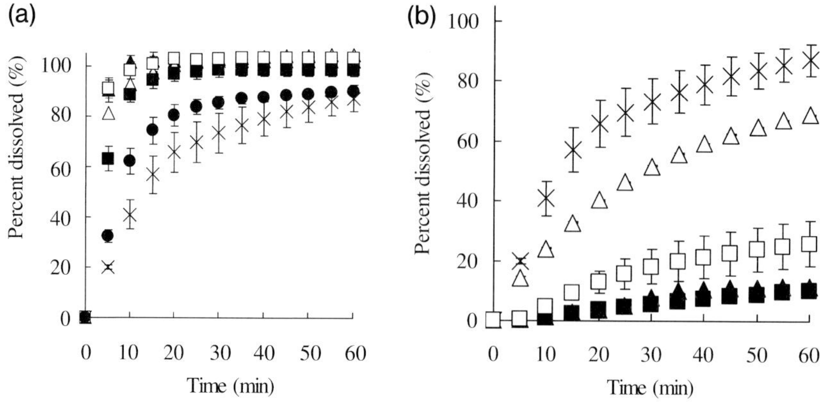

Figure 6.21. (a) Dissolution profile of TBM from solid dispersion particles with AER 200 or Sylysia 350 prepared by the spray-drying or evaporation method. × = Original TBM crystals; • = spray-dried TBM; ▲ = spray-drying solid dispersion with AER 200; ▪ = spray-drying solid dispersion with Sylysia 350; □ = evaporation solid dispersion with AER 200; ▫ = evaporation solid dispersion with Sylysia 350. (b) Dissolution profile of TBM from solid dispersion particles with AER R972 or Sylophobic 200 prepared by the spray-drying or evaporation method. × = Original TBM crystals; ▲ = spray-drying solid dispersion with AER R972; ▪ = spray-drying solid dispersion with Sylophobic 200; □ = evaporation solid dispersion with AER R972; ▫ = evaporation solid dispersion with Sylophobic 200.

lulose, having a small pore size of 4.0 nm, formed a mixture of forms II and IV in the resultant solid dispersion. The larger pore volume of porous cellulose than Sylysia 740 may be responsible for the formation of form II, although the average pore size of Sylysia 740 is as small as 2.5 nm. Another type of silastic particle, FLR, which has extremely larger pore volume, showed form II in the resultant solid dispersion. We should pay attention to the critical pore size and pore volume in using the porous silica as the drug carrier of solid dispersion [153].

The dissolution property of TBM was dramatically improved in the spray-drying solid dispersion system with hydrophilic silica (Sylysia 350 and AER 200), as shown in Fig. 6.21(a) [149]. Both the metastable crystalline form of the drug and the increased hydrophilicity of the solid dispersion particle may have contributed to this improvement. The latter effect was confirmed by measuring the drug dissolution of solid dispersions with the hydrophobic silica, Sylophobic 200 or AER R972. The spray-drying solid dispersion with the hydrophobic silica containing crystalline form II showed an extremely decreased dissolution rate (Fig. 6.21b). TBM of evaporation solid dispersion with Sylysia 350 and AER 200 showed a similar improved dissolution pattern to that of the corresponding spray-drying solid dispersion, as shown in Fig. 6.21.

The drug:carrier ratio is an important factor in designing an optimum solid dispersion system. In powder XRD analysis, the solid dispersion particles loading excess amount of drug, which was prepared in the formulation of TBM:silica =

5:1, showed much larger peaks than that prepared with the formulation of TBM:silica = 1:1. The resultant drug dissolution rate was decreased. When the spray-drying method was used, the results were almost the same [153].

From the practical point of view, the stability of metastable crystalline forms of drugs in the solid dispersion particles is an important factor in designing the final dosage forms. The metastable form of TBM in the solid dispersion particles was stable for at least 4 weeks when stored at 60 °C and 0% relative humidity (RH), while the spray-dried TBM without silica (form II) gradually changed to the stable form (form I) under the same storage conditions. Under humid storage conditions (60 °C, 75% RH), the spray-dried TBM without silica (form II) immediately converted into the stable form (form I) within 1 day, while TBM (form II) in the solid dispersions in a matrix of silica was stable for at least 1 week. In comparing their stability with respect to the type of carrier particles formulated in the solid dispersion, porous Sylysia 350 was more effective than nonporous AER 200. The same tendency was observed for the evaporation solid dispersion. As shown in Tab. 6.5, metastable form II in evaporation solid dispersion with Sylysia 350 was unchanged for up to 14 days, while metastable form III in AER 200 was converted to stable form I within the same storage period [149].

The effectiveness of porous silica as a solid dispersion carrier was confirmed using another model drug, IMC [154, 155]. IMC, whose solubility in water is 5 μg mL^{-1} [156], has a tendency to form an amorphous state. This amorphous state property of IMC was examined extensively by many workers [157, 158]. Zografi

Tab. 6.5. Stability of the crystalline form of TBM in solid dispersion particles prepared by different methods stored at 0% or 75% RH and 60 °C

RH	Solid dispersion			Evaporation	
	No	AER 200	Sylysia 350	AER 200	Sylysia 350
	II	II	II	III	II
0% 60 °C	I+II	II	II	III	II
	I+II	II	II	III	II
	I+II	II	II	I+III	II
	I+II	II	II	I+III	II
	I	II	II	I+III	II
75%	II	II	II	III	II
	I	II	II	III	II
	I	II	II	I+III	II
	I	I+II	II	I	II
	I	I+II	hallo pattern	I	hallo pattern
	I	I+II	hallo pattern	I	hallo pattern

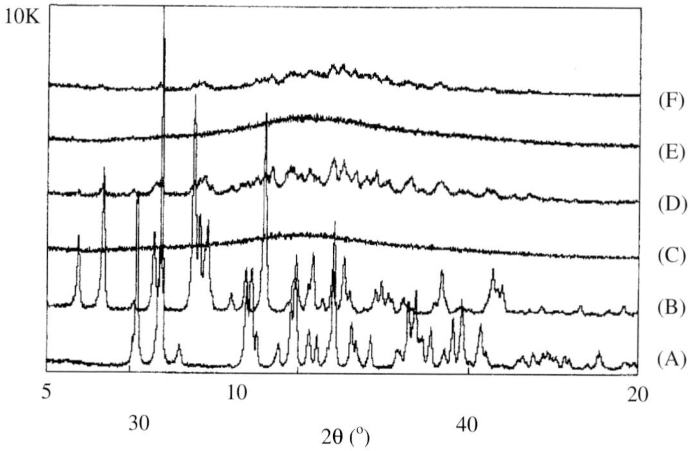

Figure 6.22. Powder XRD patterns of various types of IMC and solid dispersion particles with AER 200 or Sylysia 350. (A) Original IMC crystals (γ-form). (B) Metastable IMC crystals (α-form). (C) Amorphous IMC. (D) Spray-dried IMC. (E) Solid dispersion particles with AER1 200. (F) Solid dispersion particles with Sylysia 350.

and coworkers [159, 160] reported the interaction of IMC and PVP at the molecular level and the effect of PVP on the inhibition of crystallization of amorphous IMC in the solid dispersion system. Yoshioka and coworkers also reported the crystallization of IMC from the amorphous state above and below its glass transition temperature [161].

The solid dispersion particles of IMC were prepared with nonporous (AER 200) or porous silica (Sylysia 350) in a similar way as for TBM solid dispersion [155]. The powder XRD charts shown in Fig. 6.22 show the decreased crystallinity of IMC for spray-dried IMC and the solid dispersion particles. IMC in solid dispersion particles is almost amorphous irrespective of the type of silica formulated. In characterizing them based on the trace size of the peaks in the powder XRD charts, the crystalline form of the spray-dried IMC was a mixture of the metastable form (α-form) and stable form (γ-form), while the original IMC crystals were the stable form (γ-form). Differential scanning calorimetry (DSC) patterns of various types of IMC and IMC in solid dispersion particles are shown in Fig. 6.23. The profile of spray-dried IMC showed transformation of the amorphous part of IMC into the metastable crystalline form by heating. On the other hand, the solid dispersion particles containing amorphous IMC showed a trace endothermic peak at the lower temperature compared to the melting endothermic peak for the stable or metastable IMC crystals, which confirmed that the carrier prevented the crystallization of amorphous IMC. Comparing the small endothermic peak for the two types of solid dispersion particles with different types of silica, the area of melting peak of IMC in solid dispersion with Sylysia 350 is smaller and the position of the peak is at a lower temperature than that with AER 200. In general, the melting point of drug molecules in the pore is lower than that in the bulk state [162, 163]. Nakai and

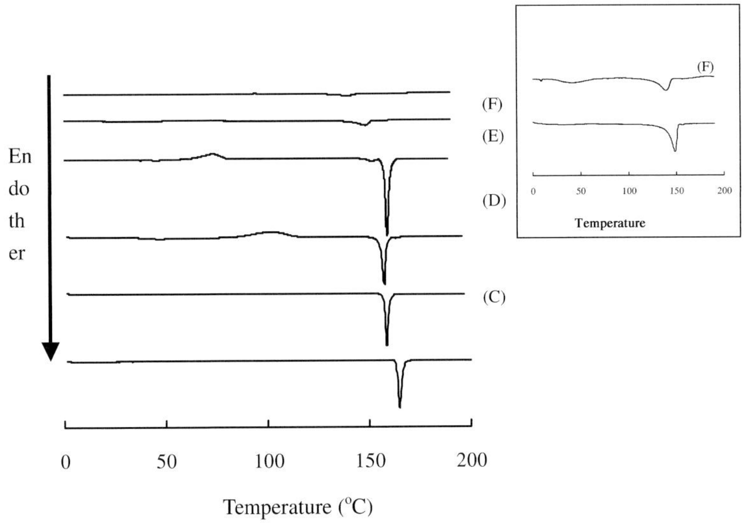

Figure 6.23. DSC patterns of various types of IMC and solid dispersion particles with AER 200 or Sylysia 350. (A) Original IMC crystals (γ-form). (B) Metastable IMC crystals (α-form). (C) Amorphous IMC. (D) Spray-dried IMC. (E) Solid dispersion particles with AER1 200. (F) Solid dispersion particles with Sylysia 350.

coworkers reported this phenomenon with porous silica or porous cellulose as the carrier in the mixing system of drug crystals and the porous materials [97, 136, 138].

Figure 6.24 shows the dissolution profile of IMC from the solid dispersion particles with AER 200 or Sylysia 350 [155]. The dissolution rate of spray-dried IMC

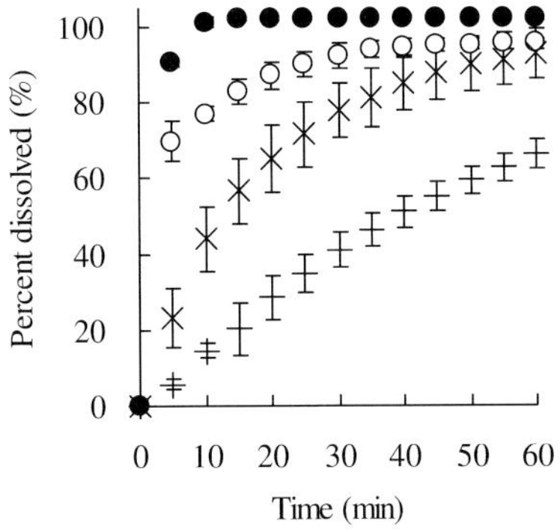

Figure 6.24. Dissolution profiles of IMC from solid dispersion particles with AER 200 or Sylysia 350. + = Original IMC crystals (γ-form). × = Spray-dried IMC. ○ = Solid dispersion particles with AER 200. • = Solid dispersion particles with Sylysia 350.

particles was faster than that of original IMC crystals because of the decrease in particle size, crystallinity and change in the crystalline form. However, 100% of spray-dried IMC could not dissolve within 60 min. On the other hand, the dissolution profile of IMC in the solid dispersions particles was remarkably improved irrespective of the type of silica formulated. This might be due to the improvement in wettability and dispersibility in the medium as well as the decrease in crystallinity of IMC in the particles, as mentioned above for the TBM solid dispersion with silica. Comparing the dissolution profiles of solid dispersion particles with AER 200 and Sylysia 350, the dissolution rate of IMC from solid dispersion particles with Sylysia 350 was faster than that with AER 200. As the drug crystallinity of the solid dispersion particles is almost the same, the difference in wettability may be responsible for the difference in the drug dissolution rate of the two different types of solid dispersion particles.

The effect of wettability on the dissolution property was clearly demonstrated with the solid dispersion particle with Sylysia 740, whose average pore size is 2.5 nm (Tab. 6.4). The dissolution rate of IMC solid dispersion with Sylysia 740 was much decreased compared with that of Sylysia 350, although Sylysia 740 was also hydrophilic silica and the drug to silica formulating ratio was the same at 1:1 [154]. The measured specific surface areas of the solid dispersion particle with Sylysia 740 and Sylysia 350 were 7.4 and 99.5 $m^2\ g^{-1}$, while those of Sylysia 740 and Sylysia 350 were 700 and 300 $m^2\ g^{-1}$, respectively. The greatly decreased specific surface area of Sylysia 740 solid dispersion implied the stuffing of pores with silica, which may lead to the reduced dispersion of the drug molecule in the pore of the carrier and covering of the silica particles with the hydrophobic drug molecule, as illustrated in Fig. 6.25. Thus, the resultant drug dissolution was decreased due to the hydrophobic property of the solid dispersion. These results may show that the pore size of silica is an important factor in obtaining the improved dissolution profile of the solid dispersion system.

The stabilizing effect of porous silica on the amorphous state of drugs was the same as observed in the case of the metastable form of TBM. In a stability test,

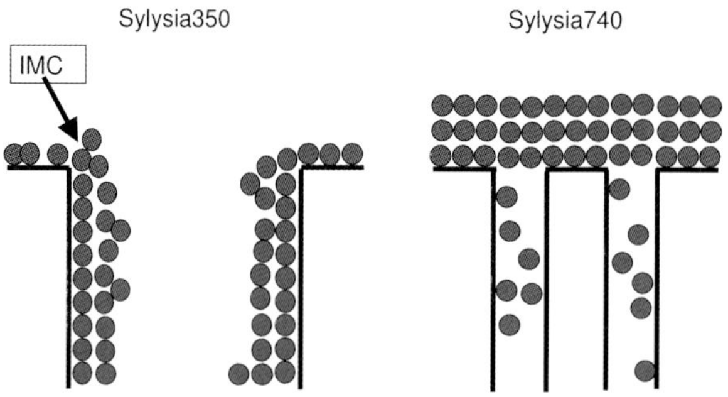

Figure 6.25. Schematic drawing of the state of IMC molecules in the pore of solid dispersions with Sylysia 350 or Sylysia 740.

amorphous IMC in the solid dispersion particles with each of the silica particles did not crystallize under storing at severe storage conditions (40 °C, 75% RH) for 2 months, while amorphous IMC without silica easily crystallized under the same conditions.

Through these two examples mentioned above, we can conclude that the porous silica particle effectively forms solid dispersion particles of poorly water-soluble drugs. Although nonporous colloidal silica has a similar carrier property to form an amorphous state of the drug in the particles, porous silica is sometimes superior to nonporous silica from the point of the resultant drug dissolution property or stability of the amorphous or metastable state of the drug.

Watanabe and coworkers [137] have reported that controlled release of IMC with nonporous silica leads to an improvement in its BA in an *in vivo* experiment. For this experiment, IMC was compounded with silica (AER 200) by cogrinding or melt-quenching. The initial dissolution rate of the coground compound was lower than the melt-quenched one, although both of them showed higher dissolution rates than a simple physical mixture of crystalline IMC and silica. The lower dissolution rate of coground IMC was explained by a stronger chemical interaction between IMC and the mechanically induced siloxane dangling bonds on the surface of silica. The resultant AUC values of coground and melt-quenched compounds were 1711 and 1519 μg h mL^{-1}, respectively, while that of the physical mixture was 751 μg h mL^{-1}. These results suggested that the initial controlled release of the drug leads to a higher BA.

6.5.2 Mesoporous Silica

Mesoporous silica is a porous silica with tightly size-controlled pores of 2–50 nm. Two types of mesoporous silica, i.e. FSM16 [164] and MCM-41 [165], have been developed by two different groups separately [166]. Both of them have the same hexagonal pore structure, although the proposed structure formation mechanism is different. FSM16 can be synthesized from a layered silicate, kanemaite, and a folding sheet mechanism was proposed. The process including the resultant structure of FSM16 is illustrated in Fig. 6.26 [166]. The pore size and specific surface area of FSM16 are 3.0 nm and around 1000 m^2 g^{-1}, respectively. Although there are several reports on mesoporous silica dealing with the preparation process and application in catalysis, few papers are available in the field of pharmaceutical engineering [166].

We have examined the usefulness of this porous particle as a carrier of the macromolecular drug insulin, because its pore size is comparable to that of the macromolecules. The simple adsorption profile of insulin on FSM16 is shown in Fig. 6.27 [167]. By assuming Langmuir-type adsorption, the maximum adsorption amount was estimated as 137 μg mg^{-1} of FSM16. The adsorption amount of insulin to Sylysia 350 or Sylysia 740 was low, although their surface area is comparable to that of FSM16 and the pore size of Sylysia 740 (2.5 nm) is similar to that of FSM16.

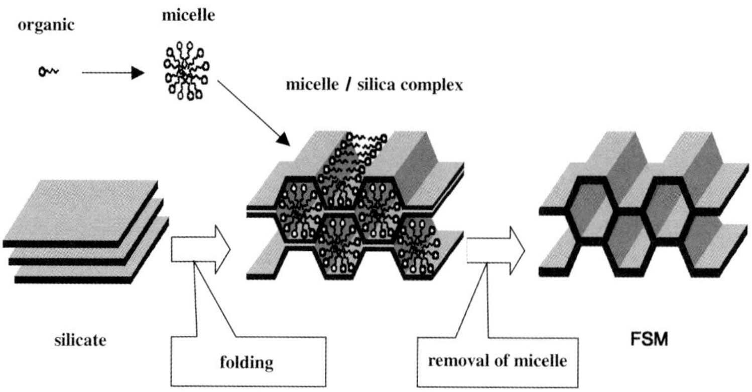

Figure 6.26. Formation and pore structure of FSM.

To increase the entrapment efficiency of insulin into the porous material, we devised a freeze–thawing method. Although the freeze–thawing method has been reported as a drug encapsulation method into liposomes, the concept of this freeze–thawing method for mesoporous silica is completely different. In this method, we used nonfrozen water formed in the pores of particles. In general, porous material has special properties such as a decreased melting point and forms nonfrozen water in the pores [162, 163]. It has also been reported that silica gel forms nonfrozen water on its surface and that nonfrozen water can be formed in the porous materials [168–170]. Morishige and coworkers [170] have observed that free water in the pores of MCM with a pore diameter of 4.2 nm was frozen abruptly around 232 K to give rise to cubic ice, while the water confined in the pores with a pore diameter of

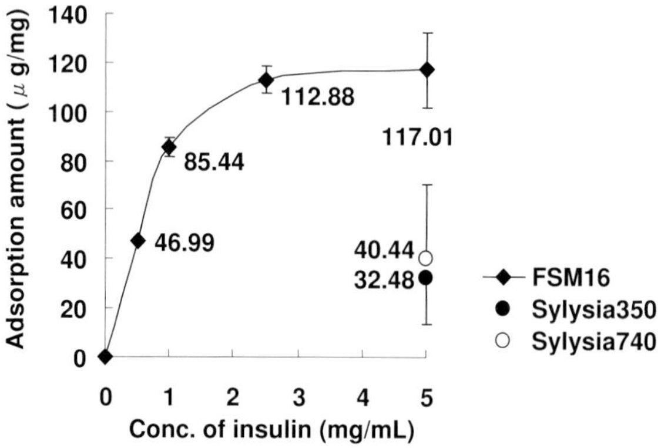

Figure 6.27. Adsorption amount of insulin on FSM16, Sylysia 350 and Sylysia 740 at various concentration of insulin solution. Adsorption conditions: temperature = 5 °C; shaking time = 24 h.

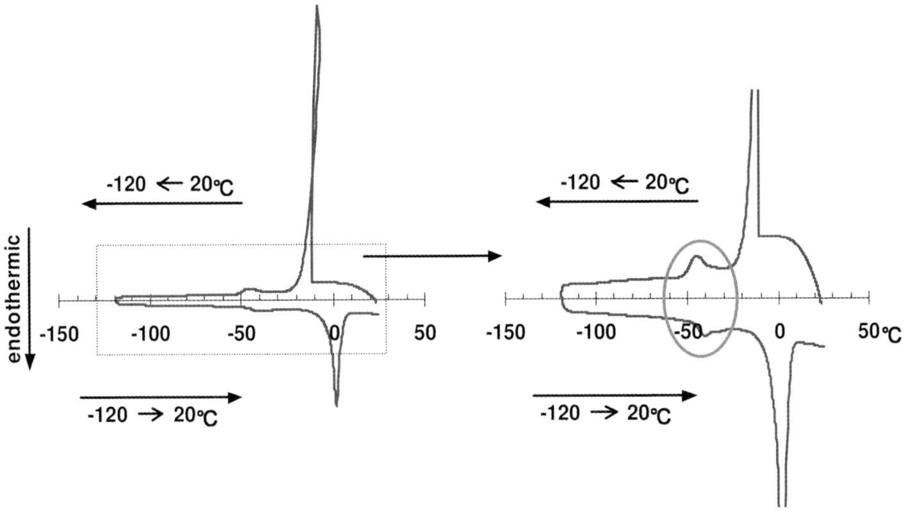

Figure 6.28. DSC profiles of FSM16 containing water.

2.4 nm was frozen very gradually at lower temperature. To confirm the formation of nonfrozen water in FSM16, we measured DSC patterns of FSM16 containing water. As shown in the DSC chart (Fig. 6.28), two clear exothermic peaks in the freezing process and two endothermic peaks in the melting process were observed [167]. The peaks observed at the lower temperature may be attributed to the freezing and melting of water in the pores. In the case of Sylysia 350, such peaks were not observed, because the pore size was much larger than FSM16. In the case of Sylysia 740, similar peaks were detected because its average pore size is as small as FSM16. However, the peaks were very small compared with that of FSM16. This may be attributed to its large pore size distribution, as observed for normal silica.

In freezing the FSM16 suspension in drug solution, the drug solution may be concentrated in the pores when the bulk water is frozen and then the freezing is stopped just before freezing of the pore water. Based on the DSC analysis which showed the pore water was frozen at around −40 °C, the freezing temperature in the freeze–thawing method was set at −30 °C. Figure 6.29 shows the increased entrapment of insulin into FSM16 using this freeze–thawing method. The entrapment amount increased by increasing the number of freezing–thawing cycles. When the freezing temperature was set at −100 instead of −30 °C, the efficiency was much reduced. This result confirmed our assumption stated above for the mechanism of drug entrapment in the freeze–thawing method. In both cases of Sylysia 350 and Sylysia 740, the entrapment amount of insulin was in the range of 50–100 $\mu g\ mg^{-1}$, even by applying this freeze–thawing method (10 times) [167].

The drug release from the insulin-loaded FSM16 was measured *in vitro*. The result showed that half of the entrapped insulin was released within 1 h (burst re-

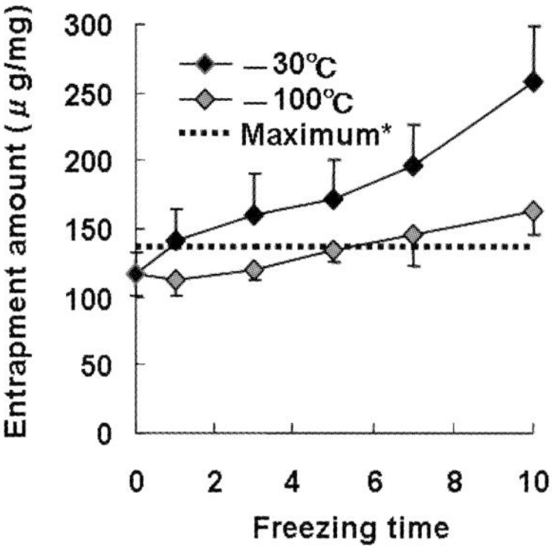

Figure 6.29. Entrapment of insulin into FSM16 with the freeze–thawing method. Initial adsorption conditions: temperature = 5 °C; shaking time = 24 h. *Maximum adsorption amount of insulin on FSM16 calculated with the Langmuir adsorption isotherm (137.0 μg mg^{-1}).

lease) followed by a very slow and sustained release (1.3 μg mg^{-1} of FSM16 day^{-1}). To utilize mesoporous silica as a drug carrier, it may be important to control the burst release. This might be achieved by modifying the entrance of the pores of FSM with some hydrophobic molecules.

To check the effectiveness of the freeze–thawing method in the encapsulation of macromolecules, three types of FITC–dextran with different molecular weights (4400, 9500 and 21 200) were selected as a model drugs [171]. When the adsorption amount of these FITC–dextran was compared under the same conditions, where 10 mg of FSM16 was dispersed in 1 mg mL^{-1} of drug solution at 5 °C, the adsorption amount of FITC–dextran depended on their molecular weight, in the order of FITC–dex4400 > FITC–dex9500 > FITC–dex21200. In applying the freeze–thawing method to the entrapment of these FITC–dextrans, the entrapment amount was increased, as shown in Fig. 6.30. As the adsorbed amount of FITC–dex9500 and FITC–dex21200 was very small in the simple adsorption process, their adsorption amounts to FSM16 with the freeze–thawing method were 6.1 and 20.7 times higher compared with a simple adsorption procedure, respectively.

FSM16 is also an excellent carrier for poorly water-soluble drugs with low molecular weight as well as usual porous silica (as discussed in the previous section). We prepared a solid dispersion of beclomethasone propionate using FSM16 as a carrier in the same manner as for the Sylysia solid dispersion [172]. The simple adsorption amount of drug to FSM16 in the dichloromethane solution was large and the maximum adsorption amount was estimated as 333.3 μg mg^{-1} of FSM16. In the case of Sylysia 350, the estimated maximum adsorption amount was 156.3 μg mg^{-1} FSM16. In the dissolution test, FSM16 solid dispersion showed a supersaturated concentration of the drug, which was 3 times higher than the saturated concentration, while Sylysia 350 solid dispersion showed almost the same drug concentration as the crystalline drug. The different drug dissolution phenomenon

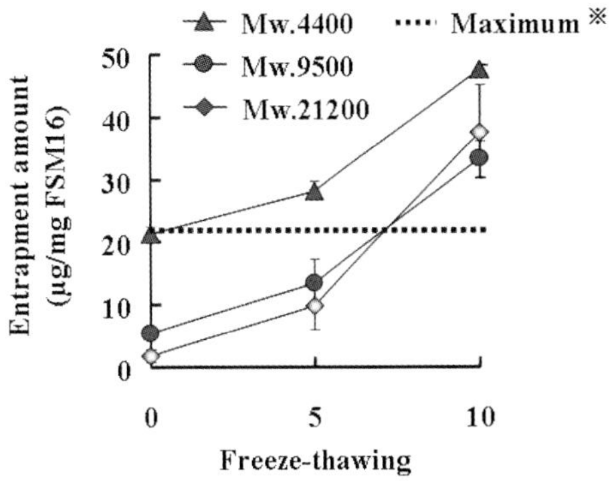

Figure 6.30. Entrapment of FITC–dextran with different molecular weights (4400, 9500 and 21 200) into FSM16 with the freeze–thawing method. Conditions of entrapment test: FITC–dex.sol., 1 mg mL^{-1}, 1 mL solvent (McIlvaine buffer, pH4.0); silica; FSM16 (10 mg); freezing temperature = −30 °C. *Maximum adsorption amount of FITC–dex4400 on FSM16 calculated with the Langmuir adsorption isotherm (22.57 μg mg^{-1}).

for FSM16 and Sylysia 350 solid dispersions suggested different adsorption modes or forces between the surface of the silica and the drug molecule.

Tozuka and coworkers [173] recently investigated the adsorption and entrapment of salicylamide molecules into FSM16. They confirmed crystalline salicylamide converted into an amorphous state on heating at 120 °C for 3 h. By measuring a shift in the fluorescence emission peak of salicylamide in the carrier, they suggested dispersion of the drug molecule into the hexagonal channels during the heating process. It was also demonstrated that the dissolution rate of the solid dispersion was higher than the crystalline one.

As mesoporous silica such as FSM16 is quite a new product, for which large-scale production processes are still being developed, the number of reports in the pharmaceutical field is small. However, data shown in this section may indicate its unique characteristics due to its extremely high surface area and tightly controlled pore size. A lot of interesting data should follow in the near future.

References

1 Fukumori, Y., Ichikawa, H. **2005**. Design of controlled release pharmaceuticals in nanoparticle coating process. *J. Soc. Powder Technol., Japan 42*, 673–581.

2 Jono, K., Ichikawa, H., Miyamoto, M., Fukumori, Y. **2000**. A review of particulate design for pharmaceutical powders and their production by spouted bed coating. *Powder Technol. 113*, 269–277.

3 Fukumori, Y., Ichikawa, H. **2003**. Fluid bed processes for forming functional particles. In *Encyclopedia of Pharmaceutical Technology*. Edited by Parikh, D. M., Marcel Dekker, New York, pp. 1–7.

4 Dashevsky, A., Kolter, K., Bodmeier, R. **2004**. Compression of pellets coated with various aqueous polymer dispersions. *Int. J. Pharmac. 279*, 19–26.

5 Lin, A. Y., Muhammad, N. A., Pope, D., Augsburger, L. L. **2003**. A study of the effects of curing and storage conditions on controlled release diphenhydramine HCl pellets coated with Eudragit NE30D. *Pharmac. Dev. Technol. 8*, 277–287.
6 Lin, A. Y., Muhammad, N. A., Pope, D., Augsburger, L. L. **2001**. Study of crystallization of endogenous surfactant in Eudragit NE30D-free films and its influence on drug-release properties of controlled-release diphenhydramine HCl pellets coated with Eudragit NE30D. *AAPS Pharmac. Sci. 3*, E14.
7 AlKhatib, H. S., Sakr, A. **2003**. Optimization of methacrylic acid ester copolymers blends as controlled release coatings using response surface methodology. *Pharmac. Dev. Technol. 8*, 87–96.
8 Liu, Y., Schwartz, J. B., Schnaare, R. L. **2003**. A multimechanistic drug release approach in a bead dosage form and *in vitro* predictions. *Pharmac. Dev. Technol. 8*, 163–173.
9 Sadeghi, F., Ford, J. L., Rubinstein, M. H., Rajabi-Siahboomi, A. R. **2000**. Comparative study of drug release from pellets coated with HPMC or Surelease. *Drug Dev. Ind. Pharm. 26*, 651–660.
10 Lippold, B. C., Monells Pages, R. **2001**. Control and stability of drug release from diffusion pellets coated with the aqueous quaternary polymethacrylate dispersion Eudragit RS30D. *Pharmazie 56*, 477–483.
11 Larsen, C. C., Sonnergaard, J. M., Bertelsen, P., Holm, P. **2003**. A new process control strategy for aqueous film coating of pellets in fluidized bed. *Eur. J. Pharmac. Sci. 20*, 273–283.
12 Ichikawa, H., Fukumori, Y., Adeyeye, C. M. **1997**. Design of prolonged-release microcapsules containing diclofenac sodium for oral suspensions and their preparation by the Wurster process. *Int. J. Pharmac. 156*, 39.
13 Ichikawa, H., Fujioka, K., Adeyeye, C. M., Fukumori, Y. **2001**. Use of ion-exchange resins to prepare 100 μm-sized microcapsules with prolonged drug-release by the Wurster process. *Int. J. Pharmac. 216*, 67–76.
14 Cole, E. T., Scott, R. A., Corror, A. L., Wilding, I. R., Petereit, H., Schminke, C., Beckert, T., Cade, D. **2002**. Enteric coated HPMC capsules designed to achieve intestinal targeting. *Int. J. Pharmac. 231*, 83–95.
15 Rudolph, M. W., Klein, S., Beckert, T. E., Petereit, H., Dressman, J. B. **2001**. A new 5-aminosalicylic acid multi-unit dosage form for the therapy of ulcerative colitis. *Eur. J. Pharmac. Biopharmac. 51*, 183–190.
16 Gupta, V. K., Beckert, T. E., Deusch, N. J., Hariharan, M., Price, J. C. **2002**. Investigation of potential ionic interactions between anionic and cationic polymethacrylates of multiple coatings of novel colonic delivery system. *Drug Dev. Ind. Pharm. 28*, 207–215.
17 Fukumori, Y. **1994**. Coating of multiparticulates using polymeric dispersions. Formulation and process consideration. In *Multiparticulate Oral Drug Delivery*, Ghebre-Sellassie, I. (Ed.). Marcel Dekker, New York, pp. 79–111.
18 Steuernagel, C. R. **1989**. Latex emulsions for controlled drug delivery. In *Aqueous Polymeric Coatings for Pharmaceutical Dosage Forms*, McGenity, J. W. (Ed.). Marcel Dekker, New York, pp. 1–62.
19 Moore, K. L. **1989**. Physical properties of Opadry, Coateric, and Surelease. In *Aqueous Polymeric Coatings for Pharmaceutical Dosage Forms*, McGenity, J. W. (Ed.). Marcel Dekker, New York, pp. 303–316.
20 Lehmann, K. O. R. **1989**. Chemistry and application properties of polymethacrylate coating. In *Aqueous Polymeric Coatings for Pharmaceutical Dosage Forms*, McGenity, J. W. (Ed.). Marcel Dekker, New York, pp. 153–246.
21 Muroi, S. **1984**. *High Polymer Latex Adhesives*. Kobunnshi-Kankokai, Kyoto, Japan.
22 Fukumori, Y., Ichikawa, H., Yamaoka, Y., Akaho, E., Takeuchi, Y., Fukuda, T., Kanamori, R., Osako,

Y. **1991**. Effect of additives on physical properties of fine ethyl cellulose microcapsules prepared by the Wurster process. *Chem. Pharmac. Bull. 39*, 164–169.

23 Fukumori, Y., Ichikawa, H., Yamaoka, Y., Akaho, E., Takeuchi, Y., Fukuda, T., Kanamori, R., Osako, Y. **1991**. Microgranulation and encapsulation of pulverized pharmaceutical powders with ethyl cellulose by the Wurster process. *Chem. Pharmac. Bull. 39*, 1806–1812.

24 Fukumori, Y., Ichikawa, H., Jono, K., Takeuchi, Y., Fukuda, T. **1992**. Computer simulation of agglomeration in the Wurster process. *Chem. Pharmac. Bull. 40*, 2159–2163.

25 Fukumori, Y., Ichikawa, H., Jono, K., Takeuchi, Y., Fukuda, T., Osako, Y. **1993**. Effect of additives on agglomeration in aqueous coating with hydroxypropyl cellulose. *Chem. Pharmac. Bull. 41*, 725–730.

26 Ichikawa, H., Jono, K., Tokumitsu, H., Fukuda, T., Fukumori, Y. **1993**. Coating of pharmaceutical powders by fluidized bed process. V. Agglomeration and efficiency in the coating with aqueous latices of copoly(EA–MMA–HEMA). *Chem. Pharmac. Bull. 41*, 1132–1136.

27 Fukumori, Y., Yamaoka, Y., Ichikawa, H., Takeuchi, Y., Fukuda, T., Osako, Y. **1988**. Coating of pharmaceutical powders by fluidized bed process. III. Aqueous coating with ethyl acrylate–methyl methacrylate–2-hydroxyethyl methacrylate copolymer and the dissolution properties of the products. *Chem. Pharmac. Bull. 36*, 3070–3078.

28 Fukumori, Y., Yamaoka, Y., Ichikawa, H., Takeuchi, Y., Fukuda, T., Osako, Y. **1988**. Coating of pharmaceutical powders by fluidized bed process. IV. Softening temperature of acrylic copolymers and its relation to film-formation in aqueous coating. *Chem. Pharmac. Bull. 36*, 4927–4932.

29 Ichikawa, H., Tokumitsu, H., Jono, K., Osako, Y., Fukumori, Y. **1994**. Coating of pharmaceutical powders by fluidized bed process. VI. Microencapsulation using blend and composite latices of copoly(EA–MMA–HEMA). *Chem. Pharmac. Bull. 42*, 1308–1314.

30 Ichikawa, H., Kaneko, S., Fukumori, Y. **1996**. Coating performance of aqueous composite latices with *N*-isopropylacrylamide shell and thermosensitive permeation properties of their microcapsule membranes. *Chem. Pharmac. Bull. 44*, 383–391.

31 Kaneko, Y., Sakai, K., Okano, T. **1998**. *Biorelated Polymers and Gels*. Academic Press, Boston, MA, pp. 26–69.

32 Ichikawa, H., Fukumori, Y. **1997**. New applications of acrylic polymers for thermosensitive drug release. *STP Pharma Sci. 7*, 529–545.

33 Wu, X. S., Hoffman, A. S., Yager, P. **1992**. Synthesis and characterization of thermally reversible macroporous poly(*N*-isopropylacrylamide) hydrogels. *J. Polym. Sci. A Polym. Chem. 30*, 2121–2129.

34 Kaneko, Y., Nakamura, S., Sakai, K., Kikuchi, A., Aoyagi, T., Sakurai, Y., Okano, T. **1998**. Deswelling mechanism for comb-type grafted poly(*N*-isopropylacrylamide) hydrogels with rapid temperature responses. *Polym. Gels. Netw. 6*, 333–345.

35 Ichikawa, H., Fukumori, Y. **2000**. A novel positively thermosensitive controlled-release microcapsules with membrane of nano-sized poly(*N*-isopropylacrylamide) gel dispersed in ethyl cellulose matrix. *J. Control. Release 63*, 107–119.

36 Kas, H. S. **1997**. Chitosan: properties, preparations and application to microparticulate systems. *J. Microencapsul. 14*, 689–711.

37 Rege, P. R., Shukla, D. J., Block, L. H. **1999**. Chitinosans as tabletting excipients for modified release delivery systems. *Int. J. Pharmac. 181*, 49–60.

38 Shu, X. Z., Zhu, K. J. **2000**. A novel approach to prepare tripolyphosphate/chitosan complex beads for controlled release drug delivery. *Int. J. Pharmac. 201*, 51–58.

39 Kawashima, Y., Handa, T., Kasai, A., Takenaka, H., Lin, S. Y., Ando, Y. **1985**. Novel method for the preparation of controlled-release theophylline granules coated with a polyelectrolyte complex of sodium polyphosphate–chitosan. *J. Pharmac. Sci. 74*, 264–268.

40 Mi, F. L., Syu, S. S., Chen, C. T., Schoung, J. Y. **1999**. Porous chitosan microsphere for controlling the antigen release of Newcastle disease vaccine: preparation of antigen-adsorbed microsphere and *in vitro* release. *Biomaterials 20*, 1603–1612.

41 Illum, L., Farraj, N., Davis, S. S. **1994**. Chitosan as a novel nasal delivery system for peptide drugs. *Pharmac. Res. 11*, 1186–1189.

42 Calvo, P., Remuñán-López, C., Vila-Iato, J. L., Alonso, M. J. **1997**. Chitosan and chitosan/ethylene oxide–propylene oxide block copolymer nanoparticles as novel carriers for proteins and vaccines. *Pharmac. Res. 14*, 1431–1436.

43 Erbacher, P., Zou, S., Bettinger, T., Steffan, A. M., Remy, J. S. **1998**. Chitosan-based vector/DNA complexes for gene delivery: biophysical characteristics and transfection ability. *Pharmac. Res. 15*, 1332–1339.

44 Hassan, E. E., Parish, R. C., Gallo, J. M. **1992**. Optimized formulation of magnetic chitosan microspheres containing the anticancer agent, oxantrazole. *Pharmac. Res. 9*, 390–397.

45 Pavanetto, F., Perugini, P., Conti, B., Modena, T., Genta, I. **1996**. Evaluation of process parameters involved in chitosan microsphere preparation by the o/w/o multiple emulsion method. *J. Microencapsul. 13*, 679–688.

46 Ganza-González, A., Anguiano-Igea, S., Oteo-Espinar, F. J., Méndez, J. B. **1999**. Chitosan and chondroitin microspheres for oral-administration controlled release of metoclopramide. *Eur. J. Pharmac. Biopharmac. 48*, 149–155.

47 Masui, S., Ichikawa, H., Fukumori, Y. **2005**. Development of non-covalently cross-linked chitosan nanoparticles and their coating performance in spouted bed spray-coating process. In *Proceedings of 8th international Symposium on Agglomeration*, Bangkok, pp. 321–325.

48 Fukumori, Y., Ichikawa, H. **2006**. Nanoparticles for cancer therapy and diagnosis. *Adv. Powder Technol. 17*, 1–28.

49 Ito, A., Honda, H., Kobayashi, T. **2003**. Cancer diagnosis and therapy using magnetite nanoparticles. *Chem. Eng., Japan 67*, 692–695.

50 Bjornerud, A., Johansson, L. O., Ahlstrom, H. K. **2001**. Pre-clinical results with clariscan (NC100150 injection); experience from different disease models. *MAGMA 12*, 99–103.

51 Kircher, M. F., Allport, J. R., Graves, E. E., Love, V., Josephson, L., Lichtman, A. H., Weissleder, R. **2003**. *In vivo* high resolution three-dimensional imaging of antigen-specific cytotoxic T-lymphocyte trafficking to tumors. *Cancer Res. 63*, 6838–6346.

52 Josephson, L., Tung, C. H., Moore, A., Weissleder, R. **1999**. High-efficiency Intracellular magnetic labeling with novel superparamagnetic–tat peptide conjugate. *Bioconjug. Chem. 19*, 186–191.

53 Zhao, M., Kircher, M. F., Josephson, L., Weissleder, R. **2002**. Differential conjugation of tat peptide to superparamagnetic nanoparticles and its effect on cellular uptake. *Bioconjug. Chem. 13*, 840–844.

54 Schellenberger, E. A., Bogdanov, Jr., A., Hogemann, D., Tait, J., Weissleder, R., Josephson, L. **2002**. Annexin V–CLIO: a nanoparticle for detecting apoptosis by MRI. *Mol. Imaging 1*, 102–107.

55 Zhang, Y., Kohler, N., Zhang, M. **2002**. Surface modification of superparamagnetic magnetite nanoparticles and their intracellular uptake. *Biomaterials 23*, 1553–1561.

56 Hogemann, D., Josephson, L., Weissleder, R., Basilion, J. P. **2000**. Improvement of MRI probes to allow efficient detection of gene expression. *Bioconjug. Chem. 11*, 941–946.

57 Akerman, M. E., Chan, W. C., Laakkonen, P., Bhatia, S. N., Ruoslahti, E. **2002**. Nanocrystal targeting *in vivo*. *Proc. Natl Acad. Sci. USA 99*, 12617–12621.

58 Tkachenko, A. G., Xie, H., Coleman, D., Glomm, W., Ryan, J., Anderson, M. F., Franzen, S., Feldheim, D. L. **2003**. Multifunctional gold nanoparticle–peptide complexes for nuclear targeting, *J. Am. Chem. Soc. 125*, 4700–4701.

59 Onishi, H., Machida, Y., Machida, Y. **2003**. Antitumor properties of irinotecan-containing nanoparticles prepared using poly(DL-lactic acid) and poly(ethylene glycol)-block-poly(propylene glycol)-block-poly(ethylene glycol). *Biolo. Pharmac. Bull. 26*, 116–119.

60 Chawla, J. S., Amiji, M. M. **2003**. Cellular uptake and concentrations of tamoxifen upon administration in poly(epsilon-caprolactone) nanoparticles. *AAPS Pharmac. Sci. 5*, E3.

61 Chawla, J. S., Amiji, M. M. **2002**. Biodegradable poly(epsilon-caprolactone) nanoparticles for tumor-targeted delivery of tamoxifen. *Int. J. Pharmac. 24*, 127–138.

62 Kataoka, K., Harada, A., Nagasaki, Y. **2001**. Block copolymer micelles for drug delivery: design, characterization and biological significance. *Adv. Drug Deliv. Rev. 47*, 113–131.

63 Cui, Z., Mumper, R. J. **2002**. Plasmid DNA-entrapped nanoparticles engineered from microemulsion precursors: *in vitro* and *in vivo* evaluation. *Bioconjug. Chem. 13*, 1319–1327.

64 Kabbaj, M., Phillips, N. C. **2001**. Anticancer activity of mycobacterial DNA: effect of formulation as chitosan nanoparticles. *J. Drug Target. 9*, 317–328.

65 Hood, J. D., Bednarski, M., Frausto, R., Guccione, S., Reisfeld, R. A., Xiang, R., Cheresh, D. A. **2002**. Tumor regression by targeted gene delivery to the neovasculature. *Science*, 296 **5577**, 2404–2407.

66 Bellocq, N. C., Pun, S. H., Jensen, G. S., Davis, M. E. **2003**. Transferrin-containing, cyclodextrin polymer-based particles for tumor-targeted gene delivery. *Bioconjug. Chem. 14*, 1122–1132.

67 Gref, R., Couvreur, P., Barratt, G., Mysiakine, E. **2003**. Surface-engineered nanoparticles for multiple ligand coupling. *Biomaterials 24*, 4529–4537.

68 Espuelas, M. S., Legrand, P., Loiseau, P. M., Bories, C., Barratt, G., Irache, J. M. **2002**. *In vitro* antileishmanial activity of amphotericin B loaded in poly(epsilon-caprolactone) nanospheres. *J. Drug Target. 10*, 593–599.

69 Tokumitsu, H., Ichikawa, H., Fukumori, Y., Block, L. H. **1999**. Preparation of gadopentetic acid-loaded chitosan microparticles for gadolinium neutron-capture therapy of cancer by a novel emulsion-droplet coalescence technique. *Chem. Pharmac. Bull. 47*, 838–842.

70 Tokumitsu, H., Ichikawa, H., Fukumori, Y. **1999**. Chitosan–gadopentetic acid complex nanoparticles for gadolinium neutron-capture therapy of cancer: preparation by novel emulsion-droplet coalescence technique and characterization. *Pharmac. Res. 16*, 1830–1835.

71 Tokumitsu, H., Hiratsuka, J., Sakurai, Y., Kobayashi, T., Ichikawa, H., Fukumori, Y. **2000**. Gadolinium neutron-capture therapy using novel gadopentetic acid–chitosan complex nanoparticles: *in vivo* growth suppression of experimental melanoma solid tumor. *Cancer Lett. 150*, 177–182.

72 Shikata, F., Tokumitsu, H., Ichikawa, H., Fukumori, Y. **2002**. *In vitro* cellular accumulation of gadolinium incorporated into chitosan nanoparticles designed for neutron-capture therapy of cancer. *Eur. J. Pharmac. Biopharmac. 53*, 57–63.

73 Oyewumi, M. O., Yokel, R. A., Jay, M., Coakley, T., Mumper, R. J. **2004**. Comparison of cell uptake, biodistribution and tumor retention of folate-coated and PEG-coated gadolinium nanoparticles in tumor-

bearing mice. *J. Control. Release 95*, 613–626.

74 Oyewumi, M. O., Liu, S., Moscow, J. A., Mumper, R. J. **2003**. Specific association of thiamine-coated gadolinium nanoparticles with human breast cancer cells expressing thiamine transporters. *Bioconjug. Chem. 14*, 404–411.

75 Oyewumi, M. O., Mumper, R. J. **2003**. Influence of formulation parameters on gadolinium entrapment and tumor cell uptake using folate-coated nanoparticles. *Int. J. Pharmac. 251*, 85–97.

76 Oyewumi, M. O., Mumper, R. J. **2002**. Engineering tumor-targeted gadolinium hexanedione nanoparticles for potential application in neutron capture therapy. *Bioconjug. Chem. 13*, 1328–1335.

77 Oyewumi, M. O., Mumper, R. J. **2002**. Gadolinium-loaded nanoparticles engineered from microemulsion templates. *Drug Dev. Ind. Pharm. 28*, 317–328.

78 Stevens, P. J., Sekido, M., Lee, R. J. **2004**. Synthesis and evaluation of a hematoporphyrin derivative in a folate receptor-targeted solid-lipid nanoparticle formulation. *Anticancer Res. 24*, 161–165.

79 Roy, I., Ohulchanskyy, T. Y., Pudavar, H. E., Bergey, E. J., Oseroff, A. R., Morgan, J., Dougherty, T. J., Prasad, P. N. **2003**. Ceramic-based nanoparticles entrapping water-insoluble photosensitizing anticancer drugs: a novel drug-carrier system for photodynamic therapy. *J. Am. Chem. Soc. 125*, 7860–7865.

80 Nigavekar, S. S., Sung, L., Llanes, Y. M., El-Jawahri, A., Lawrence, T. S., Becker, C. W., Balogh, L., Khan, M. K. **2004**. ^{3}H dendrimer nanoparticle organ/tumor distribution. *Pharmac. Res. 21*, 4764–4683.

81 Li, L., Wartchow, C. A., Danthi, S. N., Shen, Z., Dechene, N., Pease, J., Choi, H. S., Doede, T., Chu, P., Ning, S., Lee, D. Y., Bednarski, M. D., Knox, S. J. **2004**. A novel antiangiogenesis therapy using an integrin antagonist or anti-Flk-1 antibody coated ^{90}Y-labeled nanoparticles. *Int. J. Radiat. Oncol. Biol. Phys. 58*, 1215–1227.

82 Kreuter, J. **2001**. Nanoparticulate systems for brain delivery of drugs. *Adv. Drug Deliv. Rev. 47*, 65–81.

83 Vaisanen, V., Harma, H., Lilja, H., Bjartell, A. **2000**. Time-resolved fluorescence imaging for quantitative histochemistry using lanthanide chelates in nanoparticles and conjugated to monoclonal antibodies. *Luminescence 15*, 89–397.

84 Majeti, N. V., Kumar, R. **2000**. Nano and microparticles as controlled drug delivery devices. *J. Pharm. Pharmac. Sci. 3*, 234–258.

85 Akerman, M. E., Chan, W. C. W., Laakkonen, P., Bhatia, S. N., Ruoslahti, E. **2002**. Nanocrystal targeting *in vivo*. *Natl Acad. Sci. USA 99*, 12617–12621.

86 Paul, W., Sharma, C. P. **2003**. Ceramic drug delivery: a perspective. *J. Biomater. Applic. 17*, 253–264.

87 Otsuka, M., Matsuda, Y., Duncan, Y. U., Wong, J., Fox, J. L., Higuchi, W. I. **1990**. A novel skeletal drug delivery system for anti-bacterial drugs using self-setting hydroxyapatite cement. *Chem. Pharmac. Bull. 38*, 3500–3502.

88 Otsuka, M., Matsuda, Y., Suwa, Y., Fox, J. L., Higuchi, W. I. **1994**. A novel skeletal drug delivery system using self-stetting calcium phosphate cement. 2. Physicochemical properties and drug release rate of the cement-containing indomethacin. *J. Pharmac. Sci. 83 5*, 611–615.

89 Haruta, S., Hanafusa, T., Fukase, H., Miyajima, H., Oki, T. **2003**. An effective absorption behavior of insulin for diabetic treatment following intranasal delivery using porous spherical calcium carbonate in monkeys and healthy human volunteers. *Diabetes Technol. Ther. 5*, 1–9.

90 Ishikawa, F., Murano, M., Hiraishi, M., Yamaguchi, T., Tamai, I., Tsuji, A. **2002**. Insoluble powder formulation as an effective nasal drug delivery system. *Pharmac. Res. 19*, 1097–1104.

91 Yanagawa, A., Kudo, T., Mizushima, Y. **1995**. A novel particle carrier for transnasal peptide absorption. *Jpn. J. Clin. Pharmacol. Ther. 26*, 127–128.
92 Ueno, Y., Futagawa, H., Takagi, Y., Ueno, A., Mizushima, Y. **2005**. Drug-incorporating calcium carbonate nanoparticles for a new delivery system. *J. Control. Release 103*, 93–98.
93 http://www.galenisearch.com.
94 Ogawa, Y. **2005**. Novel sustained-release system for protein drugs: optimization for the application to human growth hormone and evaluation of the function. *Drug Deliv. Syst. 20*, 288.
95 Takeuchi, H., Sasaki, H., Niwa, T., Hino, T., Kawashima, Y., Uesugi, K., Ozawa, H. **1991**. Redispersible dry emulsion system as novel oral dosage form of oily drugs: *in vivo* studies in beagle dogs. *Chem. Pharmac. Bull. 39*, 3362–3364.
96 Hanawa, T., Ikoma, R., Watanabe, A., Hidaka, M., Sugihara, M. **1996**. Preparation and characterization of sealed heated mixture of ethenzamide and porous calcium silicate. *Chem. Pharmac. Bull. 44*, 1367–1371.
97 Kinoshita, M., Baba, K., Nagayasu, A., Yamabe, K., Shimooka, T., Takeichi, Y., Azuma, M., Houchi, H., Minakuchi, K. **2002**. Improvement of solubility and oral bioavailability of a poorly water-soluble drug, TAS-301, by its melt-adsorption on a porous calcium silicate. *J. Pharmac. Sci. 91*, 362–370.
98 Takashima, Y., Yuasa, H., Kanaya, Y., Nomura, I., Shinozawa, K. **1999**. Reduction of tablet coloration at tableting for oily medicine (tocopheryl nicotinate). *Int. J. Pharmac. 187*, 125–135.
99 Hwang, Y.-J., Oh, C., Oh, S.-G. **2005**. Controlled release of retinal from silica particles prepared in O/W/O emulsion: The effects of surfactants and polymers. *J. Control. Release 106*, 339–349.
100 Tenjarla, S. **1999**. Microemulsions: an overview and pharmaceutical applications. *Ther. Drug Carrier Syst. 16*, 461–521.
101 Gursoy, R. N., Benita, S. **2004**. Self-emulsifying drug delivery systems (SEDDS) for improved oral delivery of lipophilic drugs. *Biomed. Pharmacother. 58*, 173–182.
102 Charman, W. N. **2000**. Lipids, lipophilic drugs, and oral drug delivery – some emerging concepts. *J. Pharmac. Sci. 89*, 967–978.
103 Barthe, L., Woodley, J., Houin, G. **1999**. Gastrointestinal absorption of drugs: methods and studies. *Fund. Clin. Pharmacol. 13*, 154–168.
104 Rinaki, E., Valsami, G., Macheras, P. **2003**. Quantitative biopharmaceutics classification system: the central role of dose/solubility ratio. *Pharmac. Res. 20*, 1917–25.
105 Michael, S., Thole, M., Dillmann, R., Fahr, A., Drewe, J., Fricker, G. **2000**. Improvement of intestinal peptide absorption by a synthetic bile acid derivative, cholylsarcosine. *Eur. J. Pharmac. Sci. 10*, 133–140.
106 Chao, A. C., Nguyen, J. V., Broughall, M., Griffin, A., Fix, J. A., Daddona, P. E. **1999**. *In vitro* and *in vivo* evaluation of effects of sodium caprate on enteral peptide absorption and on mucosal morphology. *Int. J. Pharmac. 191*, 15–24.
107 Mesiha, M., Plakogiannis, F., Vejosoth, S. **1994**. Enhanced oral absorption of insulin from desolvated fatty acid–sodium glycocholate emulsions. *Int. J. Pharmac. 111*, 213–216.
108 Rivera, T. M., Leone-Bay, A., Paton, D. R., Leipod, H. R., Baughman, R. A. **1997**. Oral delivery of heparin in combination with sodium *N*-[8-(2-hydroxybenzoyl) amino] caprylate: pharmacological considerations. *Pharmac. Res. 14*, 1830–1834.
109 Ito, Y., Arai, H., Uchino, K., Iwasaki, K., Shibata, N., Takada, K. **2005**. Effect of adsorbents on the absorption of lansoprazole with surfactant. *Int. J. Pharmac. 289*, 69–77.
110 Ito, Y., Kusawake, T., Ishida, M., Tawa, R., Shibata, N., Takada, K. **2005**. Oral solid gentamicin preparation using emulsifier and adsorbent. *J. Control. Release 105*, 23–31.

111 RAMA PRASAD, Y. V., MINAMIMOTO, T., YOSHIKAWA, Y., SHIBATA, N., MORI, S., MATSUURA, A., TAKADA, K. **2004**. *In situ* intestinal absorption studies on low molecular weight heparin in rats using Labrasol as absorption enhancer. *Int. J. Pharmac. 271*, 225–232.

112 AMIDON, G. L., LENNERNÄS, H., SHAH, V. P., CRISON, J. R. **1995**. A theoretical basis for a biopharmaceutic drug classification: the correlation of *in vitro* drug product dissolution and *in vivo* bioavailability. *Pharmac. Res. 12*, 413–420.

113 HU, Z., TAWA, R., KONISHI, T., SHIBATA, N., TAKADA, K. **2001**. A novel emulsifier, Labrasol, enhances gastro-intestinal absorption of gentamicin. *Life Sci. 69*, 2899–2910.

114 JAIN, S. K., AWASTHI, A. M., JAIN, N. K., AGRAWAL, G. P. **2005**. Calcium silicate based microspheres of repaglinide for gastroretentive floating drug delivery: Preparation and *in vitro* characterization. *J. Control. Release 107*, 300–309.

115 STRAUB, J. A., CHICKERING, D. E., LOVELY, J. C., ZHANG, H., SHAH, B., WAUD, W. R., BERNSTEIN, H. **2005**. Intravenous hydrophobic drug delivery: a porous particle formulation of paclitaxel (AI-850). *Pharmac. Res. 22*, 347–355.

116 FORAKER, A. B., WALCZAK, R. J., COHEN, M. H., BOIARSKI, T. A., GROVE, C. F., SWAAN, P. W. **2003**. Microfabricated porous silicon particles enhance paracellular delivery of insulin across intestinal Caco-2 cell monolayers. *Pharmac. Res. 20*, 110–116.

117 AJAYAN, P. M., EBBESEN, T. W. **1997**. Nanometre-size tubes of carbon. *Rep. Prog. Phys. 60*, 1025–1062.

118 VENKATESAN, N., YOSHIMITSU, J., ITO, Y., SHIBATA, N., TAKADA, K. **2005**. Liquid filled nanoparticles as a drug delivery tool for protein therapeutics. *Biomaterials 26*, 7154–7163.

119 EAIMTRAKARN, S., RAMA PRASAD, Y. V., OHNO, T., KONISHI, T., YOSHIKAWA, Y., SHIBATA, N., TAKADA, K. **2002**. Absorption enhancing effect of Labrasol on the intestinal absorption of insulin in rats. *J. Drug Target. 10*, 255–260.

120 RAMA PRASAD, Y. V., PUTHLI, S. P., EAIMTRAKARN, S., ISHIDA, I., YOSHIKAWA, Y., SHIBATA, N., TAKADA, K. **2003**. Enhanced intestinal absorption of vancomycin with Labrasol and D-α-tocopheryl PEF 1000 succinate in rats. *Int. J. Pharmac. 250*, 181–190.

121 WONG, N., KAM, S., DAI, H. **2005**. Carbon nanotubes as intracellular protein transporters: generality and biological functionality. *J. Am. Chem. Soc. 127*, 6021–6026.

122 PANTAROTTO, D., BRIAND, J. P., PRATO, M., BIANCO, A. **2004**. Translocation of bioactive peptides across cell membranes by carbon nanotubes. *Chem. Commun.* 16–17.

123 BIANCO, A., HOEBEKE, J., GODEFROY, S., CHALOIN, O., PANTAROTTO, D., BRIAND, J. P., MULLER, S., PRATO, M., PARTIDOS, C. D. **2005**. Cationic carbon nanotubes bind to CpG oligodeoxy-nucleotides and enhance their immunostimulatory properties. *J. Am. Chem. Soc. 127*, 58–59.

124 CHAPANA, J. R., TROSZCZYNSKA, J., FIRKOWSKA, I., MORSCZECK, C., GIERSIG, M. **2005**. Multi-walled carbon nanotubes for plasmid delivery into *Escherichia coil* cells. *Lab on a Chip 5*, 536–539.

125 NIOSH/OSHA **1988**. Synthetic graphite. National Institute for Occupational Safety and Health. http://www.cdc.gov/niosh/pel88/npelname.html and http://www.cdc.gov/niosh/pel88/SYNGRAPH.html.

126 LAM, C. W., JAMES, J. T., MCCLUSKEY, R., HUNTER, R. L. **2004**. Pulmonary toxicity of single-wall carbon nanotubes in mice 7 and 90 days after intratracheal instillation. *Toxicol. Sci. 77*, 126–134.

127 WARHEIT, D. B., LAURENCE, B. R., REED, K. L., ROACH, D. H., REYNOLDS, G. A. M., WEBB, T. R. **2004**. Comparative pulmonary toxicity assessment of single-wall carbon nanotubes in rats. *Toxicol. Sci. 77*, 117–125.

128 Bianco, A., Kostarelos, K., Partidos, C. D., Prato, M. **2005**. Biomedical applications of fictionalized carbon nanotubes. *Chem. Commun.* 571–577.

129 Kasuya, D., Yudasaka, M., Takahashi, K., Kokai, F., Iijima, S. **2002**. Selective production of single-wall carbon nanohorn aggregates and their formation mechanism. *J. Phys. Chem. B 106*, 4947–4951.

130 Murata, K., Kaneko, K., Kanoh, H., Kasuya, D., Takahashi, K., Kokai, F., Yudasaka, M., Iijima, S. **2002**. Adsorption mechanism of super-critical hydrogen in internal and interstitial nanospaces of single-wall carbon nanohorn assembly. *J. Phys. Chem. B 106*, 11132–11138.

131 Murata, K., Hirahara, K., Yudasaka, M., Iijima, S., Kasuya, D., Kaneko, K. **2002**. Nanowindow-induced molecular sieving effect in a single-wall carbon nanohorn. *J. Phys. Chem. B 106*, 12668–12669.

132 Murakami, T., Ajima, K., Miyawaki, J., Yudasaka, M., Iijima, S., Shibata, K. **2004**. Drug-loaded carbon nanohorns: adsorption and release of dexamethasone *in vitro*. *Mol. Pharmac. 1*, 399–405.

133 Murakami, T., Fan, J., Yudasaka, M., Iijima, S., Shiba, K. **2006**. Solubilization of single-wall carbon-nanohorns using a PEG–doxorubicin conjugate. *Mol. Pharm. 3*, 407–414.

134 Nakai, Y., Yamamoto, K., Terada, K., Ichikawa, J. **1984**. Interaction of medicinals and porous powder. I. Anomalous thermal behavior of porous glass mixtures. *Chem. Pharmac. Bull. 32*, 4566–4571.

135 Yonemochi, E., Matsumoto, M., Oguchi, T., Yamamoto, K., Nakai, Y. **1991**. Stability of aspirin in controlled pore glass solid dispersions. *Chem. Pharmac. Bull. 39*, 1027–1031.

136 Matsumoto, K., Nakai, Y., Yonemochi, E., Oguchi, T., Yamamoto, K. **1998**. Effect of pore size on the gaseous adsorption on ethenzamide on porous crystalline cellulose and the physicochemical stability of ethenzamide after storage. *Chem. Pharmac. Bull. 46*, 314–318.

137 Watanabe, T., Ohno, I., Wakiyama, N., Kusai, A., Senna, M. **2002**. Controlled dissolution properties of indomethacin by compounding with silica. *STP Pharmac. Sci. 12*, 363–367.

138 Matsumoto, K., Nakai, Y., Yonemochi, E., Oguchi, T., Yamamoto, K. **1994**. Physicochemical characteristics of porous crystalline cellulose and formation of an amorphous state of ethenzamide by mixing. *Int. J. Pharmac. 108*, 167–172.

139 Noyes, A. A., Whitney, W. R. **1897**. The rate of solution of solid substances in their own solutions. *J. Am. Chem. Soc. 19*, 930–934.

140 Yamamoto, K., Nakano, M., Takaichi, A., Nakai, Y. **1974**. Dissolution rate and bioavailability of griseofulvin from a ground mixture with microcrystalline cellulose. *Eur. J. Pharmac. Biopharmac. 2*, 487–493.

141 Berge, M. S., Bighley, D. L., Monkhouse, S. D. **1977**. Pharmaceutical salts. *J. Pharmac. Sci. 66*, 1–19.

142 Kimura, K., Hirayama, F., Arima, H., Uekama, K. **2000**. Effect of aging on crystallization, dissolution and adsorption characteristics of amorphous tolbutamide-2-hydroxypropyl-β-cyclodextrin complex. *Chem. Pharmac. Bull. 48*, 646–650.

143 Kaneniwa, N., Ikekawa, A., Hashimoto, K. **1973**. Influence of operational variables on ball-milling of sulfadimethoxine and white alundum. *Chem. Pharmac. Bull. 21*, 676–681.

144 Serajuddin, A. T. **1999**. Solid dispersion of poorly water-soluble drugs: early promises, subsequent problems, and recent breakthroughs. *J. Pharmac. Sci. 88*, 1058–1065.

145 Chiou, W. L. **1971**. Pharmaceutical applications of solid dispersion system. *J. Pharmac. Sci. 60*, 1281–1302.

146 Chiou, W. L., Riegelman, S. **1969**. Preparation and dissolution characteristic of several fast-release solid dispersions of Griseofulvin. *J. Pharmac. Sci. 58*, 1505–1509.

147 Simonelli, A. P., Metha, S. C., Higuchi, W. I. **1969**. Dissolution

rates of high energy polyvinylpyrrolidone (PVP)–sulfathiazole coprecipitates. *J. Pharmac. Sci.* 58, 538–549.
148 Takeuchi, H., Handa, T., Kawashima, Y. **1987**. Spherical solid dispersion containing amorphous tolbutamide embedded in enteric coating polymers or colloidal silica prepared by spray-drying technique. *Chem. Pharmac. Bull. 35*, 3800–3806.
149 Takeuchi, H., Nagira, S., Hiromitsu, Y., Kawashima, Y. **2004**. Solid dispersion particles of tolbutamide prepared with fine silica particles by the spray-drying method. *Powder Technol. 141*, 187–195.
150 Burger, A. **1975**. Zur polymorphie oraler antidiabetika. 2. Mitteilung: Tolbutamide. *Sci. Pharmac. 43*, 161–168.
151 Kimura, K., Hirayama, F., Arima, H., Uekama, K. **1999**. Characterization of tolbutamide polymorphs (Burger's form II and IV) and polymorphic transition behavior. *J. Pharmac. Sci. 88*, 385–390.
152 Kimura, K., Hirayama, F., Arima, H., Uekama, K. **2000**. Effect of aging on crystallization, dissolution and adsorption characteristics of amorphous tolbutamide-2-hydroxypropyl-B-cyclodextrin complex. *Chem. Pharmac. Bull. 48*, 646–650.
153 Nagira, S. **2005**. *PhD Thesis*. Gifu Pharmaceutical University.
154 Takeuchi, H., Nagira, S., Hiromitsu, Y., Kawashima, Y. **2003**. Design of solid dispersion particles of drug with fine porous carriers. *J. Soc. Powder Technol., Japan 40*, 157–162.
155 Takeuchi, H., Nagira, S., Yamamoto, H., Kawashima, Y. **2005**. Solid dispersion particles of amorphous indomethacin with fine porous silica particles by using spray-drying method. *Int. J. Pharmac. 288*, 177–183.
156 Hancock, B.C., Parks, M. **2000**. What is the true solubility advantage for amorphous pharmaceuticals? *Pharmac. Res. 74*, 397–404.
157 Imaizumi, H., Nambu, N., Nagai, T. **1979**. Stability and several physical properties of amorphous and crystalline forms of indomethacin. *Chem. Pharmac. Bull. 28*, 2565–2569.
158 Fukuoka, E., Makita, M., Yamamura, S. **1986**. Some physical properties of glassy indomethacin. *Chem. Pharmac. Bull. 34*, 4314–4321.
159 Taylor, L. S., Zografi, G. **1997**. Spectroscopic characterization of interactions between PVP and indomethacin in amorphous molecular dispersions. *Pharmac. Res. 14*, 1691–1698.
160 Matsumoto, T., Zografi, G. **1999**. Physical properties of solid molecular dispersions of indomethacin with poly(vinylpyrrolidone) and poly(vinylpyrrolidone-*co*-vinyl-acetate) in relation to indomethacin crystallization. *Pharmac. Res. 16*, 1722–1728.
161 Yoshioka, M., Hancock, B. C., Zografi, G. **1994**. Crystallization of indomethacin from amorphous state below and above its glass transition temperature. *Pharmac. Res. 83*, 1700–1705.
162 Enüstün, B. V., Sentürk, H. S., Yurdakul, O. **1978**. Capillary freezing and melting. *J. Colloid Interface Sci. 65*, 509–516.
163 Etzler, F. M., White, P. J. **1987**. The heat capacity of water in silica pores. *J. Colloid Interface Sci. 120*, 94–99.
164 Inagaki, S., Fukushima, Y., Kuroda, K. **1993**. Synthesis of highly ordered mesoporous material from a layered polysilicate. *Chem. Commun.* 680–682.
165 Kersge, C. T., Leonowicz, M. E., Roth, W.J. **1992**. Ordered mesoporous molecular sieves synthesized by a liquid-crystal template mechanism. *Nature 710*, 359.
166 Inagaki, S. **1998**. *PhD Thesis*. Nagoya University.
167 Morimoto, Y., Yamamoto, H., Takeuchi, H., Kawashima, Y., Takahashi, H. **2001**. Entrapment of insulin into mesoporous material by using freeze-thawing method and its release property. In *Proceedings of the Autumn Research Meeting of the Society of Powder Technology of Japan*, pp. 18–19.
168 Ishikiriyama, K., Todoki, M. **1995**. Evaluation of water in silica pores

using differential scanning calorimetry. *Thermo Chim. Acta 256*, 2213–2226.

169 Ishikiriyama, K., Todoki, M., Motomura, K. **1995**. Pore size distribution (PSD) measurements of silica gels by means of differential scanning calorimetry: I. Optimization for determination of PSD. *J. Colloid Interface Sci. 171*, 92–102.

170 Morishige, K., Nobuoka, K. **1997**. X-ray diffraction studies of freezing and melting of water confined in a mesoporous adsorbent (MCM-41). *J. Chem. Phys. 107*, 6965–6969.

171 Matsuoka, M., Takeuchi, H. Unpublished data.

172 Matsuoka, M., Yamamoto, H., Takeuchi, H., Kawashima, Y., Takahashi, H. **2003**. Entrapment and release of drugs into mesoporous silica FSM. In *Proceedings of the 20th Symposium on Particulate Preparations and Designs*, 143–146.

173 Tozuka, Y., Oguchi, T., Yamamoto, K. **2002**. Adsorption and entrapment of salicylamide molecules into the mesoporous structure of folded sheets mesoporous material (FSM-16). *Pharmac. Res. 20*, 926–930.

7
NANOEGG® Technology for Drug Delivery

Yoko Yamaguchi and Rie Igarashi

7.1
Introduction

Retinoids, the natural and synthetic metabolites and analogs of vitamin A (retinol), are important regulators of epidermal proliferation and differentiation [1–6]. All-*trans* retinoic acid (ATRA, vitamin A acid) is the major naturally occurring biologically active form among retinoids. In various epithelia that normally keratinize, ATRA inhibits keratinization and induces mucous metaplasia [7, 8]. Nevertheless, ATRA has been a focus of research into topical treatments for aged skin for more than 15 years. In 1986, Klingman and coworkers [9, 10] reported that ATRA could produce smoother, less wrinkled and less pigmented skin after a few months of treatment. Melanin loss and less-wrinkled skin are, however, frequently accompanied by excess skin irritation after ATRA treatment [11]. Clinical responses predominantly comprised severe irritant dermatitis in the early stages of application (around 3 or 4 days). Such damage with a high magnitude of inflammatory events after ATRA treatment can induce chronic skin pigmentation on the area being treated, potentially resulting in imperfect repair of skin displaying a pigmented appearance. Inflammation can occur through at least two mechanisms: the acidic function (-COOH) of the terminal domain is in principle an inducer, and the presence and long-term adhesion of ATRA molecules on the stratum corneum epidermidis would presumably act as a strong irritatant. Preventing undesirable adverse effects would be expected to allow ATRA therapy to overcome the limitations of classical ATRA therapy.

In this chapter, we describe the development of a novel drug delivery system using nanotechnology with a core–shell structure using a boundary-organized nanoscale reaction. This reaction is based on the biological control of mineralization which refers to the general biochemical activity of the cells [12]. In the enclosed environments, the cells have several important functions, including spatial delineation, ion accumulation, mineral nucleation and transportation. Phospholipid and polypeptide vesicles, cellular assemblies, and macromolecular frameworks can be assembled into enclosed permeable structures that provide diffusion-limited spaces for biomineralization processes. The study of biomineralization offered valuable

Nanotechnologies for the Life Sciences Vol. 10
Nanomaterials for Medical Diagnosis and Therapy. Edited by Challa S. S. R. Kumar

ISBN: 978-3-527-31390-7

insights into the scope of materials chemistry at the organic–inorganic interface. Mann [13] began some examples that involved biomineral-inspired approaches for the synthesis of inorganic nanoparticles using boundary-organized nanoscale reaction droplets. Reverse micelles, microemulsions, vesicles and lipid bilayer films are templates for the nucleation of minerals. The synthesis of nanoparticles with a core–shell (minerals) structure requires the supramolecular assembly of structures that contain chemical reactions or phase transformations.

The conceptual framework in this study is that the preparation of ATRA nanoparticles with a core–shell structure (NANOEGG) plays a crucial role in solving the low permeation of ATRA into spaces in the stratum corneum epidermidis and the strong symptoms of irritation. Preparation of NANOEGG particles was achieved using boundary-organized nanoscale reaction droplets [13]. The strategy in which micelles are utilized as a drug carrier is already well known in the drug delivery system field. Although the normal micelles are thermodynamically stable, for human application there remains the problem of stability of micelles in blood after the injection. As a result, drugs included in micelles would be immediately released. Thus, a micelle system is occasionally not enough to control the long-term drug-release kinetics. The novel NANOEGG system is not in the equilibrium state because ATRA molecules cannot migrate from the micelle self-assembly to the continuous aqueous phase due to an inorganic coating on the surface of the micelle. It can be expected that NANOEGG will improve the potential of micelles in the drug delivery system field. This chapter provides a novel drug delivery system technology such that NANOEGG may not only prevent adverse effects, but also markedly enhance its main effect. Indeed, this technology would become an evolution of classical ATRA therapy and may enhance the potential utility in the topical drug delivery field.

In Section 7.2, the discussion focuses on the equilibrium and kinetic parameters that govern the behavior of ATRA within aqueous phase, and how the core–shell structure of NANOEGG is prepared, and the shelf stability of ATRA molecule, which is one of the improved points of NANOEGG structure, is explained. The possible implications of NANOEGG for the pharmacological mechanisms underlying the dermatological aspects of ATRA biology are then considered. In final section, as well as other aspects and drugs of NANOEGG, attention is placed on the role of NANOEGG in regeneration medicine, especially diabetes therapy medicine.

7.2 New Nanoparticles with a Core–Shell Structure: The NANOEGG System

7.2.1 Physicochemical Properties and Action of ATRA

Retinoids, the natural and synthetic metabolites and analogs of vitamin A (retinol), are important regulators of epidermal proliferation and differentiation. In recent years, discovery of the *in vitro* and *in vivo* differentiation of acute promyelocytic

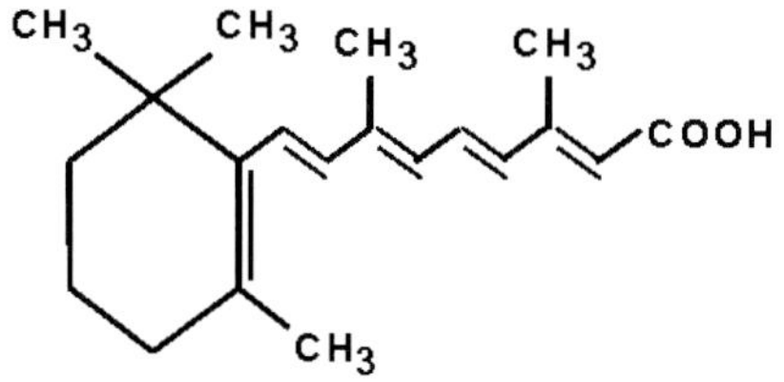

Figure 7.1. Structure of ATRA (molecular weight: 300.44).

leukemia (APL) blasts by ATRA has modified the therapeutic approach of APL, but has also led to important advances in the biology of APL and opened up new perspectives for differentiation therapy in cancer.

As a consequence of the presence of a large hydrophobic moiety in ATRA (Fig. 7.1), this compound is poorly soluble in water. This compound is comprised of three distinct structural domains: a β-ionone ring, a polyunsaturated chain and a polar end-group. The polar end-group of ATRA exists in a higher oxidation state than retinol and/or retinal. Quantitative data on the aqueous solubility of ATRA is scarce. One study used a spectrophotometric method relying on the differential absorption spectra of ATRA in water versus ethanol to measure the aqueous solubility of ATRA and found that the solubility limit of ATRA in water is 210 nM [14]. It should be noted, however, that interpretation of the data concerning ATRA may be complicated because whilst the absorption spectrum of ATRA is indeed sensitive to the polarity of the solvent, the spectrum also changes dramatically in response to variations in pH and in the ionization state of ATRA.

Self-aggregation of ATRA can have significant implications for the biological functions of this compound. For example, a reasonable explanation for the observation that the solubility of ATRA in water is higher than predicted [15] is that the observed solubility reflects self-association into micelles rather than the monomeric ATRA solubility. Thus, micelle formation may allow higher than expected aqueous concentrations of ATRA to be maintained and this concentration may be high enough to support diffusional fluxes of free ATRA sufficient for short-distance transport in cells or to allow metabolism of free ATRA. Another action of ATRA that may be affected by its self-association properties relates to the often-raised notion that at least some of the toxic effects of vitamin A are due to surface-active, "membranolytic", properties. Consideration of the chemical structure of ATRA suggests that its amphipathic nature results in "detergent-like" characteristics, and several studies have shown that the presence of ATRA affects various aspects of membrane structure and function [16, 17]. As with other detergents, ATRA may disrupt membranes both by intercalating into the lipids, thereby changing the characteristics of the bilayer, and by drawing lipids out of the bilayers into ATRA–lipid mixed micelles, leading to dissolution of the membranes. Few studies have addressed the self-association properties of ATRA. The ATRA molecules may carry an actual net charge. This feature may result in a stronger detergent-like characteristic of the ATRA and perhaps provide an explanation for the reported differences between the effects of ATRA versus other retinoids on membranes [17]. This consideration raises the question of whether the carboxyl group of ATRA is protonated or negatively charged at physiological pH and whether the self-association characteristics of ATRA affect the compound's ionization state.

The physicochemical properties of ATRA and the characteristics of its interactions with the various environments in which it is distributed *in vivo* affect its biological functions. As a consequence of the presence of a large hydrophobic moiety in ATRA, it is poorly soluble in water. However, self-aggregation of ATRA can have significant implications for the biological function of this compound. It has been reported that while the pK of monomeric ATRA in an aqueous medium is lower than 6.1, the transition from a monomeric to a micellar state results in an increase in pK to 8.5, i.e. micelle formation stabilizes the protonated form of ATRA [18]. Thus, at physiological pH and at concentrations of ATRA that are higher than the critical micellar concentration (CMC), a large fraction of ATRA is protonated; at concentrations of ATRA that are lower than the CMC, a predominant fraction of ATRA is ionized. As the aqueous solubility of the anionic ATRA is significantly higher than the solubility of the protonated form, these observations suggest that the concentrations of free ATRA molecules in aqueous spaces *in vivo* are indeed of the order of 20–50 μM.

In the presence of alkaline or physiological pH, ATRA molecules self-associate and formed micelles in aqueous solution [19]. In an alkaline environment, hydrophobic ATRA molecules abruptly change to amphiphilic molecules and when a specific concentration of ATRA is exceeded, micelles spontaneously form in water as an oriented colloidal aggregate. The CMC of ATRA was detected by the specific electron conductivity method (Fig. 7.2). Phillips defined CMC as the concentration corresponding to the maximum change in the gradient in the solution property versus concentration (ϕ–C_t) curve [20]:

$$(d^3\phi/dC_t^3)_{Ct=CMC} = 0, \quad (1)$$

where:

$$\phi = \alpha[S] + \beta[M], \quad (2)$$

where α and β are proportionality constants, C_t is the concentration of surfactant, and [S] and [M] are the concentrations of monomeric surfactant and micelle, respectively. Figures 7.2 shows the determination of CMC with surfactant in the case that the solution property ϕ is the electrical conductivity change. In an ionic surfactant system, higher concentrations are necessary to overcome the electrostatic repulsion between ionic head-groups of ionic surfactants during aggregation. As a result, the repulsive interaction between the head-groups in an ionic micelle is moderated by the strong counterion binding to the surface in the process of micelle formation. This idea is easy to understand from the fact that the slope before formation of a micelle is larger than that above the CMC in the conductivity measurements.

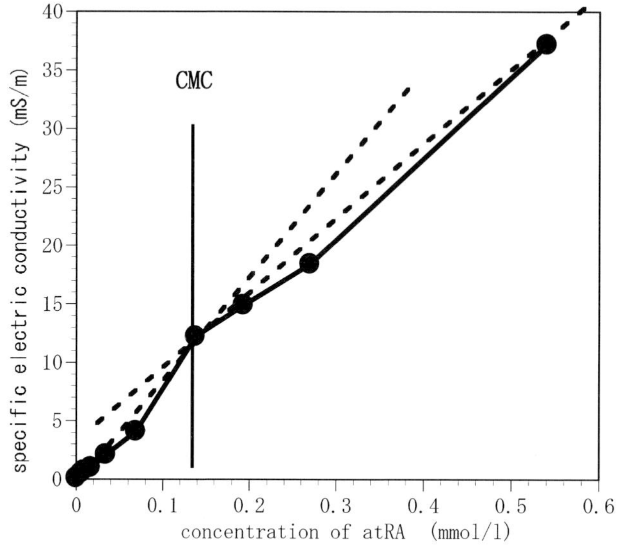

Figure 7.2. CMC of ATRA molecules in the presence of NaOH aqueous medium using the specific electric conductivity measurement. The measurement was carried out 25 °C under stirring. The dashed line corresponds to the CMC.

The CMC of ATRA is lower than 1 mM [19], but more than three orders of magnitude lower than reported CMC values for bile acids [21] and 10-fold lower than the CMC of the long-chain fatty acid palmitate [22]. This observation indicates that ATRA self-associate into micelles at substantially lower concentrations than other small amphipathic compounds.

7.2.2
NANOEGG Preparation and Characterization

Above the CMC, we synthesized inorganic-coated nanoparticles using boundary-organized nanoscale reaction droplets. In turn, the interfacial properties of organic architectures, in ATRA micelles, were used to template the nucleation and growth of inorganic minerals ($CaCO_3$). Since the surface of ATRA micelles displays numerous negative charges, oppositely charged ions (such as Ca^{2+} divalent ions) can easily thermodynamically adsorb on the surface. The interfacial properties of the ATRA micelle can thus be used to template the formation of a $CaCO_3$ shell. This procedure is shown in Scheme 7.1. The surfaces of ATRA micelles containing nonionic surfactant were coated by inorganic $CaCO_3$ with an amorphous structure. First, the mixed micelle of ATRA molecules and nonionic surfactant with polyoxyethylene function was prepared to prevent micelle sedimentation after the adsorption of divalent ions. The adsorption of divalent Ca^{2+} ions and the dissociation of surface charge of the micelle should be strongly suppressed. Finally, the micelle

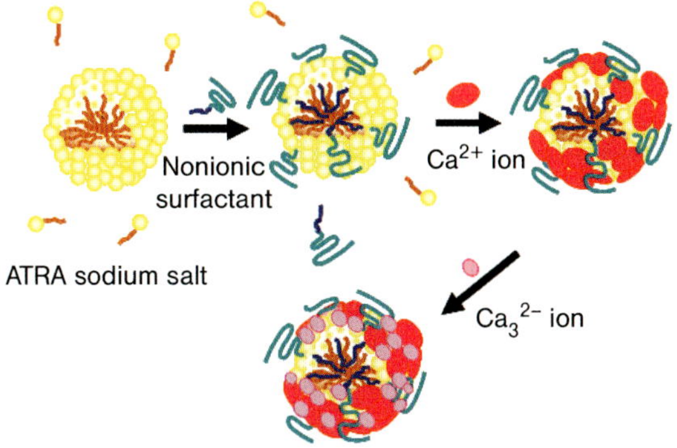

Scheme 7.1. Schematic preparation process of NANOEGG particles with a core–shell ($CaCO_3$) structure. The aqueous solution containing ATRA molecules is seen to be transparent in each step without any sedimentation.

would sediment. The presence of polyoxyethylene function on the micelle surface can maintain the hydrophilic character even if divalent ions are bound on ATRA micelle.

The solution properties of a binary surfactant mixture fall either between or outside the solution properties of the two single-surfactant solutions. Most CMCs of binary surfactant mixtures fall between the CMCs of the two components. Many of the theories concerning the CMC of binary surfactant mixtures have assumed the ideal of each component in the micellar phase [23]. An approach using a non-homologous surfactant mixture can elucidate binary mixtures quite well by using the single adjustable parameter developed by Rubingh [24]. At the CMC (C) of the binary system, the following relationships are satisfied from the mass balances for components 1 and 2:

$$\alpha C = C_1 \quad \text{and} \quad (1-\alpha)C = C_2, \tag{3}$$

where α is the net mole fraction of component 1, C_1 is the concentration of component 1 and C_2 is the concentration of component 2. Then:

$$\alpha C = \gamma_1 x C_1{}^0$$
$$(1-\alpha)C = \gamma_2(1-x)C_2{}^0, \tag{4}$$

where x is the mole fraction of component 1 in the binary surfactant phase, $C_1{}^0$ and $C_2{}^0$ are the CMCs of each single component, and γ is the activity coefficient due to nonideal mixing. If the values of $C_1{}^0$, $C_2{}^0$, γ_1 and γ_2 are available, x, C_1 and C_2 may be determined by calculation. The values of $C_1{}^0$ and $C_2{}^0$ are obtained from the CMC values of the single-surfactant solutions, but the activity coefficients are given by the regular solution theory as:

$$\gamma_1 = \exp[\beta(1-x)^2]$$
$$\gamma_2 = \exp[\beta x^2]. \quad (5)$$

At the same time, β can be evaluated by substituting Eq. (4) into (5):

$$\beta = \ln(\alpha C/xC_1{}^0)/(1-x)^2. \quad (6)$$

In general, a single parameter value of β is determined by averaging the β values against each α value over the entire composition range. The β value is an index of interaction between two surfactants. The sigh of β corresponds to positive or negative deviation from ideal, and moderate interaction between anionic and nonionic surfactants was shown for many binary surfactant systems. Thus, our micellar system between ATRA as anionic surfactant and nonionic surfactant maybe forms homogenous mixed micelles, and could not form ATRA and nonionic surfactant micelles, respectively. In the dynamic light scattering (DLS) measurement, two different diffusion coefficients of each micelle are usually detected when the different micelles are present in the system. At this case the correlation function will decay double exponentially as a function of delay time. DLS measurement was carried out on the binary ATRA and nonionic surfactant system (Fig. 7.3). The correlation function almost decayed mono-exponentially (solid line in Fig. 7.3). This is evidence for the presence of only mixed micelles being formed under our conditions.

As $CaCO_3$ is formed on the high curvature $1/R$, where R is the radius of the micelle, its structure is rather difficult in crystal state. Wide-angle X-ray scattering shows the broad scattering curve between 5° and 10° angles (data is not shown).

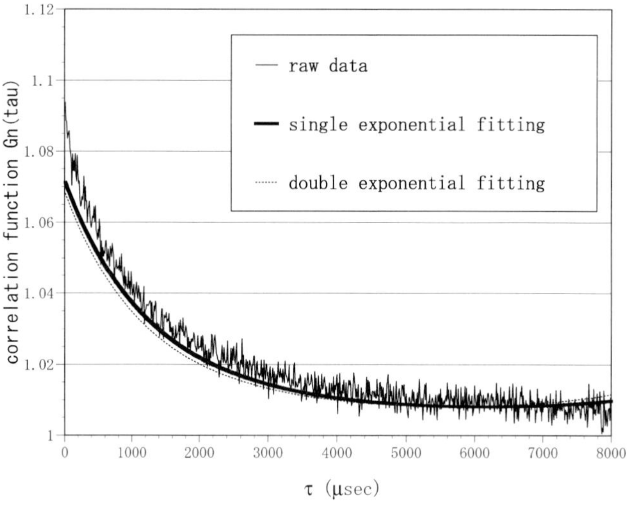

Figure 7.3. DLS measurements of ATRA sodium salt and nonionic surfactant in aqueous solution. The correlation function of ATRA sodium salt and nonionic surfactant mixed solution (45 mg L^{-1} of ATRA and 330 mg L^{-1} of nonionic surfactant) was measured at 25 °C as a function of decay time. The curve fittings were carried out by two methods, i.e. single- and double-exponential decays.

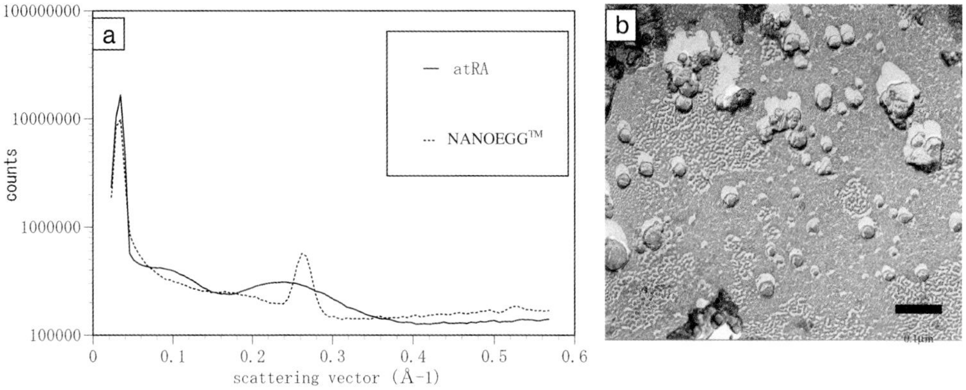

Figure 7.4. Physicochemical properties of NANOEGG in aqueous media. (a) SAXS patterns as a function of scattering vector. Solid line: ATRA micelle (1.0 wt%); dotted line: NANOEGG particles (1.0 wt% as ATRA). (b) Freeze-fracture TEM of NANOEGG aqueous solution. Bar = 0.1 μm.

High biocompatibility of the $CaCO_3$ structure is thus expected due to the amorphous coating on micelle. Thus, calcium storage in the epidermal and/or dermal region cannot take place after the external treatment.

Analysis by small-angle X-ray scattering (SAXS) reveals the presence of spherical micelles of ATRA molecules with a diameter of around 10 nm (Fig. 7.4a). This size corresponds well with the normal ionic surfactant system [13]. The SAXS profile reveals an eggshell-like structure with different electron densities in the inner structure. Discontinuous electron distribution in the inner structure is detected as a peak with a specific scattering-angle region (Fig. 7.4a). The presence of this sharp peak corresponds to a discrete thin layer of $CaCO_3$ on the surface of the ATRA micelle. This micelle displaying a core–shell (ATRA–$CaCO_3$) structure represents the NANOEGG particles. In addition, since the diameter of NANOEGG is estimated to be 13–16 nm using the scattering curve in Fig. 7.4(a), the thickness of the $CaCO_3$ layer is probably 1.5–3 nm. The presence of an egg-like core–shell structure was also confirmed using freeze-fracture transmission electron microscopy (Fig. 7.4b).

The schematic structure of the NANOEGG system is shown in Fig. 7.5. In fact, the shell-like structure of 1–2 nm width was observed outside of the spherical ATRA particles.

7.2.3
Improved Lability of ATRA in the NANOEGG System

The conjugated double bonds of the isoprenoid chain render ATRA susceptible to photodegradation, isomerization and oxidation. Consequently, naturally occurring ATRA is extremely labile. Actually, the structural integrity of ATRA must be maintained *in vivo*. The answer lies in part with the observation that most retinoids *in vivo* are associated with retinoid-binding proteins. Many of these proteins bind

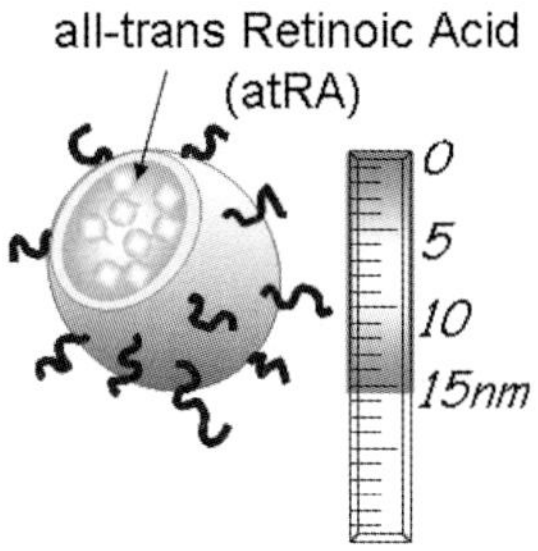

Figure 7.5. Schematic representation of a NANOEGG particle. The worm-like ribbon in the representation corresponds to the PEG function. The inside domain corresponds to ATRA molecules.

their ligands in hydrophobic pockets, thereby effectively shielding them from the aqueous environment. Binding to proteins is thus expected to protect ATRA from nonspecific oxidation and may also stabilize its isomerization state. In the same way, micelle formation of ATRA molecules can be expected to protect ATRA from the aqueous environment. The life-times of free ATRA in cytosol and in extracellular spaces, and the mechanisms by which the integrity of ATRA in these pools is maintained, are unknown. However, it has been reported that both degradation and isomerization of ATRA in water can be prevented by addition of biological antioxidants such as tocopherol [25, 26], suggesting the possibility that under at least some physiological conditions free ATRA can remain stable in cytosol. Even with the use of an antioxidant, the stability of ATRA micelles cannot be maintained over 95% of its activity for 3 years at room temperature and/or 6 months at 50 °C. Unfortunately, such a stability level of ATRA cannot be employed by pharmaceutical companies.

Figure 7.6 shows the high potential of NANOEGG for improved stability. As ATRA has a specific maximum absorbance at 340–345 nm, born of the decrease

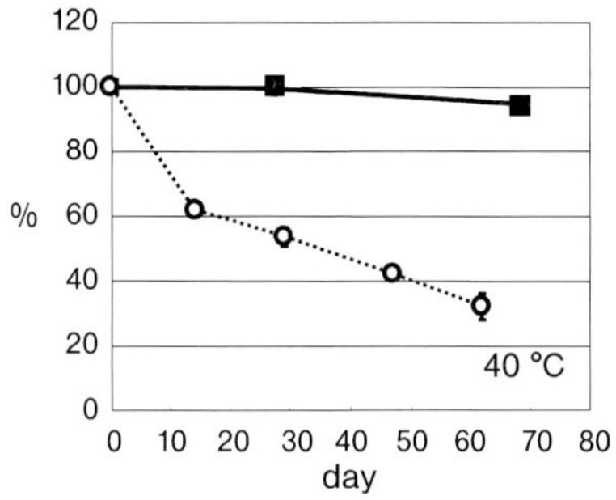

Figure 7.6. Stability of ATRA (circles) and NANOEGG (squares) at 40 °C. The ATRA was solubilized in ethanol as a negative control. Each sample was packed in the sunscreen tube.

of peak height and isomeric another peak detection in HPLC measurement are available concerning to the loss of activity. It can be seen that the peak height of NANOEGG scarcely changed for approximately 70 days in the accelerated environment at 40 °C, even without any antioxidant. It can be seen, thus, that the lability of the ATRA molecule was rather improved against temperature, as can be expected. As a result, long-term storage of ATRA ointment became possible.

7.3 NANOEGG for Dermatological Aspects

Within the epidermis, the processes of proliferation and differentiation are tightly controlled, resulting in a tissue at steady-state in which the cells that are desquamated and lost are equal to those that are produced in the germinative basal layer. Cells within the basal layer are highly proliferative and display an undifferentiated phenotype characterized by the coexpression of cytokeratin 5/14 (K5/K14) [27]. Mitosis is restricted to the basal layer and, as keratinocytes migrate into the suprabasal layers, they undergo a well-defined program of thermal differentiation, characterized by the coordinated induction of specific proteins. The initial change is the loss of K5/K14 expression and the synthesis of the K1/K10 keratins [28]. With subsequent movement into more suprabasal layers, cornified envelope substrate proteins are synthesized, including lorocrin [29], filaggrin and involucrin, together with type 1 transglutaminase – the calcium-dependent enzyme responsible for the crosslinking of the proteins. During the final stages of the differentiation process, the substrate protein crosslinking forms the resistant cornified envelopes, resulting in the cutaneous permeability barrier.

The dramatic effects of ATRA upon the skin have been known for many years. Hyperkeratinization is the result of ATRA deficiency in animals, with many epithelial sites becoming satisfied and keratinized. The historical data has been supported somewhat by more recent *in vitro* data. When keratinocytes are treated *in vitro*, ATRA inhibits terminal differentiation, suppressing the expression of K1/K10, profilaggrin, lorocrin, involucrin, transglutaminase and cornified envelope formation. The topical application of ATRA promotes keratinocyte proliferation, resulting in epidermal hyperplasia. Specifically, the thickness of the granular layer is increased and the stratum corneum is compacted, indicating effects upon differentiation in addition to proliferation. ATRA treatment not only leads to a decrease in stratum corneum thickness, but also to cell loosening and fragility, changes in lipid levels, and a subsequent decrease in the permeability barrier. As outlined, *in vivo* ATRA treatment upregulates differentiation markers.

Hyperpigmentation on the face is a anxiety-producing symptom. Photoaging refers to premature skin aging caused by repeated exposure to ultraviolet (UV) radiation from the sun for many years. Fine and coarse wrinkles, hyperpigmented macules, sallow color, dry texture, and loss of tone in habitually sun-exposed skin characterize the photoaged phenotype. Our understanding of photoaging has been greatly aided by the discovery that ATRA can repair photoaged skin, coupled with tremendous advances in the field of molecular biology, especially in the areas of how retinoic acid receptors function and how intracellular signaling is initiated by UV irradiation. For several years, ATRA and other synthetic retinoids have been widely used in the treatment of a variety of skin diseases associated with hyperproliferative processes. Retinoids induce a characteristic series of biochemical and histological modifications when applied to skin. Their effects on keratinocytes are still incompletely understood in spite of the recent discovery of nuclear ATRA receptors, which are highly expressed in human adult skin [30].

In 1986, Klingman and coworkers [9, 10] reported in the first suspicion that ATRA molecules could produce smoother, less-wrinkled and less-pigmented skin after a few months of treatment, and this has been one focus of research into topical treatments for a potent inhibitor of new melanin production [31, 7, 8]. Since the 1990s, many dermatologists have recommended the use of ATRA for a variety of nonsurgical treatments of photodamaged skin, because of a certain physiological regulation and high induction of epithelial differentiation [2–6]. The substance has been approved by the Food and Drug Administration in the US, and has been marketed as RENOVA™ and Retin-A™. Clinical responses predominantly comprised severe irritant dermatitis in the early stages of application of RENOVA and Retin-A (around 3 or 4 days) [11, 7, 8]. Such damage with a high magnitude of inflammatory events after ATRA treatment can induce chronic skin pigmentation on the area being treated, potentially resulting in imperfect repair of skin displaying a pigmented appearance.

7.3.1 Improved Irritation of ATRA in the NANOEGG System

In addition to keratinocytes and melanocytes, the epidermis also contains Langerhans cells, dendritic cells and innervating peripheral neuron cells. This means that the skin is an organ capable of responding to signals from both outside and from within the body. A predominant feature during the pathogenesis of many skin disorders is chronic inflammation, characterized by the infiltration of activated T lymphocytes. Among the factors that are critical for controlling those processes, transcription factors (such as AP-1, NF-κB, etc.) appear to be essential. Interestingly, the members of the nuclear hormone receptor superfamily are known to interact with many of these transcription factors, suggesting that ligands for these nuclear receptors many be an effective means of modulating inflammation as well as the immune response in general.

As already mentioned, ATRA causes a variable amount of irritation, more properly a heightening of cutaneous reactivity termed ATRA dermatitis, early in therapy. In the first few weeks approximately 80% of patients experience stinging, hyperesthesia or pruritus, fine scaling, dryness and mild erthema (Fig. 7.7a).

The conceptual framework in this section is that NANOEGG plays a crucial role in solving of the symptoms of irritation. After daily treatment with NANOEGG at different ATRA concentrations on the dorsal area of Wistar rats (5 weeks old, male), the induction of inflammation was visually observed. Inflammation tests are his-

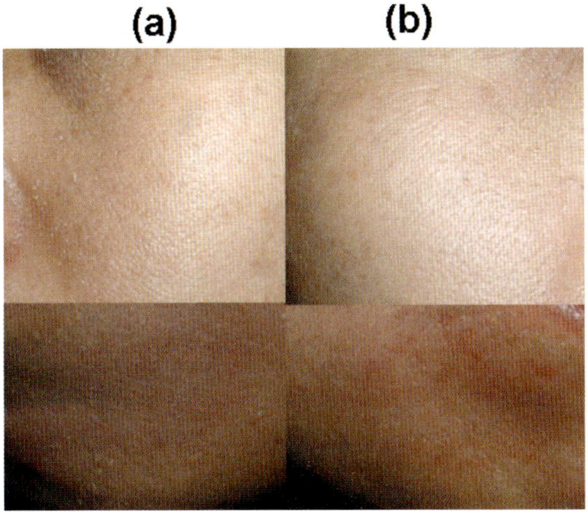

Figure 7.7. Facial features at 1 week following one time daily applications of (a) RENOVA ATRA 0.05% and (b) NANOEGG 0.05%. Note mild erthema and scaling along the jaw line and around the eye area in RENOVA treatment, while side-effects were rare in NANOEGG treatment.

torically carried out on the dorsal area of rats in cosmetic and medical companies as a standard method. It is known that this method will almost link to the degree of inflammation in the case of human skin. Hence, we also followed a rat system for the evaluation of NANOEGG. Only this experiment was carried out in a rat system. This stimulation degrees are normally numbered as three groups; 0–2: no change–fair, 2–4: stimulation, 4–6: high stimulation, which are based on visual observations. Figure 7.8 obviously shows the improvement of inflammation induced by the ATRA treatment in the case of NANOEGG.

Commercially, both Retin-A, a 0.1% ATRA cream, and RENOVA, a 0.05% ATRA cream, are marketed by Johnson & Johnson in the US. An *in vivo* experiment on the porcine dorsal area was performed for comparison with these commercial products. In the case of NANOEGG, the irritation against the porcine skin, which is known to be similar to human skin, showed the lowest level compared with other commercial products. One distinguishing feature of the human skin response to ATRA is the generation of clinical erythema. Since the erythema response of human skin to ATRA is normally dose-dependent [32], the reduced erythemogenic potential of NANOEGG should expect the reduction of irritation (Fig. 7.7b) with decreasing dose of ATRA, compared to the normal ATRA therapy.

The inflammation induced by topical ATRA treatment on skin should be caused by the elevation of AP-1 and NF-κB, and translated forms of inflammation cytokines, interleukin (IL)-1α and tumor necrosis factor (TNF)-α. Thus, the inflammation cytokines IL-α and TNF-α mRNA were measured on the skin domain treated with NANOEGG ointment (Fig. 7.9).

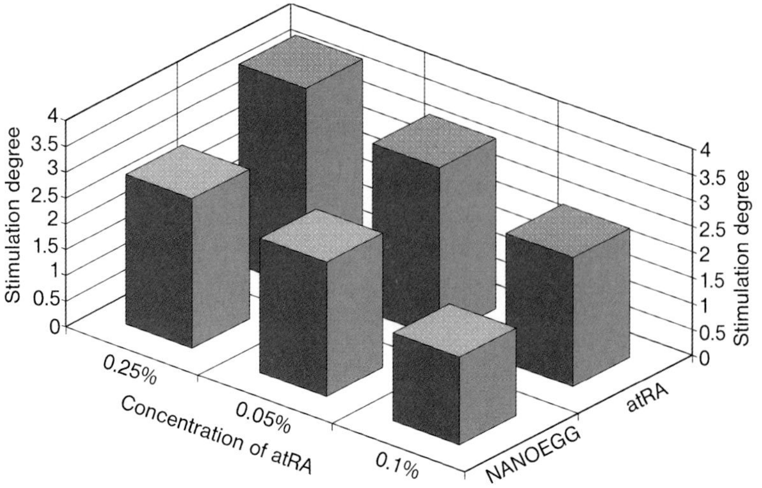

Figure 7.8. Stimulation degrees for the external administration on the dorsal area of ddY mouse of ATRA and NANOEGG in Vaseline media. Different concentrations (0.01, 0.05 and 0.25% of ATRA) were carried out as daily treatment (30 mg, 2×2 cm^2 on the dorsal area of Wistar rats, 5 weeks old, male) for 2 weeks. Stimulation degree was determined by visual observation.

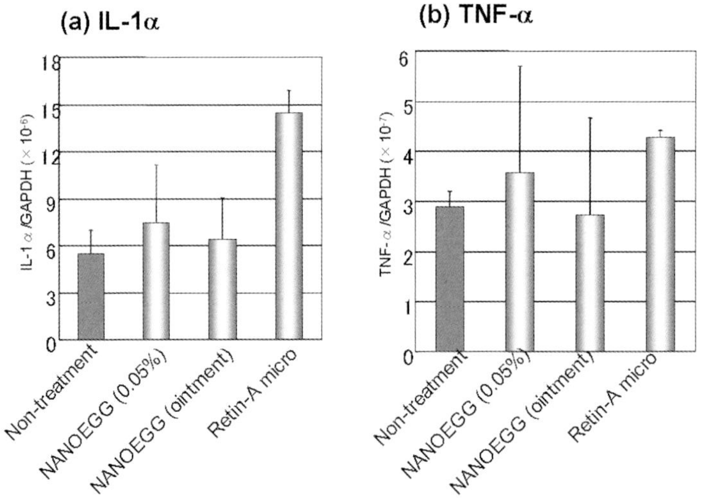

Figure 7.9. Expression of inflammation cytokines IL-1α and TNF-α mRNA on mouse skin. Each compound (NANOEGG, its base and Retin-A-Micro) was administered as 30 mg on 2×2 cm^2 for 15 days. The tissues were sacrificed 4 days after the topical administration.

7.3.2
Pharmacological Effects of the NANOEGG System

Histological improvements in the appearance of photodamaged skin following ATRA usage are associated with thickening of the epidermis and a relative reduction in melanin content [7, 8]. A study was undertaken to specifically evaluate the efficacy of NANOEGG in treating hyperpigmented lesions. Histological evaluation of ddY mouse epidermis after daily application of NANOEGG Vaseline cream for 4 days revealed more than double the increase in epidermal thickness than when using ATRA Vaseline cream (Fig. 7.10a–d). In general, a period of at least a few months is required for clinical effectiveness in treating mottled pigmentation using ATRA. Given the major increase in thickness of the epidermis in our prelim-

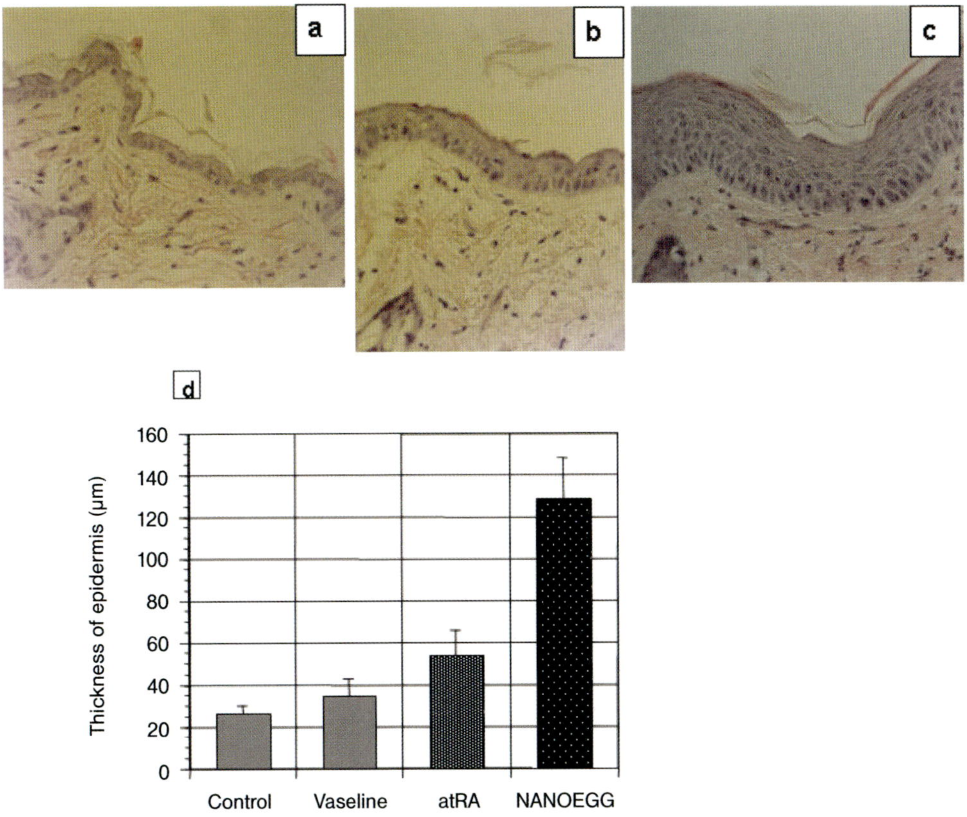

Figure 7.10. Histological and tissue analysis of the epidermis after a 4-day treatment. (a) Vehicle (Vaseline) treatment, (b) 0.1% ATRA treatment, (c) 0.1% NANOEGG treatment and (d) estimated epidermis thickness for each specimen ($n = 10$).

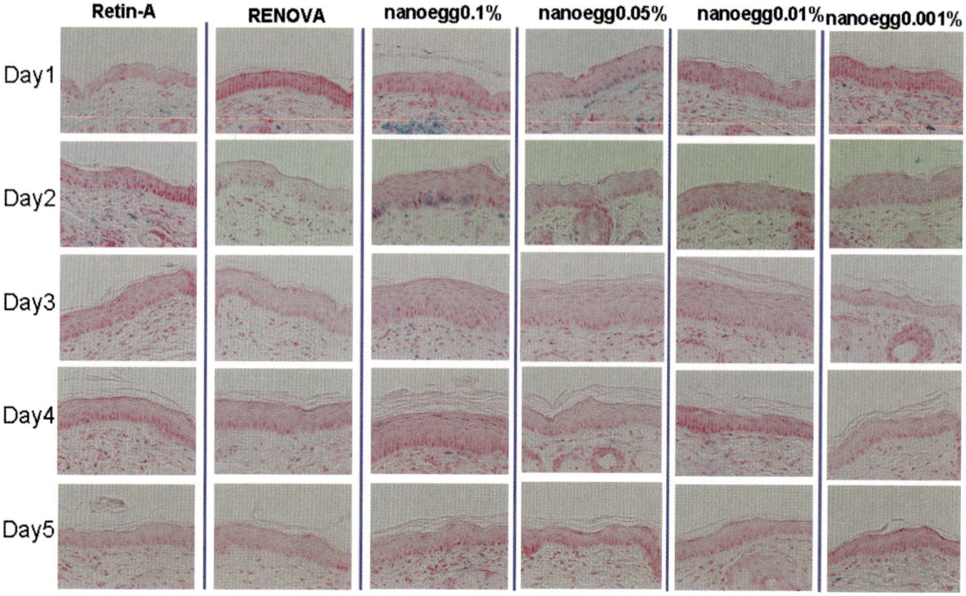

Figure 7.11. Histological evaluation of commercial products and NANOEGG 0.1, 0.05, 0.01 and 0.001% at each day after topical administration until day 5. All tissues were stained using the colloidal iron stain method to detect HA. Blue domains correspond to the presence of HA and red domains correspond to nuclear staining. The external treatments were carried out once and the tissues were sacrificed at each day until day 5. The amount of 30 mg of compound was administered in a 1-cm^2 of dorsal area of hairless mice (HR-1, male, 5 weeks old).

inary trials, reduction of melanin should rapidly be produced by NANOEGG treatment in humans.

NANOEGG-treated hairless mice underwent more progressive epidermal hyperplasia than with the commercial products at the same dose (Fig. 7.11). Even at a lower dose of ATRA (0.001%), histological evaluations suggested the effective skin regeneration of mice. Significant increases in epidermal thickness for NANOEGG treatment at all doses was revealed compared with treatment using commercial product creams. The hyperplasia of epidermis in Fig. 7.11 shows the thickened epidermal layer in all tested groups, but the NANOEGG-treated groups at each concentration of ATRA were dominant to other commercial products. The thickness of the epidermis layer in NANOEGG 0.01% treatment corresponds to that in the Retin-A (ATRA 0.1%)-treated group, thus the efficacy of NANOEGG can be supposed to be approximately 10 times that of the Retin-A commercial product. Likewise, NANOEGG may show sustained release of ATRA molecules until at least 5 days because of the observed continued hyperplasia of epidermis.

7.3.3
Expression of mRNA Heparin-binding Epidermal Growth Factor-like Growth Factor (HB-EGF) on Mouse Skin

Stoll and coworkers reported that mRNA expression of HB-EGF is induced by ATRA in human keratinocytes and skin [33]. Recently, production of HB-EGF has been shown to be one of the hallmarks of the turnover of keratinocytes [33]. Figure 7.12 shows HB-EGF mRNA expression in mouse ears in ATRA- and NANOEGG-treated groups. Daily application was performed for 4 days. Excess expression of HB-EGF in the NANOEGG-treated group was apparent compared with ATRA. This correlates well with the increased epidermal thickening for NANOEGG treatment (Fig. 7.10). Even at 4 days after the external administration, it seems that NANOEGG would gradually release tretinoin molecules from its egg-like capsule. It was confirmed whether NANOEGG possesses the controlled release ability as a drug delivery system or pulsatile release. Figure 7.13 shows the result of the expression of HB-EGF mRNA each day after a single treatment of NANOEGG on the mouse dorsal area. The small figure in Fig. 7.13 shows the concentration dependence of the expression of HB-EGF mRNA on tretinoin. With increasing concentration of NANOEGG, the production of HB-EGF mRNA was enhanced from ker-

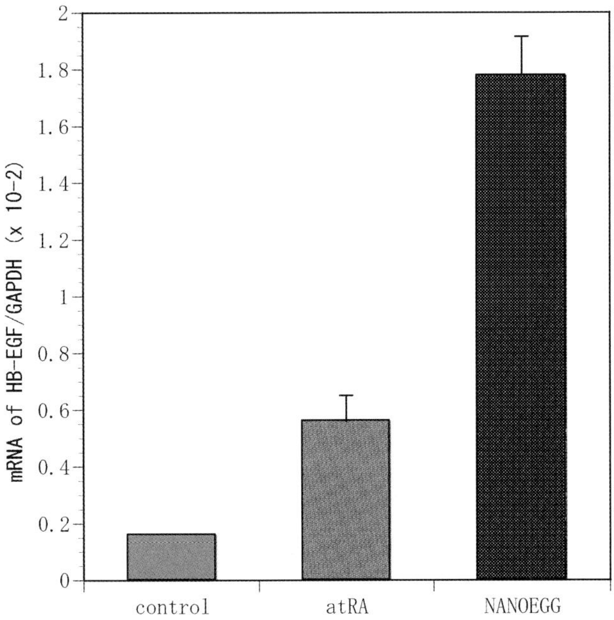

Figure 7.12. Expression of HB-EGF mRNA in mouse ears after continuous daily treatments for 4 days with ATRA or NANOEGG (0.1%) in Vaseline cream.

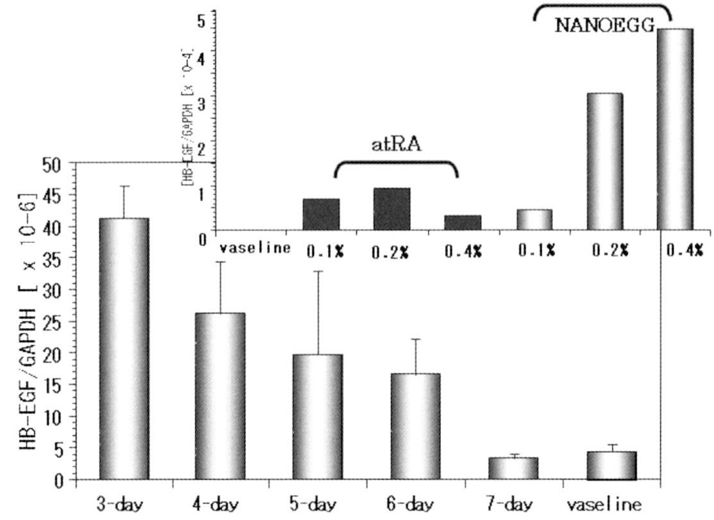

Figure 7.13. Expression of HB-EGF mRNA in mice dorsal areas at each day after 1-day treatment with NANOEGG. The small figure shows the concentration dependence of tretinoin and NANOEGG. The large figure shows the continuous expression of HB-EGF mRNA by NANOEGG as tretinoin concentration 0.2%.

atinocytes, while this was different from the case with the single treatment of tretinoin. As is obvious in Fig. 7.13, NANOEGG treatment as 0.2% tretinoin concentration could achieve expression of HB-EGF mRNA for 1 week. It is suggested that, at least here, tretinoin would gradually release from NANOEGG and as a result long-term release for around 1 week was successfully achieved by NANOEGG technology.

Also, Fig. 7.14 shows HB-EGF mRNA expression in hairless mouse dorsal tissues in Retin-A-, RENOVA- and NANOEGG-treated groups. One-day application was performed, and tissue was sacrificed and frozen in liquid nitrogen daily until day 5. Especially on the first day, excess expression of HB-EGF mRNA in the NANOEGG-treated group was apparent compared with the commercial products, RENOVA and Retin-A. Furthermore, even at the most dilute ATRA dose, the elevated expression of HB-EGF mRNA at day 1 was observed that will be expected to accelerate proliferation and differentiation of keratinocytes. The hyperplasia of the epidermis in Fig. 7.11 almost corresponds to the expression of HB-EGF mRNA in Fig. 7.14, but it would seem that a 1- or 2-day period is needed due to the thickened epidermal layer after the production of HB-EGF.

7.3.4 Proliferation and Differentiation of Keratinocytes

The mammalian epidermis is made up of multilayered epithelium consisting mainly of proliferating and differentiated, postmitotic keratinocytes. The differenti-

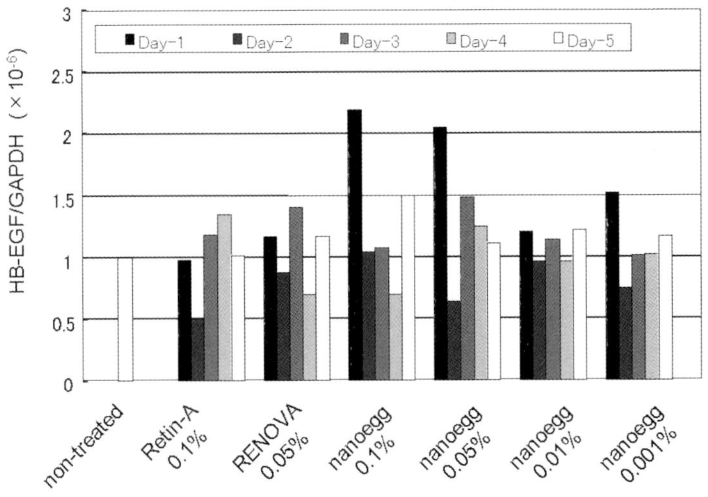

Figure 7.14. Expression of HB-EGF mRNA in hairless mice (HR-1, male, 5 weeks old) dorsal areas after 1-day treatment at day 5 with no treatment, NANOEGG (0.1, 0.05, 0.01 and 0.001%, respectively), RENOVA Retin-A. The tissues of dorsal areas were frozen using liquid nitrogen and extracted was RNA by the Isogen method.

ation is continuously replaced and recruited via transit-amplifying cells originating from stem cells, which represent a restricted number of basal keratinocytes. The continued renewal of cells in conjunction with mechanical strain poses a particular challenge to the cytoskeleton. It comes as no great surprise that epidermal keratinocytes have evolved a complex program of keratin expression along with mechanisms to alter the shape of the cytoskeleton during terminal differentiation.

As overexpression of HB-EGF mRNA was observed in NANOEGG treatment, we examined the expression of molecular markers in skin from the treated mice (5 weeks old, male) by immunofluorescence (Fig. 7.15). Cytokeratin 1 (K1) and larrikin (lord), markers of terminal differentiation in the normal epidermis layer, and cytokeratin 5 (K5), a maker of basal keratinocytes, were detected in the tissue after the treatment of atRA and NANOEGG 0.1% ointment. Expression of K5 (Fig. 7.15b and c) and larrikin (Fig. 7.15h and i) were rather enhanced in comparison with the control (wild-type mice, Fig. 7.15a), but the big difference between atRA and NANOEGG treatments was not observed, whereas the strongest expression of K1 was detected in the NANOEGG treatment (Fig. 7.15f). Excess expression of K1 might be associated with the enhanced thickening of the epidermis (Fig. 7.11b and Fig 11c). Thus, hyperplasia in the treatment of NANOEGG would mainly be due to the overexpression of HB-EGF, which could induce differentiation of keratinocytes. As a result, the differentiation of suprabasal and granule cells, which are related to the differentiation marker K1, seemed to be accelerated.

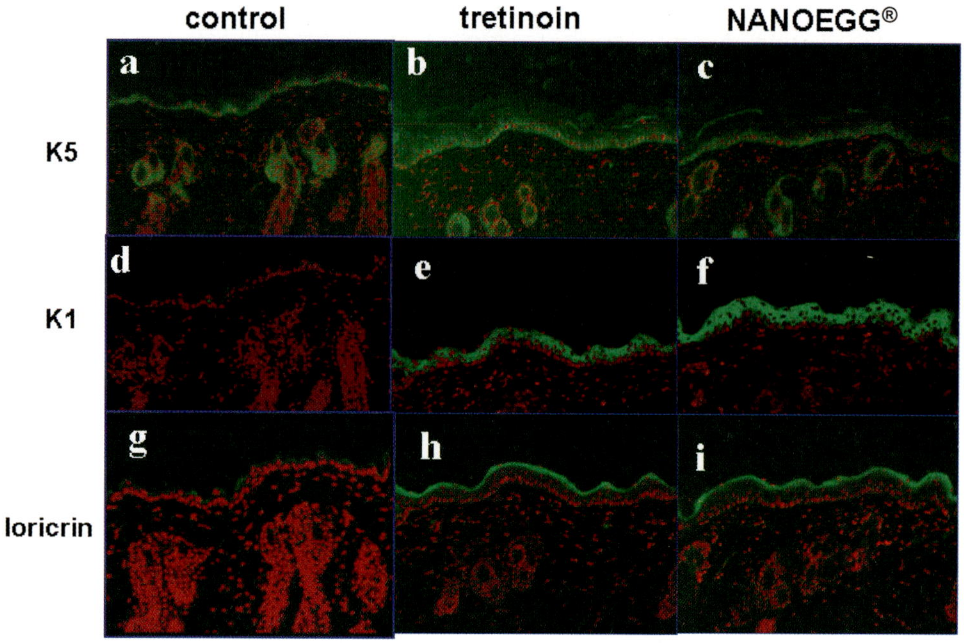

Figure 7.15. Expression of molecular markers in the epidermal layer of ddY mice. Green corresponds to antibody staining and red corresponds to nuclear staining. Dorsal skin sections from ddY mice at 4 days after the external treatment were stained with antibody against K1, K5 and lorocrin (lor). The treatments were carried out by ATRA and NANOEGG 0.1% as ATRA, respectively. The dorsal sections (1.0×1.0 cm^2) were administrated 30 mg ointment (base is Vaseline). K1 is a marker from the suprabasal layer to the stratum corneum; K5 is a marker from the basal cell; and loricrin is a marker from the granular layer to stratum corneum.

7.3.5
Production of Hyaluronic Acid (HA) in the Epidermal Layer

Another change was noteworthy – the intercellular spaces were wider and more prominent. This probably accounts for the intensified result with colloidal iron staining. Interestingly, wrinkling and skin texture may also be influenced by other epidermal factors as well as HB-EGF expression. Another histological finding of NANOEGG efficacy was obtained in this study. The influence of ATRA on epidermal differentiation is associated with the metabolism of HA by keratinocytes [36]. Tammi and coworkers reported tentative results in 1989 that HA was produced between ATRA-exposed keratinocytes [34]. The ATRA molecule leads to an accumulation of HA in the superficial layers of the epidermis by stimulating HA synthesis in keratinocytes. Deposition of HA coincides with cell proliferation and migration in several developing tissues and organs [35, 36], whereas onset of differentiation is often accompanied by reduced HA synthesis [37]. In order to evalu-

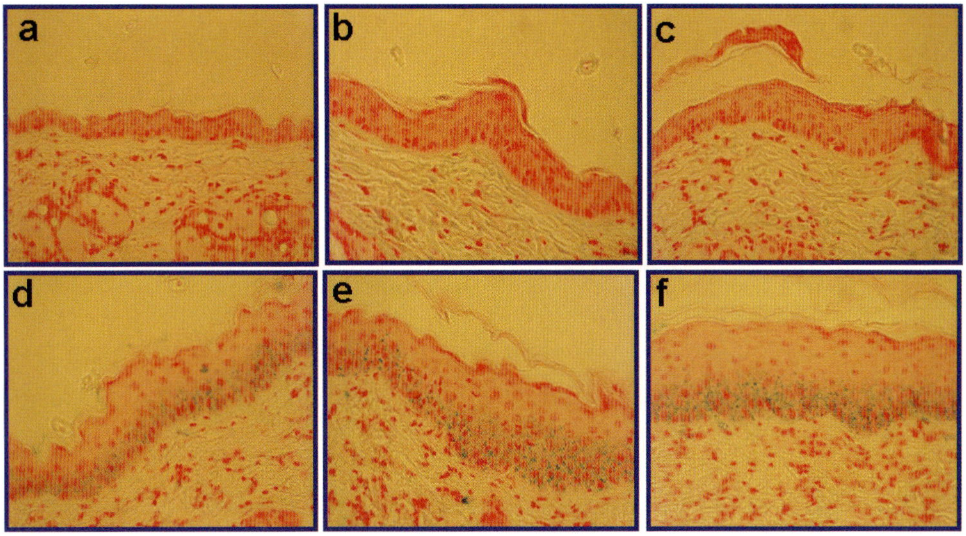

Figure 7.16. Expression of HA among keratinocytes after treatment by ATRA and NANOEGG. The dorsal tissues (ddY mouse, 5 weeks old, male) were stained using the colloidal iron stain method. The treatment of ATRA and NANOEGG was carried out once and the corresponding tissues were sacrificed 3 days after the treatment. Blue spots in the pictures correspond to HA, and they disappeared completely following the treatment with hyaluronidase (data not shown). ATRA (a) 0.1%, (b) 0.2% and (c) 0.4%; NANOEGG (d) 0.1%, (e) 0.2% and (f) 0.4%.

ate the efficacy of NANOEGG on HA production, empirical histology of the epidermis was investigated. Skin specimens treated daily for 4 days were taken from the mouse dorsal area. Specimens were prepared using colloidal iron staining to retain HA. In ATRA- and NANOEGG-treated groups, the intercellular spaces of the epidermal basal and spinous cells displayed negative and abundant presence of HA, respectively (dark blue spots correspond to accumulation of HA; Fig. 7.16a–c for ATRA treatment and Fig. 7.16d–f for NANOEGG treatment). Within the experimental period (4 days of treatment), it seems to be difficult to produce HA by ATRA treatment, at even with increasing the ATRA concentration to 0.4% (Fig. 7.16c).

Furthermore, intercellular spaces between both basal and suprabasal cells were extended wider with NANOEGG (Fig. 7.16d–f) than those with ATRA treatment (Fig. 7.16a–c). This may account for the reduced cohesion between cells compared to ATRA treatment, as HA displays a lubricating effect. Basal and suprabasal cells would therefore proliferate and migrate to the upper stratum corneum more easily. Finally, promotion of epidermal thickening accompanying melanin migration could occur with continuous application of NANOEGG on skin. In the NANOEGG system, rapid regulation of HA in the epidermis might effectively help keratinocyte growth. Production of hyaluronate in the epidermis would accelerate turnover of the epidermis, as the lubricant among cells eventually contributes to a reduction

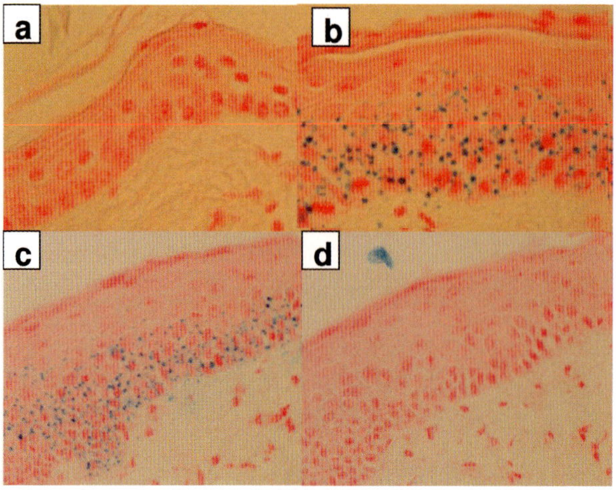

Figure 7.17. HA stain by colloidal iron. Dark-blue color domains correspond to the presence of HA. Each treatment was carried out for 4 days. (a) 0.1% ATRA in Vaseline, (b) 0.1% nano-ATRA in Vaseline, (c) same specimen as (b) but at a different area, (d) specimen (c) after treatment by hyaluronidase for 16 h and (e) change of fine wrinkles on the neck area of an aged hairless mouse (18 weeks old, male). The treatment was carried out for 4 days, with 30 mg of ATRA and NANOEGG (0.1%) in Vaseline creams.

in macular hyperpigmentation and less apparent fine wrinkles [19]. Since hyaluronidase treatment on NANOEGG-treated specimens resulted in a complete disappearance of the stained domain, this histological evaluation identified production of HA (Fig. 7.17c and d).

7.3.6
Hyperpigmentation and Fine Wrinkle Improvements by NANOEGG Treatment on Animal Skin

Photoaging involves the adverse effects of chronic UV radiation (UVR) on the skin, superimposed on the intrinsic aging process. The later sections review evidence gathered from animal and human studies regarding the ability of topical NANOEGG application to reverse many aspects of the photoaging process.

By definition, photoaging involves UVR exposure – mainly from the sun, but also from therapeutic sources of UVR. UVC (200–290 nm) is the most biologically damaging portion of the UVR spectrum, but is almost entirely absorbed by the ozone layer of the Earth's atmosphere. The strongest UV light to reach the Earth's surface is UVB (290–320 nm). UVA (320–400 nm) has the greater penetration into the skin, but is much weaker than UVB. Clinical features of photoaging include fine and coarse wrinkles, skin roughness, sallowness, mottled hyper/hypopigmentation, lentigines, telangiectasias, and skin laxity.

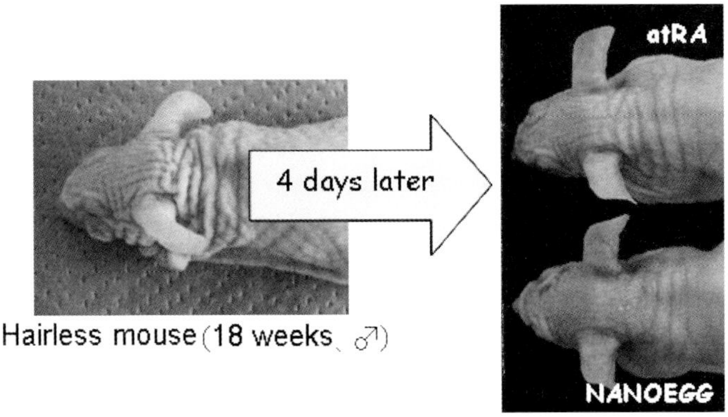

Figure 7.18. Change of fine wrinkles on the neck area of an aged hairless mouse (18-week, male). The treatment was carried out for 4 days, with 30 mg of ATRA and NANOEGG (0.1%, respectively) in Vaseline creams.

A systematic study of the photoaging process is difficult or impossible using human subjects. Animal models in which the process is accelerated are therefore desirable models. There is no naturally occurring animal model of photodamage, as diurnal animals are covered with fur, feathers or scales that protect them from UVR. The normally laboratory generated hairless mouse (HR-1) and guinea pig have been widely utilized because the animals wrinkle and produce brown spots in response to UVR within their relatively short life expectancies. To establishment fine wrinkles, first, the aged hairless mouse (HR-1, 18 weeks old) was utilized for the topical treatment of NANOEGG (Fig. 7.18). Guinea pigs (Weiser maple, 5 weeks old) were irradiated with UVA and UVB using an established protocol for 10 days to induce photodamage, and topical NANOEGG was applied at a concentration 0.05% for an additional 5 days (Fig. 7.19).

7.3.7 Clinical Trials of Fine Wrinkles and Brown Spots on the Human Face

In general, a period of at least a few months is required for clinical effectiveness in treating mottled pigmentation using ATRA cream. Given the major increase in thickness of the epidermis in our animal trials (Figs. 7.11 and 7.12), a reduction of melanin pigments should be rapidly produced by NANOEGG 0.05% treatment in humans. As a preliminary clinical trial for *in vivo* treatment of wrinkles and pigmental spots, NANOEGG therapy was performed for 1 month on human faces. The Institutional Review Board of St Marianna University permitted the clinical trial of NANOEGG ointment in human faces over 40 years old. The trial was carried out for 1 month in 30 wrinkles and 30 brown spots induced by aging and/or

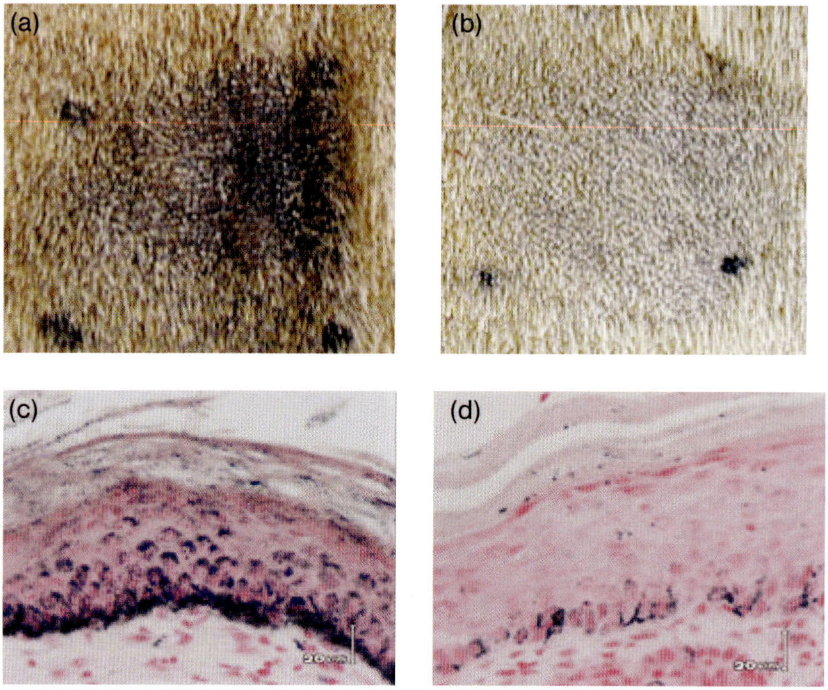

Figure 7.19. Improvement in hyperpigmentation of guinea pig dorsal skin with the topical application of NANOEGG. The establishment of brown spots was carried out by 10 days of total UVA and UVB irradiation. (a) Before treatment, (b) after the treatment of NANOEGG 0.05%, and (c) and (d) histological research corresponding to (a) and (b). The tissue was stained by melanin staining. Black granules correspond to melanin.

UV irradiation. The brown spots were also fairly decreased (Fig. 7.20). Otherwise, coarse wrinkling at the side of the eyes was consistently diminished after NANOEGG 0.05% treatment without strong irritation and inflammation (Fig. 7.20). This would certainly be due to the abundant HA accumulation in the epidermal layer at an early stage. Commercial ointment treatment could not usually achieved the decrease of hyperpigmentation after only 1 month, while the NANOEGG system could reduce the hyperpigmentation without serious irritation, as is obvious in Fig. 7.20. Actually, after treatment of NANOEGG for several days weak inflammation took place for several people. Compared with commercial products, these levels were rather weak. Accordingly, we believe that the risks due to the continuous treatment of ATRA such as erythema and irritation can prevent exactly by NANOEGG technology. Because the pharmacological effect would be gotten by the short-term treatment with the NANOEGG system. Simultaneously, the amount of water in stratum corneum also showed a statistically increase for 1 month treatment of NANOEGG (Fig. 7.21).

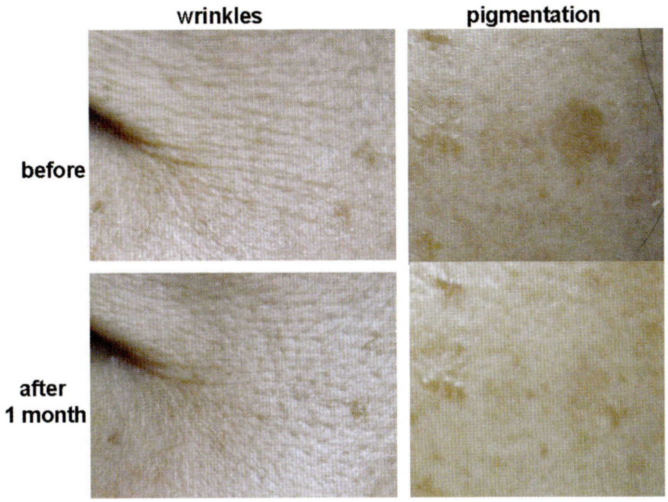

Figure 7.20. Pictures of wrinkles and photoaged hyperpigmentation on human faces (female, 48 years old). Before treatment with NANOEGG 0.05%, and after treatment for 1 month. The external daily administration was carried out one time at night, continuously.

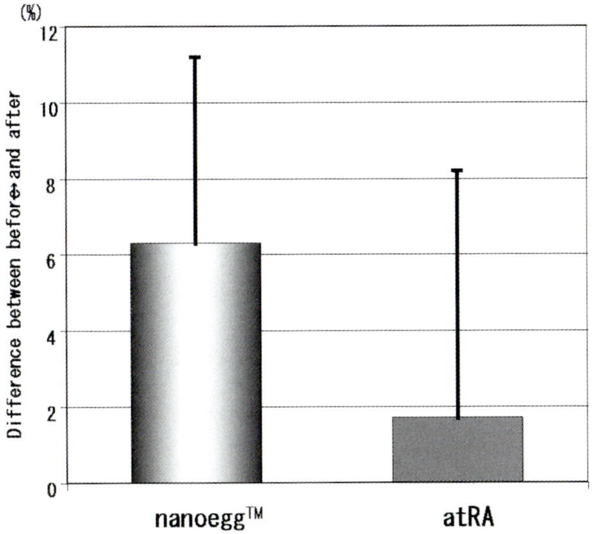

Figure 7.21. Change of amount of water in the stratum corneum of human skin. The measurements were carried out on people over 40 years old before and after treatments with NANOEGG and ATRA.

7.4
Why does NANOEGG Show the High Performance on the Improvement of Brown Spot and Wrinkles?

The superb results *in vivo* and histological evaluations obtained for NANOEGG are attributable to effective permeation into the skin. The stratum corneum is covered with lipids, natural moisturizing factors and ceramides as a barrier. In the presence of water, ceramide and other natural compounds spontaneously promote the formation of lyotropic lamella liquid crystals. When materials diffuse in such a lyotropic phase, the hydrophile–lipophile balance (HLB) of a molecule plays a significant role in the effective permeation into skin. In practice, hydrophobic ATRA would theoretically show minimal permeation through the stratum corneum epidermis. As a result, almost all of the ATRA would remain on the surface of the stratum corneum, eventually inducing irritation and inflammation. The surface of NANOEGG displays an amphiphilic character due to the coexistence of a hydrophobic domain ($CaCO_3$) and a hydrophilic PEG domain. As our NANOEGG is therefore easily dispersed in both aqueous and nonpolar media (Fig. 7.22), its permeability through the stratum corneum was substantially enhanced. Fortunately, permeability of NANOEGG can be indirectly evaluated in terms of histological staining of Ca^{2+} ions (Fig. 7.23). After treatment, red-smeared domains of biopsy specimens extended over time to the entire epidermis (Fig. 7.23b and c), while $CaCO_3$-treated subjects displayed no permeation to the inner dorsal skin (Fig. 7.23a).

Surprisingly, it is obvious that even in a quite short time (10 min, Fig. 7.23b) NANOEGG can already permeate into the skin. Not only the high permeation of NANOEGG, but also the stability of the capsule showed drastic performance in the epidermis. Since after 24 h the epidermal layer was more stained than the dermis, it indicates that NANOEGG capsules may be trapped in epidermis.

The skin is the outermost organ of the body. It is a complex membrane comprising of three major layers – epidermis, dermis and hypodermis. The epidermis is an avascular stratifying layer of epithelial cells that overlies the connective tissue layer – the dermis. The outermost layer of epidermis, i.e. the stratum corneum, is pri-

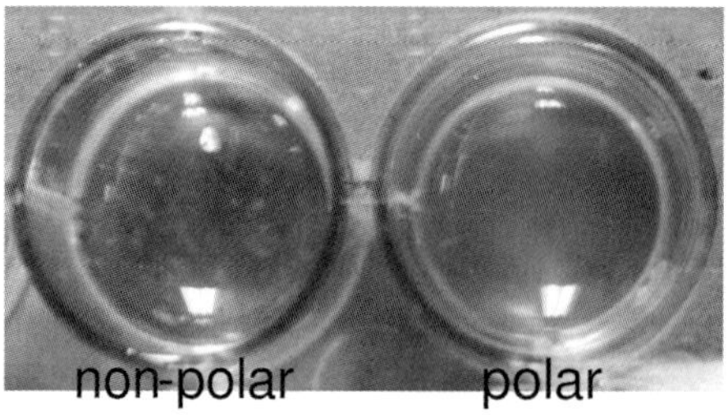

Figure 7.22. Solubility of NANOEGG 0.1% in polar (water) and nonpolar (corn oil) solvents. Both solutions showed a quite transparent appearance because of the amphiphilic property on the surface of NANOEGG.

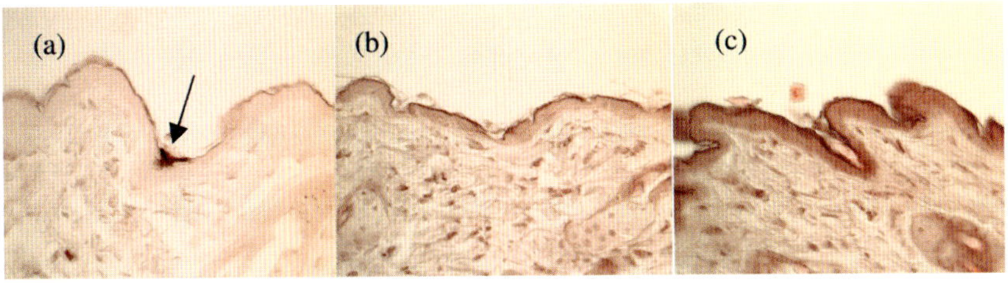

Figure 7.23. Dahl's calcium staining, which selectively traps the presence of Ca. Red smeared domains correspond to Ca distribution, particularly $CaCO_3$ [indicated by arrow as positive control (a)]. Permeation potential of NANOEGG through mouse skin as a function of time after external administration. The tissues of ddY mice were utilized for staining. Calcium was regarded as a permeation maker from the stratum corneum epidermis to the dermis region. As the NANOEGG particle is at the nanoscale, the stain in the specimen would be detected as smeared domains. Treatment with 0.1% NANOEGG Vaseline cream after (b) 10 min and (c) 24 h.

marily responsible for the barrier properties of the skin. The underlying viable epidermis is different from the stratum corneum in being physiologically more akin to other living cellular tissues, but also plays the role as second barrier, especially for ions. Following passive application, the unionized form of any compound is better absorbed than its ionized counterpart [38]. However, the penetration rates of drug molecules across skin or other epithelial surfaces are usually low due to their excellent barrier properties.

For the reasons discussed above, it can be suggested here that NANOEGG capsules could successfully permeate into skin due to passive diffusion.

7.5 NANOEGG for Other Indications

In multicellular organisms, a balance between differentiation, proliferation and cell death maintains tissue homeostasis in adult tissues and directs normal development during embryonic morphogenesis. Retinoic acid is one of the critical factors regulating the molecular events involved in these processes. The requirement for ATRA for normal development and tissue homeostasis has been known since Wolbach and Howe first reported the defects that occurred in vitamin A-deficient animals in 1926. A large literature base has since appeared describing the role of retinoids in promoting proliferation, differentiation or apoptosis *in vivo*, in a variety of cell culture systems and more recently through studies using retinoid receptor knockout strategies. In addition, these investigations have provided the mechanisms by which retinoids induce teratogenic effects and inhibit neoplastic development, particularly in cancer. Significant progress has been made in understanding the molecular mechanism by which retinoids modulate the action of negative and positive growth factors including EGF, the transforming growth factor (TGF) family, insulin, IL-1α, IL-6, IFN-γ, estrogen and vitamin D_3. Regulation by retinoids can occur at the level of expression of growth factors and cytokines, and their respective receptors/binding proteins in the signaling pathway.

Many of the biological effects and changes in gene expression induced by ATRA are mediated by six known retinoic acid receptors (RARα, RARβ and RARγ) and/or retinoid X receptors (RXRα, RXRα and RXRγ) [39–41]. It is known that each of the RAR subtypes has a specific tissue distribution pattern [42]. For example, RARγ is the most abundant retinoid receptor in the skin [43, 44], whereas RARβ is found primarily in the heart, lung and spleen. RARα is expressed at low levels in many tissue types. It follows that retinoids that activate a particular receptor subtype may elicit biological responses in specific tissues. Thus, it can be expected that retinoids would greatly improve therapeutic indices in the treatment of retinoid-responsive diseases because of receptor expression on many tissues. The full therapeutic potential of ATRA may only be realized if new technologies with vastly improved therapeutic indices can be developed.

We have been investigated the radical therapy of diabetes mellitus induced by NANOEGG. Since the ATRA molecule is soluble in water, it is impossible to inject, whereas NANOEGG is easily soluble in aqueous media. Injection of NANOEGG may systematically induce the proliferation of pancreatic β cells and differentiation of anaplastic cells in Langerhans islands and/or pancreatic ducts, resulting in the regeneration of β cells. Recent studies showed that differentiation of in different cells on pancreatic ducts could be induced by HB-EGF and, as a result, glucose tolerance was improved [45]. As already shown, the topical treatment of NANOEGG could produce abundant HB-EGF. The pancreas must also express retinoic acid receptors. HB-EGF induced by NANOEGG, thus, will be expected to regenerate pancreatic β cells in diabetic animal models. Figure 7.24 shows the change of body weight of type I diabetic rats induced by streptozotocin in the case of subcutaneous administration of NANOEGG. Obviously the loss of weight was stopped

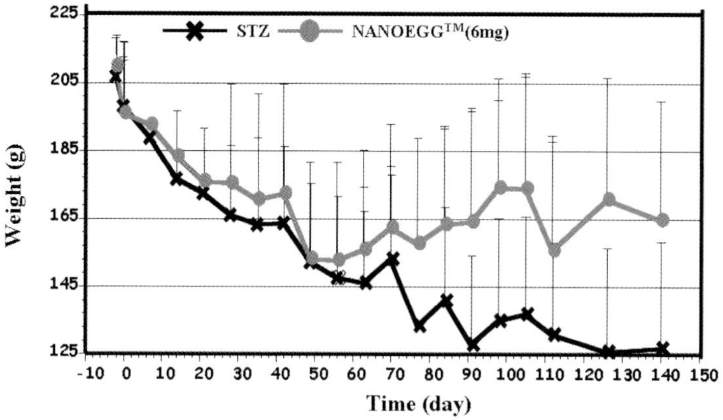

Figure 7.24. Change of body weight of Wistar rats (male) in subcutaneously administered NANOEGG (6 mg as ATRA, once a week). Model animals were induced with type I diabetes by STZ administration.

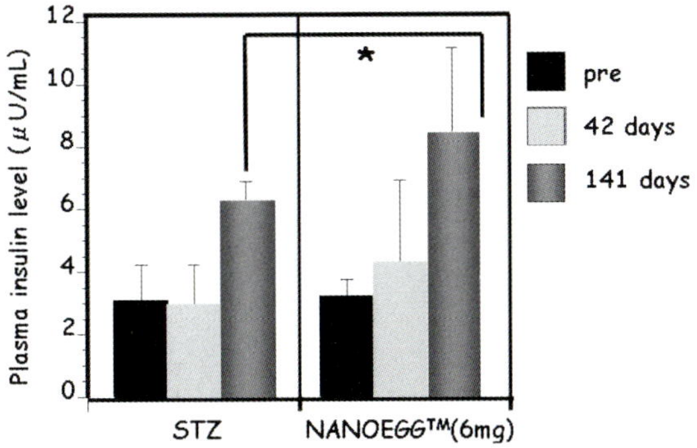

Figure 7.25. Change of insulin level in plasma after the administration of NANOEGG (6 mg as ATRA, once a week). Model animals were induced with type I diabetes by STZ administration.

in the NANOEGG-injected group around 60 days. In this case, the concentration of insulin in plasma also increased compared to the nontreated group (Fig. 7.25). Expression of transcription factor of pancreas PDX-1 in Langerhans islands relates to the differentiation of somatic stem cells to β cells [46, 47]. Figure 7.26

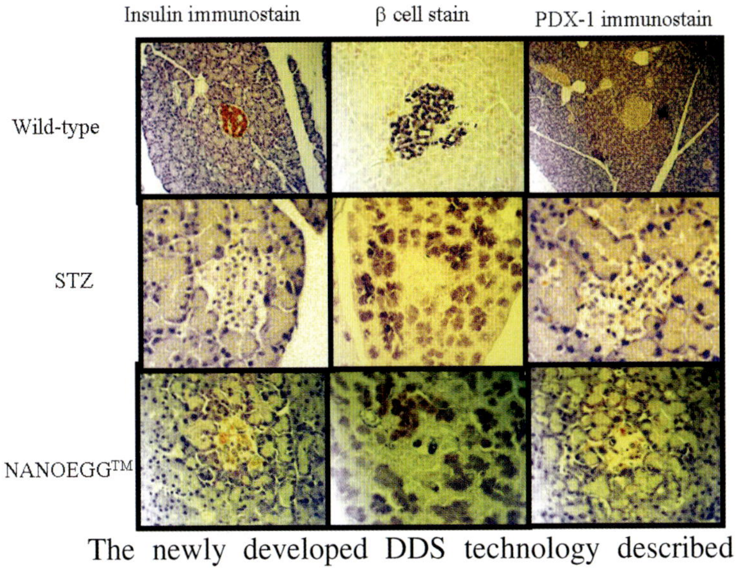

Figure 7.26. Immunostaining of insulin and transcription factor PDX-1, and β cells in Langerhans islands of rat pancreas. Model animals were prepared by the administration of STZ. Over 99% of β cells could not be observed in Langerhans islands in the case of STZ groups.

shows slight expression of PDX-1 in Langerhans islands in the group administered NANOEGG.

The administration of NANOEGG cannot only be used for the regeneration of skin, but also can be expected to be used for the regeneration therapy of β cells. New nanoshell technology NANOEGG may also be useful for other retinoid response diseases. Major advances with ATRA and/or its nanocapsule NANOEGG would be continuously in progress in clinical applications.

7.6 NANOEGG for Other Drugs

The self-assembly property in aqueous media is absolutely necessary to prepare NANOEGG. The physicochemical amphiphilic balance of the molecular structure leads to molecular association in water. ATRA can spontaneously form micelles in water with a small amount of alkaline. If drugs can form self-assemblies like micelles and their surfaces have ionic charges, the NANOEGG structure should be prepared. Even if drugs have a high molecular weight, it is possible to form the core–shell structure of the NANOEGG system. Prostaglandin and its derivatives may be able to form micelle-like structures. It would expect that NANOEGG technology will be also indicated in other drugs.

7.7 Conclusion

Up to now, clinical responses predominantly comprised severe irritant dermatitis in the early stages of application (around 3 or 4 days) of ATRA. This problem is generally managed by modifications to the dosage and schedule. Such damage with a high magnitude of inflammatory events after ATRA treatment can induce chronic skin pigmentation in the area being treated, potentially resulting in imperfect repair of skin displaying a pigmented appearance. Preventing undesirable adverse effects would be expected to allow ATRA therapy to overcome the limitations of classical ATRA therapy. Herein, we describe the development of a novel drug delivery system using nanotechnology. The conceptual framework in this study is that NANOEGG plays a crucial role in solving the low permeation of ATRA into spaces in the stratum corneum epidermis and the also the symptoms of irritation.

The newly developed drug delivery system technology described herein could help with nonsurgical treatment of photodamaged skin for which use of ATRA has been recommended. Detailed studies concerning the efficacy of NANOEGG have already been reported [19, 48, 49], suggesting not only improved permeability to the stratum corneum, but also simultaneous enhanced keratinization due to $CaCO_3$. Drastically increased epidermal thickness could be expected to result in a relative decrease in melanin content and excess expression of HA aids induction of hyperplasia, resulting in less-wrinkled skin. Moreover, the high permeability and controlled release of ATRA induces accelerated epidermal turnover. Promotion of keratinocyte proliferation and acceleration of keratinocyte differentiation are most likely the result of ATRA in regimenting treatments. Melanin granules may be washed out of the epidermis by a rapid and stronger stream of keratinocytes in the epidermis compared to topical ATRA treatment. This study clearly shows that our newly developed novel drug delivery system technology for NANOEGG offers great potential for new ATRA therapy. Histological and ultrastructural findings for empirical evaluation of NANOEGG indicate that ATRA therapy causes more than esthetic improvement, inducing histological changes in the epidermis, in all likelihood without regard to changes induced by time or sunlight.

The new nanoshell technology NANOEGG can be useful for other clinical approaches and other drugs. It would expect that drastic advances in the treatment of intractable diseases will be achieved by the NANOEGG drug delivery system.

References

1 Sporn M. B., Roberts A. B., Role of retinoids in differentiation and carcinogenesis. *Cancer Res.* **1983**, *43*, 3034–3040.

2 Mangelsdorf D. J., Evans R. M., The RXR heterodimers and orphan receptors. *Cell* **1995**, *83*, 841–850.

3 Wolbach S. B., Howe P. R., Tissue changes following deprivation and fat-soluble A vitamin. *J. Exp. Med.* **1925**, *42*, 753–777.

4 Frazier C. N., Hu C. K., Cutaneous lesions associated with a deficiently in vitamin A in man. *Arch. Intern. Med.* **1931**, *48*, 507–514.

5 Livrea M. A., *Vitamin A and Retinoids: An Update of Biological Aspects and Clinical Applications.* Birkhouser Verlag, Basel, **2000**.

6 Fisher G. J., Voorhees J. J., Molecular mechanisms of retinoid actions in skin. *FASEB J.* **1996**, *10*, 1002–1013.

7 Aydelotte M. B., The effects of vitamin A and citral on epithelial differentiation. 1. The chick oesophageal and corneal epithelia and epidermis. *J. Embryol. Exp. Morphol.* **1963**, *11*, 621–635.

8 Bellows C. G., Hardy M. H., Histochemical evidence of mucosubstances in the metaplastic epidermis and hair follicles produced *in vitro* in the presence of excess vitamin A. *Anat. Rec.* **1977**, *187*, 257–271.

9 Klingman L. H., Duo C. H., Klingman A. M., Topical retinoic acid enhances the repair of ultraviolet damaged dermal connective tissue. *Connect. Tissue Res.* **1984**, *12*, 139–142.

10 Klingman A. M., Grove G. L., Hirose R., Leyden J. J., Topical tretinoin for photoaged skin. *J. Am. Acad. Dermatol.* **1986**, *15*, 836–839.

11 Olsen E. A., Katz H. I., Levine N., Shupack J., Billys M. M., Prawer S., Gold J., Stiller M., Lufrano L., Thorne E. G., Tretinoin emollient cream: a new therapy for photodamaged skin. *J. Am. Acad. Dermatol.* **1992**, *26*, 215–224.

12 Mizuguchi K., Tsuda T., *Medical Technology, New Stain Method.* Ishiyaku, Shuppan, Japan, **1999**, pp. 122–123.

13 Moroi Y., *Micelles: Theoretical and Applied Aspects.* Plenum Press, New York, **1992**, pp. 66–73.

14 Szuts E. Z., Harosi I. H., Solubility of retinoids in water. *Arch. Biochem. Biophys.* **1991**, *287*, 297–304.

15 Li C. Y., Zimmerman C. L., Wiedmann T. S., Solubilization of retinoids by bile saltphospholipid aggregates. *Pharm. Res.* **1996**, *13*, 907–913.

16 DeBoeck H., Zidovetzki R., NMR study of the interactions of retinoids with phospholipid bilayers. *Biochim. Biophys. Acta* **1988**, *946*, 244–252.

17 Wassall S. R., Phelps T. M., Albrecht M. R., Langsford C. A., Stillwell W., ESR study of the interactions of retinoids with a phospholipids model membrane. *Biochim. Biophys. Acta* **1988**, *939*, 393–402.

18 Noy N., The ionization behavior of retinoic acid in aqueous environments and bound to serum albumin. *Biochim. Biophys. Acta* **1992**, *1106*, 151–158.

19 Yamaguchi Y., Nagasawa T., Nakamura N., Takenaga M., Mizoguchi M., Kawai S., Mizushima Y., Igarashi R., Successful treatment of photo-damaged skin of nano-scale ATRA particles using a novel transdermal delivery, *J. Control. Release* **2005**, *104*, 29–40.

20 Brecht M., Mayer U., Schlosser E., Prehm P., Increased hyaluronate synthesis is required for fibroblast detachment and mitosis. *Biochem. J.* **1986**, *239*, 445–450.

21 Small D. M., Micellar properties of sodium fusidate, a steroid antibiotic structurally resembling the bile salts. In *The Bile Acids*, Nair P. P., Kritchevsky S. (Eds.). Plenum, New York, **1971**, Vol. 1, pp. 249–355.

22 Cistra D. P., Hamilton J. A., Jackson D., Small D. A., Ionization and phase behaviour of fatty acids in water application of the Gibbs phase rule. *Biochemistry* **1988**, *27*, 1881–1888.

23 Moroi Y., Micelles, theoretical and applied aspects. *J. Phys. Chem.* **1980**, *84*, 2186–2191.

24 Heitmann P., Reactivity of sulfhydryl groups in micelles. A model for protein. *Eur. J. Biochem.* **1968**, *5*, 305–310.

25 Jones G. J., Crouch R. K., Wiggert B., Cornwall M. C., Chader G. J., Retinoid requirements for recovery of sensitivity after visual pigment bleaching in isolated photoreceptors. *Proc. Natl Acad. Sci. USA* **1989**, *86*, 9606–9610.

26 Crouch R. K., Hazard E. S., Lind T., Wiggert B., Chader G., Corson D. W., Interphotoreceptor retinoid-binding protein and α-tocopherol preserve the isomeric and oxidation state of retinol. *Photochem. Photobiol.* **1992**, *56*, 251–255.

27 Fucks E., Epidermal differentiation: the bare essentials. *J. Cell Biol.* **1990**, *111*, 2807–2814.

28 Fucks E., Keratins as biochemical markers of epithelial differentiation. *Trends Genet.* **1988**, *4*, 277–281.

29 Mehrel T., Hohl D., Rothnagel J. A., Langley M. A., Bundman D., Chenge C., Lichti U., Bisher M. E., Steven A. C., Steinart P. M., Yuspa S. H., Roop D. R., Identification of a major keratinocyte cell envelope protein, lorocrin. *Cell* **1990**, *61*, 1103–1112.

30 Kurst A., Kastner P., Petkovitch M., Zelent A., Chambon P., A third human retinoic acid receptor, hRAR-gamma. *Proc. Natl Acad. Sci. USA* **1989**, *86*, 5310–5314.

31 Sporn M. B., Roberts A. B., Role of retinoids in differentiation and carcinogenesis. *Cancer Res.* **1983**, *43*, 3034–3040.

32 Griffiths C. E. M., Finkel L. J., Tranfaglia M. G., Hamilton T. A., Voorthees J. J., An *in vivo* experimental model for effects of topical retinoic acid in human skin. *Br. J. Dermatol.* **1993**, *129*, 389–394.

33 Stoll S. W., Elder J. T., Retinoid regulation of heparin-binding EGF-like growth factor gene expression in human keratinocytes and skin. *Exp. Dermatol.* **1998**, *7*, 391–397.

34 Tammi R., Ripellino J. A., Margolis R. U., Maibach H. I., Tammi M., Hyaluronate accumulation in human epidermis treated with retinoic acid skin organ culture. *J. Invest. Dermatol.* **1989**, *92*, 326–332.

35 Brecht M., Mayer U., Schlosser E., Prehm P., Increased hyaluronate synthesis is required for fibroblast detachment and mitosis. *Biochem. J.* **1986**, *239*, 445–450.

36 Chen W. Y., Grant M. E., Schor A. M., Schor S. L., Differences between adult and foetal fibroblasts in the regulation of hyaluronate synthesis: correlation with migratory activity. *J. Cell Sci.* **1989**, *94*, 577–584.

37 Toole B. P., Trelstad R. L., Hyaluronate production and removal during corneal development in the chick. *Dev. Biol.* **1971**, *126*, 28–35.

38 Swarbrick J., Lee G., Brom J., Gensmantel P., Drug permeation through skin. II. Permeability of ionized compounds. *J. Pharm. Sci.* **1984**, *73*, 1352–1354.

39 Mangelsdorf D. J., Umesono K., Evans R. M., The retinoid receptors. In *The Retinoids*. Sporn M. B., Roberts A. B., Goodman D. S. (Eds.). Raven, New York, **1994**, pp. 319–350.

40 Giguère V., RA receptors and cellular retinoid binding proteins: complex inter-play on retinoid signaling, *Endocr. Rev.* **1994**, *15*, 61–79.

41 Chambon P., A decade of molecular biology of retinoic acid receptors. *FASEB J.* **1996**, *10*, 940–954.

42 Rees J., The molecular biology of retinoic acid receptors: orphan from good family seeks home. *Br. J. Dermatol.* **1992**, *126*, 97–104.

43 Elder J. T., Fisher G. J., Zhang Q.-Y., Eisen D., Krust A., Kastner P., Chambon P., Voorhees J. J., Retinoic acid receptor gene expression in human skin. *J. Invest. Dermatol.* **1991**, *96*, 425–433.

44 Reczek P. R., Ostowski J., Yu K.-L., Chen S., Hammer L., Roalsvig T., Starrett Jr., J. E., Driscoll, G., Whiting J. P., Spinazze P. G., Tramposch K. M., Mansuri M. M., Role of retinoic acid receptor gamma in the rhino mouse and rabbit irritation models of retinoid activity. *Skin Pharmacol.* **1996**, *8*, 292–299.

45 Kozawa J., Tokui Y., Morikawa M., Ohmoto H. L., Yuan M., Zhang J., Iwahashi H., Imagawa A., Yamagata K., Tochino Y., Shimomura I., Higashiyama S., Miyagawa J., Regenerative and therapeutic effects of heparin-binding epidermal growth factor-like growth factor on diabetes by gene transduction through retrograde pancreatic duct injection of adenovirus vector. *Pancreas* **2005**, *31*, 32–42.

46 Miyazaki S., Yamato E., Miyazaki J., Regulated expression of pdx-1 promotes *in vitro* differentiation of insulin-producing cells from embryonic stem cells. *Diabetes* **2004**, *53*, 1030–1037.

47 Taniguchi H., Yamato E., Tashiro F., Ikegami H., Ogihara T., Miyazaki J., β cell neogenesis induced by adenovirus-mediated gene delivery of transcription factor pdx-1 into mouse pancreas. *Gene Ther.* **2003**, *10*, 15–23.

48 Yamaguchi Y., Nagasawa T., Nakamura N., Kitagawa A., Matsumoto K., Takenaga M., Mizoguchi M., Igarashi R., Optical treatment new tretinoin nanoparticles with inorganic-coating. *J. Dermatol.* **2006**, in press.

49 Yamaguchi Y., Nakamura N., Nagasawa T., Kitagawa A., Matsumoto K., Soma Y., Matsuda T., Mizoguchi M., Igarashi R., Enhanced skin regeneration of all-*trans* retinoic acid by nanoegg™ formulation, *Die Pharmazie* **2006**, *61*, 117–121.

8
Polymeric Nanomaterials – Synthesis, Functionalization and Applications in Diagnosis and Therapy

Jutta Rieger, Christine Jérôme, Robert Jérôme, and Rachel Auzély-Velty

8.1
Introduction

In the last decade, polymeric nanoparticles have received increasing interest both for drug delivery purposes and as diagnostic tools. The interest in nanoparticles as drug carriers relies on the difficulties met in drug delivery. In fact, after extravascular administration of a drug, its fate is determined by the combination of several processes, i.e. absorption, distribution, metabolism and elimination (ADME). In contrast, intravenous routes circumvent the absorption process as the drug is directly available in the blood circulation. Regardless of the administration route, each of these processes depends mainly on the physicochemical properties of the drug. Therefore, drug carrier systems have been developed that allow for controlling the fate of a drug within the patient. These "drug delivery systems" cannot only influence the absorption of a drug from the gastrointestinal tract, but they also permit governing of the drug distribution within the organism. In particular, nanoparticles have received increasing interest because of their ability to deliver a wide range of drugs (or diagnostic agents) to various organs or tissues for sustained periods of time. In this chapter, two applications of nanosized polymeric colloidal carrier systems are discussed together: their use as drug delivery systems and as diagnostic tools. Indeed, for both applications most of the required features and preparation techniques are similar, if not identical.

As a remark, polymer nanoparticles are considered here as submicron carriers in the nanometer range (diameter below 1 μm) mainly prepared from natural or synthetic polymers. This definition does not take into account the morphological and structural organization of the polymer. The term "nanosphere" is used to describe nanoparticles that are constituted by a solid "homogeneous" polymeric matrix. The delivery of the therapeutics proceeds either by the diffusion through the polymer matrix or, in the case of biodegradable particles, by the degradation of the latter, or by both processes. In contrast, "nanocapsules" are nanoparticles where a polymeric membrane surrounds a cavity filled by an oily or an aqueous content. They are therefore considered as a "reservoir" system, where the diffusion of the hydro-

Nanotechnologies for the Life Sciences Vol. 10
Nanomaterials for Medical Diagnosis and Therapy. Edited by Challa S. S. R. Kumar

ISBN: 978-3-527-31390-7

philic or hydrophobic drug is controlled by the nature of the polymeric membrane. In this chapter, we focus on "frozen", not dynamic systems, i.e. systems where an exchange between individual polymer chains and polymer chains of the nano-object cannot take place. Consequently, dynamic systems such as micelles as well as liposomes are barely considered in this review. However, in Section 8.4.3.4.1, several approaches based on so-called shell crosslinked knedel-like (SCK) nanoparticles are quoted. Such SCK nanoparticles are micelles, whose outer shell is crosslinked. They can be prepared in two steps, starting from the self-assembly of amphiphilic block copolymers to form micelles, of which the shell formed by the outer block is frozen by crosslinking in a second step [1].

Polymeric nanoparticles have now been the subject of numerous studies for more than 20 years and have progressed since then. Three generations of nanoparticles may be considered.

(i) First-generation nanoparticles. Nanoparticles with no specific surface properties have been called "nanoparticles of the first generation". Indeed, whenever such kinds of nanoparticles are introduced in the human body, they are rapidly recognized as foreign bodies and, as a consequence, removed from the blood circulation. Once nanoparticles are introduced in a biological system, numerous plasma proteins adsorb at their surface, leading to the activation of the complement system. As a consequence, the colloidal drug carriers are rapidly recognized by macrophages of the mononuclear phagocyte system (MPS) and removed within seconds from the blood stream. Organs with high phagocytic activity are the liver, spleen and bone marrow. These organs possess a discontinuous, i.e. more permeable, endothelium, where the blood is directly in contact with the immune active macrophages. Therefore, nanoparticles of the first generation accumulate in and passively target the liver, spleen and bone marrow. This natural tendency to be captured by the MPS has therefore found application in the treatment of liver cancer and other liver-related diseases.

The protein adsorption on the nanoparticle surface, i.e. the key step to induce a cascade of biological processes leading to their elimination, is based on various interactions, but especially on interactions of hydrophobic domains of the proteins with hydrophobic domains present at the nanoparticle surface.

(ii) Second-generation nanoparticles. In order to target other organs than tissues with high phagocyte activity, further developments strove for avoiding the rapid adsorption of blood proteins, i.e. the activation of the complement system. This has been achieved by modifying the surface of the nanoparticles, especially by hydrophilic materials, in order to inhibit hydrophobic protein–particle interactions. The coating of the particle surface by hydrophilic chains leads to repulsion of proteins and consequently a prolonged residence time of the particles in the blood stream. These surface-modified nanoparticles are also called carriers of the "second generation", or "Stealth™" nanoparticles, as they are designed to successfully avoid MPS sequestration. The hydrophilic polymers that have been used for the surface coating of nanoparticles are synthetic polymers, particularly poly(ethylene oxide) (PEO) [2, 3], but also polysaccharides, such as heparin [4, 5] and dextran [6].

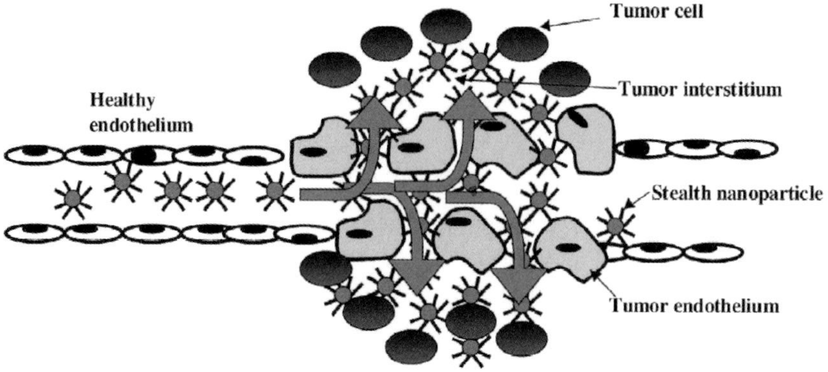

Figure 8.1. Extravasation of long-circulating (Stealth) nanoparticles in the tumor interstitium by passive diffusion or convection across the altered and hyperpermeable neoplastic endothelium.

These long-circulating colloidal systems have received much interest in the field of cancer diagnosis and treatment. Indeed, cancerous tissues are characterized by an "enhanced permeability and retention" effect [7] (Fig. 8.1). The phenomenon, that long-circulating colloidal systems are preferentially accumulated in cancerous tissues, is called "passive targeting", and is used in numerous studies both for drug delivery purposes and diagnosis [8].

(iii) Third-generation nanoparticles – active targeting. It is possible to give carriers affinity to specific tissue by decorating their surface with targeting ligands. This kind of carrier delivers a drug specifically to its pharmacological site in the organism, and thus allows us to decrease the administered quantity of drugs and to minimize side-effects. Indeed, the latter are generally the result of the presence of the drug at other tissues than at the desired one.

Targeting ligands can be monoclonal antibodies, sugars, hormones, peptides (e.g. the tripeptide, arginine–glycine–aspartic acid (RGD) [9]), vitamins (e.g. biotin [10]) or other small organic molecules (e.g. folic acid [11]). Colloidal carriers, of which the surface is decorated with targeting moieties, are also called "nanoparticles of the third generation" and today most studies tend to design such nano-objects. Quite a lot of systems have already been patented. Targeting demands optimal interaction between a targeted site and its ligand. Therefore, targeting molecules have been fixed at the end of linker molecules, such as flexible PEO chains [10].

The surface functionalization of polymeric nanoparticles is thus the key point for both targeted drug delivery and diagnosis. Indeed, this chapter focuses mainly on nanoparticles of the third generation, i.e. surface-modified nanoparticles, designed for drug delivery and diagnosis. The objective of this chapter is to discuss (i) the different ways to obtain surface-modified nanoparticles, (ii) the biological molecules used for surface modification, and (iii) the current and future applications of such polymeric nanoparticles in the field of drug delivery and diagnosis. In line with our subjects of research, we mainly report on nanospheres, rather than nanocapsules, and restrict the cited examples to approaches interesting for biomedical applications. Because of their importance for diagnosis purposes, we also report on nanoparticle composites composed of both polymer and inorganic materials (that serve as label/marker). However, metallic nanoparticles coated by polymer chains are not the subject of this chapter.

The chapter is divided into five main sections. Section 8.2 deals with polymeric materials used for the preparation of nano-sized carrier systems. In Section 8.3, the different techniques to obtain such systems are discussed. Section 8.4 describes how the surface of nanoparticles can be modified and briefly summarizes the most common techniques to characterize nanoparticle surfaces. Section 8.5 describes their application as drug delivery systems and diagnostics.

8.2 Polymer Materials Used for the Synthesis of Nanoparticles

Depending on the route of administration (oral or parenteral) and the application of polymeric nanoparticles (drug carriers or diagnostic systems), the materials used to produce the colloidal systems meet different physiological and biological requirements. Among these requirements, biocompatibility and safety are of crucial importance.

Additionally, it must be considered whether bioerosion and/or biodegradation is desired or not. Although there is no universally accepted definition for the terms bioerosion and biodegradation, bioerosion refers to solubilization of an initially water-insoluble material with or without changes in the chemical structure, while biodegradation refers to solubilization that occurs as a consequence of cleavage of main-chain bonds. The prefix "bio" is used because the erosion or degradation takes place in a biological environment, either by biocatalytic processes (fungi, enzymes, etc.) or by chemical/radical processes (hydrolysis, oxidation, UV irradiation). Degradable synthetic polymers have great potential for drug delivery purposes. They are typically degraded by chemical hydrolysis, whereas the degradation of natural polymers (i.e. polymers derived from animal or plant sources) generally requires enzymes to catalyze the hydrolysis. On the other hand, polymers used for diagnosis purposes, especially in the case of *ex vivo* (*in vitro*) tests, should not be biodegradable; therefore, nondegradable, i.e. long-term stable polymers, which are often more easy to synthesize, are used. In that way, recycling and repeated use of the device are possible. Concerning synthetic biodegradable polymers, it must be noted that not only the polymer itself used for the formulation, but also the degradation products (metabolites) must be nontoxic, biocompatible and chemically inert. The practical consequence of that is that only a limited number of nontoxic, monomeric starting materials can be really applied for the development of biodegradable nanoparticles.

In the following, the main polymers used for the preparation of nanocarriers will be described. We distinguish three groups of polymers, i.e. (i) natural polymers ("biopolymers"), (ii) synthetic polymers which are "degradable" by biological or chemical processes in the human body and (iii) "nondegradable" synthetic polymers.

8.2.1 Natural Polymers

Polysaccharides represent – besides polypeptides – the most important group of natural polymers [12]. We have chosen to focus here only on polysaccharides that display very interesting physicochemical properties, in terms of gelation characteristics, chelating properties and biological activity. Many polysaccharides show biocompatibility and biodegradability, which are the basic characteristics for using polymers as biomaterials, as reviewed by Dumitriu and coworkers [13]. Moreover, their physicochemical properties as well as their interactions with living medium can be altered by chemical modifications.

Several biocompatible polysaccharides such as chitosan, dextran, heparin and hyaluronic acid have been shown to be interesting candidates for the modification of nanoparticle surfaces. This allows, for instance, reducing nanoparticle uptake by the MPS and also, in some cases, conferring specific biological functions [14].

In addition, due to its polycationic nature, chitosan could be advantageously used as a constitutive core material of nanoparticles. This biopolymer is obtained by partial *N*-deacetylation of chitin – a natural polysaccharide found in crustaceous shells. Chitosan consists of a linear chain of (1–4)-linked 2-amino-2-deoxy-β-D-glucopyranose and 2-acetamido-2-deoxy-β-D-glucopyranose units (Fig. 8.2). It is water-soluble in acidic conditions (pH < 6) due to the existence of amino groups making it thus possible to prepare derivatives with optimized properties under homogeneous conditions. Its hydrophilicity allows covering the domain of applications in solution and in gel (after crosslinking by chemical or physical bonds). Due to its mucoadhesive properties, chitosan has been largely investigated for coating colloidal carriers administered to the gastrointestinal tract [15], or by nasal, ocular, buccal and vaginal routes. The strong mucoadhesion of chitosan can be explained by ionic interactions between this polycationic molecule and anionic substructures such as sialic moieties of the mucus gel layer on mucosa. Apart from its muco-

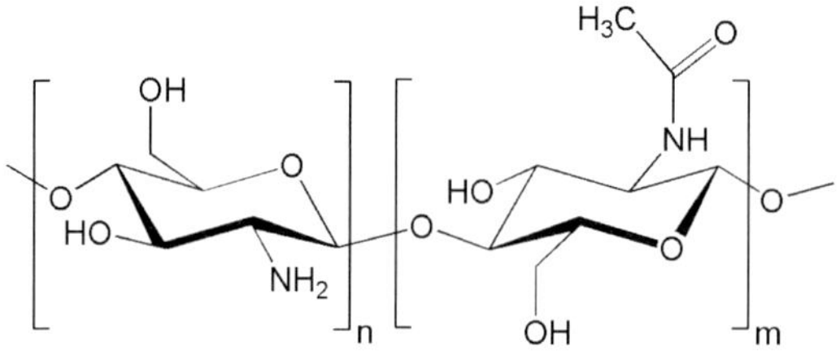

1

Figure 8.2. Chemical structure of chitosan.

adhesive properties, chitosan displays low toxicity, degradability by enzymes such as chitinase and lysozyme [13], anticoagulant properties, and antibacterial and antifungal action. It has also been demonstrated to be a promoter of wound healing in the field of surgery.

As mentioned above, taking advantage of the polycationic nature of chitosan, Alonso and coworkers [12, 16] developed chitosan nanoparticles based on ionic gelation of chitosan with sodium tripolyphosphate. The size, surface characteristics and *in vitro* release properties of these nanoparticles can be modulated by the preparation conditions and in particular by incorporation of an additional polymer such as a diblock copolymer of ethylene oxide and propylene oxide (PEO–b–PPO). The authors demonstrated that these nanoparticles have a great protein-loading capacity (protein loading up to 50%, i.e. 50 mg of protein per 100 mg of nanoparticles). Such drug-loaded chitosan-based nanocarriers have been mostly administered by mucosal routes (i.e. oral, nasal, ocular). Alonso and coworkers also investigated the nasal absorption of such chitosan nanoparticles loaded with insulin (via the glucose blood concentration) and, furthermore, studied the *in vitro* release profiles of hydrophilic drugs, such as anthracycline and doxorubicin [12], as well as of hydrophobic peptides such as cyclosporine A.

Furthermore, the polycationic character of chitosan makes it an interesting material for nonviral gene delivery. It forms polyelectrolyte complexes with the negatively charged DNA, condenses the DNA, which protects it from degradation by DNase [12, 17]. Nevertheless, the transfection rate of such chitosan–DNA complexes is very low. Therefore, more sophisticated DNA-loaded chitosan-based nanoparticles have been developed and shown to be promising gene delivery systems exhibiting better transfection rates [12].

Finally, the properties of chitosan have been modified by chemical modifications such as deacetylation, *N*-sulfation or modification by organic molecules (e.g. sugars etc.), which give rise to other applications. Very recently, polyelectrolyte complex nanoparticles have been prepared from self-complexation of amphoteric *N*-sulfated chitosan [18].

In contrast to topical (locally applied) application of chitosan-based formulations, the safety/toxicity of positively charged polysaccharides for systemic applications (e.g. intravenous administration) is currently controversial. Indeed, it has been reported that chitosan induces the opening of tight junctions between epithelial cells, enhancing their permeability [19, 20].

Exhaustive reviews on recent advances on chitosan-based micro/nanoparticles are given by several authors [21, 22].

Dextran is an α-D-1,6-glucose-linked glucan with side-chains 1–3 or 1–4 linked to the backbone units (Fig. 8.3). The branches are mostly one or two glucose units long. This biopolymer can be obtained from fermentation of sucrose-containing media by *Leuconostoc mesenteroides* bacteria. The clinical use of dextran over the past 50 years provides impressive proof of its safety and quality. Dextran may be ingested orally and is well tolerated. Due to its biocompatibility and hydrophilicity, it is often utilized as a coating material for nanoparticles. Indeed, it has been demonstrated to display protein-repulsive properties and to decrease the uptake by the

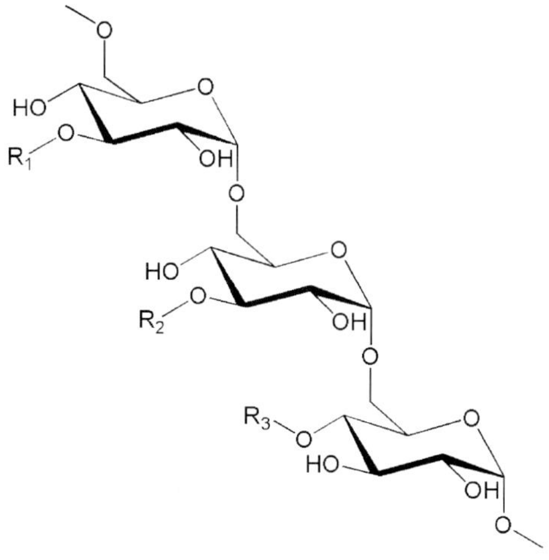

2

Figure 8.3. Chemical structure of dextran. R_1, R_2 and R_3 are positions of branching.

MPS. Moreover, the dextran macromolecule presents a large number of reactive hydroxyl groups for chemical attachment of functional molecules. Many reactions characteristic for alcohol can be used; however, due to the presence of three hydroxyl groups per glucose residue in the backbone, such reactions are not selective.

Hyaluronic acid (HA) is a linear polysaccharide composed of a repeating disaccharide unit of *N*-acetyl-D-glucosamine and D-glucuronic acid, belonging to the glycosaminoglycan family (Fig. 8.4). It is a component of the synovial fluid, cartilage, vitreous humor and extracellular matrices [13, 23]. Protein interactions with HA play crucial roles in cell adhesion, cell mobility, inflammation, wound healing and cancer metastasis. Its carboxyl groups are mostly deprotonated at physiological pH, thus conferring a polyanionic character to the polymer. Similar to chitosan, the advantage of using HA as a surface modifier in the field of drug delivery/nanoparticles relies on its bioadhesive properties, which have been particularly ex-

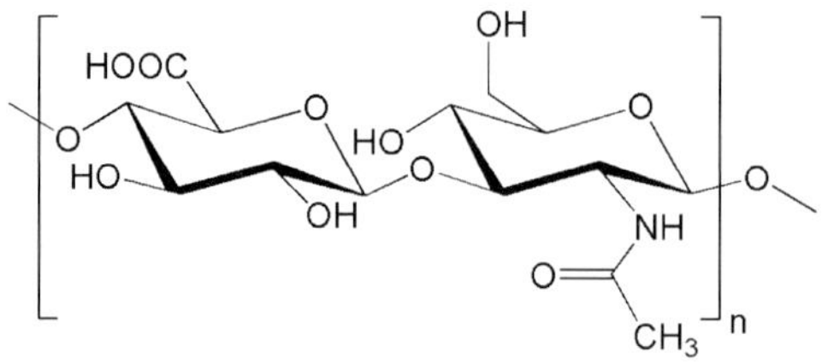

3

Figure 8.4. Repeating disaccharide units of HA.

ploited for ophthalmic applications. Indeed, as for other anionic polymers [e.g. poly(acrylic acid) (PAA)], it has been found that carboxylic groups are responsible for their adhesion to the mucus gel layer. Carboxylic acid moieties are supposed to form hydrogen bonds with hydroxyl groups of the oligosaccharide side-chains of mucus glycoproteins. It should also be emphasized, that the biological activity of HA depends on the molecular weight [24].

Chemically modified natural polymers have received increasing interest, and especially hybrid materials combining synthetic and natural polymers open up new possibilities and applications, combining the unique features of the different materials. As an example, poly(ε-caprolactone) (PCL)-grafted dextran copolymers (glycopolymers) have demonstrated amphiphilic properties, and have been used as emulsifiers and for the preparation of nanoparticles (by an emulsion-evaporation technique) [25].

8.2.2 Degradable Synthetic Polymers

In contrast to natural polymers, of which the molecular weight and distribution depend on the fabrication and extraction procedure, synthetic polymers can be tailormade. Their physical and chemical properties can be varied over a wide range, particularly by copolymerization with appropriate (functional) comonomers. Additionally, using controlled polymerization techniques, the macromolecular characteristics can be adjusted and narrow molecular weight distribution (PDI) can be reached, in contrast to most of the natural polymers. Furthermore, some synthetic polymers can be obtained in oil-in-water (o/w) emulsions, which makes the *in situ* synthesis of nanoparticles by emulsion-polymerization possible.

Fig. 8.5 presents the chemical structure of the main synthetic polymers used for the preparation of nanoparticles.

Domb and coworkers have given a complete review on "biodegradable polymers as drug carrier systems" [26]. The first and probably most important and frequently used groups of biodegradable polymers are linear polyesters. (Co)polyesters based on poly(lactic acid) [or poly(lactide) (PLA)], poly(glycolic acid) (PGA) and poly(lactide-*co*-glycolide) (PLGA) have been used for more than three decades for a variety of medical applications [26], and are considered as the best biomaterials with regard to design and performance. Indeed, they meet the biological requirements of safety and are biodegradable to nontoxic metabolites, and are approved by the Food and Drug Administration (FDA).

Since lactid acid contains an asymmetric α-carbon atom, two different optical isomers exist, D- and L-lactid acid, that give rise to morphologically distinct polymers. The polymers derived from the optically active monomers, i.e. poly(D-lactide) [(P(D-LA)] and poly(L-lactide) [(P(L-LA)] are semicrystalline materials and exhibit identical physicochemical properties, whereas the racemic P(D,L-LA) is purely amorphous and has striking different properties. Furthermore, these racemic and semicrystalline polymers exhibit different degradation rates, as the (bio)degradation is dependent on the polymer crystallinity [27].

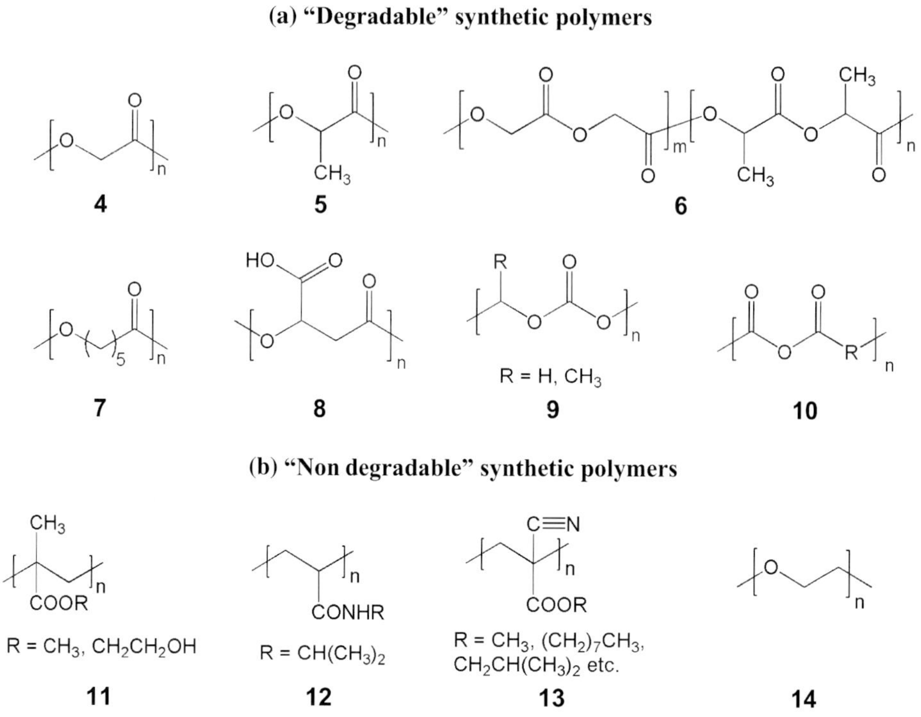

Figure 8.5. Chemical structure of (a) the main biodegradable synthetic polymers: (**4**) poly(glycolic acid), (**5**) poly(lactic acid), (**6**) poly(lactide-*co*-glycolide), (**7**) poly(ε-caprolactone), (**8**) poly(malic acid), (**9**) poly(ethylene carbonate) (R = H)/ poly(propylene carbonate) (R = CH_3) and (**10**) poly(anhydride), and (b) the main nondegradable synthetic polymers: (**11**) poly(methyl methacrylate) (R = CH_3)/ poly(hydroxyethyl methacrylate) (R = CH_2CH_2OH), (**12**) poly(*N*-isopropylacrylamide), (**13**) poly(alkylcyanoacrylate) and (**14**) poly(ethylene oxide) used as core material for the preparation of polymeric nanoparticles.

However, apart from the morphological state of the macromolecule, the biodegradation of polymeric devices is affected by many other important factors such as the chemical stability of the hydrolytically sensitive groups in the polymer backbone, the hydrophilic/hydrophobic character of the repeating units, the initial molecular weight and the molecular weight distribution. The fabrication process, size, geometry (specifically the surface area to volume ratio) and porosity of the device also have a tremendous impact on the degradation rate as well as the environmental conditions [27]. Since the hydrolytic degradation is caused by the reaction of water with labile bonds, typically ester bonds in the polymer chain, the reaction rate is intimately connected with the ability of the polymer to absorb water. Thus, devices made of PGA erode faster than identical devices made of the more hydrophobic PLA, although the ester bonds have almost the same chemical reactivity toward water in both polymers. Furthermore, as mentioned above, although P(L-LA) and P(D,L-LA) have chemically identical backbone structures and an identical degree of hydrophobicity, devices made of P(L-LA) tend to degrade much more slowly than identical devices made of P(D,L-LA). The slower rate of erosion of P(L-LA) is related to its semicrystalline morphology.

Vert and coworkers [28] demonstrated the complexity of PLA, PGA and PLGA degradation, and emphasized that the hydrolytic process depends on the size and morphology of the biomedical device. Although at first sight astonishing, it has been demonstrated that PLA microparticles degrade faster than PLA nanoparticles, and that this phenomenon relies on a diffusion mechanism [29]. Indeed, due to the large nanoparticle surface in relation to the volume, the acid (produced during the degradation) can easily diffuse out of the nanoparticle. On the contrary, within microparticles, the produced acid accumulates inside the particle as the diffusion is slower. This local decrease of the pH has an autocatalytic effect on the degradation process. Indeed, after the water uptake the polymer chains degrade in the core of the nanoparticles (corresponding to a decrease of the molecular weight), and only afterwards appears weight loss of the material due to the diffusion of the degraded polymer chains out of the bulky material.

Another example of a polyester is PCL, which is widely used in the field in biomaterials. This polymer is semicrystalline, more hydrophobic than PLA and PLGA, and hence is characterized by a slower (bio)degradation.

Furthermore, other biodegradable polyesters derived from naturally occurring, multifunctional hydroxy acids and amino acids, such as malic acid and aspartic acid, have been investigated by Lenz and Guerin [30]. Poly(malic acid) is biocompatible and degradable, and water-soluble in contrast to PLA and PCL. Biocompatibility tests indicated that poly(β-malic acid) is nontoxic and nonimmunogenic [31].

Due to the fact that most of these polyesters lack functional groups, efforts have been made to prepare biodegradable aliphatic polyesters bearing functional groups available for further modification. Such copolymers can be reached by copolymerization of novel functional monomers with conventional ones [32–36]. Their features are affected by the comonomer compositions, the polymer architecture, and the molecular weight. Copolymers have thus been synthesized in order to adjust degradation rates as well as mechanical properties. For instance, PEO-*b*-PLA block copolymers have been synthesized and used to prepare nanoparticles showing a faster degradation with respect to plain PLA nanoparticles. Indeed, the introduction of a hydrophilic polymer (PEO) favors hydration of the polyester nanoparticles, which is the key requirement for the hydrolytic degradation to take place as explained above. For the same reason, the ester functions next to the PEO segment degrade first and the PEO chains are lost rapidly.

In addition, polycarbonates, such as poly(ethylene carbonate) and poly(propylene carbonate) have been explored in the design of new polyester-related structures for the preparation of nanoparticles for drug delivery. For instance, they have been tested as biodegradable carriers for the delivery of 5-fluorouracil [37] and were found to be degraded enzymatically [38].

In addition to natural proteins, synthetic (co)poly(amides), such as poly(lysine) and poly(glutamic acids), have also been studied as drug carriers [39].

As well as the described groups of biodegradable polymers, there are a lot of other classes of biodegradable polymers used for biomaterials, such as poly(anhydrides), poly(phosphate esters), poly(phosphazenes) and poly(orthoesters). An exhaustive overview on their properties, synthesis, degradation characteristics, biocompatibility and toxicity is beyond the scope of this work, and may be found in the literature [26].

8.2.3 Nondegradable Synthetic Polymers

Polymers made of acrylic or vinylic monomers constitute an important group of nondegradable materials used for the preparation of "biostable" polymeric nanoparticles. The interest of these materials relies mainly on the ease of preparation and the availability of functional groups.

Poly(alkylcyanoacrylate) (PACA) represents an intermediate class between the synthetic biodegradable and nonbiodegradable polymers [40]; indeed, it has been shown that PACA particles are degraded by a surface erosion process [41], through enzymatic hydrolysis of the ester side-chains of the polymer. The polymer chains are therefore degraded to hydrophilic compounds and the rate of elimination is dependent of the length of the nondegradable alkyl chain [42]. It was demonstrated that materials based on PACA are well tolerated *in vivo*.

Finally, we would like to emphasize, that stimuli responsive polymers, such as poly(*N*-isopropylacrylamide) (PNIPAAm), are promising materials for the preparation of stimuli responsive colloidal carrier systems. Despite the importance of this group of materials, we are not able to discuss the materials used for nanoparticles in this chapter. There are a lot of reviews on this subject [43, 44] (see also Sections 8.5.1.3 and 8.5.2.3).

8.2.4 PEO

This section is dedicated to PEO because of its importance and frequency of use for biomaterials and, especially, nanoparticles. PEO is a hydrophilic, neutral, very flexible polymer, which is widely used for the surface modification of nanoparticles. It is FDA approved and quite an important number of PEO–drug conjugates are on the market for intravenous administration. PEO is nonbiodegradable but, due to its hydrophilicity, bioeliminable whenever its molecular weight is less than 20 000 g mol^{-1} [45].

The mechanisms of PEO–protein interactions are reported in the review by Vermette and coworkers [46]. Briefly, the protein repellence of PEO coatings has been associated to "steric repulsion" and/or "hydration"/"water structuring" of the chains. The flexibility of these PEO chains, which is particularly high in comparison to other hydrophilic polymers, is one explanation for its protein-repulsive, antifouling properties. Indeed, the reason for its flexibility must be found in the easy rotation of the ether bonds and in the absence of any bulky substituent on the PEO skeleton. The rapid and transitory change of the conformation of PEO chains is probably responsible for the poor interaction of the PEO chain with proteins. In addition, whenever a protein or another surface approaches with sufficient kinetic energy, PEO chains forming a dense brush at a surface will be compressed by the collision. This will increase the local concentration of polymer segments (corresponding to a loss of entropy of the PEO chains), enhancing the free energy and inducing the repulsion of the protein from the surface [46]. The interaction energy is thus repulsive.

A lot of works tried to understand the influence of the density and length of PEO chains at surfaces on its protein-repulsive properties. The conformation of the PEO chains changes when the distance D that separates two neighboring PEO chains tethered at the surface becomes close to or smaller than the radius of gyration of the polymer (R_g) (Fig. 8.6). In good solvents for PEO such as water, the polymer chains form "mushroom"-like structures at long distances ($D \gg R_g$), as illustrated in Fig. 8.6(A) and (B), in poor solvents flat "pancake"-like structures are expected. With decreasing distance ($D \sim R_g$), the chains start to interact with each other and approach the mushroom to brush transition (Fig. 8.6(C) and (D)). For $D < R_g$, the polymer chains strongly interact and in order to minimize the contact between them they stretch away from the surface, forming the so-called "brush" conformation [46]. It is thus clear that one of the most important parameters in determining the protein adsorption onto PEO layers is the grafting density of the PEO chains. It

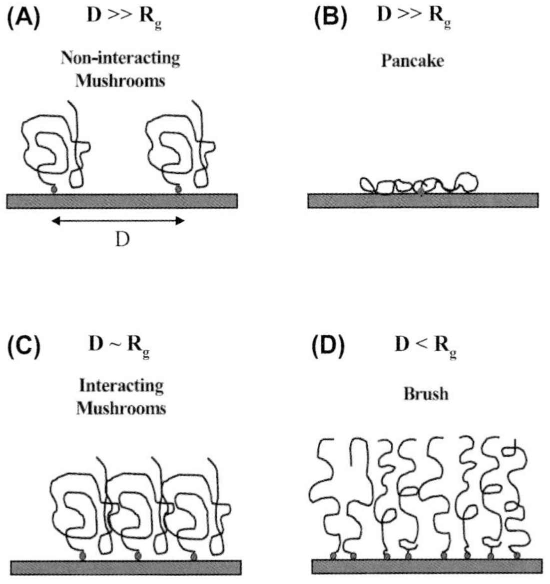

Figure 8.6. Schematic representation of polymer (PEO) structures at the interface.

has been reported that a distance d of 1.5 nm between two terminally attached PEO chains at the nanoparticle surface was found ideal for reducing protein adsorption. In addition, it has been demonstrated that rather long PEO chains (a molecular weight of 2000–5000 g mol^{-1} has been proposed as ideal molecular weight earlier [47–49]) are not necessarily a prerequisite for low protein adsorption [46].

These are the reasons why PEO is the polymer of choice for the design of nanoparticles of the second generation and third generation.

8.3 Preparation of Polymeric Nanoparticles

In the last decades, several techniques have been developed to prepare colloidal carrier systems from polymeric materials. These can be obtained either (i) by association of preformed polymers (natural, modified natural or synthetic polymers, see Section 8.2) using techniques, such as emulsion-evaporation, emulsion-diffusion and salting-out, or (ii) by (mini)emulsion or micellar polymerization of polymerizable monomers dispersed in an aqueous phase. The preparation technique must be suitable for the material with regard to solubility and stability of the polymer. In the case of emulsion polymerization, the availability of monomers polymerizable in o/w emulsion is the limiting factor.

8.3.1 Preparation of Nanospheres from Preformed Polymers

The use of preformed polymers for the preparation of nanospheres has several advantages, such as the availability of a large variety of materials with controlled and optimized macromolecular characteristics (molecular weight and polydispersity), as well as suitable physicochemical and biological properties. Indeed, in order to favor reproducibility, colloidal carriers must be synthesized from well-defined macromolecular materials. A large number of reviews are available describing in detail the different techniques to obtain colloidal carriers (e.g. Ref. [50]). In the following, we briefly discuss the most popular methods to obtain nanospheres from preformed polymers, i.e. emulsion-evaporation, emulsion-diffusion, salting-out and nanoprecipitation.

Polymers that are insoluble in water are generally used for the formation of dispersed colloidal systems in aqueous media. Thus, organic solvents are often required to dissolve the polymers – the first step to nanoparticle formation. Depending on the preparation procedure described in the following sections, the organic solvents used are either miscible or immiscible with water.

8.3.1.1 Emulsion-evaporation

Organic volatile solvents, such as chloroform and dichloromethane that are poorly miscible or immiscible with water, are suitable for the emulsion-evaporation technique, patented by Vanderhoff and coworkers [51]. First, the polymer is dissolved in the organic solvent and tiny solvent droplets are formed by emulsification in an aqueous phase containing an emulsifier [e.g. poly(vinyl alcohol) (PVA) or albumin]. Then, the crude o/w emulsion is exposed to a high-energy source, such as ultrasonic devices or homogenizers, etc. [50], and, finally, stable solid nanoparticles are formed from the emulsion droplets by slight evaporation of the organic solvent (under reduced pressure). During the evaporation process, the organic solvent diffuses from the inner core of the droplets to the external phase, maintaining a saturation of the water phase by the organic solvent. The progressive elimination of the solvents induces the precipitation of the polymer and the nanoparticles formation. The size of the droplets and also the nanoparticles can be adjusted by the nature and quantity of emulsifier, the viscosity of the dispersing phase, and stirring rate. Unfortunately, this method requires the use of large quantities of surfactants (e.g. ranging from 0.5 to 8 wt% for PVA [50]) and high energy to form stable homogeneous emulsions. When ultrasonication is used instead of high-speed homogenizers, only very polydisperse nanosuspensions could be obtained. Only hydrophobic drugs can be efficiently encapsulated, by this o/w process. As far as hydrophilic drugs are concerned, a double-emulsion (w/o/w) technique has been developed in order to obtain nanospheres of hydrophobic polymer (such as PLGA) loaded by hydrophilic biomolecules, such as proteins [52]. Therefore, an inverse w/o emulsion is first prepared from an aqueous phase, containing the hydrophilic drug, and the organic phase, containing the matrix building polymer. Then this emulsion is emulsified in a second surfactant-containing aqueous phase to form the w/o/w emulsion. Finally, the organic solvent is removed by evaporation at reduced pressure.

8.3.1.2 **Salting-out**

Solvent immiscibility and polymer precipitation can be induced through changes in temperature, pH or the addition of alcohol, but also by the addition of large quantities of salt ("salting-out"). The principle of the salting-out method [53] is to saturate the aqueous phase by electrolytes in order to reduce drastically the miscibility of the organic solvent (normally water miscible) with the aqueous phase. First, an o/w emulsion is formed between the organic phase and the surfactant [e.g. PVA, hydroxyethylcellulose or poly(vinyl pyrrolidone) (PVP)]-containing aqueous phase, which was previously saturated by the salt. Then, distilled water is added in such an amount that the total quantity of the organic solvent becomes miscible with the aqueous phase. As a result, the organic solvent diffuses into the aqueous phase, leading to the precipitation of the polymer as nanospheres. Several factors, such as stirring rate and polymer concentration, have been reported to influence the mean size of the nanoparticles. The salt is generally removed by cross-flow ultrafiltration/dialysis. This methodology allows using organic solvents of low toxicity (generally acetone) and which can be easily removed at the end of the preparation process by ultrafiltration or evaporation. However, the use of large amount of surfactants and electrolytes is necessary.

8.3.1.3 Emulsification-diffusion

The emulsification-diffusion method can be considered as a modification of the salting-out procedure, avoiding the use of salts and hence intensive purification steps [54]. Before dissolution of the polymer, the partially water-miscible organic solvent (ethyl acetate, propylene carbonate, benzyl alcohol) is saturated in water to ensure the thermodynamic equilibrium of both liquids. Then, the polymer solution is emulsified (o/w emulsion) under vigorous stirring in an aqueous solution containing a stabilizer (e.g. PVA or poloxamers, i.e. a series of copolymers composed of two PEO blocks separated by a PPO block). The subsequent addition of water to the system causes the diffusion of the organic solvent to the external aqueous phase, resulting in the formation of nanoparticles. Finally, the organic solvent is removed, depending on its boiling point, either by evaporation or crossflow ultrafiltration. The size of the nanoparticles depends on numerous factors, such as the concentration of the stabilizer (emulsifier), as well as the nature of the polymer and the stirring rate [55].

This method is only efficient for the encapsulation of lipophilic drugs. In addition, it requires the removal of large volumes of water due to the dilution-induced diffusion process. However, the advantages of this approach rely on its good reproducibility and high loading efficiencies.

8.3.1.4 Nanoprecipitation

Fessi and coworkers [56] described and patented a simple technique to obtain polymeric nanoparticles which does not require the preliminary formation of an emulsion. It relies on the use of organic solvents that are perfectly miscible with water, such as acetone, ethanol or dimethyl sulfoxide (DMSO). Furthermore, the polymer must be insoluble in the aqueous phase, but also in the mixture of both phases. This method is called the "nanoprecipitation" or "solvent displacement" technique.

Thus, the organic polymer solution is added drop-by-drop into a large volume of an aqueous phase, typically containing a surfactant (e.g. PVA, Poloxamer®). Under these conditions, the nanoparticles are formed instantaneously by the precipitation of the polymer induced by the diffusion of the organic solvent in the aqueous phase. Depending on its boiling point, the organic solvent is then eliminated by evaporation or dialysis. This technique has been modified and adjusted by various research groups [57, 58]. Polymer precipitation has also been induced by gentle progressive diffusion of water to an organic polymer solution placed in a tube of dialysis membranes [59]. The size of the nanoparticles obtained by nanoprecipitation processes is typically about 200 nm depending on the nature, miscibility and viscosity of the solvent, the polymer and its concentration in the organic solvent, and the preparation conditions.

This technique is especially interesting because of its low energy consumption and very simple handling.

As described above, most of these techniques require the use of surfactant in the aqueous phase, i.e. amphiphilic polymers such as PVA or triblock copolymers of

PEO and PPO (PEO-*b*-PPO-*b*-PEO, known as poloxamers) that exhibit interfacial activity, to guarantee the stability of the colloidal dispersions.

8.3.2
Synthesis of Nanospheres by *In Situ* Polymerization

In contrast to the techniques described above, where preformed polymers are used, nanoparticles can also be synthesized by polymerization of suitable monomers in (mini)emulsion [60, 61] or dispersion. Emulsion polymerizations employ water-insoluble monomers that are emulsified as micron-sized oil droplets (1–10 μm) in an aqueous phase stabilized by a surfactant. The initiators used in emulsion polymerizations are generally water-soluble and dissolved in the aqueous phase. Most emulsion polymerizations use a radical polymerization method. The drawback of such (macro)emulsion polymerizations is that the size of the latex particle does not correspond to the primary emulsion droplets, but rather depends on polymerization kinetic parameters. Miniemulsion polymerizations (Fig. 8.7) are a special class of emulsion polymerizations. They have many similarities, but the particle nucleation and reagent transport phenomena are different. In fact, miniemulsions consist of two immiscible liquids, a surfactant and a special cosurfactant (additive) that is only soluble in the dispersed phase. They are prepared by high-shear treatment of these mixtures, either by ultrasound or by a high-pressure microfluidizer and contain stable nanodroplets with a diameter of 30–300 nm.

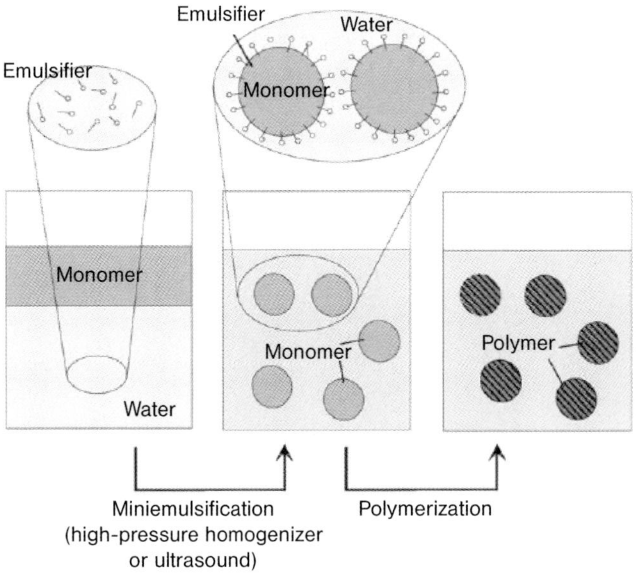

Figure 8.7. The principle of miniemulsion polymerization.

The combination of the two surfactants makes the droplets extremely stable, inhibiting the diffusion of monomers out of the miniemulsion droplets and preventing their coalescence [60]. The size of the polymer nanoparticles corresponds thus to that of the initially formed nanodroplets, which is controlled by the shear and the stabilizer system, and not [as for the (macro)emulsion] by the polymerization parameters. The active compound (drug) is generally incorporated in the dispersed phase, and therefore encapsulated in the nanoparticles during the polymerization process. More seldom, it is adsorbed onto the surface of preformed nanoparticles (after the polymerization).

Nanoparticles made of PNIPAAm, poly(*N*-vinylacetamide) (PNVA), poly(vinylamine) (PVAm) and poly(methacrylic acid) (PMAA) have been prepared according to this methodology. The corresponding vinylic and (meth)acrylic monomers are generally polymerized under free radical conditions using, for instance 2,2′-azobisisobutyronitrile (AIBN) as an initiator [62].

New processes based on the miniemulsion concept use amphiphilic polymers both as emulsifiers and surface modifiers of the final nanoparticles. For instance, the radical polymerization of styrene has been carried out in miniemulsions stabilized by amphiphilic derivatives of dextran [63]. The size of the polysaccharide-coated polystyrene particles was directly correlated to that of the initial nanodroplet and depended on the monomer concentration. The use of functional emulsifiers as surface modifiers is discussed in detail in Section 8.4.3.3.

Furthermore, other polymerization systems have also been used to prepare polymeric particles, such as dispersion or suspension polymerization. In the suspension polymerization process, the initiator is soluble in the monomer and larger particles (above 1 μm) are obtained.

In addition, dispersion polymerizations have been rediscovered in recent years for the preparation of (sub)micron-size polymer particles with narrow size distributions. This process differs notably from emulsion and suspension polymerization as it starts with a homogeneous solution of monomer(s), stabilizer(s) and initiator in a mostly organic solvent. The polymer precipitates as a colloidal dispersion during the polymerization process. As an interesting example, polystyrene core glycopolymer corona nanospheres have been obtained by free radical copolymerization of hydrophilic macromonomers and styrene (as hydrophobic comonomer) in dispersion in a polar solvent (e.g. ethanol/water mixture) [64–66] (details see Section 8.4.3.3).

One of the advantages of emulsion polymerization for the preparation of polymeric nanoparticles is its reproducibility regarding size and drug-loading rate, even at a semi-industrial level. On the other hand, the disadvantages of this approach are the possibility of residual emulsifiers, monomers, but also oligomers, and the risk of drug interaction (with the reactives) during polymerization and thus inactivation.

8.3.3
Preparation of Nanocapsules

As mentioned in the Introduction (Section 8.1), nanocapsules are built of an oily or sometimes aqueous core, surrounded by a thin polymeric wall. Similar to nanospheres, nanocapsules can be obtained from either preformed polymers or by (interfacial) polymerization of monomers at the oil–water interface. The main techniques for the synthesis of nanocapsules rely on the use of a water-miscible organic solvent, solubilizing the polymer or monomer, and the insolubility of them in both the oil and the aqueous phase. The miscibility of the organic solvent is thus the driving force for the diffusion of the polymer (or monomer) to the water–oil interface [67, 68].

In general, the polymer or monomer is first dissolved in the organic phase (consisting of the oil and a water-miscible organic solvent). Then, upon addition of the organic phase to the aqueous phase (containing a hydrosoluble surfactant), the polymer/monomer diffuses with the water-miscible organic solvent and is stranded at the interface between oil and water. As an example for interfacial polymerization, the polymerization of alkylcyanoacrylate has been initiated at the oil–water interface by hydroxyl ions present in the aqueous phase, leading to the formation of nanocapsules [69].

It should be mentioned that colloidal capsules can also be prepared by the layer-by-layer approach. This technique is based on the self-assembly of two oppositely charged species by electrostatic interactions [70, 71]. In general, the capsule wall is formed by alternating deposition of a two oppositely charged polyelectrolytes on a template core, which can be removed at the end of the process e.g. by dissolution. However, the size of the as-prepared capsules is generally in the micrometer-scale (1–5 μm) rather than in the nanoscale [72, 73].

One of the advantages of nanocapsules over nanospheres is their low polymer content and a high loading capacity for lipophilic drugs. The percentage of encapsulation is generally related to the solubility of the drug in the core phase [74].

8.4
Surface Functionalization

The surface characteristics of nanoparticles are of fundamental importance for their interaction with the environment, i.e. with living medium. In the last decade, numerous surface-modified carrier systems have thus been developed allowing the targeting of specific tissues. Polymeric materials functionalized with targeting moieties, such as sugars [75], peptides [76], folic acid [77] and antibodies [78], have received considerable interest as means to generate intelligent delivery vehicles capable of (polyvalent) specific binding interactions.

8.4.1
Functionalization with Biological (Macro)molecules

The first group of bioactive molecules considered here interacts nonspecifically with tissues. Among them, polysaccharides are of great interest, especially to confer to nanoparticles bioadhesive or mucoadhesive properties (*cf.* Section 8.2). Therefore, nanoparticles have been surface-coated by polysaccharides, such as chitosan [19] and HA [14]. It could be demonstrated that nanoparticles coated by such bioadhesive polymers, especially HA, significantly increased the ocular drug availability [79].

To overcome the fast capture of nanoparticles by the MPS, nanoparticles have been coated with dextran and heparin. Such nanoparticles circulate for an enhanced period of time in the blood stream. The polysaccharide shell probably avoided complement activation and opsonization of the nanoparticles by preventing protein adsorption [80, 81]. Aside from being long circulating, heparin-coated nanoparticles showed antithrombic activity [81].

In the 1980s, a tripeptide, RGD, was identified to promote cell attachment [9]. Consequently, RGD peptides have been attached on the surface of polystyrene nanoparticles. These nanoparticles have been shown to induce a 50-fold increase in transport across the human intestine epithelial cells compared to blank polystyrene nanoparticles [82, 83]. It has also been demonstrated that a number of RGD peptides and peptidomimetics bind preferentially to a particular integrin $\alpha_V\beta_3$, which is often overexpressed on endothelial cells in tumor neovasculature [84]. A cyclic peptide with the RGD sequence has thus been covalently attached to the surface of doxorubicin-loaded nanoparticles and it was shown that they were preferentially internalized in tumoral tissues compared to other organs, such as the liver or the spleen [85].

8.4.2
Functionalization with Specific Ligands: Specific Interaction through Biological Recognition

One of the greatest challenges is to find the optimal vector molecules or ligand to transport nanoparticles specifically to the targeted tissue. The strategy relies on the ability of the targeting agents or ligands to bind specifically to cell surface receptors triggering receptor endocytosis. The following will describe some examples of these ligands identified and used up to now for the functionalization of nanoparticles.

8.4.2.1 Mono- or Oligosaccharides (Carbohydrates)

As well documented in the literature [86–88], cell surface carbohydrates from glycoproteins and glycolipids play an essential role as recognition sites between cells or cells and microorganisms. These recognition mechanisms are essentially based on specific interactions between the oligosaccharide chains and soluble or membrane proteins called lectins. The communication network based on carbohydrate–protein interactions is crucial in a large variety of important biological phenomena such as cell growth, inflammation, cancer, viral and bacterial infections.

Taking advantage of these specific carbohydrate–lectin interactions, numerous glycomimetics have been developed for analytical, diagnostic and therapeutic purposes. In particular, sugar-mediated drug delivery allows targeting cells that possess glycoreceptors on their plasma membrane. Such a mode of drug delivery is considered as one of the most promising routes in cell-specific targeting. Indeed, membrane lectins of some cell types are able to internalize their ligands and hence the glycoconjugates that are specifically recognized by these lectins can be used as efficient carriers of drugs [89]. In particular dendritic cells of the human blood express cell surface mannose-specific lectins, i.e. specific receptors for mannose (mannose receptors) [90, 91]. In fact, these cells capture, process and present antigens to native T cells, inducing the cellular immune response [92, 93]. The possibility to target specifically dendritic cells thus makes mannose-coated nanoparticles attractive delivery systems for vaccines (see Section 8.5.1.2). Apart from this potential application, mannose-coated nanoparticles have been designed to target specifically Gram-negative bacteria, exposing mannose receptors at their surface. They could be used as carriers for antibacterial drugs [94].

In contrast to mannose, galactose interacts with hepatic cells via a Gal/GalNAc-binding mammalian lectin. Galactose conjugates have thus been synthesized, which have been used to carry antiparasitic [95] and antiviral drugs [96] specifically to liver cells. For the same purpose, polymeric nanoparticles decorated with galactose [97, 98], have been synthesized for hepatocyte-specific targeting.

It should be noted that the binding of a particular sugar to its glycoreceptor occurs in a regioselective manner [87] and thus the introduction of saccharidic ligands on polymers is generally performed by 1-*O* substitution of the sugar. Furthermore, it has been emphasized that sugar–lectin interactions depend on the "density" of the partners at a surface. Indeed, their affinity can be enhanced by multiple interactions between the binding proteins and the carbohydrate ligands, which is known as the glycoside cluster effect [99].

8.4.2.2 **Folate Receptor**

All cells require folic acid as a vitamin for essential functions. They are thus equipped with several pathways for folate internalization. Folate conjugates were shown to enter cells only via the "alternative route", i.e. via the folate receptor. This cell surface receptor is only expressed in measurable quantities on activated macrophages and at the apical surface of some polarized epithelia. In addition, the folate receptor is significantly overexpressed on the surface of many cancer cells because they require more extensive folic acid to enable their rapid proliferation. The folate receptor is thus a possible target for a number of types of cancer. Their localization on activated macrophages, but not on their quiescent or resting counterparts, makes folate conjugates promising in targeting inflammatory and autoimmune diseases because those specific macrophages cause or contribute to these diseases.

It has been shown that folate-targeted delivery cannot only enhance the drug uptake in the targeted pathologic cells, but can also reduce the drug deposition into nonpathologic cells, thereby diminishing collateral toxicity to normal tissues. This is due to the high specificity of folate for its receptors combined with the high stability of the folate-receptor complex ($K_d \sim 10^{-10}$). Consequently, such conjugates can be administered at very low (nontoxic) concentrations and still achieve a clinical response [100].

Similar to the uptake of the free vitamin, folate conjugates are taken up into cells via folate receptor-mediated endocytosis and released into the cytosol. Since folic acid is taken into cells to favor their proliferation, they are thus not delivered to lysosomes for destruction. In contrast to that, other ligands are destroyed in the latter in order to prevent continuous signalization of the cells. This feature is important when macromolecular or hydrolytically sensitive drugs have to be delivered, since most of them are inactivated by the lytic enzymes that are concentrated in lysosomes. A lot of studies on targeted drug delivery are thus based on the functionalization of nanoparticles by folic acid [11, 101–103].

8.4.2.3 **Antibodies**

Apart from ligand–receptor interactions, antigen–antibody interactions are highly specific molecular recognition processes and thus promising tools for specific targeted delivery. In fact, with the advent of monoclonal antibody technology, the utilization of antibodies increased dramatically. Monoclonal immunoglobulin G antibodies represent today a promising groups of vector molecules to transport a colloidal carrier system very specifically to the target tissue. In particular, in the field of cancer, monoclonal antibodies have been shown to be able to bind to specific tumor antigens. The ideal antigen should be expressed on all tumor cells, but not expressed on critical host cells. To date, a remarkable number of antibodies that are specific to a certain cancer type have been identified and approved by the FDA.

Unlike folic acid, which is chemically very stable (e.g. to organic solvents, acids and bases), antibodies are sensitive biomolecules and thus their introduction on the surface of nanoparticles requires the use of mild chemical ligation reactions. Apart from the interest for targeted drug delivery, antibody-decorated nanoparticles are useful tools for clinical analysis by immunoassays and medical diagnostics [104].

8.4.2.4 **Biotin**

Finally, biotin (vitamin H), a small organic biomolecule, is widely used as a versatile linker molecule to which a large variety of functional moieties can be bound via a biotin–avidin complex. Actually, biotin is known to form very stable complexes with its tetravalent ligand, avidin. The avidin–biotin complex is known as one of the strongest noncovalent biological interactions (association constant $K_a = 10^{15}$ M^{-1}). In addition, a large variety of biotinylated targeting ligands are commercially available and they can be attached to the surface of biotin-coated nanoparticles via biotin–avidin–biotin complexes (Fig. 8.8) [10].

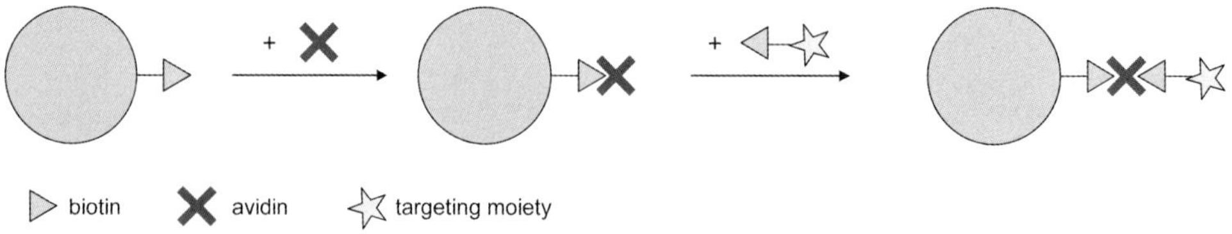

Figure 8.8. Surface functionalization via biotin–avidin–biotin complex formation.

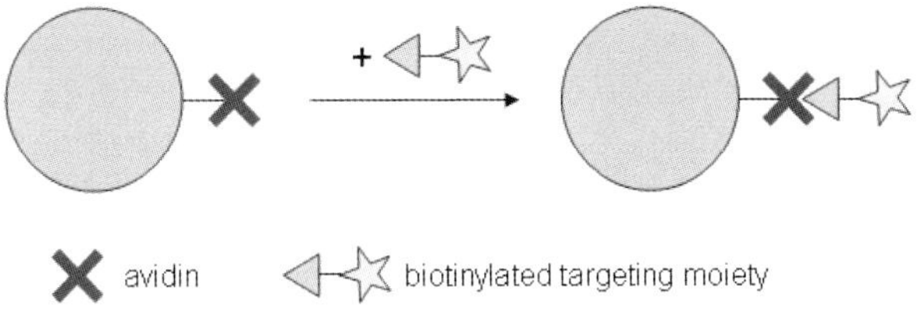

Figure 8.9. Surface functionalization of avidin-bearing nanoparticles with biotinylated molecules.

Indeed, after complex formation with one of the sites of avidin, the residual three binding sites of avidin are still available for the binding of biotin conjugates. A very versatile tool for surface modification was thus made available. It is, however, questionable whether the stability of colloidal dispersions of such nanoparticles may be maintained after the addition of avidin, as interparticular crosslinking via free avidin binding sites might take place.

To avoid this problem, it might be advantageously to attach avidin (NeutrAvidin) directly in a covalent manner to the surface of nanoparticles (Fig. 8.9). This has been developed in the work of Balthasar and coworkers (see Section 8.4.3.4.2) who prepared antibody-decorated crosslinked gelatin nanoparticles as drug carriers for the specific targeting of T lymphocytes (using biotinylated anti-CD3 antibodies).

8.4.3 Strategies for Surface Modification

Surface functionalization of nanoparticles can be achieved by various approaches. In general, the posterior attachment of bioactive molecules on the surface of preformed nanoparticles may be achieved by (i) noncovalent interaction, (ii) specific complex formation and (iii) covalent linking of the targeting moieties to the nanoparticles by chemical reactions (Fig. 8.10).

These different strategies are closely connected with each other and often combined. As mentioned above, complexing molecules such as avidin have first been covalently coupled to the nanoparticle surface before the desired biotinylated targeting moiety could be attached to the surface by avidin–biotin complex formation [102]. Figure 8.10 makes it clear that the crucial condition for successful attaching targeting moieties at the nanoparticle surface is the presence of "reactive sites", such as (i) charges, (ii) biomolecules and (iii) reactive groups, at surface of the nanoparticles. They can be introduced by different ways: by adsorption of reactive molecules on the surface of preformed nanoparticles, by preparing nanospheres from preformed polymers in the presence of "functional surfactants", or by *in situ* emulsion polymerization using functional surfactants/emulsifiers or functional monomers or functional initiators. It should be noted that these techniques can also be used to directly modify the surface by bioactive targeting probes. Therefore, the synthesis of hybrid materials, i.e. materials containing both the biologically

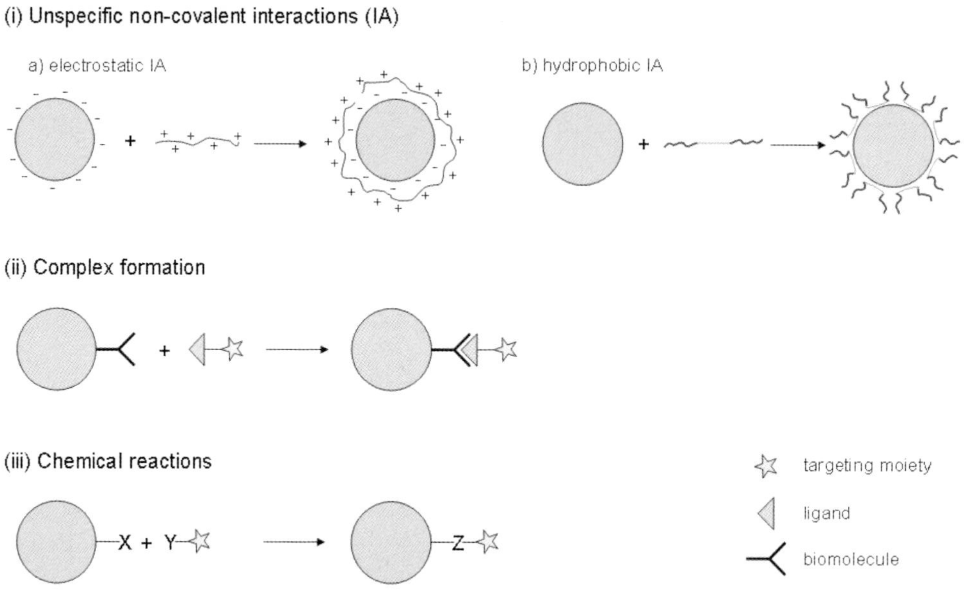

Figure 8.10. Different strategies for the conjugation of targeting moieties to nanoparticles. (i) Unspecific noncovalent interactions, adsorption of functional molecules by (a) electrostatic and (b) hydrophobic interactions. (ii) Complex formation. (iii) Covalent linking by chemical reactions.

active molecules and synthetic (polymeric) components, is often required. In this context, a major problem is maintaining the biomolecule–nanoparticle conjugates bioactive and to ensure the bioavailability of the bioactive entity. For this purpose, hydrophilic spacer molecules, such as PEO chains [10], have often been introduced between the surface and the biological ligand, thereby allowing the accessibility of the biomolecule and its interaction. Furthermore, the conjugation reactions must be carried out under mild, nondegrading reaction conditions.

The different strategies to achieve surface modifications of nanoparticles as well as the chemistry used to reach biomolecule–nanoparticle conjugates are detailed in the following sections. Finally, "molecular imprinting" of the surface of nanoparticles using template molecules is also discussed as a promising approach to modify the surface of nanoparticles.

8.4.3.1 Adsorption on Preformed Nanoparticles

Polymer adsorption on solid–liquid interfaces is a widely studied phenomenon connected with many important processes such as colloidal stabilization, flocculation, adhesion and coating [105]. Based on this concept, several works report on the adsorption of functional molecules on preformed nanoparticles [106]. The driving force for physisorption to happen is the affinity of at least part of the molecule to the nanoparticle surface.

Two kinds of adsorption should be distinguished: (i) the adsorption of polyelectrolytes or charged molecules onto oppositely charged nanoparticles and (ii) the adsorption of hydrophobic or hydrophobically modified (macro)molecules onto preformed hydrophobic polymeric nanoparticles [107].

Quite a lot of studies used electrostatic interactions to coat nanoparticles. For instance, positively charged chitosan nanoparticles loaded with proteins have been coated with sodium alginate in order to avoid a burst release, and to enhance their mechanical and thermal stability [14]. Furthermore, chitosan has been adsorbed on negatively charged PLA nanoparticles to prepare fully bioresorbable mucoadhesive nanoparticles [108].

Very recently, potential targeting probes have been adsorbed onto polymer nanoparticles by electrostatic interactions: cationized antigens [Tat(1–72)] were adsorbed on negatively charged nanoparticles [109].

On the other hand, hydrophobic nanoparticles has been surface-functionalized by using amphiphilic or hydrophobically modified macromolecules, the hydrophobic part of the macromolecule ensuring their durable adsorption and physical anchorage. Based on this approach, numerous studies have used amphiphilic block copolymers, such as Pluronics® (block copolymers based on PEO and PPO, e.g. PEO-*b*-PPO-*b*-PEO triblock copolymer also called poloxamers) as surface modifiers of hydrophobic nanoparticles [110]. The hydrophobic PPO block is the driving element for the adsorption onto the surface of nanoparticle, while the hydrophilic PEO chains expand in the aqueous environment forming a steric barrier that stabilizes the nanoparticles, prevents their aggregation and makes them stealthy to the MPS. Similarly, polystyrene nanoparticles have been surface-modified by Pluronic F-108 (PEO_{129}-*b*-PPO_{56}-*b*-PEO_{129}) end-capped by polypeptides containing the RGD sequence. Exposing cell adhesive peptides at their surface, these nanoparticles are promising devices for diagnostic purposes [83].

Apart from amphiphilic block copolymers, randomly hydrophobically modified polymers have also been used. Polystyrene-divinylbenzene (PS-DVB) particles have been coated with dextran partially substituted by phenoxy groups. Adsorption was achieved by simple incubation of the particles in the polymer solution (20 h) and the adsorbed polymer layer was then chemically crosslinked in order to avoid polymer desorption (using epichlorhydrin or butanediol diglycidyl ether). The dextran layer was shown to greatly reduce the nonspecific adsorption of bovine serum albumin (BSA) [105].

Furthermore, dextran-bearing hydrophobic phenoxy groups and comb-like copolymers of dextran-bearing pendant phenoxy groups and PEO chains (DexP-g-PEO) were synthesized [111]. They were adsorbed on polystyrene nanoparticles and the effects of the polymer composition and architecture on the protein adsorption were studied (Fig. 8.11).

It was found that the most important parameter in preventing the adsorption of BSA was the extent of the contact points between dextran and the surface, rather than the grafting density of PEO chains, in the case of DexP-g-PEO [111].

On the other hand, the naturally occurring adsorption of proteins, which is generally not desired, has also been exploited, e.g. in the case of protein delivery [109].

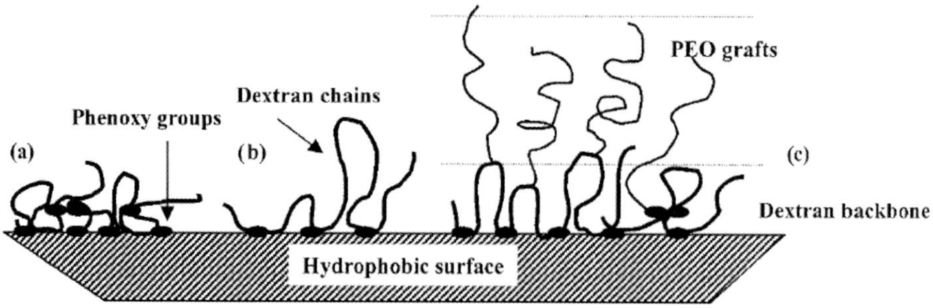

Figure 8.11. Adsorption of amphiphilic dextran (DexP) with (a) high and (b) low amounts of grafted phenoxy groups and (c) of graft DexP–g–PEO copolymer at the hydrophobic surface [111].

The advantage of surface modification via adsorption relies on the complete localization of the adsorbed molecules at the surface. However, it must be considered that the post-modification of the surface of preformed nanoparticles can alter their stability and induce their aggregation. In fact, the stability of colloidal systems relies on steric or electrostatic repulsion of the particles, so that the adsorption of material on the nanoparticle surface might diminish the interparticular repulsion and would thus induce their aggregation. Finally, the risk of desorption upon dilution and introduction into complex biological media must be considered. Therefore, most of the recent approaches rely on the covalent linking of the functional (macro)molecules to the nanoparticle's constitutive polymer (Section 8.4.3.2) or directly to the nanoparticle surface (Section 8.4.3.4).

8.4.3.2 Functional Surfactants as Stabilizers and Surface Modifiers

As explained in Section 8.3, methods for the preparation of polymeric nanoparticles generally use surfactants, which play the role of emulsifier and stabilizer. It was demonstrated that in the case of hydrophobic nanoparticles, the amphiphilic surfactant is located at the surface of the particle, i.e. at the water–hydrophobic solid interface [14, 49]. Amphiphilic copolymers conjugated with bioactive molecules may thus serve as both emulsifiers and surface modifiers. Such copolymers may be synthesized with various architectures, e.g. block [diblock (Scheme 8.1A

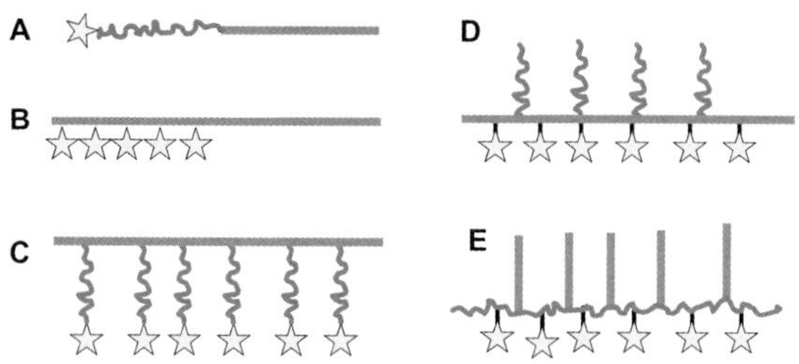

Scheme 8.1. Amphiphilic copolymers: red = hydrophobic, blue = hydrophilic, star = functional (bio)molecule.

and B) or triblock] or comb-like structures (Scheme 8.1C–E), employing controlled polymerization techniques. The functional biomolecule is rather attached on the hydrophilic part of the copolymers, in order to optimize its availability for interaction in aqueous environment. PEO has preferentially been used because of its hydrophilicity and flexibility properties (see Section 8.2.4).

8.4.3.2.1 **Functional Amphiphilic Block Copolymers** A first group of copolymers used for surface functionalization typically consists of amphiphilic block copolymers as schematically presented in Scheme 8.1A. In general, such copolymers can be obtained through four different strategies: (i) by post-polymerization functionalization, where the functional moiety is grafted to the hydrophilic end of the amphiphilic block copolymer bearing a reactive group [112], (ii) by linking the bioactive group at one end of an α,ω-bifunctional hydrophilic homopolymer, followed by the initiation of the polymerization of the second block from the other chain end, (iii) by using biologically active molecules as initiators for the sequential polymerization of the diblock copolymer (hydrophilic block being polymerized first) or (iv) by using polymerizable hydrophilic biomolecules.

The first approach (i) has mainly been applied for the functionalization of diblock copolymers by sugars and peptides. For instance, the hydrophilic end of amphiphilic PEO-*b*-P(D,L-LA) diblock copolymers has been end-capped by mannose [112], lactose [113] or peptides [114] using a reductive amination reaction. For this purpose, aldehyde (CHO)-capped copolymers and amino or aminophenyl derivatives of the biomolecule were synthesized. Then, the conjugation of both compounds was carried out in the presence of reducing agents [$NaBH(OAc)_3$ or $NaBH_3CN$] [112–114].

On the other hand, biotin [115] or protected monosaccharides [86] have been used to initiate the polymerization of the hydrophilic block (approach iii). For instance, Qi and coworkers [115] prepared nanoparticles coated by biotin from biotin-terminated PAA-*b*-poly(methyl acrylate) diblock copolymers (biotin–PAA-*b*-PMA). These functional copolymers were prepared using a biotinylated initiator for the sequential atom transfer radical polymerization (ATRP) of acrylic acid and methyl acrylate (Fig. 8.12).

Not only radical polymerizations, but also ring-opening polymerizations (ROPs) have been successfully initiated by suitably protected molecules. Yasugi and co-

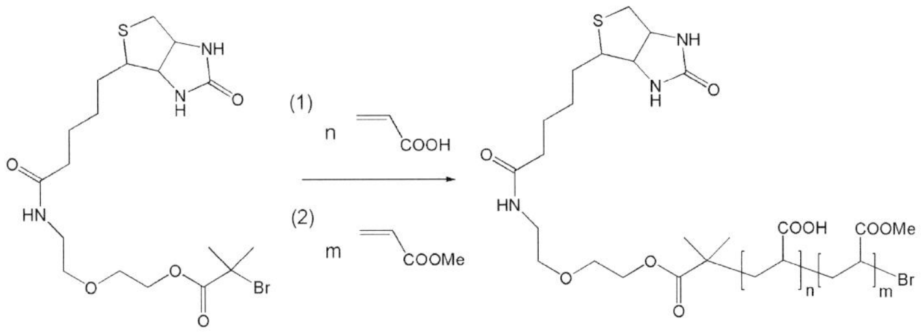

Figure 8.12. Synthesis of biotin end-capped PAA-*b*-PMA by ATRP.

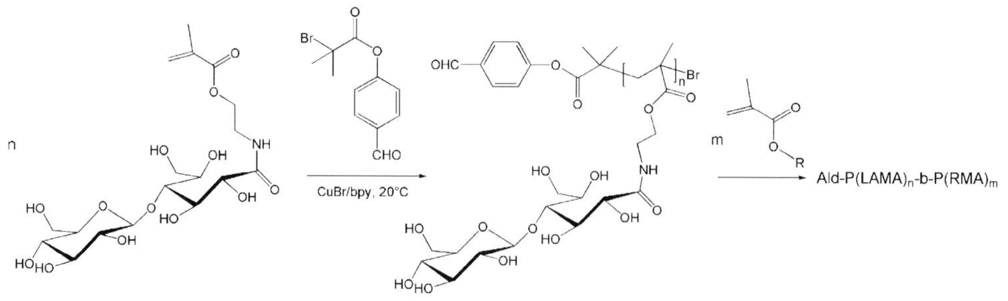

Figure 8.13. Sequential polymerization of 2-lactobionamidoethyl methacrylate (LAMA) with methacrylic monomers (R-MA) by ATRP at 20 °C.

workers [86] synthesized amphiphilic biodegradable PEO-*b*-PLA diblock copolymers that were end-functionalized by galactose. Therefore, they initiated the anionic polymerization of ethylene oxide by a metal alkoxide of a regioselectively protected galactose, followed by ROP of lactic acid.

Finally, amphiphilic functional copolymers were prepared using polymerizable carbohydrates as monomers. Armes and coworkers synthesized new sugar-modified methacrylic monomers (2-gluconamidoethyl methacrylate and 2-lactobionamidoethyl methacrylate) suitable for the preparation of sugar-modified methacrylate-based diblock (see Fig. 8.13) and triblock copolymers by ATRP starting from different (macro)initiators [116].

8.4.3.2.2 **Functional Random (Comb-like) Copolymers** The most popular pathway to amphiphilic random (comb-like) copolymers (Scheme 8.1C–E) functionalized by biomolecules relies on the synthesis of copolymers bearing groups that are prone to further chemical modification. Then, in a second step, reactive biomolecule derivatives can be grafted onto the (hydrophobic or hydrophilic) polymer backbone (called "grafting onto" approach).

For example, the pendant carboxylic acid groups of poly(methyl methacrylate-*co*-methacrylic acid) copolymers have been successfully used as reactive sites for the covalent linking of biotin molecules [117]. These random amphiphilic copolymers were efficient stabilizers and surface modifiers of PLA nanoparticles [117].

With the purpose to obtain fully biodegradable nanoparticles, biodegradable amphiphilic copolymers bearing reactive sites have been synthesized. For instance, ε-caprolactone has been randomly copolymerized with γ-substituted functional ε-caprolactone (comonomers) (bromo-, hydroxyl-, carboxylic acid-substituted), allowing the posterior reaction with biologically active compounds. Fully biodegradable surface-modified nanoparticles could be obtained by coprecipitation of PLA with these functional amphiphilic copolymers and the presence of the latter at the nanoparticle's surface was demonstrated [118].

Maruyama and coworkers also prepared biodegradable nanoparticles based on poly(D,L-LA) and poly(L-lysine)-g-polysaccharide (dextran, maltose or amylose) co-

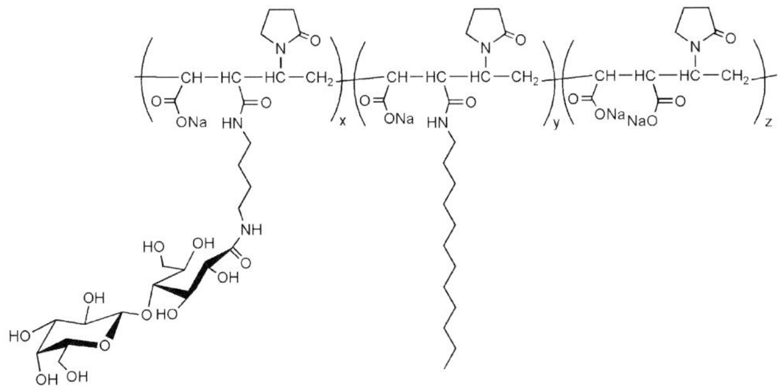

Figure 8.14. Structure of amphiphilic galactosylated copolymers Gal_x–Dod_y.

polymers either by a solvent evaporation process or a diafiltration method. These copolymers were easily prepared by a reductive amination reaction between the pendant amine function of the polypeptide and the reductive extremity of the polysaccharide. Aggregation assays using specific lectins revealed the presence of carbohydrate moieties at the nanoparticle surface. Furthermore, due to the polycationic nature of poly(lysine), the nanoparticles are positively charged. Consequently, they appear as promising candidates for the transfection of DNA (gene delivery) [119].

The efficient synthesis of amphiphilic maleic anhydride copolymers grafted by galactose units and dodecyl chains has been recently reported. (Fig. 8.14) In fact, reactive anhydride functions were introduced through copolymerization of maleic anhydride and *N*-vinylpyrrolidone in a copolymer backbone. They have then been used as reactive sites for further functionalization with *N*-(4-aminobutyl)-*O*-*β*-D-galactopyranosyl-(1–4)-D-gluconamide (an amine-functionalized galactose derivative) and dodecylamine. As illustrated in Scheme 8.1(E), amphiphilic maleic anhydride copolymers bearing pendant hydrophilic galactose moieties, as biological targeting units, and hydrophobic alkyl chains (for the interfacial activity) could be obtained [120]. These copolymers were successfully used as stabilizers and surface modifiers to produce stable nanoparticles coated with galactoses as targetable moieties on their surface, using the emulsification-diffusion technique. The presence and bioavailability of the galactose moieties at the nanoparticle surface were clearly demonstrated by lectin–sugar interactions [98].

8.4.3.3 **Emulsion, Miniemulsion or Dispersion Polymerization**

As mentioned in Section 8.3.2, polymeric nanoparticles can be prepared using emulsion, miniemulsion or dispersion polymerization. In order to modify the surface of nanoparticles, several approaches have been proposed. One relies on the miniemulsion polymerization of monomers in the presence of amphiphilic biopolymers as emulsifiers. A second approach is based on the dispersion copolymerization of a hydrophilic functional macromonomer with a hydrophobic comonomer.

According to the first strategy, the polycation chitosan [121] has been used as stabilizer to prepare chitosan-coated latexes by (mini)emulsion polymerization. While the use of chitosan alone resulted in rather large droplets and a major amount of coagulate, addition of a low-molecular-weight surfactant or a flexible polymeric costabilizer significantly improved the stabilization of the nanodroplets during the polymerization. This efficient stabilization allowed the production of well-defined chitosan-coated nanoparticles in the range of 100–300 nm.

Later, Dellacherie and coworkers coated polystyrene nanoparticles by dextran in a miniemulsion process which did not require the addition of any costabilizers and led to monodisperse nanoparticles. For this purpose, they hydrophobically modified dextran chains by randomly grafted phenoxy groups. This amphiphilic dextran showed strong interfacial activity, and could be successfully used as an emulsion stabilizer and surface modifier in miniemulsion processes to prepare polystyrene particles carrying dextran at the surface [63].

In contrast to this approach, the macromonomer method allows covalently linking biomolecules, such as monosaccharide moieties, to the surface of nanoparticles. A direct pathway to carbohydrate-functionalized nanoparticles has thus been proposed [66]. For this purpose, a hydrophilic macromonomer bearing glucose moieties has been synthesized by radical polymerization of 2-(glucosyloxy)ethyl methacrylate (GEMA) in the presence of 2-mercaptoethylamine as a chain transfer agent, followed by a peptide-like coupling reaction with 4-vinylbenzoic acid (VBA) (Fig. 8.15). Nanospheres with a polystyrene core and a GEMA oligomer corona were then obtained by free radical copolymerization of the GEMA macromonomer with styrene in an ethanol/water mixture. As mentioned in Section 8.4.2.1, such glucose-decorated nanoparticles were expected to increase the interaction with a glucose specific lectin [concanavalin A (Con A)] due to the cluster effect. Hence, investigation of the glucose-lectin interaction by the enzyme-linked lectin assay (ELLA) demonstrated that the binding activity of the carbohydrate decorated nanoparticles was less than that of the free GEMA macromonomer. It decreased even with increasing amount of glucose at the nanospheres. Steric hindrance was proposed as a possible explanation for the low bioavailabilty [66] (Fig. 8.16).

The choice of technique for the surface modification by biomolecules is thus crucial. Biological recognition assays are necessary to test the bioavailability of the biomolecules.

8.4.3.4 Covalent Linking of Functional Molecules to Preformed Nanoparticles

The surface functionalization of nanoparticles by covalent grafting of functional molecules on preformed polymeric nanoparticles is challenging (see Fig. 8.10, iii).

Such reactions require (i) the availability of functional reactive groups at the nanoparticle surface, (ii) the synthesis of biomolecules bearing reactive groups, and (iii) the use of coupling reactions that are selective and efficient. Above all, they must be smooth, not causing neither denaturation of the biomolecules nor degradation of the polymer material. These challenges led to the development of "chemical ligation", i.e. the selective covalent coupling of mutually and uniquely functional groups under mild and aqueous conditions [122]. Hitherto, only a few

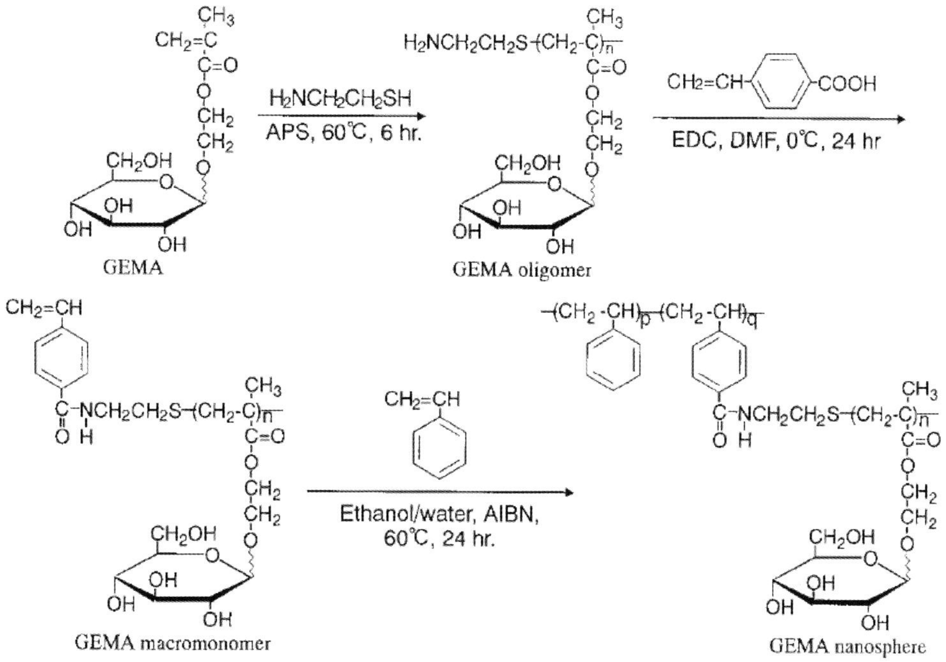

Figure 8.15. Synthesis and copolymerization of a glucose-capped macromonomer (GEMA macromonomer).

of these methods have been applied to the chemical coupling of biomolecules onto preformed nanoparticles.

In the following, we report on the universally applied amine–acid coupling and on another very selective and smooth coupling reaction, relying on the reaction of thiol groups with maleimides.

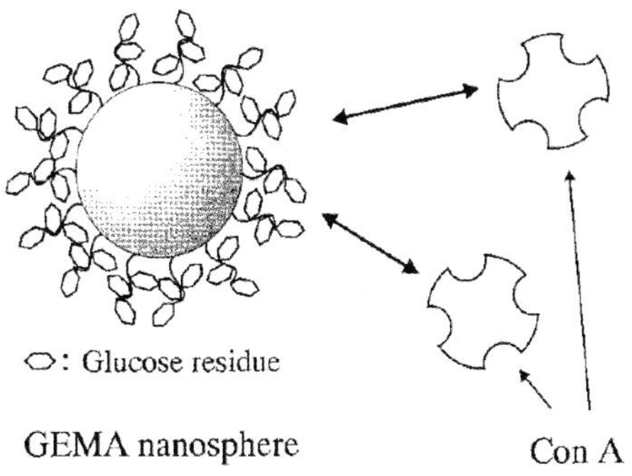

Figure 8.16. Schematic representation of a GEMA nanosphere and its interaction with Con A [66].

8.4.3.4.1 **Amine–Acid Coupling** The amine–acid coupling is one of the most universally applied and efficient coupling reactions. As an example, biomolecules bearing carboxylic acid groups have been conjugated onto NH_2-coated nanoparticles. Such nanoparticles have been prepared using amine-functionalized comonomers, either in an *in situ* copolymerization process (Section 8.3.2) [101], or by using amphiphilic copolymers that serve as surfactants and surface modifiers, e.g. in a nanoprecipitation technique (Section 8.3.1) [102]. Folic acid was then successfully conjugated to the surface using 1,3-dicyclohexylcarbodiimide (DCC).

Based on the same conjugation reaction, biomolecules bearing an amine function have been conjugated to nanoparticles exposing carboxylic acid groups. Wooley and coworkers prepared SCKs from micelles formed by poly(ε-caprolactone-*b*-acrylic acid) diblock copolymers (PCL-*b*-PAA) [123] followed by crosslinking of the PAA shell (consumption of approximately 50% of the acrylic acid groups) (Fig. 8.17, step 1). The remaining acrylic acid groups were then used for the conjugation to the amino group of a fluorescent dye [fluorescein-5-thiosemicarbazide (FTSC) (Fig. 8.17, step 2) and a biologically active peptide sequence, respectively. The latter was prepared by standard solid-phase peptide synthesis (SPPS) and extended with a flexible linker. (Fig. 8.17, step 3). The following conjugation of the peptide to the SCK nanoparticle was performed on a solid support. This technique allows attaching the peptide selectively to the surface of the SCKs, as the reaction can only take place at the interface of the SCK and the peptide-bearing resin. Moreover, by performing the SCK–peptide coupling on a solid support, any nonconjugated nanoparticles were removed by washing of the resin support. Finally, by degradation of the PCL core, fluorescent peptide-exposing nanocapsules (nanocages) could be obtained, which demonstrated good binding interactions with cells and transduction into cells [124] (Fig. 8.17, step 4).

8.4.3.4.2 **Thiol–Maleimide Coupling** The introduction of thiol groups at the surface of nanoparticles opens up a lot of new possibilities in ligand conjugation (ligation). In particular, conjugation reactions between thiols and maleimides have received increasing interest due to their specificity and reactivity. Such reactions have been found to be quantitative under physiological conditions [125]. Antibody or protein conjugation is commonly performed using bifunctional crosslinkers such as *m*-maleimidobenzoyl-*N*-hydroxysuccinimide ester (MBS) that offers two binding sites – one for primary amino groups (present in antibodies, drugs, specific peptides) and one for thiol functions (Fig. 8.18) [126].

Thus, thiolated polymer nanoparticles have been synthesized. For instance, Langer and coworkers introduced free sulfhydryl groups onto the surface of gelatin (protein) nanoparticles by the reaction of primary amino groups with 2-iminothiolane [127]. Furthermore, Nobs and coworkers developed a suitable method for the introduction of thiol functions on the surface of PLA nanoparticles. The modification of the surface involved the activation of the carboxylic acid end-groups of PLA followed by the nucleophilic attack by cysteine or cystamine in a carbodiimide reaction (providing thiol functions via an amide bond) [128].

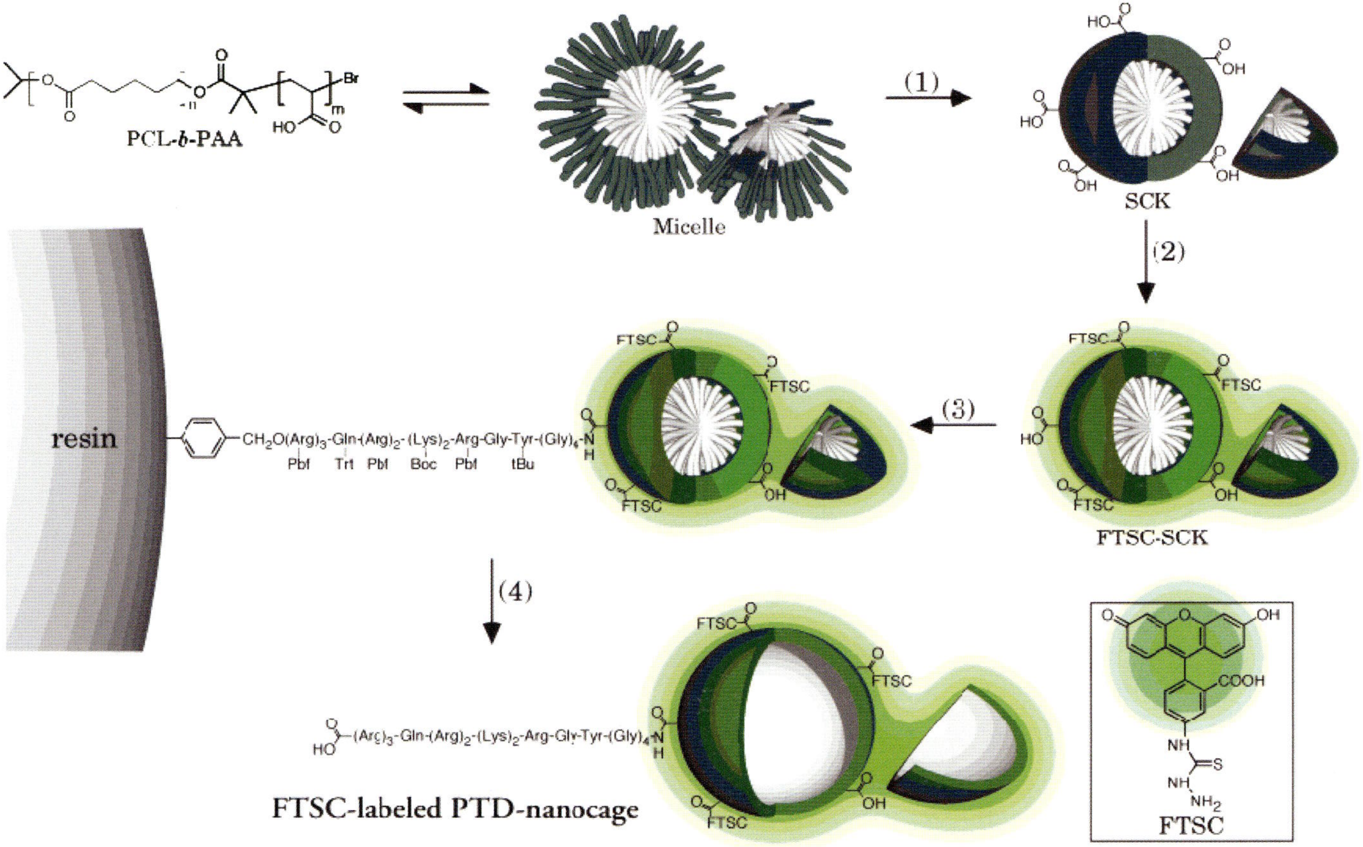

Figure 8.17. Solid-phase synthesis strategy involved coupling of the protein transduction domain (PTD) with fluorescein-labeled SCK nanoparticles, followed by cleavage from the support and excavation of the nanoparticle core domain to yield FTSC-labeled PTD nanocage bioconjugates.

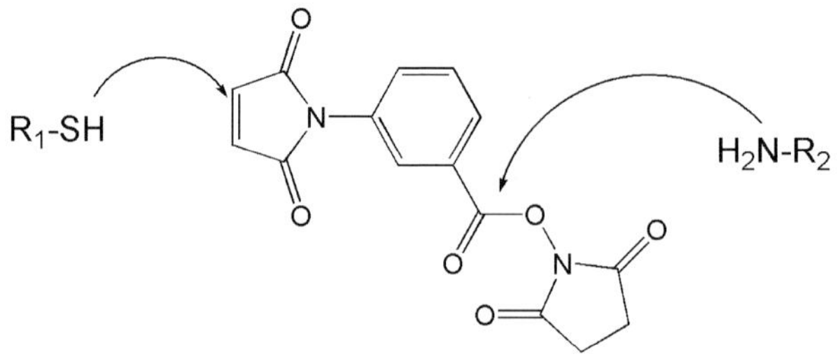

Figure 8.18. Coupling agent: bifunctional MBS.

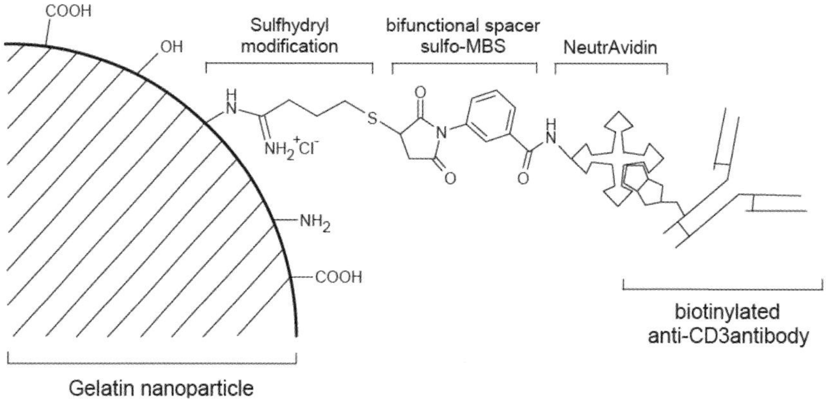

Figure 8.19. Schematic representation of antibody-loaded NeutrAvidin-modified gelatin nanoparticles. Sulfhydryl groups were introduced onto the particle surface by 2-iminothiolane followed by a conjugation reaction with NeutrAvidin using the heterobifunctional crosslinker MBS. A biotinylated anti-CD3 antibody was then attached to the particle surface by avidin–biotin complex formation.

In both cases (gelatin and PLA nanoparticles), thiol-functionalized nanoparticles were thus made available. Then, avidin (NeutrAvidin), as a model protein and linker molecule (see Section 8.4.2.4), could be successfully conjugated to the nanoparticles via MBS, as illustrated in Fig. 8.19 [129]. Balthasar and coworkers have further attached biotinylated antibodies at the surface via avidin–biotin complex formation and their bioavailability could be shown using indirect methods, such as immunoblotting or fluorimetry [130].

8.4.3.4.3 **Molecular Imprinting** In the last decade, so called molecular-imprinted polymeric materials (MIP) have gained increasing interest for biomimetic molecular recognition elements [131]. The three-dimensional arrangement of the binding functional groups on the MIP is obtained by linking the functional monomers covalently or noncovalently to the template during polymerization (Fig. 8.20).

Removal of the template from the formed polymer then generates a structure that is complementary to the template structure. Very recently, based on this prin-

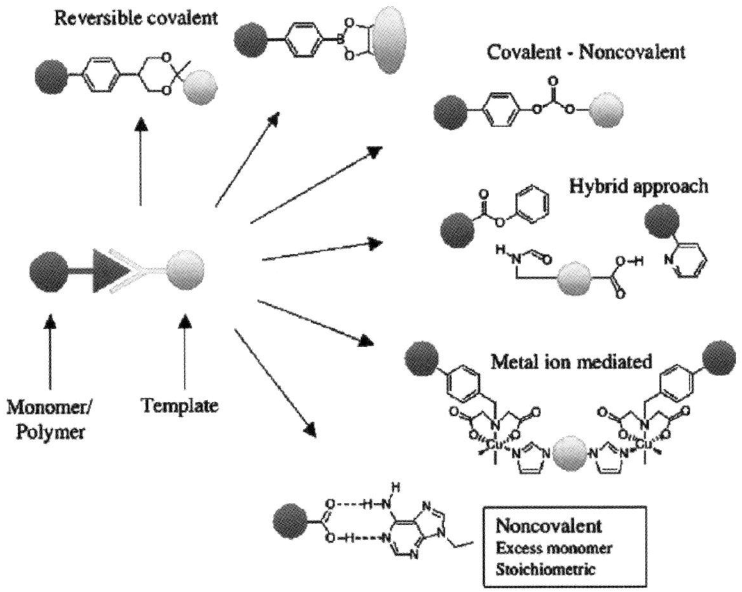

Figure 8.20. Strategies used to place binding or catalytic functional groups at defined positions in imprinted sites of network polymers.

ciple interfacial imprinting techniques have been developed to reach surface-imprinted (colloidal systems). This approach has been used for the synthesis of surface-imprinted polymeric nanoparticles. Therefore, using emulsion or precipitation polymerization techniques monomers bearing bonds to a "template molecule" have been polymerized in the presence of bioactive molecules as templates [132]. Removal of the latter leaves a polymer nanoparticle containing a memory of its shape and functionality on its surface. They are therefore synthetic analogs of biological recognition systems.

First attempts have been undertaken, and Carter and coworkers synthesized nanoparticles bearing imprints of caffeine or theophylline at their surface that show a high affinity to the template molecule (caffeine or theophylline). Such particles possessed a core–shell structure [133]. The core was prepared first by emulsion polymerization of styrene and divinyl benzene monomers (1:1). The resulting particles were then coated, in a second polymerization stage, with the imprinting monomer mixture consisting of ethylene glycol dimethacrylate and oleyl phenyl hydrogen phosphate, and caffeine (or theophylline) as noncovalent template.

8.4.4 Analytical Techniques for Surface Modification

The efficiency of the surface functionalization of nanoparticles with biomolecules, but also their bioavailability for recognition interactions, depends on many factors.

These include the architecture and composition of the polymers, the conformation of the polymer chains, and also the conditions employed for the nanoparticle formation. Therefore, numerous (indirect and direct) techniques have been developed and used to characterize the surface of nanoparticles [134]. Some of the most frequently used physicochemical techniques (Section 8.4.4.1) and biological assays (Section 8.4.4.2) are highlighted next.

8.4.4.1 Physicochemical Techniques

Physicochemical techniques can supply information both on the chemical composition of the surface and also on its physical properties, such as hydrophilicity or surface charge. In addition, the biological properties of a surface can be investigated. Thus, specific interaction reactions between biomolecules fixed on the nanoparticles and their ligands fixed on the analytical device can be revealed by physicochemical means.

8.4.4.1.1 **The ζ Potential** The ζ potential measurement of aqueous suspensions of nanoparticles is one of the most common techniques to determine surface charges and therefore surface modification. The ζ potential reflects the electrical surface potential of particles, which is influenced by the different materials located at the interface with the dispersing medium. Thus, the mobility of charged particles is monitored by applying an electrical potential. High ζ potential values, above 30 mV (positive or negative value), lead generally to stable colloidal suspensions, because electrostatic repulsion between particles prevents their aggregation.

8.4.4.1.2 **X-ray Photoelectron Spectroscopy (XPS)** Another commonly used technique is XPS, also known as electron spectroscopy for chemical analysis (ESCA), which provides information about the chemical (atomic) composition of the top layer of nanoparticles. Here, under ultra-high vacuum, the dried sample is bombarded with X-rays. When the photon is of suitable energy, it is absorbed by an atom causing ionization and the emission of a core electron (inner shell electron). Since binding energies of core electrons are characteristic for elements in a certain chemical environment, the spectrum gives information on the elemental composition of the shallow surface region. From small shifts in the binding energies, additional chemical information can be derived (e.g. the oxidation state of the element). Since photons possess a limited penetration energy, only those electrons pertaining to atoms at or near the surface (up to 10 nm) escape and can be counted. This quantitative technique gives the average composition over about 10 nm depth inside the nanoparticles. XPS at various angles allows for the determination of the composition on different depth of the sample.

8.4.4.1.3 **Time-of-Flight Secondary Ion Mass Spectroscopy (TOF-SIMS)** SIMS is a physicochemical technique of the outmost surface (10 Å). TOF-SIMS uses a pulsed primary ion beam to desorb and ionize species from a sample surface. The resulting secondary ions are accelerated into a mass spectrometer, where they are mass analyzed by measuring their TOF from the sample surface to the detector. The mass spectrum and the secondary ion images are then used to determine the composition and distribution of the sample's surface constituents. TOF-SIMS provides spectroscopy for the characterization of the surface's chemical composition, imaging for determining the distribution of the chemical species, and depth profiling for thin-film characterization. This technique thus allows to prove the chemical linkage of biomolecules to a surface via the analysis of the fragments.

8.4.4.1.4 **Electron Paramagnetic Resonance (EPR)** EPR, or electron spin resonance (ESR), is a spectroscopic technique that detects species that possess unpaired electrons. The basic physical concepts of the technique are analogous to those of nuclear magnetic resonance (NMR); however, instead of the spins of the atom's nuclei, electron spins are excited. Due to the difference in mass between nuclei and electrons, weaker magnetic fields and higher frequencies are used compared to NMR. For electrons in a magnetic field of 0.3 T, spin resonance occurs at around 10 GHz. EPR is helpful for nanoparticle characterization by using nanoparticles tagged with biological spin probes. EPR of free radicals conjugated to polymer chains has been used to discriminate between highly mobile (liquid-like) and slowly mobile (solid-like) spin labels on the basis of their magnetic relaxation times. EPR can thus provide useful information at the molecular level on the structure, mobility and organization of polymers at interfaces [135, 136].

8.4.4.1.5 **Surface Plasmon Resonance (SPR) [137]** SPR is a biophysical technique allowing us to measure biomolecular interactions in a quantitative, real-time manner. A ligand ("target") is immobilized on a special chip (SPR crystal) and a solution of the analyte ("binding partner") flows across the chip. The progress of binding is then measured by optical instruments.

This technique was applied to measure the interaction of nanoparticle–biomolecule conjugates with surfaces that had been modified by the corresponding ligand (generally a protein). As an example, for the measurement of interactions of folic acid-coated nanoparticles with the folate-binding protein, the latter was immobilized on the sensor surface [102]. It could be demonstrated that the folate nanoparticle conjugates were able to bind specifically to immobilized protein, whereas nanoparticles without folic acid-targeting moieties showed a much lower interaction (Fig. 8.21).

8.4.4.2 Biological Assays/Methods

8.4.4.2.1 **Nonspecific Interactions with Proteins** The adsorption of proteins has often been used to indirectly demonstrate the presence of a protein-repulsive coating. For this purpose, the amount of adsorbed model proteins, such as bovine- or human serum albumin (BSA or HSA), has been determined by quantification of the nonadsorbed proteins in the supernatant after centrifugation and precipitation of the nanoparticles. In a recent study the repellent properties of dextran and PEO could be demonstrated. Indeed, PCL–dextran nanoparticles adsorbed

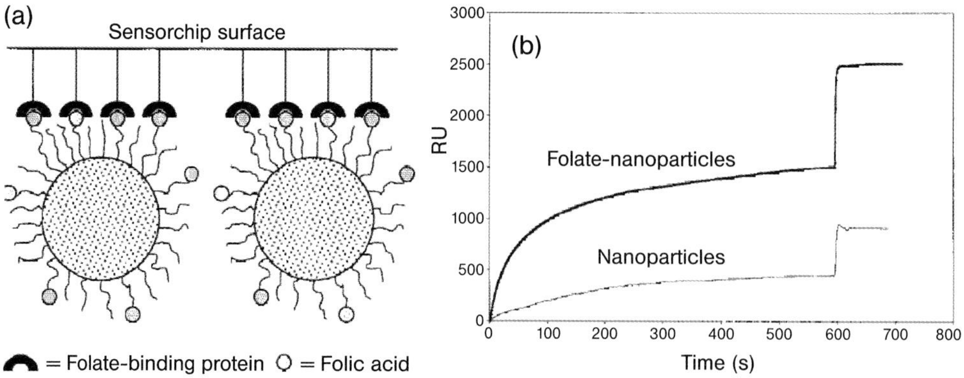

Figure 8.21. SPR on folate-coated nanoparticles.

only 0.2 mg m^{-2} BSA, which is comparable with the amount detected on the corresponding PEGylated nanoparticles taken as control [138, 139].

Other approaches tend to identify the proteins that are adsorbed most when incubating the nanoparticles with mixtures of proteins. Two-dimensional poly(acrylamide) gel electrophoresis, (2-D PAGE) has thus been used to reveal adsorption and to identify proteins and fragments.

Finally, Passirani and coworkers [5] and Chauvierre and coworkers [81] evaluated the activation of the complement system by nanoparticles, which leads to their rapid elimination from the blood circulation through the uptake by macrophages of the MPS. In fact, the key step of complement activation to take place is the adsorption of serum proteins on the surface of the nanoparticles. Thus, nanoparticles coated by different polysaccharides were incubated in normal human serum (NHS) and the activation of the complement systems determined by quantification of a key protein – complement component C3.

8.4.4.2.2 **Specific Interactions (Carbohydrates–Lectins, etc.)** Apart from physicochemical techniques, numerous biological methods have been used for the investigation of specific interactions between surface-functionalized nanoparticles and their targets, such as protein–ligand interactions.

Based on such lectin–carbohydrate interactions, the surface modification of nanoparticles by galactose could be demonstrated. Therefore, pyrene-labeled galactose-coated micelles (galactose–PEO-*b*-PLA) have been passed on a column packed with *Ricinus communis* lectin (RCA-1 lectin) immobilized beads. By fluorescence spectroscopy, they were shown to be specifically retained at the column, in comparison to non- and glucose-functionalized micelles [86].

Furthermore, numerous biological assays (based on specific biomolecular interactions) such as enzyme-linked immunosorbent assay (ELISA), ELLA and aggregation assays have been used to demonstrate the presence of biomolecules at the surface of nanoparticles.

ELISA is a biochemical test that quantifies by colorimetry a biological substance (e.g. proteins, sugars) in a biological liquid using the reaction of an antibody to its antigen. This method is based on the fixation of a first antibody to a solid device. Once the antibody is fixed and nonfixed residual free molecules are eliminated, the sample (to be quantified) is incubated, using conditions that favor antibody–protein interaction. Then, after a washing step, the complex formed is revealed by reaction with a second, detecting antibody, which is specific to another site of the protein. This antibody is typically linked to an enzyme, which serves for the quantification of the initial protein-antibody complex by reaction with a substrate and coloration of the medium by the formed product.

ELLA is a descendant of ELISA employing the lectin–carbohydrate interaction. It allows to quantify the capacity of a ligand X (e.g. sugar moieties at the surface of a nanoparticles) to inhibit the adhesion of a lectin on a reference ligand Y deposited on a solid device. Using this method, the surface functionalization of polymer nanoparticles with monosaccharides could be demonstrated via biotin–avidin sandwiching using streptavidin–horseradish peroxidase (HRP) as a detection system [98] (Fig. 8.22).

Finally, aggregation assays, based on the aggregation of carbohydrate-decorated nanoparticles by multivalent lectins, have been used to indirectly show the presence of poly- or monosaccharides at the surface of nanoparticles [119, 140] (see also Section 8.5.2.1.2). Similarly, hemagglutination inhibition assays have been developed, which are based on the inhibition of the agglutination of erythrocytes by lectins. In fact, erythrocytes are naturally decorated by saccharidic moieties. Carbohydrate-bearing polymeric particles can therefore act as inhibiting agents, as they compete with erythrocytes for the interaction with lectins [94].

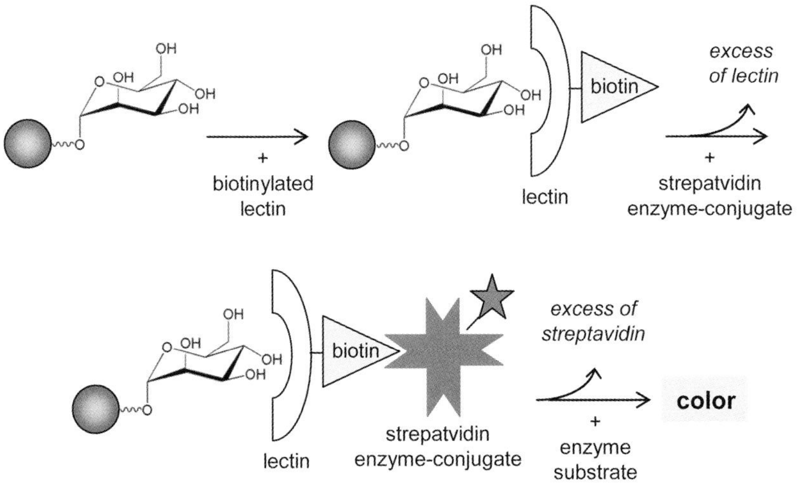

Figure 8.22. Scheme for the multistep titration of particle-fixed mannose by biotin-labeled biotin.

8.5 Applications

8.5.1 Drug Delivery Systems [141]

As already mentioned, colloidal drug delivery systems are designed to modify the pharmacokinetics and biodistribution of their associated drugs, and/or to serve as drug reservoirs (i.e. as sustained release systems). Indeed, one of the main problems of drug delivery is the poor solubility of hydrophobic drugs in aqueous media. Drug delivery systems that provide hydrophobic domains can be advantageously used to help "solubilization" of the drug. By the careful choice of the drug delivery system and the polymer material, the release profile of the drugs from the device and thus their blood concentration with time (pharmacokinetics) can be substantially controlled. Additionally, sensitive drugs can be protected from premature (enzymatic/metabolic) degradation by encapsulating them in a protecting polymer matrix.

Furthermore, colloidal drug carrier systems change the biodistribution of drugs. Due to their "large" size, colloidal drug delivery systems accumulate in diseased tissues such as tumors, which are characterized by an enhanced permeability and retention ("passive targeting"). On the other hand, the surface functionalization of particulate carriers by specific ligands should allow the specific targeting of tissues. The gain in selectivity thus leads to the concentration of the drugs at the targeted tissues, which permits to reduce the amounts of administered drug and consequently avoids side-effects resulting from the presence of the drug at undesired sites ("active targeting").

8.5.1.1 Routes of Administration

Nanoparticles can be administered via multiple routes, such as intravenous, oral, pulmonary, nasal and ocular routes, as a solid or suspension. It should be noted that most of the current systems are designed for intravenous and oral administration.

Oral administration is the most convenient route for drug delivery, improving the compliance and quality of life of the patients compared to therapy by injection or infusion. However, the oral absorption of many therapeutic agents, such as peptides [142] (e.g. insulin), proteins, oligodesoxynucleotides (ODN) and also cancer drugs, is one of the greatest challenges in the pharmaceutical field. Indeed, their bioavailability is low because of instability in the gastrointestinal tract and low permeability through the intestinal epithelium. Nanoparticles are promising carriers for such bioactive molecules, because they may protect them against enzymatic/hydrolytic degradation (e.g. by gastric or intestinal juices, which are rich in proteases such as trypsin and chymotrypsin) and they may enhance their bioavailability. Polymeric particles have been shown to cross the intestine barrier. The size of the particles as well as the nature of the polymer are critical parameters for the particle uptake by the gastrointestinal tract. Bioadhesion of nanoparticles to the mucous membrane in the gastrointestinal tract can be a tool to prolong the residence time of the drug carriers at the absorption sites and thus enhance the drug absorption. In fact, the coating of nanoparticle surfaces with hydrophilic mucoadhesive polymeric chains, such as PMAA [143] and chitosan [15, 19, 22], was shown to increase the absorption of the nanoparticles from the gastrointestinal tract.

Whenever drugs or drug delivery systems are degraded or not sufficiently absorbed after oral administration, parenteral administration, i.e. administration other than via the digestive system, is the route of choice.

Nowadays, alternative routes of administration via mucosal membranes, such as pulmonary and nasal mucosae, that circumvent the passage by the gastrointestinal tract and the liver presystemic metabolism (known as the "first-pass effect" – the first metabolic process with cytochrome P450 in the liver) are receiving a great deal of attention. Pulmonary delivery for both local and systemic treatments via aerosol inhalation has many advantages over other delivery pathways. Indeed, the lungs are characterized by a large surface area (43–102 m^2), slow mucociliary clearance and low enzymatic activity. Compared to other nasal administration, they possess a thinner, more permeable absorption barrier. Recently, various high-molecular-weight drugs have been successfully absorbed through alveolar region of the lungs, e.g. heparin, growth factors (e.g. granulocyte colony stimulating factor), peptides and proteins such as insulin [144, 145]. Micro/nanoparticles are interesting drug delivery systems for pulmonary administration as they [146] increase the systemic availability of substances by offering protection as well as exhibiting controlled release properties. The pulmonary route of application is challenging, requiring the optimal size of the drug formulation, in order to ensure the "atomization" of the drug formulation for inhalation and deposition of the aerosol particles in the alveolar region, where the drugs are absorbed best. It was found that microdrug particles (below 5 µm) were rapidly eliminated from the lung by ciliary movement and phagocytosis with macrophages [147]. Recently, polymeric nanoparticles for administration in the respiratory tract have been coated by mucoadhesive copolymers. Similar to the results of earlier studies on the intestine mucosa, chitosan-coated nanoparticles were proposed to open the tight junctions of the lung epithelium [20], enhance mucoadhesion and enable pulmonary systemic delivery [19]. Apart from the pulmonary route, nasal administration of drugs and especially of vaccines has found increasing interest. Similar to the lungs, the nasal mucosa is thin, highly permeable and incorporates a dense vascular network, and possesses a surface of "only" 50 cm^2. As an example, chitosan-coated PLGA nanoparticles have been found to enhanced the nasal transport of encapsulated tetanus toxoid [148, 149].

Numerous colloidal carrier systems have also been designed for the intravenous route of administration, especially in the case of the delivery of proteins and oligonucleotides. However, severe requirements concerning the size, size distribution and surface properties of nanoparticles are imposed. In fact, the smallest capillaries in the body are only 5–6 µm in diameter. Consequently, particles being distributed in the blood stream must be significantly smaller than 5 µm in diameter and ought not show aggregate formation in order to avoid clog formation and embolism. As mentioned in Section 8.1, the surface properties of the colloidal systems must be adapted in order to tune their biodistribution, pharmacokinetics and residence time in the vascular system before elimination by the MPS.

Compared to the intravenous route, subcutaneous/intramuscular administration imposes fewer requirements concerning particle size and size distribution. The subcutaneous route has proved to be promising in different therapeutic applications; subcutaneous injection of PLGA nanoparticles containing antitubercular drugs in mice resulted in sustained therapeutic drug levels in the plasma for 32 days and in lung/spleen for 36 days. In the field of tumor therapy, it has been demonstrated very recently that subcutaneous injection near the tumor site is the preferential route for facilitating high tumor uptake and retention, compared to intravenous or intraperitoneal injection [150]. Additionally, it should be emphasized that subcutaneous injection of nanoparticles proved to be very promising for vaccine delivery. Indeed, colloidal formulations of vaccines administered subcutaneously have been found to have strong "adjuvant activity" (defined in Section 8.5.1.2), which is usually required to cause a sufficient immune response [151, 152].

Polymeric nanoparticles have also demonstrated great potential for ophthalmic formulations. Probably the most severe disadvantage of eye-drop formulations is their rapid elimination of the instilled drug solution from the precorneal site [153]. In fact, only 1–2% of the applied dose reaches intraocular tissues. Consequently, colloidal suspensions were designed to combine ophthalmic sustained action with the ease of application of eye-drop solutions. Upon topical instillation, these particles are expected to be retained in the "cul-de-sac" and the drug to be slowly released from the particles through diffusion, chemical reaction or polymer degradation, or by an ion-exchange mechanism. Concerning the size of particles for ophthalmic purposes, Sieg and Triplett demonstrated that an upper size limit (below 10 µm) should be considered to avoid discomfort of the patients and that the retention time before washout diminishes with decreasing particle diameter. Apart from the size, the surface properties of nanoparticles have been changed in order to prevent their premature elimination. HA was found to be the polysaccharide of choice to coat polymeric nanoparticles and has been proved to enhance the ocular bioavailability of drugs, probably due to its mucoadhesive properties [79].

Finally, nanoparticles are also used for topical applications. In particular, polysaccharide-coated nanoparticles, such as chitosan-coated particles, are promising drug delivery systems for their enhanced wound-healing properties [154].

8.5.1.2 Therapeutic Applications of Nanoparticles

Nanoparticles cannot only change the distribution of drugs at the organ or tissue level, but also at the cellular level, by increasing uptake or modifying the intracellular localization of the drug. This opens up the route for a large variety of therapeutic applications. In this section we report examples of three important groups of therapeutics that can be delivered by colloidal systems, i.e. chemotherapeutics (anticancer drugs), ODNs or genes, and proteins for cancer treatment, gene therapy and vaccination.

Anticancer drugs are often poorly bioavailable and barely compatible with oral delivery, due to their poor solubility, stability and permeability across biological membranes. After intravenous administration, they are distributed throughout the body as a function of the physicochemical properties of the molecule and do not necessarily accumulate in the targeted tissues. Due to the strong toxicity of cytostatic drugs, the specific targeting of the tumor cells is extremely interesting, allowing for effective therapy by reducing side-effects. Another major problem in cancer chemotherapy is the ability of tumor cells to develop simultaneous resistance to multiple lipophilic therapeutics. This resistance has been attributed to an active drug efflux from resistant cells linked to the presence of transmembrane P-glycoprotein (P-gp), which forms transmembrane channels and pumps the drugs out of the cell. The use of nanoparticulate carriers seems a promising solution to address these problems.

In fact, as already reported in Section 8.1, cancerous tissues possess a defective vascular architecture (due to the rapid vascularization, which is necessary to serve fast-growing cancers) coupled with poor lymphatic drainage. This phenomenon is known as an "enhanced permeation and retention" effect and allows long-circulating nanoparticles (due to their large size in comparison to free drugs) to passively target cancerous tissues [7]. The coating of nanoparticles by hydrophilic polymers avoids their rapid uptake in the liver and spleen, and favors their prolonged circulation time in the blood stream allowing the nanoparticles to accumulate in tumor tissues. It has actually been shown that anticancer drugs encapsulated in such surface-modified nanoparticles accumulate preferentially in cancer cells [8, 11]. To further enhance the targeting specificity, probes that are specific to tumor cells have been conjugated to the surface of nanoparticles. One of the greatest challenges is thus defining the optimal targeting agent to selectively and successfully transport nanoparticles systems (nanoparticles) to cancerous tissue. These strategies also rely on the ability of the targeting agents or ligands to bind to the tumor cells' surface in an appropriate manner then triggering receptor endocytosis (receptor-mediated cell internalization). The therapeutic agent will hereby be delivered to the interior of the cancer cell. The folate receptor, which is overexpressed on malignant human cells, has been found to be a promising target. The folate-conjugated nanoparticles not only selectively target cancer cells, but they also improve the internalization of the encapsulated drugs within the targeted cancer cells [8]. On the other hand, monoclonal antibodies that specifically bind to the tumor antigens of a specific cancer type have been identified, and are currently used and approved by the FDA for targeted cancer treatment [11]. Thus, antibodies specific to breast cancer, etc. seem promising ligands for the covalent conjugation to nanoparticles [155].

Another challenging application of nanoparticles is their use as carriers for (antisense) nucleotides and plasmid DNA in the field of gene therapy. The ultimate goal of gene therapy is to cure both inherited and acquired disorders in a straightforward manner by removing their cause, i.e. by adding, correcting or replacing genes [156]. However, the administration of genes poses a challenge to pharmaceutical technology because of their susceptibility to enzymatic degradation (by nucleases) and their poor penetration across biological membranes (poor bioavailability). The first potential gene delivery vectors were viruses. In the last decade, however, nanoparticles, similar to liposomes, have received growing interest as condensing nonviral gene carrier systems. These synthetic colloidal carrier systems are expected to be safer, but must be optimized in terms of keeping a comparable transfection rate. Such ODN-carrying nanoparticles are generally prepared on the basis of the electrostatic interactions (ion pairing); indeed, due to the phosphodiester group, ODN are negatively charged and can therefore be adsorbed at the surface of positively charged nanoparticles (such as chitosan nanoparticles [12]) or encapsulated in the core of nanoparticles.

Nanoparticles have also been designed as delivery vehicles for proteins. Similar to oligonucleotides and genes, proteins and peptides are very sensitive compounds that need to be protected from degradation in the biological environment. Moreover, their efficiency is highly limited by their inability to cross biological barriers and to reach the target site. As such, appropriate colloidal carriers for the successful delivery of proteins in the body have been designed, either incorporating the protein into the nanocarrier [157] or else adsorbing it on the surface of the nanocarrier [109].

Nowadays, both proteins and genes are the agents of choice for vaccination. Nanoparticles are very promising carriers for subcutaneous or mucosal vaccination [149, 151]. In fact, it has been reported that due to their size, nanoparticles have general "adjuvant" properties, i.e. act in a nonspecific manner to increase the specific immunity to an antigen (as compared to that introduced by the vaccine or the antigen alone) [158].

Concerning mucosal vaccination, the use of nanoparticles coated by mucoadhesive polymers is particularly interesting, because they exhibit prolonged residence time at the mucosae and avoid a premature clearance (see Section 8.5.1.1). As an example, chitosan nanoparticles have been found successful as a nasal vaccine in some animal studies, producing significant IgG serum responses when using influenza, pertussis and diphtheria vaccines [149].

Another approach to enhance the immune response after subcutaneous injection relies on the specific targeting of dendritic cells that are involved in the immune response and have been identified as target cells for the particle-mediated immune response [93]. It has been reported that dendritic cells expose specific receptors to mannose (mannose receptor) [91]. Therefore, the functionalization of vaccine-loaded particles by mannose seems a promising approach to specifically target dendritic cells [91, 93].

In contrast to other drug delivery systems, such as drug–polymer conjugates and liposome-based formulations, nanoparticles are in clinical trials, but have not yet reached the market [159].

8.5.1.3 Triggered Release

Recently, stimuli-responsive nanoparticles have been proposed as exciting delivery systems. Such delivery systems enable the release in response to an appropriate stimulus at the target site and/or at the right moment [160]. This stimulus can be environmental, chemical or physical, such as a change in pH [161, 162], temperature [101, 163, 164], ionic strength, application of laser light [165, 166] or magnetic field [167], and/or physiological, such as a change in enzyme concentration [168]. Up to date, only few works have been dedicated to the design of stimuli-responsive nanoparticles. Due to the importance of this application, some recent promising approaches to particulate-responsive systems are highlighted here.

It is known that in some tissues/physiological fluids of the human body, the pH may be different from most of the other physiological fluids. The pH is therefore an interesting stimulus. Apart from the drop in pH in the stomach, two other sites of low pH have been reported. So, the pH in endosomes is lower than that of the cytosol by 1–2 pH units [169]. It is known that endosomes are one of the principle transporters for drugs or drug delivery systems to enter a cell (by endocytosis). Once introduced in the cytosol, the release of the drug from the drug delivery systems may thus be induced by the drop in endosomal pH as triggering mechanism [169].

Furthermore, most solid tumors can be distinguished from normal surrounding tissues by a decrease in extracellular pH due to the higher aerobic and anaerobic glycolysis in cancer cells. Drug delivery systems have thus been designed that release anticancer drugs in response to a drop in pH [170].

For instance, Soppimath and coworkers prepared pH-triggered thermally responsive polymer core–shell nanoparticles for the delivery of chemotherapeutics (doxorubicin) to tumor cells [161]. They synthesized core–shell nanoparticles self-assembled from the amphiphilic tercopolymer poly(*N*-isopropylacrylamide-*co*-*N*,*N*-dimethylacrylamide-*co*-10-undecenoic acid), P(NIPAAm-*co*-DMAAm-*co*-UA) (Fig. 8.23). The UA was used as the core building hydrophobic and pH-sensitive segment, whereas the PNIPAAm segment exhibits a low critical solution temperature (LCST) in aqueous solution (about 32 °C) and is thus thermosensitive. DMAAm was employed to adjust the LCST of the polymer. The stability of nanoparticles prepared from the tercopolymer with optimized ratios of the different monomers at 37 °C depended on the environmental pH. Indeed, at physiological pH (pH 7.4) the LCST was 38.6 °C, meaning that the nanoparticles remained in their initial shape. However, in slightly acidic environments (pH < 6.6), the LCST of the terpolymer was decreased to 35.5 °C, i.e. a temperature lower than the normal body temperature. At this pH, the release of a model anticancer drug (doxorubicin) from

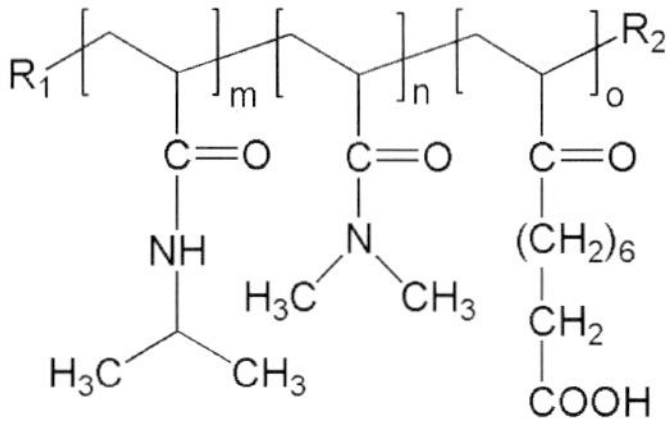

Figure 8.23. Molecular structure of P(NIPPAm-*co*-DMAAm-*co*-UA).

such nanoparticles was found to be significantly enhanced compared to the release at pH 7.4, probably due to the deformation and precipitation of the nanoparticles in acidic environment triggering the release of the entrapped anticancer drug (doxorubicin).

Recent efforts have focused on the development of optically addressable delivery systems, since irradiation with light promises to be an effective mean of releasing bioactive materials. The method relies on making the wall of polymer capsules sensitive to light by doping them with metal nanoparticles or organic dyes [171, 172]. Then, upon pulsed (below 10 ns) laser illumination, they absorb laser energy and disrupt the local environment due to a temperature increase, thus increasing the permeability of the capsule wall [166]. Such polyelectrolyte microcapsules were obtained using a layer-by-layer technique (see Section 8.3.3). This permitted for the tailoring of the composition of the wall, and the incorporation of metal nanoparticles (Fig. 8.24). In biological systems, it is desirable to trigger drug release in the near-infrared (NIR), around 800–1200 nm, as most tissues show negligible absorption in this region. Indeed, the absorption of gold nanoparticles incorporated in a polymeric capsule wall is red-shifted to the NIR (700–1500 nm) compared to the absorption of individual gold nanoparticles (around 500 nm). Such gold nanoparticles should thus absorb under *in vivo* conditions [171]. It has further been shown that fluorescein isocyanate (FITC)-labeled dextran [165] and rhodamine-labeled polystyrenesulfate (PSS-Rh) [166], convenient models for high-molecular-weight biomolecules, can be loaded into the capsules by exploiting the pH dependence of the shell permeability and then released on demand from the capsules by irradiation with 10-ns pulses of laser light at 1064 nm. These systems are thus promising vehicles for triggered topical or endoscopic drug delivery. Recently, the surface of such light-responsive polyelectrolyte/gold nanocapsules has been functionalized

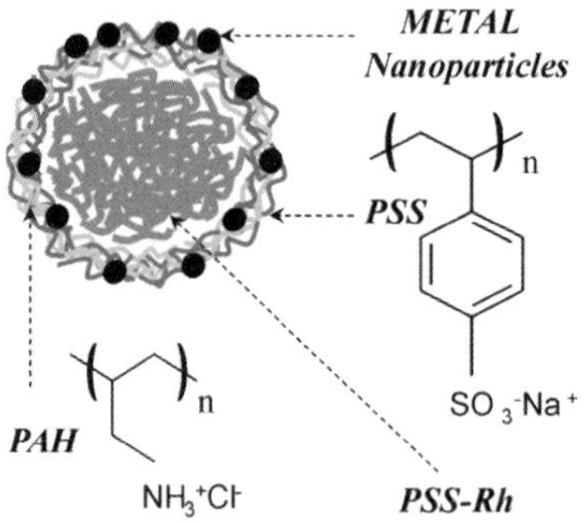

Figure 8.24. Schematic representation of a polyelectrolyte multilayer capsule incorporating PSS-Rh. The polyelectrolyte multilayer walls consist of PSS and PAH polymers and metal nanoparticles.

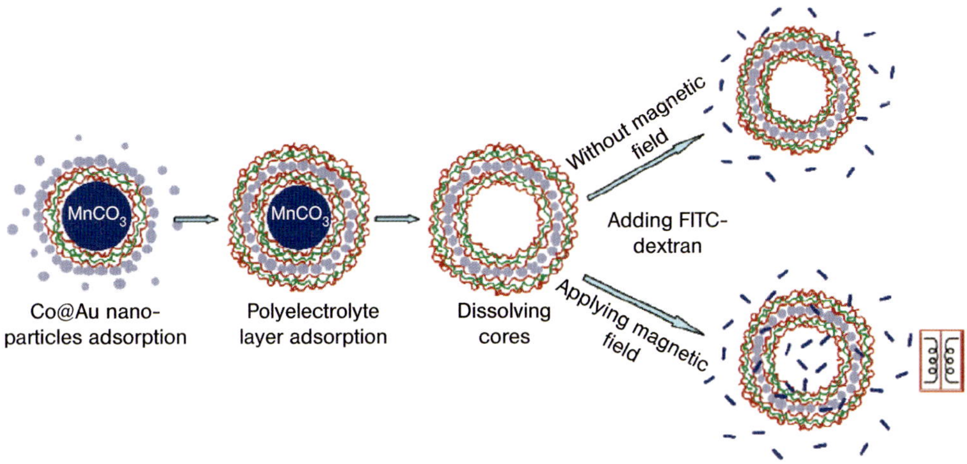

Figure 8.25. Scheme of the assembly and permeability test for microcapsules embedded with Co@Au nanoparticles under an oscillating magnetic field.

by model ligands (monoclonal immunoglobulin G antibodies), which opens new possibilities to targeted light-responsive drug delivery [165].

Similar to this work, magnetic fields has been used to trigger release from polyelectrolyte microcapsules. These capsules were designed to be more or less permeable to macromolecules depending on the application of a magnetic field. Indeed, ferromagnetic gold-coated cobalt nanoparticles (3 nm) ("Co@Au") were embedded inside the capsule wall made of bilayers of poly(sodium styrene sulfonate)/poly(allylamine hydrochloride) (PSS/PAH). It could be shown that upon application of an external alternating magnetic field, the permeability of the capsules for hydrophilic macromolecules increased significantly due to the rapid movement of the embedded Co@Au nanoparticles. Figure 8.25 illustrates the synthesis of such particles by a layer-by-layer technique and shows how dextran can be encapsulated in such particles upon application of an oscillating magnetic field inducing an enhanced permeability of the capsule wall. This process was found to be reversible and the triggered release of dextran could be demonstrated [167].

Finally, magnetites of a suitable size and magnetic properties have also been used for magnetic heating [173]. The phenomenon of magnetic hyperthermia may be exploited for colloidal drug carrier systems that are composed of magnetites embedded in a thermoresponsive polymer matrix (exhibiting LCST). In fact, the application of a magnetic field leads to the heating of the colloidal system and may induce the phase transition of the thermosensitive polymers. Consequently, the release or entrapment of a drug may be triggered. Indeed biocompatible polymer drug carriers, which released drugs in response to the application of a high-frequency magnetic field, have been reported [174].

8.5.2 Diagnosis

Polymeric nanoparticles have found great interest not only as drug delivery systems, but they have also been used as carrier systems of molecules/labels that allow for their detection *in vivo* and *in vitro*. Labeling nanoparticles allows for their (optical) imaging, and thus provides a valuable tool to follow the delivery vehicle on its journey through the body, to elucidate the real-time cellular localization of nanoparticles and to determine their *in vivo* distribution after administration. It is a powerful means to ascertain whether successful delivery to the desired organ or tissue structure can take place.

As an example, the monitoring of optically labeled drug delivery devices in the field of tumor targeting is one of the many applications in which the imaging process has been implanted successfully. Indeed, many of the same techniques used to reach delivery of drugs to cancerous tissues may also be used to target imaging agents. In fact, as targeted delivery systems approach the stage where they can be used clinically, primary assessment of the utility of a particular colloidal formulation in a particular patient may be made with imaging agents to verify that the delivery system goes rapidly to the cancerous tissues before any drug regimen is begun.

Apart from that labeled polymeric nanocarrier have found rising interest as diagnostics, i.e. in the field of medical imaging [magnetic resonance imaging (MRI), etc.] to detect morbid tissues and diseases. The interest of using polymeric nanoparticles as diagnostic tools (by encapsulating the diagnostic label) relies in (i) its size, (ii) the possibility of using biocompatible materials and (iii) the possibility of modifying the surface of the colloidal vehicle to achieve targeting devices. As explained in Section 8.1, the nanoparticles' size allows for the passive targeting of organs such as the liver or spleen, whereas the use of coating materials (e.g. PEO) permits the passive targeting of cancerous tissues (due to the enhanced permeability of blood vessels), together with an enhanced residence time (half-life time) in the blood. In addition, the surface functionalization of nanoparticles by specific probes/molecules allows the active targeting of specific cellular districts.

The following gives a nonexhaustive overview on the different types of diagnostic systems based on polymeric nanoparticles. It is structured with regard to the different labels (fluorescent dyes, contrast agents for MRI, quantum dots, gold nanoparticles, radiolabeled nanoparticles, nanoparticles for ultrasound imaging). Furthermore, their utility for *in vitro* (immunoassays, biosensors, etc.) and *in vivo* tests (MRI, etc.) is mentioned.

8.5.2.1 Fluorescence Labeling of Polymeric Nanoparticles

8.5.2.1.1 Organic Fluorescent Dyes Fluorescent labeling is a widely used and convenient tool in biology and biological imaging. In the field of drug delivery, it has been used to (i) simulate drug release (establishment of release profiles) or (ii) to localize nanoparticles and understand their fate after administration. The fluorescent label has to be chosen depending on the purpose and the physicochemical properties of the nanoparticles. In the first case (i), the fluorescent dye is used as a model drug and should therefore have similar physicochemical properties as the drug. For instance, commercially available FITC-labeled dextran ("FD-4") and tetramethylrhodamine-labeled dextran have often been used as a model for hydrophilic macromolecular "drugs" (such as proteins) to study their release profile from nanospheres [143] and nanocapsules [165].

For diagnostic applications (case ii), however, a durable encapsulation of the dye is desired, requiring good affinity of the dye for the nanoparticles material. For instance, small organic hydrophobic fluorescent molecules (rhodamine [175], fluorescein [176], etc.) are suitable for nanoparticles made of hydrophobic polymers or nanocapsules with an oily core [146]. In the case of PLGA nanoparticles labeled by lipophilic 3-(2-benzothiazolyl)-7-(diethylamino)coumarin ("coumarin 6") [177], it has been demonstrated that the nanoparticles' physical properties, such as particle size and ζ potential, were not significantly different from those of unloaded nanoparticles. As to the preparation, the small organic fluorescent molecule is generally dissolved together with the core-forming polymer during the nanoparticle preparation. These fluorescent nanoparticles thus allow the calculation of the amount of fluorescent carriers taken up by cells (*in vivo* or *in vitro*) by fluorimetry.

However, particles labeled by "free" fluorescein rapidly released this fluorescent probe in the medium used for the biological investigation [176], as a consequence of diffusion. Thus, recent developments tend focus on covalently conjugate/link fluorescent dyes to (co)polymers in order to avoid diffusion of the dyes from the polymer matrix of nanoparticles to the surrounding medium, e.g. fluorescein has been conjugated to PLGA end-capped by a carboxylic group using carbodiimide chemistry in order to diminish the diffusion from the fluorescent dye from PLGA nanoparticles [178].

8.5.2.1.2 **Quantum Dots** Semiconductor nanocrystals (also known as quantum dots) are emerging as a new class of fluorescent probes for *in vitro* and *in vivo* biomolecular and cellular imaging [179, 180]. In comparison with organic dyes and fluorescent proteins, quantum dots, whose size ranges from 1 to 10 nm in radius, have unique optical and electronic properties, including sharp emission spectra (with full width at half maximum as narrow as 25 nm) improved signal brightness and photostability [181], resistance against photobleaching (long fluorescent lifetime), and tunable size dependent emission peaks. Due to their broad excitation profiles and narrow/symmetric emission spectra, high-quality quantum dots are also well-suited for multicolor optical coding for biological assays, by combining different color quantum dots with different intensity levels. Quantum dots are mostly synthesized in nonpolar organic solvents, such as tri-*n*-octylphosphine oxide, which coordinate on the surface of quantum dots to prevent the formation of bulk semiconductors. As a result, the nanoparticles are capped with a monolayer of organic ligands and are soluble only in nonpolar organic solvents. However, for biological imaging, quantum dots must be water-soluble. To address this, different strategies have been devised including ligand exchange with thiol-functionalized molecules, and encapsulation by a layer of diblock or triblock copolymers or else in silica shells, phospholipid micelles or polymer beads. Further developments in biological applications of quantum dots aimed to functionalize the surface of quantum dots by bioaffinity ligands, such as monoclonal antibodies, peptides, oligonucleotides or carbohydrates. Thus, hydrophilic α-mannopyranosyl moieties have been linked to a phosphine oxide, which could then be used as ligand in the surface-functionalized hydrophilic quantum dots [182]. Furthermore attachment of PEG could lead to improved biocompatibility and reduced nonspecific interactions [183]. Such bioconjugated quantum dots thus have raised new possibilities for ultrasensitive and multiplexed imaging of molecular targets in living cells, animal models and, possibly, in humans.

Recent works have focused on the encapsulation of the nanocrystals in natural or synthetic polymeric materials to form "bigger" quantum dot–polymer composites in the range of some hundreds of nanometers. Such systems were expected to reduce the toxicity of quantum dots and to be suitable for further conjugation with biomolecules, while maintaining the high emission quantum yield of the quantum dots. It should be emphasized that the use of a polymeric matrix also opens up the possibility of incorporating several probes (quantum dots of different size), allowing in particular multiplexed optical coding. In the following, we will focus on quantum dot–polymer composites.

Several strategies to embed quantum dots in polymer matrices have been envisaged. Quantum dots have been incorporated either by noncovalent interactions, such as electrostatic and hydrophobic interactions, or by copolymerization of monomers with quantum dots surrounded by polymerizable ligands.

In 2003, Chen and coworkers developed an interesting method to assemble negatively charged CdSe–ZnS quantum dots into glyconanospheres through electrostatic interactions with carboxymethyldextran and poly(lysine). To enhance the long-term stability of these glyconanosphere composites built by the layer-by-layer procedure, quantum dots were cross-linked with the polysaccharide matrix by covalent amide bonds. Spherical luminescent glyconanospheres of an average diameter of 190 nm were thus obtained. The presence of glucose residues at the surface of the nanoparticles was evidenced by fluorescent imaging microscopy; indeed, upon addition of a carbohydrate-binding protein, Con A, the glyconanoparticles aggregated (Fig. 8.26(A)). As shown in Fig. 8.26(B), this aggregation was, however, prevented when free α-D-glucose was added, since glucose effectively competes with the glyconanospheres on the binding sites of Con A. These quantum dot–polysaccharide composites are thus promising tools for real-time monitoring of carbohydrate–protein (lectin) interactions that are critical steps in bacterial and viral infection [140].

On the basis of hydrophobic interactions, polymeric microbeads loaded with quantum dots could be prepared, allowing multiplexed/multicolor optical probing for biological assays. Several groups have successfully incorporated quantum dots into polymeric nanoparticles via polymerization in dispersed media [184–187]. Hydrophobic quantum dots (ZnS-capped CdSe nanocrystals) with different sizes were

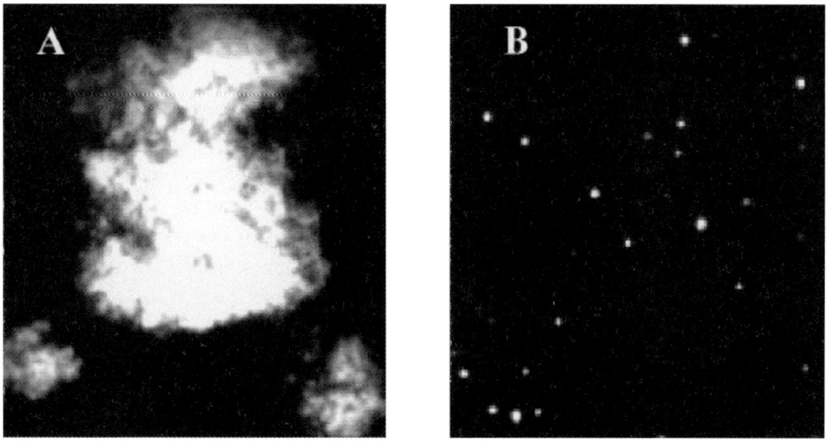

Figure 8.26. Lectin (Con A) initiated aggregation of CdSe–ZnS quantum dot luminescent glyconanospheres. (A) Luminescence image of aggregated glyconanospheres in the presence of Con A. (B) Luminescence image of the glyconanospheres in the presence of Con A and free α-D-glucose molecules. The latter compete with the glyconanospheres for the Con A binding sites and prevent nanoparticle aggregation.

thus embedded at precisely controlled ratios in the outer layer of swollen polystyrene polymer beads, previously prepared by miniemulsion polymerization of styrene, divinylstyrene and acrylic acid (98:1:1). The quantum dot-loaded particles were sealed by a silica layer, then, streptavidin molecules were covalenty coupled to the surface via the carboxylic acid groups of acrylic acid [184]. Biomolecular probes, such as oligonucleotides or antibodies, were then conjugated to the silica surface via streptavidin–biotin complex formation. The fluorescence spectra of the quantum dot-tagged beads (1.2 μm) were narrow (even narrower than those of free quantum dots) and the emission maxima remained unchanged, which indicates that the beads were highly uniform and reproducible, and that the beads were spatially separated by the beads structure. Thanks to the identification code embedded in the interior of the beads, bead identification accuracies as high as 99.9% could be reached. This approach allows combining molecular recognition and optical "barcoding" by polymeric beads, which is expected to open new opportunities in gene expression studies, high-throughput screening and medical diagnostics [184]. In comparison with bigger (150 μm × 150 μm × 150 μm) planar DNA chips, encoded-bead technology is expected to be more flexible regarding target selection (e.g. adding new genes or single-nucleotide mutations), to show faster binding kinetics (similar to that in homogenous solution) and to be less expensive to produce.

In contrast to these approaches based on the noncovalent immobilization of quantum dots in polymeric materials, O'Brien and coworkers adapted an approach previously reported by Emrick and coworkers [188] and covalently incorporated quantum dots into a polymer matrix using suspension polymerization. Thus, they prepared quantum dots surrounded by polymerizable ligands and copolymerized them with styrene using DVB as crosslinking agent. This facile procedure seems very promising for the commercialization of many bead-types with diameters ranging from 100 nm to 500 μm, where the CdS quantum dots are evenly distributed throughout the polystyrene spheres. These quantum dot–polymer composites may be used for optical biological probing/assays or combinatory chemistry applications (in solid phase organic chemistry), benefiting from quantum dots encoding [189, 190]. Employing miniemulsion polymerization, Elaissairi and coworkers synthesized quite monodisperse (100–350 nm) quantum dot-tagged colloids by copolymerization of styrene with vinyl-functionalized quantum dots [191]. Very recently, another promising approach to covalently incorporate quantum dots in latexes was proposed by Esteves and coworkers [192]. Indeed, they applied radical polymerization to miniemulsion using ATRP and initiated the miniemulsion polymerization of butyl acrylate by quantum dots functionalized by an ATRP initiator.

In conclusion, the use of fluorescent nanocrystal–polymer composites opens up new possibilities for designing luminescent surface-modified nanoparticles to deliver quantum dots specifically to the targeted tissue or cells. These luminescent quantum dots are ideal fluorophores for biological labeling because their fluorescence emission wavelength can be continuously tuned by changing the particle size and a single wavelength can be used for simultaneous excitation of different sized quantum dots. The unique properties of luminescent quantum dots thus allow multicolor experiments in cellular imaging and diagnosis, offering substantial advantages over organic dyes in multiplexed target detection.

8.5.2.2 **Contrast Agents for MRI**

MRI is based on the NMR signal of hydrogen present in body tissues (water, membrane lipids, proteins, etc.). It is currently the most important available diagnostic method and as a noninvasive technique routinely clinically used for diagnostic imaging. However, the intrinsic sensitivity and selectivity of conventional MRI techniques is very low. It has been clearly shown that the use of contrast agents, which alter the relaxivity of water, can greatly improve the sensitivity and thus the diagnostic value of MRI.

The first generation of contrast agents consists of high-spin paramagnetic ions (Gd^{3+} chelates) that are at present routinely used as MRI contrast agents. More recently, magnetic nanoparticles, with a size generally between 3 and 10 nm, have been used as contrast agents for MRI. Due to their size, these superparamagnetic nanoparticles accumulate in MPS organs (passive targeting). Third-generation magnetic nanoparticles are surface-modified by specific ligands, such as antibodies, allowing the specific targeting of cells/tissues.

Recent works tend to incorporate magnetic nanoparticles in larger polymeric nanoparticles. Such relatively "big" polymer nanoparticles are expected to passively target tumors. In addition, targeting moieties may be attached at the surface of the latter (active targeting). For this purpose, polymeric nanoparticles decorated

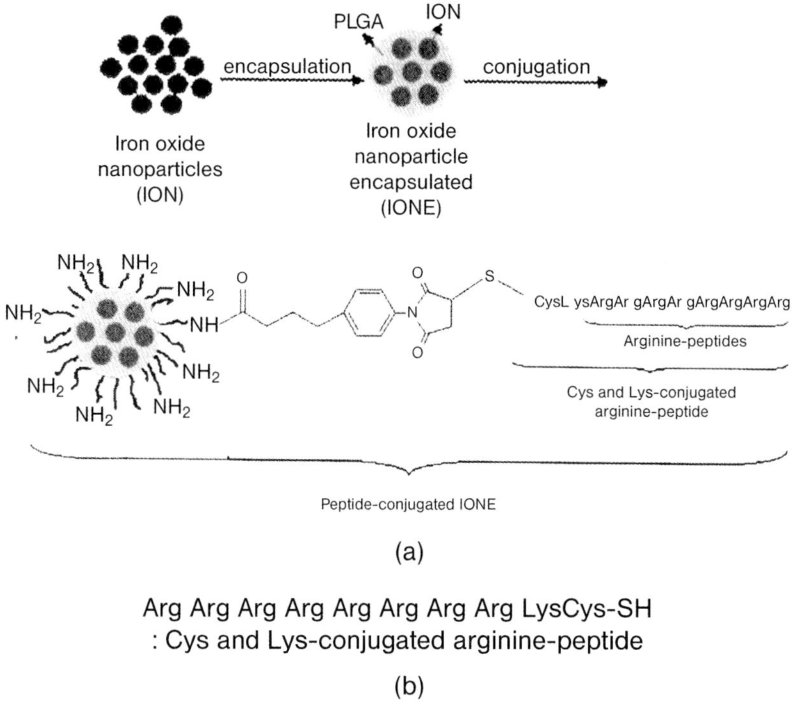

Figure 8.27. (a) Schematic diagram for preparing the γ-Fe_2O_3–PLGA–Arg–FITC nanoparticles. (b) Sequence of arginine peptide.

by targeting molecules and labeled by contrast agents have been designed. One interesting work published recently reports on the synthesis of a novel intracellular polymeric carrier as a MR molecular image diagnostic agent. Here, superparamagnetic iron oxide nanoparticles were encapsulated with peptide-conjugated PLGA using an emulsification-diffusion method. In addition, these polymer nanoparticles were labeled twice: first, by encapsulation of metallic nanoparticles for MRI and, second, by a fluorescent dye for detection by fluorescence microscopy; actually, a FTIC-conjugated arginine peptide, a "cell penetration peptide", was conjugated via its thiol group to maleimide-derivatized PLGA. Thus, nanoparticles of 110 nm diameter have been synthesized allowing for combined targeting and multiple/versatile detection [193] (Fig. 8.27).

Aside from their use in MRI, there are multiple other applications of magnetic particles encapsulated in polymer beads which are illustrated in the following.

8.5.2.3 Magnetic Nanoparticles for *In Vitro* Assays

Increasing interest has been focused on the preparation of surface-modified latexes, and their use as solid supports of biomolecules in biomedical diagnostics

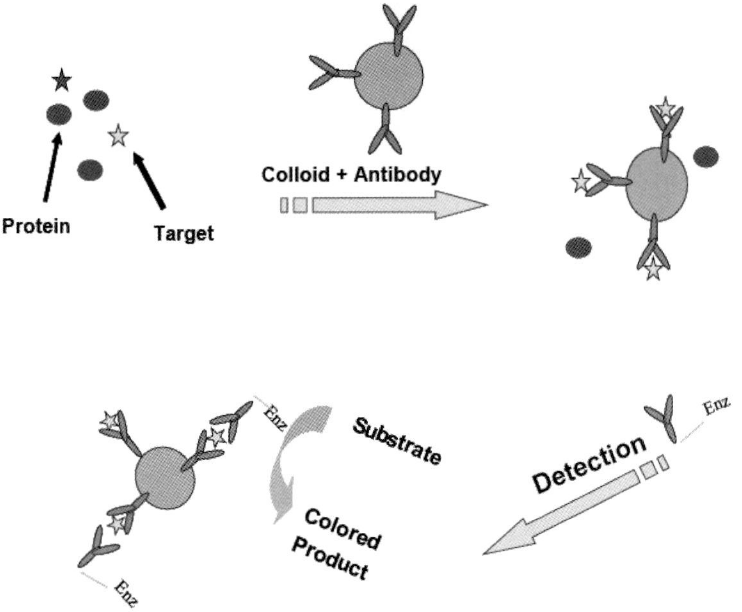

Figure 8.28. Schematic representation of the specific capture and detection of the targeted antigen (ELISA).

and purification of biological materials. The particular interest in using such colloidal systems for biomedical diagnostic systems relies on their high specific surface. Due to their size, surface-modified latex beads have been used for the capture of biological materials, their purification and concentration, and more specifically in immunoassays. In fact, the size of the nanoparticles allows their separation from the biological medium by centrifugation. Recent studies tend towards the use of magnetic latex particles. Magnetism is used here as an easy tool to separate the nanoparticles, replacing the centrifugation step applied in the case of classical non-magnetic particles. Similar to the latter, magnetic latex nanoparticles are principally used as a solid support for biomolecules involved in the specific capture of targeted biomolecules, such as antigens for immunoassays [i.e. ELISA, Fig. 8.28, and nucleic acid detection in "enzyme-linked oligosorbent assay" (ELOSA), Fig. 8.29]. For that purpose, magnetic latex particles bearing either immobilized antibodies or ODNs, complementary to the single stranded DNA of interest, are used.

Furthermore, such nanoparticles can be used for the nonspecific capture of biomolecules or viruses [194] in order to concentrate or to purify samples. In fact, this process is based on the well-controlled adsorption of biomolecules on the colloidal particles, followed by the concentration of the nanoparticles and, finally, the desorption of the adsorbed biomolecules. Thus, for the capture of nucleic acids, cationic magnetic colloids are used in order to favor attractive electrostatic interactions. Adsorption and desorption are controlled by monitoring the pH and the salinity of

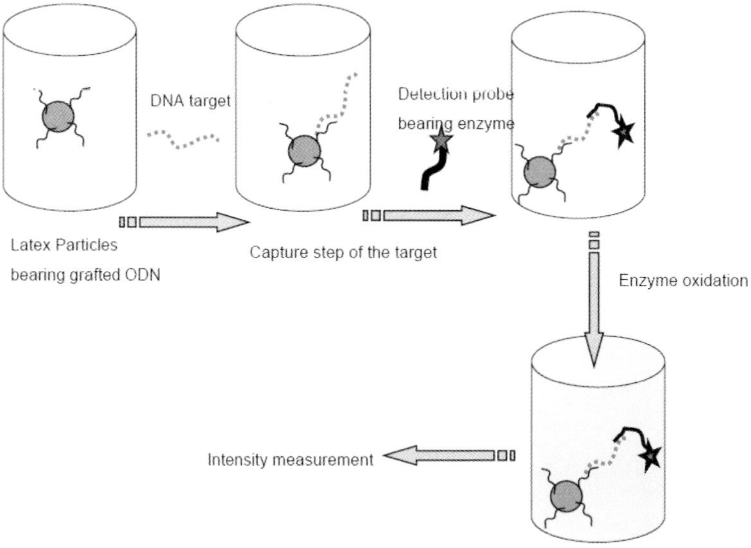

Figure 8.29. Schematic representation of the specific capture and detection of targeted DNA or RNA (ELOSA).

the medium [195]. Similarly, magnetic latex particles with a hydrophobic surface have been successfully used for the extraction, purification and concentration of proteins. Indeed, as mentioned in Section 8.1, unspecific adsorption of proteins on surfaces is mainly governed by hydrophobic attractive forces, such as van der Waals forces [196].

The synthesis of "smart" magnetic colloids has also been reported. Thus, thermosensitive magnetic latex particles have been synthesized, allowing the controlled adsorption, concentration and desorption of proteins [197]. At temperatures above the LCST, thermosensitive polymers undergo a phase transition from a hydrophilic to a hydrophobic state. Thus, nanoparticles with a thermosensitive PNIPAAm shell showed a volume phase transition temperature (T_{VPT}), below which protein adsorption was low (due to the hydrophilic character of the particle surface) and above which the adsorption was considerably high [198].

Recently, an interesting approach for the synthesis of fluorescent magnetic nanoparticles that possess reactive carboxylic acid groups at their surface was reported. First, fluorescent polystyrene nanodots (25 nm) were adsorbed onto magnetic emulsions (250 nm) via electrostatic interactions. The surface of these "hydride" particles was then sealed by adsorbing film-forming polymer nanobeads (40 nm) on their surface and heating above the grass transition temperature (T_g) [199].

A representative review about magnetic colloids, their preparation and their use in biomedical diagnostics was given by Elaissari [200]. The incorporation of magnetic nanoparticles in polymer beads is thus a promising tool in the field of diagnosis and triggered drug delivery, but they can also serve as therapeutic systems. In fact, magnetic nanoparticles have potential therapeutic applications as they can locally induce hyperthermia by application of an alternating magnetic field. This magnetically induced hyperthermia remains promising for cancer therapy aside from conventional methods, such as surgery, chemotherapy and radiotherapy [173]. Depending on the temperature, hyperthermia can be used either for immune stimulation (41–46 °C) or tumor destruction (46–56 °C).

As illustrated in Section 8.1, encapsulating magnetic nanoparticles in a submicron polymeric vehicle allows for the size-controlled "passive targeting" to tumoral tissue. Besides, they are suitable for surface functionalization by targeting biomolecules. In fact, the combination of magnetic particles in a drug-containing polymeric matrix that is sensitive to temperature is a very comprising approach. As developed in Section 8.5.1.3, the release of drugs embedded in a stimuli-responsive polymer can be induced by various stimuli, such as pH or temperature. Intracellular drug release from polymeric nanoparticles could thus be triggered by the temperature increase during the hyperthermia sequence under MRI monitoring. Instead of using thermosensitive polymers (e.g. PNIPAAm), such a mechanism could also use thermolabile bonds [174].

8.5.2.4 Electron Dense Agents for Transmission Electron Microscopy (TEM)

Organic fluorescent labels allow studying intracellular nanoparticle uptake and distribution using confocal fluorescence microscopy. More precise TEM observation requires the labeling of the nanoparticles by an electron-dense agent. For that purpose, e.g. PLGA nanoparticles have been successfully loaded with osmium tetroxide – a widely used staining agent for TEM observation [177].

Another approach relies on the labeling by gold nanoparticles. For this purpose, the surface of gold nanoparticles must be modified in order to enhance/optimize their affinity to the nanoparticles' core-forming polymer. Indeed, Qiu and coworkers successfully encapsulated gold nanoparticles surface-modified by PLA chains in PLA nanospheres [58].

8.5.2.5 Radiolabeled Nanoparticles

For a long time, radiolabeled (e.g. ^{3}H, ^{14}C) polymers have been synthesized for nanoparticles, and then the radioactivity could be quantified in order to elucidate their uptake and distribution [10, 201]. However, this method necessitates not only the synthesis of radiolabeled polymers, which require special laboratories, but also expensive equipment for the quantification.

8.6 Conclusion and Perspectives

Polymeric nanoparticles are of particular interest due to their size, the wide range of polymeric materials available, and the possibility to tailor-make both the constituting elements and the nanoparticles. Furthermore, recent developments in (polymer) chemistry, biology, biotechnology and physics have drastically enlarged the use and importance of polymeric nanoparticles. For drug delivery purposes, polymeric nanoparticles no longer possess only a protecting role, while releasing drugs in a controlled way. They are rather "Trojan" horses that allow drug delivery to a selected target, such as cancerous cells, organs or even viruses. Further trends go towards smart colloidal drug delivery systems that release drugs in response to an external trigger, such as light or a magnetic field, or even in response to an physiological internal trigger, such as pH, glucose concentration, etc.

Nanoparticles possessing targeting moieties on their surface have also found applications in diagnosis. In fact, the surface functionalization of fluorescent and magnetic colloids allows the selective detection of, for example, a tumor expressing specific antibodies at its surface. The latest developments in quantum dots technology allowing multiplexed sensing have been a revolution in the field of diagnostics.

Nowadays, the developments in polymeric nanoparticles tend towards multifunctional nanoparticles, which allow simultaneous targeting, imaging and treatment by one single system. Monitoring of the localization of the drug in a living system and the release of the drug as response to an external trigger is no longer a dream. First attempts of such combined drug delivery systems have been already proposed as "nanoclinics" [202], i.e. complex surface-functionalized polymeric nanoparticles that contain various probes for diagnostics and drugs for targeted delivery in one single unit.

References

1 Thurmond, K. B., Kowalewski, T., Wooley, K. L., Water-soluble knedel-like structures: the preparation of shell-cross-linked small particles. *J. Am. Chem. Soc.* **1996**, *118*, 7239–7240.

2 Torchilin, V. P., Long circulating microparticulate systems. *J. Microencapsul.* **1998**, *15*, 1–19.

3 Gref, R., Minamitake, Y., Peracchia, M. T., Trubetskoy, V., Torchilin, V., Langer, R., Biodegradable long-circulating polymeric nanospheres. *Science* **1994**, *263*, 1600–1603.

4 Labarre, D., Vauthier, C., Chauvierre, C., Petri, B., Müller, R., Chehimi, M. M., Interactions of blood proteins with poly(isobutylcyanoacrylate) nanoparticles decorated with a polysaccharidic brush. *Biomaterials* **2005**, *26*, 5075–5084.

5 Passirani, C., Barratt, G., Devissaguet, J.-P., Labarre, D., Interactions of nanoparticles bearing heparin or dextran covalently bound to poly(methyl methacrylate) with the complement system. *Life Science* **1998**, *62*, 775–785.

6 Österberg, E., Bergstrom, K., Holmberg, K., Schuman, T. P., Riggs, J. A., Burns, N. L., Van Alstine, J. M., Harris, J. M., Protein-rejecting ability of surface-bound dextran in end-on and side-on configurations: comparison with PEO. *J. Biomed. Mater. Res.* **1995**, *29*, 741–747.

7 Maeda, H., Wu, J., Sawa, T., Matsumara, Y., Hori, K., Tumor vascular permeability and the EPR effect in macromolecular therapeutics: a review. *J. Control. Release* **2000**, *65*, 271–284.

8 Brigger, I., Dubernet, C., Couvreur, P., Nanoparticles in cancer therapy and diagnosis. *Adv. Drug Deliv. Rev.* **2002**, *54*, 631–651.

9 Ruoslahti, E., Pierschbacher, M. D., New perspectives in cell adhesion:

RGD and integrins. *Science* **1987**, *238*, 491–497.

10 Gref, R., Couvreur, P., Barratt, G., Mysiakine, E., Surface-engineered nanoparticles for multiple ligand coupling. *Biomaterials* **2003**, *24*, 4529–4537.

11 Brannon-Peppas, L., Blanchette, J. O., Nanoparticle and targeted systems for cancer therapy. *Adv. Drug Deliv. Rev.* **2004**, *56*, 1649–1659.

12 Janes, K. A., Calvo, P., Alonso, M. J., Polysaccharide colloidal particles as delivery systems for macromolecules. *Adv. Drug Deliv. Rev.* **2001**, *47*, 83–97.

13 Dumitriu, S., Polysaccharides as biomaterials. In *Polymeric Biomaterials*, 2nd edn, Dumitriu, S. (Ed.). Marcel Dekker, New York, **2002**, pp. 1–61.

14 Lemarchand, C., Gref, R., Couvreur, P., Polysaccharide-decorated nanoparticles. *Eur. J. Pharm. Biopharm.* **2004**, *58*, 327–341.

15 Kawashima, Y., Yamamoto, H., Takeuchi, H., Kuno, Y., Mucoadhesive DL-lactide/glycolide copolymer nanospheres coated with chitosan to improve oral delivery of elcatonin. *Pharm. Dev. Technol.* **2000**, *5*, 77–85.

16 Alonso, M. J., Calvo, P., Remuñan, C., Vila, A., Jato, J. L., Application of nanoparticles based on hydrophilic polymers as pharmaceutical forms. *EU 0 860 166 A1.*

17 Hendricks, S. K., Kwok, C., Shen, M., Horbett, B. D., Ratner, B. D., Bryers, J. D., Plasma-deposited membranes for controlled release of antibiotic to prevent bacterial adhesion and biofilm formation. *J. Biomed. Mater. Res.* **2000**, *50*, 160–170.

18 Schatz, C., Bionaz, A., Lucas, J.-M., Pichot, C., Viton, C., Domard, A., Delair, T., Formation of polyelectrolyte complex particles from self-complexation of *N*-sulfated chitosan. *Biomacromolecules* **2005**, *6*, 1642–1647.

19 Yamamoto, H., Kuno, Y., Sugimoto, S., Takeuchi, H., Kawashima, Y., Surface-modified PLGA nanosphere with chitosan improved pulmonary delivery of calcitonin by mucoadhesion and opening of the intercellular tight junctions. *J. Control. Release* **2005**, *102*, 373–381.

20 Borchard, G., Luessen, H. L., De Boer, A. G., Verhoef, J. C., Lehr, C. M., Junginger, H. E., The potential of mucoadhesive polymers in enhancing intestinal peptide drug absorption. 3. Effects of chitosan-glutamate and carbomer on epithelial tight junctions *in vitro*. *J. Control. Release* **1996**, *39*, 131–138.

21 Agnihotri, S. A., Mallikarjuna, N. N., Aminabhavi, T. M., Recent advances on chitosan-based micro- and nanoparticles in drug delivery. *J. Control. Release*, **2004**, *100*, 5–28.

22 Takeuchi, H., Yamamoto, H., Kawashima, Y., Mucoadhesive nanoparticulate systems for peptide drug delivery. *Adv. Drug Deliv. Rev.* **2001**, *47*, 39–54.

23 Felt, O., Einmahl, S., Gurny, R., Furrer, F., Baeyens, V., Polymeric systems for ophthalmic drug delivery. In *Polymeric Biomaterials*, 2nd edn, Dumitriu, S. (Ed.). Marcel Dekker, New York, **2002**, pp. 377–421.

24 Balazs, E. A., Why hyaluronan has so many biological activities? In *New Frontiers in Medical Sciences: Redefining Hyaluronan*, Abatangelo, G., Weigel, P. H. (Eds.). Elsevier Science, Amsterdam, **2000**, pp. 3–10.

25 Lemarchand, C., Couvreur, P., Besnard, M., Costantini, D., Gref, R., Novel polyester-polysaccharide nanoparticles. *Pharm Res* **2003**, *20*, 1284–1292.

26 Domb, A. J., Kumar, N., Sheskin, T., Bentolila, A., Slager, J., Teomim, D., Biodegradable polymers as drug carrier systems. In *Polymeric Biomaterials*, 2nd edn, Dumitriu, S. (Ed.). Marcel Dekker, New York, **2002**, pp. 91–121.

27 Vert, M., Mauduit, L., Suming, L., Biodegradation of PLA/GA polymers: increasing complexity. *Biomaterials* **1994**, *15*, 1209–1213.

28 Grizzi, I., Garreau, H., Li, S., Vert, M., Hydrolytic degradation of devices based on poly(DL-lactic acid) size-dependence. *Biomaterials* **1995**, *15*, 305–311.

29 Park, T. G., Degradation of poly(lactic-*co*-glycolic acid) microspheres: effect of copolymer composition. *Biomaterials* **1995**, *16*, 1123 1130.

30 Lenz, R. W., Guerin, P., Functional polyesters and polyamides for medical application of biodegradable polymers. In *Polymers in Medicine: Functional Polyesters and Polyamides for Medical Applications of Biodegradable Polymers*, Chiellini, E., Giusti, P. (Eds.). Plenum Press, New York, **1983**, pp. 219–230.

31 Lee, B.-S., Vert, M., Holler, E., Water-soluble aliphatic polyesters: poly(malic acid)s. In *Biopolymers*, Doi, Y., Steinbüchel, A. (Eds.). Wiley-VCH, Weinheim, **2002**, Vol. 3a, pp. 75–103.

32 Tian, D., Dubois, P., Jérôme, R., Macromolecular engineering of polylactones and polylactides. 22. Copolymerization of epsilon-caprolactone and 1,4,8-trioxaspiro[4.6]-9-undecanone initiated by aluminum isopropoxide. *Macromolecules* **1997**, *30*, 2575–2581.

33 Detrembleur, C., Mazza, M., Halleux, O., Lecomte, P., Mecerreyes, D., Hedrick, J. L., Jérôme, R., Ring-opening polymerization of gamma-bromo-epsilon-caprolactone: a novel route to functionalized aliphatic polyesters. *Macromolecules* **2000**, *33*, 14–18.

34 Latere, J.-P., Lecomte, P., Dubois, P., Jérôme, R., 2-oxepane-1,5-dione: a precursor of a novel class of versatile semicrystalline biodegradable (co)polyesters. *Macromolecules* **2002**, *35*, 7857–7859.

35 Riva, R., Schmeits, S., Stoffelbach, F., Jérôme, C., Jérôme, R., Lecomte, P., Combination of ring-opening polymerization and "click" chemistry towards functionalization of aliphatic polyesters. *Chem. Commun.* **2005**, *42*, 5334–5336.

36 Rieger, J., Bernaerts, K. V., Du Prez, F. E., Jérôme, R., Jérôme, C., Lactone end-capped poly(ethylene oxide) as a new building block for biomaterials. *Macromolecules* **2004**, *37*, 9738–9745.

37 Kawaguchi, T., Nakano, M., Juni, K., Inoue, S., Yoshida, Y., Release profiles of 5-fluorouracil and its derivatives from polycarbonate *in vitro*. *Chem. Pharm. Bull.* **1982**, *30*, 1517–1520.

38 Kawaguchi, T., Nakano, M., Juni, K., Inoue, S., Yoshida, Y., Examination of biodegradability of poly(ethylene carbonate) and poly(propylene carbonate) in the peritoneal cavity in rats. *Chem. Pharm. Bull.* **1983**, *31*, 1400–1403.

39 Anderson, J. M., Spilizewski, K. L., Hiltner, A., Poly α-amino acids as biomedical polymers. In *Biocompatibility of Tissue Analogs*, Williams, D. F. (Ed.). CRC Press, Boca Raton, FL, **1985**, Vol. 1, pp. 67–88.

40 Webster, I., West, P. J., Adhesives for medical applications. In *Polymeric Biomaterials*, 2nd edn, Dumitriu, S. (Ed.). Marcel Dekker, New York, pp. 717–737.

41 Müller, R., Lherm, C., Herbort, P., Couvreur, P., In vitro model for the degradation of alkylcyanoacrylate nanoparticles. *Biomaterials* **1990**, *11*, 590–595.

42 Leonard, F., Kulkarni, R. K., Brandes, G., Nelson, J., Mameron, J. J., Synthesis and degradation of poly(alkylcyanoacrylates). *J. Applied Polym. Sci.* **1966**, *10*, 259–272.

43 Gil, E. S., Hudson, S. M., Stimuli-responsive polymers and their bioconjugates. *Prog. Polym. Sci.* **2004**, *29*, 1173–1222.

44 De las Heras Alarcón, C., Pennadam, S., Alexander, C., Stimuli-responsive polymers for biomedical applications. *Chem. Soc. Rev.* **2005**, *34*, 276–285.

45 Lee, J. H., Lee, H. B., Andrade, J. D., Blood Compatibility of poly(ethylene oxide) surfaces. *Prog. Polym. Sci.* **1995**, *20*, 1043–1979.

46 Vermette, P., Meagher, L., Interactions of phospholipid- and poly(ethylene glycol)-modified surfaces with biological systems: relation to physico-chemical properties and mechanism. *Coll. Surf. B Biointerfaces* **2003**, *28*, 153–198.

47 Peracchia, M. T., Stealth nanoparticles for intravenous administration. *STP Pharma. Sci.* **2003**, *13*, 155–161.
48 Otsuka, H., Nagasaki, Y., Kataoka, K., PEGylated nanoparticles for biological and pharmaceutical applications. *Adv. Drug Deliv. Rev.* **2003**, *55*, 403–419.
49 Gref, R., Lück, M., Quellec, P., Marchand, M., Dellacherie, E., Harnisch, S., Blunk, T., Müller, R. H., "Stealth" corona–core nanoparticles surface modified by polyethylene glycol (PEG): influences of the corona (PEG chain length and surface density) and of the core composition on phagocytic uptake and plasma protein adsorption. *Coll. Surf. B Biointerfaces* **2000**, *18*, 301–313.
50 Quintanar-Guerrero, D., Allémann, E., Fessi, H., Doelker, E., Preparation techniques and mechanisms of formulation of biodegradable nanoparticles from preformed polymers. *Drug Dev. Ind. Pharm.* **1998**, *24*, 1113–1128.
51 Vanderhoff, J. W., El-Aasser, M. S., Ugelstad, J., Polymer emulsification process. *US Patent 4 177 177*, **1979**.
52 Blanco, M. D., Alonso, M. J., *Eur. J. Pharm. Biopharm.* **1997**, *43*, 287–294.
53 Allémann, E., Gurny, R., Doelker, E., Development and characterization of protein-loaded poly(lactide-*co*-glycolide) nanospheres. *Int. J. Pharm.* **1992**, *87*, 247–253.
54 Fessi, H., Puisieux, F., Devissaguet, J. P., Ammoury, N., Benita, S., Nanocapsule formation by interfacial polymer deposition following solvent displacement. *Int. J. Pharm.* **1989**, *55*, R1–R4.
55 Quintanar-Guerrero, D., Fessi, H., Allémann, E., Influence of stabilizing agents and preparative variables on the formation of poly(D,L-lactic acid) nanoparticles by a emulsion-diffusion technique. *Int. J. Pharm.* **1996**, *143*, 133–141.
56 Fessi, H., Puisieux, F., Devissaguet, J. P., Process for preparing a colloidal and disperse system in the shape of nanocapsules. *Eur. Patent 274 961*, **1986**.
57 Bilati, U., Allémann, Doelker, E., Development of a nanoprecipitation method intended for the entrapment of hydrophilic drugs into nanoparticles. *Eur. J. Pharm. Sci.* **2005**, *24*, 67–75.
58 Qiu, H., Rieger, J., Gilbert, B., Jérôme, R., Jérôme, C., PLA-Coated gold nanoparticles for the labeling of PLA biocarriers. *Chem. Mater.* **2004**, *16*, 850–856.
59 Vangeyte, P., Gautier, S., Jérôme, R., About the methods of preparation of poly(ethylene oxide)-*b*-poly(ε-caprolactone) nanoparticles in water analysis by dynamic light scattering. *Colloid Surf. A Physicochem. Eng. Asp.* **2004**, *242*, 203–211.
60 Antonietti, M., Landfester, K., Single molecule chemistry with polymers and colloids: a way to handle complex reactions and physical processes. *Chem. Phys. Chem.* **2001**, *2*, 207–210.
61 Landfester, K., Polyreactions in miniemulsions. *Macromol. Rapid Commun.* **2001**, *22*, 896–936.
62 Kishida, K., Akashi, A., Sakuma, M., Suzuki, S., Kikuchi, N., Hiwatari, H., Arikawa, K., Oral Peptide delivery using nanoparticles composed of novel graft copolymers having hydrophobic backbone and hydrophilic branches. *Int. J. Pharm.* **1997**, *149*, 93–106.
63 Durand, A., Marie, E., Rotureau, E., Leonard, M., Dellacherie, E., Amphiphilic polysaccharides: useful tools for the preparation of nanoparticles with controlled surface characteristics. *Langmuir* **2004**, *20*, 6956–6963.
64 Uchida, T., Seriwaza, T., Akashi, M., Graft copolymers having hydrophobic backbone and hydrophilic branches XXI. Preparation of galactose surface-accumulated polystyrene nanospheres and their interaction with lectin. *Polymer J.* **1999**, *31*, 970–973.
65 Uchida, T., Serizawa, T., Ise, H., Akaike, T., Akashi, M., Graft copolymer having hydrophobic backbone and hydrophilic branches. 33. Interaction of hepatocytes and polystyrene nanospheres having lactose-immobilized hydrophilic

polymers on their surface. *Biomacromolecules* **2001**, *2*, 1343–1346.

66 Serizawa, T., Yasunaga, S., Akashi, M., Synthesis and lectin recognition of polystyrene core-glycopolymer corona nanospheres. *Biomacromolecules* **2001**, *2*, 469–475.

67 Gallardo, M. M., Couarraze, G., Denizot, B., Treupel, L., Couvreur, P., Puisieux, F., Study of the mechanisms of formation of nanoparticles and nanocapsules of polyisobutyl-2-cyanoacrylate. *Int. J. Pharm.* **1993**, *100*, 55–64.

68 Quintanar-Guerrero, D., Allemann, E., Doelker, H., Fessi, H., Preparation and characterization of nanocapsules from preformed polymers by a new process based on emulsification-diffusion technique. *Pharm. Res.* **1998**, *15*, 1056–1062.

69 Al Khouri, N., Fessi, H., Robot-Treupel, J. P., Devissaguet, F., Puisieux, F., An Original Procedure for preparing nanocapsules of polyalkylcyanoacrylates for interfacial polymerization. *Pharm. Acta* **1986**, *61*, 274–281.

70 Khopade, A. J., Caruso, F., Two-component, ultrathin microcapsules prepared by a core-mediated layer-by-layer approach. *Chem. Mater.* **2004**, *16*, 2107–2112.

71 Decher, G., Fuzzy nanoassemblies: toward layered polymeric multicomposites. *Science* **1997**, *277*, 1232–1237.

72 Khopade, A. J., Caruso, F., Stepwise self-assembled poly(amidoamine) dendrimer and poly(styrenesulfate) microcapsules as sustained delivery vehicles. *Biomacromolecules* **2002**, *3*, 1154–1162.

73 Schüller, C., Caruso, F., Decomposable hollow biopolymer-based capsules. *Biomacromolecules* **2001**, *2*, 921–926.

74 Fresta, M., Cavallaro, G., Giammona, G., Wehrli, E., Puglisi, G., Preparation and characterization of polyethyl-2-cyanoacrylate nanocapsules containing antiepileptic drugs. *Biomaterials* **1996**, *17*, 751–758.

75 Seymour, L. W., Duncan, R., Kopeckova, P., Kopecek, J., Potential of sugar residues attached to *N*-(2-hydroxypropyl)methacrylamide copolymers as targeting groups for the selective delivery of drugs. *J. Bioact. Compat. Polym.* **1987**, *2*, 97–119.

76 Arap, W., Pasqualini, R., Ruoslahti, E., Cancer treatment by targeted drug delivery to tumor vasculature in a mouse model. *Science* **1998**, *279*, 377–388.

77 Kono, K., Liu, M., Fréchet, J. M., Design of dendritic macromolecules containing folate or methotrexate residues. *J. Bioconjug. Chem.* **1999**, *10*, 1115–1121.

78 Seymour, L. W., Flanagan, P. A., Al-Shamkhani, A., Subr, V., Ulbrich, K., Cassidy, J., Duncan, R., Synthetic polymers conjugated to monoclonal antibodies: vehicles for tumor-targeted drug delivery. *Sel. Cancer Ther.* **1991**, *7*, 59–73.

79 Langer, K., Mutschler, E., Lambrecht, G., Mayer, D., Troschau, G., Stieneker, F., Kreuter, J., Methylmethacrylate sulfopropylmethacrylate copolymer nanoparticles for drug delivery part III: evaluation as drug delivery system for ophthalmic applications. *Int. J. Pharm.* **1997**, *158*, 219–231.

80 Passirani, C., Barratt, G., Dessaguet, J.-P., Labarre, D., Long-circulating nanoparticles bearing heparin or dextran covalently bound to poly(methyl methacrylate). *Pharm. Res.* **1998**, *15*, 1046–1050.

81 Chauvierre, C., Labarre, D., Couvreur, P., Vauthier, C., Novel polysaccharide-decorated poly(isobutyl cyanoacrylate) nanoparticles. *Pharm. Res.* **2003**, *20*, 1786–1793.

82 Gullberg, E., Particle transcytosis across the human intestinal epithelium. Model development and target identification for improved drug delivery. *Thesis*. Univeristatis Upsaliensis, **2005**.

83 Andersson, M., Fromell, K., Gullberg, E., Artursson, P., Caldwell, K. D., Characterization of surface-modified nanoparticles for *in vivo* biointeraction. A sedimentation filed flow fraction study. *Anal. Chem.* **2005**, *77*, 5488–5493.

84 Pasqualini, R., Koivunen, E., Ruoslahti, E., Alpha v integrins as receptors for tumor targeting by circulating ligands. *Nat. Biotechnol.* **1997**, *15*, 542–546.
85 Bibby, D. C., Talmadge, J. E., Dalal, M. K., Kurz, S. G., Chytil, K. M., Barry, S. E., Shand, D. G., Steiert, M., Pharmacokinetics and biodistribution of RGD-targeted doxorubicin-loaded nanoparticles in tumor-bearing mice. *Int. J. Pharmaceutics* **2005**, *293*, 281–290.
86 Yasugi, K., Nakamura, T., Nagasaki, Y., Kato, M., Kataoka, K., Sugar-installed polymer micelles: synthesis and micellization of poly(ethylene glycol)-poly(D,L-lactide) block copolymers having sugar groups at the PEG chain end. *Macromolecules* **1999**, *32*, 8024–8032.
87 Varki, A., Biological roles of oligosaccharides: all of the theories are correct. *Glycobiology* **1993**, *3*, 97–130.
88 Dwek, R. A., Glycobiology: toward understanding the function of sugars. *Chem. Rev.* **1996**, *96*, 683–720.
89 Smart, J. D., Nicholls, T. J., Green, K. L., Rogers, D. L., Cook, J. D., Lectins in drug delivery: a study of the acute local irritancy of the lectins from *Solanum tuberosum* and *Helix pomatia*. *Eur. J. Pharm. Sci.* **2000**, *9*, 93–99.
90 Waeckerle-Men, Y., Groettrupa, M., PLGA microspheres for improved antigen delivery to dendritic cells as cellular vaccines. *Adv. Drug. Deliv. Rev.* **2005**, *57*, 475–482.
91 Foged, C., Arigita, C., Sundblad, A., Jiskoot, W., Storm, G., Frokjaer, S., Interaction of dendritic cells with antigen-containing liposomes: effect of bilayer composition. *Vaccine* **2004**, *22*, 1903–1913.
92 McGreal, E. P., Miller, J. L., Gordon, S., Ligand recognition by antigen-presenting cell C-type lectin. *Curr. Opin. Immunol.* **2005**, *17*, 18–24.
93 Jilek, S., Merkle, H. P., Walter, E., DNA-loaded biodegradable microparticles as vaccine delivery systems and their interaction with dendritic cells. *Adv. Drug Deliv. Rev.* **2005**, *57*, 377–390.
94 Joralemon, M. J., Shanmugananda, M., Remsen, E. E., Becker, M. L., Wooley, K. L., Synthesis, characterization, and bioavailability of mannosylated shell cross-linked nanoparticles. *Biomacromolecules* **2004**, *5*, 903–913.
95 Trouet, A., Masquelier, M., Baurain, R., Deprez-De Campeneere, D., A covalent linkage between daunorubicin and proteins that is stable in serum and reversible by lysosomal hydrolases, as required for a lysosomotropic drug–carrier conjugate. *Proc. Natl Acad. Sci. USA* **1982**, *79*, 626–629.
96 Fiume, L., Bassi, B., Busi, C., Mattioli, A., Spinosa, G., Conjugates of 9-beta-D-arabinofuranosyladenine 5-monophosphate (ARA-AMP) with lactosaminated albumin – characterization of the drug-carrier bonds. *Biochem. Pharmacol.* **1986**, *35*, 967–972.
97 Cho, C. S., Cho, K. Y., Park, I. K., Kim, S. H., Sasagawa, T., Uchiyama, M., Akaike, T., Receptor-mediated delivery of all *trans*-retinoic acid to hepatocyte using poly(L-lactic acid) nanoparticles coated with galactose-carrying polystyrene. *J. Control. Release* **2001**, *77*, 7–15.
98 Cade, D., Ramus, E., Rinaudo, M., Auzély-Velty, R., Delair, T., Hamaide, T., Tailoring of bioresorbable polymers for elaboration of sugar-functionalized nanoparticles. *Biomacromolecules* **2004**, *5*, 922–927.
99 Woller, E. K., Cloninger, M. J., The lectin-binding properties of six generations of mannose-functionalized dendrimers. *Organic Lett.* **2002**, *4*, 7–10.
100 Antony, A. C., Folate receptor-targeted drugs for cancer and inflammatory diseases. *Adv. Drug Deliv. Rev.* **2004**, *56*, 1055–1058.
101 Nayak, S., Lee, H., Chmielelewski, J., Lyon, L. A., Folate-mediated cell targeting and cytotoxicity using thermoresponsive microgels. *J. Am. Chem. Soc.* **2004**, *126*, 10258–10259.
102 Stella, B., Arpicco, S., Peracchia, M. T., Desmaële, D., Hoebeke, J.,

RENOIR, M., D'ANGELO, J., CATTEL, L., COUVREUR, P., Design of folic acid-conjugated nanoparticles for drug delivery. *J. Pharm. Sci.* **2000**, *89*, 1452–1464.

103 PARK, E., LEE, S. B., LEE, Y. M., Preparation and characterization of methoxy poly(ethylene glycol)/poly(ε-caprolactone) amphiphilic block copolymeric nanospheres for tumor-specific folate-mediated targeting of anticancer drugs. *Biomaterials* **2005**, *26*, 1053–1061.

104 PARK, J., KUROSAWA, S., WATANABE, J., ISHIHARA, K., Evaluation of 2-methacryloyloxyethyl phosphorylcholine polymeric nanoparticle for immunoassay of C-reactive protein detection. *Anal. Chem.* **2004**, *76*, 2649–2655.

105 FOURNIER, C., LEONARD, M., LE COQ-LEONARD, I., DELLACHERIE, E., Coating polystyrene particles by adsorption of hydrophobically modified dextran. *Langmuir* **1995**, *11*, 2344–2347.

106 ILLUM, L., JONES, P. D. E., BALDWIN, R. W., DAVIS, S. S., Tissue distribution of poly(hexyl 2-cyanoacrylate) nanoparticles coated with monoclonal antibodies in mice bearing human tumor xenografts. *J. Pharmacol. Exp. Ther.* **1984**, *230*, 733–736.

107 BORGES, O., BORCHARD, G., VERHOEF, J. C., DE SOUSA, A., JUNINGER, H. E., Preparation of coated nanoparticles for a new mucosal vaccine delivery system. *Int. J. Pharm.* **2005**, *299*, 155–166.

108 MESSAI, I., DELAIR, T., Adsorption of chitosan onto poly(D,L-lactic acid) particles: a physico-chemical investigation. *Macromol. Chem. Phys.* **2005**, *206*, 1665–1674.

109 CUI, Z., PATEL, J., TUZOVA, M., RAY, P., PHILLIPS, R., WOODWARD, J. G., NATH, A., MUMPER, R. J., Strong T cell type-1 immune response to HIV-1 Tat (1–72) protein coated nanoparticles. *Vaccine* **2004**, *22*, 2631–2640.

110 REDHEAD, H. M., DAVIS, S. S., ILLUM, L., Drug delivery in poly(lactide-*co*-glycolide) nanoparticles surface modified with poloxamer 407 and poloxamine 908: *in vitro* characterization and *in vivo* evaluation. *J. Control. Release* **2001**, *70*, 353–363.

111 DE SOUSA DELGADO, A., LÉONARD, M., DELLACHERIE, E., Surface properties of polystyrene nanoparticles coated with dextrans and dextran–PEO copolymers. Effect of polymer architecture on protein adsorption. *Langmuir* **2001**, *17*, 4386–4391.

112 STUDER, P., LIMAL, D., BRETON, P., RIESS, G., Synthesis and characterization of poly(ethylene oxide)-*block*-poly(methylidene malonate 2.1.2) block copolymers bearing a mannose group at the PEO chain end. *Bioconjug. Chem.* **2005**, *16*, 223–229.

113 JULE, E., NAGASAKI, Y., KATAOKA, K., Surface plasmon resonance study on the interaction between lactose-installed poly(ethylene glycol)–poly(D,L-lactide) block copolymer micelles and lectins immobilized on a gold surface. *Langmuir* **2002**, *18*, 10334–10339.

114 YAMAMOTO, Y., NAGASAKI, Y., KATO, M., KATAOKA, K., Surface charge modulation of poly(ethyleneglycol)-poly(D,L-lactide) copolymer micelles: conjugation of charged Peptides. *Colloid Surf. B Biointerfaces* **1999**, *16*, 135–146.

115 QI, K., MA, Q., REMSON, E. E., CLARK, C. G. JR., Determination of the bioavailability of biotin conjugated onto shell cross-linked (SCK) nanoparticles. *J. Am. Chem. Soc.* **2004**, *126*, 6599–6607.

116 NARAIN, R., ARMES, S. P., Synthesis and aqueous solution of novel sugar methacrylate-based homopolymers and block copolymers. *Biomacromolecules* **2003**, *4*, 1746–1758.

117 GAUTIER, S., GRUDZIELSKI, N., GOFFINET, G., HENRY DE HASSONVILLE, S., DELATTRE, L., JÉRÔME, R., Preparation of poly(D,L-lactide) nanoparticles assisted by amphiphilic poly(methyl methacrylate-*co*-methacrylic acid) copolymers. *J. Biomater. Sci. Polym. Edn.* **2001**, *12*, 429–450.

118 GAUTIER, S., D'ALOIA, V., HALLEUX, O., MAZZA, M., LECOMTE, Ph., JÉRÔME, R., Amphiphilic copolymers of ε-caprolactone and γ-substituted ε-caprolactone. Synthesis and functionalization of poly(D,L-lactide) nanoparticles. *J. Biomater. Sci. Polym. Edn.* **2003**, *14*, 63–85.

119 Maruyama, A., Ishihara, T., Kim, J.-S., Kim, S. W., Akaike, T., Nanoparticle DNA carrier with poly(L-lysine) grafted polysaccharide copolymer and poly(D,L-lactic acid). *Bioconjug. Chem.* **1997**, *8*, 735–742.

120 Auzély-Velty, R., Cristea, M., Rinaudo, M., Galactosylated *N*-vinylpyrrolidone-maleic acid copolymers: synthesis, characterization, and interaction with lectins. *Biomacromolecules* **2002**, *3*, 998–1005.

121 Marie, E., Landfester, K., Antonietti, M., Synthesis of chitosan-stabilized polymer dispersions, capsules, and chitosan grafting products via miniemulsion. *Biomacromolecules* **2002**, *3*, 475–481.

122 Lemieux, G. A., Bertozzi, C. R., Chemoselective ligation reactions with proteins, oligosaccharides and cells. *Trends Biotechnol.* **1998**, *16*, 506–513.

123 Zhang, Q., Remsen, E. E., Wooley, K. L., Shell cross-linked nanoparticles containing hydrolytically degradable, crystalline core domains. *J. Am. Chem. Soc.* **2000**, *122*, 3642–3651.

124 Liu, J., Zhang, Q., Remsen, E. E., Wooley, K. L., Nanostructured materials designed for cell binding and transduction. *Biomacromolecules* **2001**, *2*, 362–368.

125 Dufresne, M. H., Gauthier, M. A., Leroux, J.-C., Thiol-functionalized polymeric micelles: from molecular recognition to improved mucoadhesion. *Bioconjug. Chem.* **2005**, *16*, 1027–1033.

126 Jiang, F. N., Jiang, S., Liu, D., Richter, A., Levy, J. G., Development of technology for linking photositizers to a model monoclonal antibody. *J. Immunol. Methods* **1990**, *134*, 139–149.

127 Langer, K., Coester, C., Weber, C., von Briesen, H., Kreuter, J., Preparation of avidin-labeled protein nanoparticles as carriers for biotinylated peptide nucleic acid. *Eur. J. Pharm. Biopharm.* **2000**, *49*, 303–307.

128 Nobs, L., Buchegger, F., Gurny, R., Allémann, E., Surface modification of poly(lactic acid) nanoparticles by covalent attachment of thiol groups by means of three methods. *Int. J. Pharm.* **2003**, *250*, 327–337.

129 Nobs, L., Buchegger, F., Gurny, R., Allémann, E., Poly(lactid acid) nanoparticles labeled with biologically active Neutravidin^{TM} for active targeting. *Eur. J. Pharm. Biopharm.* **2004**, *58*, 483–490.

130 Balthasar, S., Michaelis, K., Dinauer, N., Von Briesen, H., Kreuter, J., Langer, K., Preparation and characterization of antibody modified gelatin nanoparticles as drug carrier systems for uptake in lymphocytes. *Biomaterials* **2005**, *26*, 2723–2732.

131 Hilt, J. Z., Byrne, M. E., Configurational biomimesis in drug delivery: molecular imprinting of biologically significant molecules. *Adv. Drug Deliv. Rev.* **2004**, 1599–1620.

132 Silvestri, D., Borrelli, C., Guisti, P., Cristallini, C., Ciardelli, G., Polymeric devices containing imprinted nanospheres: a novel approach to improve recognition in water for clinical uses. *Anal. Chim. Acta* **2005**, *542*, 3–13.

133 Carter, S. R., Rimmer, S., Molecular recognition of caffeine by shell molecular imprinted core–shell polymer particles in aqueous media. *Adv. Mater.* **2002**, *14*, 667–670.

134 Soppimath, K., Aminabhavi, T. M., Kulkarni, A. R., Rudzinski, W. E., Biodegradable polymeric nanoparticles as drug delivery devices. *J. Control. Release* **2001**, *70*, 1–20.

135 Fournier, C., Leonard, M., Dellacherie, M., Chikihi, M., Hommel, H., Legrand, A. P., EPR spectroscopy analysis of hydrophobically modified dextran-coated polystyrene. *J. Colloid Interface Sci.* **1998**, *198*, 27–33.

136 Chauvierre, C., Vauthier, C., Labarre, D., Hommel, H., Evaluation of the surface properties of dextran-

coated poly(isobutylcyanoacrylate) nanoparticles by spin-labeling coupled with electron resonance spectroscopy. *Colloid Polym. Sci.* **2004**, *282*, 1016–1025.

137 Liedberg, B., Nylander, C., Lundström, I., Biosensing with surface plasmon resonance – how it all started. *Biosensors Bioelectron.* **1995**, *10*, RI–RIX.

138 Lemarchand, C., Couvreur, P., Besnard, M., Costantini, D., Gref, R., Novel polyester-polysaccharide nanoparticles. *Pharm. Res.* **2003**, *20*, 1284–1292.

139 Quellec, P., Gref, R., Perrin, L., Dellacherie, E., Sommer, F., Verbavatz, J. M., Alonso, M. J., Protein encapsulation within polyethylene glycol-coated nanospheres. I. Physicochemical characterization. *J. Biomed. Mater. Res.* **1998**, *42*, 45–54.

140 Chen, Y., Ji, T., Rosenzweig, Z., Synthesis of glyconanospheres containing luminescent CdSe–ZnS quantum dots. *Nano Lett.* **2003**, *3*, 581–584.

141 Barratt, G., Couarraze, G., Couvreur, P., Dubernet, C., Fattal, E., Gref, R., Labarre, D., Legrand, P., Ponchel, G., Vauthier, C., Biodegradable polymers as drug carrier systems. In *Polymeric Biomaterials*, 2nd edn, Dumitriu, S. (Ed.). Marcel Dekker, New York, pp. 753–781.

142 Sakuma, S., Hayashi, M., Akashi, M., Design of nanoparticles composed of graft copolymers for oral peptide delivery. *Adv. Drug Del. Rev.* **2001**, *47*, 21–37.

143 Sakuma, A., Sudo, R., Suzuki, N., Kikuchi, H., Akashi, M., Ishida, Y., Hayashi, M., Behavior of mucoadhesive nanoparticles having hydrophilic polymeric chains in the intestine. *J. Control. Release* **2002**, *81*, 281–290.

144 Kohler, D., Aerosole for systemic treatment. *Lung* **1990**, *168 (Suppl.)*, 677–684.

145 Garcia-Contreras, L., Morcol, T., Bell, S. J. D., Hickey, A. J., Evaluation of novel particles as pulmonary delivery systems for insulin in rats. *AAPS Pharm. Sci.* **2003**, *5*, E9.

146 Dailey, L. A., Schmehl, T., Gessler, T., Wittmar, M., Grimminger, F., Seeger, W., Kissel, T., Nebulization of biodegradable nanoparticles: impact of nebulizer technology and nanoparticle characteristics on aerosol features. *J. Control. Release* **2003**, *86*, 131–144.

147 Sharma, R., Saxena, D., Dwivedi, A. K., Misra, A., Inhalable microparticles containing drug combinations to target alveolar macrophages for treatment of pulmonary tuberculosis. *Pharm. Res.* **2001**, 1405–1410.

148 Vila, A., Sanchez, A., Tobio, M., Calvo, P., Alonso, M. J., Design of biodegradable particles for protein delivery. *J. Control. Release* **2002**, *78*, 15–24.

149 Illum, L., Jabbal-Gill, M., Hinchcliffe, M., Fisher, A. N., Davis, S. S., Chitosan as a novel nasal delivery system for vaccines. *Adv. Drug. Del. Rev.* **2001**, *51*, 81–96.

150 Reddy, L. H., Sharma, R. K., Chuttani, K., Mishra, A. K., Murthy, R. S. R., Influence of administration route on tumor uptake and biodistribution of etoposide loaded solid lipid nanoparticles in Dalton's lymphoma tumor bearing mice. *J. Control. Release* **2005**, *105*, 185–198.

151 Uchida, T., Goto, S., Foster, T. P., Size studies for subcutaneous delivery of poly(lactide-*co*-glycolide) microspheres containing ovalbumin as vaccine formulation. *J. Pharm. Pharmacol.* **1995**, *47*, 556–560.

152 Peyre, M., Fleck, R., Hockley, D., Gander, B., Sesardic, D., *In vivo* uptake of an experimental microencapsulated diphtheria vaccine following sub-cutaneous immunization. *Vaccine* **2004**, *22*, 2430–2437.

153 Zimmer, A., Kreuter, J., Microparticles and nanoparticles used in ocular delivery systems. *Adv. Drug Deliv. Rev.* **1995**, *16*, 61–73.

154 Conti, B., Giunchedi, P., Genta, I., Conte, U., The preparation and *in vivo* evaluation of the wound-healing

properties of chitosan microspheres. *STP Pharma Sci.* **2001**, *10*, 101–104.

155 Nielsen, U. B., Kirpotin, D. B., Pickering, E. M., Hong, K., Park, J. W., Shababy, M. R., Shao, Y., Benz, J. D., Marks, J. D., Therapeutic efficacy of anti-ErbB2 immunoliposomes targeted by a phage antibody selected for cellular endocytosis. *Biochim. Biophys. Acta* **2002**, *1591*, 109–118.

156 Dalgleish, A. G., Why: gene therapy? *Gene Ther.* **1997**, *4*, 629–630.

157 Rodrigues, J. S., Santos-Magalhaes, N. S., Coelho, L. C. B. B., Couvreur, P., Ponchel, G., Gref, R., Novel core (polyester)–shell (polysaccharide) nanoparticles: protein loading and surface modification with lectins. *J. Control. Release* **2003**, *92*, 103–112.

158 Warren, H. S., Leclerc, C., Adjuvants. In *Encyclopedia in Immunology*, 2nd edn, Delves, P. J., Roitt, I. M. (Eds.). Academic press, San Diego, CA, **1998**, Vol. 1, pp. 36–39.

159 Allen, T. M., Cullis, P. R., Drug delivery systems: entering the mainstream. *Science* **2004**, *303*, 1818–1822.

160 Thompson, D. H., Preface – triggering in drug delivery systems. *Adv. Drug Del. Rev.* **2001**, *53*, 245–245.

161 Soppimath, K. S., Tan, D. C.-W., Yang, Y. Y., pH-triggered thermally responsive polymer core–shell nanoparticles for drug delivery. *Adv. Mater.* **2005**, *17*, 318–323.

162 Salvage, J. O., Rose, S. F., Phillips, G. J., Hanlon, G. W., Lloyd, A. W., Ma, I. Y., Armes, S. P., Billingham, N. C., Lewis, A. L., Novel biocompatible phosphorylcholine-based self-assembled nanoparticles for drug delivery. *J. Control. Release* **2005**, *104*, 259–270.

163 Ichikawa, H., Fukumori, Y., A novel positively thermosensitive controlled-release microcapsule with membrane of nano-sized poly(*N*-isopropylacrylamide) gel dispersed in ethylcellulose matrix. *J. Control. Release* **1999**, *63*, 107–119.

164 Neradovic, D., Soga, O., Van Nostrum, C. F., Hennink, W. E., The effect of the processing and formulation parameters on the size of nanoparticles based on block copolymers of poly(ethylene glycol) and poly(*N*-isopropylacrylamide) with and without hydrolytically sensitive groups. *Biomaterials* **2004**, *25*, 2409–2418.

165 Angelatos, A. S., Radt, B., Caruso, F., Light-responsive polyelectrolyte/gold nanoparticle microcapsules. *J. Phys. Chem. B* **2005**, *109*, 3071–3076.

166 Skirtach, A. G., Dejugnat, C., Braun, D., Susha, A. S., Rogach, A. L., Parak, W. J., Möhwald, H., Sukhorukov, G. B., The role of metal nanoparticles in remote release of encapsulated materials. *Nano Lett.* **2005**, *5*, 1371–1377.

167 Lu, Z. H., Prouty, M. D., Guo, Z., Golub, V. O., Kumar, C. S. S. R., Lvov, Y. M., Magnetic switch of permeability for polyelectrolyte microcapsules embedded with Co@Au nanoparticles. *Langmuir* **2005**, *21*, 2042–2050.

168 Qiu, Y., Park, K., Environment-sensitive hydrogels for drug delivery. *Adv. Drug Del. Rev.* **2001**, *53*, 321–339.

169 Lackey, C. A., Press, O. W., Hoffman, A. S., Stayton, P. S., A biomimetic pH-responsive polymer directs endosomal release and intracellular delivery of an endocytosed antibody complex. *Bioconjug. Chem.* **2002**, *13*, 996–1001.

170 Stubbs, M., McSheehy, P. M. J., Griffiths, J. R., Bashford, C. L., Causes and consequences of tumor acidity and implications for treatment. *Mol. Med. Today* **2000**, *6*, 15–19.

171 Radt, B., Smith, T. A., Caruso, F., Optically addressable nanostructured capsules. *Adv. Mater.* **2004**, *16*, 2184–2189.

172 Skirtach, A. G., Antipov, A. A., Shchukin, D. G., Sukhorukov, G. B., Remote activation of capsules containing Ag nanoparticles and IR dye by laser light. *Langmuir* **2004**, *20*, 6988–6992.

173 Mornet, S., Vasseur, S., Grasset, F., Duguet, E., Magnetic nanoparticle

design for medical diagnosis and therapy. *J. Mater. Chem.* **2004**, *14*, 2161–2175.

174 Mueller-Schulte, D., Thermo-sensitive, biocompatible polymer carriers with a variable physical structure for treatment, diagnosis and analysis. *WO 2005042142*, **2005**.

175 Garcia-Fuentes, M., Prego, C., Torres, D., Alonso, M. J., A comparative study of the potential of solid triglyceride nanostructures coated with chitosan or poly(ethylene glycol) as carrier for oral calcitonin delivery. *Eur. J. Pharm. Sci.* **2005**, *25*, 133–143.

176 McLean, S., Prosser, E., Meehan, E., O'Malley, D., Clarke, N., Ramtoola, Z., Brayden, D., Binding and uptake of biodegradable poly-DL-lactide micro- and nanoparticles in intestinal epithelia. *Eur. J. Pharm. Sci.* **1998**, *6*, 153–163.

177 Panyam, J., Sahoo, S. K., Prabha, S., Bargar, T., Labhasetwar, V., Fluorescence and electron microscopy probes for cellular and tissue uptake of poly(D,L-lactide-*co*-glycolide) nanoparticles. *Int. J. Pharm.* **2003**, *262*, 1–11.

178 Tosi, G., Rivasi, F., Gandolfi, F., Costantino, L., Vandelli, M. A., Forni, F., Conjugated poly(D,L-lactide-*co*-glycolide) for the preparation of *in vivo* detectable nanoparticles. *Biomaterials* **2005**, *26*, 4189–4195.

179 Alivisatos, A. P., Semiconductor clusters, nanocrystals, and quantum dots. *Science* **1996**, *271*, 933–937.

180 Bruchez, M. Jr., Moronne, M., Gin, P., Weiss, S., Alivisatos, A. P., Semiconductor nanocrystals as fluorescent biological labels. *Science* **1998**, *281*, 2016–2018.

181 Chan, W. C.-W., Maxwell, D. J., Gao, X. H., Bailey, R. E., Han, M. Y., Nie, S. M., Luminescent quantum dots for multiplexed biological detection and imaging. *Curr. Opin. Biotechnol.* **2002**, *13*, 40–46.

182 Tamura, J., Fukuda, M., Tanaka, J., Kawa, M., Synthesis of hydrophilic ultrafine nanoparticles coordinated with carbohydrate cluster. *J. Carbohydrate Chem.* **2002**, *21*, 445–449.

183 Ballou, B., Lagerholm, C., Ernst, L. A., Bruchez, M. P., Waggoner, A. S., Noninvasive imaging of quantum dots in mice. *Bioconjug. Chem.* **2004**, *15*, 79–86.

184 Han, M., Xiaohu, G., Su, J. Z., Nie, S., Quantum-dot-tagged microbeads for multiplexed optical coding of biomolecules. *Nat. Biotechnol.* **2001**, *19*, 631–635.

185 Yang, X., Zhang, Y., Encapsulation of quantum nanodots in polystyrene and silica micro-/nanoparticles. *Langmuir* **2004**, *20*, 6071–6073.

186 Fleischhaker, F., Zentel, R., Photonic crystals from core–shell colloids with incorporated highly fluorescent quantum dots. *Chem. Mater.* **2005**, *17*, 1346–1351.

187 Esteves, A. C. C., Barros-Timmons, A., Monteiro, T., Trindade, T., Optical properties of the synthetic nanocomposites SiO_2/CdS/poly(styrene-*co*-maleic anhydride) and SiO_2/CdS/poly(styrene-*co*-maleimide). *J. Nanosci. Nanotechnol.* **2005**, *5*, 766–771.

188 Skaff, H., Illker, M. F., Coughlin, E. B., Emrick, T., Preparation of cadmium selenide-polyolefin composites from functional phosphine oxides and ruthenium-based metathesis. *J. Am. Chem. Soc.* **2002**, *124*, 5729–5733.

189 O'Brien, P., Cummins, S. S., Darcy, D., Dearden, A., Masala, O., Pickett, N. L., Ryley, S., Sutherland, A. J., Quantum dot-labeled polymer beads by suspension polymerization. *Chem. Commun.* **2003**, 2532–2533.

190 Li, Y., Liu, E. C. Y., Prickett, N., Skabara, P. J., Cummins, S. S., Ryley, S., Sutherland, A. J., O'Brien, P., Synthesis and characterization of CdS quantum dots in polystyrene microbeads. *J. Mater. Chem.* **2005**, *15*, 1238–1243.

191 Joumaa, N., Lansalot, M., Théretz, A., Elaissari, A., Synthesis of quantum dot-tagged submicrometer polystyrene particles by miniemulsion

polymerization. *Langmuir* **2006**, *22*, 1810–1816.

192 Esteves, A. C. C., Bombalski, L., Cusick, B., Barros-Timmons, A., Matyjaszewski, K., Trindade, T., AGET ATRP in miniemulsions from functionalized CdE (E = S, Se) q-dot's surfaces. *Polym. Prepr.* **2005**, *46*, 134–135.

193 Lee, S.-J., Jeong, J.-R., Shin, S.-C., Huh, Y.-M., Song, H.-T., Suh, J.-S., Chang, Y.-H., Jeon, B.-S., Kim, J.-D., Intracellular translocation of superparamagnetic iron oxide nanoparticles encapsulated with peptide-conjugated poly(D,L lactide-*co*-glycolide). *J. Appl. Phys.* **2005**, *97*, 10Q913.

194 Veyret, R., Elaissari, A., Marianneau, P., Sall, A. A., Delair, T., Magnetic colloids for generic capture of viruses. *Anal. Biochem.* **2005**, *346*, 59–68.

195 Elaissari, A., Rodrigue, M., Meunier, F., Herve, C., Hydrophilic magnetic latex for nucleic acid extraction, purification and concentration. *J. Magn. Magn. Mater.* **2001**, *225*, 127–133.

196 Andrade, J. D., *Protein Adsorption. Surface and Interfacial Aspect of Biomedical Polymers.* Plenum Press, New York, **1985**.

197 Elaissari, A., Bourrel, V., Thermosensitive magnetic latex particles for controlling protein adsorption and desorption. *J. Magn. Magn. Mater.* **2001**, *225*, 151–155.

198 Duracher, D., Elaissari, A., Mallet, F., Pichot, C., Adsorption of modified HIV-1 capsid p24 protein onto thermosensitive and cationic core–shell poly(styrene)–poly(*N*-isopropylacrylamide) nanoparticles. *Langmuir* **2000**, *16*, 9002–9008.

199 Lansalot, M., Sabor, M., Elaissari, A., Pichot, C., Elaboration of fluorescent and highly magnetic submicronic polymer particles via a stepwise heterocoagulation process. *Colloid Surf. Sci.* **2005**, 1267–1277.

200 Elaissari, A., Magnetic colloids: preparation and biomedical applications. *e-Polymers* **2005**, No 028.

201 Le Ray, A. M., Vert, M., Gautier, J. C., Benoit, J. P., End-chain labeling and *in vitro* stability studies of radiolabeled poly(hydroxy acid) NP. *Pharm. Res.* **1994**, *83*, 845–851.

202 Levy, L., Sahoo, Y., Kim, K.-S., Bergey, E. J., Prasad, P. N., Nanochemistry: synthesis and characterization of multifunctional nanoclinics for biological applications. *Chem. Mater.* **2002**, *14*, 3715–3721.

9
Polymeric Nanoparticles for Drug Delivery

Paraskevi Kallinteri and Martin C. Garnett

9.1
Introduction: Application of Nanoparticles for Noncancer Applications

The scientific literature contains many reviews on the therapeutic uses of nanoparticles, from formulation through to *in vitro* and *in vivo* assessment of activity, and for various routes of delivery, including oral, lung, mucosal and parenteral. Therapeutic development of nanoparticulate delivery systems has been dominated by applications for cancer because of the potential advantages in localization in cancer tissues and hence in targeting advantages to drugs which lack specificity. However, there are a variety of more subtle reasons why nanoparticle therapeutics should be useful for other delivery routes and diseases. These include protection of the drug, enhancing circulation half-life, acting as a slow release system and compartmentalization of the delivery system either by preventing the drug reaching certain tissues or by enhancing uptake into particular cells/tissues. These potential advantages have led to work on nanoparticles in a number of other areas including delivery to local sites such as the eye and lung, the delivery of peptides and proteins via a number of alternative routes, including oral, nasal and pulmonary routes, and for treatments where cells of the immune system can be readily targeted by nanoparticles e.g. vaccine delivery, AIDS, antifungal treatment and tuberculosis. However, we have been unable to find any recent reviews covering the noncancer applications as a group, the distinctive reasons why these should be useful targets for polymeric nanoparticles or why nanoparticles may produce more effective delivery systems.

In this chapter, we have attempted to bring together a number of different areas. First, to understand the physiology and anatomy underlying the diseases which may be treatable using nanoparticulates and the way that nanoparticles are handled by the body. The effect of the route of application has also been considered here. Second, to review the main work that has been carried out with polymeric nanoparticle formulations for this range of applications and assess their future potential. This second area of work has been arranged into individual diseases or groups of diseases which would benefit from similar formulations or similar

Nanotechnologies for the Life Sciences Vol. 10
Nanomaterials for Medical Diagnosis and Therapy. Edited by Challa S. S. R. Kumar

ISBN: 978-3-527-31390-7

principles of delivery for the nanoparticles. Finally, we draw some brief overall conclusions.

One of the first areas to consider in assessing the potential of nanoparticles as delivery systems are the potential physiological barriers to transport of nanoparticles and how physiological factors can be best exploited to maximize the advantages of nanoparticulates.

9.1.1 Physiological and Uptake of Particles

In general, nanoparticles cannot simply partition across membranes, or cells, so uptake is limited to specific transport pathways through cells and the paracellular route passing between cells. The paracellular route poses a problem for the passage of nanoparticles through epithelia and endothelia because of the presence of tight junctions in most of these tissues. The tight junctions typically restrict the gap between cells to about 4–6 nm in endothelia and 2 nm in epithelia, and would therefore be expected to prevent the passage of macromolecules and nanoparticles past these barriers [1]. In addition the presence of a basement membrane underlying these tissues, with a fibrous mesh thought to be around 15 nm between strands, would also be expected to restrict passage of nanoparticles [2].

9.1.1.1 Routes of Tissue and Cellular Uptake of Particles

Although unable to partition through membranes and gain direct access into cells, there are a variety of endocytic mechanisms for the uptake of macromolecules and small particles into cells. These include phagocytosis of large particles by specialized cells such as macrophages and neutrophils [3], and uptake of macromolecules and smaller particles by a variety of mechanisms, which probably include a nonspecific pinocytosis as well as receptor-mediated uptake involving clathrin [4] or uptake via caveolae [5]. Endocytosis may offer two major drug delivery advantages: (i) a preferential uptake to macrophages and other cells associated with the immune system, and (ii) access to the endosomal/lysosomal compartments of cells where the acidic and degradative environment offers a useful drug release mechanism.

More recently, evidence is beginning to accumulate that the endothelium may be less of a barrier to nanoparticle delivery systems than once believed. It was proposed some years ago that the extravasation of macromolecules into lymphatic tissues was mediated by a process of transcytosis in which macromolecules were endocytosed on one side of the cell and exocytosed on the other through a vesicular system [6]. Recent evidence suggests that this process may be mediated by caveolae and involves some specific transport [7]. Some nanoparticles have been reported able to exploit this transcytosis process to pass across endothelia for the brain [8], lymph nodes [9] and bone marrow [10], although it is not yet clear how many tissues can be accessed by this route nor how selective it is for particular tissues. Too little work has been done in this area for this to be reflected in the development of drug delivery systems for specific applications, except as directed towards therapy of brain tumors [8]. However, it offers prospects to widen the range of diseases, which may be accessible to nanotherapeutics.

9.1.1.2 Uptake by Macrophages and Lymphoid Tissues

Delivery to macrophages and other cells of the immune system could allow access to a range of conditions. A number of parasites and diseases are known to inhabit the endosomal compartment of macrophages, e.g. malaria and tuberculosis [11]. In addition, both macrophages and other cells of the immune system are involved in antigen processing, so serve as a port of entry for vaccine antigens.

The macrophages are the main component of the mononuclear phagocytic system (MPS). Due to the preferential uptake of particulates by macrophages, particles tend to accumulate in the main tissues of the MPS such as liver, spleen and lymph nodes. For nanoparticles less than 250 nm, the spleen tends to be less important as a site for uptake [12]. This uptake is potentiated by opsonization [13] – the coating of particulates by blood proteins occurring either specifically through antigen recognition or nonspecifically mainly through hydrophobic interactions. The surface properties of nanoparticles are therefore very important and hydrophilic coatings by polymers such as polysaccharides or poly(ethylene glycol) (PEG) reduce both opsonization and uptake by the MPS. These coatings are usually achieved either by coating with PEG containing surfactants which adsorb to the surface of particles or by the use of PEG copolymers incorporated into the nanoparticles. The hydrophilic coatings also stabilize the particles against aggregation [14]. A further property of the coatings in reducing protein adsorption is that certain blood components can adsorb preferentially to the coated surfaces and this can result in adsorption of a protein, mediating transcytosis to specific organs such as the brain [8].

A further consequence of the MPS uptake of particulates is that, eventually, most particulate preparations do end up in the liver for detoxification and this has the potential to cause liver toxicity. This is particularly important because there is no opportunity for elimination of drug through the kidney until drug has been released from the particle, either by slow release from the particle or by metabolism at its target site or the liver. However, once more this offers a possible drug delivery opportunity by providing a generalized slow release system for drugs mediated by liver metabolism.

9.1.1.3 Mucosal-associated Lymphoid Tissues (MALT)

The mucosae have an important role as an interface between the outside world and the body. They are thus a key element of the defense of the body, both from the point of view of acting as a barrier to the outside world, while at the same time being uniquely placed to sample the environment. Lymphatic tissue is found at a variety of mucosal sites including the bronchi (BALT), nose (NALT) and gut (GALT) [15]. These lymphoid tissues constitute an efficient way of inducing protective immune responses, both humoral and cellular. Moreover, the stimulation of one mucosal site can result in dissemination of response to other mucosal sites. MALT constitutes 80% of immunocytes and functions independently from the systemic system. The lymphoid tissues contain a number of specialized cells, which include fixed macrophages, and also cells like dendritic cells, which act as mobile scouts sampling the environment. These lymphoid tissues, as will be seen below, also seem to act as conduits by which particles may pass through to other tissues.

9.1.2 Routes of Delivery

9.1.2.1 Oral

The gut at first sight appears an unpromising route for nanoparticle delivery systems. The presence of a very acid environment in the stomach, high concentrations of degradative enzymes and a thick layer of mucus above an epithelial layer are all significant physiological barriers. Also, it is well known that macromolecules are poorly absorbed in the gut. However, reports of orally administered particles being present in the lymphatics and circulation have been documented for many years. There have been a number of recent and comprehensive reviews collating the evidence supporting this route of particle uptake. These include specific consideration of the physical barriers and their relevance to oral absorption [16], how particles are taken up across the epithelium and into the lymphatics [17], specific mechanisms and routes of trancytosis [18], and the role of polymers comprising the nanoparticles in influencing uptake [19]. Consequently, only a brief summary of these aspects of oral particulate delivery will be presented here.

Mucus does appear to operate as a barrier to uptake, particularly for larger particles (above 300 nm). Penetration of mucus by nanoparticles is also affected by surface characteristics, with hydrophilic particles penetrating more easily. There are several potential routes of nanoparticle uptake in the gut. Paracellular transport is not expected to be significant as there are tight junctions in the gut as in most other epithelial tissues. However, there have been reports of particles up to 50–100 nm penetrating by this route in the presence of modifiers such as chitosan or calcium ions. Polyacrylate and starch have also been reported to enhance paracellular transport. The process of persorption has also been described in the gut, where the tips of villi become denuded of epithelial cells allowing larger particles access to the underlying mucosa. However, it is not thought that this route of uptake is particularly prominent.

There has been intensive study of the lymphoid tissue within gut as a possible portal of entry for particles. Peyer's patches consisting of multiple lymphoid follicles are the most widely discussed, but are not the sole lymphoid tissue within the gut. A significant number of isolated lymphoid follicles and lymphocyte-filled villi also exist. However, the degree to which these various lymphoid tissues contribute to particle uptake is widely debated. Similarly, it is unclear the extent to which nonlymphoid epithelium is involved in nanoparticle uptake. The principal route of uptake is often assumed to be the M cells in Peyer's patches, but it may be that only a small proportion of M cells are involved.

Uptake of particles involves both trancytosis across the epithelial layer and translocation to other tissues. Peyer's patches, as well as containing M cells also have a more porous basement membrane and are closely associated with efferent lymphatics. These characteristics would account for the reported route of translocation of nanoparticles via the mesenteric lymph ducts. It is also possible that particles may be shuttled to distant mucosal sites following uptake by immune cells.

The uptake of particles by Peyer's patches has, like passage through mucus, been found to be dependent on size. Uptake and translocation to mesenteries and liver seems to be greatest for particle of 50 nm. However, immune responses are most effectively stimulated by particles of 4 μm, which correlates with the observation that larger particles tend to be found in dendritic cells. The surface characteristics of particles have also been reported to be important for both uptake and translocation.

Overall, studies show that there are clearly routes of nanoparticle uptake, but the extent of uptake is under debate due to the wide range of uptake rates reported. It is thought that in general uptake rates are lower than for typical small drug molecule administration. Consequently it is likely that nanoparticle delivery systems will be most appropriate for immune delivery, delivery to intestinal lymph and drugs which are poor for oral delivery because of poor solubility or permeability characteristics, e.g. potent and labile biological macromolecules.

9.1.2.2 **Nasal**

The nasal epithelium has been investigated as a delivery route for conventional drugs, peptides and proteins, and vaccines. A useful description of the anatomy of the nose relevant to drug delivery can be found in reviews by Illum [20] and Jones [21]. The nasal epithelium has a relatively large surface area because of the presence of microvilli and has the advantage that it avoids first-pass metabolism to the liver. However, the nasal mucosa has a significant level of degradative enzymes. Like the gut, nasal mucosa is covered by a layer of mucus, which poses a barrier to delivery mainly because of the rate of clearance into the nasopharynx and gut. The epithelium is well vascularized.

In humans, there is a limited amount of macroscopically visible nasal lymphoid tissue, which is confined to the nasopharynx and tonsils. However, antigen-presenting cells (APCs), and B and T lymphocytes are present within the mucosa.

9.1.2.3 **Pulmonary**

Delivery to the lung is an attractive route because of the easy access and administration of formulations, and the large surface area of the lung provided by the alveoli, estimated to be about 140 m^2 of internal surface area.

The lung structure is that of a multibranching tree with the airways dividing further at each branch. The airways divide repeatedly into primary bronchi, lobar, segmental bronchi and bronchioles until reaching the terminal bronchiole leading to 15–20 alveoli. The walls of the entire respiratory tract are covered by a mucus blanket about 5 μm thick. The mucus is a mucopolysaccharide which can trap particles for subsequent removal by the ciliated cells of the bronchi. This happens by a continual upwards movement of mucus known as the mucociliary escalator.

The alveoli mainly consist of thin squamous cells about 5 μm thick (type I cells). There are also a few thicker type II cells responsible for secreting the surfactant coating the surface of the lungs. The capillaries are closely associated with the alveolar cells and partly form the wall of the alveoli. The alveolar wall therefore consists of alveolar cells, basement membrane and capillary endothelial cells held together by connective tissue. The alveolar membrane is covered by a thin (15 nm) layer of surfactant. Due to the tight junctions joining the alveolar epithelia and the capillary endothelium, penetration of macromolecules from the alveolar space into the capillary circulation is limited, so it would be expected that penetration of nanoparticles would be even more limited. However, it is clear that there is transport of materials across lung endothelium and epithelium by caveolae [22], so this may also be a route for transport of small nanoparticles as well.

Alveolar macrophages may be found either fixed within the connective tissue of the alveoli or free within the mucus layer. They can leave the lung either via the mucus through the mucociliary escalator and out through the sputum or, alternatively, leave via the lymphatics within the lung. This may therefore be another route of transfer of materials from within the airways of the lung into the tissues.

Delivery of particles to the lung is dependent on a number of physical processes, which are diameter dependent. Particles larger than 5 μm are deposited by inertial impaction on the trachea walls following a change in direction of air flow. Settling is proportional to the square of the particle diameter and is less important for small particles. Particles less than about 500 nm in diameter are deposited largely by Brownian diffusion. So, overall, particles in the size range 5 μm down to 500 nm largely avoid impaction on the airways and are large enough to deposit by sedimentation, while those below 500 nm can only deposit by Brownian motion. In general, optimum pulmonary penetration is found with monodisperse aerosols of 2–3 μm diameter. Extremely small aerosols (below 100 nm diameter) also appear to deposit very efficiently through Brownian diffusion, but such fine aerosols are very difficult to produce. Only particles that contact the mucus layer can be deposited and thus be available for either drug release into the mucus or uptake into the macrophages, or possibly the epithelial cells. There may therefore be some possibility of exploiting these various transport mechanisms for drug delivery systems.

A more complete description of pulmonary structure and its effects on drug delivery can be found in Washington and coworkers [23].

9.1.2.4 **Transdermal/Subcutaneous**

One of the main functions of the skin is to act as a barrier to the entry of macromolecules and particles. The stratum corneum, consisting of eight to 16 layers of flattened, stratified and keratinized dead cells is largely responsible for the barrier function of the cell. Due to the barrier function of the skin, there is also a complex relationship with the immune system. Langerhans or dendritic cells are specialized APCs, which constantly monitor the environment by taking up antigens and processing them. They are an integral part of the immune system, and are involved in migration from the epidermis to the regional lymph nodes, resulting in the induction and maintenance of cutaneous immunity sensitization or stimulation of the immune system [24]. These cells could therefore take up and transport particles to the lymph nodes and lymphatics.

In addition to topical application of particulates, the intradermal or subcutaneous route of injection delivers particles to the extracellular space, where they can be taken up by the lymphatics. This route therefore gives a potential route for delivery to the lymphatics, and in particular to the lymph nodes [25].

In summary, therefore, there are a number of routes with potential for delivery of nanoparticles for a variety of therapeutic applications. Work carried out on these applications is detailed below.

9.2 Drug Delivery

9.2.1 Ocular Delivery

9.2.1.1 Anatomy of the Eye

Current ocular drug delivery is by administration of eye-drops, suspensions, ointments, gels, subconjunctival and intraocular injections, and, more recently, implants. There are, however, physiological and anatomical features of the eye that prevent effective therapy. Looking in detail at the eye (Fig. 9.1), there are anterior and posterior sections.

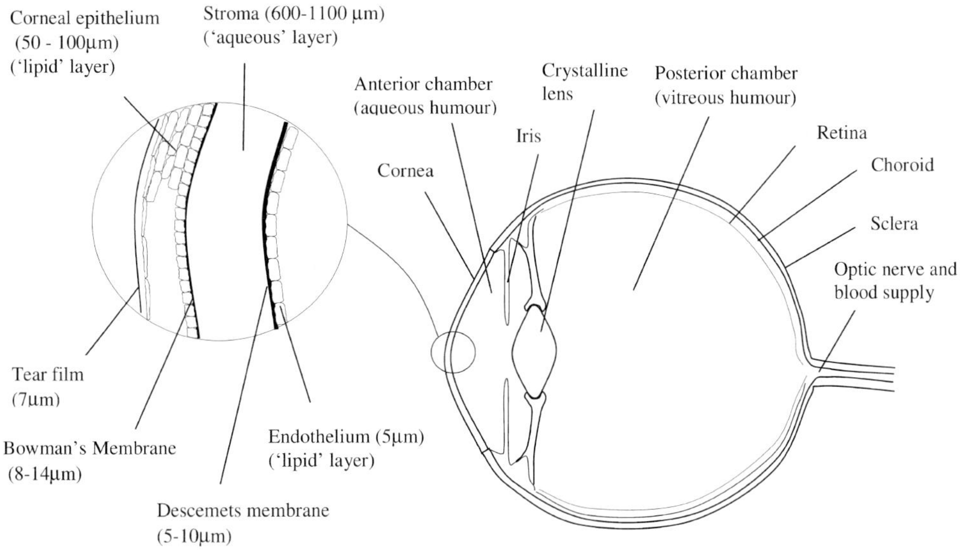

Figure 9.1. Anatomy of the eye. The general anatomy of the eye is shown on the right, with an inset on the left showing the detailed structure of the cornea.

The anterior section includes the lens and the cornea. The posterior segment consists of three layers, i.e. the sclera, choroid and retina, surrounding the vitreous cavity, which is filled by the vitreous humor [26].

The first barrier to drug uptake is the cornea comprising three parts. The outer part is the epithelium, consisting of five to six layers of tightly packed cells restricting the passage of hydrophilic and ionized compounds, with little penetration via the paracellular route. The middle part is the hydrophilic stroma restricting passage of lipophilic compounds. Due to a relatively open structure, drugs with a molecular size up to 50 000 can diffuse in normal stroma. The third part is a monolayer of endothelial cells. Effective drugs therefore need to combine both hydrophilic and hydrophobic properties to be able to pass through the cornea. Formulation pH adjustment can improve the trans-corneal drug accumulation.

It has been reported that less than 5% of the applied eye-drop reaches the intraocular tissues [26–28]. The percentage dose of the drug absorbed through the cornea depends very much upon the time that the instilled drop remains on the corneal surface, which is mainly dependent on the lachrymal system of the eye. The lachrymal glands secrete tears, which are distributed over the eyes by the blinking reflex of the eyelids and collected in the lower conjuctival sac. From there, the tears are drained into the lachrymal sac through the puncta and the lachrymal duct. Eventually, the fluid reaches the nasopharynx and, finally, the gastrointestinal tract. Consequently, blinking and tear secretion stimulated after the eye-drop instillation are responsible for the fast washout of the drug from the precorneal area, while nasolacrymal drainage can lead to serious side-effects through uptake into the blood circulation. A good example is the β-blocker, timolol, which is used for the treatment of the wide-angle glaucoma and can cause side-effects to the heart if transported to the systemic circulation via nasolacrymal drainage.

The conjunctiva, a thin vascularized mucus membrane, which lines the inner surface of the eyelids and covers the anterior part of the sclera up to the cornea is also responsible for a large amount drug uptake. This uptake route adds to the systemic side-effects [28].

In the posterior section, the sclera maintains the shape of the eyeball and the choroid is a vascular layer that provides the blood supply that supports the retinal cells. The retina is separated from the choroid by Bruch's membrane.

9.2.1.2 Pathology

Ocular formulations aim to treat either inflammatory external eye infections (i.e. conjunctivitis, blepharitis, keratitis sicca) or intraocular diseases like glaucoma, uveitis, etc. The latter can be classified to anterior (iritis, iridocyclitis), intermediate (behind the iris and lens in the region of ciliary body and pars plana), posterior (retinitis, choroiditis, optic neuritis) and diffuse (all parts of the eye).

9.2.1.3 Drug Delivery

Ocular delivery has a low efficiency due to the cornea's low permeability to drugs, rapid tear turnover and nasolacrymal drainage. Diseases of the posterior segment are treated by intravitreous or subconjunctival injections, which are quite invasive and are able to cause inflammatory reactions.

There is a need for production of new formulations able to ensure increased stability of the drug and longer elimination half-life through sustained release. Nanoparticles and nanospheres are attractive as alternative delivery systems for the treatment of eye disorders because they are characterized by increased stability and longer elimination half-life in the tear fluid (20 min) in comparison to conventional drugs applied topically to the eye (1–3 min).

Ideally, particles need to be biodegradable, biocompatible, nontoxic, sterile, have a sustained release at a desirable rate, easy manufacturing procedure and be smaller than 10 μm so as to avoid any scratching or discomfort to the patient. Other important factors influencing the efficiency of such carriers are the charge, the drug lipophilicity and/or the carrier.

A number of polymers can be used to prepare particles (nanoparticles or nanospheres), which can be classified mainly into two categories: acrylate derivatives like poly(butyl cyanoacrylate) (PBCA) [29], PEG–polyethyl-2-cyanoacrylate (PECA) [30], poly[methoxy poly(ethylene glycol)cyanoacrylate-*co*-hexadecyl cyanoacrylate] (PEG–PHDCA) [31], copolymers of poly(ethylacrylate, methyl methacrylate and chlorotrimethyl-ammonioethyl methacrylate) [Eudragit®] [32–34] and the positively charged chitosan [35–37]. Poly(lactic acid) (PLA) [38], poly(D,L-lactic-*co*-glycolic) acid (PLGA) [39] and poly(ε-caprolactone) (PCL) [40] have been tested, too. Particles have been made using the mucoadhesive poly(acrylic acid) (PAA) and poly(itaconic acid) (PIA) [41], while hyaluronic acid (HA) [40] has been treated as a coating material for nanospheres made out of PCL (Fig. 9.2). Enhanced polymer–cornea affinity is the main aim to increase the particle residence time in the eye.

The mechanism of action is different for each of these polymers. PBCA, PAA, PIA and HA are characterized as mucoadhesive because they attach to the precor-

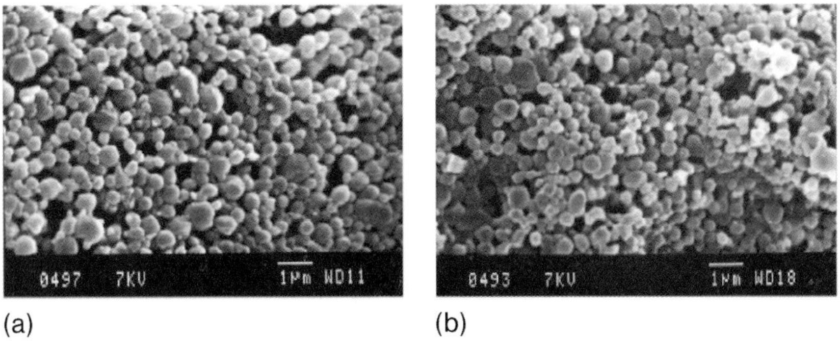

Figure 9.2. Scanning electron microscopy photographs of PCL nanospheres positively charged by stearylamine (SA) (a) or BKC (b) and coated with HA 0.025% (PCL/SA/HA ads and PCL/BKC/HA ads) Bar = 1 μm; original magnification ×10 000. (Reprinted from Ref. [40], © 2002, with permission from Elsevier.)

neal mucin layer via noncovalent bonds [40]. PEG molecules interact via hydrogen bonds with the mucin macromolecules present on the ophthalmic surface and may induce reversible opening of the tight junctions of the conjunctival tissue (allowing paracellular transport of drug molecules across ophthalmic tissues) [30]. Positively charged Eudragit™ and chitosan interact strongly with the negatively charged sialic acid residues in mucus. PLA and PLGA are generic materials for particle preparation, with FDA approval.

The physicochemical and surface characteristics are important in efficient drug accumulation into the eye. Other important factors are the preparation method and the presence of surfactants. Most of the particles produced using the materials mentioned above have a size range between 35 [Eudragit RL100, poly(acrylic acid) (PAA)] and 280 nm [PBCA, chitosan, PCL–benzalkonium chloride (BKC)] with an average size around 100 nm. The particle size mainly depends on the preparation method. According to de Campos and coworkers [35], the production of chitosan nanoparticles is dependent upon the chitosan concentration (decreased concentration leads to decreased size) and the acetonitrile/water volume (increasing the ratio leads to size decrease). Ibuprofen-loaded Eudragit RL100 and RS100 nanoparticles are prepared by the quasi-emulsion solvent diffusion method. Thus, the particle size is reduced as the polymer concentration or the volume of ethanol decreases [32]. Giannavola and coworkers [38] studied the incorporation of acyclovir into PLA nanoparticles using the nanoprecipitation method using various nonionic surfactants (Triton X-100, Tween 80, Brij 96, Pluronic F68). The particle size decreased as the polymer molecular weight increased while Tween 80 was the most efficient in decreasing the size and maintaining particle stability. Fresta and coworkers [30] produced similar PECA nanospheres by micellar polymerization using Pluronic F68.

Nanoparticles are preferred to microparticles because Giordano and coworkers [42] reported that the latter can cause a localized reaction confined to the inferior retina involving macrophages and multinucleated giant cells. Also, there was a nonuniform drug distribution within the vitreous cavity due to the accumulation of the particulate systems at the inferior retina [43]. Calvo and coworkers [44] reported that the *in vivo* corneal uptake of indomethacin-loaded PCL colloidal particles was higher than microparticles after topical instillation into the albino rabbit eye. Qaddumi and coworkers [39] drew the same conclusion studying the uptake of PLGA nanoparticles of 100 nm, 800 nm and 10 μm on primary cultured rabbit conjunctival epithelial cells (RCECs) The smaller (100 nm) particles exhibited the highest uptake.

The surface charge of the particles is important for particle adhesion to cornea. Positively charged colloids are able to deliver drugs to the eye due to their interaction with the negatively charged cornea. Positively charged chitosan nanoparticles or microspheres are much more effective than negatively charged particles due to the strong electrostatic interaction of the former with the negatively charged sialic acid residues in mucus [45]. The particulate nature is also important in increasing the intraocular penetration of drugs and decreasing the systemic absorption [46]. The importance of the cationic surface was shown by studying indomethacin containing nanocapsules coated with either poly(L-lysine) (PLL) or chitosan, resulting in completely different drug kinetics profiles [47]. Chitosan-coated nanocapsules significantly increased the indomethacin concentration in the cornea and aqueous humor 30 min and 1 h after the instillation to the eye in comparison to the uncoated and PLL-coated nanocapsules. The bioavailability [area under the concentration–time curve (AUC)] of indomethacin from chitosan-coated nanocapsules was 7- to 8-fold higher in the cornea and aqueous humor respectively, while the values for PLL-coated capsules were almost 4-fold higher than the Idocollyre® in both cornea and aqueous humor.

Drug incorporation and drug release are the main limiting factors for these systems. The drug–polymer affinity, the drug hydrophilic/lipophilic balance and solubility are some of the main obstacles and challenges to efficient ocular nanoparticle formulations. A great example is cyclosporin A (CyA) – an endecapeptide used in a variety of immune-mediated ocular surface phenomena like vernal conjunctivitis, dry eye syndrome, prevention of corneal allograft rejection [36]. Its high lipophilicity reduces corneal uptake and many formulations (e.g. oil solutions, complexation with cyclodextrins, micelles, etc.) were unsuitable for a variety of reasons. However, Calvo and coworkers [48] achieved a 50% incorporation of CyA in the oily phase of Mygliol nanocapsules surrounded by PCL where the final drug concentration was 10 mg mL^{-1}. These nanocapsules were taken up by corneal epithelial cells, so the drug level at the cornea was increased 5 times more than that obtained using the conventional 10 mg mL^{-1} CyA oily solution. Even here, drug retention at the ocular mucosa was poor, so it was considered useful only for the treatment of extraocular diseases. Chitosan particles were more promising carriers since the drug loading was approximately 9%, but they were characterized by rapid drug release (62% in 15 min in sink conditions). Even so 2- to 6-fold increase of CyA was found in cornea and conjunctival after topical instillation of these carriers. It was also noteworthy that the CyA amount found in cornea was higher than that in conjunctiva because drug-loaded carriers are cleared faster from the conjunctiva either due to the uptake by macrophages or to the passage to the blood circulation [35].

The antivirals, aciclovir and ganciclovir, have been in the focus of research since they are used for the treatment of herpes simplex infections and their ocular administration faces some problems. Aciclovir is used for Herpes simplex keratitis with the spread of the virus, at the most severe cases, in to the stromal cells, thus damaging them. However, the topical administration of the drug is difficult due to the low corneal penetration, and its poor water and lipid bilayer solubility [38].

The incorporation of aciclovir into PLA and PEG–PLA nanospheres was attempted in the presence of Tween 80 (0.5% w/v). The loading capacity was 2–5.9% in the former and 7.7% in the latter. The drug loading increased as the polymer molecular weight decreased for the PLA spheres, while it exhibited a further increase after the PEG insertion. This probably happened because the drug interacted with the PEG moiety, which retained the drug close to the particle surface. The drug release showed a burst effect and biphasic kinetics. Drug release reduced as the polymer molecular weight increased, while the presence of PEG did not offer any advantage in the release rate. In fact, the drug release was faster than the uncoated particles, which indicated a different drug distribution in the polymeric matrix.

Fresta and coworkers [30] studied the drug loading in PECA or PEG–PECA nanospheres in the presence of Pluronic F68, and showed that the drug entrapment was not affected by the presence of either PEG or cyclodextrins, or the concentration of surfactant used. PEG-coated spheres released aciclovir slower than uncoated PECA nanospheres, while the presence of cyclodextrin did not improve the release rate. The aciclovir release showed the same profile as that observed using the PLA nanospheres.

Ocular bioavailability tests showed that using PLA nanospheres, the effective levels of aciclovir in the aqueous humor at 6 h were (1 μg of aciclovir mL^{-1} aqueous humor) in comparison to the free drug formulations (no drug was detected 6 h later). PEG-coated PLA nanospheres were more effective than the uncoated PLA nanospheres and the free drug formulation, with 1.8- and 12.6-fold increase, respectively [38]. Similar results were reported after the instillation of aciclovir-loaded PEG–PECA nanospheres to the eye, which showed a 25-fold increase in comparison to free drug suspensions. Both research groups attributed the higher degree of success to mucoadhesive properties because of the polyoxyethylene presence on the nanosphere surface.

Ganciclovir is used for the treatment of more acute viral infections like the human cytomegalovirus (HCMV) retinitis, which is the major cause of visual loss in AIDS patients. Intravitreal administration of the drug is quite effective with a half-life of about 13 h, so frequent injections are needed to maintain the therapeutic efficacy. On top of that, the administration route imposes a high risk of cataract development, retinal detachment and endophthalmitis [49–50].

Another Food and Drug Administration (FDA)-approved antiviral drug is fomivirsen, which exhibits a 55-h half-life after intravitreal administration [51]. Despite its resistance to the nucleases, the administration of this drug is problematic due to its poor penetration through cell membranes because it is a polyanion. Albumin nanoparticles have been investigated for the entrapment of those drugs and the study of the intraocular disposition after their intravitreal injection to rats. Ganciclovir-loaded albumin nanoparticles were prepared by either adding drug after the particle preparation or during the preparation procedure. Drug loading and release was 15 μg ganciclovir mg^{-1} nanoparticles and 60% in 24 h for the first preparation, while it was 27 μg ganciclovir mg^{-1} nanoparticles and 40% in 24 h for the latter. The first formulation was more active and inhibited the expression of the HCMV early antigens at a lower concentration than the conventional drug solution after their incubation on a cell line.

Formivirsen was entrapped into albumin nanoparticles made in the same way as the ganciclovir, and resulted in 3.35 and 5.24 μg mg^{-1} nanoparticles, respectively. The oligonucleotide release was 100% after 8 h, while the latter formulation exhibited sustained release for up to 5 days. The release of both drugs show the same biphasic release profile with burst release as described earlier. According to the literature [51, 52], the albumin molecules have fusogenic properties enabling the transfer of the oligonucleotides to the nucleus of the cells. The intraocular disposition of biotin-labeled albumin nanoparticles was studied by intravitreal injection of 900 μg of particles per 5 μl. Two weeks later it was shown that the carriers diffused through the vitreous space, with most of them located in a thin layer overlying the retina as well as in adjacent sites to the blood aqueous barrier and the ciliary body. There was no evidence of nanoparticles in the inner retinal layers like the visual cells and the neuronal interplay area.

Tamoxifen (nonsteroidal estrogen receptor modulator) for the treatment of uveoretinitis [31] has been formulated into PEG-coated PHDCA nanoparticles. The drug loading and release were not reported but it was found that the intraocular injection of 0.25 μg of tamoxifen/10 μl incorporated in PEG–PHDCA particles was efficient in reducing the uveoretinitis induced to rats while the free tamoxifen had no effect on the inflammation. According to the reported results in the rats carrying uveoretinitis, the nanoparticles were dispersed through the anterior and posterior segments of the eye 8 h after intravitreal injection. After 24 h, the particles passed through the edematous retina, and accumulated in the subretinal space and within the retinal pigment epithelium. Particles were not found in the choroid, but a high amount was detected in the anterior chamber of the eye. the particles were still detected in the retinal pigment epithelium 3–9 days after the injection.

The nonsteroidal anti-inflammatory drugs, ibuprofen and flurbiprofen, were formulated into RS100 and RL100 acrylate nanosuspensions to treat miosis induced by surgical manipulation, e.g. cataract extraction [32, 34]. Approximately 92% of flurbiprofen incorporation into both types of nanoparticles was achieved. Drug release from RS100 particles was slower than that from RL100 particles because the latter contain a higher amount of quaternary ammonium group which makes the nanoparticle matrix more permeable. Drug release studies showed no burst release. The flurbiprofen-loaded RS100 formulation was found in the aqueous humor and antagonized successfully the miosis caused because of a surgical trauma.

Ibuprofen incorporation was as high as flurbiprofen in RS100 particles (approximately 90%). Most of the drug was released after 24 h, but even though the drug concentration in the aqueous humor was higher than that of the free drug solution, the reduction of miosis was not significant [33].

Brimonidine (α_2-adrenoreceptor antagonist) has been incorporated into PAA and polyitaconic acid (PIA) [41] nanoparticles with a loading capacity of 3.6 and 2.7 mg per 10 mg of nanoparticles respectively at pH 6.5. This corresponds to 80–85 and 70–75% loading efficiency in these systems, and 98% of the drug was retained for a period of 5 weeks at room temperature.

An alternative way to increase the residence time of the drug in the eye is the loading of nanocapsules into disposable soft contact lenses [53]. Nanocapsules were made with octadecyltrimethoxysilane (OTMS) in presence of Brij 97 (final size 13 nm) and loaded with lidocaine. OTMS creates a silica shell around the particles. The capsules were added to the polymerization medium, for lens formation of 1 mm thickness from poly(2-hydroxyethyl methacrylate) (pHEMA). The final particle content in the gel was 25%. When the gels were soaked in water, the drug was released almost completely after 7–8 days with burst release.

The mechanism of action is described herein. The drug diffuses from the particles through the lens matrix. A tear film is trapped between the cornea and lens; therefore, drug molecules will remain longer (30 min) in the post-lens tear film than in the case of eye-drops (2–5 min). This will enhance the influx of the drug through the cornea and reduce the systemic escape of the drug. Even so, there is still a fraction of the drug that will be lost due to tear drainage and absorption through the conjunctiva. According to these researchers, loading the lens with 0.024 mg of timolol will be enough to release therapeutic levels of the drug for 4 days.

The mechanism of interaction of various particles was studied either using primary cell lines or *in vivo*. Qaddoumi and coworkers [39] investigated the uptake mechanism of PLGA nanoparticles (100 nm) by primary cultured RCECs. After using a series of inhibitors for different specific uptake mechanisms located on the cell membrane, the group concluded that particle endocytosis takes place independently of both clathrin heavy chain and caveolin-1, although PLGA uptake may in part occur via clathrin-mediated processes. However, some endocytic process must be occurring because the conjunctival epithelium is a very strict barrier [54] and the paracellular pore radius is only 5 nm [55].

Chitosan nanoparticles are taken up by conjunctival epithelial cells more effectively than corneal epithelial cells because the conjunctival epithelium covers a larger surface area, and the concentration of mucin is higher there [56]. Chitosan nanoparticles can be transported by both paracellular and transcellular pathways because they are able to open the tight junctions between the epithelial cells due to the interactions between the positively charged groups of the polymer and the negative sites of the cell membrane and tight junctions. However, in conjunctiva, chitosan nanoparticles are located mostly in the cells rather than in the intercellular spaces. This happens because the conjunctival epithelium is more heterogeneous than that of cornea and contains goblet cells and APCs as well as epithelial cells. Thus, the particles could be transported to the APCs (Langerhans cells and macrophages) or even a specific cell receptor might be involved in the transport to some epithelial cells [45].

9.2.1.4 Tolerability

As potential candidates for ocular drug delivery, most of the systems described above were well tolerated without any sign of irritation or inflammation to the animal model tested, apart form the PIA nanoparticles, which were proved highly cytotoxic. Approximately 90% loss of corneal epithelial cells viability was observed 30 min after the incubation of the PIA nanoparticles with the cells.

9.2.1.5 Future Prospects for Nanoparticles in Ocular Delivery

Polymeric nanoparticles seem promising carriers for drug delivery to the eye. Some particles have shown adequate drug loading, prolonged site residence and good tolerability, but there are many more challenges to be faced yet. Drug loading, sustained release, storage stability and shelf-life are the main problems for many formulations. From a manufacturing point of view, the difficulty of producing sterile dispersions is also problematic. No nanoparticulate systems have yet solved all these problems and reached the market.

9.2.2 Macrophage-related Diseases

9.2.2.1 Leishmaniasis

Leishmaniasis is a disease occurring mostly in tropical and subtropical countries. Leishmanial promastigotes invade macrophages and survive in the phagolysosomal compartments of the host cells [57]. Primaquine, an antimalarial drug, has demonstrated some activity against visceral leishmaniasis, but it is highly toxic against red blood cells. PACA nanoparticles without drug showed some activity against *Leishmania donovani* infection in rats [58]. Primaquine-loaded poly(isohexyl cyanoacrylate) (PIHCA) nanoparticles were tested for their anti-infection activity *in vitro* using the macrophage-like J774G8 cell line. PIHCA nanoparticles can be phagocytosed by Kupffer cells and spleen macrophages; hence, they can be potentially used against visceral leishmaniasis [59]. The nanoparticles were not toxic to the J774G8 cells at concentrations up to 48 $\mu g\ mL^{-1}$ for 48 h of incubation. Primaquine-loaded PIHCA nanoparticles showed a 21-fold increase of antileishmanial activity, while the two components, i.e. primaquine and nanoparticles, acted synergistically compared to the mixture of free drug and nanoparticles at equivalent concentrations.

Primaquine was also incorporated in poly(D,L-lactide) nanoparticles and was administered intravenously to healthy and infected BALB/c mice with the aim to evaluate tolerance [60]. The particles were formed in presence of phospholipids and Poloxamer (1%) and the final drug-loaded carriers were 150–200 nm, while the ζ potential was -14.6 mV. The efficiency of primaquine was 85–94% using an initial drug concentration 0.5 $mg\ mL^{-1}$.

The acute lethal toxicity of primaquine after intravenous administration to healthy mice was reduced after incorporation of the drug in the particles. For example, LD_{50} of free primaquine was 17.5 mg of drug kg^{-1}, while for drug-loaded particles it was 26.9 $mg\ kg^{-1}$, corresponding to 536 mg PLA kg^{-1}. The lower toxicity is attributed to the rapid clearance of the particles to the MPS system so that the drug showed activity in the infected macrophages.

Neither free drug nor primaquine-loaded particles showed any lethal toxicity after injection of 10 $mg\ kg^{-1}$ 3 times in a 5-day period to infected BALB/c mice. As reported previously, the primaquine-loaded nanoparticles were 3.3 times more effective than the free drug in the suppression of the amastigotes of *L. donovani* in the liver of BALB/c mice [61].

Another drug used for the treatment against *Leishmania* is pentamidine, which is not fully effective and it has toxic side-effects [62]. Pentamidine has been incorporated onto the surface of methacrylate nanoparticles based on the ionic interactions with the free carboxyl groups of the polymer. Complete binding of pentamidine was obtained after mixing the drug (7 $\mu g\ mL^{-1}$ nanoparticle suspension). The particle size was approximately 330 nm. Methylglucamine antimoniate was used as the reference antileishmanial drug. The drug-loaded carriers suppressed the parasite burden by 77%, which was close to that achieved administering the reference drug (86%). The mean suppression by free drug was 35% while unloaded particles had no effect.

The pentamidine-loaded methacrylate particles were found to be effective against *Leishmania infantum* infection of BALB/c mice [63]. Parasite suppression of 50% was obtained after 1.06 mg of free drug kg^{-1} and 0.17 mg of pentamidine-loaded particles kg^{-1}. The latter ED_{50} was comparable to that achieved using liposomal amphotericin B (0.256 mg kg^{-1}).

Paul and coworkers [64] studied the physicochemical properties of pentamidine-loaded methacrylate nanoparticles and shown that the optimum stabilization of the drug on the particle surface was pH 7.5, where both drug and polymer are highly ionized. They found out that at the lysosomal pH of 5, 50% of the drug is released. Following the fate of the drug-loaded vesicles in the liver Kupffer cells of infected BALB/c mice, the authors found that phagocytotic vacuoles containing nanoparticles were fused with primary lysosomes to form secondary lysosomes. Half of the pentamidine was released in the lysosome due to its acidic pH. However, the drug is still ionized, so it cannot pass through the lysosomal membrane. The parasitophorous vacuole (pH 4.7–5.2) is fused with the secondary lysosome and the drug is still retained in the vacuole. Despite the fact that nanoparticles cannot be internalized by the parasites, the released pentamidine resulted in parasite growth suppression.

Another group incorporated amphotericin B in PLGA nanoparticles (size 166 nm), and evaluated the leishmanicidal potency of those particles on macrophages *in vitro* as well as the effect of trehalose on the multiplication of promastigotes and the macrophage activation [65]. Amphotericin B is sometimes used for the treatment of visceral leishmaniasis when the usual antimonial drugs are noneffective [66]. Liposomal amphotericin is used to reduce the toxicity and increase the drug efficacy. However, the amphotericin-loaded nanoparticles did not exhibit any advantage over the free amphotericin B in treating the infected macrophages, probably because the majority of the particles were washed away so there was only a limited amount endocytosed by the macrophages. Moreover, trehalose reduced promastigote multiplication. It has been shown previously that *L. donovani* promastigotes interact with the mannose/fucose receptors on human monocyte-derived macrophages in order to invade the host cells [67]. The presence of trehalose was shown to be toxic to the macrophages in a concentration higher than 50%. The sugar was tolerated in a concentration of 1 mg mL^{-1} by both infected and noninfected macrophages, but infected macrophages showed higher tolerance than the noninfected ones. This happened because lower amounts of specific receptors were available on the infected macrophages rather than the noninfected ones. Also, both infected and noninfected macrophages were activated by the presence of trehalose, while a greater effect was obtained for the infected ones. Thus, the sugar can alter the fate of *L. donovani* in the cells.

There is still a need for the development of new molecules with antileishmanial activity due to the toxic effects of the current drugs or due to their lack of efficiency [68]. Based on a previous report that the chalcones are quite effective against *L. donovani* [69], a group of researchers incorporated 2′,6′-dihydroxy-4′-methoxychalcone (DMC) extracted from *Piper aduncum* in PLA nanoparticles [70]. Pluronic F68 (1%) was used as surfactant to facilitate the particle formulation. The size of empty and loaded-nanoparticles was 130 and 168 nm, respectively, and the encapsulation efficiency was approximately 92%. BALB/c mice infected with *L. amazonensis* promastigotes were injected intraperitoneally with either empty particles (1 mg), DMC–PLA particles (200 μg DMC mg^{-1} PLA), glucantime (200 μg) or phosphate-buffered saline alone on days 42 and 48 after infection. It was shown that DMC–PLA particles were as effective as glucantime (first choice drug for the treatment of leishmaniasis) in reducing the number of parasites into the cells, making the drug-loaded particles promising agents for antileishmanial treatment.

Many other attempts to develop new antileishmanial agents have been reported [71–73]. One of these is quercetin, which belongs to the flavonoid family and is metabolized in the colon – it exhibits mostly antioxidant, anti-inflammatory, antihepatotoxic and antiulcer properties [71]. It has been formulated in different carriers, like liposomes, niosomes, microspheres and nanocapsules (PLA). It has been shown that quercetin inhibits the growth of *L. donovani* promastigotes and intracellular amastigotes both *in vitro* and *in vivo*, while it leads *L. donovani* promastigotes to apoptosis through inhibition of DNA topoisomerase II inhibition [74]. Quercetin EC_{50} was 3 mg kg^{-1} body weight; therefore, the different formulations were administered subcutaneously to hamsters after 30 days of their infection at a dose of 300 μg per 0.5 ml of vesicles suspension every 3 days for a total of 6 doses in 15 days. The final administered dose was equivalent to the EC_{50} of quercetin. The highest efficiency was obtained after the quercetin-loaded nanocapsules, which demonstrated 87% reduction of spleen parasite burden compared to the 25% achieved with the free drug. As for the rest of the formulations tested, the efficacy was 68, 51 and 44% for drug loaded-niosomes, liposomes and microspheres, respectively.

The same set of experiments was carried out with the carriers mentioned above using another potential antileishmanial agent named harmine (7-methoxy 1-methyl β-carboline), previously shown to be effective at Parkinson's disease and related neurological/psychiatric diseases [72]. Harmine has also exhibited activity against *Trypanosome cruzi*, while it can be effective against AIDS and tumors. It is believed that harmine condenses chromatin [75] and inhibits DNA topoisomerase I [76]. The effective dose of harmine was found to be 25 μg kg^{-1} body weight in 24 h after incubation of *L. donovani in vitro*. After the subcutaneous injection of the harmine-loaded particles, the reduction of the spleen parasite load was by 44% for the free drug, and 61, 67 and 79% for liposomes, niosomes and nanocapsules, respectively. One reason for the highest efficacy of the nanocapsules was the fact that they were the smallest formulation and their composition enabled them to circulate in the blood stream longer in comparison to the other type of vesicles, probably due to the presence of Tween 80 as a capsule component.

The same group carried out a similar piece of work on arjunglucoside, a pentacyclic triterpene glycoside of the saponin group, in nanogels of 90 nm or PLA nanoparticles (250 nm) for similar reasons [73]. The nanogel consisted of *N*-isopropyl-acrylamide (NIPAAm) and *N*-vinyl-pyrrolidone (VP). The drug incorporation efficiency was 80 and 60% for nanogel and PLA nanoparticle, respectively. After the subcutaneous injection of the two formulations in infected hamsters, they both exhibited a similar reduction in the spleen parasite load, which was recorded to be 75 and 79% for the nanogel and the nanoparticles, respectively. The effective dose of the drug was 4 mg kg^{-1} body weight. *In vitro* release of drug from nanogels was accompanied with an initial burst release of 50% and a total release of 75% after 25 h, while the drug release from PLA nanoparticles was 40% initially and it remained mostly constant up to 25 h.

Particles with neoglycoproteins having either glucose, mannose or fucose moieties grafted on the vesicle surface would enable more effective macrophage targeting according to comparative studies between liposomes, niosomes, microspheres and nanoparticles as presented by Basu and coworkers [77].

9.2.2.2 **Other Parasitic Infections**

Unloaded poly(isobutyl cyanoacrylate) (PIBCA) nanoparticles demonstrated antitrypanosomal activity after their *in vitro* and *in vivo* tests on *Trypanosoma brucei* [78]. More specifically, after *in vitro* treatment of *T. brucei* with different concentrations of PIHCA, the parasitic mobility disappeared in the presence of 1.2 μg mL^{-1}. Mice pretreated with 1.2 μg mL^{-1} and infected with trypanosomes survived until 30 days later, but they were not completely cured. The above nanoparticles were not effective against *Trypanosoma vaginalis* or *Entamoeba histolytica*.

Schistosomiasis is another serious public health problem in tropical countries. Praziquantel is the drug of choice, but the poor water solubility and the fast metabolism make long-lasting therapy hard to achieve. PLGA polymer was used to prepare nanoparticles with the emulsion-solvent evaporation method and a variety of factors were considered in order to prepare a formulation with optimum physicochemical properties [79] (Fig. 9.3). Those factors were PLGA and surfactant content in the formulation, time of sonication, ratio of the volume of aqueous to organic phase, and praziquantel content. Sonication (20 min) led to a particle size of 255 nm with polydispersity index of 0.22 and a monomodal distribution.

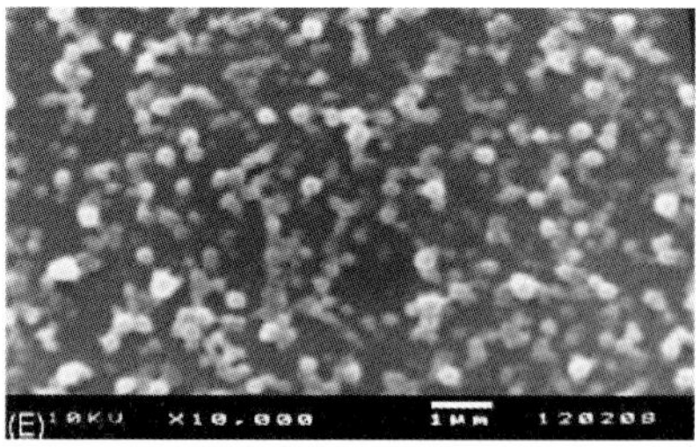

Figure 9.3. PLGA nanoparticles prepared with 20% of praziquantel. (Reprinted from Ref. [79], © 2005, with permission from Elsevier.)

Using 12.5 mg of PLGA polymer, the particles were of spherical shape without agglomeration.

As the polymer concentration (12.5, 25 and 50 mg) increased, the particle size increased and the particle shape deviated from the spherical pattern. As the surfactant content increased, the particle size reduced and the best formulation was obtained using 0.7% of surfactant. Also, the rate of evaporation of the organic solvent should be as slow as possible, so as the volume of the organic phase is reduced and the viscosity increases, the droplet size equilibrium will not change instantaneously and the particles will have the time to be formed in a good spherical shape of small size without agglomeration.

Praziquantel encapsulation efficiency was constant (approximately 75%) over the range of initial amount of the drug used from 10 to 30%. As the drug content increased, the size of the particles increased due to the increase of the dispersion viscosity. *In vitro* release of praziquantel was studied using particles prepared in the presence of 10 and 30% theoretical loadings; 100% of the drug was found in the dispersion medium in 2 h. As for the drug-loaded particles, 6 and 20% of drug was released from nanoparticles after 24 h from 10 and 30% drug-loaded particles. It is concluded that highest drug release is obtained with the highest drug loading.

An Antimalarial nanoparticle formulation has been reported by Legrand and coworkers [80]. Nanocapsules were prepared using PLA–PEG copolymers (PLA:PEG molecular weight ratios of 45:5 and 45:20) and Miglyol 810 to encapsulate halofantrine – a very hydrophobic antimalarial drug. Drug incorporation was better then 99.5% with 25% drug by weight of nanocapsules. Ther particles were stable for more than 10 months at 4 °C and had a size of 175–220 nm.

Drug release was slow in the presence of Tween 80 (used to allow solubility of drug in water), but rapid in the present of serum proteins. The nanocapsules were long circulating and when administered to mice infected with *Plasmodium berghei* showed a reduction in parasite infection within a short period, which was maintained for several days. The nanocapsule treatment was much more rapid in onset than with the free drug. The toxicity of the encapsulated drug was also much reduced in comparison to free drug.

9.2.3 Antifungal

9.2.3.1 Treatment

Drugs used in fungal infections are polyene antifungals (amphotericin, nystatin), imidazole antifungals (ketoconazole, miconazole), triazole antifungals (fluconazole, itraconazole), and others like griseofulvin, caspofungin, flucytosine and terbinafine [66]. Some of those drugs exhibit limitations either of absorption via the oral route or high toxicity. For example, polyene antifungals are not absorbed when given orally. They are used for oral, oropharyngeal and perioral infections by local application in the mouth. Amphotericin is highly toxic and mostly nephrotoxic, but lipid formulations (Abelcet®, AmBisome® and Amphocil®) have been produced reducing its toxicity.

Also, ketoconazole is characterized as highly hepatotoxic, but it is absorbed well when it is given orally. Itraconazole is another drug associated with liver damage.

9.2.3.2 **Drug Delivery Systems**

Only a few attempts have been reported using nanoparticles to improve the therapeutic prospects of the above mentioned drug molecules by reducing their limitations. Amphotericin B (used against infections by *Candida albicans*) was launched in the market as lipid formulations that are expensive. Thus, Tiyaboonchai and coworkers [81] have incorporated the antifungal drug in polyethylenimine (PEI)–dextran sulfate (DS) nanoparticles produced with the complex coacervation method (Fig. 9.4).

This method has the advantage of being simple and low cost without the need for organic solvents. It is based on the electrostatic interaction of the two oppositely charged molecules. Due to the poor water solubility of amphotericin B and low absorption from the gastrointestinal tract, the drug is administered parenterally. Particle size and size distribution are crucial parameters for parenteral formulations. The pH of PEI solutions, the charge and mass ratio of the two polymers as well as the zinc concentration influenced the particle size. The optimal conditions for am-

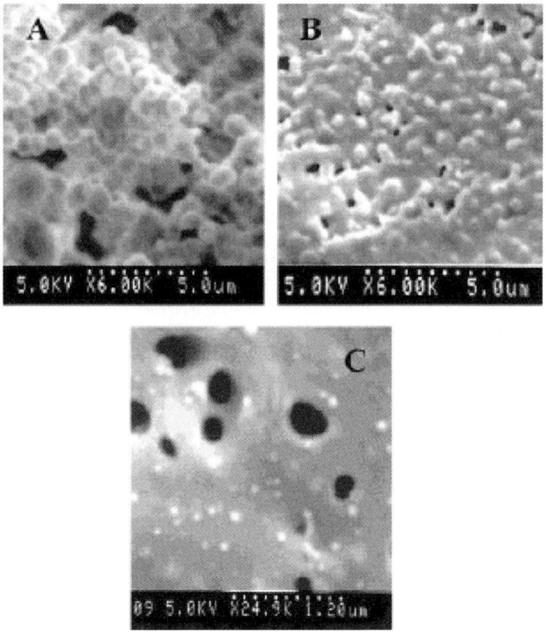

Figure 9.4. Scanning electron microscopy micrographs of unloaded nanoparticles formed with pH 7 PEI solution and a PEI:DS mass ratio of 1:1, and washed in (A) water and (B) 5% w/v mannitol. (C) Scanning electron microscopy micrograph of amphotericin B particles formed with pH 8 PEI solution and a PEI:DS mass ratio of 2:1, and washed in 5% mannitol. (Reprinted from Ref. [81], © 2001, with permission from Wiley.)

photericin B nanoparticle formation was the use of a PEI solution of pH 8, PEI:DS polymer ratio 2:1 and 25 μm zinc sulfate. Entrapment efficiency was about 85%. The particles produced had an average size of approximately 260 nm with a range of 100–600 nm. Mannitol was used as a cryoprotectant during the lyophilization procedure making the particles easily redispersable, which was not the case when mannitol was not present.

In vitro dissolution studies showed a rapid release of the drug, which, according to the authors, would be clinically useful due to the poor drug solubility and thus, the sustained release effect.

After incubating the drug-loaded nanoparticles with human cells, amphotericin B-loaded vesicles exhibited 100-fold lower toxicity compared to a reduction in the antifungal activity of the molecule of only 2-fold.

A different approach was to prevent the adhesion of *C. albicans* so to prevent the start of the infection [82]. This was based on using poly(propyl cyanoacrylate) nanoparticles in the presence of anionic, cationic or nonionic surfactants to promote adsorption onto the blastospore surface and, hence, reduce blastospore adherence to buccal epithelial cells. The adherence of blastospores that had been treated with nanoparticles produced in presence of docusate sodium was 73% lower than that of untreated blastospores. This phenomenon was reported to be due to the steric hindrance that the particles cause after their adherence on the spore's surface.

Molina and coworkers [83] improved the therapeutic efficacy of a sterol biosynthesis inhibitor, DO870, by incorporating it into PEG–PLA nanoparticles. This inhibitor was used successfully against the Y and CL strains of *Trypanosome cruzi* in Chagas' disease, but its development has been discontinued [84]. Also, ketoconazole- and itraconazole-loaded particles were used for comparison. Particle sizes in the range 100–200 nm were achieved and entrapment efficiencies were 90, 87 and 92% for DO870, itraconazole and ketoconazole, respectively. The drug-loaded nanoparticles were administered to infected mice either orally or intravenously and were well tolerated by the mice for the treatment period of 93 days. In contrast, for the group of mice treated with free DO870, 100% death was observed at the day 93, postinfection period.

After administration of DO870-loaded particles via the intravenous route (1.5–3.0 mg kg^{-1} day^{-1}) or the oral route (5 mg kg^{-1} day^{-1}) no reappearance of parasites in the blood was observed. The cure rate for those formulations was approximately 80% in mice infected with the CL strain of *T. cruzi*. For the Y strain, infected mice received an intravenous administration of 3 mg kg^{-1} day^{-1}. The cure rate of DO870-loaded particles was 60%, while there was no positive influence of the ketoconazole or itraconazole-loaded spheres.

Nisin is a bacteriosin produced by *Lactococcus lactis* and is used as a food preservative, but it is unstable and so it was incorporated into nanoparticles [85]. Those particles were made using PLA with the method of supercritical fluids. Using supercritical or compressed gas techniques to make nanoparticles is very attractive due to the omission of surfactants or stabilizers that may cause protein denaturation or toxic effects, the process flexibility, the high product yield and, possibly,

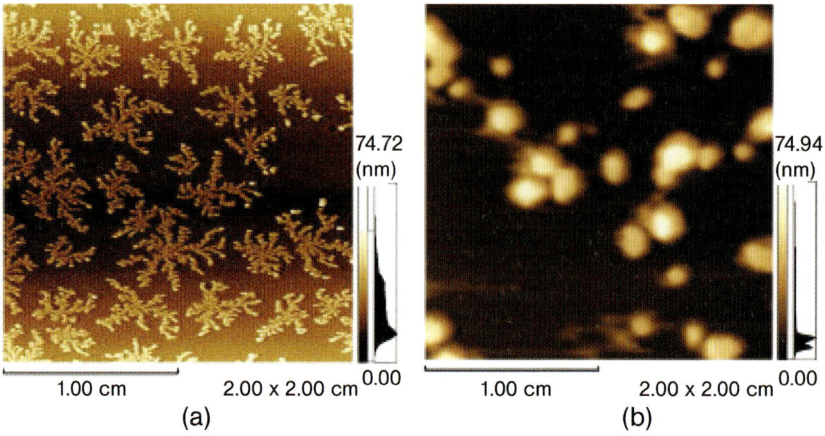

Figure 9.5. Atomic force micrographs of chitosan nanoparticles at pH 5.0: chitosan nanoparticles (A) and copper-loaded nanoparticles (B). (Reprinted from Ref. [86], © 2004, with permission from Elsevier.)

efficient protein encapsulation. The optimal ratios for particle preparation were: dimethylsulfoxide:dichloromethane 50:50 where the nisin solubility was 60 mg mL^{-1}, and a PLA solution of 10 mg mL^{-1} containing 0.5 or 2 mg mL^{-1} nisin. The optimal preparation conditions were: 1 ml min^{-1} organic solution injection into the precipitation vessel, 288 K and 15 MPa, 1500 NL (normal liters) h^{-1} CO_2 flow rate and 1 h CO_2 washing after the particle preparation. The process yield was approximately 80% and the remaining DMSO and DCM were less than 300 and 15 p.p.m., respectively. Biological studies showed that nisin was entrapped in the particles in its active form so the efficacy of the preparation procedure was demonstrated. However, the nisin-loaded particles had a weaker antibacterial activity attributed to the delay of protein release from the spheres.

Finally, we should mention the recently reported antibacterial activity of chitosan nanoparticles and copper-loaded chitosan nanoparticles [86] (Fig. 9.5). The particle preparation took place in presence of tripolyphosphate (TPP) with anionic gelation at room temperature. Absorption of copper ions on the particle surface affected the physicochemical properties of the particles. The particle sizes were 4 and 275 nm and the ζ potentials were 51 and 96 mV for the chitosan and copper-loaded chitosan nanoparticles, respectively.

Bacteria can adhere on the chitosan surface either in the particle or the molecular form in 30 min. According to the literature, chitosan possess antimicrobial activity against a number of Gram-negative and Gram-positive bacteria [87–88]. Chitosan nanoparticles and copper-loaded chitosan nanoparticles showed stronger antibacterial activity than chitosan alone or doxycycline. Chitosan nanoparticles surround the bacteria after 30 min. This leads to the cell degradation in 60 min and finally the cells begin to fragment after 3 h. A possible mechanism of action is that either it chelates with nutrients and so inhibits the bacteria growth or chitosan interacts with the anionic groups of the cell surface and forms polyelectrolyte complexes with bacterial surface compounds. Hence, they form an impermeable layer around the cell, which prevents the transport of essential solutes in the bacterial cell. Also, it was shown that the nanoparticle nature of chitosan was responsible for the higher antimicrobial activity.

In the case of copper-loaded nanoparticles, copper was adsorbed on the chitosan particles and passes through the pores of the vesicles towards the inner surface of the particles, where it is chelated. The antimicrobial mechanism of action of copper is that copper is reduced from Cu^{2+} to Cu^{1+} in the bacteria. The O_2^- and H_2O_2 produced by such redox reactions cause cytotoxicity by inhibition of DNA synthesis and thus reduction of cell viability.

9.2.4 Tuberculosis

9.2.4.1 Physiology and Pathology

Mycobacterium tuberculosis is the causative organism of tuberculosis, which occurs mainly in the lungs, although it can be disseminated to other organs. Bacteria reach the deep lung and are phagocytosed by alveolar macrophages. There, the bacteria will be either destroyed, replicate within the macrophages or remain latent indefinitely. If replication is not prevented the bacilli will multiply and eventually cause the macrophage to rupture.

Tuberculosis is transmissible between people and is most prevalent in places where poor hygienic conditions are found, e.g. during war, famine, homelessness, people lacking adequate medical care, etc. It continues to be found worldwide and causes about 2 million deaths per year. Treatment is long and inadequate or incomplete treatment promotes the development of resistant strains of tuberculosis.

9.2.4.2 Treatment

Tuberculosis is treated in two phases. (i) An initial phase of 2 months, which comprises daily administration of a combination of at least three of the drugs rifampicin (RIF), isoniazid (INH), pyrazinamide (PZA) or ethambutol according to the patient tolerance or bacterial strain resistance. (ii) A continuation phase of 4 months using two drugs, mainly INH and RIF. The treatment is usually oral, but sometimes treatment is parenteral. INH, RIF and PZA are associated with liver toxicity, so hepatic function and renal function should be checked before the treatment commences. Visual acuity should be tested before induction of ethambutol to the therapeutic scheme. Patient noncompliance due to daily multidrug dosing is a significant drawback in tuberculosis therapy.

The main aim of microparticles or nanoparticles for antituberculosis therapy is to reduce the drug systemic toxicity and dosage whether by oral or pulmonary delivery. According to Pandey and coworkers [89], using nanoparticles is preferable to microspheres because of "the high drug loading minimizing the consumption of polymers, their ability to pass through various barriers due to their small size eliciting better therapeutic response".

9.2.4.2.1 **Oral** Polymeric nanoparticles for oral delivery have been prepared using PLGA polymer [90–92]. The three drugs, RIF, INH and PZA were coencapsulated and exhibited a high drug encapsulation efficiency of 56.9, 66.3 and 68%, respectively with a particle size range of 186–290 nm. After a single oral administration (therapeutic dose of RIF: 12 mg kg^{-1} + INH 10 mg kg^{-1} + PZA 25 mg kg^{-1}) of these particles to mice with experimental tuberculosis, therapeutic levels in plasma were maintained for 4 days in the case of RIF, and for up to 9 days for INH and PZA. Therapeutic concentrations in the tissues higher than the mean inhibitory concentration (MIC) were found for up to 11 days for INH. The free drugs or mixture of free drugs with empty PLGA nanoparticles, administered as a one single oral dose, were cleared rapidly since no drug was detected in the plasma after 12–24 h. According to Pandey and coworkers [90], PLGA polymers are adhesive to the intestinal mucosa so the nanoparticles can be adsorbed directly by intracellular or paracellular routes. More specifically, the nanoparticles can be taken up either by transcytosis via M cells, or intracellular uptake and transport via the epithelial cells lining the intestinal mucosa or uptake via Peyer's patches [93]. Increased lung accumulation was not observed with multiple dosing (five doses at 10 day intervals), but no tubercle bacilli could be detected in the tissues. It was also shown that reducing the oral administration of the previously mentioned formulation by one-third, RIF remained in the circulation for 5 days while INH and PZA remained for 12 days. The drug tissue levels were higher than the MIC up to 14 days in guinea pigs [91]. Even with two-thirds of the therapeutic dose of PLGA-NP, bacilli could not be detected after five doses of treatment.

In order to increase the therapeutic efficacy of the PLGA nanoparticles, the lectin, wheat germ agglutinin (WGA), was incorporated onto the particle surface [92] to interact with specific receptors on intestinal and alveolar epithelium. This lectin has very low immunogenicity, thus making these particles potential candidates for oral and aerosol drug delivery. After a single oral administration of drug-loaded WGA–PLG nanoparticles to guinea pigs with tuberculosis, RIF was still found in the blood circulation 7 days later, and INH and PZA after 13 days. The therapeutic levels in the tissues were maintained higher than the MIC for 15 days and nanoparticle formulations did not show any hepatotoxicity.

9.2.4.2.2 **Pulmonary** During oral administration, only a fraction of the total dose of drugs reaches the lungs and even this fraction is cleared quickly so that frequent doses of antitubercular drugs are necessary [89]. Bearing in mind those problems as well as the fact that the pulmonary route leads the drug directly to the most affected organ, the lungs, nanoparticle administration has also been attempted via nebulization or aerosolization. Pulmonary administration is particularly attractive because of the direct targeting of alveolar macrophages, which are used by mycobacteria as a site for their prolonged survival. Lung delivery will also reduce drug systemic toxicity, therefore improving patient compliance. The lungs offer an enormous surface area for absorption, a favorable environment for proteins, avoidance of first-pass metabolism and better patient acceptability than an injection [94].

PLGA nanoparticles loaded with RIF, INH and PZA with a mass median aerodynamic diameter (MMAD) of 1.88 ± 0.01 μm were used for inhalation as a single dose every 10 days in guinea pigs [95, 96]. The drug plasma concentration was detected from 6 h onwards until 6 days for RIF, and until 8 days for INH and PZA. The tissue drug concentration at levels higher than MIC was seen for up to 11 days. When the WGA lectin was incorporated on the surface of those nanoparticles [4] (MMDA 2.8 ± 1.4 μm), the formulation showed improved potency. After one dose to guinea pigs the INH and PZA plasma levels were retained up to 13 and 14 days, respectively, whereas the RIF levels were detected for up to 6 days. The tissue drug levels higher than MIC were estimated up to 15 days and no hepatotoxicity was observed.

PLGA polymer has limitations as a carrier for lung delivery because of the degradation products of the polymer which can be accumulated in the lung tissue. The polymer induced a mild inflammation lasting for 2–3 weeks [97], but with no obvious consequence on lung function. Bulk PLGA degradation creates an acidic environment, which can damage pH-sensitive drugs such as peptides and proteins [94].

New biomaterials have also been used for drug delivery via aerosolization. Fu and coworkers [94] synthesized the polyether anhydride, sebacic acid (SA)–PEG copolymer, consisting of FDA-approved materials. The PEG content of this polymer leads to the decrease of aerodynamic diameter as well as to increased degradation times. These characteristics give the flexibility of producing particles of different properties for different parts of the lung.

Dailey and coworkers [98] prepared nanoparticles with the branched polyester, diethylaminopropylamine–poly(vinyl alcohol)-g-poly(lactide-co-glycolide) (DEAPA–PVAL-g-PLGA). The nanoparticles included some polyions [carboxymethylcellulose (CMC), dextran sulfate, DNA] in order to modify the physicochemical properties and to study the formulation with the best stability. The greatest advantage of these polymers was that they could be assembled into particles in the absence of surfactant, to reduce possible effects on lung function. It was shown that the positively charged particles interacted efficiently with lung cells, unfortunately only the anionic particles, which did not show any interaction with cells, could be nebulized efficiently.

Alginate, a biodegradable FDA-approved natural polymer, has also been investigated. Nanoparticles made after cation-induced controlled gelification of alginate were of approximately 235.5 nm diameter and the drug encapsulation efficiency was 80–90% for RIF, and 70–90% for INH and PZA. After aerosolization the MMAD was 1.1 ± 0.4 μm [99]. A single dose of particles loaded with RIF, INH and PZA was administered to guinea pigs. The drugs were detected in the plasma from 3 h onwards. RIF was found in the plasma up to 10 days, and INH and PZA for 14 days. The drug tissue levels were higher than MIC up to 15 days. Thus, overall, alginate particles appeared earlier in the plasma, and RIF was present in the serum for longer than WGA–PLGA nanoparticles with similar retention of tissue drug levels. Again, hepatotoxicity was not observed using the alginate nanoparticles. All these formulations were capable of eliminating the mycobacteria after administration of five doses once every 10 days.

9.2.4.2.3 Subcutaneous Administration PLGA nanoparticles loaded with RIF, INH and PZA, and administered via subcutaneous injection to mice, showed sustained release maintaining therapeutic drug levels for up to 36 days in the lungs and the spleen and up to 32 days in the plasma [100]. This resulted in undetectable colony-forming units, while the subcutaneous injection of the free drugs did not reduce the bacterial presence in the organs of infected mice.

9.2.4.3 Future Prospects

From the results reported so far, it seems that the formulation of the three main antitubercular drugs into nanoparticles is very promising for the effective treatment of the disease using either the oral or the pulmonary pathway. The drug loading was high and inhalable formulations were produced from polymer nanoparticles. The use of ligand-bearing particles or particles made with natural polymers promoting cell binding and uptake showed prolonged therapeutic efficacy. A significant reduction in dosage from 45 administrations to five was achieved without compromising performance. The reduction of the dosing scheme is very encouraging because it contributes to patient convenience. The problems that still have to be tackled are mainly the improvement of inhalable formulations, and the cost for the large-scale production of those particles and final products, which will have to exhibit long shelf-life.

9.2.5 AIDS

9.2.5.1 Pathology

HIV is a retrovirus with two primary types: HIV-1 and HIV-2. There are many strains of both types and all mutate rapidly, which has made it particularly difficult for researchers to find an effective vaccine or treatment for the virus. HIV infection is often mostly or entirely asymptomatic (without symptoms) and the most common signs, which include fever, fatigue, rash and lymphadenopathy (swollen lymph nodes), are often mistaken for mononucleosis, flu or similar, comparatively harmless diseases. Eventually, full-blown AIDS develops in the vast majority of cases.

9.2.5.2 Treatment

The infection caused by the HIV cannot be cured, but drugs are used to slow down the progression of the disease [66]. Drugs for HIV are toxic and expensive, but they increase life expectancy considerably. The aim of the treatment is to reduce the plasma viral load as much as possible and as long as possible before the immune system is irreversibly damaged. The treatment scheme should be chosen taking into account the drug toxicity, patient convenience and tolerance. Using a combination of drugs can halt the drug resistance. This drug combination should have a synergistic therapeutic effect, but not an additive toxic effect. The suggested treatment is the combination of two nucleoside reverse transcriptase inhibitors with either a non-nucleoside reverse transcriptase inhibitor or one or two protease inhibitors.

Nucleoside analogs or nucleoside reverse transcriptase inhibitors were the first substances used for the HIV treatment. They are DNA chain terminators or competitive inhibitors of the virus-associated reverse transcriptase. Such nucleoside analogues are zidovudine [azidothymidine (AZT)], abacavir, didanosine, lamivudine, stavudine, tenofovir and zalcitabine.

The second group of molecules used for HIV treatment are protease inhibitors, and include amprenavir, indinavir, lopinavir, nelfinavir, ritonavir and saquinavir. They can block the replication of HIV in chronically infected cells. They are metabolized by P450 enzyme systems, and are associated with lipodystrophy and metabolic effects.

The third category of anti-HIV drugs is made up of the non-nucleoside reverse trancriptase inhibitors efavirenz and nevirapine.

9.2.5.3 Nanoparticle Delivery Systems

Due to the high dosage scheme in order to achieve antiviral activity and the high toxicity of anti-HIV drugs, there have been attempts to entrap some of these drugs into polymeric nanoparticles to make the treatment more tolerable for the patient and to effectively reduce the drug dosage.

At first, the potential of the antiviral activity of zalcitabine or saquinavir loaded into nanoparticles was studied by incubating HIV-infected primary human macrophages *in vitro* and comparison with the free drug activity on the same cells [101]. The problem with zalcitabine is the rapid viral resistance, while saquinavir is a poorly soluble drug with low bioavailability. Poly(hexyl cyanoacrylate) (PHCA) was used as the polymer of choice to make nanoparticles, which entrapped 15–20% of zalcitabine and 50–60% of saquinavir, respectively. The particle size was approximately 200 and 475 nm, respectively. After the incubation of the drug-loaded nanoparticles with the macrophages, the antiviral activity of zalcitabine did not show any advantage by incorporating the drug into the polymeric carriers, while the activity of saquinavir showed 10-fold improvement. This can be explained on the basis that the zalcitabine molecule itself enters the cell through diffusion and through some transport mechanisms. The activity of this drug is depended on its intracellular conversion to the corresponding 5′ mono-, di- and triphosphate derivatives [102].

Later, AZT bound to hexylcyanoacrylate nanoparticles was administered intravenously to rats to estimate the targeting feasibility of these nanoparticles to macrophages [103]. Polysorbate 80 (1%)-coated nanoparticles loaded with AZT were used as well to study the influence of the surfactant on the uptake by the brain with the aim of treating the dissemination of the virus to the brain (microglia). Indeed, 8 h postinjection, 60% of AZT was found in the reticuloendothelial system (RES) or-

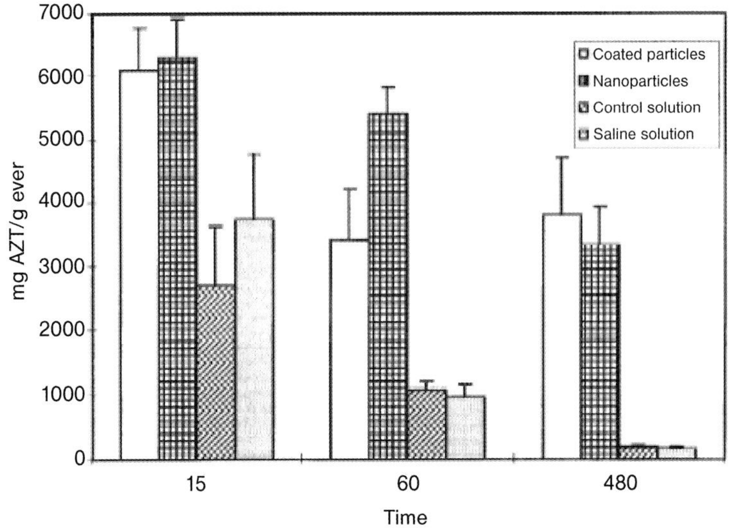

Figure 9.6. Liver concentrations of AZT (mg of AZT g^{-1} liver) after intravenous injection of Polysorbate-80-coated AZT nanoparticles, AZT nanoparticles, an AZT control solution (with emulsifier) and a saline AZT solution (without emulsifier). (Reprinted from Ref. [103], © 1998, with permission from Elsevier.)

gans, while only 12% of the drug injected in its free form was found in the same organs (Fig. 9.6). No trend was obtained in the other organs mainly due to the large fluctuations observed.

Polysorbate-80-coated nanoparticles showed a significant decrease in the liver accumulation, prolonged half-life and significant increase in the brain 1 h after intravenous injection. The increase of the surfactant coated nanoparticles was 35% higher compared to the uncoated particles and 45% compared to the unbound AZT, so there is the possibility of reducing the AZT dose to reduce the AZT side effects.

The same drug was formulated in nanospheres made by PIHCA aiming to concentrate AZT in the intestinal epithelium and associated immunocompetent cells which are known to be one of the major reservoirs of HIV [104]. PIHCA was used due to the controlled release properties in the gastrointestinal tract and its tendency to interact with the intestinal mucosa. The nanospheres were administered by intragastric intubation to rats. The carrier size was approximately 250 nm and the ζ potential -23 mV. The release of AZT was estimated in different media; a burst release of 35% of AZT was observed in water or USP XIII-simulated gastric medium containing pepsin. In the presence of pancreatin, 80% of AZT was released 8 h later, probably due to the presence of esterases.

AZT accumulation was 4.4 and 5.9 times higher in intestinal mucosa 30 and 90 min later, respectively, in comparison to the control systems. Similarly, 67% and 64% of the initial dose of AZT was found in the gastrointestinal tract, while only

15 and 11% of the drug was found, respectively, after the administration of drug solution.

The drug accumulation from the particles was 4- and 28-fold higher in stomach 30 and 90 min postadministration, respectively and around 5.5-fold higher in intestine. AZT concentration was maintained constant in the intestine, while it was very low in cecum and colon. Additionally, nanoparticles resulted in higher AZT concentrations in the mucus when compared to the solution (59 and 60.5 nmol AZT g^{-1} organ for the nanoparticles at 30 and 90 min, respectively, compared to 8.1 and 10.6 nmol g^{-1} organ for the solution). Moreover, 4-fold AZT increase was achieved in Peyer's patches while a very low concentration was found in the lymphatics.

HIV protease inhibitors are characterized by poor pharmacokinetic characteristics and bioavailability problems, which were addressed by the use of nanoparticles. Thus, the HIV protease inhibitor, CGP-57813, was incorporated into pH-sensitive nanoparticles made by Eudragit S100 or L100-55 (approximately 14% drug loading, 250 nm size) [105]. The difference between the two types of polymers lay in the part of the gastrointestinal tract where they were soluble. Also, the influence of the presence of food in the gastrointestinal tract in the effective delivery of the HIV protease inhibitor was studied after the oral administration (25 mg CGP 57813 mL^{-1}) of the particles to dogs. According to these studies, Eudragit L100-55 particles did not show any improvement in bioavailability in fasted dogs and only a small increase was obtained in fed dogs, probably because of the rapid dissolution of the polymer in the intestinal pH, which led to the precipitation of the compound.

The presence of food had a more pronounced effect on CGP 57813 bioavailability, while no detectable plasma levels were reported in fasted dogs. The same series of experiments were carried out in mice with opposite results. Eudragit L100-55-loaded particles were more favorable in increasing the bioavailability of the protease inhibitor, indicating that the optimal formulation depends strongly on the animal species [106].

Eudragit L100-55 was studied for improvement of the solubility and bioavailability of HIV-1 protease inhibitor CGP 70726 after oral administration to dogs in the presence or absence of food [107]. Not only nanoparticles, but microspheres were studied here to investigate the influence of the size. The latter did not seem to make any significant difference in the performance of those pH-sensitive systems, but the presence of food reduced the bioavailability especially in the case of nanoparticles. This is probably due to the pH alterations in the gastrointestinal tract in presence of food, which resulted in fast release and precipitation of the drug in the stomach.

Saquinavir is a HIV-1 and HIV-2 protease inhibitor, which is well tolerated, but suffers from low oral bioavailability [108]. This is because it undergoes hepatic metabolism, it exhibits poor water solubility and thus a very low absorption, and it is unable to cross the intestinal barrier due to the multidrug resistance transporter, P-glycoprotein. Therefore, saquinavir was complexed with hydroxypropyl-β-cyclodextrin (HPβCD) and incorporated in nanoparticles made by either PIBCA or PIHCA polymers. Only 2.4 and 2.9 μg of saquinavir mg^{-1} of polymer, respectively, were incorporated in to the nanoparticles mentioned earlier. However, in the presence of 10% HPβCD, the entrapped saquinavir was 45 and 50 μg mg^{-1} of particles for PIBCA and PIHCA, respectively. The drug loading reached a plateau when the HPβCD–saquinavir complex attained 5 and 7.5 mg mL^{-1} for PIBCA and PIHCA, respectively, which corresponds to a 20-fold increase. The ζ potentials of unloaded nanoparticles were −36.9 and −37.1 mV for PIBCA and PIHCA, respectively. These values became more positive as the cyclodextrin concentration increased. Apparently, PIHCA exhibited higher drug loading because it was more hydrophobic. This study showed that these nanoparticles could potentially reduce the dose of saquinavir for the treatment of HIV patients.

Berton and coworkers [109] tried to protect a cytotoxic phosphorothioate oligonucleotide, GEM91 in polymeric nanoparticles consisting of PLA. Antisense oligonucleotides (AS-ODNs) are used to block different replication phases of the virus life cycle and phosphorothioate analogs are less sensitive to nucleases than phosphodiesters. Another serious obstacle for the successful antiviral activity of these oligonucleotides is their uptake into appropriate cellular compartments. The results indicated that the PLA formulation facilitated the delivery of the incorporated oligonucleotides to both HeLa $P_{4-2}CD_4^+$ and CEM (human lymphoid T cells) cell lines at nanomolar concentrations. [The P_{4-2} indicators cells are HIV-1-susceptible HeLa CD_4^+ cells carrying the bacterial *lacZ* gene driven by the HIV-1 long terminal repeat (LTR). β-Galactosidase expression is induced by the LTR transactivation by the viral Tat protein produced during infection.]

Models used to test the antiviral activity were: (i) cells containing the Tat activation region (TAR) of the HIV-1-LTR, which controls the transcription of the β-galactosidase reporter gene. Incubation of cells with the oligonucleotide-loaded nanoparticles at the time of virus infection resulted in a reduction in β-galactosidase production 48 h later. This indicates that these antisense carrier systems have the ability to inhibit the early events of the viral cycle life. (ii) Acutely infected CEM cells were treated with the oligonucleotide carriers and it was showed that the HIV-1 reverse transcriptase activity was reduced significantly and kept at low levels for the duration of the experiment. GEM91 alone (100 nm) did not have any impact on the HIV-infected cells, while it caused 90% inhibition after incorporation into the particles.

Another way to enable the delivery of AS-ODNs into cells is by complex formation with protamine, which was studied using primary human macrophages and CD_4^+ T cells [110]. Protamine complexation shields the negative charge of the ODN and protects it from degradation. The mean particle size was 150–180 nm and the ζ potential was positive for protamine:AS-ODN ratios above 1.5 and negative for protamine:AS-ODN ratios below 0.5. Complete complexation occurred when protamine:AS-ODN ratio was above 1.25. High internalization rates were obtained after the treatment of primary human macrophages and T cells with protamine/AS-ODN nanoparticles with no any sign of cytotoxicity up to 5 μM concentration.

By tracking both components of the complex by fluorescent labeling and incubating them with primary human macrophages, it was shown that the AS-ODN was released in the cell 24 h after cellular uptake. Complexes comprised of phosphorothioate (PTO) and protamine treated in the same way as the protamine/AS-ODN mentioned earlier, showed that the particles were stable even after 48 or 72 h following their cellular uptake. The specific inhibitory effect of protamine/anti-Tat AS-ODN nanoparticles was about 30% at a concentration of 2 µM, in contrast to protamine/PTO complexes, which did not show any significant inhibition. The latter happened due to the very slow release of the PTO from its carriers indicating that the dissociation of the antisense compound from the complex was an essential process for antisense activity.

9.2.5.4 Vaccines and AIDS

Apart from the improvement in delivery of anti-AIDS drugs incorporated into nanoparticles, research has been focused on development of anti-HIV vaccines. AIDS is characterized by immunosupression due to the overproduction of immunosuppressive cytokine interferon (IFN)-α and the regulating HIV-1 Tat protein released in the extracellular compartment of acutely infected lymphoid tissue [111]. Tat reduces the immune reactivity of still uninfected T cells and further induces overproduction of IFN-α by APCs. Tat toxoid is the version of Tat that is detoxified, but still immunogenic. This is the antigen used to produce anti-Tat antibodies. Anti-Tat vaccination is aimed at mucosal immunity since the virus entry to the body is through the mucosal membranes, which constitutes the 70% of lymphoid tissues of an organism. Therefore, the induction of mucosal immunity was attempted towards Tat protein in mice by either intranasal or oral route using either an oily adjuvant, chitosan nanoparticles or PLGA microparticles. None of these formulations was found to be more advantageous over the other and it seems that all of them were effective enough to cause the production of anti-Tat IgA antibodies. It was shown that cell-mediated immunity was caused as the stimulation indices obtained after the treatment of splenocytes of anti-Tat-immunized mice with Tat protein or Tat toxoid were higher than those of nonimmunized mice.

Using Tat toxoid may not be the optimum antigen because some important epitopes could have been damaged due to the preparation procedure [112]. In more detail, Tat protein is a small protein consisting of 86–101 amino acids and encoded by two exons. There are five domains, but the three most important are the amino-terminal domain (1–21 amino acids), the cysteine rich domain (22–37 amino acids), which is the trans-activation domain, and the basic domain (49–72 amino acids), which contains the nuclear localization signals. That basic domain is responsible for the transactivation of HIV to the other cells and of cellular processes altering the intracellular signaling of various cell types [113, 114]. The biologically active Tat (1–72) protein, which was confirmed to be immunogenic and nonimmunosuppressive, was adsorbed on the surface of anionic nanoparticles. The latter were made by the emulsification of wax (oil phase) and sodium dodecyl sulfate (SDS, anionic surfactant) dissolved in water. Tat was adsorbed on the particles (100 nm) produced by its basic domain and the final formulation was administered subcutaneously to mice on days 0 and 14. Immune responses recorded from mice immunized with the particle formulation were compared to those obtained from mice immunized either with alum Tat (T_h2 control) with alum adjuvant and Tat (T_h1 control) with lipid A as adjuvant. There were strong antibody responses (IgG and IgM) and the IgG titer from the Tat-immunized mice was approximately 3-fold higher than that in "naive" mice, even after 10 000 dilution of the particle formulation. The Tat-coated nanoparticles caused the production of IFN-γ to the same level as the Tat with lipid A as adjuvant, which indicates that the specific formulation induces an enhancement of T_h1 immune response and, thus, is considered as a promising vaccine product.

Another novel nontoxic polyelectrolyte formulation is composed of polylysine modified with imidazole side-chains condensing HIV-2 *env* DNA into nanoparticles [115]. The size of the resulting nanoparticles was approximately 150 nm and it was considered ideal for targeting clathrin-coated pit uptake into the cell. The complexation with cationic polymer prevents DNA degradation in the lysosomal compartment and the imidazole side-chains optimize the escape to the cytoplasm of the target cell. The polyelectrolyte complexes induced higher levels of IgA, IgM and IgG antibodies by the intradermal route to BALB/c mice (Fig. 9.7).

Kawamura and coworkers [116] used concanavalin A-polystyrene nanospheres (Con A-NS) to capture HIV-1 envelope antigen gp120 due to the high affinity that the lectin exhibits for the HIV-1 antigen. In this study, dendritic cells were the targets for the immune response since they are unique major APCs capable of stimulating "naive" T cells in the primary immune response and more potent APCs

Figure 9.7. Comparison of HIV-2 gp120-specific antibodies in mice immunized with a polylysine nanoparticle formulation. Serum from mice was evaluated using samples taken 28 days after the third DNA immunization by the intradermal route. IgG subclasses (A) and antibody isotypes (B) were evaluated in mouse serum samples. ELISA results are shown using serum from mice immunized with polylysine nanoparticles containing DNA encoding HIV-2 gp140 (solid bars), naked DNA encoding gp140 (diagonal lines) and plasmid vector DNA formulated with polylysine nanoparticles (stippled bars). (Reprinted from Ref. [115], © 2003, with permission from Elsevier.)

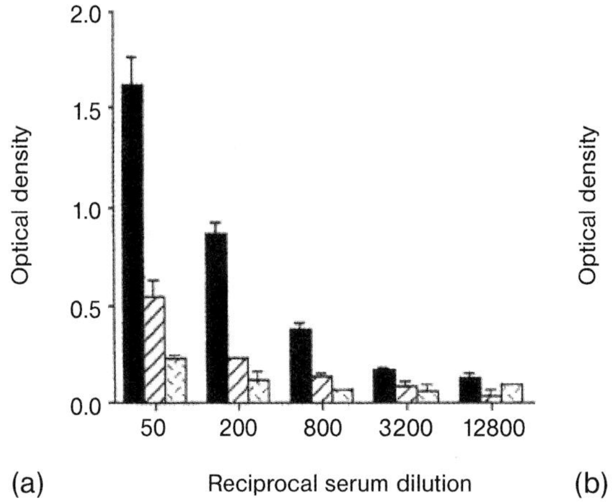

than monocytes/macrophages or B cells. This is due to the high level of expression of major histocompatibility complex (MHC) and costimulatory molecules such as CD40, CD80 and CD86. They cause the secretion of T_h1 cytokines (interleukin-12, IFN-α). BALB/c mice were immunized intranasally with either gp120, or p24 or HIV-NS suspension on days 0, 7, 14 and 42. After that, a low level of gp120-specific IgA was detected in the vaginal samples of the HIV-NS immunized mice. Con A-NS were taken by pulmonary dendritic cells 24 h after intranasal administration. Phagocytosis was partially responsible for the uptake of Con A-NS and gp120-NS. Thus, approximately a 100-fold increase of the gp120-NS uptake was observed in comparison to gp120 alone. T cells from mice immunized with gp120-NS produced much more IFN-γ than those immunized with gp120, which indicates that the gp120-NS are more advantageous in inducing T_h1 responses.

However, according to Miyake and coworkers [117], the mouse is not a representative model for developing a HIV-1 vaccine. That group tested inactivated simian/human immunodeficiency virus KU-2-capturing nanospheres (SHIV-NS) in macaques, while Con A-NS were used as control. Two groups of three macaques in each group were given a series of six immunizations in a week with either Con A-NS or SHIV-NS intranasally. Vaginal anti-HIV-gp120 IgA and IgG antibodies were detected in all SHIV-NS-immunized macaques, but not in the Con A-NS-immunized macaques. After intravaginal challenge with the virus SHIV-KU2, one of the three macaques of each group was infected. The population of $CD4^+$ T cells was less in the Con A-NS and "naive" macaques, while it remained constant in the SHIV-NS-immunized mammals. The two uninfected macaques were rechallenged with the intravenous injection of SHIV-KU2, which led to infection of all macaques. A significant decrease of RNA viral loads was observed in SHIV-NS-immunized macaques 3 and 8 weeks after their rechallenge with the virus. The peripheral $CD4^+$ T cell population decreased at the beginning of the infection and recovered to about 30–50% of the preinfected levels. Also, the intravenously infected SHIV-NS macaques showed a rapid antibody response and the highest levels of anti-gp120 antibodies, which means that gp120 specific memory cells were acquired.

9.2.6
Vaccines

Vaccines are a form of active immunity because they cause the production of antibodies and cellular responses in the patient [66]. Vaccines can be:

- Live attenuated form of a virus or bacteria.
- Inactivated preparations of the virus or bacteria.
- Extracts of or detoxified exotoxins produced by a microorganism.

The immunization after administration of live attenuated vaccines is generally achieved with a single dose and lasts for long time, but not as long as if it was produced from the natural infection. Inactivated vaccines need more than one dose for adequate immunity to be achieved. The duration of immunity varies from months to years. Extracts of or detoxified exotoxins are more immunogenic if adsorbed onto an adjuvant (i.e. aluminum hydroxide). They require a series of injections followed by booster doses.

9.2.6.1 Delivery Route

The most common way of administering vaccines is by injecting them intramuscularly or subcutaneously. Of course this is not a pleasant way, especially for children. Therefore, the formulation of vaccines to exploit other available routes (i.e. oral, intranasal) is under investigation. Also, many vaccines in the form of peptides are difficult to administer due to low immunogenic response or the toxicity of the adjuvants used. Nanoparticles have been tested as potential carriers to increase the immune response or for alternative routes of administration.

9.2.6.1.1 **Systemic** Again as reported in previous sections, chitosan and PLGA are the main polymers of choice for nanoparticle formulation. A number of parameters like polymer hydrophobicity, particle size and the use of adjuvants were evaluated for the best immunization responses. Raghuvanshi and coworkers [118] used a mixture of nanoparticles and microparticles prepared with either PLA or PLGA using the water/oil/water (w/o/w) emulsification technique to entrap tetanus toxoid (TT) in the particles. The mean size of nanoparticles and microparticles were 630 nm and 4 μm, respectively. TT was released from the particles with a burst release (20%).

The immunization responses were recorded after intramuscular injection of a mixture of either, PLA (45 kDa) nanoparticles and microparticles (1/1) or PLGA (50:50) nanoparticles and microparticles (1:1) to rats. Immune responses from polymer-entrapped TT particles were higher than those obtained with saline TT and lasted for 5 months. However, a single injection of the particles, either one type or the physical mixture of particles, resulted in immune responses lower that those achieved after two doses of alum-adsorbed TT.

Low-molecular-weight PLGA particles elicited higher and faster immune responses in comparison to high-molecular-weight PLGA due to the lower T_g of the polymer. Thus, the polymeric matrix was softening and released the entrapped TT near the periphery of the particle matrix more rapidly, so the antigens were presented quickly to the APCs. Immunization with PLA particles elicited significantly higher anti-TT antibody titers than PLGA particles (antibody titers were 2-fold higher from PLA than PLGA particles). This is believed to be because the PLA polymer is more hydrophobic than the PLGA and so the APCs are attracted more to the PLA particles.

Coadministration of alum (adjuvant) at the same time as the particles improved serum immune responses still further. High antibody titers were detected 15 days postimmunization using PLGA and alum, which was faster than that obtained with the particles alone. PLA microparticles administered with alum proved almost as effective as a two-dose immunization with alum-adsorbed TT only. The antibody titers were not only high, but were also maintained for almost 150 days. This increased effect is probably due to the adsorption of the TT by the alum, enabling the antigen to be presented to the APCs, resulting in high antibody response. Also, it was shown that Al^{3+} cations neutralize the negatively charged protein and make it more hydrophobic facilitating the attraction to APCs [119].

The desirable physicochemical properties that particles should possess to develop an optimum vaccine delivery system able to permeate the skin were investigated by other groups. Kohli's group [120] used latex nanoparticles of various sizes (50, 100, 200 and 500 nm) and surface charge (positively charged, neutral and negatively charged particles). Only negatively charged particles of size 50 and 500 nm permeated through the skin. The authors assumed that the contradictory phenomenon of the permeability of negative particles through the skin is due to repulsive forces between negatively charged lipids within the skin and particles at the surface. These forces might result in a temporary initiation of channels in the skin, allowing for particle permeation. On this basis, it was suggested that there might be a threshold charge, which must be reached to allow adequate repulsion of lipids to permit permeation of species through the skin, although this mechanism has not been confirmed yet.

According to Newman and coworkers [121], PLGA nanoparticles are taken up preferably by dendritic cells after intradermal administration of the particles in mice. Based on this finding, the same group studied the *in vitro* optimization of PLGA particle delivery for activation of T cells using murine bone marrow-derived dendritic cells [122]. Also, the influence of the coadministration of an immunomodulator [monophosphoryl-lipid A (MPLA)] was evaluated. The PLGA nanoparticles contained a human MUC1 lipopeptide, BLP25 prepared with the double-emulsion technique (mean size: 287 nm, peptide loading: 1% w/w). Particle uptake was found to depend on the incubation time and particle concentration. The optimum incubation conditions used were 2 mg of nanoparticles with 1×10^7 dendritic cells (day 7 culture) in 20 ml medium for 24 h in a Petri dish. Finally, it was shown that after incubation of dendritic cells with PLGA particles, dendritic cells exhibited an increase in the expression of MHC class II and CD86 compared to untreated cells. This phenomenon was increased further after the coincubation of PLGA particles and the immunomodulator, MPLA. Particle size is an important parameter for the maturation of dendritic cells according to results reported after the incubation of PLGA microparticles (approximately 10 μm) with dendritic cells, which did not increase the expression of MHC class II and CD86 [123].

PLGA nanoparticles were then used to incorporate either the hepatitis B core antigen (HBcAg) only or HBcAg plus the immunomodulator, MPLA, in order to examine their influence on the T_h1 immune responses [124]. PLGA particles were prepared with the emulsification method, and the loading efficiency of HBcAg was 50.8 and 51.0% in the absence and presence of MPLA, respectively. When MPLA was incorporated in the particles, the loading efficiency was approximately 45%. The average size of all formulations was approximately 265–270 nm. Particles (10 mg) containing 1 μg of HBcAg and 20 μg of MPLA were injected subcutaneously to mice. It was shown that the mice immunized with HBcAg + MPLA nanoparticles exhibited the strongest HbcAg-specific T cell proliferation. The incorporation of MPLA in the HBcAg nanoparticles increased the stimulation index almost 4 times compared to the unencapsulated HBcAg. Also, the high level of IFN-γ production from the primed T cells due to the immunization with HBcAg + MPLA nanoparticles indicated a predominant T_h1 immune induction.

Again, the particle size importance was emphasized by those authors because particles of size smaller than 500 nm induced higher immune responses than particles of mean size greater than 2 μm [125].

Due to the fact that dendritic cells are the most important APCs involved in antigen uptake and presentation to antigen-specific T cells, the state of maturity of dendritic cells was evaluated as to the nanosphere uptake and the dendritic cell responses [126]. However, both immature and mature dendritic cells exhibited the same ability to take up polystyrene nanospheres or antigen-loaded nanospheres in a dose- and time-dependent manner. Phagocytosis was the suggested mechanism of nanosphere uptake. The particulate nature of the antigen-loaded nanoparticles was responsible for the enhanced immune responses by dendritic cells in comparison to soluble antigens. Thus, when low amounts of ovalbumin (OVA) were adsorbed on the nanosphere surface, strong antigen-primed T cell proliferation and production of IFN-γ were induced *in vitro*. The antigen adsorption/loading on the particle surface means that lower amounts of antigens will be needed to induce immunity in the future.

Nanoparticles have also been used for DNA vaccine formulations. Cui and coworkers [127] have tried to develop chitosan-based nanoparticles containing plasmid DNA (pDNA) as a potential approach to genetic immunization by topical application. The pDNA was either added during the preparation procedure or added on preformed cationic chitosan/CMC nanoparticles. Different ratios of chitosan:CMC and chitosan oligomers (lower molecular weight than that of chitosan: 102 kDa) were used. The particle size range was between 90 and 270 nm for almost all of the ratios tested. A chitosan:CMC ratio of 1:1 (w/w) was chosen for pDNA coating studies because of the relatively small size (179 nm) and positive ζ potential (+44 mV) of the particles produced. Chitosan oligomer:CMC ratios of 3:1 and 4:1 were chosen for pDNA coating studies due to the particle small size (121 and 93 nm, respectively) and positive ζ potential (+24 and +25 mV respectively). The incorporation efficiency of pDNA on the chitosan oligomer/CMC complexes was almost 100%, which was expected using positively charged nanoparticles.

The final pDNA-coated chitosan/CMC or chitosan oligomers/CMC complexes selected for the genetic immunization by topical application were negatively charged. The latter is based on previous results reported by the same group [128], suggesting that the positively charged particles or complexes produce lower immune responses and gene expression in comparison to negatively charged ones. A number of particle specifications were tested. Also, "naked" DNA was administered topically as control. Only pDNA (300 μg mL^{-1}) coated on chitosan oligomer/CMC nanoparticles (300/100 w/w, μg mL^{-1}) caused a 32-fold increase of the IgG titer in mice as compared to that obtained after immunization using "naked" pDNA alone applied topically. None of the other formulations tested demonstrate any influence in comparison to the administration of the "naked" pDNA alone.

The same group carried out further work using pDNA-coated nanoparticles to induce immune responses after topical application to the skin [129]. The difference in this study was the type of the nanoparticles. They were not made with chitosan but with a mixture of emulsifying wax/Polysorbate 60 in a ratio 20/1 with hexadecyltrimethyl-ammonium bromide (CTAB) as a surfactant (cationic) (mean size 100 nm, ζ potential about 25 mV). No allergic, inflammatory or toxic effects have been observed with these systems in mice after their delivery via the intramuscular, subcutaneous and topical route. Also, dioleoyl phosphatidylethanolamine (DOPE) and cholesterol were part of the nanoparticle composition as endosomolytic agents. DOPE causes disruption of the endosomal membrane because it changes to the hexagonal conformation in the acidic environment of the endosome. *In vitro* studies showed a 7-fold increase of the transfection efficiency compared to nanoparticles without DOPE, but the effect of the cholesterol incorporation was not statistically significant. Also, pDNA remained functional after coating onto the preformed engineered cationic nanoparticles. Mannan cholesterol was also incorporated into the nanoparticles because human and mice dendritic cells have mannose receptors, which stimulated robust T_h1 and cytotoxic T lymphocyte responses [130–132]. Negatively charged nanoparticles were also used for these formulations (Fig. 9.8).

It was shown that pDNA-coated nanoparticles and pDNA-coated particles with DOPE and the mannan ligand caused 6- and 16-fold enhancement of IgG titer, respectively, compared to that of "naked" DNA. *In vitro* and *in vivo* studies proved that the incorporation of DOPE in the nanoparticles improved both the transfec-

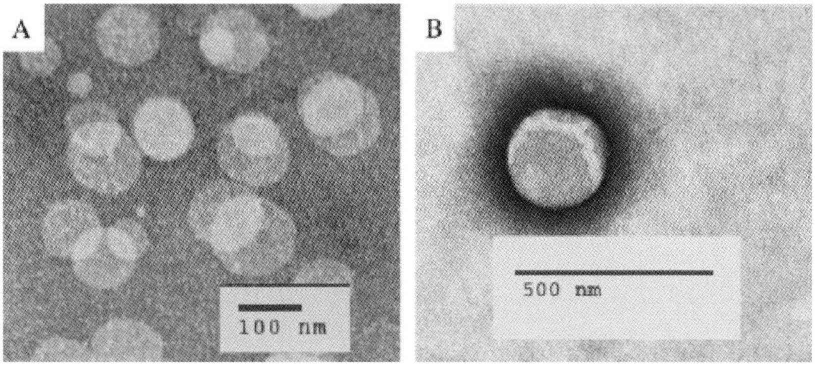

Figure 9.8. Transmission electron micrographs. (A) Mannan-coated cationic nanoparticles and (B) pDNA-coated nanoparticles. Spherical and homogeneous cationic nanoparticles were engineered directly from the oil droplets of a clear microemulsion composed of emulsifying wax (2 mg), DOPE (100 µg) and CTAB (15 mM) in 1 mL water at 55 °C, cooling to room temperature during gentle stirring. Chol-mannan was added. Mannan-coated nanoparticles were purified by gel permeation chromatography, prior to the addition of pDNA. pDNA (CMV-β-galactosidase) was coated on the surface of the cationic nanoparticles (1 mL) to obtain a final pDNA concentration of 50 µg mL^{-1}. (Reprinted from Ref. [133], © 2003, with permission from Elsevier.)

tion efficiency and the overall immune response. Surprisingly, the mannan-coated nanoparticles showed only a modest effect on enhancing the immune response. This was subsequently shown to be due to the reduced binding of mannan caused by the presence of pDNA on the particle surface. Thus, maybe the topical route is not the most efficient to target the dendritic cells using the mannan ligand. In these studies, pDNA doses as low as 4–5 μg applied topically to chemically untreated skin resulted in significant and measurable humoral and proliferative immune responses.

The route of injection has also been investigated. The same type of nanoparticles was administered either (i) via topical immunization with application of the formulation over the skin without applying pressure, (ii) via subcutaneous injection or (iii) via jet injection [133]. It was shown that the intradermal jet injection of pDNA-coated nanoparticles led to the highest antibody titer of all groups. The titer obtained with pDNA-coated nanoparticles delivered by jet injection was over 20 and 65 times higher than that obtained after subcutaneous or the topical route, respectively. After the administration of the "naked" DNA via the routes mentioned above, the IgG titers after jet injection and subcutaneous injection were almost the same, and both titers were significantly greater than after topical application of the "naked" DNA only. Also after the subcutaneous injection of pDNA-coated nanoparticles, the IgG titer in sera was 10-fold higher in comparison to DNA only. Intradermal injection of the same particles increased the IgG titer in sera 200-fold compared to DNA alone.

Various adjuvants have been investigated for promotion of DNA vaccine effectiveness. When the pDNA was coadministered with cholera toxin (CT) (10 or 100 μg) via the topical route, the IgG titer increased 4- and 20-fold, respectively, compared to pDNA alone. The IgG titer demonstrated a more than 300-fold increase after the topical administration of pDNA-coated nanoparticles with 100 μg of CT compared to "naked" DNA alone. Another known adjuvant, lipid A, was coadministered subcutaneously in mice with either pDNA or pDNA-coated nanoparticles [134]. A 16-fold increase of the IgG titer was achieved after immunization with "naked" pDNA in presence of lipid A (50 μg) compared to pDNA alone. In the case of delivery of pDNA-coated nanoparticles with lipid A (50 μg), the IgG titer showed a 16- and 250-fold increase compared to pDNA nanoparticles without lipid A or pDNA alone in absence of lipid A, respectively. Therefore, lipid A (subcutaneous) and CT (topical route) are potential adjuvants to further improve immune responses using the novel cationic nanoparticle-based DNA vaccine delivery system described.

9.2.6.1.2 **Oral** The main reason to develop oral vaccines is that the mucosal surfaces are the entry point for many pathogens to the body [135]. However, purified antigens given orally are not effective due to their degradation in the gut and because the antigens give only short-lived low-titer immune responses. A major obstacle to mucosal vaccination is the absence of nontoxic but potent adjuvants, which are able to enhance the poor immunogenicity of antigens delivered via mucosal routes. In order to protect the antigens and change their immune potency, nanoparticles have been formulated loaded with the mucosal antigens and help them to reach the desirable sites of action – the M cells in the Peyer's patches.

PLGA nanoparticles were made with the double-emulsification method incorporating *Helicobacter pylori* lysates with a loading efficiency of 67% and a mean particle size of 320 nm [135]. Oral immunization of mice took place in three doses at weeks 0, 1 and 2, and another booster dose was given at week 8. The adjuvant, CT, was given in a mixture with either the *H. pylori* lysates or the *H. pylori* lysate-loaded PLGA nanoparticles. *H. pylori* lysate-loaded PLGA nanoparticles induced high immune responses at week 9, after the booster dose at week 8. A mixture of *H. pylori* with 10 μg of CT induced high immune responses at week 4 and was enhanced significantly after the booster at week 8. A mixture of *H. pylori* with CT enhanced the immune response significantly higher than the *H. pylori*-loaded PLGA particles. Apart from IgA, the major IgG subclasses produced were IgG1, IgG2b and lower levels of IgG2a. The synthesis of those antibodies was supported by T_h2 cell-secreted cytokines induced by CT. This means that the *H. pylori* loaded nanoparticles resembled the action of CT since both a mixture of *H. pylori* with CT and the *H. pylori*-loaded PLGA particles induced the production of the same antibodies after oral immunization.

The low entrapment efficiency of peptides/proteins in PLGA nanoparticles, the unavoidable use of organic solvents and the emulsification preparative technique are obstacles that demand alternative solutions. Therefore, Jung and coworkers [136] evaluated the adsorption of TT on particles made with the branched polymer poly(sulfobutyl-polyvinyl alcohol)-*g*-(lactide-*co*-glycolide) (SB-PVAL-*g*-PLGA) using a solvent displacement technique. The particle size was in the range from 100 to 200 nm and different degrees of sulfobutylation produced particles with different ζ potentials ranging from -3.2 to -22 mV (for a degree of substitution of 43%). The amount of TT adsorbed on the particle surface started from 6.5 μg mg^{-1} polymer in the case of PVAL-*g*-PLGA up to 56.8 μg mg^{-1} for the 43% substituted polymer. Increasing surface hydrophilicity and/or surface charge density resulted in a higher TT adsorption onto the particle surface. The adsorption is a result of the electrostatic interactions between the negatively charged particle surface and positively charged protein residues. According to adsorption isotherm data, a monolayer adsorption model describes the interaction of TT with the particle surface. The antigenicity of the TT was influenced only slightly making the delivery system a potent one for mucosal immunization.

In another attempt to improve the formulation characteristics and preparation procedure, mucoadhesive cationic and anionic materials like alginate, carrageenens and pectin [137] were used. Also a different method was tried in order to omit the harmful organic solvent during the preparation procedure and to create a friendlier environment in the interior/core of the nanoparticles. According to this, the anionic solution (core) was introduced in the form of a mist into the cationic solution (corona), which resulted in instantaneous particle formation [138]. The antigen is part of the core and the shell according to the nature of the protein/peptide entrapped and the particle composition. The ζ potential was positive and the entrapment efficiency varied (it could reach even almost 50%). By using polydextran aldehyde, crosslinking could occur and, thus, the particles were stabilized even more. The 100% crosslinked particles released only about 20% OVA after 24 h incubation in presence of 3% NaCl as dissolution medium, while approximately 40% was released after 5 days incubation from the same particles in a medium of pH 1.83. Also, the crosslinked nanoparticles provoked high immune responses while the noncrosslinked ones did not cause any response after oral immunization. This was the case for particles having either OVA or TT incorporated. The OVA-loaded nanoparticles show a dramatic difference in the immune response compared to that obtained with OVA in solution and OVA in a mixture with empty nanoparticles. Concluding, this system seems to offer a higher versatility in developing protein-loaded carriers for oral vaccination.

The hydrophilic polymer chitosan, due to its mucoadhesive properties, is very popular in the field of vaccine development. The cationic nature of the polymer ensures electrostatic interactions with negatively charged proteins (i.e. BSA, TT, CT) according to the pH of the preparation solutions during the nanoparticle formation and the p*I* of each protein [139]. The loading efficiency was estimated as almost 90, 50 and 50% for BSA, TT and CT, respectively, when the proteins were dissolved in the TPP solution (pH 8.3) and the particle formation took place with a chitosan solution of pH 5.0. Poly(ethylene oxide-*co*-propylene oxide) (PEO–PPO) polymer was introduced to the nanoparticles during the preparation procedure in order to modify the particle size and ζ potential. Thus, lower entrapment efficiency of BSA was obtained due to the lower amount of chitosan available when PEO–PPO was present. BSA release from 25% CS nanoparticles or 20% CS/PEO–PPO nanoparticles was slow and prolonged without a burst release. A burst release was exhibited by 40% BSA-loaded particles, probably due to adsorbed BSA molecules on the carrier surface. TT release from 14% TT-loaded CS particles at pH 5 was approximately 20% after 18 days and the toxoid was still antigenically active.

From a formulation point of view, coating of OVA-adsorbed chitosan nanoparticles with sodium alginate increased both the stability of protein adsorbed on the particle surface and the particle stability in simulated intestinal fluid at 37 °C [140] (Fig. 9.9).

The loading capacity with OVA on the chitosan nanoparticles ranged from 30 to 50%, but significant desorption of OVA occurred during the coating procedure, especially if the latter took place at pH 5.5. Thus, the coating procedure was carried out at pH 7.4 due to compromised results between loading capacity and coating efficiency. Another drawback of the preparation procedure was the high polydispersity of the particle population produced, with a mean average size of approximately 650 nm. Despite those disadvantages, the alginate coating offered protection against the degradation of chitosan and OVA in the simulated intestinal fluid as it showed a 60% release of OVA after 7 h of particle incubation at 37 °C.

The introduction of lectins on the particle surface was also shown to enhance the uptake of antigen-loaded nanoparticles by M cells or other epithelial cells of the intestinal wall [141, 142].

DNA vaccines have also been incorporated into nanoparticle formulations for oral delivery. *Toxoplasma gondii* GRA1-pDNA was incorporated into chitosan nano-

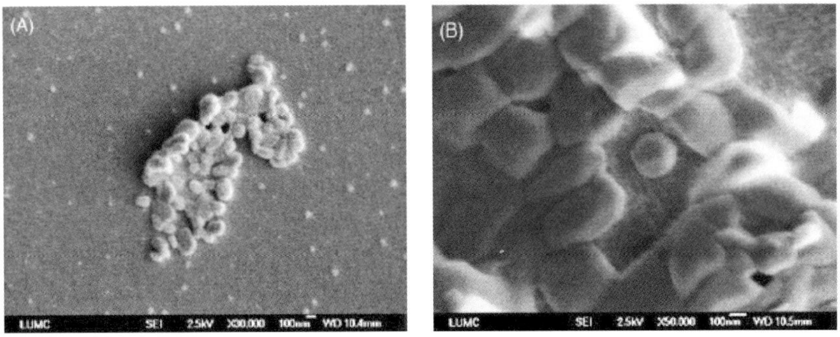

Figure 9.9. Scanning electron micrographs of chitosan nanoparticles. (A) After freeze-drying and resuspending in water. (B) After the coating procedure with sodium alginate. (Reprinted from Ref. [140], © 2005, with permission from Elsevier.)

particles of mean size of 400 nm and ζ potential of 27 mV [143]. The incorporation into the polymeric carriers (more than 98%) protected the plasmid from the degradation of DNase I. The interaction of pDNA with the chitosan molecules in the formulation was strong enough so DNA did not escape into the dissolution medium 8 days after the carrier incubation in pH 7.3 at 25 °C. However, the plasmid-loaded nanoparticles did not induce any significant response 1 month postintragastric administration of the formulation in mice. Therefore, mice were boosted with intragastric administration of chitosan nanoparticles and, indeed, a higher response was obtained from mice immunized with either GRA1 microparticles or GRA1-pDNA-loaded nanoparticles. The latter response was enhanced more after a second round of immunization with intramuscular administration of pDNA, although, GRA1-loaded microparticles demonstrated the highest immune responses compared to GRA1-pDNA-loaded nanoparticles. The difference between the two types of formulations is that the GRA1-microparticles raised/caused a mixed T_h1/T_h2 response, while the GRA1-pDNA-loaded nanoparticles induced the secretion of IgG1, which is associated with T_h2-type responses. The latter is unusual as T_h1 immune responses were expected to be obtained as reported previously by the same and other research groups.

In another study it was shown that the pDNA of a house dust mite allergen, Der p1, was incorporated in chitosan nanoparticles efficiently enough to be able to cause immune responses (IgG2a production) to Der p1 and the Der p1-derived peptides after oral administration in mice [144]. The intramuscular administration of those particles could not raise such responses. However, the orally induced immune responses could be boosted about 13 weeks postfeeding by intramuscular injection of "naked" DNA.

9.2.6.1.3 **Intranasal** The advantages of drug delivery through the nasal cavity have already been highlighted, but the most important feature is that the drug delivery system bypasses the liver. The required qualities for a drug delivery system appropriate for intranasal delivery, such as particle hydrophobicity, size and ζ potential, were investigated more thoroughly by Tobio and coworkers [145]. TT-loaded PLA and PLA–PEG nanoparticles were prepared with the double-emulsification method and the final size was less than 200 nm. The ζ potential of PLA and PLA–PEG particles was −50 and −30 mV, respectively. The encapsulation efficiency was about 35% regardless of the particle composition. PLA–PEG particles showed a prolonged TT release in comparison to the more hydrophobic PLA particles. At 24 and 48 h postintranasal administration of the toxoid-loaded PLA–PEG nanoparticles in rats, TT was found in a 10-fold higher concentration in blood and lymph nodes compared to TT levels obtained after PLA intranasal particle administration. The accumulation of TT in the lymph nodes after administration of PLA–PEG vesicles was almost 2-fold higher than that recorded in blood 24 and 48 h after intranasal administration. Also, the TT accumulation in the lymph nodes was significantly higher than that in organs like the liver, spleen, lungs and small bowel 24 and 48 h postadministration. Therefore, the suggested hypothesis was that a part of PLA–PEG nanoparticles was taken up by the M cells of the NALT and another part passed to the submucosal layer and then to the lymphatics and the blood. Also, some of the particles could have been taken up by the BALT and GALT. This hypothesis can be supported by the fact that the free toxoid was cleared from the blood rapidly and absorption by the organs was very much lower compared to the particles.

Another study demonstrated the potential of using PLGA as a carrier for the entrapment of bovine parainfluenza type 3 virus (BPI-3) for vaccination of young calves [146]. However, preliminary experiments were carried out by intranasal inoculation in mice using two particle types: PLGA, where BPI-3 was incorporated in the particle matrix, and poly(methyl methacrylate) (PMMA), where the antigen was adsorbed on the particle surface. The latter formulation was not successful in inducing any immune response in contrast to BPI-3-loaded PLGA particles.

The use of particles made from high-molecular-weight chitosan have already been described. Vila and coworkers [147] investigated the feasibility of using lower molecular weight chitosan (23 and 38 kDa molecular weight) to formulate nanoparticulate vaccine carriers incorporating TT. The nanoparticles had a size of approximately 350 nm and ζ potential of +40 mV, while the TT loading efficiency was 50–60%. Burst release occurred, but the release profile was prolonged and the TT was antigenically active. Indeed, it was shown that the TT-loaded nanoparticles significantly enhanced either the humoral (IgG) or mucosal (IgA) immune responses compared to those achieved by the soluble vaccine. Also, the immune responses were not affected significantly by the dose of the antigen-loaded low-molecular-weight chitosan nanoparticles for the range used between 70 and 200 μg.

An alternative to the previous chitosan formulations was the development of chitosan-coated emulsions where OVA and CT were adsorbed on the emulsion surface [148]. Chitosan nanoparticles were prepared for comparison, and the two types of formulations were administered intranasally and intraperitoneally in rats. The particle sizes achieved for the nanoparticles and the chitosan-coated emulsions were in the range of 0.4–3 and 0.4–0.7 µm, respectively. The ζ potential was positive due to the chitosan presence, and it was approximately 35 and 15 mV, respectively. The adsorbed OVA was very high in both formulations (85 and 100%, respectively) and there was no release of OVA detected after 3 h of incubation in phosphate-buffered saline (pH 7.2) at 37 °C. Nanoparticles induced significantly higher IgG response in comparison to control (OVA only, or nanoparticles only) administered either intraperitoneally or intranasally regardless of the particle size. Nanoparticles of 0.4 and 1 µm exhibited significantly higher IgA response than those of 3 µm.

Chitosan-coated emulsions did not elicit IgG production of any significance compared to control after intraperitoneal administration irrespective of the particle size, while the IgA levels were similar to those obtained with the nanoparticles after intraperitoneal administration. However, chitosan-coated emulsions showed a significant increase of both IgG and IgA levels compared to control after intranasal administration regardless of the particle size. Thus, the chitosan-coated emulsions are considered as another approach for vaccine formulation for intranasal delivery.

Some work has also been carried out on DNA vaccines for intranasal delivery. Cui and coworkers [149] worked on cationic emulsions made of the emulsifying wax CTAB and/or Brij 78 where pDNA was adsorbed on the surface of the final products. The positive ζ potential of the particles is attributed to CTAB presence. Due to its potential toxicity, the amount used is being reduced and partly replaced by Brij 78. IgG responses caused by pDNA on the Brij 78 and CTAB nanoparticles were 18- and 28-fold higher than those recorded with pDNA alone. Also, the IgA levels increased 25- and 30-fold more than pDNA alone. It is worth noting that the amount used for the intranasal immunization in this study was 1.25 µg compared to 50 µg used by another group [150]. This system would probably enable immunization with significantly lower doses of pDNA.

9.2.7
Diabetes

Diabetes is classified as insulin- and noninsulin-dependent diabetes type I or II, respectively [66]. Type I diabetes is also known as diabetes mellitus (IDDM) and it is caused because of a deficiency of insulin following autoimmune destruction of pancreatic β cells. Patients with type I diabetes require administration of insulin. Type II diabetes (NIDDM) is due to insufficient secretion of insulin or to peripheral resistance to the action of insulin. Type II diabetes can be controlled by diet alone, but oral antidiabetic drugs or insulin can be used if needed.

9.2.7.1 Treatment
Insulin is a polypeptide hormone of complex structure and is the required treatment for IDDM and ketoacidosis. Insulin used for therapeutic purposes can be extracted from pig pancreas, or, alternatively, human sequence insulin can be produced either semisynthetically by enzymatic modification of porcine insulin or biosynthetically by recombinant DNA technology from bacteria or yeast.

It is inactivated by gastrointestinal enzymes and has to be administered by subcutaneous injection. Fat hypertrophy can occur due to subcutaneous injections, but can be minimized by rotating the injection sites. Soluble insulin is administered for urgent treatment, for fine control in serious illness and in the perioperative period.

Drug administration via injections is not the most convenient or desirable route for the patient; therefore, alternative routes of insulin administration, mainly oral or intranasal, have been investigated. These have utilized complexation of insulin with polymeric materials into self-assembled nanoparticles. A brief overview of the current research towards these objectives follows.

9.2.7.2 **Delivery Routes**

9.2.7.2.1 **Oral** PIBCA and chitosan have been the polymers of choice for insulin formulation into nanoparticles. PIBCA was shown by Damgè and coworkers [151–152] to be able to deliver a sufficient amount of active insulin after oral administration of insulin-loaded PIBCA nanocapsules to fasted, streptozotocin-induced diabetic rats and they decreased the blood glucose level from 300 to the normal 125 mg dL^{-1}. Indeed, PIBCA nanocapsules were found to protect insulin in the gastric environment both *in vitro* in reconstituted gastric and intestinal medium compared to phosphate-buffered saline as control, and *in vivo* (intragastric administration to rats; insulin dose: 57 and 2.8 IU kg^{-1}) [153]. In the intestine, 75% of insulin was released, although most of the capsules were degraded after 30 min according to results deduced from the *in vitro* release of insulin in reconstituted intestinal medium. The remaining intact nanocapsules were localized on the intestinal mucosa and passed through the submucosal layers.

In another study, the same polymer was used to prepare nanoparticles and not nanocapsules, incorporating the insulin at the very beginning of the polymerization procedure and using a pluronic surfactant as stabilizer [154]. The desired particle size was less than 100 nm and was achieved by using an appropriate concentration of pluronic acid (2.0%) in contrast to nanocapsules of 265 nm used in the previously mentioned study. Insulin-loaded nanoparticles were administered subcutaneously or orally to streptozotocin-induced diabetic rats. A prolonged hypoglycemic effect of the hormone was observed up to 72 h postinjection. A similar pattern was observed after oral delivery of insulin-loaded nanoparticles with the hypoglycemic effect starting 2 h postadministration, while a less prominent effect was shown by the same dose of insulin-loaded nanocapsules as reported by Damgè and coworkers [151]. The enhanced effect in the case of nanoparticles could be due to the smaller particle size, leading to faster intestinal absorption.

Chitosan is used to enhance the absorption of insulin by the intestinal mucosa due to its mucoadhesive properties and transient opening of the tight junctions between the epithelial cells. Pan and coworkers [155] made insulin-loaded chitosan nanoparticles by ionotropic gelation of chitosan with tripolyphosphate anions. Insulin association was found up to be approximately 80%, and the electrostatic interactions between the acidic groups of insulin and the amino groups of chitosan

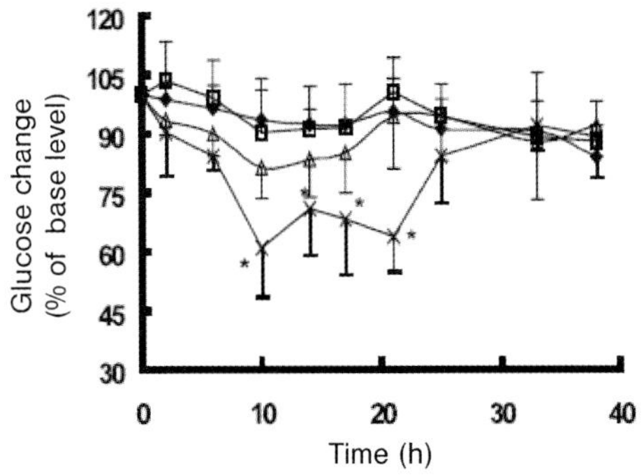

Figure 9.10. Hypoglycaemic effect of oral administration of: control (drinking saline without oral administrating anything, ♦); insulin-chitosan solution (△); insulin solution (□); 14 IU kg^{-1} insulin-loaded chitosan nanoparticles suspended in pH 5.5 saline (×). Data represents the mean ± SD, $n = 8$ per group. Statistically significant difference from control ($^{*}P < 0.01$). (Reprinted from Ref. [155], © 2002, with permission from Elsevier.)

were highly contributory to this. Insulin was rapidly released from nanoparticles in pH 7.4 and 4.0, but it was slower at pH 5.8, probably due to lower insulin solubility at this pH. After oral administration of insulin-loaded chitosan nanoparticles at a dosage of 14 IU kg^{-1}, there was no significant blood glucose decrease observed for the first 6 h, but the hypoglycemic effect was very prominent 10 h later (post-administration) in comparison to the insulin control solution and lasted for 10 h from the onset of the hypoglycemia (Fig. 9.10). Increasing the insulin-loaded nanoparticle dosage to 21 IU kg^{-1}, the blood glucose dropped to normal levels for more than 8 h. These results show that the chitosan nanoparticles facilitated the intestinal absorption of insulin.

The presence of Poloxamer 188 in the nanoparticle formulation could have affected the *in vivo* behavior of insulin-loaded nanoparticles because it can reduce the intestinal peristalsis and so prolong the retention of nanoparticles in the intestinal tract. Also, the surfactant can reduce the opsonization and thus the particle clearance from the RES due to the hydrophilic groups on the particle surface.

The successful incorporation of insulin in the nanoparticles depends strongly on the formulation conditions and pH is a very important parameter of the procedure. Optimization of the formulation process will lead to highly efficient nanoparticles in delivering insulin after oral administration [156]. Thus, insulin was premixed with either pentasodium TPP anions or the chitosan solution prior to nanoparticle formulation and the particles produced were designated as TPP-np or CS-np, respectively [155] (Fig. 9.11). The particle preparation was carried out in a pH range of 2.3–6.3. Up to that maximum of pH 6.3, the particle size was not affected significantly by the pH changes, but beyond that value, particle agglomeration was observed.

When the initial insulin concentration was 0.88 mg mL^{-1}, the association efficiency of insulin was pH-dependent. Maximum association efficiency was 62.99

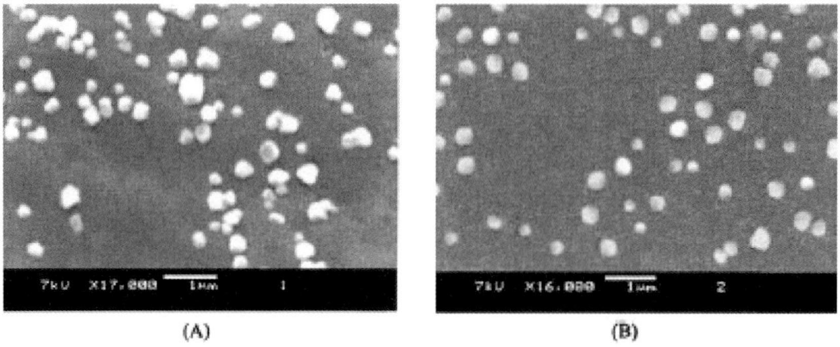

Figure 9.11. Scanning electron microscopy micrographs of (A) TPP-np and (B) CS-np prepared at pH 5.3 with an insulin-loading concentration of 4.28 U mL^{-1}. Nanoparticles were prepared by ionotropic gelation of chitosan with TPP anions; TPP-np were obtained by premixing insulin with TPP solution, and CS-np by premixing insulin with chitosan solution, prior to nanoparticle formation. (Reprinted from Ref. [156], © 2002, with permission from Wiley.)

and 57.67 at pH 6.1 for the TPP-np and CS-np nanoparticles, respectively. Small changes around pH 6 led to big variations of association efficiency in both types of formulations. This is not the case for more acidic environments. The association efficiency of insulin was improved significantly by increasing insulin-loading concentrations. Regardless of the insulin concentration, the maximum association efficiency was achieved at pH 6.1. Insulin-loading concentration did not affect the mean particle size. The loading efficiency (amount of insulin incorporated per milligram of nanoparticle) was not affected by the pH of the formulation process.

Although, insulin was released rapidly (100%) from the particles made at pH 6.1 even if the association efficiency was approximately 80%, it was very much slower (10–20%) from particles made at pH 5.3 (association efficiency approximately 50%). At pH 5.3, the association of insulin to chitosan occurs via stronger electrostatic interactions and it is pH dependent, while at higher pH seems that the association is of a hydrophobic nature.

Lim's group also evaluated the uptake of chitosan molecules and chitosan nanoparticles by Caco-2 cells, and their ability to enhance the insulin transport into these cells [157]. They show that nanoparticle uptake was dependent on time, temperature and loading concentration. It was a saturable event and more likely to be taken up by clathrin-mediated adsorptive endocytosis.

In contrast, chitosan polymer molecules were taken up by endocytosis through caveolae. The chitosan polymer was more effective at disrupting the intercellular tight junctions than chitosan nanoparticles, so the former facilitated the insulin transport via the paracellular pathway, being more effective than the particles. Their results agree with those reported by Dyer and coworkers [158], where the insulin-loaded nanoparticles given intranasally showed a lower hypoglycemic effect in comparison to chitosan solutions in sheep and rats.

After particle optimization for different pH range and insulin-loading concentrations, *in vivo* evaluation of two chosen formulations [made at pH 5.3 (f5.3) and 6.1 (f6.1)] followed in streptozotocin-induced diabetic rats [159]. Particles were administered orally at two insulin doses: 50 or 100 IU kg^{-1}. It was shown that the 100 IU kg^{-1} insulin of f5.3 demonstrated a higher hypoglycemic effect lasting up to 11 h. The f6.1 nanoparticles were less efficient even if the hypoglycemic action started 2 h postadministration in comparison to f5.3 particles where blood glucose dropped only after 10 h.

9.2.7.2.2 **Nasal** The intranasal administration of insulin has been attempted using chitosan nanoparticles or more recently nanocomplexes with branched polyesters. Chitosan is by far the most used polymer in research in the delivery of small or larger molecules via the oral, nasal or pulmonary route due to the previously mentioned properties of mucoadhesion and transient opening of the tight junctions of the epithelial cells. Urrusuno and coworkers [160] studied the potential of chitosan nanoparticles as a formulation to increase the availability of insulin after nasal instillation to rabbits. The particles were made with the ionotropic gelation method using two types of chitosan (0.1% CS-210Cl and 0.2% CS-110Cl) with TPP in a ratio chitosan:TPP 6:1. The particle size was 300–400 nm and the ζ potential varied from 25 to 54 mV. Insulin association efficiency was greater than 87% and loading efficiency was approximately 55%. After nanoparticle instillation to rabbits, the blood glucose level dropped to 60% of basal levels at 1 h post-administration of insulin-loaded CS-210Cl nanoparticles. This formulation demonstrated the strongest hypoglycemic effect. The same activity was obtained using the insulin-loaded CS-110Cl nanoparticles (two types of chitosan were used in the form of HCl salt, CS-110Cl and CS-210Cl, and their differences were molecular weight, below 50 and 130 respectively, deacetylation degree, 87 and below 70% respectively, and intrinsic viscosity, 10 and 20–200, respectively) (Fig. 9.12). In contrast, the administration of 5 IU kg^{-1} insulin control solution (pH 4.3) resulted in a decrease of blood glucose levels of less than 15% at 30 min postinstillation. This is an indication that insulin was released from the nanoparticles in its active form, which meant that the formulation preparation did not affect the peptide. Moreover, these authors showed that chitosan in nanoparticle form decreased blood glucose more significantly than the chitosan solution, a finding that is different to that reported by other groups [157].

The pH of chitosan solutions plays an important role in their ability to act as absorption enhancers. The *in vivo* effect was investigated by comparing insulin-loaded nanoparticles with insulin solutions following nasal instillation at pH 6.4 and 4.3. The hypoglycemic effect of insulin solution at pH 6.4 was negligible due to slow solubility and formation of high-molecular-weight aggregates. When insulin-loaded chitosan nanoparticles were administered intranasally at the same pH, a reduction of blood glucose levels was recorded for 1.5 h. Even if the hypoglycemic effect of insulin from the nanoparticles was lower at pH 6.4 than 4.3, the increase in the response to the hormone-loaded nanoparticles and the insulin/chitosan solutions was the same: 18.6% at pH 6.4 and 17.4% at pH 4.3.

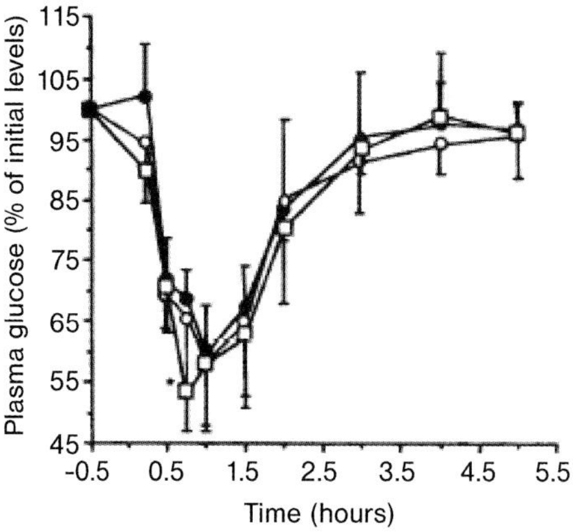

Figure 9.12. Plasma glucose levels achieved in rabbits following nasal administration (at pH 4.3) of: insulin-loaded chitosan 210 Cl nanoparticles suspended in acetate buffer, 0.16 mg kg^{-1} chitosan (●) and 0.35 mg kg^{-1} chitosan (□), and insulin-loaded chitosan 110 Cl nanoparticles suspended in acetate buffer (○) ($n = 6$). (Mean ± SD $n = 6$.) *Statistically significant differences from insulin-loaded chitosan 210 Cl nanoparticles suspended in acetate buffer, 0.16 mg kg^{-1} chitosan ($P < 0.05$). (Reprinted from Ref. [160], © Plenum Publishing Corporation with permission of Springer Science and Business Media.)

Insulin/chitosan solutions and insulin-loaded chitosan nanoparticles were studied for their ability to improve the bioavailability of insulin in two animal models [157]. Again particles were made by the same gelation method used by Urrusuno and coworkers [159]. In this study, insulin-loaded chitosan nanoparticles were used as well as postloaded insulin/chitosan nanoparticles. The empty (nonloaded) nanoparticles had a mean particle size around 250 nm and a ζ potential of about 29 mV. All nanoparticles exhibited a size less than 1 μm. The result was that in the rat model the chitosan nanoparticles were not advantageous in comparison to the chitosan solutions in the overall hypoglycemic effect.

Regarding the response in the sheep model, the insulin/chitosan solution was more effective than the insulin-loaded and postloaded insulin chitosan nanoparticles. However, the best acting formulation was the insulin/chitosan powder, which is assumed to remain longer (115 min) in the nasal cavity of the sheep than the chitosan solution (45 min).

Another promising approach to develop a carrier system for insulin delivery exploiting the intranasal or the oral route was one based on the complexation between polymer/peptide according to the hydrophobic and electrostatic interactions of the two parts [161]. Therefore, a hydrophilic charged-modified poly(vinyl alcohol) backbone was produced with covalently bound diethylamine groups. L-Lactide groups were grafted onto the backbone imparting a hydrophobic character to the previously hydrophilic molecule. The nanocomplexes produced were of a range of sizes between 200 and 500 nm according to the backbone composition and number of grafted lactic acid groups. Increasing the amount of lactic acid groups, the complexes tend to be smaller and more compact. The ζ potential ranged from +3 mV at a low substitution to +35 mV at the highest substitution. The insulin complexation was higher with high degrees of amine substitution or by a combination of medium charge density and a higher lactic acid content. When the initial insulin concentration was 1.25 mg mL^{-1}, approximately 98% of insulin was found in the complexes.

9.2.7.2.3 **Pulmonary** Drug delivery via the pulmonary route is, of course, preferable to injections because it is noninvasive and systemic absorption is expected to be at higher rates since the lung provides a large surface area and enzymic degradation is relatively low. PBCA nanoparticles were used to compare the pharmacological potential between pulmonary and subcutaneous delivery of insulin-loaded particles [162]. The mean size of the particles was 255 nm and the insulin association efficiency was 79%. Burst release phenomena accompanied the release profile of insulin at pH 7 in saline at 37 °C. The particles were administered intratracheally to normal rats and an increase in the reduction of blood glucose level was observed as the insulin dose increased from 5 to 20 IU kg^{-1}, while the minimum glucose level was reached in 4, 4 and 8 h for 5, 10 and 20 IU kg^{-1}, respectively. The hypoglycemic effect of insulin-loaded nanoparticles at doses 10 and 20 IU kg^{-1} was prolonged compared to that obtained with the insulin solutions (Fig. 9.13). However, the hypoglycemic effect achieved after subcutaneous administration of 5 IU kg^{-1} insulin-loaded nanoparticles was much higher than that obtained after intratracheal delivery of the same nanoparticles. According to these authors, this phenomenon is attributed to the ability of normal rats to adjust the blood glucose level.

An idea for pulmonary delivery of insulin-loaded chitosan nanoparticles was the microencapsulation of those particles into microspheres made by lactose or mannitol by spray-drying [163]. Indeed, it was shown that the microspheres produced were mostly spherical with the appropriate aerodynamic properties for good deliv-

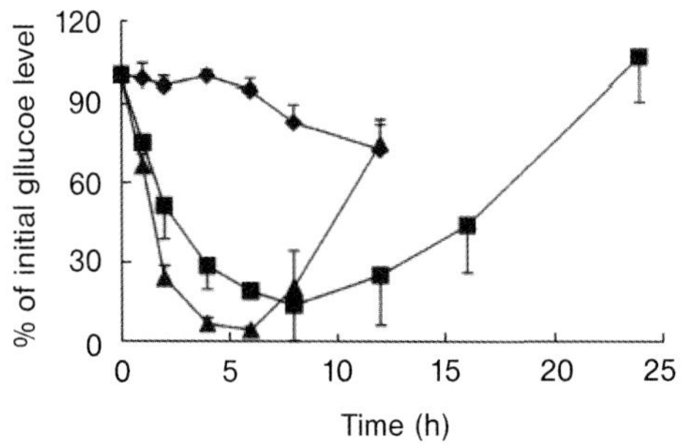

Figure 9.13. Hypoglycaemic effect of a single intratracheal administration of insulin-loaded nanoparticles of 20 IU kg^{-1} (■) and insulin solution of 20 IU kg^{-1} (▲) to normal rats fasted overnight. The glucose concentration at time zero served as the basis for comparison (%). Results are means for five or six animals. The control (♦) is phosphate buffer solution (pH 7). (Reprinted from Ref. [162], © 2001, with permission from Elsevier.)

ery, but their morphology was strongly influenced by the nanoparticle content. The microspheres with the best properties were those made with mannitol:nanoparticles 80:20 and the nanoparticles were made with chitosan:TPP: 6:1. The insulin-loaded chitosan/TPP nanoparticles were of approximately 350 nm size, and had a ζ potential of +40 mV and a protein loading capacity 65–80%. After 15 min incubation in phosphate-buffered saline (pH 7.4) at 37 °C, 75–80% of insulin was released from either nanoparticles or nanoparticles encapsulated into microspheres. Also, the nanoparticles could be recovered from microspheres after their contact with water with no significant changes in their physicochemical properties. Therefore, the microspheres containing nanoparticles would be able to be delivered to the deep lung and thereafter the aqueous environment would release the nanoparticles and subsequently the entrapped insulin.

9.2.7.2.4 **Parenteral Delivery (Subcutaneous, Intravenous, Intraperitoneal)** In addition to the high instability and degradation of insulin in the gastrointestinal tract, it also exhibits a short half-life when administered by subcutaneous injections. Its incorporation in to nanoparticles was therefore also investigated to sustain the hypoglycemic effect. Barichello and coworkers [164] evaluated the use of Pluronic gels (20% and 30% Pluronic concentration used), PLGA nanoparticles and their combination for parenteral delivery of peptides and proteins having short half-lives, using insulin as a model molecule. The important characteristic in using Pluronic gels is the enhanced protein stability into the gel matrix with complete recovery of full insulin activity when the gel is dissolved in excess buffer. The drawback is the loss of gelation ability in the presence of inorganic salts used to control the pH in such gels. Insulin was released more slowly from gels with higher concentration of Pluronic (20 and 30% Pluronic concentrations in the gels were used) while the possible mechanism is erosion and probably some diffusion due to zero-order release kinetics.

PLGA nanoparticles were produced with an insulin content around 60% and particle size 128 nm. After subcutaneous injection of insulin-loaded PLGA nanoparticles, a constant hypoglycemic effect was observed with a slow recovery of the serum glucose levels during the 2 h postadministration period. Subcutaneous injection of insulin solution only demonstrated an acute hypoglycemic effect of insulin with a peak 1 h later; however, when insulin loaded in the Pluronic gel was injected, the impact of the hormone was more prolonged. The same profile was obtained after nanoparticle-gel injection with an effect up to 6 h later. The bioavailability of the peptide from the nanoparticle-gel formulation increased almost 3-fold to that estimated after the subcutaneous injection of insulin solution only.

A sustained hypoglycemic effect up to 4 h after subcutaneous injection to diabetic rats was achieved using nanoparticles made with the oppositely charged PEI and DS stabilized by crosslinking with zinc [165]. PEI solution of pH 9 was mixed with DS in a ratio of approximately 2:1 with 25 μM of zinc as a stabilizer in the presence of insulin in the polymer mixture. Ninety percent of insulin was entrapped in to particles of size 250 nm and of ζ potential +30 mV. However, 70% of particle-bound insulin was dissociated from the particles in 10 mM phosphate buffer in 5 min, which suggests that insulin was adsorbed on the particle surface through apolar interactions. The interaction of insulin with PEI caused conformational changes to insulin at low pH, but not at pH 9. Moreover, a hypoglycemic effect was induced in diabetic rats regardless of polymer ratio, indicating preservation of insulin biological activity.

Simple mixing of cholesterol-bearing pullulan with insulin resulted in complex formation (size of 20–30 nm) that did not demonstrate any particular advantage to the blood glucose reduction in comparison to free insulin solution after intravenous injection to normal fasting rats [166]. Insulin was stabilized in those complexes, but it was replaced with BSA after nanoparticle incubation in the presence of the latter protein (50 mg mL^{-1}) for 1 h at 37 °C.

9.2.7.2.5 **Other Formulations** A very promising technique for enhancement of insulin incorporation into nanoparticles is the use of gas antisolvent techniques or supercritical fluids [167]. This method is considered advantageous for labile pharmaceutical molecules and polymers due to mild operation conditions and a reduction in the amount of organic solvent used. The remaining organic solvents in the final preparation are much reduced and the ability of drug entrapment higher as entrapment is not dependent on the drug partitioning between the liquid phases. Supercritical carbon dioxide precipitation was applied to a mixture of PLA (molecular weight 102 000)/insulin or PLA/PEG/insulin organic solutions (DMSO:dichloromethane 50:50) resulting in polymeric nanoparticles with a mean size of 400–600 nm. The residual dichloromethane was only 8 p.p.m., less than that of 400 and 600 p.p.m. reported by the US and European Pharmacopoeia, respectively. The residual DMSO was 300 p.p.m.

Insulin loading was 90% and it was affected by the presence of PEG in the nanoparticle composition. By increasing the PEG content or the PEG molecular weight, a decrease of insulin loading was observed. High insulin loading was achieved using PEG molecules of less than 1900 molecular weight The content and molecular weight of PEG used influenced the insulin release from those particles. Using PEGs of higher molecular weight of 1900 or a high concentration of PEG, insulin was released with a burst release phenomenon, which is not the case with PEGs smaller than 1900. Less than 3% of insulin was released from particles with PEG of molecular weight 350, 750 or 1900. Additionally, 80% of the peptide activity was retained, as an induced-hypoglycaemic effect was caused in mice by the insulin extracted from the nanoparticles.

A self-regulating insulin delivery system was developed by Zhang and coworkers based on insulin release from membranes embedded with insulin-loaded nanoparticles. A decrease in the pH of the microenvironment is caused when the system senses an increase in glucose concentration [168]. When the pH of the microenvironment decreases, the particle size in the matrix decreases and insulin is released. Glucose oxidase (GOD) embedded in the membrane was used as a glucose sensor. GOD converts glucose to gluconic acid causing the pH to decrease. Due to the low amount of oxygen available for the amount of glucose to be oxidized and because of toxic hydrogen peroxide formation as a side-product, catalase is coentrapped in/

on to the membrane breaking down the hydrogen peroxide into oxygen and water. The GOD incorporated in to the membrane retained 80% of its activity in comparison to free enzyme and the addition of catalase favored the oxidation rate of glucose.

The nanoparticles were made with the pH sensitive polymer poly(NIPAAm-*co*-methacrylic acid) and the insulin was released after 5–15 min from the onset of hyperglycemia. The responsiveness of the system to glucose levels was evaluated by increasing the amount of glucose in the surrounding medium. It was found that the insulin permeability increased 3-fold as the glucose concentration increased from 50 to 200 mg mL^{-1}. In general, it was shown that the glucose concentration fluctuations stimulated the insulin release in a rapid and reversible way.

9.3 Conclusions

This chapter has presented most of the ongoing research using polymeric nanoparticles for noncancer applications. The most important diseases have been discussed in some detail, but nanoparticles have been evaluated on a few other noncancer diseases as well, such as arthritis, osteoporosis, problems with arteries, etc. Most of the applications reported in this chapter have displayed very promising therapeutic results with only a few exceptions, and the advantages and limitations of using polymeric nanoparticles have been reported in each case examined.

The most obvious advantages of incorporating drugs into nanoparticles are the reduced toxicity of highly toxic drugs, the protection against environmental conditions, the reduction of the drug dose to give the prospect of better patient compliance and versatility in delivery route. The latter advantage arises because the characteristics of the final formulation, which can favor the use of alternative delivery routes over conventional ones (e.g. pulmonary or nasal delivery instead of subcutaneous injection).

PLGA polymer and chitosan have been the most used polymers. In general, chitosan seems to be more favorable than PLGA, especially when the particles are destined to interact with mucosal surfaces (pulmonary, nasal, ocular, oral/gastrointestinal tract interaction), because it seems to enable the paracellular transport of the nanoparticles. Also, chitosan particles can be made into nanoparticles using methods that do not need the use of organic solvents (important because solvents remain in the particles at low levels and can be irritant or toxic in some cases). In addition, PLGA can be disadvantageous because its degradation products can create an acidic environment, damaging pH-sensitive proteins or peptides.

The drug release profile is one factor that requires further development. With some drugs and applications, the rapid rate of drug release can be a limiting factor (e.g. PLGA almost always shows a significant initial burst release). Thus, there is a need for polymer development to produce particles with sustained drug release and which retain the essential properties of polymer delivery systems, such as biodegradability and biocompatibility.

Finally, in order to reach the clinic and the market, these polymeric formulations will need to be produced in a large scale, have to exhibit a long shelf-life, and to be characterized by reasonable manufacturing cost and formulation stability. There is still a problem of producing sterile dispersions for ocular delivery, too. However, with the promise already shown in the formulations discussed above, it seems likely that the necessary resources will be found to resolve these remaining issues.

References

1 Diamond, J. M. The epithelial junction: bridge gate and fence, *Physiologist* **1977**, *20*, 10–18.

2 Inoue, S. Ultrastructure of basement membranes, *Int. Rev. Cytol.* **1989**, *117*, 57–98.

3 van Oss, C. J. Phagocytosis: an overview, *Methods Enzymol.* **1986**, *132*, 3–15.

4 van Deurs, B., Peterson, O. W., Olsnes, S., Sandvig, K. The ways of endocytosis, *Int. Rev. Cytol.* **1989**, *117*, 131–177.

5 Anderson, R. G., Kamen, B. A., Rothberg, K. G., Lacey, W. W. Potocytosis: sequestration and transport of small molecules by caveolae, *Science* **1992**, *255*, 410–411.

6 Ghitescu, L., Fixman, A., Simionescu, M. and Simionescu, N. Specific binding sites for albumin restricted to plasmalemmal vesicles of continuous capillary endothelium: receptor mediated transcytosis, *J. Cell Biol.* **1986**, *102*, 1304–1311.

7 Schnitzer, J. E. Caveolae: from basic trafficking mechanisms to targeting transcytosis for tissue specific drug and gene delivery *in vivo*, *Adv. Drug Deliv. Rev.* **2001**, *49*, 265–280.

8 Kreuter, J. Nanoparticulate systems for brain delivery of drugs, *Adv. Drug Deliv. Rev.* **2001**, *47*, 65–81.

9 Lind, K., Kresse, M., Debus, N. P., Müller, R. H. A novel formulation for superparamagnetic iron oxide (SPIO) particle enhancing MR lymphography: comparison of physicochemical properties and the *in vivo* behaviour, *J. Drug Target.* **2002**, *10*, 221–230.

10 Gibaud, S., Demoy, M., Andreux, J. P., Weingarten, C., Gouritin, B., Couvreur, P. Cells involved in the capture of nanoparticles in hematopoietic organs, *J. Pharm. Sci.* **1996**, *85*, 944–950.

11 Agrawal, A. K., Gupta, C. M. Tuftsin bearing liposomes in treatment of macrophage based infections, *Adv. Drug Deliv. Rev.* **2000**, *41*, 135–146.

12 Moghimi, S. M., Porter, C. J. H., Muir, I. S., Illum, L., Davis, S. S. Non-phagocytic uptake of intravenously injected microspheres in rat spleen: influence of particle size and hydrophilic coating, *Biochem. Biophys Res. Commun.* **1991**, *177*, 861–866.

13 Absolom, D. R. Opsonins & dysopsonins: an overview, *Methods Enzymol.* **1986**, *132*, 281–318.

14 Stolnik, S., Illum, L., Davis, S. S. Long circulating microparticulate drug carriers, *Adv. Drug Deliv. Rev.* **1995**, *16*, 195–214.

15 Holmgren, J., Capron, P. B. P. A., Francotte, M., Kilian, M., Kraehenbuhl, J. P., Lehner, T., Seljelid, R. European Commission COST/STD Initiative, Report of the expert panel VI. Concerted efforts in the field of mucosal immunology, *Vaccine* **1996**, *14*, 644–664.

16 Norris, D. A., Puri, N., Sinko, P. The effect of physical barriers and properties on the oral absorption of particulates, *Adv. Drug Deliv. Rev.* **1998**, *34*, 135–154.

17 Hussain, N., Jaitley, V., Florence, A. T. Recent advances in the understanding of uptake of microparticulates across the gastrointestinal

lymphatics, *Adv. Drug Deliv. Rev.* **2001**, *50*, 107–142.

18 Florence, A. T., Hussain, N. Transcytosis of nanoparticle and dendrimer delivery systems: evolving vistas, *Adv. Drug Deliv. Rev.* **2001**, *50*, S69–S89.

19 Jung, T., Kamm, W., Breitenbach, A., Kaiserling, E., Xiao, J. X., Kissel, T. Biodegradable nanoparticles for oral delivery of peptides: is there a role for polymer to affect mucosal uptake, *Eur J. Pharm. Biopharm.* **2000**, *50*, 147–160.

20 Illum, L. Nasal delivery. The use of animal models to predict performance in man, *J. Drug Target.* **1996**, *3*, 427–442.

21 Jones, N. The nose and paranasal sinuses physiology and anatomy, *Adv. Drug Deliv. Rev.* **2001**, *51*, 5–19.

22 Gumbleton, M. J. Caveolae as potential macromolecule trafficking compartments within alveolar epithelium, *Adv. Drug Deliv. Rev.* **2001**, *49*, 281–300.

23 Washington, N., Washington, C., Wilson, C. G. *Physiological Pharmaceutics: Barriers to Drug Absorption*, 2nd edn. Taylor & Francis, London, **2001**.

24 Jakob, T., Ring, J., Udey, M. C. Multistep navigation of Langerhans/dendritic cells in and out of the skin, *J. Allergy Clin. Immunol.* **2001**, *108*, 688–696.

25 Hawley, A. E., Davis, S. S., Illum, L. Targeting of colloids to lymph nodes: influence of lymphatic physiology and colloidal characteristics, *Adv. Drug Deliv. Rev.* **1995**, *17*, 129–148.

26 Mainardes, R. M., Urban, M. C. C., Cinto, P. O., Khalil, M. N., Chaud, M. V., Evangelista, R. C., Gremiao, M. P. D. Colloidal carriers for ophthalmic drug delivery, *Curr. Drug Targets* **2005**, *6*, 363–371.

27 Lang, J. C. Ocular drug delivery conventional ocular formulations, *Adv. Drug Deliv. Rev.* **1995**, *16*, 3943.

28 Alonso, M. J., Sanchez, A. The potential of chitosan in ocular drug delivery, *J. Pharm. Pharmacol.* **2003**, *55*, 1451–1463.

29 Salgueiro, A., Egea, M. A., Espina, M., Valls, O., Garcia, M. L. Stability and ocular tolerance of cyclophosphamide-loaded nanospheres, *J. Microencapsul.* **2004**, *21*, 213–223.

30 Fresta, M., Fontana, G., Bucolo, C., Cavallaro, G., Giammona, G., Puglisi, G. Ocular tolerability and *in vivo* bioavailability of poly(ethylene glycol) (PEG)-coated polyethyl-2-cyanoacrylate nanosphere-encapsulate acyclovir, *J. Pharm. Sci.* **2001**, *90*, 288–297.

31 De Kozak, Y., Andrieux, K., Villarroya, H., Klein, C., Thillaye-Goldenberg, B., Naud, M. C., Garcia, E., Couvreur, P. Intraocular injection of tamoxifen-loaded nanoparticles: a new treatment of experimental autoimmune uveoretinitis, *Eur. J. Immunol.* **2004**, *34*, 3702–3712.

32 Pignatello, R., Bucolo, C., Spedalieri, G., Maltese, A., Puglisi, G. Flurbiprofen-loaded acrylate polymer nanosuspensions for ophthalmic application, *Biomaterials* **2002**, *23*, 3247–3255.

33 Pignatello, R., Bucolo, C., Ferrara, P., Maltese, A., Puleo, A., Puglisi, G. Eudragit RS100 nanosuspensions for the ophthalmic control delivery of ibuprofen, *Eur. J. Pharm. Sci.* **2002**, *16*, 53–61.

34 Pignatello, R., Bucolo, C., Puglisi, G. Ocular tolerability of Eudragit RS100 and RL100 nanosuspensions as carriers for ophthalmic controlled drug delivery, *J. Pharm. Sci.* **2002**, *91*, 2636–2641.

35 de Campos, A. M., Sanchez, A., Alonso, M. J. Chitosan nanoparticles: a new vehicle for the improvement of the delivery of drugs to the ocular surface. Application to cyclosporin A, *Int. J. Pharm.* **2001**, *224*, 159–168.

36 Lallemand, F., Felt-Baeyens, O., Besseghir, K., Behar-Cohen, F., Gurny, R. Cyclosporine A delivery to the eye: a pharmaceutical challenge, *Eur. J. Pharm. Biopharm.* **2003**, *56*, 307–318.

37 Rabinovich-Guilatt, L., Couvreur, P., Lambert, G., Dubernet, C. Cationic vectors in ocular drug

delivery, *J. Drug Target.* **2004**, *12*, 623–633.
38 Giannavola, C., Bucolo, C., Maltese, A., Paolino, D., Vandelli, M. A., Puglisi, G., Lee, V. H. L., Fresta, M. Influence of preparation conditions on acyclovir-loaded Poly-D,L-lactic acid nanospheres and effect of PEG coating on ocular drug bioavailability, *Pharm. Res.* **2003**, *20*, 584–590.
39 Qaddoumi, M. G., Hovhannes, G. J., Davda, J., Labhasetwar, V., Kim, K. J., Lee, V. H. L. Clathrin and caveolin-1 expression in primary pigmented rabbit conjunctival epithelial cells: role in PLGA nanoparticle endocytosis, *Mol. Vision* **2003**, *9*, 559–68.
40 Barbault-Foucher, S., Gref, R., Russo, P., Guechot, J., Bochot, A. Design of poly-ε-caprolactone nanospheres coated with bioadhesive hyaluronic acid for ocular delivery, *J. Control. Release* **2002**, *83*, 365–375.
41 De, T. K., Bergey, E. J., Chung, S. J., Rodman, D. J., Bharali, D. J., Prasad, P. N. Polycarboxylic acid nanoparticles for ophthalmic drug delivery: an *ex vivo* evaluation in human cornea, *J. Microencapsul.* **2004**, *21*, 841–855.
42 Giordano, G. G., Refojo, M. F., Arroyo, M. H. Sustained delivery of retinoic acid from microspheres of biodegradable polymer in PVR, *Invest. Ophthalmol. Vis. Sci.* **1993**, *34*, 2743–2751.
43 Colthurst, M. J., Williams, R. L., Hiscott, P. S., Grierson, I. Biomaterials used in the posterior segment of the eye, *Biomaterials* **2000**, *2*, 649–665.
44 Calvo, P., Alonso, M. J., Vila-Jato, J. L., Robinson, J. R. Improved ocular bioavailability of indomethacin by novel ocular drug carriers, *J. Pharm. Pharmacol.* **1996**, *48*, 1147–1152.
45 de Campos, A. M., Diebold, Y., Carvalho, E. L. S., Sanchez, A., Alonso, M. J. Chitosan nanoparticles as new ocular drug delivery systems: *in vitro* stability, *in vivo* fate and cellular toxicity, *Pharm. Res.* **2004**, *21*, 803–810.
46 Calvo, P., Vila-Jato, J. L., Alonso, M. J., Comparative *in vitro* evaluation of several colloidal systems, nanoparticles, nanocapsules, and nanoemulsions, as ocular drug carriers, *J. Pharm. Sci.* **1996**, *85*, 530–536.
47 Calvo, P., Vila-Jato, J. L., Alonso, M. J. Evaluation of cationic polymer-coated nanocapsules as ocular drug carriers, *Int. J. Pharm.* **1997**, *153*, 41–50.
48 Calvo, P., Sanchez, A., Martinez, J., Lopez, M. I., Calonge, M., Pastor, J. C., Alonso, M. J. Polyester nanocapsules as new topical ocular delivery systems for cyclosporin A, *Pharm. Res.* **1996**, *13*, 311–315.
49 Heinemann, M. H. *Am. J. Ophthalmol.* **1989**, *107*, 643–644.
50 Cochereau-Massin, I., Lehoang, P., Lautier-Frau, M., Zerdoun, E., Zazoun, L., Robinet, M., Marcel, P., Leport, C. Ocular toxoplasmosis in human immunodeficiency virus-infected patients. *Ophthalmology* **1991**, *988*, 1348–1355.
51 Irache, J. M., Merodio, M., Arnedo, A., Camapanero, M. A., Mirshahi, M., Espuelas, S. Albumin nanoparticles for the intravitreal delivery of anticytomegaloviral drugs, *Mini-Rev. Med. Chem.* **2005**, *5*, 293–305.
52 Simoes, S., Slepushkin, V., Pires, P., Gaspar, R., Pedroso de Lima, M. C., Duzgunes, N. *Biochim. Biophys. Acta* **2000**, *1463*, 459–469.
53 Gulsen, D., Chauban, A. Ophthalmic drug delivery through contact lenses, *IOVS* **2004**, *45*, 2342–2347.
54 Saha, P., Kim, K. J., Lee, V. H. A primary culture model of rabbit conjunctival epithelial cells exhibiting tight barrier properties, *Curr. Eye Res.* **1996**, *15*, 1163–1169.
55 Horibe, Y., Hosoya, K., Kim, K. J., Ogiso, T., Lee, V. H. Polar solute transport across the pigmented rabbit conjuctiva: size dependence and the influence of 8-bromo cyclic adenosine monophosphate, *Pharm. Res.* **1997**, *14*, 1246–1251.
56 Nichols, B. A., Chiappino, M. L., Dawson, C. R. Demonstration of the mucous layer of the tear film by elec-

tron microscopy, *Invest. Ophthalmol. Vis. Sci.* **1985**, *24*, 464–473.

57 Gaspar, R., Opperdoes, F. R., Preat, V., Roland, M. Drug targeting with polyalkylcyanoacrylate nanoparticles: *in vitro* activity of primaquine-loaded nanoparticles against intracellular *Leishmania donovani*, *Ann. Trop. Med. Parasit.* **1992**, *86*, 41–49.

58 Fouarge, M., Osuna, A., Couvreur, P., Roland, M., Vranckx, H. Development of dehydroemetine nanoparticles for the treatment of visceral leishmaniasis, *J. Microencapsul.* **1989**, *6*, 29–34.

59 Lenaerts, V., Nagelkerke, J. F., Van Berkel, T. J. C., Couvreur, P., Grislain, L., Roland, M., Speiser, P. *In vivo* uptake of polyisobutylcyanoacrylate nanoparticles by rat liver, Kupffer, endothelial and parenchymal cells, *J. Pharm. Sci.* **1984**, *73*, 980–982.

60 Rodrigues, Jr., J. M., Fessi, H., Bories, C., Puisieux, F., Devissaguet, J.-Ph. Primaquine-loaded poly(lactide) nanoparticles: physicochemical study and acute tolerance in mice, *Int. J. Pharm.* **1995**, *126*, 253–260.

61 Rodrigues, Jr., J. M., Croft, S. L., Fessi, H., Bories, C., Devissaguet, J. Ph. The activity and ultrastructural localization of primaquine-loaded poly(D,L-lactide) nanoparticles in *Leishmania donovani* infected mice, *Trop. Med. Parasitol.* **1994**, *45*, 223–228.

62 Fusai, T., Deniau, M., Durand, R., Bories, C., Paul, M., Rivollet, D., Astier, A., Houin, R. Action of pentamidine-bound nanoparticles against *Leishmania* on an *in vivo* model, *Parasite* **1994**, *1*, 319–324.

63 Durand, R., Paul, M., Rivollet, D., Houin, R., Astier, A., Deniau, M. Activity of Pentamidine-loaded Methacrylate nanoparticles against *Leishmania infantum* in a mouse model, *Int. J. Parasitol.* **1997**, *27*, 1361–1367.

64 Paul, M., Durand, R., Boulard, Y., Fusai, T., Fernandez, C., Rivollet, D., Deniau, M., Astier, A. Physicochemical characteristics of pentamidine-loaded polymethacrylate nanoparticles: implication in the intracellular drug release in *Leishmania* major infected mice, *J. Drug Target.* **1998**, *5*, 481–490.

65 Venier-Julienne, M. C., Vouldoukis, I., Monjour, L., Benoit, J. P. *In vitro* study of the antileishmanial activity of biodegradable nanoparticles, *J. Drug Target.* **1995**, *3*, 23–29.

66 *British National Formulary 43*, **2003**.

67 Ofek, I., Sharon, N. Lectinophagocytosis: a molecular mechanism of recognition between cell surface sugars and lectins in the phagocytosis bacteria, *Infect. Immun.* **1988**, *56*, 539–547.

68 Desjeux, P. Leishmaniasis: public health aspects and control, *Clin. Dermatol.* **1996**, *14*, 417–423.

69 Chen, M., Christensen, S. B., Theander, T. G., Kharazmi, A. Antileishmanial activity of licochalcone A in mice infected with *Leishmania major* and in hamsters infected with *Leishmania donovani*, *Antimicrob. Agents Chemother.* **1994**, *38*, 1339–1344.

70 Torres-Santos, E. C., Rodrigues, J. M., Jr., Moreira, D. L., Auxiliadora, M., Kaplan, C., Rossi-Bergmann, B. Improvement of *in vitro* and *in vivo* antileishmanial activities of 2′,6′-dihydroxy-4′-methoxychalcone by entrapment in poly(D,L-lactide) nanoparticles, *Antimicrob. Agents Chemother.* **1999**, *43*, 1776–1778.

71 Sarkar, S., Mandal, S., Sinha, J., Mukhopadhyay, S., Das, N., Basu, M. K. Quercetin: critical evaluation as an antileishmanial agent *in vivo* in hamsters using different vesicular delivery modes, *J. Drug Target.* **2002**, *10*, 573–578.

72 Lala, S., Pramanick, S., Mukhopadhyay, S., Bandyopadhyay, S., Basu, M. K. Harmine: evaluation of its antileishmanial properties in various vesicular delivery systems, *J. Drug Target.* **2004**, *12*, 165–175.

73 Tyagi, R., Lala, S., Verma, A. K., Nandy, A. K., Mahato, S. B., Maitra, A., Basu, M. K. Targeted delivery of

arjunglucoside I using surface hydrophilic and hydrophobic nanocarriers to combat experimental leishmaniasis, *J. Drug Target.* **2005**, *13*, 161–171.
74 Mittra, B., Saha, A., Chowdhury, R., Pal, A., Mandal, C., Mukhopadhyay, S., Bandyopadhyay, S., Majumber, H. K. Luteolin – an abundant dietary component is a potent antileishmanial agent that acts by inducing topoisomerase-II mediated kinetoplast DNA cleavage leading to apoptosis, *Mol. Med.* **2000**, *6*, 527–541.
75 Molero, M. L., Hazen, M. J., Perez-Gorrono, A. I., Stockert, J. C. Simple beta-carboline alkaloids as nucleic acid fluorochromes, *Acta Histochem.* **1995**, *97*, 165–173.
76 Sobhani, A. M., Ebrahim, S. A., Mohmoudian, M. An *in vitro* evaluation of human DNA topoisomerase I inhibition by *Peganum harmala* L. seeds extract and its beta-carboline alkaloids, *J. Pharm. Pharm. Sci.* **2002**, *5*, 19–23.
77 Basu, M. K., Lala, S. Macrophage specific drug delivery in experimental leishmaniasis, *Curr. Mol. Med.* **2004**, *4*, 681–689.
78 Lherm, C., Couvreur, P., Loiseau, P., Boriest, C., Gayral, P. Unloaded polyisobutylcyanoacrylate nanoparticles: efficiency against bloodstream trypanosomes, *J. Pharm. Pharmacol.* **1987**, *39*, 650–652.
79 Mainardes, R. M., Evangelista, R. C. PLGA nanoparticles containing praziquantel: effect of formulation variables on size distribution, *Int. J. Pharm.*, **2005**, *290*, 137–144.
80 Legrand, P., Mosqueira, V., Loiseau, P., Bories, C., Barratt, G. Les nanocapsules á temps de circulation prolongé: intérêt dans le traitement du paludisme sévère par l'halofantrine, *Ann Pharm Fr.* **2003**, *61*, 196–202.
81 Tiyanboonchai, W., Woiszwillo, J., Middaugh, C. R. Formulation and characterization of Amphotericin-B–polyethylenimine–dextran sulfate nanoparticles, *J. Pharm. Sci.* **2001**, *90*, 902–914.
82 McCarron, P. A., Donnelly, R. F., Canning, P. E., McGovern, J. G., Jones, D. S. Bioadhesive, non-drug-loaded nanoparticles as modulators of candidal adherence to buccal epithelial cells: a potentially novel prophylaxis for candidosis, *Biomaterials* **2004**, *25*, 2399–2407.
83 Molina, J., Urbina, J., Gref, R., Brener, Z., Júnior, J. M. R. Cure of experimental Chagas' disease by the bis-triazole DO870 incorporated into "stealth" polyethyleneglycol–polylactide nanospheres, *J. Antimicrob. Chemther.* **2001**, *47*, 101–104.
84 Urbina, J. A. Chemotherapy of Chagas' disease: the how and the why, *J. Mol. Med.* **1999**, *77*, 332–338.
85 Salmaso, S., Elvassore, N., Bertucco, A., Lante, A., Caliceti, P. Nisin-loaded poly-L-lactide nanoparticles produced by CO_2 anti-solvent precipitation for sustained antimicrobial activity, *Int. J. Pharm.* **2004**, *287*, 163–173.
86 Qi, L., Xu, Z., Jiang, X., Hu, C., Zou, X. Preparation and antibacterial activity of chitosan nanoparticles, *Carbohydr. Res.* **2004**, *339*, 2693–2700.
87 Ueno, K., Yamaguchi, T., Sakairi, N., Nishi, N., Tokura, S. *Adv. Chitin Sci.* **1997**, *2*, 156–161.
88 Jeon, Y. J., Park, P. J., Kim, S. K. Anti microbial effect of chitooligosaccharides produced by bioreactor, *Curbohydr. Polym.* **2001**, *44*, 71–76.
89 Pandey, R., Khuller, G. K. Antitubercular inhaled therapy: opportunities, progress and challenges, *J. Antimicrob. Chemother.* **2005**, *55*, 430–435.
90 Pandey, R., Zahoor, A., Sharma, S., Khuller, G. K. Nanoparticle encapsulated antitubercular drugs as a potential oral drug delivery system against murine tuberculosis, *Tuberculosis* **2003**, *83*, 373–378.
91 Sharma, A., Pandey, R., Sharma, S., Khuller, G. K. Chemotherapeutic efficacy of poly (DL-lactide-*co*-glycolide) nanoparticle encapsulated antitubercular drugs at sub-therapeutic dose against experimental tuberculosis, *Int.*

J. Antimicrob. Agents **2004**, *24*, 599–604.

92 Sharma, A., Sharma, S., Khuller, G. K. Lectin-functionalized poly(lactide-*co*-glycolide) nanoparticles as oral/aerosolised antitubercular drug carriers for treatment of tuberculosis, *J. Antimicrob. Chemother.* **2004**, *54*, 761–766.

93 Gelperina, S., Kisich, K., Iseman, M. D., Heifets, L. The potential advantages of nanoparticle drug delivery systems in chemotherapy of tuberculosis, *Am. J. Respir. Crit. Care Med.* **2005**, *17*, 1487–1490.

94 Fu, J., Fiegel, J., Krauland, E., Hanes, J. New polymeric carriers for controlled drug delivery following inhalation or injection, *Biomaterials* **2002**, *23*, 4425–4433.

95 Lipworth, B. J. Targets for inhaled treatment. *Respir. Med.* **2000**, *94 (Suppl. D)*, S13–S16.

96 Pandey, R., Sharma, A., Zahoor, A., Sharma, S., Khuller, G. K., Prasad, B. Poly (DL-lactide-*co*-glycolide) nanoparticle-based inhalable sustained drug delivery system for experimental tuberculosis, *J. Antimicrob. Chemother.* **2003**, *52*, 9881–986.

97 Grayson, A. C., Voskerician, G., Lynn, A. Differential degradation rates *in vivo* and *in vitro* of biocompatible poly(lactic acid) and poly(glycolic acid) homo- and co-polymers for a polymeric drug-delivery microchip, *J. Biomater. Sci. Polym. Ed.* **2004**, *15*, 1281–304.

98 Dailey, L. A., Kleemann, E., Wittmar, M., Gessler, T., Schmehl, T., Roberts, C., Seeger, W., Kissel, T. Surfactant-free, biodegradable nanoparticles for aerosol therapy based on the branched polyesters, DEAPA–PVAL-g-PLGA, *Pharm. Res.* **2003**, *20*, 2011–2019.

99 Zahoor, A., Sharma, S., Khuller, G. K. Inhalable alginate nanoparticles as antitubercular drug carriers against experimental tuberculosis, *Int. J. Antimicrob. Agents* **2005**, *26*, 298–303.

100 Pandey, R., Khuller, G. K. Subcutaneous nanoparticle-based antitubercular chemotherapy in an experimental model, *J. Antimicrob. Chemother.* **2004**, *54*, 266–268.

101 Bender, A. R., Briesen, H., Kreuter, J., Duncan, I. B., Rubsamen-Waigmann, H. Efficiency of nanoparticles as a carrier system for antiviral agents in human immunodeficiency virus-infected human monocytes/macrophages *in vitro*, *Antimicrob. Agents Chemother.* **1996**, *40*, 1467–1471.

102 Hao, Z., Cooney, D. A., Hartman, N. R., Perno, C. F., Fridland, A., DeVico, A. L., Sarngadharan, M. G., Broder, S., Johns, D. G. Factors determining the activity of 2′,3′-dideoxynucleosides in suppressing human immunodeficiency virus *in vitro*, *Mol. Pharmacol.* **1988**, *34*, 431–435.

103 Löbenberg, R., Araujo, L., von Briesen, H., Rodgers, E., Kreuter, J. Body distribution of azidothymidine bound to hexyl-cyanoacrylate nanoparticles after i v. injection to rats, *J. Control. Release* **1998**, *50*, 21–30.

104 Dembri, A., Montisci, M. J., Gantier, J. C., Chacun, H., Ponchel, G. Targeting of 3′-azido-3′-deoxythymidine (AZT)-loaded poly(isohexylcyanoacryalte) nanospheres to the gastrointestinal mucosa and associated lymphoid tissues, *Pharm. Res.* **2001**, *18*, 467–473.

105 Leroux, J. C., Cozens, R. M., Roesel, J. L., Galli, B., Doelker, E., Gurny, R. pH-sensitive nanoparticles: an effective means to improve the oral delivery of HIV-1 protease inhibitors in dogs, *Pharm. Res.* **1996**, *13*, 485–487.

106 Leroux, J. C., Cozens, R., Roesel, J. L., Galli, B., Kubel, F., Doelker, E., Gurny, R. Pharmacokinetics of a novel HIV-1 protease inhibitor incorporated into biodegradable or enteric nanoparticles following intravenous and oral administration to mice, *J. Pharm. Sci.* **1995**, *84*, 1387–1391.

107 De Jaeghere, F., Allemann, E., Kubel, F., Galli, B., Cozens, R., Doelker, E., Gurny, R. Oral bioavailability of a poorly water soluble

HIV-1 protease inhibitor incorporated into pH-sensitive particles: effect of the particle size and nutritional state, *J. Control. Release* **2000**, *68*, 291–298.

108 Boudad, H., Legrand, P., Lebas, G., Cheron, M., Duchêne, D., Ponchel, G. Combined hydroxypropyl-*β*-cyclodextrin and poly(alkylcyanoacrylate) nanoparticles intended for oral administration of saquinavir, *Int. J. Pharm.* **2001**, *218*, 113–124.

109 Berton, M., Turelli, P., Trono, D., Stein, Cy. A., Allémann, E., Gurny, R. Inhibition of HIV-1 in cell culture by oligonucleotide-loaded nanoparticles, *Pharm. Res.* **2001**, *18*, 1096–1101.

110 Dinauer, N., Lochmann, D., Demirhan, I., Bouazzaoui, A., Zimmer, A., Chandra, A., Kreuter, J., von Briesen, H. Intracellular tracking of protamine/antisense oligonucleotide nanoparticles and their inhibitory effect on HIV-1 transactivation, *J. Control. Release* **2004**, *96*, 497–507.

111 Le Buanec, H., Vetu, C., Lachgar, A., Benoit, M. A., Gillard, J., Paturance, S., Aucouturier, J., Gane, V., Zagury, D., Bizzini, B. Induction in mice of anti-Tat mucosal immunity by the intranasal and oral routes, *Biomed. Pharmacother.* **2001**, *55*, 316–320.

112 Cui, Z., Patel, J., Tuzova, M., Ray, P., Phillips, R., Woodward, J. G., Nath, A., Mumper, R. J. Strong T cell type-1 immune responses to HIV-1 Tat (1–72) protein-coated nanoparticles, *Vaccine* **2004**, *22*, 2631–2640.

113 Frankel, A. D., Pabo, C. O. Cellular uptake of the Tat protein from human immunodeficiency virus, *Cell* **1988**, *55*, 1189–1193.

114 Li, C. J., Ueda, Y., Shi, B., Borodyansky, L., Huang, L., Li, Y. Z. Tat protein induces self-perpetuating permissivity for productive HIV-1 infection, *Proc. Natl. Acad. Sci. USA* **1997**, *94*, 8116–8120.

115 Locher, C. P., Putnam, D., Langer, R., Witt, S. A., Ashlock, B. M., Levy, J. A. Enhancement of a human immunodeficiency virus *env* DNA vaccine using a novel polycationic nanoparticle formulation, *Immunol. Lett.* **2003**, *90*, 67–70.

116 Kawamura, M., Wang, X., Tomofumi, U., Sato, K., Ueno, M., Akagi, T., Hiraishi, K., Matsuyama, T., Akashi, M., Baba, M. Induction of dendritic cell-mediated immune responses against HIV-1 by antigen-capturing nanospheres in mice, *J. Med. Virol.* **2005**, *76*, 7–15.

117 Miyake, A., Akagi, T., Enose, Y., Ueno, M., Kawamura, M., Horiuchi, R., Hiraishi, K., Adachi, M., Serizawa, T., Narayan, O., Akashi, M., Baba, M., Hayami, M. Induction of HIV-specific antibody response and protection against vaginal SHIV transmission by intranasal immunization with inactivated SHIV-capturing nanospheres in macaques, *J. Med. Virol.* **2004**, *73*, 368–377.

118 Raghuvanshi, R. S., Katare, Y. K., Lalwani, K., Ali, M. M., Singh, O., Panda, A. K. Improved immune response from biodegradable polymer particles entrapping tetanus toxoid by use of different immunization protocol and adjuvants, *Int. J. Pharm.* **2002**, *245*, 109–121.

119 Naim, J. O., van Oss, C. J., Wu, W., Giese, R. F., Nickerson, P. A. Mechanism of adjuvancy: I – metal oxide as adjuvants, *Vaccine* **1997**, *11*, 1183–1193.

120 Kohli, A. K., Alpar, H. O. Potential use of nanoparticles for transcutaneous vaccine delivery: effect of particle size and charge, *Int. J. Pharm.* **2004**, *275*, 13–17.

121 Newman, K. D., Elamanchili, P., Kwon, G. S., Samuel, J. Uptake of poly(D,L-lactic-*co*-glycolic acid) microspheres by antigen-presenting cells *in vivo*, *J. Biomed. Mater. Res.* **2002**, *60*, 480–486.

122 Elamanchili, P., Diwan, M., Cao, M., Samuel, J. Characterization of poly(D,L-lactic-*co*-glycolic acid) based nanoparticulate system for enhanced delivery of antigens to dendritic cells, *Vaccine* **2004**, *22*, 2406–2412.

123 Sun, H., Pollock, K. G., Brewer, J. M. Analysis of the role of vaccine adjuvants in modulating dendritic cell

activation and antigen presentation *in vitro*, *Vaccine* **2003**, *21*, 849–55.

124 Chong, C. S. W., Cao, M., Wong, W. W., Fischer, K. P., Addison, W. R., Kwon, G. S., Tyrell, D. L., Samuel, J. Enhancement of T helper type 1 immune responses against hepatitis B virus core antigen by PLGA nanoparticle vaccine delivery, *J. Control. Release* **2005**, *102*, 85–99.

125 Nixon, D. F., Hioe, C., Chen, P. D., Bian, Z., Kuebler, P., Li, M. L., Qiu, H., Li, X. M., Singh, M., Richardson, A., McGee, P., Zamb, T., Koff, W., Wang, C. Y., O'Hagan, D. Synthetic peptides entrapped in microparticles can elicit cytotoxic T cell activity, *Vaccine* **1996**, *14*, 1523–1530.

126 Wang, X., Uto, T., Sato, K., Ide, K., Akagi, T., Okamoto, M., Kaneko, T., Akashi, M., Baba, M. Potent activation of antigen-specific T cells by antigen-loaded nanospheres, *Immunol. Lett.* **2005**, *98*, 123–130.

127 Cui, Z., Mumper, R. J. Chitosan-based nanoparticles for topical genetic immunization, *J. Control. Release* **2001**, *75*, 409–419.

128 Cui, Z., Mumper, R. J. Dendritic cell-targeted genetic vaccines engineered from novel microemulsion precursors, *Mol. Ther.* **2001**, *3*, S352.

129 Cui, Z., Mumper, R. J. Topical immunization using nanoengineered genetic vaccines, *J. Control. Release* **2002**, *81*, 173–184.

130 Toda, S., Ishii, N., Okada, E., Kusakabe, K. I., Arai, H., Hamajima, K., Gorai, I., Nishioka, K., Okuda, K. HIV-1-specific cell-mediated immune responses induced by DNA vaccination were enhanced by mannan-coated liposomes and inhibited by anti-interferon-γ antibody, *Immunology* **1997**, *92*, 111–117.

131 Gu, X. G., Schmitt, M., Hiasa, A., Nagata, Y., Ikeda, H., Sasaki, Y., Akiyoshi, K., Sunamoto, J., Nakamura, H., Kuribayashi, K., Skiku, H. A novel hydrophobized polysaccharide/oncoprotein complex vaccine induces *in vitro* and *in vivo* cellular and humoral immune responses against HER2-expressing murine sarcomas, *Cancer Res.* **1998**, *58*, 3385–3390.

132 Tan, M. C., Mommaas, A. M., Drijfhout, J. W., Jordens, R., Onderwater, J. J., Verwoerd, D., Mulder, A. A., van der Heiden, A. N., Scheidegger, D., Oomen, L. C., Ottenhoff, T. H., Tulp, A., Neefjes, J. J., Koning, F. Mannose receptor-mediated uptake of antigens strongly enhances HLA antigens class II-restricted antigen presentation by cultured dendritic cells, *Eur. J. Immunol.* **1997**, *27*, 2426–2435.

133 Mumper, R. J., Cui, Z. Genetic immunization by jet injection of targeted pDNA-coated nanoparticles, Methods **2003**, *31*, 255–262.

134 Cui, Z., Mumper, R. J. The effect of co-administration of adjuvants with a nanoparticle-based genetic vaccine delivery system on the resulting immune responses, *Eur. J. Pharm. Biopharm.* **2003**, *55*, 11–18.

135 Kim, S. Y., Doh, H. J., Jang, M. H., Ha, Y. J., Chung, S., Park, H. J. Oral immunization with *Helicobacter pylori*-loaded poly(D,L-lactide-*co*-glycolie) nanoparticles, *Helicobacter* **1999**, *4*, 33–39.

136 Jung, T., Kamm, W., Breitenbach, A., Klebe, G., Kissel, T. Loading of tetanus toxoid to biodegradable nanoparticles from branched poly(sulfobutyl-polyvinyl alcohol)-g-(lactide-*co*-glycolide) nanoparticles by protein absorption: a mechanistic study, *Pharm. Res.* **2002**, *19*, 1105–1113.

137 Prokop, A., Kozlov, E., Newman, G. W., Newman, M. J. Water-based nanoparticulate polymeric system for protein delivery: permeability control and vaccine application, *Biotechnol. Bioeng.* **2002**, *78*, 459–466.

138 Prokop, A. Micro-particulate and nano-particulate polymeric delivery system. Vanderbilt University, US patent pending, **1997**, also *PCT application WO9918934A1.*

139 Calvo, P., Remuñan-López, C., Vila-Jato, J. L., Alonso, M. J. Chitosan and chitosan/ethylene oxide–

propylene oxide block copolymer nanoparticles as novel carriers for proteins and vaccines, *Pharm. Res.* **1997**, *14*, 1431–1436.
140 Borges, O., Borchard, G., Verhoef, J. C., de Sousa, A., Junginger, H. E. Preparation of coated nanoparticles for a new mucosal vaccine delivery system, *Int. J. Pharm.* **2005**, *299*, 155–166.
141 Russell-Jones, G. J. Oral vaccine delivery, *J. Control. Release* **2000**, *65*, 49–54.
142 Russell-Jones, G. J., Veitch, H., Arthur, L. Lectin-mediated transport of nanoparticles across Caco-2 and OK cells, *Int. J. Pharm.* **1999**, *90*, 165–174.
143 Bivas-Benita, M., Laloup, M., Versteyhe, S., Dewit, J., Braekeller, J. D., Jongert, E., Borchard, G. Generation of *Toxoplasma gondii* GRA1 protein and DNA vaccine loaded chitosan particles: preparation, characterization and preliminary *in vivo* studies, *Int. J. Pharm.* **2003**, *266*, 17–27.
144 Chew, J. L., Wolfowicz, C. B., Mao, H. Q., Leong, K. W., Chua, K. Y. Chitosan nanoparticles containing plasmid DNA encoding house dust mite allergen, Der p 1 for oral vaccination in mice, *Vaccine* **2003**, *21*, 2720–2729.
145 Tobio, M., Gref, R., Sánchez, A., Langer, R., Alonso, M. J. Stealth PLA–PEG nanoparticles as protein carriers for nasal administration, *Pharm. Res.* **1998**, *15*, 270–275.
146 Shephard, M. J., Todd, D., Adair, B. M., Po, A. L. W., Mackie, D. P., Scott, E. M. Immunogenicity of bovine parainfluenza type 3 virus proteins encapsulated in nanoparticle vaccines, following intranasal administration to mice, *Res. Vet. Science* **2003**, *74*, 187–190.
147 Vila, A., Sánchez, A., Janes, K., Behrens, I., Kissel, T., Vila-Jato, J. L., Alonso, J. M. Low molecular weight chitosan nanoparticles as new carriers for nasal vaccine delivery in mice, *Eur. J. Pharm. Biopharm.* **2004**, *57*, 123–131.
148 Nagamoto, T., Hattori, Y., Takayama, K., Maitani, Y. Novel chitosan particles and chitosan-coated emulsions inducing immune response via intranasal vaccine delivery, *Pharm. Res.* **2004**, *21*, 671–674.
149 Cui, Z., Mumper, R. J. Intranasal administration of plasmid DNA-coated nanoparticles results in enhanced immune responses, *Pharm. Pharmacol.* **2002**, *54*, 1195–1203.
150 Klavinskis, L., Barnfield, C., Gao, L., Parker, S. Intranasal immunization with plasmid DNA–lipid complexes elicits mucosal immunity in the female genital and rectal tracts, *J. Immunol.* **1999**, *162*, 254–262.
151 Damgè, C., Michel, C., Aprahamian, M., Couvreur, P. New approaches for oral administration of insulin with polyalkyl-cyanoacrylate nanocapsules as a drug carrier, *Diabetes* **1988**, *37*, 246–251.
152 Damgè, C., Michel, C., Aprahamian, M., Couvreur, P., Devissaguet, J. P. Nanocapsules as carriers for oral peptide delivery, *J. Control. Release* **1990**, *13*, 233–239.
153 Aboubakar, M., Couvreur, P., Pinto-Alphandary, H., Gouritin, B., Lacour, B., Farinotti, R., Puisieux, F., Vauthier, C. Insulin-loaded nanocapsules for oral administration: *in vitro* and *in vivo* investigation, *Drug Dev. Res.* **2000**, *49*, 109–117.
154 Mesiha, M. S., Sidhom, M. B., Fasipe, B. Oral and subcutaneous absorption of insulin poly(isobutylcyanoacrylate) nanoparticles, *Int. J. Pharm.* **2005**, *288*, 289–293.
155 Pan, Y., Li, Y. J., Zhao, H. Y., Zheng, J. M., Xu, H., Wei, G., Hao, J. S., Cui, F. D. Bioadhesive polysaccharide in protein delivery system: chitosan nanoparticles improve the intestinal absorption of insulin *in vivo*, *Int. J. Pharm.* **2002**, *249*, 139–147.
156 Ma, Z., Yeoh, H. H., Lim, L. Y. Formulation pH modulates the interaction of insulin with chitosan nanoparticles, *J. Pharm. Sci.* **2002**, *91*, 1396–1404.

157 Ma, Z. and Lim, L. Y. Uptake of chitosan and associated insulin in Caco-2 Cell monolayers: a comparison between chitosan molecules and chitosan nanoparticles, *Pharm. Res.* **2003**, *20*, 1812–1819.

158 Dyer, M. A., Hinchcliffe, M., Watts, P., Castile, J., Jabbal-Gill, I., Nankervis, R., Smith, A., Illum, L. Nasal delivery of insulin using novel chitosan based formulations: a comparative study in two animal models between simple chitosan formulations and chitosan nanoparticles, *Pharm. Res.* **2002**, *19*, 998–1008.

159 Ma, Z., Lim, T. M., Lim, L. Y. Pharmacological activity of peroral chitosan-insulin nanoparticles in diabetic rats, *Int. J. Pharm.* **2005**, *293*, 271–180.

160 Fernández-Urrusuno, R., Calvo, P., Remuñán-Lopez, C., Vila-Jato, J. L., Alonso, M. J. Enhancement of nasal absorption of insulin using chitosan nanoparticles, *Pharm. Res.* **1999**, *16*, 1576–1581.

161 Simon, M., Wittmar, M., Bakowsky, U., Kissel, T. Self-assembling nanocomplexes from insulin and water-soluble branched polyesters, poly[(vinyl-3-(diethylamino)-propylcarbamate-*co*-(vinyl acetate)-*co*-(vinyl alcohol)]-graft-poly(L-lactic acid): a novel carrier for transmucosal delivery of peptides, *Bioconjug. Chem.* **2004**, *15*, 841–849.

162 Zhang, Q., Shen, Z., Nagai, T. Prolonged hypoglycemic effect of insulin-loaded polybutylcyanoacrylate nanoparticles after pulmonary administration to normal rats, *Int. J. Pharm.* **2001**, *218*, 75–80.

163 Grenha, A., Seijo, B., Remuñán-Lopez, C. Microencapsulated chitosan nanoparticles for lung protein delivery, *Eur. J. Pharm. Sci.* **2005**, *25*, 427–437.

164 Barichello, J. M., Morishita, M., Takayama, K., Nagai, T. Absorption of insulin from Pluronic F-127 gels following subcutaneous administration in rats, *Int. J. Pharm.* **1999**, *1884*, 189–198.

165 Tiyaboonchai, W., Woiszwillo, J., Sims, R. C., Middaugh, C. R. Insulin containing polyethylenimine–dextran sulfate nanoparticles, *Int. J. Pharm.* **2003**, *255*, 139–151.

166 Akiyoshi, K., Kobayashi, S., Shichibe, S., Mix, D., Baudys, M., Kim, S. W., Sunamoto, J. Self-assembled hydrogel nanoparticle of cholesterol-bearing pullulan as a carrier of protein drugs: complexation and stabilization of insulin, *J. Control. Release* **1998**, *54*, 313–320.

167 Elvassore, N., Bertucco, A., Caliceti, P. Production of insulin-loaded poly(ethylene glycol)/poly(L-lactide) (PEG/PLA) nanoparticles by gas antisolvent techniques, *J. Pharm. Sci.* **2001**, *90*, 1628–1636.

168 Zhang, K., Wu, X. Y. Modulated insulin permeation across a glucose-sensitive polymeric composite membrane, *J. Control. Release* **2002**, *80*, 169–178.

10
Solid Lipid and Polymeric Nanoparticles for Drug Delivery

José Luis Pedraz, Gorka Orive, Manoli Igartua, Alicia R. Gascón, Rosa M. Hernández, Maria Angeles Solinis, and Amaia Esquisabel

10.1
Introduction

Over the past few years, significant effort has been devoted to design and develop nanoparticles and nanosystems for drug delivery. Scientists have understood that apart from the synthesis of the drug molecule, the efficient release of the latter from the drug delivery system is essential if a suitable therapeutic efficacy is to be achieved. Therefore, the development of effective drug delivery systems which could transport and deliver the drug at the right time, in a safe and reproducible way, and only to the target where it is needed is becoming the "holy grail" of pharmaceutical researchers [1, 2].

The idea that nanotechnology could be used as a tool for efficient drug delivery has recently emerged since nanoparticles can be designed with different structures and compositions favoring a wide range of therapeutic applications [3]. Nanoparticles do not only differ in their relative size, but also in their biopharmaceutical properties and therapeutic applications. In general, the therapeutic product [drug, peptide, protein, DNA, small interfering RNA (siRNA), etc.] is either entrapped, adsorbed, attached, dissolved or encapsulated into the particle, allowing the precise control over drug release profiles [4]. Nanoparticles are less than 1000 nm in size and they present higher intracellular uptake compared with microparticles, which makes nanoparticles excellent candidates for targeted drug delivery to specific intracellular compartments.

One focus of research is the technological design and development of the nanoparticles assuming that the latter can present very different compositions and biological properties. However, a more interesting and effective way to design these nanosystems would be to rationally fabricate them based on a full understanding of the pathobiological characteristics of the disease under study and the biological microenvironment where the nanoparticles are to suppose to work. For example, if the intracellular release of the drug is required, a deep knowledge of the mecha-

Nanotechnologies for the Life Sciences Vol. 10
Nanomaterials for Medical Diagnosis and Therapy. Edited by Challa S. S. R. Kumar

ISBN: 978-3-527-31390-7

nisms that regulate the uptake of the particles, intracellular trafficking, retention and sorting pathways will be necessary [5]. Furthermore, the biopharmaceutical and technological properties of the nano drug delivery systems are also major issues to be considered. In fact, the therapeutic dose to be administered and the duration of drug delivery required at the target site are key factors in the pharmaceutical design of the nanoparticles in order to obtain an efficient treatment.

The present chapter describes two different types of nanoparticles suitable for continuous drug delivery. The selection of these nanoparticles is based on their extensive application for drug delivery purposes. The basic principles of solid lipid nanoparticles (SLNs) and polymeric nanoparticles will be presented in detail. The aim of this chapter is to describe the production processes and the main parameters related to their characterization. Furthermore, a wide range of therapeutic applications of both types of nanoparticles will be discussed in detail.

10.2 SLNs

10.2.1 Introduction

SLNs are colloidal carrier systems made from solid lipids with an average diameter in the nanometer range, introduced at the beginning of the 1990s as a drug delivery system alternative to existing colloidal carriers. Incorporation of a drug into a carrier system can protect it against degradation, the release can be controlled and it also offers possibilities of targeting. There is, however, a need for further, improved particulate carrier systems, which should fulfill as much as possible the following main requirements [6]:

- Easy to produce.
- Applicable to as many drugs as possible.
- Physically stable.
- Being composed of well-tolerated excipients that are accepted by the regulatory authorities.
- Feasibility of large-scale production.
- Production lines should be able to be qualified and acceptable by regulatory authorities.

The SLN is a particulate drug carrier system developed with the aim of combining the advantages of other innovative carrier systems such as lipid emulsions, liposomes and polymeric micro/nanoparticles, minimizing the associated problems. Excellent tolerability and the possibility of qualified industrial large-scale production are clear advantages of SLNs. Main disadvantages are the coexistence of alternative colloidal structures and, in general, low drug-loading capacity.

10.2.2 Composition

SLNs are particles made from solid lipids (usually lipids in solid state at room temperature and also at body temperature), water and stabilized by surfactant(s); for certain preparation methods a cosolvent, which is generally removed, is also used.

In general, physiological lipids such as triglycerides (e.g. tristearin), partial glycerides (e.g. Imwitor), fatty acids (e.g. stearic acid), steroids (e.g. cholesterol) and waxes (e.g. cetyl palmitate) are used. This physiological lipid matrix is more biocompatible, thus decreasing the danger of acute and chronic toxicity, and increasing their toxicological safety. There are a few exceptions and some authors have prepared SLNs with different types of molecules, such as amphiphilic cyclodextrins [7] and calixarenes [8, 9].

Most of the lipids used represent a mixture of several chemical compounds. The general lipid composition will have different crystallinities and capacities for accommodating foreign molecules. The composition might therefore vary from different suppliers and even for different batches. However, small differences in the lipid composition (e.g. impurities) might have a considerable impact on the quality of SLN dispersion [10] (e.g. by changing the ζ potential, retarding crystallization processes, etc.).

In addition to the lipid composition, the influence of lipid content on particle size has been studied, showing that increasing the lipid content over 5–10% in most cases results in larger particles (including microparticles) and broader particle size distributions [11]. The other main SLN ingredient is the stabilizing agent; a large variety of ionic and nonionic emulsifiers of different molecular weight have been used to stabilize the lipid dispersions and to prevent particle agglomeration. The most frequently used compounds include different kinds of poloxamer, polysorbates, lecithin and bile salts. The choice of the emulsifier depends on the administration route and is more limited for parenteral administrations [10]. The emulsifiers selected and their concentration have a great impact on the quality and stability of the SLNs dispersion [12–14]. It has been found that the combination of emulsifiers might prevent particle agglomeration more efficiently than the use of a single surfactant. Another important point to consider is the influence of the emulsifier on drug incorporation; stabilizing agents are not localized exclusively on the lipid surface, but also in the aqueous phase in different forms, which might serve as an alternative location to accommodate the drug molecules [10].

As it has been reported [6, 10, 15, 16], the status of excipients for SLNs has to be discussed as a function of the administration routes. SLNs can be produced with regulatory accepted excipients or at least with material able to be degraded in the body to physiological compounds or to products used for parenteral nutrition. Therefore, they are not problematic at all for topical and oral administration. The full range of surfactants and lipids used in dermal products, tablets and capsules can be exploited. Even such "nasty" surfactants with regard to parenteral administration such as sodium dodecyl sulfate can be applied to stabilize the suspension. They possess excellent dispersing properties and are accepted up to a certain concentration in oral products. The situation is slightly different for parenteral administration – to our knowledge, no solid lipids have been administered parenterally; therefore, they would require a toxicity study before their use. However, the glycerides used for nanostructured lipid carrier (NLC) production can be selected with this purpose, since they are composed of fatty acids already present in the oils of emulsions for parenteral nutrition [6].

10.2.3 Production Processes

The four main procedures existing for the preparation of lipid nanoparticles dispersions are briefly described in this section. Later, scaling-up feasibility and secondary production steps such as drying and sterilization will be reviewed.

10.2.3.1 Preparation Techniques

10.2.3.1.1 High-shear Homogenization and Ultrasound High-shear homogenization and ultrasound are dispersing techniques which were initially used for the production of solid lipid nanodispersions [17, 18]. Both methods are widespread and easy to handle. The disadvantages of these techniques are due to the presence of microparticles and the fact that metal contamination has to be considered when ultrasound is used.

10.2.3.1.2 High-pressure Homogenization (HPH) HPH has emerged as a reliable and powerful technique for the preparation of SLNs. Homogenizers of different sizes are commercially available from several manufacturers at reasonable prices. The two basic production methods for SLNs are the hot homogenization technique and the cold homogenization technique. In both cases the drug is incorporated in the lipid melt. The hot homogenization technique is carried out at temperatures above the melting point of the lipid. The drug-containing melt is dispersed under stirring in a hot aqueous surfactant solution to the same temperature. Then the obtained pre-emulsion is homogenized. The primary product is a hot oil/water (o/w) nanoemulsion that is cooled down to room temperature, leading to solid lipid nanoparticles.

Cold homogenization has been developed to overcome the following three problems of the hot homogenization technique: temperature-induced drug degradation, drug distribution into the aqueous phase during homogenization and complexity of the crystallization step of the nanoemulsion. This technique minimizes thermal exposure of the sample. The drug-containing lipid melt is rapidly cooled and the solid lipid ground to lipid microparticles which are dispersed in a cold surfactant solution yielding a presuspension. Then this presuspension is homogenized at or below room temperature leading to solid lipid nanoparticles.

10.2.3.1.3 Microemulsion Microemulsion-based SLNs preparation techniques have been developed by Gasco [19]. Emulsions are made by stirring the melted lipid and a mixture of water, cosurfactant(s) and the surfactant heated to the same temperature as the lipid. A transparent, thermodynamically stable system is formed when the compounds are mixed in the correct ratio. Finally, this microemulsion is dispersed in a cold aqueous medium (2–3 °C) under stirring, thus resulting in the formation of SLNs.

10.2.3.1.4 **Solvent Emulsification/Evaporation** Sjöström and Bergenståhl described in 1992 a production method to prepare nanoparticles in o/w emulsions [20]. The lipophilic material is dissolved in a water-immiscible organic solvent that is emulsified in an aqueous phase to give an o/w emulsion. Upon evaporation of the solvent a nanoparticle dispersion is formed by precipitation of the lipid in the aqueous medium. An important advantage of this method is the avoidance of heat during the preparation, which makes it suitable for the incorporation of highly thermolabile drugs. However, problems might arise due to solvent residues in the final dispersion.

10.2.3.2 Scaling-up, Sterilization and Drying

10.2.3.2.1 **Scaling-up** The possibility of qualified industrial large-scale production must be provided for the introduction of a product to the market. HPH production for SLNs and scaling-up feasibilities have been widely investigated [21–24]. Moreover, production lines for HPH already exist in the pharmaceutical industry and have been even used for the production of parenteral products. The HPH lines used for parenteral nutrition can be qualified and accepted by the regulatory authorities. Based on this premise, no regulatory hurdles are expected in the use them for SLNs carriers systems [6]. A system has been developed and scale-up feasibility has been investigated for the production via microemulsions [25].

10.2.3.2.2 **Sterilization** SLN dispersions can be sterilized or prepared aseptically using already established techniques in the pharmaceutical industry. Aseptic production, filtration, γ-irradiation and heating are normally used in order to achieve sterility. Filtration sterilization of dispersed systems requires high pressure and is not applicable to particles larger than 0.2 μm. SLN dispersions can be sterilized by filtration similar to emulsions for parenteral nutrition. It is very important to filter them in liquid state, since this allows particles with a size larger than the pores in the filter to be filtered [10, 15, 25].

10.2.3.2.3 **Drying** It is expected that the solid state of SLNs will present a better chemical and physical stability than aqueous lipid dispersions. Transformation into a solid form will prevent crystal growth by Ostwald ripening and avoid hydrolysis reactions.

Lyophilization is a widely used process in the pharmaceutical field to remove water from samples. This technique involves two necessary and additional transformations that may be the source of additional stability problems – freezing of the sample and evaporation of water under vacuum. The addition of cryoprotectants to the sample will be necessary in order to decrease SLN aggregation and to obtain a better redispersion of the dry product. Typical cryoprotective agents are sorbitol, mannose, trehalose, glucose and polivinylpyrrolidone. The lyophilization process has been optimized with regard to the operating conditions, lipid concentration, type and concentration of cryoprotectant, and redispersing conditions [26–28].

Spray-drying might be an alternative procedure to lyophilization. The influence of lipid type and concentration, carbohydrate type and concentration, redispersion medium, and spraying medium has been investigated by Freitas and coworkers [29]. An evaporative drying process with a nitrogen stream at low temperatures has been evaluated and compared to lyophilization by Marengo and coworkers [30]. The advantages of this process are the avoidance of freezing and the energy efficiency resulting from the higher vapor pressure of water.

10.2.4
Drug Incorporation, Loading, Incorporation Efficiency, Nanoparticle Recovery and Drug Release

10.2.4.1 Drug Incorporation

In different studies, which were later reviewed by Müller [15], Menhert proposed that there are basically three different models for the incorporation of active ingredients into SLNs (Fig. 10.1):

- *Homogeneous matrix model*: consisting of a homogeneous matrix with molecularly dispersed drug or drug being present in amorphous clusters.
- *Drug-enriched shell model*: an outer shell enriched with active compound.
- *Drug-enriched core model*: a core enriched with active compound. This leads to a membrane controlled release governed by the Fick law of diffusion.

The structure obtained is a function of the formulation composition (lipid, active compound, surfactant) and of the production conditions (hot versus cold homogenization). A large number of drugs with a great variety of lipophilicity and different structures have been studied with regard to their incorporation into SLNs. However, few data exist on the localization site and the physical state of the drug mole-

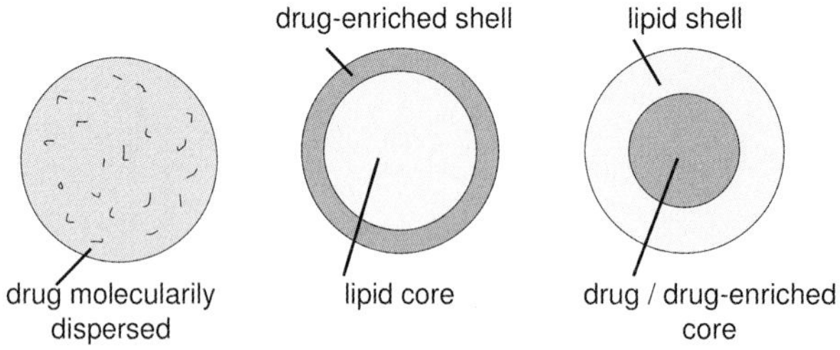

Figure 10.1. Three drug incorporation models. (Adapted from Ref. [15], with permission from Elsevier.)

cule. Drug incorporation implies the localization of the drug in the solid lipid matrix. Micelle-forming surfactant molecules will be present in different forms, and may lead to colloidal species such as micelles, mixed micelles and liposomes, that are known to solubilize drugs and are, therefore, alternative drug incorporation sites [10].

10.2.4.2 Drug Loading

SLNs were first developed for the administration of lipophilic drugs, although they have been also applied for the encapsulation of hydrophilic drugs. One of the main drawbacks of particulate drug carriers is drug-loading capacity, which is limited to approximately 25% with regard to the lipid matrix. The drug-loading capacity of SLNs is limited by the solubility of drug in the lipid melt, miscibility of the melted drug and lipid, chemical and physical structure of the matrix, and the polymorphic state of the lipid matrix [15]. The prerequisite to obtain a sufficient loading capacity is a sufficiently high solubility of the drug in the lipid melt. To enhance the solubility in the lipid melt one can add solubilizers, especially in the case of hydrophilic drugs.

The structure of the lipid is important because if the lipid matrix consists of especially similar molecules (i.e. tristearin or tripalmitin), a perfect crystal with few imperfections is formed and cannot accommodate large amounts of drug. Therefore, the use of more complex lipids (mono-, di- and triglycerides with different chain lengths) is more sensible for higher drug loading.

Crystalline structure – related to the chemical nature of the lipid – is a key factor to determine whether a drug will be expelled or firmly incorporated. The transition to highly ordered lipid particles is also the reason for drug expulsion. Directly after production, lipids crystallize; if the crystallinity index increases during the storage, then the drug will be expelled from the lipid matrix and it can then neither be protected from degradation nor released in a controlled way [31]. Consequently, intensive characterization of the physical state of the lipid particles is highly essential in order to get a controlled optimization of drug incorporation and loading.

10.2.4.3 Determination of Nanoparticle Recovery and Drug Incorporation Efficiency

These are general characterization parameters that can be applied to any type of nanoparticle, including SLNs.

The nanoparticle (NP) recovery, which is also referred to as nanoparticle yield in the literature, can be calculated using:

$$\text{nanoparticle recovery (\%)} = \frac{\text{mass of nanoparticle recovered} \times 100}{\text{mass of drug and excipients}}. \tag{1}$$

An additional important *in vitro* characterization parameter is the determination of the drug incorporation efficiency in nanoparticle formulations. Drug incorporation efficiency is expressed both as drug content (% w/w), also referred to as drug loading in the literature, and drug entrapment efficiency (%); represented by:

$$\text{drug loading (\% w/w)} = \frac{\text{mass of drug in nanoparticle}}{\text{mass of nanoparticle recovered}} \times 100 \tag{2}$$

$$\text{drug entrapment efficiency (\%)} = \frac{\text{mass of drug in nanoparticle}}{\text{mass of drug used in formulation}} \times 100. \tag{3}$$

Two different methods have been suggested for the determination of drug loading and entrapment efficiency. The first involves the solubilization of nanoparticles by dispersing a measured amount of them in a suitable medium under agitation. The second method is based on the estimation of the differences between the total amount of the drug added to the formulation and the unentrapped amount detected in the supernatant of the nanoparticle dispersion. The amount of drug is analyzed by an appropriate analytical technique.

10.2.4.4 **Drug Release**

The effect of formulation parameters and production conditions on the release profile from SLNs was intensively investigated by Mehnert and zur Mühlen [32, 33] by the study of the model drugs tetracaine, etomidate and prednisolone. A burst drug release was obtained with tetracaine and etomidate SLNs; in contrast, prednisolone SLNs showed a prolonged release. This demonstrated the principle suitability of the SLNs system for prolonged drug release. More interestingly, they showed that it was possible to modify the release profiles as a function of lipid matrix, surfactant concentration and production parameters (e.g. temperature).

Müller and coworkers [34] reviewed in detail the release of active compounds from SLNs and summarized that the higher the solubility in the water phase during production, the more pronounced is the burst effect. The solubility increases with increasing production temperature and increasing surfactant concentration (the latter only when the surfactant solubilizes the active compound). Consequently, little or no burst will be obtained when SLNs are produced at low temperatures, low surfactant concentration or in surfactant-free medium.

10.2.5
Related Structures and Stability

Potential problems associated with SLNs such as limited drug-loading capacity, adjustment of drug release profile and potential drug expulsion during storage are avoided or minimized by the new generation of lipid nanoparticles, the NLCs, although the term SLNs is sometimes used to describe different types of lipidic matricial structures [such as NLCs and lipid–drug conjugates (LDCs)] regardless of their composition and arrangement. Using spatially incompatible lipids leads to special structures of the lipid matrix and, thus, three types of NLCs [35] (see Fig. 10.2):

(i) *The imperfect type.* A potential problem in SLNs is the formation of a perfect crystal. Using spatially different lipids leads to imperfections in the crystal to accommodate the drug.

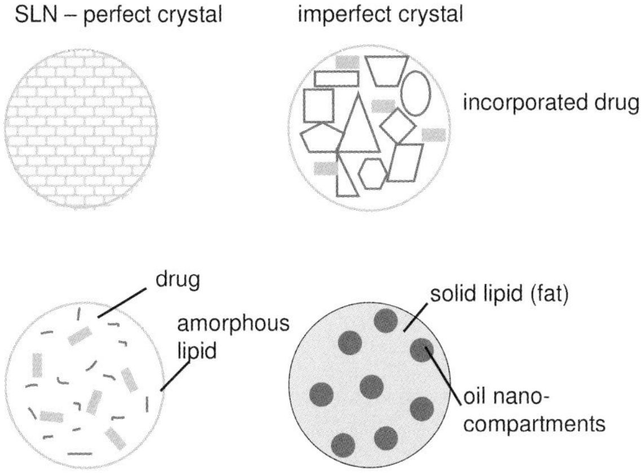

Figure 10.2. The three types of NLCs compared to the relatively ordered matrix of SLNs (upper left); NLCs types: imperfect type (upper right), amorphous type (lower left) and multiple type (lower right). (Adapted from Ref. [34], with permission from Elsevier.)

(ii) *The amorphous (structureless) type.* Drug expulsion is caused by an ongoing crystallization process of the solid lipid towards a perfect crystal. The particles are solid, but crystallization upon cooling is avoided by mixing special lipids.
(iii) *The multiple type.* System comparable to w/o/w emulsions since it is an oil-in-solid lipid-in-water dispersion. The solid lipid matrix contains tiny liquid oil nanocompartments. Many drugs show a higher solubility in oils than in solid lipids so that they can be dissolved in the oil and still be protected from degradation by the surrounding solid lipids.

Recent studies concluded that neither SLNs nor NLCs lipid nanoparticles showed any advantage with respect to the incorporation rate or retarded accessibility to the drug compared with conventional nanoemulsions. It is has been shown that the liquid lipid forms a half drop on the solid platelet [36–38]. SLNs are useful for the incorporation of lipophilic (soluble) drugs. Aiming to increase the drug-loading capacity of hydrophilic drugs, the structure of LDCs has been recently suggested as more adequate [16].

LDC nanoparticles present drug-loading capacities of up to 33% [39, 40]. Here, an insoluble drug–lipid conjugate bulk is prepared either by salt formation (e.g. with a fatty acid) or by covalent linking (e.g. to esters or ethers). In the salt formation process, the free drug base and fatty acid are dissolved in a suitable solvent. The solvent is then consequently evaporated under reduced pressure. For the covalent linking, the drug (salt) and a fatty alcohol react in the presence of a catalyst, and the LDC bulk is then purified by recrystallization. The obtained LDC bulk is then processed with an aqueous surfactant solution to a nanoparticle formulation using HPH.

The physical stability of SLN dispersions has been investigated intensively, e.g. by measurements of particle size [photon correlation spectroscopy (PCS), laser diffraction (LD)], charge (ζ potential) and thermal analysis [differential scanning calorimetry (DSC)], as reviewed later in this chapter. In addition, as noted above, transformation of SLNs into a solid form by drying will have a better chemical and physical stability than aqueous lipid dispersions.

10.2.6 Analytical Characterization of SLNs

An adequate characterization of SLNs is a prerequisite for the control of the quality of the product. Several parameters have to be considered in the characterization of lipid nanoparticle formulations which have direct impact on the stability and release kinetics [10, 15]:

(i) Particle size and ζ potential.
(ii) Degree of crystallinity and lipid modification.
(iii) Coexistence of additional colloidal structures (micelles, liposomes, supercooled melts, drug nanoparticles) and dynamic phenomena.

10.2.6.1 Particle Size

Particle size is predominantly used to evaluate the colloidal size range. This parameter is crucial in the development and optimization of preparation processes as well as in the evaluation of dispersion stability.

The most widely used method to characterize the size of SLNs is PCS. This method measures the fluctuation of the intensity of the scattered light which is caused by Brownian motion. PCS is a good tool to characterize nanoparticles, but it is not available for the detection of larger microparticles. They can be visualized by means of LD measurements. This method is based on the dependency of the diffraction angle on the particle radius (Fraunhofer spectra). Smaller particles cause more intense scattering at high angles compared with the larger ones. Difficulties may arise both in PCS and LD measurements for samples which contain several populations of different size. Therefore, additional techniques might be useful. The Coulter counter method and light microscopy may be considered to detect trace amounts of microparticles in SLN dispersions. Electron microscopy, in contrast to PCS and LD, provides direct information on the particle shape and structure. However, possible artifacts may be caused by the sample preparation.

Atomic force microscopy (AFM) has also been applied to image the morphological structure of SLNs [41, 42]. Advantages of AFM are the simplicity of sample preparation as no vacuum is needed during operation and that the sample does not need to be conductive. Therefore, it has the potential for the direct analysis of the originally hydrated, solvent-containing samples. A disadvantage of this method is the required fixation of the particles (by removal of water), which changes the status of emulsifier and might also cause polymorphic transitions of the lipid.

Particle sizing by field-flow fractionation (FFF) is based on the different effect of a perpendicular applied field on particles in a laminar flow. The separation principle corresponds to the nature of the perpendicular field and may, for example, be based on different mass (sedimentation FFF), size (cross-flow FFF) or charge (electric-field FFF). Mäder and coworkers have been applied recently cross-flow FFF to investigate nanoemulsions, SLNs and nanostructure lipid carriers [38].

10.2.6.2 The ζ Potential

The surface charges and the strength and extension of the electrical field around the particles play an important role in the manual repulsion of nanoparticles, and thus in their stability against aggregation. Therefore, the measurement of the ζ potential allows for predictions about the storage stability of colloidal dispersion. In general, particle aggregation is less likely to occur for charged particles (high ζ potential) due to electric repulsion. However, this rule cannot strictly be applied for systems which contain steric stabilizers, because the adsorption of steric stabilizers will decrease the ζ potential due to the shift in the shear plane of the particle [10].

10.2.6.3 Crystallinity and Polymorphism and Colloidal Structures

Particle size measurements alone are not sufficient for the characterization of SLN dispersions. The degree of crystallinity and lipid modifications are strongly correlated with drug incorporation and release rates. DSC and X-ray techniques are the most widely used for the characterization of crystallinity and polymorphism of solid lipid particles. DSC uses the fact that different lipid modifications possess different melting points and melting enthalpies. By means of X-ray scattering it is possible to assess the length of the long and short spacing of the lipid lattice [15]. The coexistence of additional colloidal structures (micelles, liposomes, mixed micelles, supercooled melts, drug nanoparticles) has to be taken into account for all SLN dispersions. Nuclear magnetic resonance (NMR) and electron spin resonance (ESR) are powerful tools for investigating dynamic phenomena and the characteristics of nanocompartments in colloidal lipid dispersions. Both methods are sensitive to the simultaneous detection of different colloidal species, do not require preparatory steps and, due to the noninvasiveness, repeated measurements of the same sample are possible. Similar results to the ERS experiments can be obtained with fluorescence measurements [36]. Rheometry has been used for the characterization of the viscoelastic properties of SLN formulations [43].

10.2.7 Applications

Since the development of lipid microparticles by Speiser and coworkers at the beginning of the 1980s [44] and the later evolution in the 1990s towards SLNs, these lipidic particulate systems have been applied to encapsulate different drugs aiming to get sustained release of the entrapped drug, to improve drug stability by protecting the drug from degradation or to improve the bioavailability of poorly soluble drugs. SLNs can be administered by different routes: parenteral, oral, ocular, pulmonar, rectal, etc., as recently reviewed by Wissing and coworkers [16]. SLNs appear to be a promising sustained release for orally administered lipophilic drugs [45, 46], showing increased bioavailability and prolonged plasma peaks. In addition, these nanoparticles could be directly administered (as an aqueous dispersion) or formulated in different dosage forms, such as tablets or capsules. Regarding topical application, SLNs are considered as a good alternative to liposomes, possessing similar film-forming properties after application onto the skin [15]. These can be presented either in creams, gels or ointments, or topically applied as highly concentrated lipid dispersions [10]. Moreover, SLNs have been found to target drugs to particular skin layers and to sustain drug release into the skin.

When thinking about SLN administration one should bear in mind the *in vivo* fate after their administration. As widely reported in the literature, nanoparticles with a hydrophobic surface administered by different routes that will reach the blood stream will be rapidly taken up by the mononuclear phagocytic system (MPS). As a result, several approaches have been developed in order to increase the circulation time of the nanoparticles, and their targeting to organs and tissues other than the liver, lung and spleen [47]. In order to increase nanoparticle circulation time it has been stated that these particles should be 100 nm or less and have a hydrophilic surface. The approaches used to avoid unwanted uptake by macrophages include adsorption of surfactants to the nanoparticle surface, formation or inclusion with block copolymers with hydrophilic and hydrophobic domains (poloxamers and poloxamines) or grafting of a hydrophilic polymer such as poly(ethylene glycol) (PEG) [48].

In a recent study, Göppert and Müller [49] have investigated the surface modification of SLNs by the use of different poloxamers and poloxamines, and the influence of such surface modification on the adsorption of different proteins to SLNs assessed by two-dimensional polyacrylamide gel electrophoresis. They were looking for the type of poloxamer/poloxamine which would render the surface more hydrophilic, thus allowing the adsorption of albumin or apolipoproteins, giving rise to stealth SLNs and a more prolonged blood circulation time. They found that SLNs stabilized with low-molecular-weight Poloxamer 184 and Poloxamer 235 showed interestingly high adsorption of apolipoprotein E (ApoE), which mediates the uptake through the blood–brain barrier and, thus, the delivery to the brain. Interestingly, they have also reported that nanoparticles surface modified with high-molecular-weight Poloxamine 908 are able to circulate longer in the blood despite the high adsorption protein patterns found in this study, concluding that in order to avoid uptake by the MPS it is important to characterize the type of proteins that are adsorbed onto SLNs surface; if dysopsonins (such as albumin and apolipoproteins) are adsorbed and the absence of immunoglobulins and complement-activating proteins on the surface is avoided, a long circulation time of the nanoparticles might be expected.

Table 10.1 summarizes some of the main applications described for SLNs.

10.2.7.1 **Gene Therapy**

Gene therapy is a rapidly advancing field with great potential for the treatment of genetic and acquired systemic diseases. Present delivery systems can be divided

Tab. 10.1. Some examples of drugs and genes encapsulated into SLNs.

Application	Drug/gene	Administration route	Reference
Gene therapy	*β*-galactosidase expression plasmid	–	50
	dimeric HIV-1 Tat peptide (TAT2)	lung (inhalation)	51
	green fluorescent protein (GFP) plasmid	–	52
Peptides and proteins	gonadorelin	oral–parenteral	53
	calcitonin	oral	54
	insulin	oral	55
	[D-Trp-6]LHRH	parenteral	56
	thymopentin	parenteral	57
	lysozyme	oral, nasal, parenteral (immunization)	58
	cyclosporin A	oral	46, 59
	sodium cromoglycate	–	60
Low soluble drugs	tobramycin	ocular	61
	ketoconazole	topical	62
	clobetasol propionate	–	63
	clotrimazole	topical	64
	THP-adriamycin	parenteral	65
	ibuprofen	oral	66
	all-*trans* retinoic acid (anticancer drugs)	parenteral	67
	paclitaxel	parenteral	68
	progesterone	–	60
	doxorubicin	parenteral	69
	bupivacaine	parenteral	70
	5-fluoro-2′-deoxyuridine (FUdR) derivative	parenteral	71
	AZT and derivatives	parenteral	72, 73
	etoposide	parenteral	74
	acyclovir	–	75
	camptothecin	oral	45
	ascorbyl palmitate	topical	76
	piribedil	oral	77
Topical/cosmetics	vitamin A	topical	78
	coenzyme Q10	topical	79
	vitamin E	topical	80
	sunscreens: *n*-dodecyl-ferulate	topical	81
	perfumes	topical	82
	α-lipoic acid	topical	83

into virus-based, plasmid-based, and composites of both virus-based and plasmid-based systems. Plasmid-based delivery systems for so-called nonviral gene therapy are being developed as an alternative to virus-based systems. The isolated plasmid by itself can be administered locally, yielding expression in the injected tissue. Formulating the plasmid with synthetic gene delivery systems can increase the transfection efficiency.

In recent years, SLNs have been developed as potential carriers for a number of drugs, but there are only a few reports of the use of SLN delivery of genes [51, 84, 85]. However, there are a large number of publications about cationic liposomes for gene therapy; in spite of that, no marketed products have been developed. SLNs and liposomes formulated from the same cationic lipids showed equipotent *in vitro* transfection efficiencies. It is not the colloidal structure in which the cationic lipids are arranged, but the cationic lipid composition the seems to govern gene transfer efficiency. As SLNs can be produced in large scale and under favorable technological parameters, they may become a valuable addition to the well-established repertoire of nonviral transfection agents lead by cationic liposomes [85].

Olbrich and coworkers [50] showed that cationic SLNs were able to transfect mammalian cells (COS-1) *in vitro.*

For over a decade, cationic lipids have been used for gene transfer both in cell culture and in animals [86, 87]. A cationic lipid is a positively charged amphiphile with a hydrophilic head and a hydrophobic tail that self-associates in aqueous solution to form either micelles or bilayer liposomes. This results in particles which can interact with the negative charges on a polynucleotide, such as DNA. The goal of cationic lipid-mediated gene transfer is to deliver a plasmid of DNA to a cell such that it becomes transcribed and translated into a desired protein/peptide [88]. The sequence of events involve in cationic lipid-mediated gene transfer include, but are not exclusive to: (i) the formation of the cationic lipid into a nanoparticle or liposome, providing a multivalent surface charge that is (ii) attached via electrostatics to the negative charges on the DNA phosphate backbone. This mixture forms a small particle. If these particles have an excess of positive charge they will (iii) bind to the negative charges on the surface of cells. The complexes become (iv) internalized though a vesicular pathway, followed by (v) the release of DNA form the particle into the cell cytoplasm. The release of DNA is thought to occur concomitantly with the release from the cationic lipid. Then some fraction of the released DNA is (vi) successfully trafficked by, as yet, an unknown mechanism to the nucleus where is transcribed and later translated to protein. These cellular barriers to gene transfer are reviewed in depth by Meyer and coworkers [89].

SLNs must incorporate cationic lipids in order to facilitate DNA binding. When SLNs are produced with cationic lipids, a matrix lipid and, in most cases, additional surfactants are required. The resulting particles consist of a lipid core that presents cationic lipids on its surface. The cationic components are likely to be organized in raft-like monolayers that allow interaction between the modified SLN surface and DNA. Recent studies revealed the relation between transfection activity and SLN composition [85]. A large number of cationic lipids with low toxicity and exhibiting different abilities to mediate gene transfer have been synthesized and studied for gene delivery [90–96]. In addition to *N*-[1-(2,3-dioleyloxy)-propyl]-*N*,*N*,*N*-trimethyl ammonium chloride (DOTMA) and 1,2-dioleoyloxy-3-(trimethylammonio)propane (DOTAP) (two of the most used cationic lipids), which are both two-chained amphiphiles whose acyl chains are linked to the propyl ammonium group (through ether and ester bonds, respectively), numerous new lipids have become commercially available for transfection purposes. Although a direct correlation between the nature of the cationic lipids and their ability to mediate transfection and to develop toxicity has been established, the nature of this dependency has not yet been completely clarified [97].

The incorporation into nanoparticles of colipids such as DOPE and others improves the ability to transfect cells. This fact has been attributed to the ability of dioleoyl-L-α-phosphatidylethanolamine (DOPE) to facilitate the formation of the complexes in conjunction with cationic lipids and to its tendency to undergo a transition from a bilayer to a hexagonal configuration under acidic pH, which facilitates fusion with or destabilization to target membranes. More recently, it was suggested that DOPE can also play a role in facilitating the disassembling of the lipid-based DNA formulations after internalization and escape of DNA from endocytotic vesicles. Cholesterol has also been employed as a colipid to prepare cationic liposomes, resulting in the formation of more stable but less efficient complexes than those containing DOPE [97].

Another approach to circumvent the problem of low efficiency of transfection is to incorporate peptides that are capable of penetrating the plasma membrane. Such peptides are called protein transduction domains (PTDs) or cell-penetrating peptides (CPPs). The most well-known CPPs are penetratin, corresponding to the third helix of the Antennapedia homeodomain, Tat(48–60), derived from HIV-1 Tat protein and oligoarginines [98]. Thorén and coworkers [98] have studied the interaction of different CPPs with phospholipids vesicles in order to better understand the mechanism of cellular uptake. Nonendocytotic uptake was only observed for the arginine-rich peptides TatP59W and R7W. Studies of the leakage from dye-loaded vesicles indicate that none of the assayed peptides (penetratin, R7W, TatP59W and TatLysP59W) forms membrane pores and that vesicles fusion is not accompanied by leakage of the aqueous content of the vesicles. The authors suggest that the discovered variations in propensity to destabilize phospholipid bilayers between the peptides investigated, in some cases to induce fusion, may be related to their different cellular uptake properties. Hyndman and coworkers [99] have demonstrated that the incorporation a protein transduction domain of the HIV-1 into gene delivery lipoplexes improves gene transfer, suggesting that the endocytosis uptake pathway is involved. The mechanism for the CPP-facilitated cellular uptake is unknown [100, 101]. Zieger and coworkers [102] have shown that membrane-associated heparan sulfate is involved in the uptake of HIV-1 protein.

The attachment of ligands to target the particles for cell-specific uptake via highly internalizing receptor can be a very useful strategy for the treatment of some diseases. Pedersen and coworkers [103] prepared SLNs with Compritol ATO 888 with a size of approximately 100 nm an a ζ potential of +15 mV which were able to condense DNA, they are very stable under physiological conditions and they display low cytotoxicity in cell culture. In addition to binding to DNA, the SLNs could simultaneously bind substantial amounts of streptavidin directly via electrostatic interactions. The SLN:DNA:streptavidin complexes are stable and are capable of binding biotinlylated ligands, which can interact with surface receptors.

10.2.7.2 **Peptide and Protein Delivery**

Over the last few years, and thanks to the development of the biotech industry, a great number of bioactive molecules and vaccines based on peptides, proteins and oligonucleotides have been discovered, showing great promise as therapeutic agents. However, the administration of these molecules is often limited because of their poor stability, low oral bioavailability, short *in vivo* half-lives and limited ability to cross cell membranes. In order to overcome such disadvantages, a suitable design of sustained release carrier systems is needed to enter the therapeutic market [104]. Peptide and protein nanoparticles can be administered by different routes, depending on the application intended. If they are to be administered by the oral route, formulation of peptides and proteins into a suitable drug carrier is a relevant task, especially due to epithelial barriers of the gastrointestinal tract, and gastrointestinal degradation by the acidic pH of the stomach and digestive enzymes [105].

The most commonly used particulate drug carriers for the administration of peptide and protein drugs have traditionally been poly(lactic acid) (PLA), poly(glycolic acid) (PGA) and their copolymers, poly(lactide-*co*-glycolide) (PLGA). However, there are only a few of products on the market based on PLGA microparticles and, to the best of our knowledge, no nanoparticulate product based on this kind of polymers has reached the market, probably because of the cytotoxicity of polymers and the difficulties for the scaling-up of the nanoencapsulation processes [15].

Among the different particulate drug carriers proposed as alternative materials, lipids appear to be suitable matrix materials for sustained release formulations of peptide and proteins, presenting good biocompatibility properties and being able to form different colloidal drug carriers, as microemulsions, SLNs, lipospheres, NLCs or microparticles.

In fact, one of the advantages of SLNs compared to PLGA nanoparticles is their better tolerability. Müller and coworkers [106] compared the *in vitro* toxicity of PLA, PLGA and SLN nanoparticles in order to determine the toxicological acceptance as an intravenous formulation. They found that the effective dose to reduce viability of the cells to 50% was around 0.30% for PLA polymers, 0.15% for PLGA and above 10% for SLNs, proving that SLNs are the least cytotoxic preparation.

Schöler and coworkers [107] have recently studied the cytotoxic properties of SLNs intended for parenteral administration, analyzing the viability and activation of macrophages [production of interleukin (IL)-6, IL-12 and tumor necrosis factor (TNF)-α as a function of the lipid type used and SLN particle size]. No activation of peritoneal was observed when triglycerides, cetylpalmitate or paraffin were used for the lipid matrices, although a concentration-dependent cytotoxicity was found for

SLNs. This is the reason why it is essential to select properly the lipid matrices of SLNs to be used for parenteral administration. As previously summarized in Tab. 10.1, SLNs have been applied to the encapsulation of different peptide and proteins aiming a controlled release of the entrapped protein, to overcome the gastrointestinal barriers for the oral administration of the peptide or even an adjuvant capacity of the particulate carrier system.

Olbrich and coworkers [108] have described the adjuvant capacity of antigens adsorbed or entrapped in SLNs, inducing an immune response comparable to that of Freund's incomplete adjuvant. However, this adjuvant capacity was found to be strongly dependent on the SLN size: SLNs bigger than 100 nm exhibited a strong adjuvant capacity, whereas for SLNs smaller than 100 nm this adjuvant capacity was quite low or even negligible. In addition, SLNs may offer a sustained release of the antigen, which can be continuously presented to the immune system contributing to an optimized immune response and making these systems appropriate for the administration of vaccines.

Morel and coworkers [56] first adapted the techniques they were using for the preparation of microemulsions for the encapsulation of the peptidic drug [D-Trp-6]LHRH. They obtained lipospheres by a warm multiple water/oil/water (w/o/w) microemulsion using stearic acid as lipid matrix. The encapsulation efficiency was about 90% and the drug was sustained release following a pseudo-zero-order kinetic. Later, the same research group [57] applied the same encapsulation method (w/o/w microemulsion) and the o/w microemulsion for the formulation of thymopentin. In order to increase the incorporation of hydrophilic drugs into lipospheres, lipophilic ion-pairs of the drug with hexadecylphosphate were prepared in this warm o/w microemulsion technique. As expected, this later technique allowed the incorporation of a much higher amount of the drug than the w/o/w multiple microemulsion technique (5.2 versus 1.7%). Moreover, the percentage of the drug released from lipospheres prepared by both methods was practically identical (10% in 6 h).

One of the most interesting studies on the feasibility of the encapsulation of peptide drugs into SLNs was published in 1997, when Almeida and coworkers [58] studied the influence of production parameters of peptide SLNs using lysozyme as model protein. These researchers applied the cold HPH technique for the encapsulation of this model peptide, studying different parameters that could affect the formation of these SLNs: the type of lipid used, the time of exposure to different temperatures, pressure and number of homogenization cycles. They showed that lysozyme was able to withstand the formulation conditions needed to prepare SLNs, without loosing its activity and integrity. The entrapment efficiency of hydrophilic drugs of these SLNs is usually low (they obtained encapsulation efficiencies between 43.2 and 59.2%), and depends on the lipid mixture employed and the homogenization conditions. However, every protein may behave differently, and its encapsulation must be studied in depth and optimized accordingly.

As commented above, some of the peptidic drugs that have been successfully introduced to the market in particulate drug carrier form are luteinizing hormone-releasing hormone (LHRH) analogs. In order to improve the formulation by means of improving drug stability during polymer degradation, Hu and coworkers [53] prepared SLNs to encapsulate gonadorelin. In this case, SLNs were obtained by a novel solvent diffusion method in an aqueous system. Using this technique, encapsulation efficiency increased up to 69.4%. In addition, gonadorelin showed a slow release profile after a burst release period of 6 h in which 24% of the drug was released, after that burst release almost 4% of gonadorelin was sustained-released every day during the 14 days of the study.

Another procedure that has been applied for the preparation of SLNs containing peptides is the w/o/w multiple emulsion technique. The group of Alonso [54, 55, 109] have modified this technique to develop surface-modified lipid nanoparticles for the encapsulation of different peptidic model drugs. As previously reviewed in this chapter, different polymers can be used to modify the surface properties of lipid nanoparticles. In the first study, poloxamer and PEG–stearate were used to form a coating on the surface, and thus protect orally administered nanoparticles from the effect of gastrointestinal fluids. They established that coating lipid nanoparticles with PEG–stearate prevents them from aggregation and reduced pancreatin-induced degradation, making them suitable for oral administration. In a later study, Prego and coworkers [109] coated lipid nanoparticles with chitosan, reporting that this type of coating can switch their ζ potential from negative to positive, and confers on them the capacity of enhancing the *in vitro* intestinal absorption of calcitonin, assayed in Caco-2 cells – results that were corroborated after the oral administration of calcitonin in rats. Next, this group [54] studied the release profiles of these PEG–stearate- and chitosan-coated nanoparticles. Both types of nanoparticles exhibited an initial burst release (lower for chitosan-coated nanoparticles) followed by a more prolonged slow release in which 40% of calcitonin was released during the 6 h of the study, for both PEG–stearate- and chitosan-coated nanoparticles. Moreover, and as was the case for PEG–stearate nanoparticles, coating with chitosan also protected lipid nanoparticles from the acidic and intestinal environment. Recently, they have determined the interaction of these surface-modified nanoparticles (PEG–stearate and chitosan) with Caco-2 cells, concluding that PEG–stearate did not affect the permeability of Caco-2 cells monolayers unlike chitosan nanoparticles.

Cyclosporin is another of the peptidic drugs that has been successfully incorporated into SLNs [59, 46]. It is an undecapeptidic hydrophobic drug, insoluble in water and widely used for the prevention of xenograft rejection following organ transplantation. Cyclosporin was encapsulated into SLNs aiming to improve oral bioavailability and thus reducing toxic side-effects, maintaining at the same time good, sustained plasma levels.

10.2.7.3 **Low-soluble Drugs**

Despite having good therapeutic effects, many drugs fail in clinical situations due to their poor water solubility. Although many techniques have been employed to improve the oral absorption of poorly soluble drugs, little information is available in the literature on the improvement in the oral bioavailability of poorly soluble drugs by incorporation into SLNs. Like other formulations, such as microemulsions or submicron emulsions, reduction in the particle size is a key factor for improving the peroral performance of poorly soluble drugs. Due to their small particle size, SLNs may exhibit bioadhesion to the gastrointestinal tract wall or enter the intervillar spaces, thus increasing their residence time in the gastrointestinal tract. Another advantage of SLN formulations is the lipid protection of the drug from chemical and degradation, thereby delaying the *in vivo* metabolism. Good physical stability also plays an important key in the oral absorption of the incorporated drugs [110].

Incorporation of drugs into SLNs opens the perspective of enhanced and/or less-variable bioavailability and prolonged plasma levels [77, 111], which is postulated due to a controlled, optimized release in combination with general adhesive properties of small particles [112]. Zimmermann and Müller [113] evaluated the influence of artificial gastrointestinal media on the physical stability of SLN formulations consisting of different lipids and various surfactants/stabilizers with respect to ionic strength and pH. They showed that it is possible to produce SLNs stable in the gastrointestinal tract by optimizing the surfactant/mixture for each lipid *in vitro*. The stabilizing properties obviously depend on the specific interaction of the lipid matrix with the emulsifier, e.g. anchoring of the stabilizer on the lipid surface and density on the surface.

On the other hand, knowledge about enzymatic degradation velocity of SLNs is essential. Olbrich and Müller [114] studied the effects of different surfactants on the degradation velocity. These authors showed that the degradation velocity is substantially affected by the stabilizer used for the preparation of the SLNs. Some stabilizers such as cholic acid sodium salt have degradation accelerating effects, other such as Poloxamer 407 distinctly slow down the degradation velocity. Degradation velocity can be thus modulated by changing the surfactant ratio. Müller and coworkers [115] had previously showed that the degradation velocity of SLNs in solutions of pancreatic lipase/colipase depends on the composition on the lipid matrix. In general, degradation velocity increased with decreasing length of the fatty acid chain length when using glycerides as lipid matrix [116]. In addition, the degradation of SLNs based on waxes (e.g. cetylpalmitate) was found to be slower compared to glyceride matrices.

El-Gibaly and coworkers [117] encapsulated allopurinol into sustained-release solid lipospheres elaborated by melting wax components and hexaconasol, a new hydrophobic wax modifier. The drug was dispersed in the respective molten wax under continuous stirring using a magnetic stirrer. In this study, SLNs were intended for use in a suspension formulation and other oral dosage forms. A significant decrease of plasma uric acid levels and hepatic impairment in male rats was observed after oral administration of SLS suspension of one of their formulations, compared to suspensions of pure allopurinol.

All-*trans* retinoic acid (ATRA) has been limited in clinical use due to its poor aqueous solubility. ATRA has been formulated into SLNs [110] elaborated by HPH with Compritol 888 ATO and soy lecithin/Pluronic F 68 or soy lecithin/Tween 80 as emulsifiers in order to increase its oral bioavailability. After oral administration to male rats, SLNs produced a significant improvement in the bioavailability of ATRA compared with ATRA solution. Compared with the ATRA emulsion, which also produced an improvement in oral absorption, SLNs exhibit a high physical stability.

10.2.7.4 Topical and Transdermal Administration

SLNs are being investigated as drug carrier system for topical application. These carriers are composed of physiological and biodegradable lipids of low systemic toxicity and also low cytotoxicity [118]. SLNs for topical application to the skin are made up from lipids such as glyceryl behenate (Compritol 888 ATO), glyceryl monostearate (Inwitor 900), glyceryl palmtostearate (Precirol ATO 5), triglycerides (trimyristin, tripalmitin, tristearin) or the wax cetyl palmitate [119].

The generally low lipid content and the poor viscosity of lipid nanodispersions render these preparations, as they are, less suitable for dermal drug application. The handling of the preparation by the patient is improved by SLN incorporation into ointments, creams and gels. Alternatively, ready-to-use preparations may be obtained by one-step production, increasing the lipid phase to at least 30%. However, increasing the lipid frequently results in an unwanted increase in particle size. Surprisingly, it has been found that very concentrated (30–40%) semisolid cetyl palmitate formulations preserve the colloidal particle size [34]. If SLNs are incorporated into vehicles, interactions with the vehicle constituents may induce physical instabilities such as dissolution or aggregation of lipid particles. It is important to follow the particle size and the solid character of the particles during storage.

Particle size of the SLNs influences drug penetration, as has been shown for nanoemulsions, in such a manner that when decreasing particle size, drug penetration and systemic activity of drug increase [120]. Similar effects for particle size reduction on penetration into the skin were found for polymeric particles [121].

Occlusion properties which can enhance the penetration of drugs through the stratum corneum by increased hydration have been reported [120, 122]. Occlusion properties are due to the formation of a film on the skin which enhances the penetration of drugs through the stratum corneum.

SLNs can provide a sustained drug release due to the solid matrix of the particles [78]. Sustained drug release becomes important in dermal application concerning drugs that are irritating at high concentrations. Furthermore, it provides the possibility to supply an active agent over a prolonged period of time and can reduce systemic absorption. Controlled triggered release of drugs is feasible due polymorphic transitions of the lipids induced by water evaporation from the dosage form after application to the skin. Furthermore, electrolytes present in the upper skin surface can initiate polymorphic transitions accompanied by drug expulsion due to the formation of a stable polymorph [123].

Common disadvantages of SLNs are their particle growth, their unpredictable gelatin tendency, their unexpected dynamic of polymorphic transitions and their inherent low incorporation rate because of the crystalline structure of the solid lipid [10, 124, 125]. It has been claimed that this last drawback can be overcome by oil-loaded solid nanolipids (also described as NLCs) [34, 35, 123]. Liquid lipids solubilize the drug to a much higher extent than solid lipids. In a preferred scenario, the liquid lipids form inner droplets in the solid nanoparticles. In this model, the NLC nanoparticles would provide a high incorporation rate (because of the liquid lipid) and a controlled release (because of the outer solid lipid).

Souto and coworkers [62, 64] have prepared SLNs and NLCs for topical delivery of clotrimazole and ketoconazole. The authors show that these lipid nanoparticles are useful as modified release formulations for lipophilic drugs over a prolonged period of time.

10.2.7.5 Cosmetic Applications for SLNs

SLNs are also considered a promising carrier system for cosmetic active ingredients due to their numerous advantages. These kind of delivery systems (i) provide protection to labile compounds against chemical degradation, as is the case of retinol and tocopherol, (ii) can provide sustained release of the active ingredients, (iii) act as occlusives, e.g. they can be used in order to increase the water content of the skin and (iv) show a ultraviolet (UV)-blocking potential, i.e. they act as physical sunscreens on their own and can be combined with molecular sunscreens in order to achieve improved photoprotection [126].

SLNs have been shown that they act as active carriers for sunscreens [127]. Song and Liu [128] prepared SLNs as carriers for 3,4,5-trimethoxibenzoylchitin, a new UV-absorbing macromolecule and vitamin E; the nanoparticles act both as physical sunscreens themselves and as carriers in order to enhance the effect of UVB protection. The incorporation of vitamin E appears to have a better effect on UVB absorption.

10.3 Polymeric Nanoparticles

10.3.1 Introduction

Polymeric nanoparticles are small colloidal particles ranging in size from 10 to 1000 nm, which are made of nonbiodegradable or biodegradable polymers. Depending on the method used for their preparation, two different types of nanoparticles can be obtained: nanospheres and nanocapsules. Nanospheres have a matrix-type structure, where active compounds can be absorbed at their surface, entrapped or dissolved in the matrix. Nanocapsules, which are reservoir systems, have a polymeric shell and an inner core. In this case, the active substances are usually dissolved in the core, but may also be adsorbed at their surface. Among the polymeric nanoparticles currently under investigation for controlled drug delivery and drug-targeting applications, those receiving most attention are probably the nanoparticles based on synthetic polymers such as PLA, PGA and PLGA. These polymers are known for both their biocompatibility and resorbability through natural pathways. Additionally, the degradation rate and accordingly the drug release rate can be manipulated by varying the ratio of PLA (increased hydrophobicity) to PGA (increased hydrophilicity).

10.3.2 Nanoparticle Preparation Methods

Nanoparticles can be prepared by a number of methods, which are classified into two main categories depending on whether the polymer is formed by *in situ* polymerization of monomers or by dispersion of the preformed polymers.

10.3.2.1 Nanoparticles Prepared by *In Situ* Polymerization of Monomers

The polymerization methods can be classified into two groups based on whether nanospheres or nanocapsules are formed. Nanospheres are mostly prepared by emulsion polymerization, whereas nanocapsules are obtained by interfacial polymerization performed in emulsions or microemulsions.

10.3.2.1.1 Emulsion Polymerization The polymerization is usually initiated by the reaction of an initiator with the monomer molecules that are dissolved in the continuous phase of an o/w or w/o emulsion. Couvreur and coworkers [129, 130] reported the production of biodegradable poly(alkyl cyanoacrylate) (PACA) nanospheres (40–250 nm diameter) by a simple emulsification polymerization procedure. The nanospheres were obtained by mechanically emulsifying alkylcyanoacrylate monomers in an aqueous acidic medium in the presence of a non ionic surfactant (e.g. Polysorbate 20, Poloxamer 188) and stabilizers like Dextran 70. The polymerization is spontaneously initiated by the hydroxide ions present in water, under vigorous mechanical stirring at ambient temperature. The NP suspension is then purified by ultracentrifugation or by resuspending the particles in an isotonic surfactant-free medium. The drug is dissolved in the polymerization medium either before the addition of the monomer or at the end of the polymerization reaction, so that it can be either incorporated into the matrix or adsorbed at the surface of the nanospheres. A wide variety of drugs have been efficiently incorporated into PACA nanospheres including cytostatic agents, a peptide growth hormone and several antibiotics [131–133].

Methylidene malonates are other monomers that give biodegradable polymers and polymerize according to a mechanism similar to that of alkylcyanoacrylates [134]. Other polymers proposed for the production of nanospheres by emulsion polymerization include polyglutaraldehyde, poly(vinyl pyridine) and polystyrene; however, their lack of biodegradability compromises their clinical use [135, 136].

10.3.2.1.2 Interfacial Polymerization In this procedure an ethanolic phase containing an oil or a nonmiscible organic solvent, the monomers and the drug to be encapsulated is dispersed in an aqueous external phase containing a surfactant. The ethanol rapidly diffuses out of the organic phase giving tiny oil droplets. Due to their interfacial properties, the monomer molecules spontaneously locate at the surface of the oil nanodroplets at the water/oil interface, leading to the formation of nanocapsules [137]. This method has been used for the encapsulation of oily soluble products into PACA nanocapsules. In order to entrap water-soluble molecules, the process was adapted by addition of the monomer to the oily phase of a previously prepared microemulsion [138, 139].

10.3.2.2 Nanoparticles Prepared from Preformed Polymers

The nanoparticles prepared by *in situ* polymerization suffer from two main drawbacks: (i) the presence of toxic residues (unreacted monomers, initiators and surfactant molecules) whose elimination is time-consuming and not always efficient, and (ii) the possible interaction of monomer molecules with the active substance during the polymerization process, leading to the denaturation and inactivation of the drug. Therefore, new encapsulation techniques involving the dispersion of already polymerized materials have been developed to avoid these problems. A major advantage of these methods over the previously described techniques is that the polymers are well characterized and the nanoparticle preparation conditions will not determine their physicochemical characteristics.

10.3.2.2.1 **Emulsification/Solvent Evaporation–Extraction Method** In this method, the polymer is dissolved in a volatile organic solvent like dichloromethane, chloroform or ethyl acetate. The drug is dissolved or dispersed into the polymer solution, and this mixture is further emulsified by high-speed homogenization or sonication into an aqueous solution containing a suitable emulsifier like poly(vinyl alcohol) (PVA), polysorbate, poloxamer, etc. After the formation of a stable o/w emulsion, the organic solvent is either extracted by the continuous phase (solvent extraction), diffuses into the same and evaporates by increasing the temperature/under pressure or by continuous stirring (solvent evaporation) or is removed by a combination of both, leading to the formation of nanoparticles. At the end of the procedure, the solidified particles are usually collected by centrifugation, washed and dried.

The emulsification/solvent evaporation–extraction method has been used for the production of nanospheres with a wide range of polymers including PLGA, poly(ε-caprolactone) (PCL) and poly(hydroxybutyrate) (PHB). Although this method was proposed for the encapsulation of lipophilic compounds [140, 141], a modification of this technique has been used for encapsulating a model protein, bovine serum albumin (BSA), achieving encapsulation efficiencies up to 70% [142]. An aqueous solution of BSA was emulsified in a PLGA solution in dichloromethane by sonication. This w/o emulsion was then added to an aqueous PVA solution resulting in a w/o/w emulsion which is sonicated again. Polymer hardening and nanoparticle formation is induced by solvent evaporation-extraction upon addition of an aqueous isopropanolic solution.

More recently, Freitas and coworkers [143] have developed a novel ultrasonic flow-through cell for the production of PLA or PLGA nanoparticles with a mean diameter of 500 nm. The equipment consisted of a glass tube for the conduction of the sonicated fluid, which was installed in a steel jacket excited by a transducer and filled with pressurized water for the transmission of sounds waves. This novel technology can avoid the contamination of the fluid from the environment and is well suited for aseptic continuous nanoparticle production.

10.3.2.2.2 **Emulsification/Solvent Diffusion Method** This method uses partially water-soluble solvents like benzyl alcohol or propylene carbonate instead of chlorinated solvents that could degrade certain drugs and proteins. The polymer and active compound are dissolved in the solvent and emulsified in the aqueous phase containing the stabilizer. Water is added to the emulsion to allow the diffusion of the solvent into the water and leading to the formation of the nanoparticles. Once the nanoparticles are formed, they can be collected by centrifugation or the solvent can be removed by dialysis [144].

10.3.2.2.3 **Salting-out Method** The salting-out method was first reported by Bindschaedler and coworkers in 1988 [145]. In this case, an o/w emulsion is formed by addition of an aqueous phase saturated with electrolytes, and containing PVA as stabilizing agent to an acetone solution of polymer and the active compound. The miscibility of both phases is prevented by the saturation of the aqueous phase with electrolytes according to a salting-out phenomenon. Subsequently, water is added until the volume is sufficient to disrupt the equilibrium between the two phases and to allow diffusion of the acetone into the water, which results in polymer precipitation and the formation of nanoparticles. Finally, this suspension is purified by cross-flow filtration and lyophilization. One disadvantage of this procedure is the use of salts that are incompatible with many bioactive compounds.

10.3.2.2.4 **Direct Precipitation-based Method** The nanoprecipitation method developed by Fessi and coworkers [146] represents an easy and reproducible technique that allows us to obtain nanoparticles without a previous emulsification step. The process is based on the drop-wise addition of the polymer dissolved in water-miscible solvents such as acetone, ethanol or methanol to an aqueous medium under stirring. The polymer precipitation gives rise to nanoparticle formation. The solvent is then removed by evaporation under reduced pressure. This technique is mostly suitable for the encapsulation of hydrophobic compounds due to the rapid migration and therefore loss of water-soluble drugs into the aqueous phase. Molpeceres and coworkers [147] encapsulated cyclosporin A into PCL nanoparticles based on this method. The polymer and drug were dissolved in acetone and this organic phase was injected trough a needle into an aqueous medium containing Poloxamer 188. Nanoparticle formation could be visualized by the Tyndall effect.

10.3.3 Characterization of Polymeric Nanoparticles

Nanoparticles are usually characterized in terms of size, morphology, charge, constituent properties, drug content and *in vitro* drug release. The techniques used are similar to those described for SLNs in Sections 10.2.4 and 10.2.6.

10.3.4 Pharmaceutical Applications of Nanoparticles

Polymeric nanoparticles are promising candidates for the delivery of a broad number of peptide and protein drugs for diagnostic and therapeutic applications, since they are advantageous in a number of ways. On the one hand, the solid matrix of particulate carriers protects the incorporated drugs against enzymatic and hydrolytic degradation. On the other hand, they present tissue-targeting capacities, thereby increasing the bioavailability of drugs at the site of action and simultaneously reducing both the total dose and the side effects associated with the drug. Furthermore, they can be used to modulate the immune responses against encapsulated antigens due to their ability to efficiently target professional antigen-presenting cells (APCs), and to facilitate appropriate processing and presenting antigens to T cells. One additional advantage of particulate carriers is that their surface properties can be modified in order to evade the macrophages of the reticuloendothelial system (RES) or in such a way as to improve the uptake and transport across mucosal barriers.

10.3.4.1 Protein Delivery

Advances in biotechnology and biochemistry had led to the discovery of numerous bioactive molecules, some of which are peptides and proteins. These macromolecules are characterized by poor solubility, limited chemical stability *in vitro* and *in vivo* after administration, and poor bioavailability. Indeed, they are usually administered by the parenteral route and frequent, high-dose injections are required to circumvent their extremely rapid clearance in the body. One approach for improving the therapeutic index of these macromolecules could be the development of nanoparticulate carriers able to maintain appropriate drug blood levels for long periods of time. Csaba and coworkers [148] have developed a new nanoparticulate system consisting on a blend nanomatrix of PLGA and a poly(ethylene oxide) (PEO) derivative for the encapsulation of insulin providing a more stable environment to the encapsulated macromolecules. These new nanoparticles release the insulin in a constant rate over a time period of 2 weeks with a negligible burst effect typically observed for proteins encapsulated in PLGA micro/nanoparticles. In another study reported by Barrichelo and coworkers [149], different bioactive agents and insulin were encapsulated into PLGA nanoparticles using the nanoprecipitation method. Insulin was preferentially bound to the surface of PLGA nanoparticles. Nevertheless, a strong hypoglycemic effect of the insulin was observed after administration of the nanoparticles suspension to the ileum loop of male Wistar rats, indicating that insulin was absorbed.

More recently nanoparticles are being investigated as drug carriers for proangiogenic growth factors proposed as a novel approach for the therapy of various ischemia-related pathophysiological conditions. Proangiogenic growth factors have shown promising results in preclinical studies using protein- and gene-based therapies. However, their success in clinical trials is hindered by the lack of an optimal delivery strategy that would provide sustained and localized levels of the growth factors in the diseased tissue [150]. Davda and coworkers [151] evaluated the efficacy of sustained release biodegradable nanoparticles, formulated with PLGA, for the delivery of vascular endothelial growth factor protein (VEGF), a potent proangiogenic agent. Nanoparticles encapsulating VEGF, which were formulated using a double-emulsion solvent evaporation technique, demonstrated sustained release of the growth factor in bioactive form. Furthermore, the growth factor encapsulated in nanoparticles demonstrated greater and more sustained effect compared with a solution on endothelial cell proliferation, migration and morphogenesis, which are key elements of blood vessel outgrowth. The greater efficacy of encapsulated VEGF was due to the ability of nanoparticles to maintain the growth factor level in culture for a sustained period of time. The data thus suggest that nanoparticles can be used as an effective delivery system for growth factors to induce therapeutic angiogenesis.

A new method to prepare heparin-functionalized PLGA nanoparticles for the controlled release of growth factors has been recently reported by Chung and coworkers [152]. The system is composed of PLGA as a hydrophobic core, Pluronic F-127 as a hydrophilic surface layer and heparin as the functionalized moiety. The incorporation of heparin is based on its high specific binding for various growth factors, which enables them to crosslink their receptors and to be protected from proteolytic degradation. The release of VEGF from the nanoparticles (below 200 nm) showed a linear profile without initial burst over 1 month. The authors proposed that these nanoparticles can be used as a growth factor delivery system in tissue engineering scaffolds as well as sustained release systems of various heparin-binding growth factors.

Interferon (IFN)-α is another macromolecule that has been encapsulated in order to simplify its administration and improve its therapeutic effects. The currently approved therapies require the injection of repeated high nonphysiological doses due to the short half-life of the free macromolecule [153]. Nevertheless, the potential of IFN formulated in these controlled release systems has been limited by the reduction of its biological activity during the encapsulation and/or release process [154]. Sanchez and coworkers [155] have used Poloxamer 188 as a stabilizing agent for the encapsulation of IFN-α into biodegradable micro/nanoparticles. PLGA/poloxamer blend microspheres were able to provide significant amounts of active IFN-α for up to 96 days. These new delivery systems might improve the effectiveness of IFN-α and the quality of life of patients.

10.3.4.2 Protein Delivery by Mucosal Routes

In recent years, considerable research has been done using nanoparticles for the delivery of protein and peptide drugs by mucosal routes. After oral administration the drug carriers are expected to remain in the gastrointestinal tract while protecting the entrapped peptide drugs from enzymatic degradation until they are absorbed. Carino and coworkers [156] developed an oral nanosphere formulation to protect insulin from degradation and facilitate systemic uptake by the oral route. This formulation was shown to have 11.4% of the efficacy of intraperitoneally delivered zinc insulin and was able to control plasma glucose levels when faced with a simultaneous administered glucose challenge.

The same concept could be also applied to the pulmonary route, which has been considered as a promising way to improve delivery of insulin with particulate systems. The nebulized PLGA nanospheres significantly reduced the blood glucose levels of fasted guinea pigs and the hypoglycemia was prolonged over 48 h compared to the nebulized aqueous insulin solution as a reference (6 h). This result could be attributed to the sustained release of insulin from the nanospheres deposited widely on to the whole lung [157]. When developing polymeric nanoparticles, controversy still exists on physicochemical factors governing nanoparticle uptake and transport across mucosal barriers, including size, size distribution, hydrophobicity and surface properties. Many studies on size effects have demonstrate that size is an important parameter controlling the internalization of nanoparticles into the epithelia of the gastrointestinal tract and, as a rule of thumb, sizes smaller than 500 nm are required [105]. Apart from particle size, surface properties seem to influence the uptake by intestinal epithelia. Summarizing numerous absorption studies of polymeric nanoparticles in intestinal tissues, it can be concluded that a combination of both nanoparticles surface charges and increased hydrophobicity of the matrix material seem to affect gastrointestinal uptake in a positive sense [158–160]. In addition, different research groups have demonstrated that increased nanoparticle internalization can be achieved by conferring mucoadhesive properties to them by coating their surface with mucoadhesive polymers such as chitosan and carbopol. Takeuchi and coworkers [161] reported the preparation of elcatonin-loaded PLGA nanospheres coated with chitosan. They found that, following the oral or pulmonary administration in rats and guinea pig, the reduction in calcium concentration obtained with mucoadhesive nanoparticles was more effective and prolonged in comparison with that obtained with noncoated systems. These results indicate that chitosan nanospheres adhere to the mucus layer in the gastrointestinal tract and lung tissues, due to the mucoadhesive properties of chitosan, and release the drug over a longer period of time. In another study by Vila and coworkers [162], it was demonstrated that the coating of tetanus toxoid-containing PLA nanoparticles with PEG or chitosan improved their stability in physiological fluids, and enhanced the transport across the intestinal and nasal mucosae, thereby confirming the usefulness of mucoadhesive nanoparticulate systems for the delivery of peptide drugs.

Nanoparticles have also been used in the induction of oral tolerance, since successive and extended exposure of the immune system to the antigen in the intestine is indispensable for inducing peripheral immune tolerance. Kim and coworkers reported that a single administration of PLGA nanoparticles entrapping type II collagen could induce oral tolerance more efficiently than repeated administration of intact protein [163]. In a subsequent study, they prepared PLGA nanoparticles entrapping PEG-conjugated immunodominant peptides of type II collagen for oral tolerance induction in collagen-induced arthritis. The single intragastric administration of these nanoparticles induced the production of IL-4 and

IL-10 in CD4$^+$ T cells of Peyer's patches, which was comparable to that in mice fed 6 times with peptide solution. Taking into account that IL-4 and IL-10 play a critical role in arthritis suppression, they conclude that oral administration of nanoparticles might block arthritis progression through this mechanism [164].

10.3.4.3 Vaccine Adjuvants

Nanoparticles containing entrapped or adsorbed antigens have been intensively investigated as vaccine adjuvants alternatives to the currently used aluminum salts [165, 166]. A major drawback with current vaccination regimes lies in the method of administration, which generally employs the parenteral route, which might lead to noncompliance. Thus, alternative routes of vaccine administration have been tested: nasal, oral, intradermal and vaginal. Carcaboso and coworkers [167] have demonstrated the adjuvant properties of PLGA nanoparticles containing encapsulated Spf66 antigen. The systemic immune response obtained following nasal administration with nanoparticles was superior to that induced by the same dose of peptide solution; however, in this study, the best responses were obtained with 1-μm particles. This latter formulation greatly improves and maintains higher antibody levels compared to conventional alum adjuvant and to the administration of the particles by others routes (subcutaneous, oral).

In recent studies, Coolí and coworkers [168] have investigated the effect of size and charge on the permeation of nanoparticles through the skin as the first step in designing a transdermal vaccine delivery system. The results showed that only 50- and 500-nm fluorescent particles that were negatively charged were able to permeate the pig skin. This provides evidence of the potential of nanoparticles as delivery vectors for antigens and DNA for the purpose of transdermal vaccination protocols.

In general, vaccination against major diseases requires a humoral immune response; however, in the case of intracellular viral, bacterial and parasitic infections a cellular response is needed [169]. It is known that aluminum hydroxide can preferentially induce T_h2 immune responses [170, 171] and deposits the antigen only for 2–3 weeks [172]. Although aluminum hydroxide can induce the production of antibodies, it has little effect on eliciting CD4$^+$ T_h1 cells (defined by their production of IL-2 and IFN-γ cytokines, that induce cell-mediated immune responses) or CD8$^+$ T cell response. Polymeric nanoparticle delivery systems play an interesting role in the design of new vaccines since it have been demonstrated that they can elicit a T_h1/T_h2 combined response. According to the results reported by Schöll and coworkers [173], the subcutaneous administration of the major allergen of birch pollen loaded into PLGA nanoparticles modulated an ongoing T_h2 response in the BALB/c mouse model. This response was demonstrated by downregulation of IgG1, and production of IFN-γ and IL-10, suggesting that PLGA nanoparticles can be used for formulations of allergen extracts or derivatives for the "few-shot" treatment of type 1 allergy.

Furthermore, it has been suggested that PLGA nanoparticles are suitable for simultaneous targeting of immunoadjuvants and antigens to APCs, and can reduce the effective adjuvant dose significantly [174]. Chong and coworkers [175] investigated the immune-enhancing effects of codelivery hepatitis B core antigen

(HBcAg) and monophospholipid A (MPLA) in a murine model. In this study, a single subcutaneous immunization with a vaccine formulation containing MPLA and HBcAg coencapsulated in PLGA nanoparticles promoted a stronger T_h1 cellular immune response with IFN-γ production than those induced by the antigen alone, mixed with MPLA or HBcAg-loaded nanoparticles. Such response is critical for the control of viral replication and the elimination of chronic hepatitis B, indicating that the simultaneous delivery of antigens and immune modulators in a single particulate formulation may be an interesting strategy for the development of effective hepatitis B virus therapeutic vaccines.

References

1 P. Basu. Technologies that deliver. *Nat. Med.* **2003**, *9*, 1100–1101.

2 G. Orive, A. R. Gascón, R. M. Hernández, A. Dominguez-Gil, J. L. Pedraz. Drug delivery in biotechnology: present and future. *Curr. Opin. Biotechnol.* **2003**, *14*, 659–664.

3 V. Labhasetwar. Nanotechnology for drug and gene therapy: the importance of understanding molecular mechanisms of delivery. *Curr. Opin. Biotechnol.* **2005**, *16*, 674–680.

4 G. Orive, A. R. Gascón, R. M. Hernández, A. Dominguez-Gil, J. L. Pedraz. New approaches in the delivery of pharmaceuticals. *Trends Pharmacol. Sci.* **2003**, *24*, 207–210.

5 A. T. Jones, M. Gumbleton, R. Duncan. Understanding endocytic pathways and intracellular trafficking: a prerequisite for effective design of advanced drug delivery systems. *Adv. Drug Deliv. Rev.* **2003**, *55*, 1353–1357.

6 R. H. Müller, C. M. Keck. Challenges and solutions for the delivery of biotech drugs – a review of drug nanocrystal technology and lipid nanoparticles. *J. Biotechnol.* **2004**, *113*, 151–170.

7 A. Dubes, H. Parrot-Lopez, W. Abdelwahed, G. Degobert, H. Fessi, P. Shahgaldian, A. W. Coleman. Scanning electron microscopy and atomic force microscopy imaging of solid lipid nanoparticles derived from amphiphilic cyclodextrins. *Eur. J. Pharm. Biopharm.* **2003**, *55*, 279–282.

8 J. Gualbert, P. Shahgaldian, A. W. Coleman. Interactions of amphiphilic calix[4]arene-based solid lipid nanoparticles with bovine serum albumin. *Int. J. Pharm.* **2003**, *257*, 69–73.

9 P. Shahgaldian, E. Da Silva, A. W. Coleman, B. Rather, M. J. Zaworotko. Para-acyl-calix-arene based solid lipid nanoparticles (SLNs): a detailed study of preparation and stability parameters. *Int. J. Pharm.* **2003**, *253*, 23–38.

10 W. Mehnert, K. Mäder. Solid lipid nanoparticles: production, characterization and applications. *Adv. Drug Deliv. Rev.* **2001**, *47*, 165–196.

11 B. Siekmann, K. Westesen. Melt-homogenized solid lipid nanoparticles stabilized by the nonionic surfactant tyloxapol. *Pharm. Pharmacol. Lett.* **1994**, *3*, 194–197.

12 R. Cavalli, O. Caputo, E. Marengo, F. Pattarino, M. R. Gasco. The effect of the components of microemulsions on both size and crystalline structure of solid lipid nanoparticles (SLN) containing a series of model molecules. *Pharmazie* **1998**, *53*, 392–396.

13 R. H. Müller, W. Mehnert, J. S. Lucks, C. Schwarz, A. zur Mühlen, H. Weyhers, C. Freitas, D. Rühl. An alternative colloidal carrier system for controlled drug delivery. *Eur. J. Pharm. Biopharm.* **1995**, *41*, 62–69.

14 M. Uner, S. A. Wissing, G. Yener, R. H. Muller. Influence of surfac-

tants on the physical stability of solid lipid nanoparticle (SLN) formulations. *Pharmazie* **2004**, *59*, 331–332.

15 R. H. Müller, K. Mäder, S. Gohla. Solid lipid nanoparticles (SLN) for controlled drug delivery – a review of the state of the art. *Eur. J. Pharm. Biopharm.* **2000**, *50*, 161–177.

16 S. A. Wissing, O. Kayser, R. H. Müller. Solid lipid nanoparticles for parenteral drug delivery. *Adv. Drug Deliv. Rev.* **2004**, *56*, 1257–1272.

17 P. Speiser. Lipidnanopellets als Trägersystem für Arzneimittel zur peroralen Anwendung. *European Patent EP 0167825*, **1990**.

18 A. J. Domb. Lipospheres for controlled delivery of substances. *US Patent, USS 5,188,837*, **1993**.

19 M. R. Gasco. Method for producing solid lipid microspheres having a narrow size distribution. *US Patents 5,250,236*, **1993**.

20 B. Sjöström, B. Bergenståhl. Preparation of submicron drug particles in lecithin-stabilized o/w emulsions I. Model studies of the precipitation of cholesteryl acetate. *Int. J. Pharm.* **1992**, *88*, 53–62.

21 A. Dingler, S. Gohla. Production of solid lipid nanoparticles (SLN): scaling up feasibilities. *J. Microencapsul.* **2002**, *19*, 11–16.

22 S. H. Gohla, A. Dingler. Scaling up feasibility of the production of solid lipid nanoparticles (SLN). *Pharmazie* **2001**, *56*, 61–63.

23 V. Jenning, A. Lippacher, S. H. Gohla. Medium scale production of solid lipid nanoparticles (SLN) by high pressure homogenization. *J. Microencapsul.* **2002**, *19*, 1–10.

24 R. H. Müller, A. Dingler, T. Schneppe, S. Gohla. Large scale production of solid lipid nanoparticles (SLN) and nanosuspensions (DissoCubes). In *Handbook of Pharmaceutical Controlled Release Technology*, Wise, D. (Ed.). Marcel Dekker, New York, **2000**, pp. 359–376.

25 E. Marengo, R. Cavalli, O. Caputo, L. Rodriguez, M. R. Gasco. Scale-up of the preparation process of solid lipid nanospheres. Part I. *Int. J. Pharm.* **2000**, *205*, 3–13.

26 C. Dulieu, D. Bazile. Influence of lipid nanocapsules composition on their aptness to freeze-drying. *Pharm. Res.* **2005**, *22*, 285–292.

27 H. Heiati, R. Tawashi, N. C. Phillips. Drug retention and stability of solid lipid nanoparticles containing azidothymidine palmitate after autoclaving, storage and lyophilization. *J. Microencapsul.* **1998**, *15*, 173–184.

28 E. Zimmermann, R. H. Müller, K. Mäder. Influence of different parameters on reconstitution of lyophilized SLN. *Int. J. Pharm.* **2000**, *196*, 211–213.

29 C. Freitas, R. H. Müller. Spray-drying of solid lipid nanoparticles (SLN™). *Eur. J. Pharm. Biopharm.* **1998**, *46*, 145–151.

30 E. Marengo, R. Cavalli, G. Rovero, M. R. Gasco. Scale-up and optimization of an evaporative drying process applied to aqueous dispersions of solid lipid nanoparticles. *Pharm. Dev. Technol.* **2003**, *8*, 299–309.

31 C. Freitas, R. H. Müller. Correlation between long-term stability of solid lipid nanoparticles (SLN™) and crystallinity of the lipid phase. *Eur. J. Pharm. Biopharm.* **1999**, *47*, 125–132.

32 A. zur Mühlen, C. Schwarz, W. Mehnert. Solid lipid nanoparticles (SLN) for controlled drug delivery – drug release and release mechanism. *Eur. J. Pharm. Biopharm.* **1998**, *45*, 149–155.

33 A. zur Mühlen, W. Mehnert. Drug release and release mechanism of prednisolone loaded solid lipid nanoparticles. *Pharmazie* **1998**, *53*, 552–555.

34 R. H. Müller, M. Radtke, S. A. Wissing. Solid lipid nanoparticles (SLN) and nanostructured lipid carriers (NLC) in cosmetic and dermatological preparations. *Adv. Drug Deliv. Rev.* **2002**, *54*, S131–S155.

35 R. H. Müller, M. Radtke, S. A. Wissing. Nanostructured lipid matrices for improved microencapsulation of drugs. *Int. J. Pharm.* **2002**, *242*, 121–128.

36 K. Jores, W. Mehnert, K. Mäder. Physicochemical investigations on solid lipid nanoparticles and on oil-loaded solid lipid nanoparticles: a nuclear magnetic resonance and electron spin resonance study. *Pharm. Res.* **2003**, *20*, 1274–1283.

37 K. Jores, A. Haberland, S. Wartewig, K. Mader, W. Mehnert. Solid lipid nanoparticles (SLN) and oil-loaded SLN studied by spectrofluorometry and raman spectroscopy. *Pharm. Res.* **2005**, *22*, 1887–1897.

38 K. Jores, W. Mehnert, M. Drechsler, H. Bunjes, C. Johann, K. Mäder. Investigations on the structure of solid lipid nanoparticles (SLN) and oil-loaded solid lipid nanoparticles by photon correlation spectroscopy, field-flow fractionation and transmission electron microscopy. *J. Control. Release* **2004**, *95*, 217–227.

39 C. Olbrich, A. Gessner, O. Kayser, R. H. Muller. Lipid–drug-conjugate (LDC) nanoparticles as novel carrier system for the hydrophilic antitrypanosomal drug diminazenediaceturate. *J. Drug Target.* **2002**, *10*, 387–396.

40 C. Olbrich, A. Gessner, O. Kayser, R. H. Müller. Lipid–drug conjugate (LDC) nanoparticles as an alternative carrier system with high drug content. *Proc. Int. Symp. Control. Release Bioact. Mater.* **2000**, 295–296.

41 M. Igartua, P. Saulnier, B. Heurtault, B. Pech, J. E. Proust, J. L. Pedraz, J. P. Benoit. Development and characterization of solid lipid nanoparticles loaded with magnetite. *Int. J. Pharm.* **2002**, *233*, 149–157.

42 A. zur Mühlen, E. zur Mühlen, H. Niehus, W. Mehnert. Atomic force microscopy studies of solid lipid nanoparticles. *Pharm. Res.* **1996**, *13*, 1411–1416.

43 E. B. Souto, S. A. Wissing, C. M. Barbosa, R. H. Müller. Comparative study between the viscoelastic behaviors of different lipid nanoparticle formulations. *J. Cosmet. Sci.* **2004**, *55*, 463–471.

44 T. Eldem, P. Speiser, A. Hincal. Optimization of spray-dried and -congealed lipid micropellets and characterization of their surface morphology by scanning electron microscopy. *Pharm. Res.* **1991**, *8*, 47–54.

45 S. C. Yang, J. B. Zhu, Y. Lu, B. W. Liang, C. Z. Yang. Body distribution of camptothecin solid lipid nanoparticles after oral administration. *Pharm. Res.* **1999**, *16*, 751–757.

46 T. Bekerman, J. Golenser, A. Domb. Cyclosporin nanoparticulate lipospheres for oral administration. *J. Pharm. Sci.* **2004**, *93*, 1264–1270.

47 L. Brannon-Peppas, J. O. Blanchette. Nanoparticle and targeted systems for cancer therapy. *Adv. Drug Deliv. Rev.* **2004**, *56*, 1649–1659.

48 G. Storm, S. O. Belliot, T. Daemen, D. D. Lasic. Surface modification of nanoparticles to oppose uptake by the mononuclear phagocyte system. *Adv. Drug Deliv. Rev.* **1995**, *17*, 31–48.

49 T. M. Goppert, R. H. Müller. Protein adsorption patterns on poloxamer- and poloxamine-stabilized solid lipid nanoparticles (SLN). *Eur. J. Pharm. Biopharm.* **2005**, *60*, 361–372.

50 C. Olbrich, U. Bakowsky, C. M. Lehr, R. H. Müller, C. Kneuer. Cationic solid-lipid nanoparticles can efficiently bind and transfect plasmid DNA. *J. Control. Release* **2001**, *77*, 345–355.

51 C. Rudolph, U. Schillinger, A. Ortiz, K. Tabatt, C. Plank, R. H. Müller, J. Rosenecker. Application of novel solid lipid nanoparticle (SLN)-gene vector formulations based on a dimeric HIV-1 TAT-peptide *in vitro* and *in vivo*. *Pharm. Res.* **2004**, *21*, 1662–1669.

52 C. Erni, C. Suard, S. Freitas, D. Dreher, H. P. Merkle, E. Walter. Evaluation of cationic solid lipid microparticles as synthetic carriers for the targeted delivery of macromolecules to phagocytic antigen-presenting cells. *Biomaterials* **2002**, *23*, 4667–4676.

53 F. Q. Hu, Y. Hong, H. Yuan. Preparation and characterization of solid lipid nanoparticles containing peptide. *Int. J. Pharm.* **2004**, *273*, 29–35.

54 M. Garcia-Fuentes, D. Torres, M. J. Alonso. New surface-modified lipid nanoparticles as delivery vehicles for salmon calcitonin. *Int. J. Pharm.* **2005**, *296*, 122–132.

55 M. Garcia-Fuentes, D. Torres, M. J. Alonso. Design of lipid nanoparticles for the oral delivery of hydrophilic macromolecules. *Colloids Surf. B Biointerfaces* **2002**, *27*, 159–168.

56 S. Morel, M. R. Gasco, R. Cavalli. Incorporation in lipospheres of [D-Trp-6]LHRH. *Int. J. Pharm.* **1994**, *105*, R1–R3.

57 S. Morel, E. Ugazio, R. Cavalli, M. R. Gasco. Thymopentin in solid lipid nanoparticles. *Int. J. Pharm.* **1996**, *132*, 259–261.

58 A. J. Almeida, S. Runge, R. H. Müller. Peptide-loaded solid lipid nanoparticles (SLN): influence of production parameters. *Int. J. Pharm.* **1997**, *149*, 255–265.

59 E. Ugazio, R. Cavalli, M. R. Gasco. Incorporation of cyclosporin A in solid lipid nanoparticles (SLN). *Int. J. Pharm.* **2002**, *241*, 341–344.

60 R. Cortesi, E. Esposito, G. Luca, C. Nastruzzi. Production of lipospheres as carriers for bioactive compounds. *Biomaterials* **2002**, *23*, 2283–2294.

61 R. Cavalli, M. R. Gasco, P. Chetoni, S. Burgalassi, M. F. Saettone. Solid lipid nanoparticles (SLN) as ocular delivery system for tobramycin. *Int. J. Pharm.* **2002**, *238*, 241–245.

62 E. B. Souto, R. H. Müller. SLN and NLC for topical delivery of ketoconazole. *J. Microencapsul.* **2005**, *22*, 501–510.

63 F. Q. Hu, H. Yuan, H. H. Zhang, M. Fang. Preparation of solid lipid nanoparticles with clobetasol propionate by a novel solvent diffusion method in aqueous system and physicochemical characterization. *Int. J. Pharm.* **2002**, *239*, 121–128.

64 E. B. Souto, S. A. Wissing, C. M. Barbosa, R. H. Müller. Development of a controlled release formulation based on SLN and NLC for topical clotrimazole delivery. *Int. J. Pharm.* **2004**, *278*, 71–77.

65 N. Hodoshima, C. Udagawa, T. Ando, H. Fukuyasu, H. Watanabe, S. Nakabayashi. Lipid nanoparticles for delivering antitumor drugs. *Int. J. Pharm.* **1997**, *146*, 81–92.

66 A. Lamprecht, J. L. Saumet, J. Roux, J. P. Benoit. Lipid nanocarriers as drug delivery system for ibuprofen in pain treatment. *Int. J. Pharm.* **2004**, *278*, 407–414.

67 S. J. Lim, C. K. Kim. Formulation parameters determining the physicochemical characteristics of solid lipid nanoparticles loaded with all-*trans* retinoic acid. *Int. J. Pharm.* **2002**, *243*, 135–146.

68 R. Cavalli, O. Caputo, M. R. Gasco. Preparation and characterization of solid lipid nanospheres containing paclitaxel. *Eur. J. Pharm. Sci.* **2000**, *10*, 305–309.

69 A. Fundaro, R. Cavalli, A. Bargoni, D. Vighetto, G. P. Zara, M. R. Gasco. Non-stealth and stealth solid lipid nanoparticles (SLN) carrying doxorubicin: pharmacokinetics and tissue distribution after i.v. administration to rats. *Pharmacol. Res.* **2000**, *42*, 337–343.

70 S. Toongsuwan, L. C. Li, B. K. Erickson, H. C. Chang. Formulation and characterization of bupivacaine lipospheres. *Int. J. Pharm.* **2004**, *280*, 57–65.

71 J. X. Wang, X. Sun, Z. R. Zhang. Enhanced brain targeting by synthesis of 3′,5′-dioctanoyl-5-fluoro-2′-deoxyuridine and incorporation into solid lipid nanoparticles. *Eur. J. Pharm. Biopharm.* **2002**, *54*, 285–290.

72 H. Heiati, R. Tawashi, N. C. Phillips. Solid lipid nanoparticles as drug carriers: II. Plasma stability and biodistribution of solid lipid nanoparticles containing the lipophilic prodrug 3′-azido-3′-deoxythymidine palmitate in mice. *Int. J. Pharm.* **1998**, *174*, 71–80.

73 R. Löbenberg, L. Araujo, H. von Briesen, E. Rodgers, J. Kreuter. Body distribution of azidothymidine bound to hexyl-cyanoacrylate nanoparticles after i.v. injection to rats. *J. Control. Release* **1998**, *50*, 21–30.

74 L. Harivardhan Reddy, R. K. Sharma, K. Chuttani, A. K. Mishra, R. S. R. Murthy. Influence of administration route on tumor uptake and biodistribution of etoposide loaded solid lipid nanoparticles in Dalton's lymphoma tumor bearing mice. *J. Control. Release* **2005**, *105*, 185–198.

75 G. Lukowski, P. Pflegel. Electron diffraction of solid lipid nanoparticles loaded with aciclovir. *Pharmazie* **1997**, *52*, 642–643.

76 J. Kristl, B. Volk, M. Gasperlin, M. Sentjurc, P. Jurkovic. Effect of colloidal carriers on ascorbyl palmitate stability. *Eur. J. Pharm. Sci.* **2003**, *19*, 181–189.

77 M. Demirel, Y. Yazan, R. H. Müller, F. Kilic, B. Bozan. Formulation and *in vitro–in vivo* evaluation of piribedil solid lipid micro- and nanoparticles. *J. Microencapsul.* **2001**, *18*, 359–371.

78 V. Jenning, M. Schäfer-Korting, S. Gohla. Vitamin A-loaded solid lipid nanoparticles for topical use: drug release properties. *J. Control. Release* **2000**, *66*, 115–126.

79 H. Bunjes, M. Drechsler, M. H. J. Koch, K. Westesen. Incorporation of the model drug ubidecarenone into solid lipid nanoparticles. *Pharm. Res.* **2001**, *18*, 287–293.

80 A. Dingler, R. P. Blum, H. Niehus, R. H. Müller, S. Gohla. Solid lipid nanoparticles (SLN™/Lipopearls™) – a pharmaceutical and cosmetic carrier for the application of vitamin E in dermal products. *J. Microencapsul.* **1999**, *16*, 751–767.

81 E. B. Souto, C. Anselmi, M. Centini, R. H. Müller. Preparation and characterization of *n*-dodecyl-ferulate-loaded solid lipid nanoparticles (SLN®). *Int. J. Pharm.* **2005**, *295*, 261–268.

82 S. A. Wissing, K. Mäder, R. H. Müller. Solid lipid nanoparticles (SLN™) as a novel carrier system offering prolonged release of the perfume Allure. *Proc. Int. Symp. Control. Release Bioact. Mater.* **2000**, 311–312.

83 E. B. Souto, R. H. Müller, S. Gohla. A novel approach based on lipid nanoparticles (SLN®) for topical delivery of alpha-lipoic acid. *J. Microencapsul.* **2005**, *22*, 581–592.

84 K. Tabatt, M. Sameti, C. Olbrich, R. H. Müller, C. M. Lehr. Effect of cationic lipid and matrix lipid composition on solid lipid nanoparticle-mediated gene transfer. *Eur. J. Pharm. Biopharm.* **2004**, *57*, 155–162.

85 K. Tabatt, C. Kneuer, M. Sameti, C. Olbrich, R. H. Müller, C. M. Lehr, U. Bakowsky. Transfection with different colloidal systems: comparison of solid lipid nanoparticles and liposomes. *J. Control. Release* **2004**, *97*, 321–332.

86 K. L. Brigham, B. Meyrick, B. Christman, M. Magnuson, G. King, L. C. Berry, Jr. *In vivo* transfection of murine lungs with a functioning prokaryotic gene using a liposome vehicle. *Am. J. Med. Sci.* **1989**, *298*, 278–281.

87 P. L. Felgner, T. R. Gadek, M. Holm, R. Roman, H. W. Chan, M. Wenz, J. P. Northrop, G. M. Ringold, M. Danielsen. Lipofection: a highly efficient, lipid-mediated DNA-transfection procedure. *Proc. Natl Acad. Sci. USA* **1987**, *84*, 7413–7417.

88 L. S. Uyechi-O'Brien, F. C. Szoka. Mechanisms for cationic lipids in gene transfer. In *Pharmaceutical Gene Delivery Systems*, Rolland, A., Sullivan, S. M. (Eds.), Marcel Dekker, New York, **2003**, pp. 79–108.

89 K. E. B. Meyer, L. S. Uyechi, F. C. Szoka. Manipulating the intracellular trafficking of nucleic acids. In *Gene Therapy for Diseases of the Lung*, Brigham, K. L. (Ed.), Marcel Dekker, New York, **1997**, pp. 135–180.

90 J. H. Felgner, R. Kumar, C. N. Sridhar, C. J. Wheeler, Y. J. Tsai, R. Border, P. Ramsey, M. Martin, P. L. Felgner. Enhanced gene delivery and mechanism studies with a novel series of cationic lipid formulations. *J. Biol. Chem.* **1994**, *269*, 2550–2561.

91 C. M. Gorman, M. Aikawa, B. Fox, E. Fox, C. Lapuz, B. Michaud, H.

Nguyen, E. Roche, T. Sawa, J. P. WienerKronish. Efficient *in vivo* delivery of DNA to pulmonary cells using the novel lipid EDMPC. *Gene Ther.* **1997**, *4*, 983–992.

92 E. R. Lee, J. Marshall, C. S. Siegel, C. W. Jiang, N. S. Yew, M. R. Nichols, J. B. Nietupski, R. J. Ziegler, M. B. Lane, K. X. Wang, N. C. Wan, R. K. Scheule, D. J. Harris, A. E. Smith, S. H. Cheng. Detailed analysis of structures and formulations of cationic lipids for efficient gene transfer to the lung. *Hum. Gene Ther.* **1996**, *7*, 1701–1717.

93 T. Paukku, S. Lauraeus, I. Huhtaniemi, P. K. Kinnunen. Novel cationic liposomes for DNA-transfection with high efficiency and low toxicity. *Chem. Phys. Lipids* **1997**, *87*, 23–29.

94 I. Solodin, C. S. Brown, M. S. Bruno, C. Y. Chow, E. H. Jang, R. J. Debs, T. D. Heath. A novel series of amphiphilic imidazolinium compounds for *in-vitro* and *in-vivo* gene delivery. *Biochemistry* **1995**, *34*, 13537–13544.

95 J. Wang, X. Guo, Y. Xu, L. Barron, F. C. Szoka, Jr. Synthesis and characterization of long chain alkyl acyl carnitine esters. Potentially biodegradable cationic lipids for use in gene delivery. *J. Med. Chem.* **1998**, *41*, 2207–2215.

96 C. J. Wheeler, P. L. Felgner, Y. J. Tsai, J. Marshall, L. Sukhu, S. G. Doh, J. Hartikka, J. Nietupski, M. Manthorpe, M. Nichols, M. Plewe, X. W. Liang, J. Norman, A. Smith, S. H. Cheng. A novel cationic lipid greatly enhances plasmid DNA delivery and expression in mouse lung. *Proc. Natl Acad. Sci. USA* **1996**, *93*, 11454–11459.

97 M. C. Pedroso de Lima, S. Simoes, P. Pires, H. Faneca, N. Duzgunes. Cationic lipid–DNA complexes in gene delivery: from biophysics to biological applications. *Adv. Drug Deliv. Rev.* **2001**, *47*, 277–294.

98 P. E. Thorén, D. Persson, P. Lincoln, B. Nordén. Membrane destabilizing properties of cell-penetrating peptides. *Biophys. Chem.* **2005**, *114*, 169–179.

99 L. Hyndman, J. L. Lemoine, L. Huang, D. J. Porteous, A. C. Boyd, X. Nan. HIV-1 Tat protein transduction domain peptide facilitates gene transfer in combination with cationic liposomes. *J. Control. Release* **2004**, *99*, 435–444.

100 M. Silhol, M. Tyagi, M. Giacca, B. Lebleu, E. Vives. Different mechanisms for cellular internalization of the HIV-1 Tat-derived cell penetrating peptide and recombinant proteins fused to Tat. *Eur. J. Biochem.* **2002**, *269*, 494–501.

101 S. R. Schwarze, K. A. Hruska, S. F. Dowdy. Protein transduction: unrestricted delivery into all cells? *Trends Cell Biol.* **2000**, *10*, 290–295.

102 A. Ziegler, P. Nervi, M. Durrenberger, J. Seelig. The cationic cell-penetrating peptide Cpp(TAT) derived from the HIV-1 protein TAT is rapidly transported into living fibroblasts: optical, biophysical, and metabolic evidence. *Biochemistry* **2005**, *44*, 138–148.

103 N. Pedersen, S. Hansen, A. V. Heydenreich, H. G. Kristensen, H. S. Poulsen. Solid lipid nanoparticles can effectively bind DNA, streptavidin and biotinylated ligands. *Eur. J. Pharm. Biopharm.* **2006**, *62*, 155–162.

104 S. Könnings, A. Göpferich. Lipospheres as delivery systems for peptides and proteins. In *Lipospheres in Drug Targets and Delivery. Approaches, Methods and Applications*, Nastruzzi, C. (Ed.). CRC Press, Boca Raton, FL, **2005**, pp. 67–86.

105 T. Jung, W. Kamm, A. Breitenbach, E. Kaiserling, J. X. Xiao, T. Kissel. Biodegradable nanoparticles for oral delivery of peptides: is there a role for polymers to affect mucosal uptake? *Eur. J. Pharm. Biopharm.* **2000**, *50*, 147–160.

106 R. H. Müller, S. Maaßen, H. Weyhers, F. Specht, J. S. Lucks. Cytotoxicity of magnetite-loaded polylactide, polylactide/glycolide

particles and solid lipid nanoparticles. *Int. J. Pharm.* **1996**, *138*, 85–94.
107 N. Schöler, H. Hahn, R. H. Müller, O. Liesenfeld. Effect of lipid matrix and size of solid lipid nanoparticles (SLN) on the viability and cytokine production of macrophages. *Int. J. Pharm.* **2002**, *231*, 167–176.
108 C. Olbrich, R. H. Müller, K. Tabatt, O. Kayser, C. Schulze, R. Schade. Stable biocompatible adjuvants – a new type of adjuvant based on solid lipid nanoparticles: a study on cytotoxicity, compatibility and efficacy in chicken. *Altern. Lab. Anim.* **2002**, *30*, 443–458.
109 C. Prego, M. Garcia, D. Torres, M. J. Alonso. Transmucosal macromolecular drug delivery. *J. Control. Release* **2005**, *101*, 151–162.
110 L. D. Hu, X. Tang, F. D. Cui. Solid lipid nanoparticles (SLNs) to improve oral bioavailability of poorly soluble drugs. *J. Pharm. Pharmacol.* **2004**, *56*, 1527–1535.
111 L. Penkler, R. H. Müller, S. Runge, V. Ravelli. Pharmaceutical cyclosporine formulation with improved biopharmaceutical properties, improved physical quality and greater stability, and method for producing said formulation. *WO 99/56733*, **1999**.
112 G. Ponchel, M. J. Montisci, A. Dembri, C. Durrer, D. Duchene. Mucoadhesion of colloidal particulate systems in the gastro-intestinal tract. *Eur. J. Pharm. Biopharm.* **1997**, *44*, 25–31.
113 E. Zimmermann, R. H. Müller. Electrolyte- and pH-stabilities of aqueous solid lipid nanoparticle (SLN™) dispersions in artificial gastrointestinal media. *Eur. J. Pharm. Biopharm.* **2001**, *52*, 203–210.
114 C. Olbrich, R. H. Müller. Enzymatic degradation of SLN – effect of surfactant and surfactant mixtures. *Int. J. Pharm.* **1999**, *180*, 31–39.
115 R. H. Müller, D. Rühl, S. A. Runge. Biodegradation of solid lipid nanoparticles as a function of lipase incubation time. *Int. J. Pharm.* **1996**, *144*, 115–121.
116 C. Olbrich, W. Mehnert, R. H. Müller. Development of an *in vitro* degradation assay for solid lipid nanoparticles. *Proc. 2nd World Meeting APGI/APV*, **1998**, 627–628.
117 I. El-Gibaly, S. K. bdel-Ghaffar. Effect of hexacosanol on the characteristics of novel sustained-release allopurinol solid lipospheres (SLS): factorial design application and product evaluation. *Int. J. Pharm.* **2005**, *294*, 33–51.
118 R. H. Müller, D. Rühl, S. Runge, K. Schulze-Forster, W. Mehnert. Cytotoxicity of solid lipid nanoparticles as a function of the lipid matrix and the surfactant. *Pharm. Res.* **1997**, *14*, 458–462.
119 M. Schäfer-Korting, W. Mehnert. Delivery of lipophilic compounds with lipid nanoparticles. Applications in dermatics and for transdermal therapy. In *Lipospheres in Drug Targets and Delivery. Approaches, Methods and Applications*, Nastruzzi, C. (Ed.). CRC Press, Boca Raton, FL, **2005** pp. 127–142.
120 T. de Vringer, H. A. de Ronde. Preparation and structure of a water-in-oil cream containing lipid nanoparticles. *J. Pharm. Sci.* **1995**, *84*, 466–472.
121 A. Rolland, N. Wagner, A. Chatelus, B. Shroot, H. Schaefer. Site-specific drug delivery to pilosebaceous structures using polymeric microspheres. *Pharm. Res.* **1993**, *10*, 1738–1744.
122 V. Jenning, G. E. Hildebrand, A. Gysler, R. H. Müller, M. Schäfer-Korting, S. Gohla. Solid lipid nanoparticles (SLN™) for topical application: occlusive properties. *Proc. Int. Symp. Control. Release Bioact. Mater.* **1999**, 405–406.
123 V. Jenning, A. F. Thunemann, S. H. Gohla. Characterisation of a novel solid lipid nanoparticle carrier system based on binary mixtures of liquid and solid lipids. *Int. J. Pharm.* **2000**, *199*, 167–177.
124 K. Westesen, H. Bunjes, M. H. J. Koch. Physicochemical characterization of lipid nanoparticles and evalua-

tion of their drug loading capacity and sustained release potential. *J. Control. Release* **1997**, *48*, 223–236.

125 K. Westesen, B. Siekmann. Investigation of the gel formation of phospholipid-stabilized solid lipid nanoparticles. *Int. J. Pharm.* **1997**, *151*, 35–45.

126 S. A. Wissing, R. H. Müller. Cosmetic applications for solid lipid nanoparticles (SLN). *Int. J. Pharm.* **2003**, *254*, 65–68.

127 S. A. Wissing, R. H. Müller. A novel sunscreen system based on tocopherol acetate incorporated into solid lipid nanoparticles. *Int. J. Cosmet. Sci.* **2001**, *23*, 233–243.

128 C. Song, S. Liu. A new healthy sunscreen system for human: solid lipid nannoparticles as carrier for 3,4,5-trimethoxybenzoylchitin and the improvement by adding Vitamin E. *Int. J. Biol. Macromol.* **2005**, *36*, 116–119.

129 P. Couvreur, B. Kante, M. Roland, P. Goit, P. Bauduin, P. Speiser. Polycyanoacrylate nanocapsules as potential lysosomotropic carriers: preparation, morphology and sorptive properties. *J. Pharm. Pharmacol.* **1979**, *31*, 331–332.

130 P. Couvreur, M. Roland, P. Speiser. Biodegradable submicroscopic particles containing a biologically active substance. *US patent 4,329,332*, **1982**.

131 C. Chavany, T. Le Doan, P. Couvreur, F. Puisieux, C. Helene. Polyalkylcyanoacrylate nanoparticles as polymeric carriers for antisense oligonucleotides. *Pharm. Res.* **1992**, *9*, 441–449.

132 C. E. Soma, C. Dubernet, D. Bentolila, S. Benita, P. Couvreur. Reversion of multidrug resistance by co-encapsulation of doxorubicin and cyclosporin A in polyalkylcyanoacrylate nanoparticles. *Biomaterials* **2000**, *21*, 1–7.

133 K. Krauel, T. Pitaksuteepong, N. M. Davies, T. Rades. Entrapment of bioactive molecules in poly(alkylcyanoacrylate) nanoparticles. *Am. J. Drug Del.* **2004**, *2*, 251–259.

134 F. Lescure, C. Seguin, P. Breton, P. Bourrinet, D. Roy, P. Couvreur. Preparation and characterization of novel poly(methylidene malonate 2.1.2.)-made nanoparticles. *Pharm. Res.* **1994**, *11*, 1270–1277.

135 J. Kreuter. *Colloidal Drug Delivery Systems*. Marcel Dekker, New York, **1994**.

136 C. Vauthier-Holtzscherer, S. Benabbou, G. Spenlehauer, M. Veillard, P. Couvreur. Methodology for the preparation of ultra-dispersed polymer systems. *STP Pharm. Sci.* **1991**, *1*, 109–16.

137 M. Gallardo, G. Couarraze, B. Denizot, L. Treupel, P. Couvreur, F. Puisieux. Study of the mechanisms of formation of nanoparticles and nanocapsules of polyisobutyl-2-cyanoacrylate. *Int. J. Pharm.* **1993**, *100*, 55–64.

138 S. Watnasirichaikul, T. Rades, I. G. Tucker, N. M. Davies. Effects of formulation variables on characteristics of poly(ethylcyanoacrylate) nanocapsules prepared from w/o microemulsions. *Int. J. Pharm.* 1–2, **2002**, *235*, 237–246.

139 T. Pitaksuteepong, N. M. Davies, I. G. Tucker, T. Rades. Factors influencing the entrapment of hydrophilic compounds in nanocapsules prepared by interfacial polymerisation of water-in-oil microemulsions. *Eur. J. Pharm. Biopharm.* **2002**, *53*, 335–342.

140 L. Mu, S. Feng. Vitamin E TPGS used as emulsifier in the solvent evaporation/extraction technique for fabrication of polymeric nanospheres for controlled release of paclitaxel (Taxol®). *J. Control. Release* **2002**, *80*, 129–144.

141 R. Gref, P. Quellec, A. Sanchez, P. Calvo, E. Dellacherie, M. J. Alonso. Development and characterization of CyA-loaded poly(lactic acid)–poly(ethylene glycol) PEG micro- and nanoparticles. Comparison with conventional PLA particulate carriers. *Eur. J. Pharm. Biopharm.* **2001**, *51*, 111–118.

142 I. Gutierro, R. M. Hernández, M. Igartua, A. R. Gascón, J. L. Pedraz. Size dependent immune response after subcutaneous, oral and intranasal

administration of BSA loaded nanospheres. *Vaccine* **2002**, *21*, 67–77.
143 S. Freitas, G. Hielscher, H. P. Merkle, B. Gander. Continuous contact- and contamination-free ultrasonic emulsification – a useful toll for pharmaceutical development and production. *Ultrason. Sonochem.* **2006**, *13*, 76–85.
144 J. C. Leroux, E. Alléman, E. Doelker, R. Gurny. New approach for the preparation of nanoparticles by an emulsification-diffusion method. *Eur. J. Pharm. Biopharm.* **1995**, *41*, 14–18.
145 C. Brindschaedler, R. Gurny, A. W. Doelker. Process for preparing a powder of water-insoluble polymer which can be redispersed in a liquid phase, the resulting powder and utilization thereof. *Patent WO 88/08011*, **1988**.
146 H. Fessi, J. P. Devissaguet, F. Puisieux, C. Thies. Procédé de préparation de systèmes colloidaux dispersibles d'une susbstance sous forme de nanaoparticles. *French Patent 2,608,988*, **1986**.
147 J. Molpeceres, M. Guzman, M. R. Aberturas, M. Chacon, L. Berges. Application of central composite deigns to the preparation of polycaprolactone nanocapsules. *J. Pharm. Sci.* **1996**, *85*, 206–213.
148 N. Csaba, L. González, A. Sánchez, M. J. Alonso. Design and characterization of new nanoparticulate polymer blends for drug delivery. *J. Biomater. Sci. Polym. Ed.* **2004**, *15*, 1137–1151.
149 J. M. Barrichello, M. Morishita, K. Takayama, T. Nagai. Encapsulation of hydrophilic and lipophilic drugs in PLGA nanoparticles by the nanoprecipitation method. *Drug Dev. Ind. Pharm.* **1999**, *25*, 471–476.
150 J. Davda, V. Labhasetwar. An update on angiogenesis therapy. *Crit. Rev. Eukaryot. Gene Expr.* **2001**, *11*, 1–21.
151 J. Davda, V. Labhasetwar. Sustained proangiogenic activity of vascular endothelial growth factor following encapsulation in nanoparticles. *J. Biomed. Nanotech.* **2005**, *1*, 74–82.
152 Y. Chung, G. Tae, S. H. Yuk. A facile method to prepare heparin-funcionalized nanoparticles for controlled release of growth factors. *Biomaterials* **2006**, in press.
153 A. Kozlowski, J. M. Harris. Improvements in protein PEGylation: pegylated interferons for treatment of hepatitis C. *J. Control. Release* **2001**, *72*, 217–224.
154 J. L. Cleland, A. J. S. Jones. Stable formulations of recombinant human growth hormone and interferon-gamma for microencapsulation in biodegradable microspheres. *Pharm. Res.* **1996**, *13*, 1464–1475.
155 A. Sánchez, M. Tobío, L. González, A. Fabra, M. J. Alonso. Biodegradable micro- and nanoparticles as long-term delivery vehicles for interferon-alpha. *Eur. J. Pharm. Sci.* **2003**, *18*, 221–229.
156 G. P. Carino, J. S. Jacob, E. Mathiowitz. Nanosphere based oral insulin delivery. *J. Control. Release* **2000**, *65*, 261–269.
157 Y. Kawashima, H. Yamamoto, H. Takeuchi, S. Fujioka, T. Hino. Pulmonary delivery of insulin with nebulized DL-lactide/glycolide copolymer (PLGA) nanospheres to prolong hypoglycemic effect. *J. Control. Release* **1999**, *62*, 279–287.
158 D. A. Norris, P. J. Sinko. Effect of size, surface charge and hydrophobicity on the translocation of polyestyrene microspheres through gastrointestinal mucin. *J. Appl. Polym. Sci.* **1997**, *63*, 1481–1492.
159 A. M. Hillery, A. T. Florence. The effect of adsorbed poloxamer 188 and 407 surfactants on the intestinal uptake of 60-nm polystyrene particles after oral administration in the rat. *Int. J. Pharm.* **1996**, *132*, 123–154.
160 S. K. Sahoo, J. Panyam, S. Prabha, V. Labhasetwar. Residual polyvinyl alcohol associated with poly(D,L-lactide-*co*-glycolide) nanoparticles affects their physical properties and cellular uptake. *J. Control. Release* **2002**, *82*, 105–114.
161 H. Takeuchi, H. Yamamoto, Y. Kawashima. Mucoadhesive nano-

particulate systems for peptide drug delivery. *Adv. Drug Deliv. Rev.* **2001**, *47*, 39–54.

162 A. Vila, M. Sanchez, M. Tobío, P. Calvo, M. J. Alonso. Design of biodegradable particles for protein delivery. *J. Control. Release* **2002**, *78*, 15–24.

163 W. U. Kim, W. K. Lee, J. W. Ryoo, S. H. Kim, J. Kim, J. Youn, S. Y. Min, E. Y. Bae, S. Y. Hwang, S. H. Park, C. S. Cho, J. S. Park, H. Y. Kim. Suppression of collagen-induced arthritis by single administration of poly(lactic-*co*-glycolic acid) nanoparticles entrapping type II collagen: a novel strategy for induction of oral tolerance. *Arthritis Rheum.* **2002**, *46*, 1109–1120.

164 W. Lee, J. Park, S. Jung, Ch. Yang, W. Kim, H. Kim, J. Park, J. Park. Preparation and characterization of biodegradable nanoparticles entrapping immunodominant peptide conjugated with PEG for oral tolerance induction. *J. Control. Release* **2005**, *105*, 77–88.

165 P. Elamanchili, M. Diwan, M. Cao, J. Samuel. Characterization of poly(D,L-lactic-*co*-glycolic acid) based nanoparticulate system for enhanced delivery of antigens to dendritic cells. *Vaccine* **2004**, *22*, 2406–2412.

166 M. J. Shephard, D. Todd, B. M. Adair, A. L. W. Po, D. P. Mackie, E. M. Scott. Immunogenicity of bovine parainfluenza type 3 virus proteins encapsulated in nanoparticle vaccines, following intranasal administration to mice. *Res. Vet. Sci*, **2003**, *74*, 187–190.

167 A. M. Carcaboso, R. M. Hernández, M. Igartua, J. E. Rosas, M. E. Patarroyo, J. L. Pedraz. Potent, long lasting systemic antibody levels and mixed T_h1/T_h2 immune response after nasal immunization with malaria antigen loaded PLGA microparticles. *Vaccine* **2004**, *22*, 1423–1432.

168 A. K. Coolí, H. O. Alpar. Potential use of nanoparticles for transcutaneous vaccine delivery: effect of particle size and charge. *Int. J. Pharm.* **2004**, *275*, 13–17.

169 N. L. Letvin, B. R. Bloom, S. L. Hoffman. Prospects for vaccines to protect against AIDS, tuberculosis and malaria. *J. Am. Med. Ass.* **2001**, *285*, 606–611.

170 J. M. Brewer, M. Conacher, C. A. Hunter, M. Mohrs, F. Brombacher, J. Alexander. Aluminum hydroxide adjuvant initiates strong antigen-specific T_h2 responses in the absence of IL-4- or IL-13-mediated signaling. *J. Immunol.* **1999**, *163*, 6448–54.

171 T. R. Mosmann, R. L. Coffman. T_H1 and T_H2 cells: different patterns of lymphokine secretion lead to different functional properties. *Annu. Rev. Immunol.* **1989**, *7*, 145–73.

172 R. K. Gupta, E. H. Relyveld, E. B. Lindblad, B. Bizzini, S. Ben-Efraim, C. K. Gupta. Adjuvants – a balance between toxicity and adjuvanticity. *Vaccine* **1993**, *11*, 293–306.

173 I. Schöll, A. Weissenböck, E. Förster-Waldl, E. Untersmayr, F. Walter, M. Willheim, G. Boltz-Nitulescu, O. Scheiner, F. Gaborw, E. Jensen-Jarolim. Allergen-loaded biodegradable poly(D,L-lactic-*co*-glycolic) acid nanoparticles down-regulate an ongoing T_h2 response in the BALB/c mouse model. *Clin. Exp. Allergy* **2004**, *34*, 315–321.

174 M. Diwan, M. Tafaghodi, J. Samuel. Enhancement of immune responses by co-delivery of a CpG oligodeoxynucleotide and tetanus toxoid in biodegradable nanospheres *J. Control. Release* **2002**, *85*, 247–262.

175 C. S. W. Chong, M. Cao, W. W. Wong, K. P. Fischer, W. R. Addison, G. S. Kwon, D. L. Tyrell, J. Samuel. Enhancement of T helper type 1 immune responses against hepatitis B virus core antigen by PLGA nanoparticle vaccine delivery. *J. Control. Release* **2005**, *102*, 85–99.

11
Intelligent Hydrogels in Nanoscale Sensing and Drug Delivery Applications

J. Zach Hilt

11.1
Introduction

This chapter highlights recent activities in the field of intelligent hydrogels, specifically in sensing and drug delivery micro/nanotechnologies. This is a relatively undeveloped field, but there is high promise and interest in the area, which has led to rapid growth. Here, some selected examples of the cutting-edge research being conducted are presented and, where appropriate, the reader is directed to key reviews within the field. In the past, numerous research groups have utilized hydrogels as functional components in biomedical applications, such as in biomaterials and biosensors, but only recently have hydrogels begun to be applied at the micro/nanoscale.

Example applications of hydrogels at the small scale include work by Ito and collaborators [1–3] patterning pH-sensitive and thermosensitive hydrogels for potential use in various microdevices. In other studies by Matsuda and coworkers [4–8], hydrogels have been micropatterned using a surface polymerization technique to create regions with different physicochemical properties to control the direction of cell adhesion and cellular behavior. In addition, Peppas and coworkers micropatterned poly(ethylene glycol) (PEG)-based hydrogels for application in biomedical devices [9]. Several other groups have focused on developing microdevices utilizing the mechanical response of environmentally sensitive hydrogels for microactuation. Beebe and coworkers [10, 11] have micropatterned pH-responsive hydrogels inside microfluidic channels to create flow controls that could respond to the ambient environmental conditions.

The application of intelligent hydrogels in micro/nanoscale sensing and drug delivery applications are highlighted within this chapter. First, in Section 11.2, the field of intelligent hydrogels is introduced and several example systems are highlighted, including ionic, temperature responsive, biohybrid and imprinted hydrogels. Section 11.3 focuses on sensor applications of intelligent hydrogels. Section 11.4 introduces drug delivery applications of intelligent hydrogels, such as in microfabricated devices and nanoscale structures.

Nanotechnologies for the Life Sciences Vol. 10
Nanomaterials for Medical Diagnosis and Therapy. Edited by Challa S. S. R. Kumar

ISBN: 978-3-527-31390-7

11.2
Intelligent Hydrogels

The molecular structure of polymer networks can be designed to result in preprogrammed and intelligent interactions with their environment. Of particular interest, environmentally responsive hydrogels have been synthesized that are capable of sensing and responding to changes to external stimuli such as changes to the pH, specific analytes and temperature, and recent reviews have highlighted the extensive research focused on developing new and applying current environmentally sensitive hydrogels [12–15]. The response mechanism of these hydrogel systems results from the chemical structure of the polymer network, such as the functionality of side-chain groups, branches and crosslinks.

11.2.1
Ionic Hydrogels

In ionic hydrogels containing weakly acidic or basic pendent groups, differentials in water sorption can result from ionization of these pendent groups depending on the solution pH and ionic composition. In the ionized state, these hydrogels act as semipermeable membranes to the counterions influencing the osmotic balance between the hydrogel and the external solution through ion exchange, depending on ion–ion interactions. For ionic gels containing weakly acidic pendent groups, the equilibrium degree of swelling increases as the pH of the external solution increases, while the degree of swelling increases as the pH decreases for gels containing weakly basic pendent groups.

11.2.2
Temperature-responsive Hydrogels

Temperature-responsive hydrogels are some of the most widely studied responsive hydrogel systems, with most systems based on poly(*N*-isopropyl acrylamide) (PNIPAAm) and its derivatives. The response to changes in temperature is due to a reversible volume-phase transition with a change in the temperature and these systems have been studied for a variety of applications, including in drug delivery and tissue engineering [13, 16]. This type of behavior is related to polymer phase separation as the temperature is raised above a critical value known as the lower critical solution temperature (LCST), e.g. PNIPAAm exhibits a LCST around 33 °C. Networks showing lower critical miscibility temperature are in a collapsed state above the LCST and the networks swell upon lowering the temperature below the LCST.

11.2.3
Biohybrid Hydrogels

Biohybrid hydrogels can be created by integrating biological entities with synthetic hydrogels, and these systems have the potential to synergistically combine the well-evolved biological mechanisms (e.g. high affinity and specificity of binding) and the tailorable hydrogel properties (e.g. mechanical stability and environmentally responsive nature). For example, research groups have immobilized enzymes within the network structure of hydrogels. Activated glucose oxidase has been incorporated into pH-sensitive cationic hydrogels. The glucose oxidase converts glucose into gluconic acid, lowering the pH of the local environment and causing the hydrogel network to swell in the case of a cationic gel [17]. In other work, Miyata and coworkers [18] prepared biohybrid hydrogels containing grafted antigen and corresponding antibody within the hydrogel network and demonstrated these systems to be responsive to a specific antigen. Furthermore, Wang and coworkers [19] have prepared hybrid hydrogels containing hydrophilic monomers and coiled-coil protein domains, which were demonstrated to exhibit a temperature-dependent swelling response based on the change in protein structure.

11.2.4 Imprinted Hydrogels

Another class of intelligent hydrogels is based on molecularly imprinted polymers (MIPs), which are prepared using template-mediated polymerization techniques that create recognition domains able to specifically bind template molecules with high affinity. Although MIPs have been studied for more than three decades, imprinted hydrogel systems have only recently gained attention [20–23]. These systems are designed and synthesized to create chemical functionality and structure that is organized in a precise three-dimensional configuration, and these have potential application where controlled recognition properties to various biological analytes and physiological processes are required.

11.3 Sensor Applications

By tailoring the response properties of hydrogel systems, they can be optimized for application in sensor devices. In particular, environmentally responsive hydrogels have been applied as sensing elements for development of novel sensor platforms. For example, hydrogels have been utilized as actuation elements where the mechanical response of the network was applied to actuate various transduction elements. In other examples, hydrogel matrices have been used for optical sensing platforms and electrical sensing platforms. In the following, selected examples are highlighted.

11.3.1 Actuation Detection

The mechanical response of hydrogels resulting from network swelling with changes in ambient environmental conditions can be used to actuate a transducing element to create a sensor platform. For example, Grimes and coworkers [24, 25] demonstrated wireless pH sensors utilizing the actuation response of pH-responsive hydrogels integrated with magnetoelastic thick films. The sensor device functioned by monitoring the change in resonance frequency due to applied mass load of the magnetoelastic sensor device. In other research, Han and coworkers [26] demonstrated a constant-volume hydrogel osmometer as a novel sensor platform. The concept was illustrated with a device where a pH-responsive hydrogel was confined between a rigid semipermeable membrane and the diaphragm of a miniature pressure sensor, where changes in the osmotic swelling pressure of the hydrogel resulting from changes pH were accurately measured via the pressure sensor. Although the device was of macroscale in dimensions, the design can be easily miniaturized for microscale or even nanoscale sensor development.

Recently, microelectromechanical system (MEMS) sensor platforms have been applied in a wide variety of applications. Gerlach and coworkers [27] developed piezoresistive sensors which measured the swelling of hydrogel systems by monitoring the deflection of the silicon membrane within the sensor chip (Fig. 11.1). Specifically, two systems, i.e. a network based on a poly(vinyl alcohol) (PVA) and poly(acrylic acid) (PAA) blend and a network based on PNIPAAm, were applied in

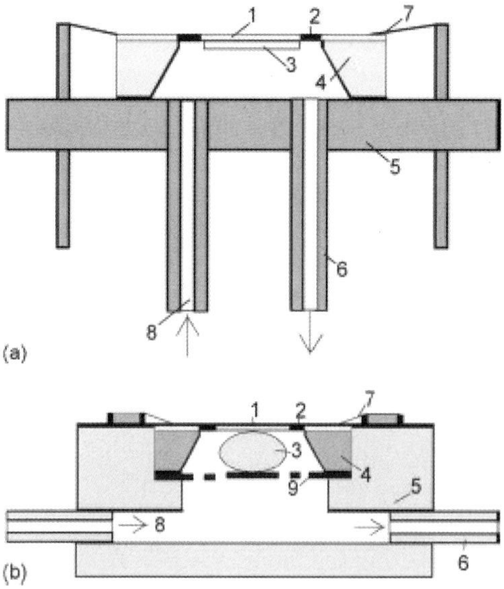

Figure 11.1. Operational principle of hydrogel-based sensors: (a) with PVA/PAA hydrogel layer, deposited onto the bending plate and (b) with PNIPAAm foil piece in a cavity. (1) Bending plate; (2) mechano-electrical transducer (piezoresistive bridge); (3) swellable hydrogel; (4) Si chip; (5) socket; (6) tube; (7) interconnect; (8) solution; (9) grate [27].

this sensor platform to develop pH and organic solvent concentration sensors, respectively. In other work, a MEMS sensor based on a capacitive pressure sensing technique and an uncrosslinked poly(2-hydroxyethyl methacrylate) (PHEMA) hydrophilic polymer was demonstrated [28]. An inductor–capacitor (LC) LC circuit was utilized to enable wireless detection of the sensor response.

MEMS sensor platforms based on micro/nanocantilevers have also been of high interest, as a result of their ultrahigh sensitivity. For example, environmentally responsive hydrogels have been integrated with silicon microcantilevers to develop an ultrasensitive bioMEMS sensor platform (Fig. 11.2). Specifically, a pH microsensor was demonstrated based on a methacrylic acid based pH-responsive hydrogel [29, 30] and this was the first demonstration of a microscale MEMS sensor device where actuation is controlled by an intelligent polymer network. In similar work, Thundat and coworkers [31] have demonstrated a variation on this sensor platform by integrating hydrogels responsive to CrO_4^{2-} with commercial silicon microcantilevers to create CrO_4^{2-} sensors. More recently, another variation has been demonstrated where hydrogels containing benzo-18-crown-6 coated on microcantilevers to create Pb^{2+} sensors [32].

In other research, Richter and collaborators [33] investigated the suitability of a quartz crystal microbalance as a transducer element for hydrogel-based liquid sensors. A blend of PAA and PVA was polymerized onto the sensor surface, and the system was demonstrated to have response time of 500 ms for a pH change from 1.8 to 3.1. Ionic hydrogels, microparticles [34] and thin films [35, 36] have also been applied for the detection of CO_2 gas by measuring the pH decrease that occurs when CO_2 diffuses through a gas-permeable membrane and into an electrolyte solution. A commercially available pressure sensor was used for the transduction of the swelling event and a schematic of the device is included in Fig. 11.3.

11.3.2
Optical Detection

There have been various optical-based detection schemes applied to hydrogel-based systems, and a few of these are highlighted in the following. For example, researchers have demonstrated a multianalyte hydrogel biosensor array platform which consists of analyte specific features that are indexed by shape [37]. The platform was based on lithographically patterned PEG diacrylates that contained biomolecules for oligonucleotide and cell-based sensing applications.

In other research, McShane and coworkers have developed a novel hydrogel microsphere sensor platform based on polyelectrolyte-coated calcium alginate microspheres (Fig. 11.4) [38, 39]. In particular, glucose oxidase was encapsulated with an oxygen-quenched ruthenium compound, allowing for the detection of glucose concentrations. The polyelectrolyte multilayer films were nanoscale in thickness (around 10–100 nm), and were used to stabilize enzyme entrapment and control of substrate diffusion.

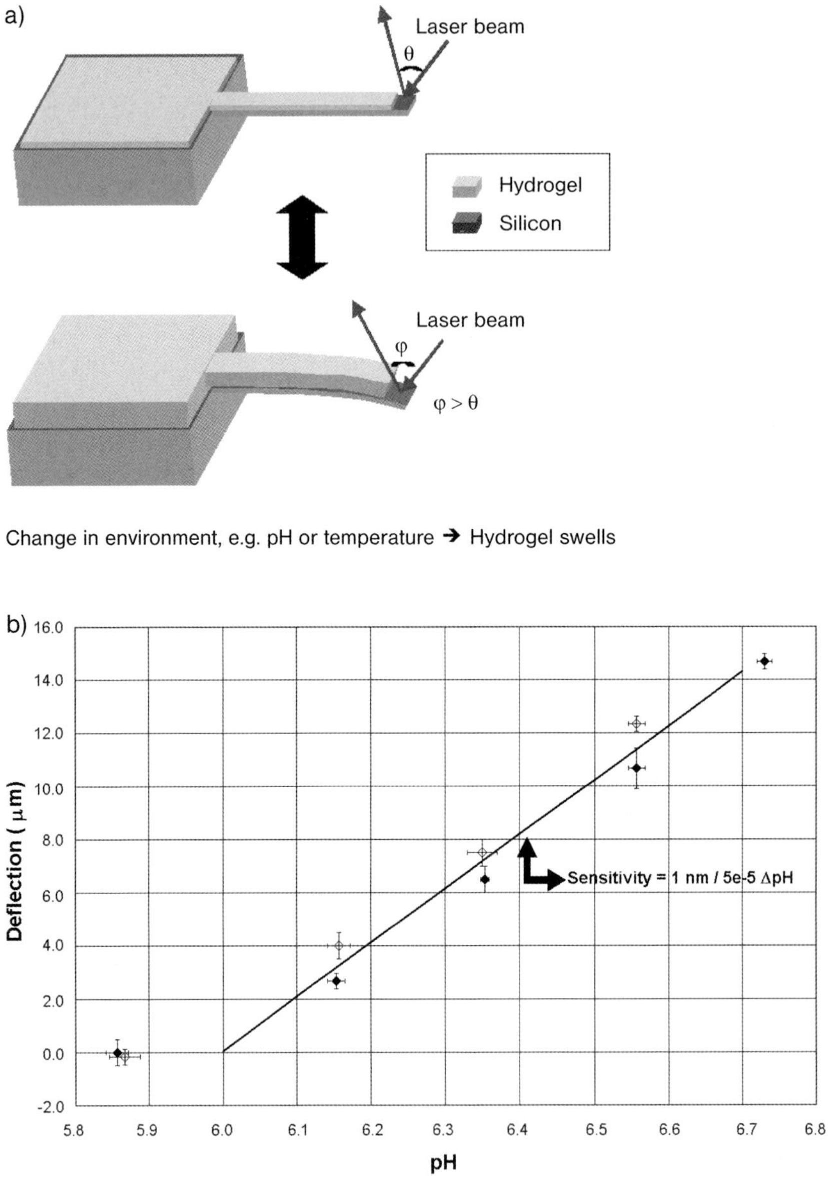

Figure 11.2. Hydrogel as a sensing element in a bioMEMS sensor platform. (a) A schematic of the bioMEMS sensor platform based on a microcantilever patterned with an environmentally responsive hydrogel. (b) A detailed examination of the equilibrium bending response versus pH (constant ionic strength of 0.5 M) is shown [30].

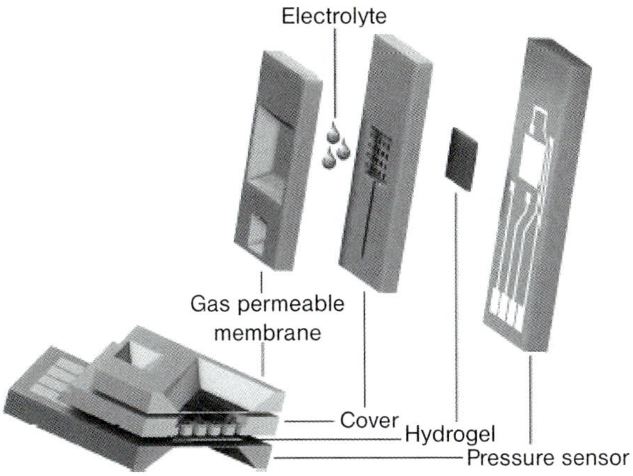

Figure 11.3. Cross-section and exploded view of the hydrogel-based CO2 sensor [35] (permission pending).

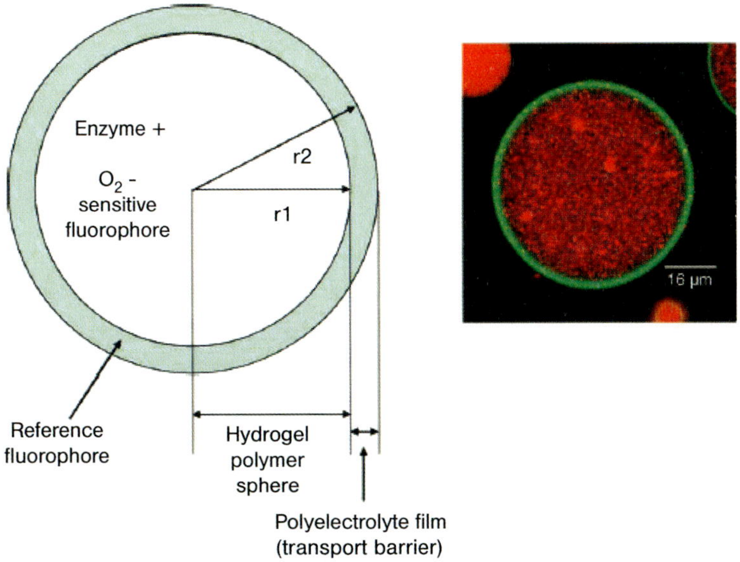

Figure 11.4. Illustration of nanoengineered microsphere optical glucose sensors. (a) A functional schematic of the microsphere sensor. (b) Confocal laser scanning micrograph of an actual prototype glucose sensor (red fluorescence = O_2 indicator in alginate microsphere, green fluorescence = reference fluorescence in polyelectrolyte film) [39].

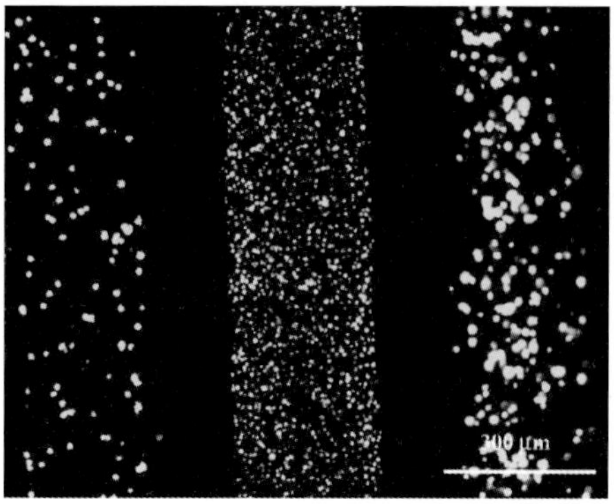

Figure 11.5. A multiphenotypic microdevice containing (left to right) hepatocytes, macrophages and endothelial cells stained with calcein AM [41].

Other researchers have applied hydrogels microstructures as three-dimensional scaffolds for the encapsulation of living cells [40–42], and these structures have potential advantages in the development of cell-based sensors for detecting chemical and biological toxins, and for assaying cellular responses to target compounds (e.g. drug screening). For example, a multiphenotypic whole-cell microsensor platform (Fig. 11.5) was demonstrated that could monitor cell viability via optical methods [41]. This platform enabled the comparison of the toxic effect of concanavalin A on macrophages and hepatocytes relative to the relatively unaffected endothelial cells.

By incorporating enzymes within hydrogel networks, biosensing elements can be fabricated. These biohybrid structures can be advantageous by allowing the precise control over the micro/nanoenvironment of the enzymes. In addition, these biohybrid structures can be patterned at the micro/nanoscale, allowing for their integration into sensor devices [43–45]. Pishko and coworkers [43, 44] have applied photolithography techniques to pattern hydrogel arrays containing immobilized enzymes, such as alkaline phosphatase, acetylcholinesterase and urease. The enzymes were conjugated to pH-sensitive fluorophores, allowing for optical detection of the changes in microenvironment pH due to the enzyme-catalyzed reactions. In addition, Crooks and coworkers [45] have demonstrated a microfluidic biosensor based on arrays of hydrogel-entrapped enzymes (micropatches). This platform was applied to simultaneously detect different concentrations of the same analyte (e.g. glucose) and multiple analytes in real time (Fig. 11.6).

Nanoscale probes encapsulated by biologically localized embedding (PEBBLEs) have been developed by Kopelmann and collaborators [46], and these sensing and imaging probes range from 20 to 600 nm in diameter, and are often constructed of hydrogel networks (e.g. polyacrylamide). For information on recent activities in this area, the reader is referred to a recent review of the topic [46].

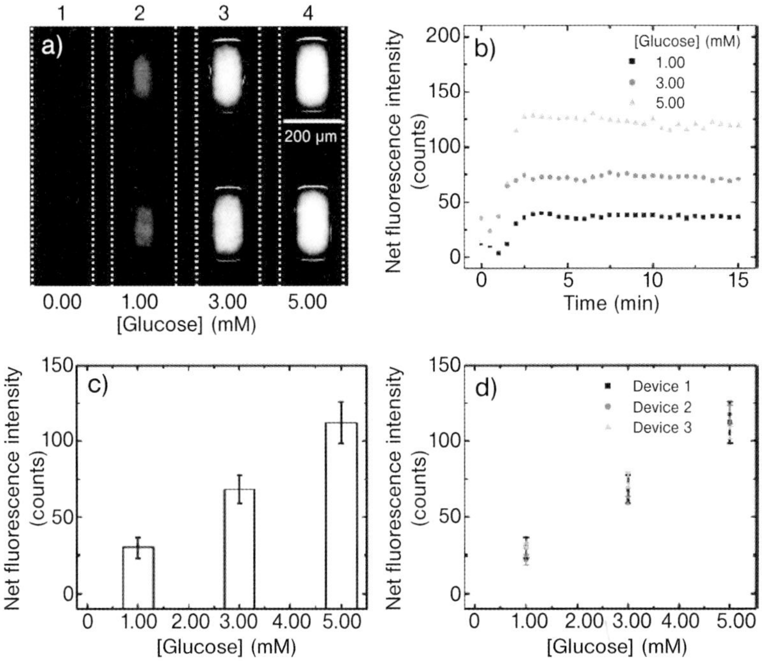

Figure 11.6. Biosensor based on hydrogel-containing microchannels. (a) Fluorescence micrograph obtained 15 min after solutions containing 0.10 mM Amplex Red plus different concentrations of glucose (shown at the bottom of each channel) were introduced into each of the four channels. The flow rate was 1.0 $\mu L\ min^{-1}$. Each micropatch contained both glucose oxidase and hydrogen peroxidase. The fluorescence emission was integrated for 0.7 s. The dashed white lines indicate the positions of channel walls. (b) Time-dependent net fluorescence intensity profiles collected from the hydrogel micropatches shown in the top row of (a). The net fluorescence intensity was obtained by subtracting the intensity of the micropatch in channel 1 (no glucose present) from the fluorescence intensities arising from the micropatches in channels 2–4. (c) Graph showing the average net fluorescence intensity as a function of the glucose concentration for the three micropatches present in each channel of the device shown in (a). The error bars represent 1σ for the three micropatches. (d) Plot of net fluorescence intensity as a function of glucose concentration for three independently prepared microfluidic devices. The error bars represent 1σ for the three micropatches in each channel of each device. Fluorescence micrographs were obtained with a Photometrics 16-bit gray scale CCD camera [45].

11.3.3 Electrical Detection

Several research groups have patterned biohybrid hydrogels containing immobilized oxidoreductase enzymes, such as glucose oxidase, lactate oxidase and alcohol oxidase, onto electrodes to create biosensors for monitoring various analyte levels [47–50]. For example, Jimenez and coworkers [50] fabricated enzymatic microsensors that employed polyacrylamide as a entrapment matrix for immobilization of enzyme recognition elements, including glucose oxidase and urease, that was patterned onto a pH-sensitive ion selective field-effect transistor (FET). In other work, Sheppard and coworkers developed miniature conductimetric pH sensors based on the measurement of the conductivity of pH-responsive hydrogels that were photolithographically patterned onto planar interdigitated electrode arrays [51–53]. The sensor monitored the changes in the electrical conductivity of the hydrogel membrane that resulted with its swelling/collapsing. In related work, Guiseppi-Elie and coworkers [54] demonstrated chemical and biological sensors that applied conducting electroactive hydrogel composites as recognition elements and utilized electrochemical detection.

In the above sensor applications, the majority of patterning applications of hydrogels have relied on UV photolithography and, thus, have been limited to microscale applications. For the application of hydrogels in nanoscale sensing applications, it is critical that nanopatterning techniques are developed, and this is a new area receiving much research attention. For example, Libera and coworkers [55] have applied electron-beam crosslinking methods to pattern amine-terminated PEG thin films on silicon substrates with lateral dimensions of order of 200 nm (Fig. 11.7). It was demonstrated that the amine groups remained functional after electron-beam exposure, enabling the covalent attachment of proteins of interest.

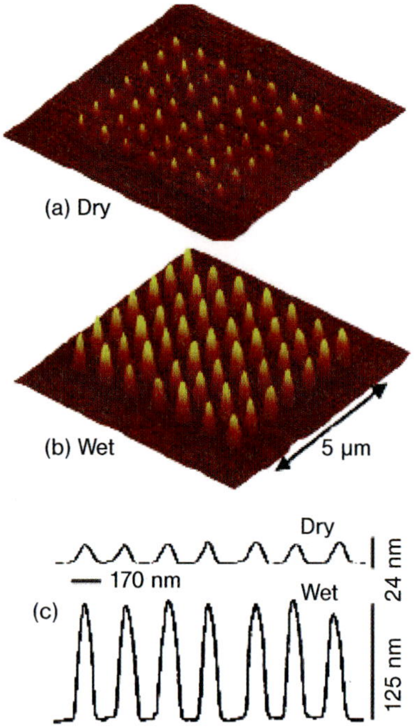

Figure 11.7. AFM images of a 5 μm × 5 μm array of amine-terminated PEG hydrogels with an inter-gel spacing of 715 nm. (A) Dry, (B) hydrated and (C) height profiles of a row of nanogels which swell by a factor exceeding 5 times [55].

11.4
Drug Delivery Applications

For the application of hydrogels as intelligent carriers in controlled drug delivery, researchers have optimized their properties by engineering their physical and chemical properties at the molecular level, such as permeability for sustained release applications, environmentally responsive nature for pulsatile release applications, surface functionality for targeted or stealth release (PEG coatings) and biodegradability for bioresorbable applications [12, 15, 56, 57]. In particular, environmentally responsive hydrogels have been applied in a wide variety of controlled drug delivery applications, since they allow for release that is controlled by the conditions of the environment. For example, temperature-responsive hydrogels have been widely used to create drug delivery systems exhibiting a pulsatile release profile in response to temperature changes [13, 16]. In addition, pH-responsive hydrogels have been applied in numerous controlled release applications, such as

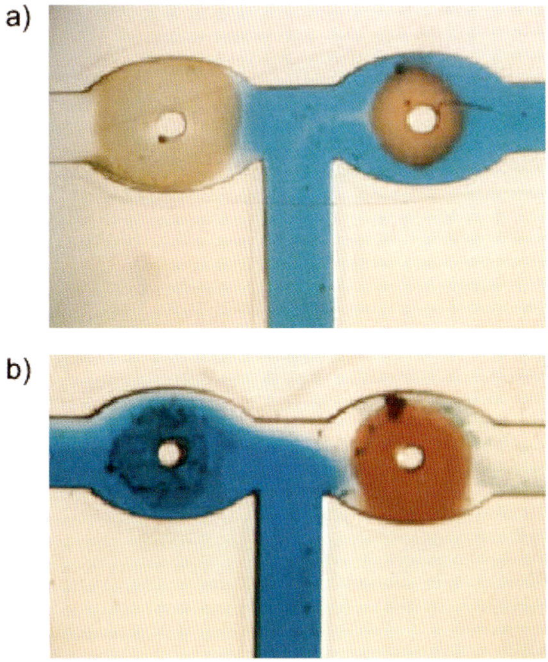

Figure 11.8. Two valves formed at a T-junction in a microfluidics device, one made of a gold–colloid nanocomposite hydrogel and the other a gold–nanoshell nanocomposite hydrogel. The channels are 100 μm wide. (a) When the entire device was illuminated with green light (532 nm, 1.6 W cm^{-2}), the gold colloid valves opened while the nanoshell valve remained closed. (b) However, when the device was illuminated with near infrared light (832 nm, 2.7 W cm^{-2}), the opposite response was observed. In both cases, the valves opened within 5 s [65].

PEG-containing ionic networks that have been applied for the oral delivery of proteins, including insulin [58, 59] and calcitonin [60, 61].

In therapeutic applications, polymeric micro/nanotechnologies have found widespread application in the form of implantable devices, functional particles and tissue engineering constructs. The reader is directed to Ref. [62] for detailed information on the application of hydrogel nanoparticles. In the following, the application of hydrogels as functional components of devices is highlighted, and there is also a brief mention of nanoshell hydrogel structures.

11.4.1 Micro/nanoscale Devices

In a recent review, polymeric systems for implantable drug delivery systems have been highlighted [63]. In recent years, several controlled drug delivery devices where a target release is controlled by hydrogel valves have been proposed [64–67]. Optomechanically responsive nanocomposite hydrogels have been developed based on poly(*N*-isopropylacrylamide-*co*-acrylamide) and particles with distinct and strong optical-absorption profiles (gold colloids and nanoshells) [64, 65]. These nanocomposite hydrogels were photopatterned as valves in a microfluidics device and their wavelength dependent actuation was demonstrated (Fig. 11.8). Recently, Daunert and collaborators [66] developed novel biohybrid hydrogel systems that exhibited stimuli responsive swelling due to Ca^{2+} and applied these as valves in a microdevice (Fig. 11.9). Madou and coworkers [67] developed electro-active polymers for application as microvalves potentially for controlled drug delivery.

11.4.2 Nanoscale Macromolecular Structures

In recent years, there has been increased interest in the practical application of organic chemistry, and its molecular-level control, for the preparation of nanostructured macromolecular structures with tailored properties and functions [68]. A prime example has been the work of Wooley and coworkers [69–72], where well-defined nanostructured materials have been created by organizing polymers into micellar assemblies followed by stabilization through intramolecular crosslinking of the chain segments that compose the polymer micelle shell [shell crosslinked knedel-like (SCK)]. In Fig. 11.10, a schematic of the synthetic approach for preparing SCK polymer assemblies is provided. These SCK nanostructures have great potential as nanoscale intelligent drug delivery carriers, such as their ability to be tailored to be entirely hydrophilic and responsive to environmental conditions [70], be functionalized for targeted drug delivery applications (e.g. cancer cell targeting) [71], and be mineralized on their surface to further control dissolution and permeability properties for controlled drug delivery applications [72].

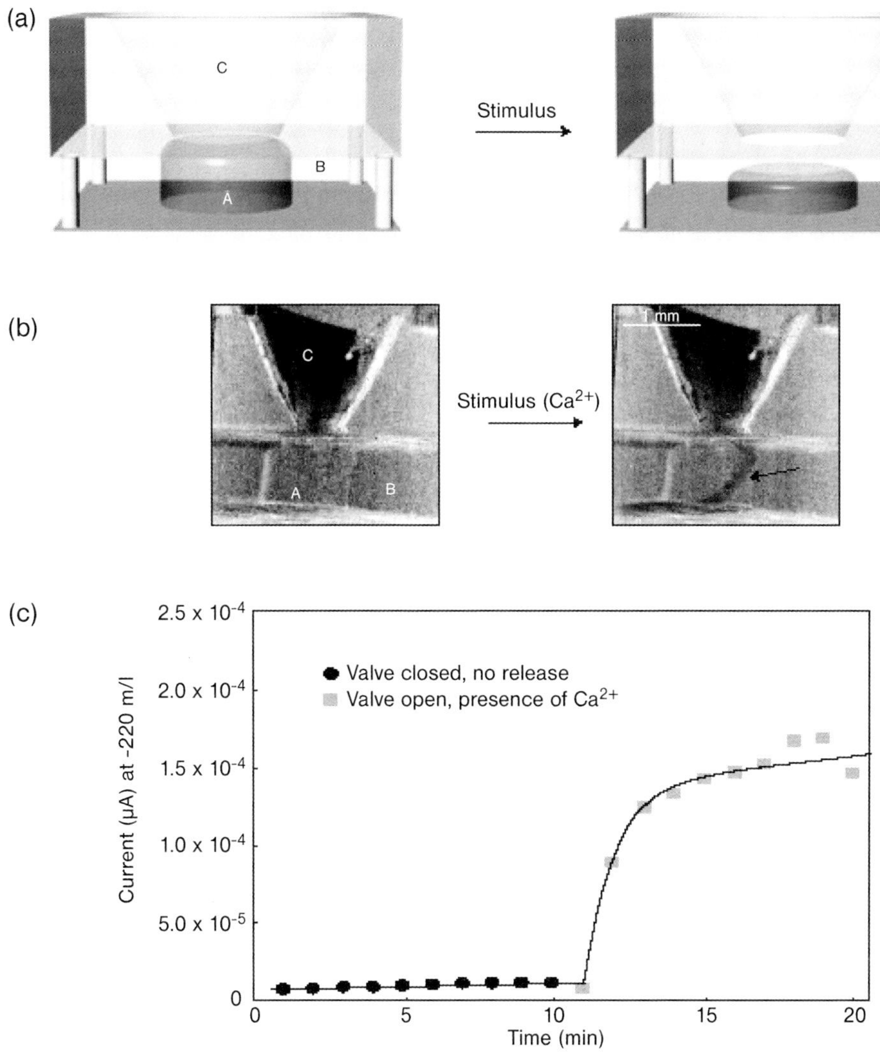

Figure 11.9. Incorporation of hydrogels in microfluidic systems. (a) Schematic of microactuator 'plunger' configuration. The stimuli-responsive hydrogel (A) shrinks in the presence of a stimulus in the bulk solution (B) allowing release from a reservoir (C). (b) The release of a solution containing blue dextran and an electrochemical probe [hexaamine ruthenium chloride(III)] in the presence of a stimulus (Ca^{2+}). Arrow denotes release plume. (c) Electrochemical response of probe during the release event [66].

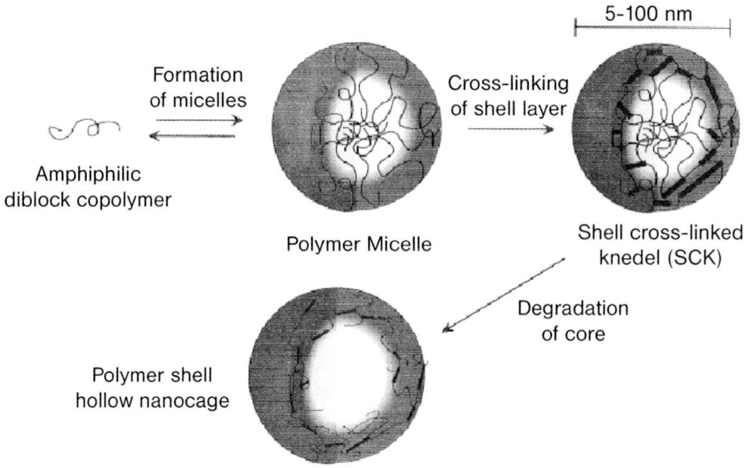

Figure 11.10. The general synthetic approach for the preparation of SCK polymer assemblies involves a combination of self-assembly and covalent stabilization, providing robust nanostructured materials from supramolecular, dynamic precursors [69].

11.5 Conclusions

This chapter has highlighted the recent activities in the field of intelligent hydrogels, with a focus on the applications in sensing and drug delivery micro/nanotechnologies. The field of intelligent hydrogels was introduced and several example systems (e.g. ionic, temperature-responsive, biohybrid and imprinted hydrogels) were highlighted. Selected sensor and drug delivery applications of intelligent hydrogels were introduced and briefly discussed. Although this is a new field, the potential is clear with many expected applications where intelligent hydrogel systems will positively impact the fields of sensing and drug delivery.

References

1 Ito, Y., Photolithographic synthesis of intelligent microgels. *J. Intell. Mater. Syst. Struct.* **1999**, *10*, 541–547.
2 Chen, G., Imanishi, Y., Ito, Y., Photolithographic synthesis of hydrogels. *Macromolecules* **1998**, *31*, 4379–4381.
3 Chen, G., Ito, Y., Imanishi, Y., Micropattern immobilization of a pH-sensitive polymer. *Macromolecules* **1997**, *30*, 7001–7003.
4 Nakayama, Y., Anderson, J., Matsuda, T., Laboratory-scale mass production of a multi-micropatterned grafted surface with different polymer regions. *J. Biomed. Mater. Res. (Appl. Biomater.)* **2000**, *53*, 584–591.
5 DeFife, K., Colton, E., Nakayama, Y., Matsuda, T., Anderson, J., Spatial regulation and surface chemistry control of monocyte/macrophage adhesion and foreign body giant cell

formation by photochemically micropatterned surfaces. *J. Biomed. Mater. Res.* **1999**, *45*, 148–154.

6 Higashi, J., Nakayama, Y., Marchant, R., Matsuda, T., High-spatioresolved microarchitectural surface prepared by photograft copolymerization using dithiocarbamate: surface preparation and cellular responses. *Langmuir* **1999**, *15*, 2080–2088.

7 Nakayama, Y., Nakamata, K., Hirano, Y., Goto, K., Matsuda, T., Surface hydrogelation of thiolated water-soluble copolymers on gold. *Langmuir* **1998**, *14*, 3909–3915.

8 Nakayama, Y., Matsuda, T., Surface macromolecular architectural designs using photo-graft copolymerization based on photochemistry of benzyl *N,N*-diethyldithiocarbamate. *Macromolecules* **1996**, *29*, 8622–8630.

9 Ward, J., Bashir, R., Peppas, N. A., Micropatterning of biomedical polymer surfaces by novel UV polymerization techniques. *J. Biomed. Mater. Res.* **2001**, *56*, 351–360.

10 Beebe, D. J., Moore, J. S., Bauer, J. M., Yu, Q., Liu, R. H., Devadoss, C., Jo, B., Functional hydrogel structures for autonomous flow control inside microfluidic channels. *Nature* **2000**, *404*, 588–590.

11 Beebe, D. J., Moore, J. S., Yu, Q., Liu, R. H., Kraft, M. L., Jo, B., Devadoss, C., Microfluidic tectonics: a comprehensive construction platform for microfluidic systems. *Proc. Natl Acad. Sci. USA* **2000**, *97*, 13488–13493.

12 Peppas, N. A., Bures, P., Leobandung, W., Ichikawa, H., Hydrogels in pharmaceutical formulations. *Eur. J. Pharm. Biopharm.* **2000**, *50*, 27–46.

13 Jeong, B., Kim, S., Bae, Y., Thermosensitive sol-gel reversible hydrogels. *Adv. Drug Deliver. Rev.* **2002**, *54*, 37–51.

14 Miyata, T., Uragami, T., Nakamae, K., Biomolecule-sensitive hydrogels. *Adv. Drug Deliver. Rev.* **2002**, *54*, 79–98.

15 van der Linden, H., Herber, S., Olthuis, W., Bergveld, P., Stimulus-sensitive hydrogels and their applications in chemical (micro)analysis. *Analyst* **2003**, *128*, 325–331.

16 Sershen, S., West, J., Implantable, polymeric systems for modulated drug delivery. *Adv. Drug Deliver. Rev.* **2002**, *54*, 1225–1235.

17 Podual, K., Doyle, F. J., Peppas, N. A., Glucose-sensitivity of glucose oxidase-containing cationic copolymer hydrogels having poly(ethylene glycol) grafts. *J. Control. Release* **2000**, *67*, 9–17.

18 Miyata, T., Asami, N., Uragami, T., A reversibly antigen-responsive hydrogel. *Nature* **1999**, *399*, 766–769.

19 Wang, C., Stewart, R. J., Kopecek, J., Hybrid hydrogels assembled from synthetic polymers and coiled-coil protein domains. *Nature* **1999**, *397*, 417–420.

20 Byrne, M. E., Oral, E., Hilt, J. Z., Peppas, N. A., Networks for recognition of biomolecules: Molecular imprinting and micropatterning poly(ethylene glycol)-containing films. *Polym. Adv. Technol.* **2002**, *13*, 798–816.

21 Peppas, N. A., Huang, Y., Polymers and gels as molecular recognition agents. *Pharm. Res.* **2002**, *19*, 578–587.

22 Byrne, M. E., Park, K., Peppas, N. A., Molecular imprinting within hydrogels. *Adv. Drug Deliver. Rev.* **2002**, *54*, 149–161.

23 Hilt, J. Z., Byrne, M. E., Configurational biomimesis in drug delivery: molecular imprinting of biologically significant molecules. *Adv. Drug Deliver. Rev.* **2004**, *56*, 1599–1620.

24 Ruan, C., Ong, K. G., Mungle, C., Paulose, M., Nickl, N. J., Grimes, C. A., A wireless pH sensor based on the use of salt-independent micro-scale polymer spheres. *Sensors Actuators B* **2003**, *96*, 61–69.

25 Ruan, C., Zeng, K., Grimes, C. A., A mass-sensitive pH sensor based on a stimuli-responsive polymer. *Anal. Chim. Acta* **2003**, *497*, 123–131.

26 Han, I., Han, M., Kim, J., Lew, S., Lee, Y. J., Horkay, F., Magda, J. J., Constant-volume hydrogel osmometer: a new device concept for miniature

biosensors. *Biomacromolecules* **2002**, *3*, 1271–1275.

27 Gerlach, G., Guenther, M., Sorber, J., Suchaneck, G., Arndt, K., and Richter, A., Chemical and pH sensors based on the swelling behavior of hydrogels. *Sensors Actuators B* **2005**, 111–112, 555–561.

28 Strong, S., Wang, A., McConaghy, C., Hydrogel-actuated capacitive transducer for wireless biosensors. *Biomed. Microdev.* **2002**, *4*, 97–103.

29 Bashir, R., Hilt, J. Z., Gupta, A., Elibol, O., Peppas, N. A., Micromechanical cantilever as an ultrasensitive pH microsensor. *Appl. Phys. Lett.* **2002**, *81*, 3091–3093.

30 Hilt, J. Z., Gupta, A. K., Bashir, R., Peppas, N. A., Ultrasensitive bioMEMS sensors based on microcantilevers patterned with environmentally responsive hydrogels. *Biomed. Microdev.* **2003**, *5*, 177–184.

31 Zhang, Y., Ji, H., Brown, G. M., Thundat, T., Detection of CrO_4^{2-} using a hydrogel swelling microcantilever sensor. *Anal. Chem.* **2003**, *75*, 4773–4777.

32 Liu, K., Ji, H., Detection of Pb^{2+} using a hydrogel swelling microcantilever sensor. *Anal. Sci.* **2004**, *20*, 9–11.

33 Richter, A., Bund, A., Keller, M., Arndt, K., Characterization of a microgravimetric sensor based on pH sensitive hydrogels. *Sensors Actuators B* **2004**, *99*, 579–585.

34 Herber, S., Olthuis, W., Bergveld, P., A swelling hydrogel-based P_{CO2} sensor. *Sensors Actuators. B* **2003**, *91*, 378–382.

35 Herber, S., Bomer, J., Olthuis, W., Bergveld, P., van den Berg, A., A miniaturized carbon dioxide gas sensor based on sensing of pH-sensitive hydrogel swelling with a pressure sensor. *Biomed. Microdev.* **2005**, *7*, 197–204.

36 Herber, S., Eijkel, J., Olthuis, W., Bergveld, P., van den Berg, A., Study of chemically induced pressure generation of hydrogels under isochoric conditions using a microfabricated device. *J. Chem. Phys.* **2004**, *121*, 2746–2751.

37 Meiring, J., Schmid, M., Grayson, S., Rathsack, B., Johnson, D., Kirby, R., Kannappan, R., Manthiram, K., Hsia, B., Hogan, Z., Ellington, A., Pishko, M., Willson, C., Hydrogel biosensor array platform indexed by shape. *Chem. Mater.* **2004**, *16*, 5574–5580.

38 Brown, J., Srivastava, R., McShane, M., Encapsulation of glucose oxidase and an oxygen-quenched fluorophore in polyelectrolyte-coated calcium aginate microspheres as optical glucose sensor systems. *Biosensors Bioelectron.* **2005**, *21*, 212–216.

39 Brown, J., McShane, M., Modeling of spherical fluorescent glucose microsensor systems: design of enzymatic smart tattoos. *Biosensors Bioelectron.* **2006**, *21*, 1760–1769.

40 Zguris, J., Itle, L., Koh, W., Pishko, M., A novel single-step fabrication technique to create heterogeneous poly(ethylene glycol) hydrogel microstructures containing multiple phenotypes of mammalian cells. *Langmuir* **2005**, *21*, 4168–4174.

41 Itle, L., Pishko, M., Multiphenotypic whole-cell sensor for viability screening. *Anal. Chem.* **2005**, *77*, 7887–7893.

42 Liu, V., Bhatia, S., Three-dimensional photopatterning of hydrogels containing living cells. *Biomed. Microdev.* **2002**, *4*, 257–266.

43 Yadavalli, V., Koh, W., Lazur, G., Pishko, M., Microfabricated protein-containing poly(ethylene glycol) hydrogel arrays for biosensing. *Sensors Actuators B* **2004**, *97*, 290–297.

44 Koh, W., Pishko, M., Immobilization of multi-enzyme microreactors inside microfluidic devices. *Sensors Actuators B* **2005**, *106*, 335–342.

45 Heo, J., Crooks, R., Microfluidic biosensor based on an array of hydrogel-entrapped enzymes. *Anal. Chem.* **2005**, *77*, 6843–6851.

46 Buck, S., Xu, H., Brasuel, M., Philbert, M., Kopelman, R., Nanoscale probes encapsulated by biologically localized embedding (PEBBLEs) for ion sensing and imaging in live cells. *Talanta* **2004**, *63*, 41–59.

47 Sirkar, K., Pishko, M. V., Amperometric biosensors based on oxidoreductases immobilized in photopolymerized poly(ethylene glycol) redox polymer hydrogels. *Anal. Chem.* **1998**, *70*, 2888–2894.

48 Munoz, A., Mas, R., Galan-Vidal, C. A., Dominiguez, C., Garcia-Raurich, J., Alegret, S., Thin-film microelectrodes for biosensing. *Quim. Anal.* **1999**, *18*, 155–157.

49 Jobst, G., Moser, I., Varahram, M., Svasek, P., Aschauer, E., Trajanoski, Z., Wach, P., Kotanko, P., Skrabal, F., Urban, G., Thin-film microbiosensors for glucose–lactate monitoring. *Anal. Chem.* **1996**, *68*, 3173–3179.

50 Jimenez, C., Bartrol, J., de Rooij, N. F., Koudelka, M., Use of photopolymerizable membranes based on polyacrylamide hydrogels for enzymatic microsensor construction. *Anal. Chim. Acta* **1997**, *351*, 169–176.

51 Sheppard, Jr., N. F., Lesho, M. J., McNally, P., Francomacaro, A. S., Microfabricated conductimetric pH sensor. *Sensors Actuators B* **1995**, *28*, 95–102.

52 Lesho, M. J., Sheppard, Jr., N. F., Adhesion of polymer films to oxidized silicon and its effect on performance of a conductometric pH sensor. *Sensors Actuators B* **1996**, *37*, 61–66.

53 Sheppard, Jr., N. F., Tucker, R. C., Salehi-Had, S., Design of a conductimetric pH microsensor based on reversibly swelling hydrogels. *Sensors Actuators B* **1993**, *10*, 73–77.

54 Brahim, S., Wilson, A. M., Narinesingh, D., Iwuoha, E., Guiseppi-Elie, A., Chemical and biological sensors based on electrochemical detection using conducting electroactive polymers. *Microchim. Acta* **2003**, *143*, 123–137.

55 Hong, Y., Krsko, P., Libera, M., Protein surface patterning using nanoscale PEG hydrogels. *Langmuir* **2004**, *20*, 11123–11126.

56 Peppas, N. A., Hydrogels and drug delivery. *Curr. Opin. Colloid* **1997**, *2*, 531–537.

57 Peppas, N. A., Wood, K. M., Blanchette, J. O., Hydrogels for oral delivery of therapeutic proteins. *Expert Opin. Biol. Ther.* **2004**, *4*, 881–887.

58 Lowman, A. M., Morishita, M., Kajita, M., Nagai, T., Peppas, N. A., Oral delivery of insulin using pH-responsive complexation gels. *J. Pharm. Sci.* **1999**, *88*, 933–937.

59 Morishita, M., Lowman, A. M., Takayama, K., Nagai, T., Peppas, N. A., Elucidation of the mechanism of incorporation of insulin in controlled release systems based on complexation polymers. *J. Control. Release* **2002**, *81*, 25–32.

60 Torres-Lugo, M., Garcia, M., Record, R., Peppas, N. A., Physicochemical behavior and cytotoxic effects of p(methacrylic acid-g-ethylene glycol) nanospheres for oral delivery of proteins. *J. Control. Release* **2002**, *80*, 197–205.

61 Torres-Lugo, M., Garcia, M., Record, R., Peppas, N. A., pH-sensitive hydrogels as gastrointestinal tract absorption enhancers: transport mechanisms of salmon calcitonin and other model molecules using the Caco-2 cell model. *Biotechnol. Prog.* **2002**, *18*, 612–616.

62 Nayak, S., Lyon, L., Soft nanotechnology with soft nanoparticles. *Angew. Chem. Int. Ed.* **2005**, *44*, 7686–7708.

63 Sershen, S., West, J., Implantable, polymeric systems for modulated drug delivery. *Adv. Drug Deliv. Rev.* **2002**, *54*, 1225–1235.

64 Sershen, S., Westcott, S., Halas, N., West, J., Temperature-sensitive polymer–nanoshell composites for photothermally modulated drug delivery. *J. Biomed. Mater. Res.* **2000**, *51*, 293–298.

65 Sershen, S., Mensing, G., Ng, M., Halas, N., Beebe, D., West, J., Independent optical control of microfluidic valves formed from optomechanically responsive nanocomposite hydrogels. *Adv. Mater.* **2005**, *17*, 1366–1368.

66 Ehrick, J., Deo, S., Browning, T., Bachas, L., Madou, M., Daunert, S., Genetically engineered protein in

hydrogels tailors stimuli-responsive characteristics. *Nat. Mater.* **2005**, *4*, 298–302.

67 Low, L., Seetharaman, S., He, K., Madou, M., Microactuators toward microvalves for responsive controlled drug delivery. *Sensors Actuators B* **2000**, *67*, 149–160.

68 Hawker, C., Wooley, K., The convergence of synthetic organic and polymer chemistries. *Science* **2005**, *309*, 1200–1205.

69 Wooley, K., Shell crosslinked polymer assemblies: nanoscale constructs inspired from biological systems. *J. Polym. Sci. A Polym. Chem.* **2000**, *38*, 1397–1407.

70 Ma, Q., Remsen, E., Kowalewski, T., Schaefer, J., Wooley, K., Environmentally-responsive, entirely hydrophilic, shell cross-linked (SCK) nanoparticles. *Nano Lett.* **2001**, *1*, 651–655.

71 Pan, D., Turner, J., Wooley, K., Folic acid-conjugated nanostructured materials designed for cancer cell targeting. *Chem. Commun.* **2003**, 2400–2401.

72 Perkin, K., Turner, J., Wooley, K., Mann, S., Fabrication of hybrid nanocapsules by calcium phosphate mineralization of shell cross-linked polymer micelles and nanocages. *Nano Lett.* **2005**, *5*, 1457–1461.

12 Nanoshells for Drug Delivery

Melgardt M. De Villiers and Yuri M. Lvov

12.1 Introduction

Nanomedicine, especially the field of nanopharmaceuticals (drugs and drug delivery systems), describes the preparation of nanoscale assemblies, which can be relatively simple nanoemulsions, nanoparticles or polymer conjugates (of proteins or drugs), or complex multicomponent systems containing drugs, proteins or genes, arrays of targeting ligands and/or signal systems to enable *in vitro* or *in vivo* detection. Therefore, nanopharmaceutics is defined as the science and technology of nanometer-sized complex drug delivery systems, consisting of at least two components, one of which is the active ingredient. In this field the concept of "nanoscale" is seen to range from 1 to 1000 nm. Currently just one nanoparticle product – Abraxane® (an albumin nanoparticle containing paclitaxel) – has been approved, but many more are being developed and are in phase I, II or III of the drug development process. This means that this class of drug delivery systems is rapidly growing, and is moving from the development of individual building blocks to multifunctional, often biomimetic and bioresponsive systems [1, 2].

These more complex nanosized drug delivery systems are either self-assembling or involve covalent conjugation of multicomponent systems, e.g. drug, protein and polymer. The bioresponsive and/or biomimetic materials used to create such drug delivery systems typically include synthetic or semisynthetic polymers, and/or natural materials such as lipids, polymers and proteins. One nanosystem that is being proposed as a drug carrier is nanoshells or nanocapsules because these novel "nanoparticles" can address the three principal goals of drug delivery research today, i.e. more specific drug delivery and targeting, greater safety and biocompatibility, and faster development of new, safe medicines. Current research in nanoshell drug delivery could lead to, amongst others, vectors that will overcome the biological barriers for effective gene delivery, cancer targeting, brain delivery and the combination of the potential of antibody targeting with nanoparticle technology. This would improve drug targeting to the whole body or cellular and subcellular localization of drugs, proteins and genes [2].

Nanotechnologies for the Life Sciences Vol. 10
Nanomaterials for Medical Diagnosis and Therapy. Edited by Challa S. S. R. Kumar

ISBN: 978-3-527-31390-7

The nanoshells most studied as potential nanopharmaceuticals are metallic nanoparticles composed of a dielectric (e.g. silica) core coated with an ultrathin metallic (e.g. gold) layer and nanoshells formed by electrostatic layer-by-layer molecular self-assembling (E-LbL). Here, the two types of nanoshells are compared and their application in drug delivery illuminated. Although several reviews and chapters have appeared describing the properties of these nanoshells separately, this chapter focuses on the differences between the two types of nanoshells as it applies to drug delivery. As, to date, metallic nanoshells have found limited application in drug delivery the bulk of the chapter describes the assembly, characterization and properties of E-LbL self-assembled polymeric or polymeric/nanoparticulate nanoshell drug delivery systems.

12.2
Metallic Nanoshells

In the past few years, silica–gold nanoshells have emerged as powerful building blocks for devices in which electromagnetic waves can be controlled at the nanometer length scale [1]. Due to this unique property, Halas and West demonstrated in a series of clever experiments how silica–gold nanoshells are uniquely suitable for use in whole-blood immunoassays, optically triggered drug delivery and targeted photothermal destruction of cancer cells [2]. The use of metallic nanoparticles dates back to the Renaissance when artists handcrafted vibrantly colored church windows and glass vases by dissolving minute amounts of noble metal impurities in a glass melt to induce precipitation of nanometer-size metallic clusters [3]. Gustav Mie provided the theory explaining this phenomenon [4]. This theory predicts that metallic nanoclusters strongly absorb visible light at a well-defined plasmon resonance frequency that depends on the particle size and shape, the presence of other particles, and the dielectric environment [5]. Due to this phenomenon the silica–gold nanoshells offer enormous flexibility to tune the resonance frequency by varying the relative dimensions of the silica core and gold shell [6, 7]. In contrast to solid-core metallic nanoparticles, the resonance of a silica–gold nanoshell particle can easily be positioned in the near-infrared (NIR) region between 800 and 1300 nm, where absorption by biomatter is low. Together with the high degree of biocompatibility of these nanoshells, low bioabsorption opens the door to a wide variety of biological applications.

12.2.1
Synthesis of the Nanoshells

Numerous methods have been reported for preparing metallic nanoshells. For example gold nanoshells with a gold sulfide core and a gold shell are formed by combining specific volumes of 2 mM $HAuCl_4$ and 1 mM Na_2S. The progress of the reaction is monitored using an ultraviolet (UV)/visible spectrophotometer to observe the extinction spectrum of the solution from 400 to 1050 nm [8, 9]. As

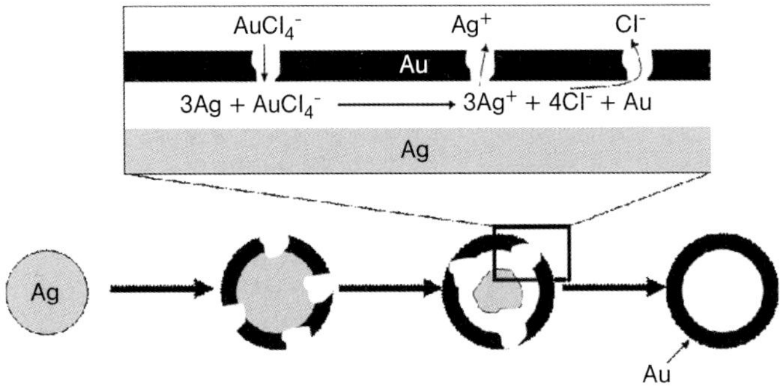

Figure 12.1. Schematic representation of the production of gold nanoshells by templating against silver nanoparticles [adapted from Ref. 10].

the nanoshells formed, the extinction spectra exhibit a peak that red-shifts into the IR, then halts and begin to blue-shift into the visible spectrum. The peak narrows and increase in magnitude as this occurs. Mercaptoproprionic acid is added to halt this shift by halting the growth of the gold shell when the extinction peak is centered around 1050 nm. The solution then is adjusted to pH 10.5 with 1 M NaOH, centrifuged at 3000 r.p.m. for 4×20 min and stored at 4 °C. The size and polydispersity of the resulting nanoshells are determined by evaporating a drop of the nanoshell solution onto a carbon film on a copper grid and viewing the nanoshells via transmission electron microscopy (TEM).

Sun and coworkers demonstrated a procedure based on replacement reactions for generating highly crystalline nanoshells from various metals [10]. The major steps involved are shown in Fig. 12.1 with gold/silver combination as an example. Since the standard reduction potential of the $AuCl_4^-/Au$ redox pair is higher that that of the Ag^+/Ag redox pair silver nanoparticles are immediately oxidized to silver ions when mixed with and aqueous $HAuCL_4$ solution. Elemental gold is thus confined in the vicinity of the template surface where it will nucleate and grow into small clusters and eventually will evolve into a shell around the silver template. The reaction initiates at facets with the highest surface free energy. As a result the thin shell formed initially is incomplete, and therefore both the $HAuCL_4$ and AgCl will diffuse across the layer until the silver template is completely dissolved. The wall of each gold nanoshell can then be reconstructed into a highly crystalline structure via processes such as Ostwald ripening. Since stoichiometrically one gold atom is generated when three silver atoms are oxidized the thickness of the gold nanoshell in only one-ninth of the lateral dimension of the silver template.

In an alternative preparation method, Caruso and coworkers employed the LbL adsorption of polyelectrolytes and charged gold colloids to build shell-like structures around colloidal template particles whose surfaces have been derivatized with appropriately charged groups [11]. However, the gold nanoparticles prepared by all these methods are characterized by relatively low yields, problems with surface roughness, polycrystallinity, nonuniformity in shell thickness, poorly defined composition and difficulty in removing colloidal templates without breaking the shells [12].

12.2.2
Application in Nanomedicine

In one study, Halas and West showed how NIR resonant nanoshells could be used to enable fast whole-blood immunoassays [13]. For conventional blood immunoassays, optical tests are performed at visible wavelengths. As a purification step needs to be performed to separate out a variety of unwanted biomaterials that absorb visible light, the whole procedure can take several hours or days. In the proposed immunoassay procedure nanoshells are conjugated with antibodies that act as recognition sites for a specific analyte. The analyte causes the formation of dimmers, which modify the plasmon-related absorption feature in a known way. The presence of analyte can then be determined by a fast absorption measurement in the water window, circumventing the time-intensive purification step.

Gold nanoshells can also be incorporated into temperature-sensitive hydrogels to synthesize a new type of composite material that collapses on laser irradiation [2]. Upon irradiation plasmon excitations are quickly damped and the electron kinetic energy is converted into heat through electron–phonon interactions. This fast damping is usually undesirable, but here the efficient light-to-heat conversion in metallic nanoshells is used to shrink the volume of the hydrogel from a remote location. The absorption cross-section of a nanoshell is about a million times larger than that of a typical molecular chromophore and hydrogel collapse thus occurs at relatively low pump-power densities. By incorporating nanoshells with different resonance frequencies, one can selectively collapse specific hydrogel volumes. Such remotely addressable hydrogels may find application in drug delivery and microfluidic valves or pumps.

For example, composites of thermally sensitive hydrogels and optically active nanoparticles have been developed for the purpose of photothermally modulated drug delivery [2]. Copolymers of *N*-isopropylacrylamide (NIPAAm) and acrylamide (AAm) exhibit a lower critical solution temperature (LCST) that is slightly above body temperature. When the temperature of the copolymer exceeds the LCST, the hydrogel collapses, causing a burst release of any soluble material held within the hydrogel matrix. When gold–gold sulfide nanoshells, a new class of nanoparticles designed to strongly absorb NIR light, were incorporated into poly(NIPAAm-*co*-AAm) hydrogels temperature changes in the hydrogel could be induced with light. Light at wavelengths between 800 and 1200 nm, which is transmitted through tissue with relatively little attenuation, was absorbed by the nanoparticles and converted to heat. Using this system, significantly enhanced drug release from composite hydrogels was achieved in response to irradiation by light at 1064 nm as shown in Fig. 12.2. This system controlled the release of methylene blue and proteins of varying molecular weight.

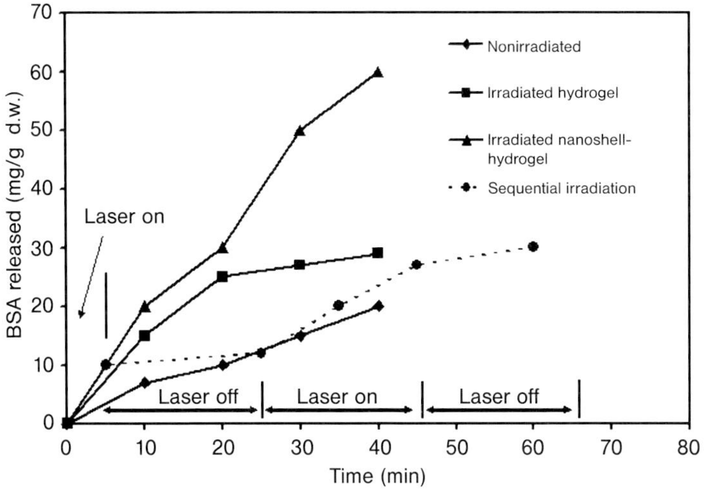

Figure 12.2. Release of BSA from nonirradiated and irradiated hydrogel with and without nanoshells. Irradiation was at 1064 nm at 164 mJ pulse^{-1}, 7 ns pulse length and 10 Hz repetition rate. (Adapted from Ref. [2].)

The nanoshell composite hydrogels can also release multiple bursts of protein in response to repeated NIR irradiation [2]. If the entire drug load is not released during the initial irradiation sequence, additional bursts of release of the drug can be elicited by subsequent irradiation. Once the laser irradiation is stopped, the driving force for the convective transport of material out of the hydrogel matrix is removed. During this time, the drug release is driven by diffusion and the amount released is much less than that generated by irradiation. The hydrogel will begin to swell as soon as the laser is turned off, returning to its equilibrium state. A second irradiation sequence delivered at this time will cause the hydrogel to collapse again, resulting in another burst of release of the "drug" molecule. Such a release pattern for bovine serum albumin is shown in Fig. 12.2. This type of release profile may be useful in insulin therapy as well as in other applications where controlled pulsatile release of a drug is necessary.

Additionally, it has been speculated that metallic nanoshells could play a role in future cancer treatments. These particles are small enough to find their way through the human circulatory system on injection. Bioactive molecules can be attached to the nanoshell surface to cause selective binding or accumulation of these particles within a tumor. Using a NIR laser, carcinoma tissue can then be destroyed by local thermal heating around the nanoshells. For example by tuning the nanoshells to strongly absorb light in the NIR, where optical transmission through tissue is optimal, a distribution of nanoshells at depth in tissue can be used to deliver a therapeutic dose of heat by using moderately low exposures of extracorporeally applied NIR light [14]. In this study, human breast carcinoma cells incubated with nanoshells *in vitro* were found to have undergone photothermally induced morbidity on exposure to NIR light (820 nm, 35 W cm^{-2}), as determined by using a fluorescent viability stain. Cells without nanoshells displayed no loss in viability after the same periods and conditions of NIR illumination. Likewise, *in vivo* studies under magnetic resonance guidance revealed that exposure to low doses of NIR light (820 nm, 4 W cm^{-2}) in solid tumors treated with metal nanoshells reached average maximum temperatures capable of inducing irreversible tissue damage ($\Delta T \sim 38$ °C) within 5 min. Controls treated without nanoshells demonstrated significantly lower average temperatures on exposure to NIR light ($\Delta T < 10$ °C). These findings demonstrated good correlation with histological findings. Tissues heated above the thermal damage threshold displayed coagulation, cell shrinkage, and loss of nuclear staining, which are indicators of irreversible thermal damage. Control tissues appeared undamaged.

Due to all these positive developments, the design and fabrication of new types of plasmonic metallic nanostructures have seen a flurry of activity. In particular, the unique properties of nanoshells seem to promise a golden future for metallic nanostructures in drug delivery and it will be fascinating to see what other applications arise in the near future [12–14].

12.3 Nanoshells Formed by Polyion E-LbL Self-assembly

This nanoencapsulation method involves the formation of an outer nanothick shell around a core that is stable, permeable, compatible and allows the release of the core material through the shell. In the last decade, E-LbL self-assembly has been developed as a practical and versatile nanoencapsulation method to form nanoshells. The core templates may be "passive" (such as 50–300 nm latex or silica), which later will be dissolved, or "active" and functional (such as drug micro/nanocrystals). Tailoring of the different components of individual particles becomes important in order to develop these functionalized colloids, i.e. to combine several properties in one core–shell structure. Due to these advantages E-LbL assembly has the capacity to employ a great variety of substances as shell constituents as well as core material. Only general aspects of the method had been elaborated to demonstrate its potential, and it still has to be further developed and better understood [15–20].

12.3.1 Preparation of E-LbL Nanoshells

The sequential adsorption of oppositely charged colloids was reported in a seminal paper in 1966 by Iler [21]. The technique of E-LbL self-assembly of thin films by means of alternate adsorption of oppositely charged linear polyions was then further developed in earnest starting in the early 1990s [22–25]. The basis of the

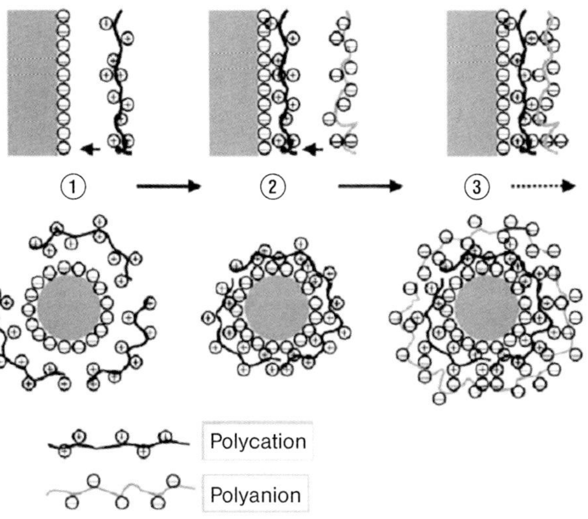

Figure 12.3. The procedure of E-LbL self-assembly on two-dimensional substrates and three-dimensional micro/nanotemplates. Particles with negative surface charge is coated with a layer of polycation (step 1). This reverses the surface charge, which is then coated with an anionic polyelectrolyte (step 2). The original surface charge change is restored and the surface is ready for further assembly (step 3). (Adapted from Refs. [20, 22].)

method involves resaturation of polyion adsorption, resulting in the reversal of the terminal surface charge of the film after deposition of each layer (Fig. 12.3) [20, 22].

As a standard approach for film preparation on a solid support, the following steps are employed [22, 24, 26]:

(i) Take aqueous solutions of polyion, nanoparticles or protein at a concentration of 0.1–1 mg mL^{-1} and adjust the pH in such a way that the components are oppositely charged.
(ii) Take a substrate carrying a surface charge [e.g. plates or polymer films covered by a layer of cationic poly(ethylenimine) (PEI) which may be readily attached to many surfaces].
(iii) Carry out alternate immersion of the substrate in the component's solutions for 10 min with 1 min of intermediate water rinsing. To rinse a sample use a solution with pH that keeps the polyions ionized.
(iv) Dry the sample using a stream of nitrogen (note that drying may hinder the assembly process and it is not necessary for the procedure).

The method provides the possibility of designing ultrathin multilayer films with a precision better than 1 nm of defined molecular composition. To date, this method has been used with more than 50 different charged macromolecules. The polyions predominately used in the assembly are:

- Polycations: PEI, poly(dimethyldiallylammonium chloride) (PDDA), poly(allylamine) (PAH), polylysine, chitosan.
- Polyanions: poly(styrene sulfonate) (PSS), poly(vinylsulfate), poly(acrylic acid) (PAA), dextran sulfate, sodium alginate, gelatin, chondroitin, heparin, DNA.

These charged materials can be combined with enzymes, antibodies, viruses and inorganic nanoparticles to produce multifunctional shells in both two- and three-dimensional nanoassembly processes. The architecture of these shells can be designed with nanometer precision (in cross-section) to meet different requirements such as thickness, biocompatibility, controlled permeability, targeting and optical or magnetic properties.

The only crucial factor for successful deposition is the surface charge reversal upon deposition of layers, which can be achieved by choice of proper deposition conditions. Since then various polyelectrolyte species could be adsorbed onto the surface of solid or liquid materials by means of electrostatic adsorption, forming layered structures with unique properties. It has been established that films can contain more than 1000 polyelectrolyte multilayers [27]. The universal character of the method does not impose any restriction on the type of polyelectrolyte. The multilayers can also produce diverse shapes when various materials beside polyelectrolytes, such as organic, inorganic nanoparticles and crystals, biomolecules, lipids and viruses, are used in the coating process. Such a coating produces complicated laminated structures. The use of polymers as the coating component is often advantageous in comparison with employment of their low-molecular-weight analogs. Mechanical strength, elasticity, electrical, optical and other properties make them unique building blocks for the creation of composite materials. In addition, the incorporation of proteins and nucleic acids in multilayer films may lead to the application as biosensors and in biotechnology [28–30].

The latter may even provide the base for development of ultrathin multistep chemical catalysts or photosynthesis systems mimicking plants. Applications can also be found in the fabrication of optical devices [31] and gas separation membranes [32]. The efficient use of this unique multilayer coating is interlinked with investigations of their properties. Although the methods for studying multilayer properties are straightforward, they are very often not applicable or are time consuming because of the low amount of material studied and the possible influence of the surface used as a support for layer growth. To eliminate the first factor, one should drastically increase the total surface of the multilayers, which can be done by using colloidal particles as templates [33]. Dissolution of the colloidal core could avoid the second objection. The derived hollow capsules allow the study of polyelectrolyte multilayers at the liquid–liquid interface, which seems to be very difficult while working on the solid support [23, 34].

These developments show that after the first publications on nanoshell formation in 1992–1999 [15–17], the structure of nanoshells has been characterized and the procedures to increase the functionality of the nanoshells have been elaborated through the efforts of several research groups [18, 22, 30]. For example, pore openings in these polyion multilayers were first discovered by Mendelsohn and coworkers [35], and then later applied for enzyme loading into nanoshells by Lvov and Caruso [18]. This growth in our knowledge regarding E-LbL nanoshell fabrication, structure and properties has led to noteworthy achievements that have many advantages. However, many practical clinical applications in nanomedicine remain to be developed.

12.3.1.1 Proving the Nanoshells

For the time-dependent monitoring of the assembly *in situ*, a quartz crystal microbalance (QCM) is most often used because of its proven suitability [22, 36, 37]. First of all, the kinetics of the adsorption process can be delineated by the QCM technique, which is indispensable for establishing proper assembly conditions (e.g. saturation adsorption time). Multilayer assembly is generally characterized by means of the QCM technique in two ways: (i) after drying a sample in a nitrogen stream we measure the resonance frequency shift and calculated an adsorbed mass by the Sauerbrey equation or (ii) by monitoring of the resonator frequency during the adsorption process onto one side of the resonator which is in permanent contact with the polyion solutions. Frequency shifts of about 800 Hz are seen for every adsorption cycle in solution QCM, which is more than that detected, for example, for a dried film of PSS/PAH. This difference is ascribed to the strong hydration of the layer that had just been adsorbed. The bound water is included in the film and is removed after drying. This means that most polyion films swell by 40–60% before drying and that only 5–10% of the water remains in polyion films after drying.

It is assumed that polyion adsorption occurs in two stages: quick anchoring to a surface and slow relaxation. To reach a surface charge reversion during linear polyion adsorption one needs a concentration greater than 10^{-5} M [36]. However, the dependence of polyion layer thickness on concentration is not great because in the concentration range of 0.1–5 mg mL^{-1} the PSS/PAH pair yielded a similar bilayer thickness. A further decrease in polyion concentration (using 0.01 mg mL^{-1}) decreased the layer thickness of the adsorbed polyion. Other the other hand, an increase in the component concentrations to 20–30 mg mL^{-1} may result in the nonlinear (exponential) enlargement of the growth rate with adsorption steps, especially if an intermediate sample rinsing is not long enough [38].

In addition, at the beginning of the alternate assembly process one often sees nonlinear film growth [36, 39]. As shown in Fig. 12.4, in the first two to three layers, smaller amounts of polyion are adsorbed as compared with further assembly, when the film mass and thickness increase linearly with the number of adsorption cycles. Tsukruk and coworkers [40] explained this as an island-type adsorption of the first polyion layer on a weakly charged solid support. In the following two to three adsorption cycles these islands spread and cover the entire surface, and further multilayer growth occurs linearly. If a substrate is well charged then a linear growth with repeatable steps begins earlier.

In addition to measuring weight changes with a QCM, following changes in the UV spectra is another simple method to control LbL assembly on glass or quartz slides. After every other layer one can measure the sample UV spectra and use Beer's law (absorbance is proportional to the material mass) to judge the amount

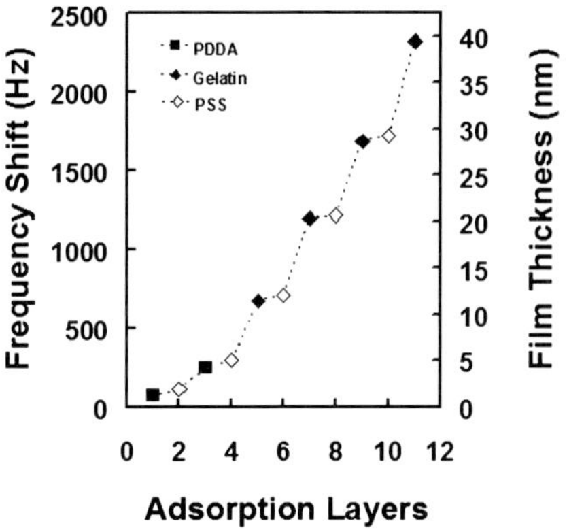

Figure 12.4. Frequency shift and film thickness of each assembly layer for PDDA + $(PSS/PDDA)_2$ + $(PSS/gelatin)_4$ adsorption on QCM electrodes. The first four-layer precursor is about 4 nm thick. The averaged frequency shift of every gelatin layer is 483 Hz, corresponding to a thickness of 8 nm.

of adsorbed polymer and whether the assembly process linear with number of adsorbed layers. Figure 12.5 shows the UV spectra for three, five, seven and nine bilayers of PSS/PAH deposited on quartz slide. There is a linear increase of absorbency with an increase in the number of layers; therefore, the mass of the film was increasing linearly too. The absorbance maximum at 225 nm corresponds to the absorbency of benzyl rings of PSS.

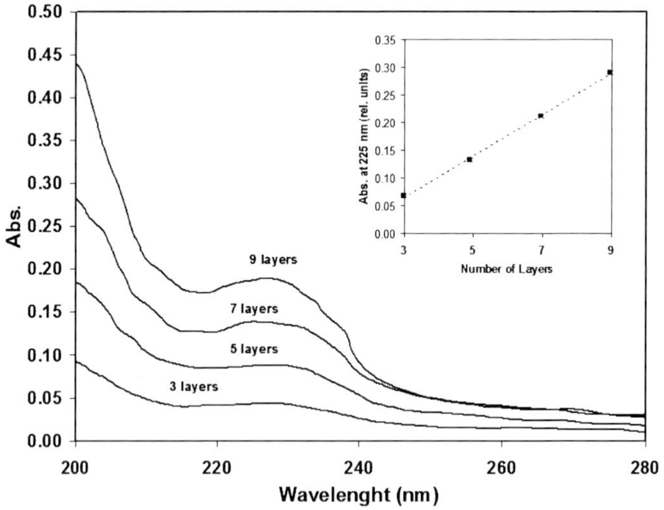

Figure 12.5. The increase in absorbance with an increase in the number of PSS/PAH layers deposited on a glass slide. The insert show the linear increase in layer mass.

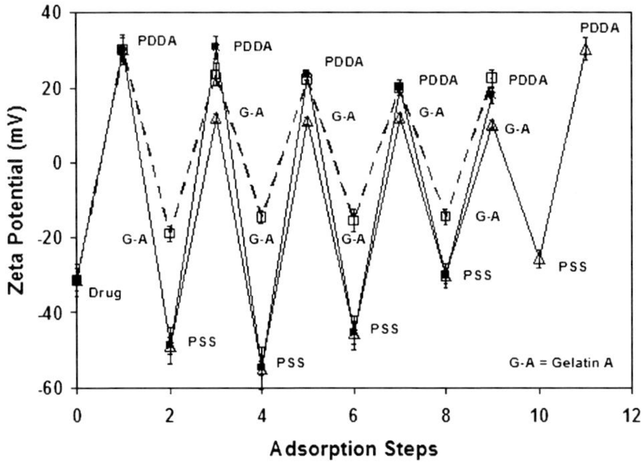

Figure 12.6. Changes in the ζ potential of the coated dexamethasone particles as a function of the number of adsorption steps for capsule composition of dexamethasone core/(PDDA/PSS)$_4$/PDDA (solid line and solid squares), dexamethasone core/(PDDA/gelatin A)$_4$/PDDA (broken line and open squares) and dexamethasone core/PDDA/(PSS/gelatin A)$_4$/(PSS/PDDA)$_1$ (solid line and open triangles).

Another method to monitor the assembly process is to ensure the reversal of charge after each polyion coating as shown in Fig. 12.6 [41]. For this the ζ potential of the suspended nanoshells is measured after each layer has been applied. If the solid support (e.g. drug crystal) with negative surface charge is, for example, incubated in a solution containing a cationic polyelectrolyte, a layer of polycation is adsorbed. As the adsorption is carried out at a relatively high concentration of polyelectrolytes, a number of ionic groups remain exposed at the interface with the solution and thus the surface charge is effectively reversed. The reversed surface charge prevents further polyion adsorption. Solid supports or microtemplates are then rinsed with pure water or washed by centrifugation, respectively, to remove excess free polyions. The surface is then immersed in a solution of anionic polyelectrolytes. Again, a layer is adsorbed, but now the original surface charge (negative) is restored and the surface is ready for further assembly. These two steps are repeated alternately until a layer of the desired thickness is obtained. More than two components can be used in the assembly as long as one condition, i.e. a proper alternation of positive and negative charge, is observed [20, 22, 41].

More detail structural information can be obtained from X-ray and neutron reflectivity data. X-ray or neutron reflectivity measurements of polyion films show patterns with profound intensity oscillations, the so-called Kiessig fringes, due to the interference of radiation beams reflected from solid support/film and air/film interfaces [42]. From the periodicity of these oscillations one can calculate the film thickness (with the help of the Bragg-like equation and taking into account refraction phenomena which are essential at small-angles). Growth steps for a bilayer of 1.1–2.0 nm are typical for alternate linear polyion assembly and a thickness of one layer often equals half of this value [43]. These values correspond to a polyion cross-section and show that in one cycle of excessive adsorption we have approximately one monolayer coverage of the substrate. The nanoparticle/polyion bilayer thickness is determined by the diameter of the particle. Model fitting of X-ray data gives a surface roughness of the polyion film of order 1 nm, while atomic force microscopy (AFM) and scanning electron microscopy (SEM) data revealed a surface roughness of 1–2 nm [42]. Polyion films are insoluble in water and in many organic solvents and are stable to 250–280 °C [44].

The polycation/polyanion bilayer thickness depends on the charge density of the polyions. It was shown that more than 10% of polyion side-groups have to be ionized for a stable reproducible multilayer assembly via alternate electrostatic adsorption [45]. High ionization of polyions results in a smaller step of film growth (1–2 nm) and lower ionization gives a larger growth step (3–6 nm). It can be reached either by adding salt to a polyion solution (as discussed above for strong polyelectrolytes, such as PDDA and PSS) or by varying the pH for weak polyelectrolytes [46].

12.3.1.2 **Influence of the Core on Nanoshell Properties**

So far it has been shown that the procedure of E-LbL nanoshell formation is a multistep process. Although the further properties of capsules depend strongly on the choice of polyelectrolytes employed and adsorption conditions, such as ionic strength, temperature, solvent composition, number of layers, etc., an extremely important step in determining the success of the experiment is the proper choice of the cores type [27]. This is especially important when fabricating intact capsules consisting only of the material used during the coating – the process of core dissolution should result in 100% elimination of the core without affecting the polyelectrolyte multilayers. In fact, the molecular weight of core components is typically 100 times more than that of the polymers forming the shell and the task of complete core removal seems to be complicated from a chemical point of view. At present, cores that have been exploited to template hollow capsules can be classified into three groups differing by dissolution properties and chemical interaction with polyelectrolyte components of the shell [27].

The first class is made up of organic cores made of water-insoluble oligomers including the widely studied melamine formaldehyde (MF) cores dissolvable at low pH and in some organic solvents, polystyrene (PS) cores soluble in tetrahydrofuran (THF) and biofriendly poly(lactic acid)/poly(lactic-*co*-glycolic acid) (PLA/PLGA) soluble in acetone/*N*-methyl-2-pyrrolidinone mixture. The second class is made up cores that dissolves into small molecules and ions. These can be either ionic or molecular crystals soluble in acidic or basic conditions or in an organic solvent. At present, different carbonate particles ($CaCO_3$, $CdCO_3$ and $MnCO_3$) [47] and SiO_2 particles [48] have been used for polyelectrolyte multilayer templating. The main advantage of exploiting such inorganic particles is the absence of osmotic stress upon dissolution and complete elimination of the core. The third class of cores is made up of those subjected to strong oxidation. A biological cell is a typical example of this kind of cores. For example, the assembly of polyelectrolyte multilayers can be performed using fixed erythrocyte cells as templates [49, 50]. The removal of the cell cores can be achieved by oxidation with sodium hypochlorite solution. The main effect of changing the core is that the employment of a different core material will result in different permeability properties of the shell.

12.3.1.3 Barrier Properties of E-LbL Assembled Nanoshells

The barrier properties of nanoshells formed by E-LbL depend on film thickness, ionic strength and charge of the permeating molecule, temperature annealing, resealing by additional layers, and chemical modification. If the permeability of the polyelectrolyte multilayer is provided by diffusion through the entangled polymer network, it should scale with the inverse of the layer thickness. However, most studies show that the permeability decreases with increasing layer number much faster than expected for a straightforward thickness increase. Only from approximately eight layers onwards does the permeability multiplied by the shell thickness become constant, indicating that the permeability is now controlled by the thickness increase and the diffusion-limiting region relates to the properties of the polyelectrolyte layer [51]. Normally, the deeper layers are denser, resulting in a 5-fold reduction of the estimated diffusion coefficient, while the loose structure of the interfacial layers leads to a very slow increase in the dissolution time. This means that only the presence of the internal dense layers can slow down the dissolution time. For thinner walls, the drastic dependence on shell thickness may be explained either by the existence of pores that are successively closed by further layer deposition or by a thickness-dependent diffusion coefficient. Diffusion dependent on layer depth was indeed observed when the diffusion of polar labels in planar polyelectrolyte films was studied [51].

Another parameter that can influence the multilayers structure is the ionic strength [27]. It has been shown that the multilayer structure is affected if the salt concentration is changed once the film is built up. Polyelectrolyte multilayer vesicles can be subjected to temperature treatment that significantly influences their properties. For example, at temperatures up to 95 °C the polyelectrolyte capsules keep their integrity, but undergo irreversible structural changes [52]. The resulting structure is characterized by decreasing capsule diameter with simultaneously increasing shell thickness as revealed by scanning force microscopy (SFM). From thermodynamic point of view this effect can be explained by approaching the equilibrium state of polyelectrolyte complexes. In another example hollow capsules were fabricated by LbL deposition of oppositely charged diblock copolymers each containing a PNIPAAm block and a charged negative or positive block (20 mol%) [53]. PNIPAAm is known to undergo a phase transition at a temperature of 32 °C (the so-called LCST), after which it is not soluble. This transition is rather sharp and completely reversible upon cooling. The obtained capsules exhibit changes in morphology and permeability at elevated temperatures. However, this process is only partially reversible in the multilayers. Relaxation requires more than 1 month, which limits their thermosensitivity to one heating circle.

Chemical modification can be another way to induce the excessive charge into the polyelectrolyte multilayers and change other characteristics of the film. One method proposed is using PAA, partially modified by Fisher esterification with different alcohols, as a multilayer constituent [54]. Depending on the nature of the derivatizing alcohol, the hydrophobicity of the film could be tuned. The hydrophobicity of ester groups was shown to result in advancing water contact angles to more than 100°. Crosslinking of these hydrophobic films via heat-induced amidation stabilized coatings over a wide pH range, but did not significantly influence their permeability. It has been proposed that crosslinking of the reactive groups in the multilayers is sometimes the only possibility of making films composed of weak polyelectrolytes stable at a wide range of pH and ionic strength. One example is PAA/PAH multilayers, which readily decompose upon a shift of pH or ionic strength, that can be crosslinked in order to gain stability [55]. In contrast, nanoshells composed of PSS/PAH multilayers have semipermeable properties [26]. They are permeable for small molecules, such as dyes and ions, while under most conditions high-molecular-weight compounds are excluded. One of the explanations for this is the much smaller size of the pores in the multilayer film in comparison with the hydrodynamic radius of the permeating molecule.

Filled capsules can also serve as microreactors [56]. This is advantageous because for macromolecules there is an advantage in encapsulating enzymes and proteins in general because their inaccessibility for inhibitors, proteases (which are polymers and cannot permeate the capsule wall) and, of course, for bacteria. This means the activity of enzymes encapsulated is higher as compared with typical values of chemically immobilized enzymes. In addition, the native conformation of proteins such as hemoglobin does not change upon encapsulation due to contact with the nanoshell because there was no change registered in the position of a so-called Soret band, which is very sensitive to the changes in the heme conformation. All these studies showed that the possibility exists to control and reversibly change the capsule permeability for both low- and high-molecular-weight molecules as shown in Fig. 12.7. This can be desirable for many applications, including drug delivery. This means that the exploration of the permeability properties of capsules and multilayers must be further developed because it promises many possibilities as drug carriers, biosensors, micro-reactors and catalysts, construction materials, etc. [56].

12.3.2 Controlled Release of Active Pharmaceutical Ingredients Encapsulated by E-LbL Assembled Nanoshells

A major challenge in the development of carrier systems of submicron dimensions lies in the field of advanced drug formulations, especially when it comprises the elaboration of delivery systems capable of providing sustained release of bioactive materials [27]. Mainly, these bioactive compounds are small molecules with different solubility and diffusion coefficients. If we consider only physical entrapment without any covalent binding in order to develop a delivery system, one has to encapsulate the active molecules within the shell proving certain release character-

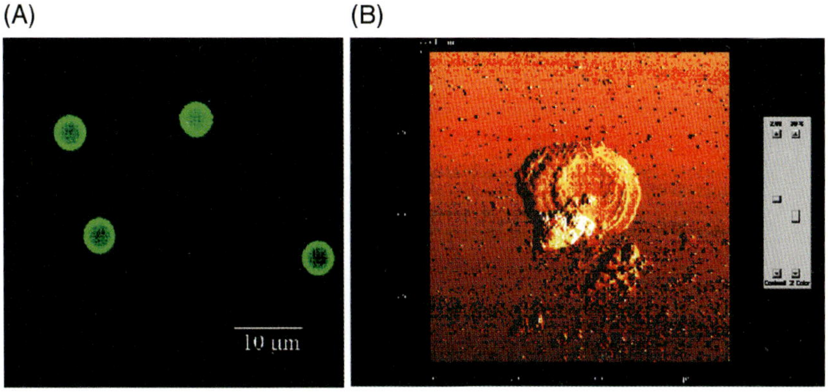

Figure 12.7. (A) Polyelectrolyte microcapsules with (PSS/PAH)$_5$ wall composition loaded with FITC-labeled glucose oxidase (confocal image). (B) AFM tipping mode image of the same broken dry capsule on mica; release of the encapsulated material is visible. (Adapted from Ref. [56].)

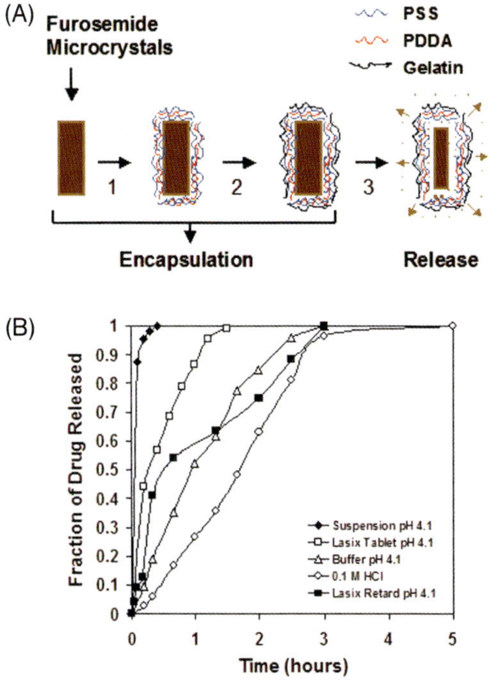

Figure 12.8. (A) Illustration of furosemide microcrystal encapsulation and release study. In step 1, precursor layers of (PSS/PDDA)$_2$ are assembled onto positively charged furosemide microcrystals. In step 2, (PSS/gelatin)$_{2-6}$ layers are added. In step 3, drug release in aqueous solution was monitored at different pH values. (B) Dissolution profiles of (PSS/PDDA)$_2$ + (PSS/gelatin)$_4$-coated furosemide microparticles compared to uncoated particles and a commercially available tablet in physiologically relevant media using the dissolution test described in the USP 24. (Adapted from Ref. [22].)

istics. The potential use of polyelectrolyte capsules with drug entrapped in the nanoshell for controlled drug delivery currently requires more study and is not well established. In contrast, microencapsulation of drug microparticles is a well-established technique for prolonging release. When microcapsules are coated with appropriate antigens, they can also be targeted to specific regions in the body. This can lead to lowered overall dosage requirements, increased drug concentrations in the necessary regions and reduced side-effects. Polymer- and liposome-based systems have been used for drug encapsulation, mostly as unordered drug–polymer conjugates [57–60].

The E-LbL self-assembly technique based on alternate adsorption of oppositely charged components was developed to add nanometer-thick films to surfaces [15, 17, 35, 61, 62], offering the opportunity to design controlled release systems by encapsulating micron-scale cores with a very thin outer shell. The core must be insoluble under some conditions, such as low pH, and soluble under the conditions at which controlled release is to take place. The release rate generally depends on the thickness of the encapsulating shell and the material used in the coating. Thicker shells lead longer release times.

12.3.2.1 Nanoshell Permeability for Low-molecular-weight Compounds

In the first report on controlled release, fluorescent dye microcrystals were used as a model system for controlled release studies [24]. PSS and PAH were used to form a polyelectrolyte shell on the fluorescein core. Increasing the number of layers decreased the shell permeability and resulted in prolonged dye–core dissolution. Encapsulation of ibuprofen also resulted in prolonged release at different pH values [63]. The ibuprofen dissolution time from capsules with walls built from 15 bilayers of chitosan–dextran was 40 s at pH 7.4, compared to 10 s with no coating. Therefore, prolongation of the release was minimal.

To determine whether encapsulation by E-LbL assembly can substantially increase drug release time, the technique was used to assemble polypeptides and polyions on microcrystals of 5-(aminosulfonyl)-4-chloro-2-[(furanylmethyl)amino] benzoic acid, commonly known as furosemide [22]. Furosemide is a diuretic and antihypertension drug that is practically insoluble in water. Although the therapeutic effect is fast and intense after oral administration of furosemide, the oral bioavailability of the drug from an immediate release dosage form is poor and highly variable [64]. These problems can potentially be overcome by developing a modified release dosage form. Ai and coworkers encapsulated furosemide microcrystals with polyions and gelatin to control the release of the drug in aqueous solutions (Fig. 12.8) [22]. In step 1, precursor layers of $(PSS/PDDA)_2$ are assembled onto positively charged furosemide microcrystals. In step 2, $(PSS/gelatin)_{2-6}$ layers are added. In step 3, drug release in aqueous solution was monitored at different pH values. Charged linear polyions and gelatin were alternatively deposited on 5-μm drug microcrystals through E-LbL self-assembly. Sequential layers of PDDA and PSS were followed by adsorption of two to six gelatin/PSS bilayers with corresponding capsule wall thicknesses ranging from 45 to 115 nm. They then determined furosemide release from the E-LbL encapsulated crystals under two physiological pH conditions, i.e. pH 1.4 (stomach) and pH 7.4 (blood). At both pH values, the release rate of furosemide from the encapsulated particles was reduced by 50–300 times (for capsules coated with two to six bilayers) compared to uncoated furosemide. The results provide a method of achieving prolonged drug release through self-assembly of polymeric nanoshells on drug microcrystals.

In a study that further expanded the application of core–shell structures fabricated by E-LbL self-assembling for drug delivery, Pargaonkar and coworkers reported the controlled release of dexamethasone from microcrystals encapsulated with a polyelectrolyte shell [41]. The E-LbL self-assembly process was used to produce dexamethasone particles layered with $PDDA^+$, $(PDDA/PSS)_4/PDDA$, $(PDDA/gelatin A)_4/PDDA$, dexamethasone core/$(PDDA/gelatin B)_4/PDDA$ or dexamethasone core/$PDDA/(PSS/gelatin A)_4/(PSS/PDDA)_1$. The nanothin shells were characterized by QCM measurements, microelectrophoresis, microcalorimetry, confocal microscopy and SEM. The *in vitro* release of dexamethasone from the microcapsules suspended in water or carboxymethylcellulose (CMC) gels, measured using vertical Franz-type diffusion cells, showed that the assembly of multiple polyelectrolyte layers around these monodispersed cores produced a polyelectrolyte multilayer shell around the drug microcrystals which allowed for controlled release depending on the composition and the number of layers.

Ye and coworkers showed that indomethacin microcrystals can be directly encapsulated with polysaccharides sodium alginate and chitosan multilayers through LbL self-assembly [65]. The retention of the drug microcrystal was found to gradually decrease due to its partial dissolution in the deposition solution. It was very significant that increasing the deposition temperature from 20 to 60 °C reduced the release rate efficiently, due to the increase in multilayer thickness and formation of a more perfect multilayer film. This finding provides a new and simple method to control the permeability of the LbL assembled multilayer films.

12.3.2.2 Nanoshell Permeability for High-molecular-weight Compounds

DNA and polynucleotides (polyuridylic and polyadenylic acids) can be readily assembled in alternation with polycations (PEI, PAH, polylysine) [66]. Alternate adsorption of 0.1 mg mL^{-1} DNA at pH 5.2 with polycations gave multilayers with a DNA/PEI bilayer thickness of 4.4 nm and DNA/PAH bilayer thickness of 3.6 nm. Fourier-transform IR spectra confirmed the native double-stranded DNA conformation in DNA/PEI and DNA/PAH multilayers. Coating DNA/polyion films on medical implants may have applications in local gene therapy. In other studies, proteins including lysozyme, horseradish peroxidase, albumin, bacteriorhodopsin, immunoglobulins, glucoamylase, glucose oxidase (GOx), catalase, glucose isomerase and diaphorase were used at concentrations of 0.1–2 mg mL^{-1} for LbL assembly [20]. As the surface structure of the solid support can affect the stability of proteins, precursor films of alternate PEI/PSS are normally used as standard surfaces.

Proteins immobilized in multilayers with strong polyions, such as PSS, PEI and PDDA, are insoluble in buffers in a pH range between 3 and 10. Protein multilayers with weak polyions are partially soluble in solutions with a pH close to the isoelectric point of one of the components, but such multilayers can be stabilized with crosslinking agents. Assembled proteins are in most cases not denatured [67, 68].

Nano-organized encapsulation of protein microcores such as insulin nanoparticles in the presence of high concentration of neutral polymers (PEG) was also elaborated with a LbL assembly. Uncoated insulin PROMAXX microparticles formed by controlled phase separation from hydrophilic compounds undergo to a fast dissolution if the PEG concentration is decreased [69]. Insulin release from PROMAX was extended with LbL encapsulation. After the complex of insulin in the core and the first layer of oppositely charged polymer is formed, the microparticle is stabilized and adding new polyelectrolyte layers can be continued. Balancing strong interaction of the first polyelectrolyte layer with protein microcore and easing this interaction by depositing the second oppositely charge polyelectrolyte (polyanion/polycation for positive cores at pH 5.8 and polycation/polyanion for negative cores at pH 7.0) allowed us to control complexation of the encapsulated proteins and to reach a sustained insulin release. Fine tuning of the release profile was reached by using the third and forth polyelectrolyte layer addition.

Therefore, the general idea of controllable complex formation is as follows. Adsorption of the first polyelectrolyte layer results in strong complex formation and very slow release. An addition of the second, oppositely charged polyelectrolyte layer results in relaxed complex and quicker release. The third oppositely charged layer again gives slower release, etc. Just growing thickness of the capsule walls within five to 10 bilayers (30–60 nm) did not slow insulin release from the microparticles. With this, the concept formulated in a Max Planck Institute research group [23, 24, 28] defining LbL multilayer as a tight diffusion barrier with adjustable thickness in the range of five to 12 bilayers was converted to a new approach where the main role in the controlled release from protein microaggregates is given to adjustable interpolyelectrolyte complex formation controlled by alternate polycation/polyanion coating of two to three monolayers.

E-LbL can also increase the stability of macromolecules as demonstrated for membrane-disrupting peptide that are easily degraded *in vivo* [70]. The peptides are important because when conjugated to peptide hormones they have been shown to specifically destroy primary tumors and metastases in mouse models. Consequently, the encapsulation and sustained systemic release of these peptides could further improve treatment efficacy by protecting the peptides from degradation. When silica nanoshells are coated by E-LbL with polyelectrolyte layers of gelatin B or CMC carrying the peptide drug, Phor21-βCG(ala), the release kinetics of the embedded peptide drug, can be controlled and its potency to destroy breast cancer cells can be enhanced *in vitro*. The silica–peptide nanoshells produced by this process had a diameter of 450 nm, and the adsorption efficacy was 20% and was linear with an increasing numbers of layers. Up to 34% of the embedded Phor21-βCG(ala) was released in a linear fashion from the CMC multilayers over a period of 20 h. The release kinetics was dependent on the pH. *In vitro* toxicity to human breast cancer cells using gelatin B and CMC silica–peptide nanoshells showed that Phor21-βCG(ala) was released from the multilayers, and the peptide retained its potency in destroying human breast cancer cells and did not cause aggregation of the peptide drug. This showed that E-LbL assembled silica–peptide nanoshells may be used not only for sustained release of a peptide cancer drug to treat primary tumors and metastases, but also to increase the stability of the active ingredient.

Taken together, all these studies demonstrate the successful controlled delivery of large biomolecules not only from a core encapsulated with a nanoshell, but also from the nanoshell where the active molecule was used in the construction of the nanoshell via the E-LbL process.

12.3.3
E-LbL Assembled Nanoshells as Protective and Functional Barriers

Nanoshells prepared by E-LbL self-assembly can be used as a new type of protective microcontainer, capable of preventing oxidation of encapsulated compounds by low-molecular-weight oxidizing agents [29, 30, 34]. These researchers developed protective polyelectrolyte microcapsules that effectively prevents the oxidation of encapsulated bovine serum albumin by a low-molecular-weight agent, H_2O_2 (Fig. 12.9). Two approaches for designing protective capsule microcontainers were demonstrated. First, the "passive armor" approach is composed of a sacrificial reducing agent as a shell constituent, while the "active armor" approach includes the catalyst for H_2O_2 decomposition deposited onto the shell as the outer layer. In the latter case, the protective material is not consumed during the H_2O_2 treatment, thus prolonging the protection activity of the microcapsule. The designed microcontainers combine the protective function with the controlled release of the encapsulated substance and, moreover, can possess magnetic activity to perform magnetically adjusted delivery of the encapsulated material in aggressive media. Protective polyelectrolyte capsules can find applications as delivery and depot systems in medicine, drug industry and biotechnology. These results demonstrated the possibility of using developed microcontainers for preserving the bioactivity of different encapsulated enzymes such as urease, chymotripsin, etc.

Another novel use of E-LbL nanoassembly is using biocompatible nanoparticulate TiO_2 multilayers to coat photosensitive materials to increase their photostability. The added benefit of this process is that due to surface modification, an increase the dissolution rate and possibly the bioavailability of a poorly water-soluble drug can be achieved. The photostability of nifedipine microcrystals (35 μm) coated with a nanoshell composed of multiple bilayers of positively charged PDDA and negatively charged nanosized TiO_2 particles (20–25 nm) was increased because even with one TiO_2 layer the shelf-life of nifedipine was increased by 30 h independent of the intensity of the light exposure, as shown in Fig. 12.10. With an increase in the number of TiO_2 layers, the photostability of the drug was enhanced even more. In addition, a TiO_2 monolayer decreased the contact angle by 20° for water

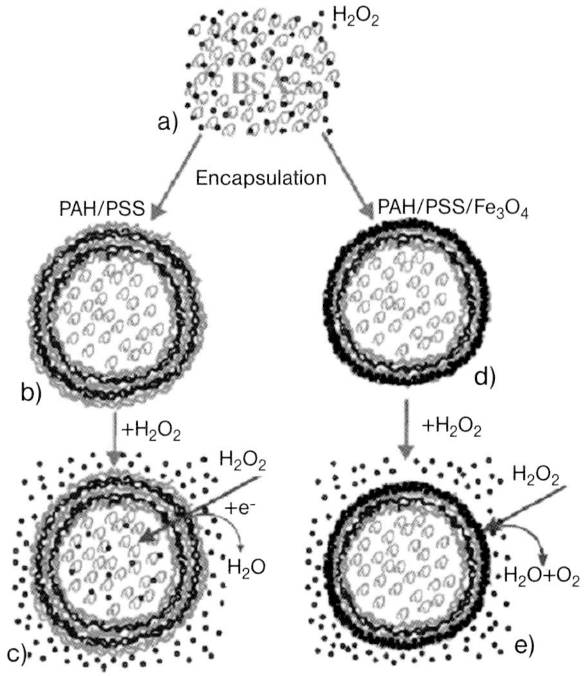

Figure 12.9. Schematic overview of the "passive" and "active" protection approaches for nanoengineered polyelectrolyte capsules. For "passive" shells (b and c), part of the H_2O_2 is reduced by the PAH/PSS shell material. "Active" ones (d and e) combine catalytic and redox mechanisms to provide a more efficient protection barrier. The magnetic activity of polyelectrolyte capsules doped with Fe_3O_4 is also preserved after (and during) H_2O_2 treatment. (Adapted from Ref. [33].)

and 33° for the dissolution medium as compared with uncoated nifedipine surfaces. This increase in wettability due to a decrease in contact angle increased the dissolution rate of nifedipine microcrystals coated with one PDDA/TiO_2 bilayer 13-fold after 10 min, 5-fold after 1 h and 2-fold after 12 h when compared to uncoated microcrystals. It is assumed that TiO_2 increased the photostability because the nanoparticulate multilayers act as a potential filter protecting the drug from damaging light rays reaching the drug crystals. The dissolution rate was increased because the hydrophilic TiO_2 nanoparticles increased the aqueous wettability of the drug crystals, thereby preventing aggregation in the dissolution medium. This ensured that the maximum drug surface area was exposed to the dissolution medium.

The increased dissolution observed for TiO_2-coated drug particles showed that in addition to protecting the drug load, E-LbL nanoshells can also assist in changing the physicochemical properties of drug cores. This was also illustrated for dexamethasone where sonication during the layering process helped to reduce the particle size of the drug, thereby increasing the dissolution rate of this practically water-

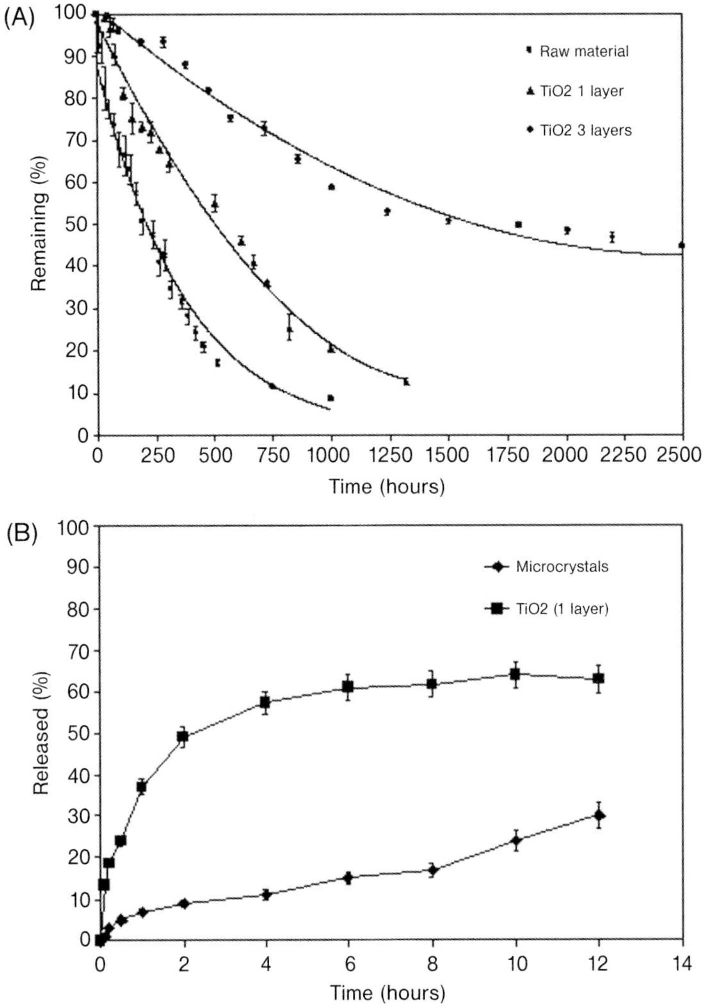

Figure 12.10. (A) Decrease in the photo-instability of nifedipine microcrystals when LbL coated with nanosized TiO_2 particles where exposed to an illuminance of 12 W m^{-2} corresponding to a light dose of 30 klux. (B) *In vitro* release profiles for nifedipine showing the increase in the dissolution rate of the drug when coated with one layer of TiO_2 nanoparticles.

insoluble drug, while also increasing the suspension stability [41]. For negatively charged micronized dexamethasone particles the effective adsorption of a first layer of PDDA during sonication as evidenced by microelectrophoresis measurement of the reversal in charge caused enhanced dispersability of the dexamethasone particles because of the colloidal stabilization produced by the positively charged PDDA coating combined with a significant reduction particles size to below 2 μm. Stabilizing of the practically monodispersed particles also reduced the

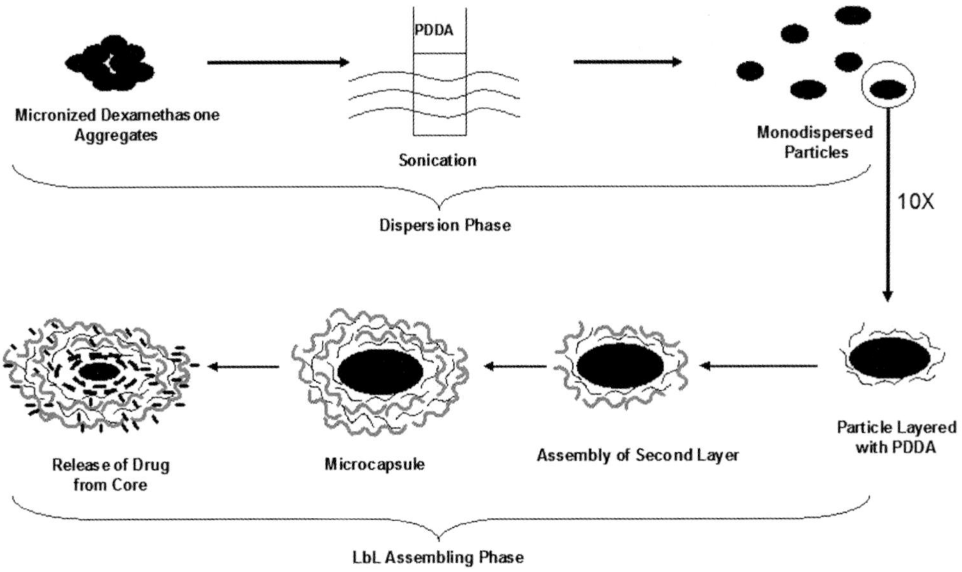

Figure 12.11. Illustration of the monodispersion of micronized dexamethasone drug particles by E-LbL encapsulation followed by the subsequent controlled release of the drug through the insoluble porous shell.

Ostwald maturation of the colloidal particles of the scarcely soluble dexamethasone, thereby preserving the reduction in particles size and the integrity and the shape of the original crystals. A schematic of this process is shown in Fig. 12.11.

12.3.4
Magnetic Nanoshells

By using the E-LbL assembly it is also possible to include magnetic nanoparticles (such as magnetite or cobalt) into the shell, thereby making the entire capsule magnetic. The example in Fig. 12.12 shows a 400-nm diameter capsule composed of a glucose oxidase core covered with a shell composed of two bilayers of 12-nm diameter magnetite alternating with cationic PEI. Deposition of magnetite nanoparticles provided a magnetic momentum that allowed the nano/bioreactors to be self-stirred and even be separated by the application of an external magnetic field [71].

In a further development based on this work, ferromagnetic cobalt nanoparticles coated with gold (Co@Au) were included in the capsule shell. With these particles, the application of a low-frequency rotating magnetic field rotated these particles, eventually providing shell distortion and release of the capsule content (Fig. 12.13) [72]. While looking at these functional capsules it is important to underline that the effect is not due to hypothermal heating because this effect works at much

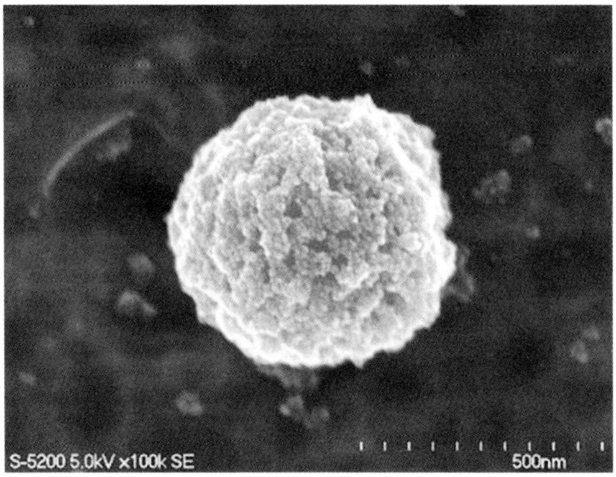

Figure 12.12. A 400-nm diameter GOx core coated with $(PSS/PEI)_2 + (magnetite/PEI)_2$ shells. The 12-nm diameter magnetite nanoparticles are visible on the surface.

higher frequencies of the magnetic field. However, a magnetic field to modulate the permeability of polyelectrolyte microcapsules prepared by LbL self-assembly was also explored. For this purpose 5-nm diameter ferromagnetic Co@Au nanoparticles were embedded inside capsule walls. The final 5-μm diameter microcapsules had wall structures consisting of four bilayers of PSS/PAH, one layer of Co@Au and five bilayers of PSS/PAH. Applying an external alternating magnetic field of 100–300 Hz and 1200 Oe rotated the embedded Co@Au nanoparticles. This rotation subsequently disturbed and distorted the capsule wall, and drastically increased its permeability for macromolecules like fluorescein isothiocyanate (FITC)-labeled dextran. The capsule permeability change was estimated by taking the capsule interior and exterior fluorescent intensity ratio using confocal laser scanning microscopy. Capsules with one layer of Co@Au nanoparticles and 10

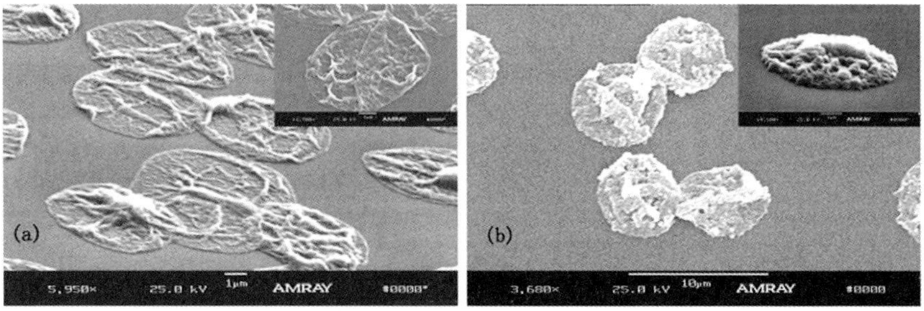

Figure 12.13. SEM images of (a) hollow capsules with $(PSS/PAH)_{11}$ and (b) magnetic capsules with one layer of embedded Co@Au $[(PSS/PAH)_4(PSS/Co@Au)_1(PSS/PAH)_6]$ (both in the dry and collapsed state).

polyelectrolyte bilayers were optimal for magnetically controlling permeability. In this study the authors provided a theoretical explanation for the permeability control mechanisms. What is important to realize is that "switching on" of these microcapsules using a magnetic field makes this method a good candidate for controlled drug delivery in biomedical applications.

12.3.5 Nano-organized Shells with Functions other than a Adjustable Diffusion Barrier

12.3.5.1 Colloidal Stabilization

The above discussions have focused on the concept of nanoshell assembly based on the possibility to design multilayer walls with controllable diffusion which may include active defense of the capsule interior. One of the advantages of this approach is using in mild cooperative electrostatic interaction not involving covalent bonding that may disturb drug molecules structure (especially for enzymatic drugs). One of disadvantages of this technology is the necessity of a multistep deposition process which often may be reached only after 10–16 sequential adsorption steps. During development of this technique, we found that not only slow drug release is in demand, but colloidal stabilization and faster release for poorly soluble drugs are also important. In such an application, one does not need many adsorption steps that produce a thick nanoshell and we can convert submicron insoluble drug particles to stable colloids with controllable fast release only with two to three deposition steps as shown in Fig. 12.11.

12.3.5.2 Interpolyelectrolyte Complex Formation

Working with soft protein microcores (such as insulin), the crucial importance of interpolyelectrolyte complexation between the shell polyelectrolyte layers and the protein core was shown [69]. In this case, the shell grows "roots" into the core and for controlled release the optimization of this complex formation is more important than just increasing of number of polymer layers in the shell wall [69]. To illustrate this, nano-organized encapsulation of protein microcores in the presence of high concentrations of a neutral polymer (PEG) was elaborated using the E-LbL process. This is important because it was found that uncoated insulin microparticles formed by controlled phase separation from hydrophilic compounds undergo fast dissolution if the PEG concentration is decreased. For the same insulin, when E-LbL encapsulation was used, the microparticle was stabilized after complexation of the insulin core with the first layer of oppositely charged polymer. This meant that the addition of new polyelectrolyte layers was easier. However, balancing the strong interaction of the first polyelectrolyte layer with the protein microcore was crucial, and the controlled release depended on the second and subsequent layers because this interaction was decreased by depositing the second oppositely charge polyelectrolyte. This allows for the control of complexation of the encapsulated proteins with the first polyelectrolyte layer until sustained release of the insulin is achieved. The general idea of controllable complex formation can be summarized as follows. First, adsorption of the first polyelectrolyte layer results in strong complex formation and very slow release. Addition of the second, oppositely charged polyelectrolyte layer results in a relaxed complex and quicker release. The third oppositely charged layer again gives slower release, etc. Therefore just increasing the thickness of the capsule walls within five to 10 bilayers (30–60 nm) did not slow insulin release from the microparticles. With this, the concept formulated earlier [69] where the LbL multilayer was considered as a tight diffusion barrier with adjustable thickness is now converted to a new approach where the main role in the controlled release from protein microaggregates is governed by adjustable interpolyelectrolyte complex formation controlled by alternate polycation/polyanion coating of as few as two to three monolayers.

12.3.5.3 **Biomimetic Approach**

The concept of using E-LbL shells to act as a nonbiological (engineered) replica allows the reproduction of the shape and maybe even some organization features of biological cells and viruses. Ai and coworkers [73] demonstrated the E-LbL nanocoating of blood platelets. This nanocoating included an antigen outermost layer for targeting these cells to antibody-coated regions in a capillary that simulated a blood vessel. Using this approach, other small biological cores may also be reproduced through shell formation. For example, the nonbiological replication of the shape and dimensions of a virus with E-LbL nanoassembly is a feasible goal to develop, for example, a viral-like drug delivery vehicle. Figure 12.14 gives preliminary results for the design of a nanoparticulate shell replica of bacteriophage Sd that has an average diameter of 78 nm. As can be seen for the transmission electron microscopy (TEM) images, the nanocapsule E-LbL assembly may be a good instrument for designing artificial virus systems to serve as intercellular drug carriers. In addition, with this nano-architecture, the E-LbL method can be use to reproduce some features of the virus structure, such as certain protein or lipid layers, in the replica shell, making this drug nanocarrier very similar to the virus. This means that treatment with such replicas will follow the same biological path as the viral infection.

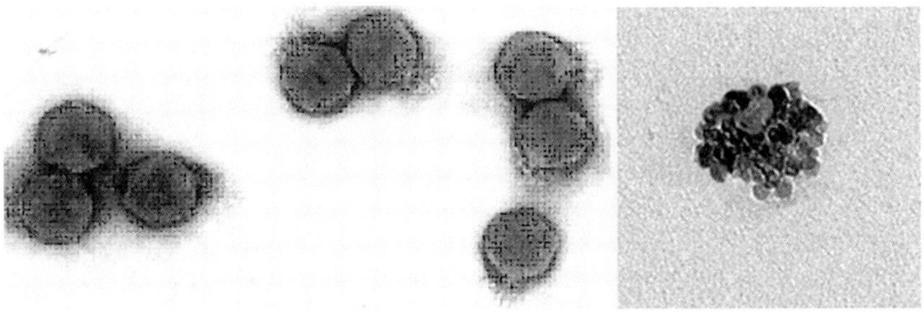

Figure 12.14. TEM images of bacteriophage Sd used as a template for the formation of a 8-nm silica nanoparticle shell (right image with the icosahedra shape), overall diameter $D = 78$ nm, clearly showing the small tail or "basal plate". The DNA core diameter is 68 nm and protein shell thickness is about 5 nm.

12.4 Conclusion

Nanoshells present a unique class of nano/microparticles with a wide range of potential application in nanomedicine. The most exciting include the possibility of engineering very small and/or very thin structures that through experimentation can be developed into reproducible and reliable platforms that integrate micro/nanotechnologies for the advanced delivery and targeting of drugs. In addition they can be used to immobilize and copy cells or viruses, and to trap, embed and protect small and macromolecules on surfaces. Although this field is still in its infancy, many ongoing developments (and the products produced) offer some unique opportunities for possible clinical applications that still need to be explored. Concurrently exploring of these technologies can also lead to the development of very sensitive *in vivo* testing methods and targeted *in vivo* diagnostic systems. The ultimate goal is to combine delivery, sensing and targeting into a single multifunctional nanoshell.

These novel possibilities should ensure that the future for nanoshell technologies remains bright. As we learn more about the construction and permeability properties of these nanothick shells, their applications as drug carriers, biosensing devices, microreactors, etc., are becoming clearer. This is especially true if one looks at recent research results that have uncovered the effect of and the controlled use of variables such as pH, ionic strength and temperature to modulate not only the fabrication of nanoshells, but also to control the permeability of these shells. Progress in the understanding of these principles of multilayer construction, interaction of charges within the shell and competition of various interactions within the crowded environment of polyelectrolyte layers is vital for the future progress in the area of responsive metallic and polyelectrolyte nanoshells.

In addition, answering the fundamental questions of the effect of self-assembly conditions and the strength of intermolecular adhesion within nanoshells and their effect on the rate of macromolecular rearrangements in responsive films and the permeation rate of solute molecules within or from nanoshells may enable the rational design of nanoshells with specific response characteristics. Hopefully, unraveling these fundamental properties may lead to new strategies in the construction of responsive coatings, e.g. those that respond to multiple stimuli and deliver multiple active molecules in a controlled way, thus producing novel drug delivery systems.

Last, but not least, we speculate that nanoshells could play a role in the future treatment of specific diseases such as cancers. These particles can be designed in such a way that they are small enough to find their way through the human circulatory system after injection. Bioactive molecules can be attached to the nanoshell surface, trapped within the shell or covered by the shell to cause selective binding or accumulation of these particles within a tumor. Using external sources such as magnetic fields or heating with a NIR laser, carcinoma tissue can then be destroyed by local effects such as thermal heating around the nanoshells.

To conclude, nanotechnology as represented by nanoshells can provide numerous advances for medicine. It might revolutionize methods used in medical science, enabling future medicine to become even more successful in its objective to save lives. We believe that the examples mentioned here represent a small fraction of the future advances that will come from nanoshells. We also believe that although the two methods to prepare nanoshells have the same foundation, there is no evidence that the future developments obtained using the two methods will be equivalent. The presence of some trends and research data leads us to believe that the versatility of polyelectrolyte LbL nanoencapsulation currently makes its wide application in drug delivery perhaps more promising. However, it will be fascinating to see what new applications arise in the future for both these systems.

References

1 S. A. Maier, P. G. Kik, H. A. Atwater, S. Meltzer, E. Harel, B. E. Koel, A. R. G. Local detection of electromagnetic energy transport below the diffraction limit in metal nanoparticle plasmon waveguides, *Nat. Mater.* **2003**, *2*, 229–232.

2 S. R. Sershen, S. L. Westcott, N. J. Halas, J. L. West. Temperature-sensitive polymer–nanoshell composites for photothermally modulated delivery, *J. Biomed. Mater. Res.* **2000**, *51*, 293–298.

3 K. Nassau. *The Physics and Chemistry of Color.* Wiley, New York, **2001**.

4 G. Mie. Contributions to the optics of turbid media, especially colloidal metal solutions, *Ann. Phys. (Leipzig)* **1908**, *25*, 377–445.

5 U. Kreibig, M. Vollmer. *Optical Properties of Metal Clusters.* Springer, Berlin, **1995**.

6 S. J. Oldenburg, R. D. Averitt, S. L. Westcott, N. J. Halas. Nano-engineering of optical resonances, *Chem. Phys. Lett.* **1998**, *288*, 243–247.

7 E. Prodan, A. Lee, P. Nordlander. The effect of a dielectric core and embedding medium on the polarizability of metallic nanoshells, *Chem. Phys. Lett.* **2002**, *360*, 325–332.

8 R. D. Averitt, S. L. Westcott, N. J. Halas. Ultrafast optical properties of gold nanoshells, *J. Opt. Soc. Am. B* **1999**, *16*, 1824–1832.

9 R. D. Averitt, D. Sarkar, N. J. Halas. Plasmon resonance shifts of Au-coated Au2S nanoshells: insight into multicomponent nanoparticle growth, *Phys. Rev. Lett.* **1997**, *78*, 4217–4220.

10 Y. Sun, B. T. Mayers, Y. Xia. Template-engaged replacement reaction: a one-step approach to the large-scale synthesis of metal nanostructures with hollow interiors, *Nano Lett.* **2002**, 2, 481–485.

11 F. Caruso, M. Spasova, V. Salguirino-Maceira, L. M. Liz-Marzan. Multilayer assemblies of silica-encapsulated gold nanoparticles on decomposable colloid templates, *Adv. Mater.* **2001**, *13*, 1090–1094.

12 Y. Sun, B. Mayers, Y. Xia. Metal nanostructure with hollow interiors, *Adv. Mater.* **2003**, *15*, 641–646.

13 L. R. Hirsch, A. Jackson, A. Lee, N. J. Halas, J. L. West. A whole blood immunoassay using gold nanoshells, *Anal. Chem.* **2003**, *75*, 2377–2381.

14 L. R. Hirsch, R. J. Stafford, J. A. Bankson, S. R. Sershen, B. Rivera, R. E. Price, J. D. Hazle, N. J. Halas, J. L. West. Nanoshell-mediated near-infrared thermal therapy of tumors under magnetic resonance guidance, *Proc. Natl Acad. Sci. USA* **2003**, *100*, 13549–13554.

15 Y. M. Lvov, G. Decher, H. Möhwald. Assembly, structural characterization

and thermal behavior of layer-by-layer deposited ultrathin films of polyvinylsulfate and polyallylamine, *Langmuir* **1993**, *9*, 481–486.

16 Y. M. Lvov, K. Ariga, I. Ichinose, K. Kunitake. Assembly of multicomponent protein films by means of electrostatic layer-by-layer adsorption, *J. Am. Chem. Soc.* **1995**, *117*, 6117–6123.

17 G. Decher. Fuzzy nanoassemblies: toward layered polymeric multicomposites, *Science* **1997**, *227*, 1232–1237.

18 Y. M. Lvov, F. Caruso. Biocolloids with ordered urease multilayer shells as enzymatic reactors, *Anal. Chem.* **2001**, *73*, 4212–4217.

19 J. B. Tieke, F. van Ackern, L. Krasemann, A. Toutianoush. Ultrathin self-assembled polyelectrolyte multilayer membranes, *Eur. Phys. E* **2001**, *5*, 29–39.

20 H. Ai, S. A. Jones, Y. M. Lvov. Biomedical applications of electrostatic layer-by-layer nano-assembly of polymers, enzymes and nanoparticles, *Cell Biochem. Biophys.* **2003**, *39*, 23–43.

21 R. K. Iler. Multilayers of colloidal particles, *J. Colloid Interface Sci.* **1966**, *21*, 569–594.

22 H. Ai, S. A. Jones, M. M. de Villiers, Y. M. Lvov. Nano-encapsulation of furosemide microcrystals for controlled drug release, *J. Control. Release* **2003**, *86*, 59–68.

23 G. B. Sukhorukov, E. Donath, S. Davis, H. Lichtenfeld, F. Caruso, V. I. Popov, H. Möhwald. Step-wise polyelectrolyte assembly on particle surfaces-a novel approach to colloid design, *Polym. Adv. Technol.* **1998**, *9*, 759–767.

24 A. A. Antipov, G. B. Sukhorukov, E. Danoth, H. Möhwald. Sustained release properties of polyelectrolyte multilayer capsules, *J. Phys. Chem. B* **2001**, *105*, 2281–2284.

25 I. Suzuki, T. Ishizaki, H. Ihoue, J. Anzai. Modification of polyelectrolyte layered assembly using an active ester of azobenzene carboxylate, *Macromolecules* **2002**, *35*, 6470–6474.

26 G. B. Sukhorukov, E. Danoth, E. Moya, S. Susha, A. Voigt, A. Hartmann, H. Mohwald. Microencapsulation by means of stepwise adsorption of polyelectrolytes, *J. Microencapsul.* **2000**, *17*, 177–185.

27 A. A. Antipov, G. B. Sukhorukov. Polyelectrolyte multilayer capsules with tunable permeability, *Adv. Colloid Interface Sci.* **2004**, *111*, 46–61.

28 A. Voigt, N. Buske, G. B. Sukhorukov, A. A. Antipov, S. Leporatti, H. Lichtenfeld, H. Baumler, E. Donath, H. Mohwald. Novel polyelectrolyte multilayer micro- and nanocapsules as magnetic carriers, *J. Magn. Magn. Mater.* **2001**, *225*, 59–66.

29 R. Ghan, T. Shutava, A. Patel, V. John, Y. M. Lvov. Enzyme-catalyzed polymerization of phenols within polyelectrolyte microcapsules, *Macromolecules* **2004**, *37*, 4519–4524.

30 T. Shutava, Z. Zheng, V. John, Y. M. Lvov. Microcapsule modification with peroxidase-catalyzed phenol polymerization, *Biomacromolecules* **2004**, *5*, 914–921.

31 M. Gao, C. Lesser, S. Kirstein, H. Mohwald, A. L. Rogach, H. Weller. Electroluminescence of different colors from polycation/CdTe nanocrystal self-assembled films, *J. Appl. Phys.* **2000**, *87*, 2297–2302.

32 P. Stroeve, V. Vasquez, M. A. Coelho, J. F. Rabolt. Gas transfer in supported films made by molecular self-assembly of ionic polymers, *Thin Solid Films* **1996**, 284–285, 708–712.

33 D. G. Shchukin, T. Shutava, E. Shchukina, G. B. Sukhorukov, Y. M. Lvov. Modified polyelectrolyte microcapsules as smart defense systems, *Chem. Mater.* **2004**, *16*, 3446–3451.

34 T. Shutava, M. Prouty, D. Kommireddy, Y. M. Lvov. pH responsive decomposable layer-by-layer nanofilms and capsules on the basis of tannic acid, *Macromolecules* **2005**, *38*, 2850–2858.

35 J. Mendelsohn, C. Barrett, V. Chan, A. Pal, A. Mayes, M. Rubner. Fabrication of microporous thin films from polyelectrolyte multilayers, *Langmur* **2000**, *16*, 5017–5023.

36 M. Sano, Y. M. Lvov, T. Kunitake. Formation of ultrathin polymer layers on solid substrates by means of polymerizationinduced epitaxy and alternate adsorption, *Annu. Rev. Mater. Sci.* **1996**, *26*, 153–187.

37 Y. M. Lvov, K. Ariga, T. Kunitake. Layer-by-layer assembly of alternate protein/polyion ultrathin films, *Chem. Lett.* **1994**, 2323–2326.

38 D. Elbert, C. Herbert, J. Hubbell. Thin polymer layers formed by polyelectrolyte multilayer techniques on biological surfaces, *Langmuir* **1999**, *15*, 5355–5362.

39 G. Decher, Y. M. Lvov, J. Schmitt. Proof of multilayer structural organization of polycation/polyanion self-assembled films, *Thin Solid Films* **1994**, *244*, 772–777.

40 V. Tsukruk, F. Rinderspacher, V. Bliznyuk. Self-assembled multilayer films from dendrimers, *Langmuir* **1997**, *13*, 2171–2176.

41 N. Pargaonkar, Y. M. Lvov, N. Li, J. H. Steenekamp, M. M. De Villiers. Controlled release of dexamethasone from microcapsules produced by polyelectrolyte layer-by-layer nanoassembly, *Pharm. Res.* **2005**, *22*, 826–835.

42 Y. M. Lvov, R. R. Price, J. V. Selinger, A. Singh, M. S. Spector, J. M. Schnur. Imaging nanoscale patterns on biologically derived microstructures, *Langmuir* **2000**, *16*, 5932–5935.

43 Y. M. Lvov, K. Ariga, M. Onda, I. Ichinose, T. Kunitake. A careful examination of the adsorption step in the alternate layer-by-layer assembly of linear polyanion and polycation, *Colloids Surf. A* **1999**, *146*, 337–346.

44 M. Onda, Y. M. Lvov, K. Ariga, T. Kunitake. Sequential reaction and product separation on molecular films of glucoamylase and glucose oxidase assembled on an ultrafilter, *J. Ferment. Bioeng.* **1996**, *82*, 502–506.

45 N. G. Hoogeveen, M. A. C. Stuart, G. J. Fleer, M. R. Boehmer. Formation and stability of multilayers of polyelectrolytes, *Langmuir* **1996**, *12*, 3675–3681.

46 D. Yoo, S. S. Shiratori, M. F. Rubner. Controlling bilayer composition and surface wettability of sequentially adsorbed multilayers of weak polyelectrolytes, *Macromolecules* **1998**, *31*, 4309–4318.

47 A. A. Antipov, D. Shchukin, Y. Fedutik, A. I. Petrov, G. B. Sukhorukov, H. Mohwald. Carbonate microparticles for hollow polyelectrolyte capsules fabrication, *Colloids Surf. A Physicochem. Eng. Asp.* **2002**, *224*, 535–541.

48 G. Ibarz, L. Dahne, E. Donath, H. Mohwald. Controlled permeability of polyelectrolyte capsules via defined annealing, *Chem. Mater.* **2002**, *14*, 4059–4062.

49 B. Neu, A. Voigt, R. Mitlohner, S. Leporatti, I. L. Radchenko, E. Donath, H. Mohwald. Biological cells as templates for hollow microcapsules, *J. Microencapsul.* **2001**, *18*, 385–395.

50 S. Moya, L. Dahne, A. Voigt, S. Leporatti, E. Donath, H. Mohwald. Polyelectrolyte multilayer capsules templated on biological cells: core oxidation influences layer chemistry, *Colloids Surf. A Physicochem. Eng. Asp.* **2001**, 183–185, 27–40.

51 R. VonKlitzing, H. Mohwald. A realistic diffusion model for ultrathin polyelectrolyte films, *Macromolecules* **1996**, *29*, 6901–6906.

52 S. Leporatti, C. Gao, A. Voigt, E. Donath, H. Mohwald. Shrinking of ultrathin polyelectrolyte multilayer capsules upon annealing: a confocal laser scanning microscopy and scanning force microscopy study, *Eur. Phys. J. E Soft Matter* **2001**, *5*, 13–20.

53 K. Glinel, G. B. Sukhorukov, H. Mohwald, V. Khrenov, K. Tauer. Thermosensitive hollow capsules based on thermoresponsive polyelectrolytes, *Macromol. Chem. Phys.* **2003**, *204*, 1784–1790.

54 J. Dai, A. W. Jensen, D. K. Mohanty, J. Erndt, M. L. Bruening. Controlling the permeability of multilayered polyelectrolyte films through derivatization, cross-linking, and hydrolysis, *Langmuir* **2001**, *17*, 931–937.

55 A. I. Petrov, A. A. Antipov, G. B. Sukhorukov. Base–acid equilibria in polyelectrolyte systems: from weak polyelectrolytes to interpolyelectrolyte complexes and multilayered polyelectrolyte shells, *Macromolecules* **2003**, *36*, 10079–10086.

56 Y. Lvov, A. Antipov, A. Mamedov, H. Mohwald, G. Sukhorukov. Urease encapsulation in nanoorganized microshells, *Nano Lett.* **2001**, *1*, 125–128.

57 K. Leong, B. Brott, R. Langer. Bioerodible polyanhydrides as drug-carrier matrices. I: characterization, degradation, and release characteristics, *J. Biomed. Mater. Res.* **1985**, *9*, 941–955.

58 B. Jeong, Y. Bae, D. Lee, S. Kim. Biodegradable block copolymers as injectable drug-delivery systems, *Nature* **1997**, *388*, 860–862.

59 L. Mounkes, W. Zhong, G. Cipres-Palacin, T. Heath, R. Debs. Proteoglycans mediate cationic liposome–DNA complex-based gene delivery *in vitro* and *in vivo*, *J. Biol. Chem.* **1998**, *273*, 26164–26170.

60 V. Junyaprasert, A. Mitrevej, N. Sinchaipanid, P. Boonme, D. Wurster. Effect of process variables on the microencapsulation of vitamin a palmitate by gelatin-acacia coacervation, *Drug. Dev. Ind. Pharm.* **2001**, *27*, 561–566.

61 S. Keller, H.-N. Kim, T. Mallouk. Layer-by-layer assembly of intercalation compounds and superlattices on surfaces: towards molecular "beaker" epitaxy, *J. Am. Chem. Soc.* **1994**, *116*, 8817–8821.

62 J. Schlenoff. Redox-active polyelectrolyte multilayers, *Adv. Mater.* **1998**, *10*, 347–351.

63 X. Qiu, S. Leporatti, E. Donath, H. Mohwald. Studies on the drug release properties of polysaccharide multilayers encapsulated ibuprofen microparticles, *Langmuir* **2001**, *17*, 5375–5380.

64 H. Beyers, S. Malan, J. van der Watt, M. M. De Villiers. Structure–solubility relationship and thermal decomposition of furosemide, *Drug. Dev. Ind. Pharm.* **2000**, *26*, 1077–1083.

65 S. Ye, C. Wang, X. Liu, Z. Tong. Deposition temperature effect on release rate of indomethacin microcrystals from microcapsules of layer-by-layer assembled chitosan and alginate multilayer films, *J. Control. Release* **2005**, *106*, 319–328.

66 G. B. Sukhorukov, H. Mohwald, G. Decher, Y. M. Lvov. Assembly of polyelectrolyte multilayer films by consecutively alternating adsorption of polynucleotides and polycations, *Thin Solid Films* **1996**, *284*, 220–223.

67 J. Kong, Z. Lu, Y. M. Lvov, R. Desamero, H. Frank, J. Direct electrochemistry of cofactor redox sites in bacterial photosynthetic reaction center protein, *J. Am. Chem. Soc.* **1999**, *120*, 7371–7372.

68 F. Caruso, K. Nikura, N. Furlong, Y. Okahata. Assembly of alternating polyelectrolyte and protein multilayer films for immunosensing, *Langmuir* **1997**, *13*, 3427–3433.

69 J. Rashba-Step, R. Darvari, Q. Lin, J. Kelly, T. Shutava, Y. Lvov, T. Scott. Surface modification of PROMAXX microparticles. In *Proceedings 33rd Annual Controlled Release Society Meeting*, Vienna, **2006**, pp. 126–129.

70 C. Leuschner, W. Hansel. Membrane disrupting lytic peptides for cancer treatments, *Curr. Pharm. Des.* **2004**, *10*, 2299–2310.

71 M. Fang, P. Grant, M. McShane, G. Sukhorukov, V. Golub, Y. M. Lvov. Magnetic bio/nanoreactor with multilayer shells of glucose oxidase and inorganic nanoparticles, *Langmuir* **2002**, *18*, 6338–6344.

72 Z. Lu, M. Prouty, Z. Guo, V. Golub, C. Kumar, Y. M. Lvov. Magnetic switch of permeability for polyelectrolyte microcapsules embedded with Co@Au nanoparticles, *Langmuir* **2005**, *21*, 2042–2050.

73 H. Ai, M. Fang, S. Jones, Y. Lvov. Electrostatic layer-by-layer nanoassembly on biological microtemplates: platelets, *Biomacromolecules* **2002**, *3*, 560–564.

13
Bionanoparticles and their Biomedical Applications

L. Andrew Lee, Hannah N. Barnhill, and Qian Wang

13.1
Introduction

Bionanotechnology is a newly emerging field in which novel nanomaterials are developed from biological building blocks. Primary building materials, DNA and peptides (or peptidomimetics), have been extensively studied as starting materials for nanomaterial synthesis [1–4]. Other basic elements derived from Nature's own designs include the virus and virus-like particles, ferritins, and other self-assembled protein cages such as heat shock protein (Hsp) cages [5] and some enzyme complexes [6]. These biogenic systems self-assemble based on multiple noncovalent interactions to become highly organized scaffolds with robust physical properties. These bionanoparticles (BNPs), in particular, offer fascinating structural features and sophisticated chemistries, yet are under the control of malleable genetic information. These qualities are exploited to tailor the BNPs at the atomic and molecular scales with specific functionalities (i.e. biomedical applications, supramolecular chemistry, etc.). Moreover, Hsp cages and ferritin average 12 nm in diameter, and the different viral cages span from 15 [7] to 160 nm [8], offering an extensive array of sizes.

Distinctive features of BNPs, in comparison to synthetic nanoparticles, make these biomaterials attractive for the following reasons:

- Monodispersed particles with uniform size distributions.
- Three-dimensional structures characterized at atomic or near-atomic levels.
- Genetic control over the composition and surface properties.
- High stability and organization of self-assembled architecture in nanometer ranges.
- Economic large-scale production in gram and kilogram quantities.

The aim of this chapter is to provide an overview in BNP programming and its current research in biomedical applications. There is a growing interest in BNPs as new biomaterials for directing cellular processes, such as cell growth and differentiation. Multiple ligands and peptides can be anchored to the biomaterials with

Nanotechnologies for the Life Sciences Vol. 10
Nanomaterials for Medical Diagnosis and Therapy. Edited by Challa S. S. R. Kumar

ISBN: 978-3-527-31390-7

predetermined nanometer spacing to act as homing signals for tissue-specific targeting, and these precise adornments on the nanosystems can even be transferred to more complex schemes for host immune evasion or activation. Notable nanosystems already in clinical uses as vaccines are the recombinant chimeric hepatitis B virus (HBV) particles [9] and the virus-like particles of human papillomavirus [10, 11]. The highly ordered and repetitive structures of BNPs facilitate pattern recognition by the immune systems and, consequently, are of a great benefit in protective immunity induction [12, 13]. Additionally, both genetic and chemical tools can be used to mold the scaffolds, which ultimately allows the precise control over the spatial layout of functional groups at the molecular level.

The different methods involved in manipulating the viruses and ferritins without affecting the self-assembly process is covered in section 13.2. In the following section, there is particular emphasis on controlling the orientation and density of ligands decorated on the surface of biomolecular shells via chemical and genetic methods. Then the following sections in this chapter have been divided and devoted to the various programmed functionalities of the protein-based nanoparticles: cell targeting, gene/drug delivery, bioimaging, vaccine development, immune response modulation and, lastly, the future directions of BNP research.

13.2
BNPs

Viruses provide a wide array of shapes such as rods and spheres, and a variety of sizes spanning from tens to hundreds of nanometers. These protein structures are evolutionary tested, multifaceted systems with highly ordered spatial arrangements, and natural cell-targeting and genetic information-storing capabilities. The years of dissecting the details of virus infection, replication and assembly pathways have imparted a wealth of information on the stabilities and functionalities of these materials. The structural information provided by X-ray crystallography, nuclear magnetic resonance and previous mutagenesis studies lay the firm, primary foundation for viral vector redesign. Intricately fashioned, multifunctional BNPs for various biomedical applications have spun off from viral vector-based gene therapy and vaccine development founded on the polyvalent antigen display on virus coat proteins. Virus-based assemblies are, and continue to be, a major point in the nexus of bionanotechnology.

Ferritin, another primary building block in bionanoscience, is a highly conserved protein complex that spans approximately 12–13 nm in diameter as a tetracosameric protein shell. The interior shell measures approximately 7–8 nm in diameter and encapsulates the mineralized iron core. This protein shell is endowed with astounding thermal and pH stabilities, along with tremendous resistance to denaturation in high ion concentrations to act as protein templates for inorganic material synthesis. The biomineralization with a variety of other metal atoms in apoferritin, the hollow protein shell without the iron core, exemplifies this concept of using such a biological template for inorganic nanoparticle synthesis [14–16].

Although research on viruses and ferritin outweighs the other protein cages, new systems such as chaperones [5, 17] and carboxysomes [18] have sprung up as possible alternative protein cages for bionanosciences. The characterizations of these systems are in much earlier phases compared to the preceding nanosystems of viruses and ferritin, but each individual system is a potential novel nanomaterial for future chemistries and genetic reprogramming. These platforms, derived from protein-based systems like viruses and ferritin, offer a high degree of spatial organization with well-characterized self-assembly motifs – a quality that can be of major advantage in BNPs for controlling functional group density and orientation. Many of these protein shells permit biological modifications by genetic insertions of foreign peptide sequences and orthogonal chemistries to alter the native protein to incorporate multiple functionalities.

Viruses and other BNPs have been previously employed as vaccine carriers and gene therapy vectors [19–23], but the potential applications of viruses and BNPs for chemical reactions and material synthesis have not been systematically explored until recently. Current research topics in BNP chemistry can be broadly classified as host–guest chemistry (including biomineralization and phage display), controlled self-assembly and bioconjugate chemistry.

BNP-based inorganic materials development has advanced greatly over the past few years, pioneered by S. Mann, T. Douglas (together with M. Young) and A. M. Belcher. Mann and coworkers have prepared magnetic nanoparticles with apoferritin as nanoreactors by biomimetic syntheses [14]. Douglas, Young and coworkers have made important contributions in the syntheses of inorganic nanoparticles with cowpea chlorotic mottle virus (CCMV) and other protein cages as templates [15, 24–28] or catalysts [16]. Belcher and coworkers' work on using filamentous bacteriophage M13 to bind and align nanocrystals in an ordered array is another example of harnessing the logic of biological synthesis for nanomaterial development [6, 29, 30]. Genetically modified M13 have been used as templates to align inorganic, organic and biological nanosized materials into nanowires [31, 32], nanorings [33], nanofibers [34], films [35, 36] and other nanostructures [29, 37–39].

In addition to the organic reactions of ferritin and adenovirus [40–44], there have been many recent developments in the chemoselective organic modifications of BNPs. Finn and coworkers have extensively quantified the organic chemical reactions of viruses as molecular entities [45–48]. Cowpea mosaic virus (CPMV) has been demonstrated to be a robust platform for conjugation with a variety of molecules, including fluorescent dyes [45–48], poly(ethylene glycol) (PEG) chains [49], stilbene derivatives [45], biotin [47, 48], DNA, peptides [50], antibodies [45] and carbohydrates [51]. This strategy permits the covalent installation of functional groups in multiples of 60 at well-defined locations. Following CPMV, the chemical reactivities of many other viruses have been studied, including CCMV [52], Nudaurelia capensis ω virus (NωV) [53], tobacco mosaic virus (TMV) [54], small Hsp

[5], turnip yellow mosaic virus (TYMV) [55, 56] and bacteriophage MS2 [57]. In short, BNPs provide chemists and material scientists with conveniently accessible scaffolds whose structure and functionality can be genetically programmed and manipulated.

These protein shells are treated as complex chemical compounds that can be utilized as vehicles for drug/gene delivery [58–60], two-dimensional ordered arrays [35], nanowire synthesis [31], depositions on films or polymers or even biocomposite material synthesis [29, 32, 34, 37–39]. The precise manipulation of these platforms relies heavily on the multidisciplinary integration of organic synthesis, molecular, structural and cell biology, and bio-organic chemistry to devise, functionalize and analyze these complex macromolecular structures. These disciplines are unified under a unique theme of re-engineering the self-organizing biological systems in the nanometer range with molecular specificity for a strategic purpose – gene or drug delivery, eliciting an immune response or *in vivo* bioimaging.

13.3 Genetic and Chemical Alterations of BNPs

13.3.1 Chemical Modifications

Although a few organic reactions of ferritin and adenovirus have been reported [40–44], it was not until recently that the chemoselective organic modification of BNPs has been studied systematically. In all the cases, the accessibility is the key to the reactivity of a functional residue on BNPs. In other words, if a functional side-chain is exposed on the surface (either interior or exterior) or is accessible to the reactant, it generally can be modified.

13.3.1.1 Conventional Bioconjugation Methods for Selective Modifications

The conventional way to modify the BNP relies on the protein chemistry, particularly the reactivity of the functional groups of the side-chains. The amino group of lysine residues (Lys), the thiol group of cysteine residues (Cys), the carboxylic groups of glutamic acid (Glu) and aspartic acid (Asp), and the phenol groups of tyrosines (Tyr) are among the best for chemical modification (Fig. 13.1) [61]. If accessible Lys, Cys, Glu/Asp and Tyr can be found or created, they should be able to be derivatized. In addition, orthogonal reaction conditions are generally required to modify a group of residues selectively without interference with the other functional groups.

CPMV, as a prototype of icosahedral viruses for organic reactions, is now well understood from the studies of Finn and Johnson groups over the past 5 years [45–48, 51, 62, 63]. The particle has been found to be highly rigid in the X-ray crystal structure, such that residues are shown to be hindered and remain inaccessible to chemical reagents in solution.

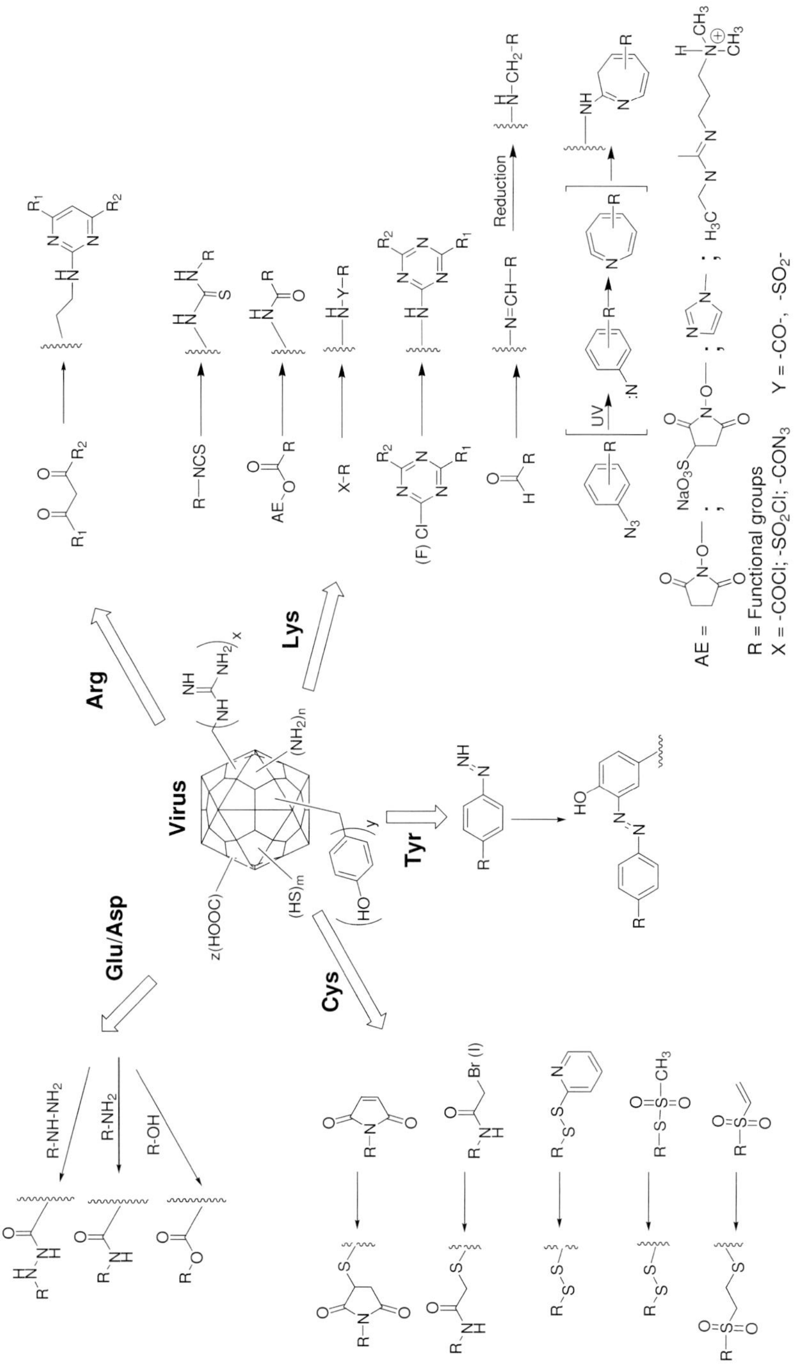

Figure 13.1. Chemical modifications toward multiple functional groups on BNPs.

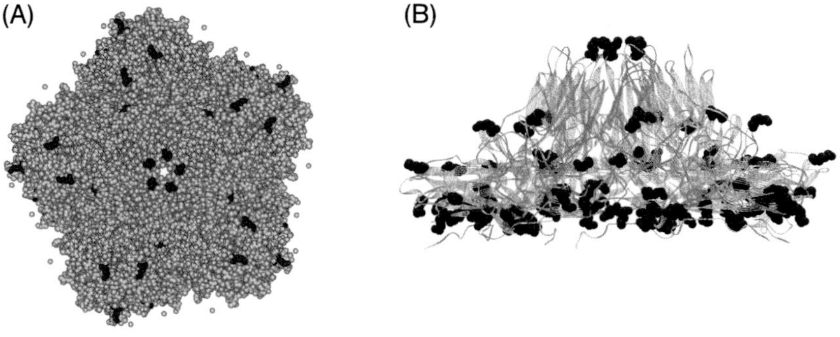

Figure 13.2. Structure of the pentameric units of CPMV coat protein with lysines marked in blue. (A) Top view of the space-filling model showing the exterior surface-exposed lysines. (B) Side view of the ribbon diagram of the pentamer with all lysines highlighted. Most of the lysines locate at the interior surface of the protein cell to bind to the RNA inside.

13.3.1.1.1 **Lysine Reactivity** Figure 13.2 shows the space-filling and ribbon diagrams of the outside surface of the CPMV pentameric unit. Only five lysine residues appear to be exposed to the solvent on the exterior, whereas at least 10 are found on the interior surface, presumably involved in electrostatic interactions with the packaged RNA genome and therefore unreactive with external reagents. In initial studies, fluorescent dyes were employed as probes to monitor the reactivities of CPMV. The exposed lysines of wild-type CPMV were reacted with fluorescein *N*-hydroxysuccinimide (NHS) ester **1** and isothiocyanate **2**, which are reagents selective for reactions with available lysine residues (Scheme 13.1) [48].

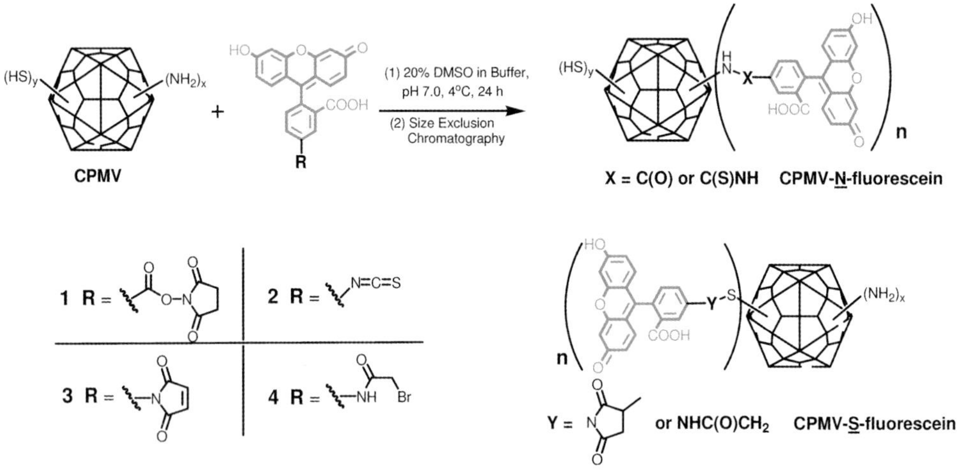

Scheme 13.1. Chemical modification of CPMV at reactive lysines and cysteines (virus shown in a schematic manner).

The particles were very stable, which can withstand the organic reagents and the conditions. The integrity of the modified viral particles was confirmed by sucrose gradient sedimentation, transmission election microscopy (TEM) and fast protein liquid chromatography (FPLC) analysis. Covalently modified virions were separated from excess dye reagents by multiple passages through size-exclusion columns until dye was undetectable in the wash solution and the relevant absorbance ratios for the virus samples were constant. Nonspecific dye adsorption to the virus had not been observed. The stoichiometries were determined by absorption measurements on solutions of labeled particles by comparison of the intensities of dyes (495 nm for fluorescein) to viruses (260 nm), each having nonoverlapping bands with well-established molar absorptions.

At neutral pH, wild-type CPMV was found to be readily labeled by NHS esters at room temperature, up to a ratio of between 60 and 70 dye molecules per virion, in a dose-dependent fashion through a reagent ratio (dye:viral protein) of 200:1 (Fig. 13.3B). Pushing the reaction with greater amounts of **1** (up to

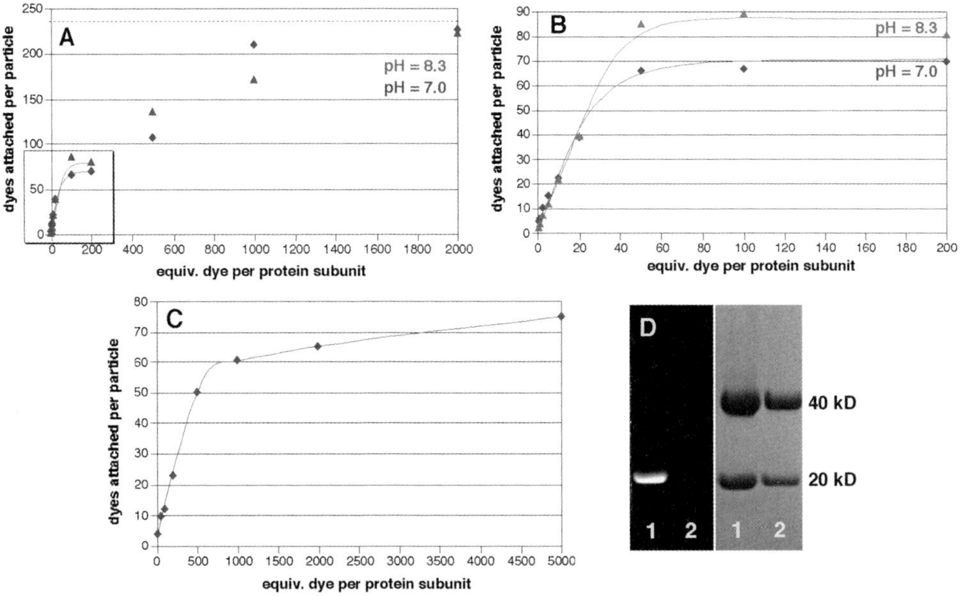

Figure 13.3. Relationship of the ratio of reactants (Scheme 13.1) to the number of attached dyes per CPMV particle. (A) Results of reactions using fluorescein NHS ester **1**, showing the full range of ratios of the reactants used. (B) Expansion of the boxed area in (A). (C) Results of reactions using fluorescein isothiocyanate (FITC) **2**. (D) Sodium dodecyl sulfate–polyacrylamide gel electrophoresis (SDS–PAGE): lanes 1, CPMV-*N*-fluorescein prepared using reagent **2**, containing approximately 50 dyes per particle; lanes 2, underivatized wild-type CPMV. Left (black background), visualized directly under UV illumination showing the attachment of fluorescein to the small subunit; right (lighter background), stained with Coomassie blue to reveal both subunits. (Reprinted from Ref. [48], © 2002, with permission from Elsevier.)

dye:protein = 4000:1) gave a maximum loading at both pH 7.0 and 8.3 of about 240 dyes per virion, indicating that four lysine residues per asymmetric unit are accessible under forcing conditions (Fig. 13.3A). The isothiocyanate reagent proved to be less reactive and thus more selective, requiring approximately 1000 equivalents to get a loading of 60 dyes per virus particle (Fig. 13.3C). Further increasing the amount of isothiocyanate dye by a factor of 5 resulted in only a modest increase in the number of dye molecules attached per virion. Electrophoresis of the resulting particles under denaturing conditions showed predominant lysine reactivity at lower loading (50 dyes per particle using isothiocyanate **2**) to be associated with the small subunit (Fig. 13.3D).

NHS esters and isothiocyanates are very efficient regents to modify accessible lysines on BNP. For example, fluorescent dye **1** has also been applied to derivatize the lysines of CCMV [52] and the small Hsp (MjHsp) cage from *Methanococcus jannaschii* [5]. The latter has been used in selective attachment and release of chemotherapeutic agents [64]. A similar strategy has been applied to study the differentiated reactivities of lysine residues of NωV virus-like particles (VLPs) during a pH-induced conformational change [53]. NωV is a single-stranded RNA icosahedral insect virus, whose capsid is composed of 240 copies of the 70-kDa subunit protein. The VLPs of NωV are readily produced using a recombinant baculovirus system. At pH 7.6 the coat protein assembled into a stable ("procapsid") particle, which is 480 Å in diameter and quite porous. Upon lowering the pH to 5.0, a concerted reorganization into a 410-Å diameter mature capsid structure occurs. The

Figure 13.4. (A) Cryo-electron microscopy analysis results of Nanogold-modified CPMV with the density of gold labeled with a golden color. The electron densities of gold clusters were generated by subtracting density computed with the native CPMV X-ray structure from the density of Nanogold-derivatized CPMV cysteine mutants. (B) A pentameric section of the gold densities superimposed on the atomic model of CPMV showing that the gold is attached at the site of designed cysteine mutation. (Reprinted from Ref. [46], © 2002, with permission from Wiley-VCH.)

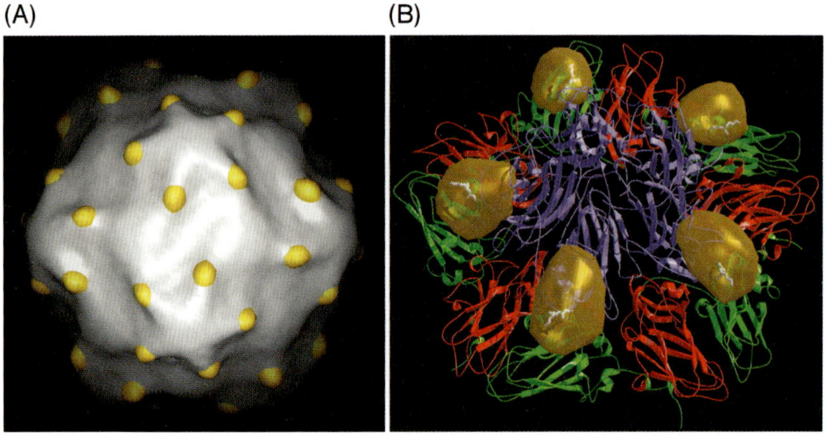

pH-induced contraction of NωV is one of the largest relative changes known to occur in virus particles. Since both the procapsid and capsid forms of NωV VLPs are stable at pH 7.6, this system offers a rare opportunity to study the chemical reactivities of such large assemblies in two dramatically different states. With fluorescein derivatives **1** and **2**, approximately 240 dye units can be attached per VLP in the mature capsid form. As expected, procapsid VLPs were significantly more reactive than their capsid counterparts under identical conditions [53]. This result clearly demonstrated the importance of accessibility of a functional group to its reactivity.

13.3.1.1.2 **Cysteine Reactivity** The reactivity of cysteines of CPMV has also been carefully studied. The crystal structure of CPMV displays no free cysteine residue exposed on the exterior surface of the capsid. When wild-type CPMV was treated with thiol-selective reagents such as N-bromoacetamide **3** and maleimide **4** (Scheme 13.1), the reactions were very slow and give alkylation of thiol residues located exclusively on the *interior* surface of the protein capsid. There were no obvious reactions after 6 h of incubation with **3** and **4** [46, 51]. Additional amino acids can be inserted into a few solvent-exposed sites without interfering the ability of the resulting mutant virus to propagate in the host plant [20, 65–67]. Taking advantage of the biological nature of the virus, addressable cysteine residues were genetically introduced on the exterior surface of CPMV, using standard cloning techniques. These sites, the βB–βC and $\beta C'$–$\beta C''$ loops of the small subunit and the βE–βF loop of the large subunit, are color-marked in Fig. 13.5. Each of the virus mutants contain a cysteine residue inserted as part of an added small loop or as a point mutation, and thus each particle contains 60 such insertions arrayed in icosahedral symmetry on the 30-nm diameter capsid. The altered sequences are genetically stable through multiple rounds of infection, harvesting, and reinoculation. The average purification yield of the mutant viruses is comparable to wild-type, but the presence of β-mercaptoethanol (BME) or tris(2-carboxyethyl)phosphine (TCEP) was necessary throughout the isolation procedure to avoid crosslinking of particles when they were pelleted by ultracentrifugation or stored after purification.

The thiol groups of the introduced cysteine residues of the mutant viruses are more exposed to the surface than the native cysteines of CPMV. Compared with the wild-type virus, the new inserted cysteines demonstrated much higher reactivity. All the thiol groups could be derivatized with very low concentration of the maleimide or bromoacetamide electrophiles at neutral pH within 6 h at 4 °C (Scheme 13.1). More importantly, the different sites of attachment could be programmed by genetic mutagenesis based on the structure information. For example, when mutant virus was reacted with monomaleimido-Nanogold®, derivatized particles were flash frozen and examined by cryo-electron microscopy and a three-dimensional image reconstruction was computed. In Fig. 13.4, the electron densities of the gold clusters are clearly visible at the positions of the inserted cysteine residues [46]. This provided an example of the engineering of chemically reactive functional groups at designated positions on the icosahedral protein template by genetic methods.

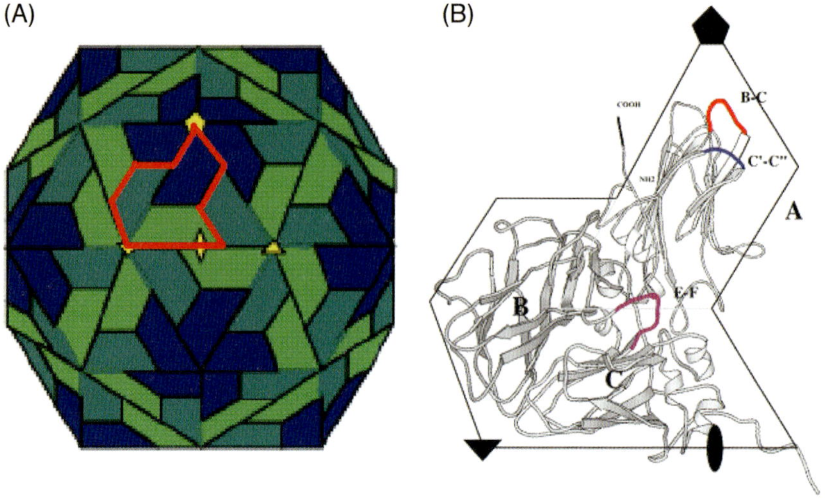

Figure 13.5. CPMV structure. (A) A diagrammatic representation of CPMV showing the distribution of the two subunits that comprise the "asymmetric unit", 60 copies of which form the icosahedral particle. The trapezoids in red and green represent the two domains of the large subunit clustered around the 3-fold symmetry axes and the blue trapezoid represents the small subunit clustered about the 5-fold symmetry axes. (B) Ribbon diagram of the two subunits of the CPMV coat protein, with the sites of mutational insertion highlighted in red (βB–βC loop) and purple (βE–βF loop). (Reprinted from Ref. [48], © 2002, with permission from Elsevier).

It is an interesting observation that in general there is no cysteine exposed to the exterior environment for any native virus or other BNPs. While that may be a result of evolution to avoid nonspecific aggregation, it offers a unique opportunity to selectively modify the BNPs. Genetic introduction of accessible cysteine very often brings in a unique reactive site, which can be derivatized chemoselectively and regioselectively. In addition to CPMV, such a technique has also been applied to CCMV [52, 68] and MjHsp [5].

13.3.1.1.3 **Reactivity on Carboxylic Groups (Glutamate And Aspartate)** At neutral pH and mild conditions, amines can be used to derivatize surface-exposed carboxylic groups upon activation. A cocatalyzed system, 1-ethyl-3-(3-dimethylaminopropyl)carbodiimide (EDC) and NHS, is commonly used in the modification of the carboxylic groups of BNPs. For example, horse spleen ferritin (HSF) has been modified with long-chain aliphatic amine activated by EDC/NHS. The resulted particles can be dissolved in nonaqueous solutions [41, 69]. Similarly, CCMV [52], TMV [54] and TYMV [55] can also be addressed on the exterior surface.

13.3.1.1.4 **Orthogonal Modification of BNPs** Based on conventional bioconjugation methods, it is possible to attach multiple, distinct functionalities on BNPs with orthogonal reactions. For example, the cysteine-inserted CPMV particles maintain the native reactive lysines. Therefore, one can selectively modify the lysines with NHS ester (or isothiocyanate) and the cysteines with maleimides. With this method, blue fluorescent antibody and PEG have been attached to CPMV cysteine mutants [45]. Scheme 13.2 shows two other examples of dual modification of BNPs [70, 71].

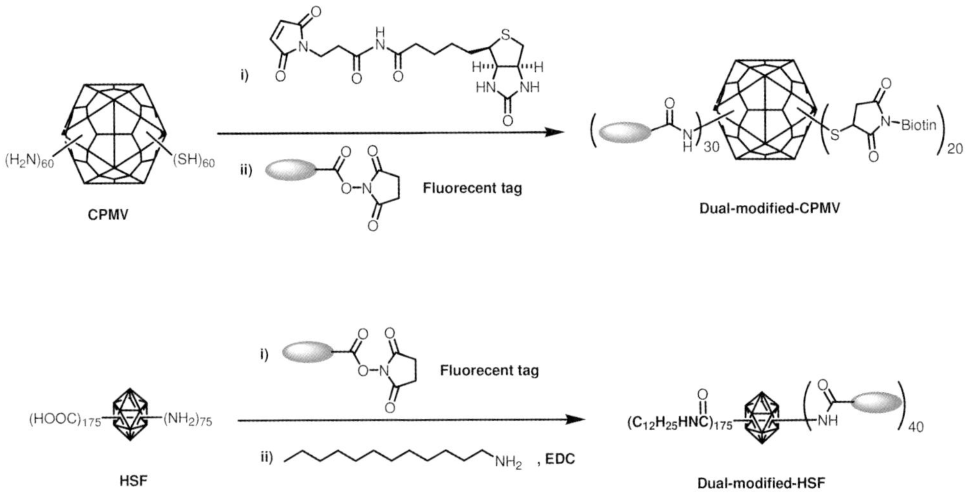

Scheme 13.2. Dual modification of CPMV and HSF with orthogonal reactive lysines and cysteines.

13.3.1.2 **"Click Chemistry" for Bioconjugation of BNPs**

The copper-catalyzed azide–alkyne cycloaddition (CuAAC) reaction, discovered in 2002 [72, 73], has emerged as an excellent method for connecting diverse building blocks in organic synthesis. It is a classic example of "click chemistry" coined by Sharpless and his coworkers [73, 74]. As the azide and alkyne groups are each almost entirely unreactive with proteins, nucleic acids, acids, bases and water, the reaction is well suited to the formation of covalent bonds to biological molecules with no side-reactions. In particular, shortly after the discovery of the CuAAC reaction, many other new catalytic systems were been reported [72, 75–77], which further promoted the application of this reaction in bioconjugation process. Finn and coworkers pioneered in using this reaction for the bioconjugation of plant virus [78]. CPMV was successfully labeled at all 60 identical protein asymmetric units of the capsid (Scheme 13.3A). Tris(carboxylethyl)phosphine (TCEP), a water-soluble reducing agent, was used to reduce Cu(II) to Cu(I) at 4 °C. Addition of ligand **5** drastically enhanced the reaction rate and an almost quantitative amount of modified proteins could be recovered after the reaction. The azide moiety could be attached to lysine, cysteine or tyrosine residues [62, 78]. Different fluorescent compounds

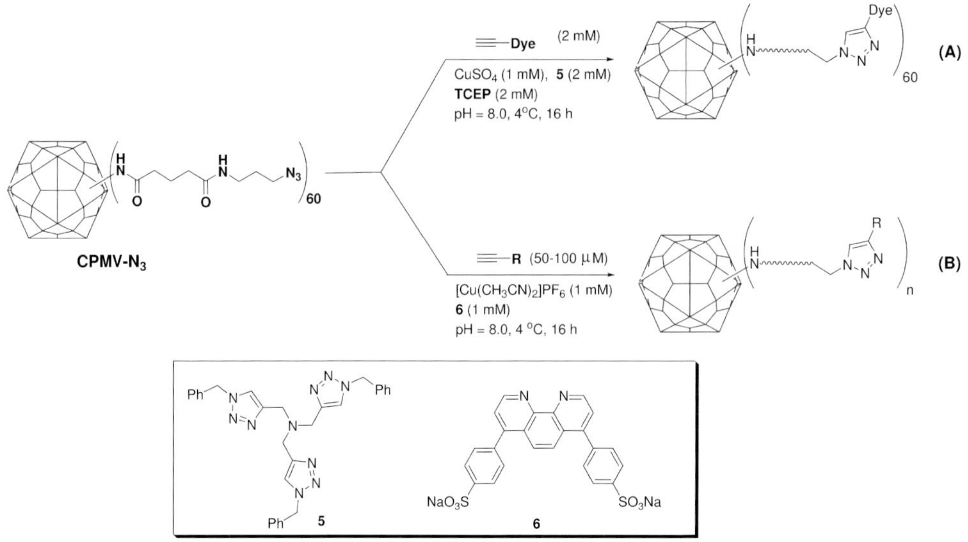

Scheme 13.3. Bioconjugation by azide–alkyne cycloaddition to derivatized CPMV particles through the Cu(I)-catalyzed azide–alkyne coupling reaction under different catalytic conditions [77, 78].

contained acetylene groups were anchored on viral surfaces with this reaction, while only millimolar concentrations of dye reactants were required [78, 79]. Using a new catalyst **6** [77], the reactivity of the reaction has been improved significantly so that micromolar protein can be connected to mid-micromolar concentrations of small molecules, polymers and proteins, all in high yield and with excellent purity (Fig. 13.3B) [80].

The ligation strategy developed by Finn and coworkers was confirmed to be remarkably reliable and suitable for most of bio-platforms and has been followed by other groups for different purposes. For example, Tirrell and coworkers incorporated non-natural azido-amino acids into the *Escherichia coli* cell membrane protein OmpC, which were successfully modified with biotin-alkyne via a Cu(I)-mediated 1,3-dipolar cycloaddition [75, 81]. Schultz and coworkers introduced azido-amino acids or alkyne-amino acids into proteins in yeast [82, 83] and the pIII protein of M13 filamentous phage [84]. These were sequentially reacted with fluorescent dyes or polyethylene glycols via the CuAAC reaction. Recently, two useful fluorogenic click reactions have been reported independently by the groups of Fahrni and Wang (Scheme 13.4) [85, 86]. Wang and coworkers synthesized 3-azidocoumarins (**7**), which show no or very weak fluorescence due to the quenching effect from the 3-azido groups. Upon coupling with arylalkynes, most of the triazole products strongly fluoresce [86]. The mild reaction conditions allowed the combinatorial screening of the best azidocoumarin–alkyne pairs on the basis of fluorescent emis-

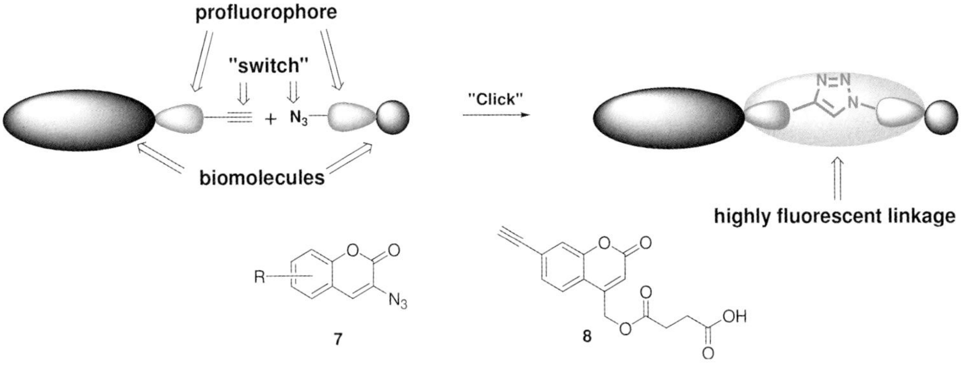

Scheme 13.4. Schematic illustration of the fluorogenic "click" reactions.

sion. Similarly, the fluorescence of **8**, synthesized by the Fahrni group, can be greatly enhanced by the triazole formation [85].

As this reaction tolerates most of functional groups and the azidocoumarin will only attack the acetylenes [62, 78], the location of the acetylene groups can be predetermined by detailed proteomic study. Then, the CuAAC reaction with azidocoumarins can anchor different kinds of functionalities on predefined positions of BNPs and the fluorescent signals from the product can be used to monitor the reaction efficiency.

13.3.1.3 **New Developments in Tyrosine Modification**

The electron donating effect of the hydroxyl group makes the phenol group of tyrosine a good nucleophile towards electronphilic attack at the *ortho* position of the OH group. Using diazonium salts ($Ar{-}N{\equiv}N^+$), tyrosine can be selectively derivatized under mild conditions [61]. This reaction has been applied to modified TMV on surface tyrosines [54]. However, the reactivity of the reaction is reduced when the diazonium reagents without electron-withdrawing group on the aromatic rings are used. To solve this shortcoming, Francis and coworkers further improved the reaction with sequential derivations to render the tyrosine residue more susceptible to sophisticated modifications [57]. As shown in Scheme 13.5, the nitro-substituted diazonium salts afforded excellent tyrosine modification with MS2 bacteriophage. The resulting particles were reduced with sodium dithionite and reoxidized to *o*-iminoquinone. A further Diels–Alder reaction with acrylamides was completed in 2 h at room temperature with conversion levels exceeding 90% [57]. This modified protocol affords a versatile orthogonal pathway for bionanoparticle modification at tyrosines.

The unique structural feature of tyrosine can support multifaceted reactions other than simple nucleophilic or electrophilic substitution reactions with amino, thiol or carboxylic groups. Many new bioconjugation pathways have been revealed or re-elaborated recently, which opened new venues toward the selective modifica-

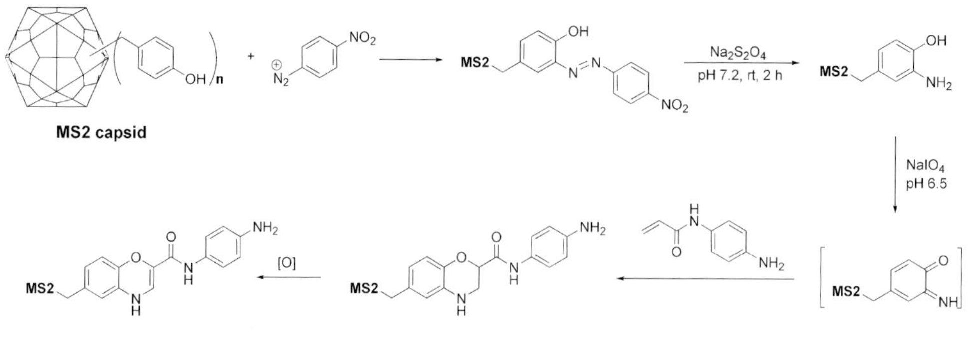

Scheme 13.5. Sequential functionalization of bacteriophage MS2.

tion of BNPs. For example, selective alkylation of protein tyrosines can be achieved by π-allylpalladium complexes (Scheme 13.6A) [87] and the *ortho* position of the hydroxyl group of tyrosine can be addressed with Mannich-type coupling reactions (Scheme 13.6B) [88].

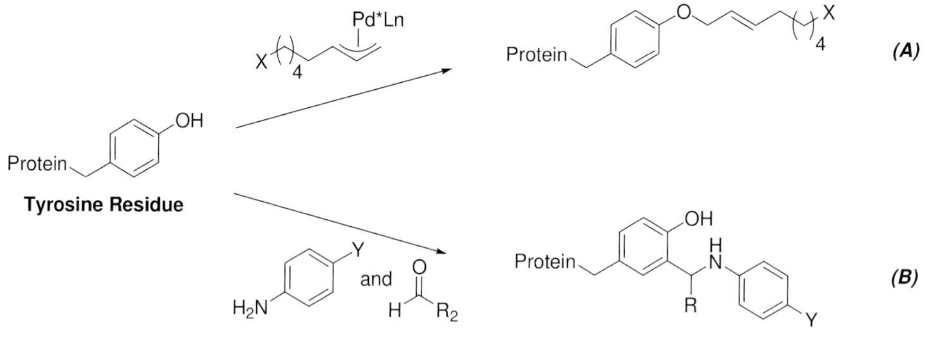

Scheme 13.6. New reactions in the selective modification of protein tyrosine residues.

13.3.2
Genetic Alterations

Many of the viruses in isolated forms are complex macromolecular assemblies of metabolically inert molecules, which can be chemically modified. Alternatively, the virus can be genetically reprogrammed in its hosts with foreign peptides to express an antigen [89, 90] or to alter the affinity of the recombinant viral particle for different cell surface receptor [59, 91]. Furthermore, single-amino-acid substitution mutagenesis allows the site-specific incorporation of reactive amino acids, such as lysines or cysteines, or non-natural amino acids (NAAs) [92] on the virus coat protein for regioselective chemical modifications. Using such methods, Schultz and his group have incorporated PEG [83], alkyne-modified amino acids [93] and photoisomerizable amino acids into the proteins [94]. *In vivo* and *in vitro* protein expression systems derived from cell lysates have also been used to drive viral protein synthesis with the NAAs [93, 95]. To that end, molecular cloning techniques are well integrated into the generation of hybrid BNPs with novel biological, chemical and physical properties.

13.3.2.1 Heterologous Peptide Insertions

The structural information provided by X-ray crystallography and NMR studies can be hallmarks for discovering strategic locations when designing a recombinant virus particle. Many of the BNPs have their structures resolved at near-atomic resolution, facilitating the generation of the recombinant nanoparticles. Often the outer surface exposed loops between major secondary structures (β-sheets and α-helices) or amino/carboxy-termini of the coat protein can be prime candidate sites for insertional mutagenesis. These alterations have ranged from single-amino-acid substitutions [47] to entire protein domain incorporations [96, 97].

The biological, physical, and structural properties of CPMV have been well characterized [98, 99]. The virus resists temperatures of up to 60 °C and is stable at extremely low pH levels for extended periods [65], providing the system with an extended shelf-life. The structure of the nonenveloped plant virus has been determined at 2.8-Å resolution [100], indicating that the virus displays a picorna-like $T = 1$ $(P = 3)$ protein shell (termed a "capsid"). Each capsid is composed of 60 copies of the asymmetric units and each unit contains three jelly-roll β-sandwich folds formed by two polypeptides (identified as "small" subunit, A domain and "large" subunit, B + C domains in Fig. 13.5).

The asymmetric units are assembled in an icosahedral surface lattice around the single-stranded viral genomic RNA to form the virus particle of approximately 30 nm in diameter. The two different RNA molecules are required for infection, which are packaged by identical capsid structures, giving virions of differing densities and molecular weights (5.16×10^6 and 5.98×10^6 Da, correspondingly). The viral genes have been cloned to a robust vector driven by CMV 35S promoter [101], which eases the transfection process by allowing direct infection with the cDNA clone rather than with RNA transcripts. Thus, the virus can be easily and inexpensively isolated from in yields of 1–2 g of virus per kilogram of infected leaves by using a simple and convenient procedure [102].

A series of peptide insertions on different positions of the virus revealed that the coat protein accomodates inserts of up to 30 amino acids with little effect on virus host range [103]. Moreover, among all the recombinant vectors synthesized, increases in viral coat protein isoelectric point had an adverse effect on the ability of the virus to spread systemically [103]. In vaccine development studies, short peptide inserts on the virus with a variety of foreign antigenic sequences have been successfully engineered on the surface of the virus with gp41 of HIV type 1 [67, 104] and VP2 protein of mink enteritis virus (MEV) [105]. These chimeric viral particles properly displayed the epitopes to elicit neutralizing antibodies against the viruses and confer protective immunity in mink against a lethal challenge of MEV. In particular, the large subunit contains a highly exposed βB–βC loop on

Figure 13.6. TYMV particle and its asymmetric unit highlighted in yellow.

the surface (Fig. 13.5), which appears to be uninvolved in intersubunit assembly and exhibits high variability in viruses within the comoviridae family [106]. A chimeric CPMV particle incorporating a 12-mer insert from the CD46 receptor on the exposed βB–βC loop was shown to inhibit measles virus entry into neurons in the brains of treated mice and prevented a brain infection when the mice were pretreated with the chimeric particles [107].

Similar protein structures within a family of viruses can be compared to reveal permissible mutational sites and identify critical residues for gene encapsidation or supramolecular assembly. TYMV (Fig. 13.6) is an RNA plant virus within the family of tymoviridae, which contains at least 20 different known species, among which three have been determined at near-atomic resolution. Selective replacements on TYMV with the homologous regions of another tymovirus, belladonna mottle virus (BeMV), had not affected the infectivity in Chinese cabbages [108]. Six of 10 such recombinants were fully viable and gave symptoms in the plants. According to this study, the amino-terminus region was particularly amendable to short peptide substitutions. The first 9 amino acids were successfully replaced with 9 amino acids from E-71 major merozoite surface antigen of *Plasmodium falciparum* to generate chimeric TYMV particles [108]. However, the study indicated that these residues reacted poorly to the antibodies raised against the E-71 epitope and the antigenic inserts were weakly immunogenic [108], suggesting that these inserts were less accessible to the surface.

In the structural comparison of the three related viruses, TYMV, physalis mottle virus (PhyMV) and desmodium yellow mottle virus (DYMoV) (Fig. 13.7), the residues His68 and His/Ser180 have been identified in the crystal structures to adopt similar configurations [109]. Bink and coworkers suggest that these two residues are involved in the RNA encapsidation or decapsidation by the virus, as mutations of the two histidines to alanines showed an absence of systemic symptoms in plants, but had not affected capsid assembly when virus coat proteins were overexpressed in *E. coli* cells [109]. The comparative analysis also revealed conserved

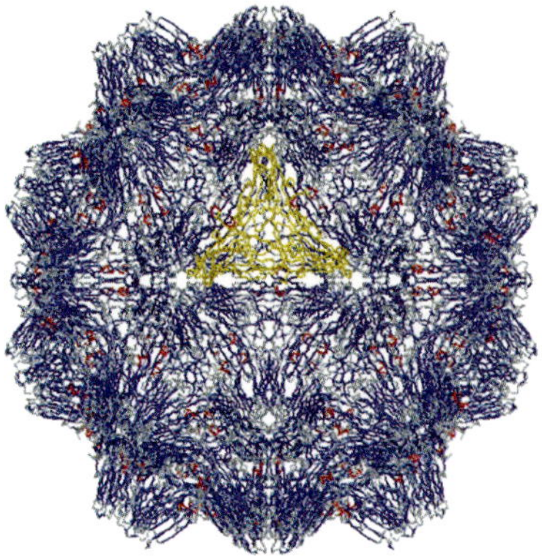

13.3 *Genetic and Chemical Alterations of BNPs* | 573

(A) (B)

(C)

Figure 13.7. Asymmetric unit (a) TYMV with H68, 180 in yellow (b) DYMoV with H68 and S180 in red, and (c) PhyMV with H69 and S181 in green.

regions throughout the coat protein gene and highly variable loops on the viral coat protein. A systematic peptide insert study on TYMV, similar to studies in CPMV, may provide valuable information on potential permutation sites.

An exceptional behavior of TYMV is its ability to release its genomic contents without completely losing its entire capsid structure. The empty vesicles can be generated via high pressures [110] or deep-freeze/thaw methods [111] and these unique structures have been visualized by cryo-electron microscopy as intact particles in solution after decapsidation. The particles offer the unique opportunity to decorate the interior cavity of about 18 nm in diameter.

TMV is a rod shaped plant virus measuring 300 nm in length and 18 nm in diameter, and assembles in a highly ordered fashion with both amino- and carboxy-termini exposed to the surface of the particle (Fig. 13.8).

The virus is highly immunogenic in mammalian hosts, which is ideal for adapting TMV-based vectors for antigen display. An initial study by Haynes and co-workers demonstrated the feasibility of incorporating immunogenic peptides as fusion proteins on the plant virus capsids [112]. Short peptide fragments of up to 21 residues had been repeatedly fused to the carboxyl-terminus of TMV using

Figure 13.8. Ribbon diagram of TMV CP. Amino- and carboxy-terminal residues are marked in blue and red, respectively. Residues Ser154 and Gly155 marked as green spheres.

a leaky "UAG" stop codon without losing viral replication or assembly [113, 114]. By exploiting the suppressible amber stop codon, a mixed pool of fused coat proteins and native coat proteins are synthesized, which can then assemble together to form the rod-like structures [113, 114]. In other studies, a variety of short inserts were made between Ser154 and Gly155 (see Fig. 13.3) using polymerase chain reaction (PCR)-based site-directed mutagenesis [115, 116]. Similar to CPMV chimeras, the isoelectric points of the TMV chimeric particles influenced the virus infectivity and systemic spreading of the recombinant virus through the plants [115]. Longer peptide sequences of up to 25 amino acids had also been fused to the carboxy-terminus by deleting 4–6 amino acids at the carboxyl end [117].

In lieu of crystallography data, other studies can provide the necessary structural information for designing a fusion peptide on the virus. Potato virus X (PVX), which has no crystallographic data, has structural [118] and serological [119] evidence suggesting that the amino-terminal domain is displayed on the surface of the virus. Based on this evidence, one team utilized PVX as foreign peptide display vector by fusing a 27-kDa green fluorescent protein (GFP) to the viral coat protein [96]. The strategy involved incorporating a 16-residue peptide derived from foot and mouth disease virus peptide 2A (FDMV 2A) at the GFP carboxy-terminus, followed by the amino-terminus of the viral coat protein gene. The linker peptide sequence, FDMV 2A, mediates a processing event that signals the cleavage of the peptides at the carboxy-terminal glycine residue [120]. This strategy allowed the generation of a heterogeneous pool of fused and free forms of viral coat proteins, which had been necessary to form virus-like rod structures in PVX, as well as in TMV [113]. Subsequently, a similar study showed the plant vector assembled as rod-like structures with a single-chain antibody fused to the viral coat protein using a mixture of native coat proteins with modified coat proteins [121]. Apparently, the fusion of larger peptides on the viral coat protein is limited by the steric constraints and the chimeric particles fails to assemble to rod-like structures without the presence of the native viral coat proteins [121]. PVX vector also facilitated the expres-

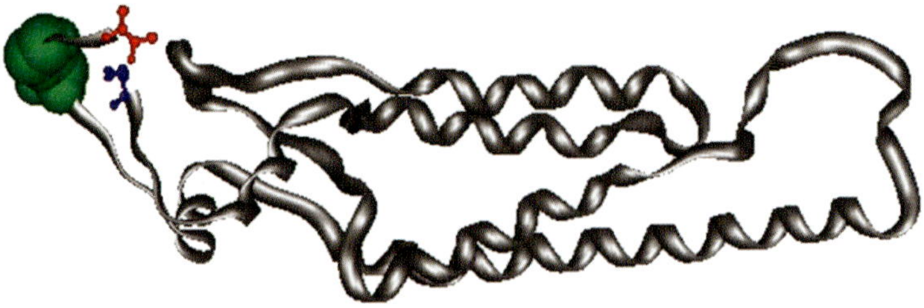

sion of an unstable peptide derived from the sequence of microbicidal yeast killer toxin (KT) by direct attachment to the viral coat protein [122]. The purified recombinant virus fused with the 10 amino acids from the yeast KT had shown enhanced antimicrobial activity against a variety of plant and human pathogens [122]. The authors suggest that the higher efficacy observed in virus-fused peptides may be due to the increased stability of the fused KP in solution when compared to the chemically synthesized KP [122].

Ferritins serve as an iron storage particle, ubiquitously found as highly ordered protein cages in higher eukaryotes [123]. The bioparticles have been demonstrated to accommodate polypeptides and proteins fused to the amino- and carboxy-termini to display the polypeptides in the interior and exterior of the protein shell, respectively [124]. A silver nucleating polypeptide fused to the carboxy-terminus had been used to sequester silver metals within the confines of the protein cage, demonstrating the potential of the ferritin cages to template inorganic materials [124].

Both site-directed and random mutagenesis are practical means of generating chimeric BNPs. However, the rate at which chimeric particles are generated in site-directed mutagenesis cannot rival the rate of chimeric particles generated by random mutagenesis. One common system, the phage display library, utilizes the natural ability of the biological system to express random polypeptides fused to the viral protein. The polypeptide is then isolated through a series of selections based on functionality or binding affinity [125]. The directed evolution of the phage system has been investigated thoroughly over the years [126] and utilized as a display platform for a variety of polypeptides (antibodies [127] and peptide ligands [125] with altered functionalities). Belcher's group exploited this feature of M13 phage to synthesize ordered nanostructures, directing the growth and assembly of the nanoparticles into one-dimensional arrays [31, 32, 36, 128]. A series of polypeptides were screened on the phage template to yield nucleating peptides for semiconductors and ferromagnetic alloys [31]. The study demonstrates that in biological systems, substrate-specific peptides can be achieved through the modification of templates.

Similar to phage display systems, a BNP can be subjected to random mutagenesis to generate variants, which can then be selected based on functionality. This combinatorial approach would be an untapped, powerful advantage in BNPs, which would require overcoming two major issues. First, the mutations of polypeptide inserts must be in the context of the BNPs as a supramolecular unit. The screening of the mutants is based on functionality and its capacity to self-assemble, which is problematic in the frame of phage display. An example is the peptide screening system designed directly on adeno-associated virus (AAV) that resulted in altered vector tropism, redirecting the selected AAV vector to primary human coronary artery endothelial cells [129]. Multiple mutation sites on the exterior of the virus coat protein had been identified and with the use of a helper virus, a series of mutant AAVs were produced. In addition, many BNPs are incompatible with bacterial expressions for rapid protein synthesis and screening. Advances in inducible protein expression and cell-free protein synthesis systems have been integrated in this field to generate many of the plant viruses.

13.3.2.2 NAA Substitutions

The advantage of generating proteins with novel functional groups encoded by the genetic template is the production of a homogenous protein unit with novel physical, chemical, and biological functionalities. Exogenous chemical agents can attach to nonspecific residues of the protein, leading to a heterogenous particle, whereas the NAA incorporation takes advantage of the natural biosynthetic translation machinery to yield a modified protein. Currently, two major methodologies exist in the production of proteins with NAAs. One method incorporates NAAs directly into the proteins *in vivo* by introducing a new tRNA–tRNA synthetase pair [82, 84, 92, 93]. The tRNA synthetase specifically aminoacylates the tRNA with the NAA, after which the charged tRNA is used in the translation process to precisely decode the RNA template. The method was used in conjunction with phage display to generate proteins with an alkyne functional group attached to the surface which was then conjugated to a variety of chemical compounds via "click chemistry" [84]. The other method involves an *in vitro* biosynthetic pathway with bacterial cell lysates and mammalian cell lysates. Over the years, Sisido and coworkers have optimized the system with a versatile tRNA aminoacylation technique [95, 130–133] to incorporate a blue-laser-excitable fluorescent amino acid [134] and multiple NAAs on a single protein using a four codon/anticodon tRNA [133].

13.3.2.3 Protein Expression Systems

Ultimately, the display of polypeptides on viruses for epitope presentation has its limitations. In some cases, foreign sequence insertions in the viral coat protein can result in loss of infectivity, replication or protein folding. Two major themes have evolved to address this limitation in virus systems. The heterologous peptide sequence can be chemically conjugated to the virus scaffold by using a bifunctional linker [80] or an alternative expression system can be explored.

Since the loss of infectivity or replication in a virus is not always correlated with the assembly pathway, recombinant virions can be produced from a variety of other protein expression systems, such as the *E. coli* expression system, *Arabidopsis thaliana* protoplast, baculovirus expression and wheat germ embryo cell extract. The generation of these reactive mutants utilizes many of the protein expression technologies developed over the years to greatly expand the repertoire of programming a protein with novel functionalities. The primary route of expression still relies on the original host cell for virus expression. However, the mutations leading to the loss of infectivity eliminates the possibility of propagation and production of the virus. The bacterial expression system is another possible option or better-suited production of some viral protein shells. Recently, the bacterial expression system has been modified to incorporate NAAs with high sequence specificity. These unnatural amino acids, such as propargylglycine, consist of an alkyne group that reacts with azide with a Cu(I) catalyst to form a triazole ring complex [78, 84, 93].

However, in other viruses, the proteins synthesized from the prokaryotes fail to assemble correctly without the proper post-translational modifications made in eukaryotic systems, ultimately requiring an economic eukaryotic protein strategy.

Plant protoplasts can also be used to directly transfect with viral RNA for the production of many types of plant viruses without the necessity of retaining the natural infection pathway. The cell-free wheat germ embryo extracts have become another possible peptide synthesis factory with several advantages over the previous protein expression systems, particularly in terms of the production of cytotoxic peptides and maintaining correct eukaryotic post-translation modifications. However, until the cost and production efficiency of the cell-free system can rival or even closely match the preceding systems, it is likely to remain as the last resort to synthesize viral coat proteins.

13.4
BNPs in Therapeutics

As described in previous sections, BNPs have several advantages over synthetic platforms, such as their ease of isolation, uniform size and defined structures. The large surface area and well-defined reactivities allow regioselective expression of polyvalent targeting units, which is extremely important for cell binding or recognition. In particular, the polyvalent display of cell-binding ligands can enhance the binding affinity and specificity dramatically. For example, Manchester and coworkers have used mutant CPMV in antiviral applications [107]. A well-characterized interaction between measles virus (MV) and its cellular receptor, CD46, were chosen for the anti-MV study. Since a specific region of CD46 has been previously identified to mediate the interaction with MV and the infection could be blocked by competition with short peptides from CD46 corresponding to the MV-interacting domains [135, 136], CPMV chimeras displaying the inhibitory peptide had been generated, which efficiently inhibited MV infection of HeLa cells *in vitro*, while wild-type CPMV did not. Furthermore, CPMV CD46 protected mice from mortality induced by an intracranial challenge with MV. The CD46 peptide presented in the context of CPMV was also up to 100-fold more effective than the solution CD46 peptide at inhibiting MV infection *in vitro* [107]. These results highlighted the polyvalent effect with BNPs as display scaffolds. In addition, the benefits of BNPs include:

(i) They represent very stable self-assembled architectures at the nanometer level with many size ranges, which are otherwise difficult to produce by standard synthetic methods in the laboratory.
(ii) They are inexpensive to isolate in large quantities. Both CPMV and TYMV can be grown in plants and purified in gram quantities with a half-day procedure.
(iii) Their structures have been characterized at near-atomic resolution.
(iv) The infectious cDNA clones of viruses are available as high-yield expression

vectors. Thus, their composition and surface properties can be precisely controlled using molecular biology techniques.
(v) In-capsid cavity can be used to encapsulate fluorescent dyes or drugs to avoid the nonspecific binding being observed with other systems.
(vi) The large surface area and well-defined reactivity allow regioselective expression of polyvalent targeting units, which is extremely important for the requirement of weak-binding ligands (e.g. boronic acid and carbohydrates) or the demand of special geometrical arrangement.
(vii) Orthogonal cell-targeting mechanisms can be engineered simultaneously on one BNP platform. Similarly, multiple detection functionalities (e.g. optical, magnetic resonance imaging, etc.) can be programmed.

13.4.1
Cell Targeting

Targeting the specific diseased cell types would localize the therapeutic agent, reducing potential side-effects and increasing the therapeutic efficacy. A few strategies have evolved over the years in arming cell-targeting moieties on various systems, including BNPs. One involves taking advantage of the natural affinity of the BNPs to target the cells. In other cases, genetic modifications on the BNPs with short peptide fragments redirect the system towards different cell surface receptors. Short peptide sequences from ligands can be genetically engineered on the BNPs. Portions of antibodies can be chemically conjugated to the protein cages to confer novel cell-targeting capability. Finally, small molecules are attached to the particles to modulate the affinity of the nanosystems for different cell types [137].

One strategy is to use the pre-existent cell-targeting motifs on the noninfectious replicas for therapeutic purposes, such as gene delivery or bioimaging. Many viruses of Polyomaviridae family generate intact VLPs, solely constructed of the major coat protein, VP1, without the two minor coat proteins (VP2 and VP3) [138]. VP1, when expressed in insect cells [139–142], yeast [143] and *E. coli* [144, 145], self-assembles as protein cages, and naturally targets a cell surface glycoprotein with a terminal $\alpha 2,3$-linked *N*-acetyl neuraminic acid [138, 146], and is internalized by the cells via $\alpha_4\beta_1$ integrin receptors [147, 148]. Human JC polyomavirus, which in its native form infects human oligodendrocytes in the brain [149], was engineered as VLPs to deliver therapeutic genes to human fetal glial cells [150]. HBV, a human liver-specific virus, contains three overlapping envelope genes in a single open reading frame, encoding for small, medium and large proteins in its 3.2-kb genome [91]. The large protein subunit of HBV can be isolated as an aggregate form of a phospholipoprotein vesicle with an average size of 80 nm, with a targeting motif for human hepatocytes specified by the sequence located in the amino-terminus of the large subunit [151]. These hybrid vesicles have been demonstrated as safe vehicles for delivery of genes with high *ex vivo* and *in vivo* transfection efficiencies, and high targeting specificity to human hepatocyte-derived cells [91, 151].

A cell-targeting system based primarily on natural binding motifs would severely limit its potential therapeutic applications. Redirecting the protein shells to other cell types by inserting peptide ligands or portions of ligands have been shown to be effective in programming altered affinities. In one study, urokinase plasminogen activator (uPA) sequences had been genetically inserted into VP1 proteins of polymaviruses to direct the recombinant particles to uPA receptor (uPAR) expressing cells [139]. In HBV nanoparticles, its native biorecognition motif was replaced with the epidermal growth factor (EGF) moiety to direct the particles to EGF receptor overexpressing cells [152]. Similarly, when an integrin receptor-targeting sequence had been fused to a small Hsp, the protein cage exhibited cell-binding capability *in vitro* [153].

Another docking concept involves attaching an antibody on the surface of BNP to change its tropism. The murine polyomavirus-like particles were engineered with eight glutamic acid residues and one cysteine residue in one of the exterior loops to attach a portion of the anti-tumor antibody B3 [154]. The antibody fragment was modified at the carboxy-terminus with peptide sequences (Arg_8CysPro), which associates with the mutant VLP via electrostatic interactions, and the complex is further stabilized by the formation of a disulfide linkage. This coupling reaction yielded polyoma VLPs with 30–40 antibody fragments bound to the surface, allowing the modified VLPs to bind to the breast carcinoma cells with high efficiencies [154]. Alternatively a bifunctional crosslinker had been used to conjugate the antibodies, which can effectively target specific cells within a mixed population [153].

The conjugation of antibodies on the BNPs can be difficult and costly to manufacture. Facile chemical modifications with small molecules can be designed to modify the surface of BNPs for cell-specific targeting. CPMV, TYMV, TMV and many other viral platforms have demonstrated robust chemical modifications directed via conventional bioconjugation techniques and alternative methods (see Section 13.3.1).

13.4.2
Gene Delivery

Gene therapy is still a promising frontier in medicine with unparalleled potential to combat genetic diseases, cancer or viral infections. Many of the retroviruses efficiently package, deliver and integrate into the host chromosomal DNA, but the wide range of cell infectivity provides little cell specificity. In addition, the labor-intensive design and high production costs in obtaining tropism-modified recombinant retroviral vectors have diverted attention to safer and more economic gene delivery systems with VLPs, which are innocuous counterparts of the original virus. The noninfectious particles in many ways mimic the functions of the original virus, but lack the essential components of the viral genome to self-propagate in the host, reducing its potential safety hazards. HBV nanoparticles and polyoma VLPs are capable of packaging a therapeutic gene and efficiently delivering it to the target cells and organs *in vitro* and *in vivo* [152, 155–157]. These particles consist of proteins produced in bacterial or yeast expression systems, which are also easily programmable by genetic and chemical methods to adapt various cell-targeting ligands, receptors or carbohydrates.

Since the initial proposal in 1970 to develop polyomavirus as a potential gene delivery vector by Osterman and coworkers [158], various methods have been established to introduce genes into a variety murine, monkey and human tissues [159–161]. Circular DNA sequences of up to 17.7 kb can be encapsulated *in vitro* by polyomavirus VP1 [159], and have been used to deliver exogenous DNA to human brain cells and fetal kidney epithelial cells [155]. Atomic force microscopy images indicated that polyoma VLPs aggregated around the heterologous DNA to form loosely associated structures and DNA transfer was mediated by cell surface sialic acid residues [60]. The polyoma VLPs were also adapted to deliver plasmids expressing short hairpin RNAs and synthetic small interfering RNAs to human lymphoblastoid cells and HeLa cells to downregulate gene expression [162].

Regardless of the vehicle, all effective gene delivery agents deal with complicated issues of targeting appropriate cells or tissue, efficient packaging, transferring, precisely integrating the therapeutic gene in the host genome, and properly expressing the therapeutic gene in the host genome with economic production and safety considerations [152].

13.4.3
Bioimaging

For *in vivo* or *in vitro* imaging (such as diffusion fluorescent tomography), it is important to have high local concentrations with no quenching of fluorescence to enhance the imaging contrast. Since BNPs can be genetically or chemically modified in a chemoselective manner, high-loading fluorescent dyes can be loaded with a precisely designed geometrical distribution on the surface of BNPs and inside the cage of BNPs. The rigid and highly ordered structures of the protein structures of BNPs "fix" the attached imaging agents at designed positions on the surface. Therefore, the attached dye molecules have no mobility to interact or aggregate to each other, which often quench the fluorescence. The observation that no fluorescence quenching of the virus–dye conjugates occurred even at a high local concentration of the dyes has been evidently demonstrated [55, 56].

Fluorescent probes are the most common imaging reagent used in BNP labeling. For example, using fluorescent dye-modified CPMV, Manchester and her coworkers have studied the systemic trafficking of CPMV in mice via the oral route [163]. The pattern of localization of CPMV particles to mouse tissues following oral or intravenous dosing was then determined by confocal fluorescent microscopy and viral RNA detection. For several days following oral or intravenous inoculation, CPMV was found in a wide variety of tissues throughout the body, including the spleen, kidney, liver, lung, stomach, small intestine, lymph nodes, brain and bone marrow. CPMV particles were detected after cardiac perfusion, suggesting that the particles entered the tissues [163]. Fluorescent dye-labeled CPMV has also been employed for intravital vascular imaging [164]. The CPMV can be labeled with high densities of Alexa Fluor or fluorescein dyes, showing no measurable quenching. The resulting exceptionally bright particles were used to visualize the vasculature and blood flow in living mouse and chick embryos to a depth of up to 500 μm. Therefore, the intravital visualization of human fibrosarcoma-mediated tumor angiogenesis using fluorescent CPMV provides a means to identify arterial and venous vessels, and to monitor the neovascularization of the tumor microenvironment [164]. In another study, the lateral mobility of fluorescent labeled murine polyoma virus-like particles bound to living cells and artificial lipid bilayers was studied by single fluorescent particle tracking using total internal reflection fluorescence microscopy [165].

To minimize the background and enhance the deep-tissue penetration ability, near-infrared (NIR) fluorescent dyes are often used for *in vivo* imaging. Significant efforts have been placed on the development of efficient bioconjugation methods for the attachment of NIR fluorescent agents to BNPs. As shown in Fig. 13.9, cyanine NIR-782 dye was attached to CPMV with over 40 dye molecules per viral particle, making a local concentration of around 1.8 mM. The purified viral–dye hybrid has been employed as a probe for NIR fluorescence imaging. Using tissue-like phantoms, fluorescent tomographic data have been obtained through a multichannel frequency domain system. The spatial maps of fluorescence quantum yield were detected with a finite element-based reconstruction algorithm [166]. In addition, a new class of carbocyanine dyes has been synthesized and conjugated to CPMV by the "click" reaction of azides and alkynes [79].

Magnetic imaging complexes or other probes can also be used to decorate BNPs. For example, luminescent semiconductor nanocrystals (quantum dots) were employed to modify CPMV [167]. Using CPMV mutants expressing available 6-histidine sequences inserted at loops on the viral coat protein [168], it was shown that CPMV particles were specifically immobilized on NeutrAvidin functionalized substrates in a controlled fashion via metal-affinity coordination. Two linking chemistries were employed to decorate CPMV with CdSe–ZnS core–shell quantum dots to target the histidine or lysine residues on the exterior virus surface and utilize biotin–avidin interactions. In the first case, quantum dots are immobilized on the surface-tethered CPMV via electrostatic attachment to avidin previously bound to the virus particle. In the second case, chemical modification of the surface lysine residues with biotin groups and the biotinylated CPMV is discretely immobilized onto the substrate via NeutrAvidin–biotin interactions. The biotin units on the upper exposed surface of the immobilized CPMV then serve as capture sites for avidin-derivatized quantum dots [167]. Similar conjugation chemistry has been used to produce virus–carbon nanotube [169] and virus–metal nanoparticle complexes [170], which have potential as biological sensors. For example, networks of gold nanoparticles and bacteriophage have recently been engineered to preserve the cell-targeting and internalization properties mediated by the specific peptide display [171]. In addition, the gold nanoparticles acted as signal reporters for fluorescence and dark-field microscopy and NIR surface-enhanced Raman scattering (SERS) spectroscopy [171]. In all these cases, BNPs

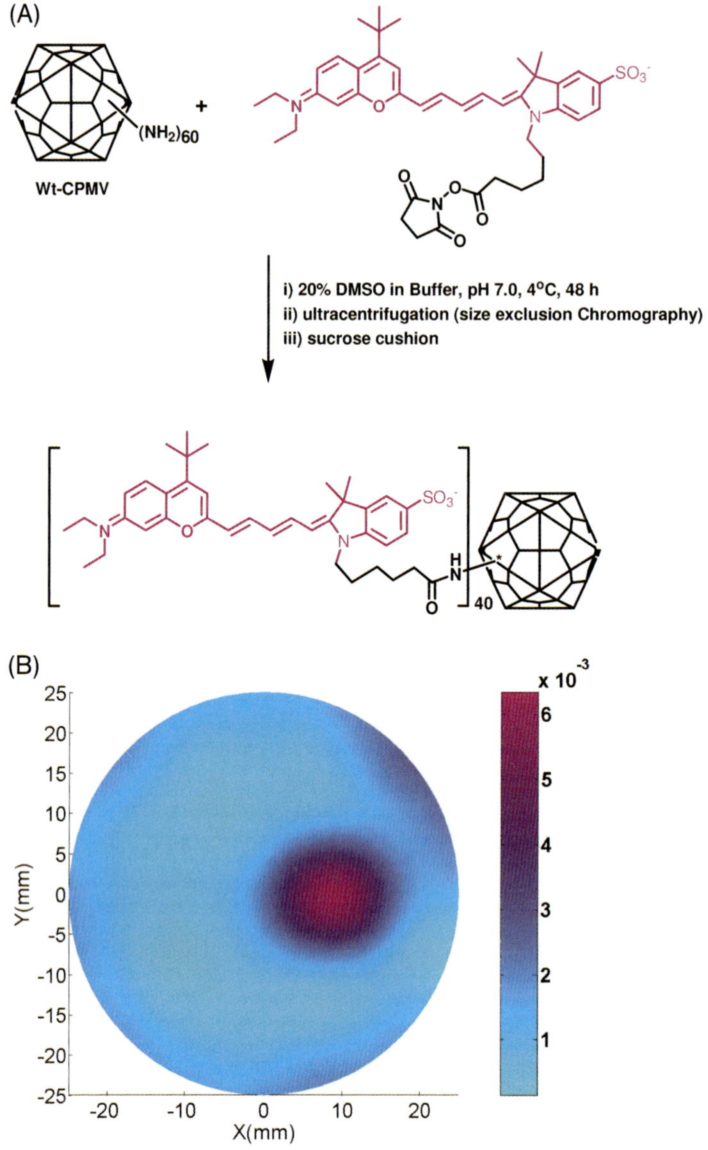

Figure 13.9. (A) Attachment of NIRF-782 to CPMV. (B) Reconstruction image of fluorescent quantum yield of dye-modified CPMV. The left and bottom axes illustrate the spatial scale in millimeters, which the color scale records the value of the quantum yield.

served as an excellent scaffold to modulate the organization of reporters for biosensing or bioimaging.

13.4.4
Drug Encapsulation and Release

The interior cavities of BNPs are hollow spaces that can encapsulate other elements for drug delivery by genetic and chemical modifications. Covalently attached small molecules are tethered to the BNPs, preventing leakage from the interior, and circumventing drug degradation and avoiding nonspecific binding, until a signal or low endosomal pH within the cell releases the drug from the carrier. Recent studies with polyoma VLPs and Hsp demonstrated the feasibility of packaging chemical compounds within the protein cage. In the case with polyoma VLPs, Schmidt and coworkers inserted the first WW domain of mouse formin binding protein 11 (FBP 11) to the amino-terminus of VP1 to attach proline-rich ligands (bearing the consensus sequence PPLP) to the inner surface of the VLPs [172]. In a similar study with polyoma VLPs, a stretch of 49 amino acids of the inner core protein from polyomavirus VP2 protein had been fused to GFP or covalently attached to methotrexate (MTX) [173]. The amino acids specifically anchored GFP and MTX to VP1, resulting in VLPs with GFP or MTX enclosed by VP1 coat proteins [173]. The encapsulated MTX retained similar cytotoxicity in the cells, and destroyed MTX-resistant cell by circumventing MTX transport.

Flenniken and coworkers covalently modified the Hsp cage interior with antitumor drugs by genetically introducing cysteine residues at the inner surface and selectively attaching the chemical compound to the reactive cysteines with a pH-sensitive linker [64]. This Hsp assembles into a 24-subunit spherical structure with an octahedral symmetry, which is 12 nm in diameter and has a porous protein shell that allows free small-molecular exchange between the interior and bulk solution [5]. The (6-maleimidocaprol) hydrazone derivative of doxorubicin was linked to the interior surface of this Hsp via coupling of maleimide and cysteine (Scheme 13.7) [64]. The quantitative analysis by absorbance spectroscopy indicated

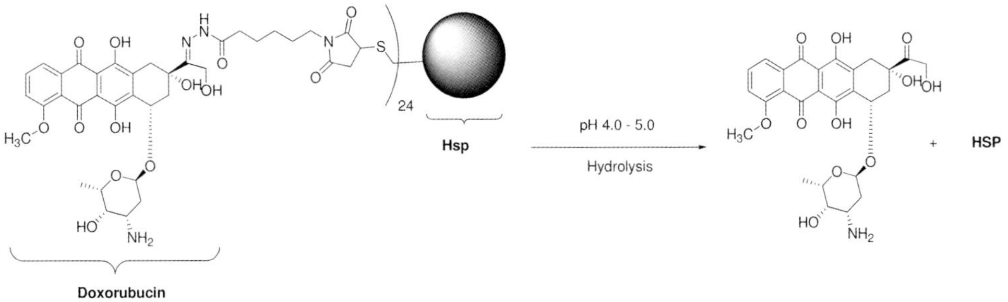

Scheme 13.7. Controlled release of doxorubicin from the interior of a small Hsp cage [64].

that 24 doxorubicin moieties were encapsulated and, under acidic conditions, doxorubicin was selectively released through the hydrolysis of hydrazone linkage (Scheme 13.7). This study demonstrates that a therapeutic agent could be housed within the interior of a BNP cage to realize its controlled release. Therefore, a BNP system has the potential to serve as a versatile drug delivery system.

13.5
Immune Response

13.5.1
Vaccine Development

The virus surface consists of highly organized repeating motifs that are ideally suited for eliciting an immune response. Although this is problematic for gene therapy or drug delivery, the polyvalent display on the BNPs can be extremely advantageous for vaccine development. In particular, plant viruses show great potential for production of pharmaceuticals in plants. The small size of plant viral genomes, the ease with which they can be manipulated and the simplicity of the infection process make the plant viral vectors an attractive alternative as transgenic systems for the displaying antigenic proteins. CPMV, TMV, PVX and alfalfa mosaic virus (AlMV) have all demonstrated enormous potential to incorporate recombinant peptide sequences to confer protective immunity and to combat against viral and bacterial infections [65, 174].

The immunological analysis of plant virus-based chimeras has been one of the most thoroughly documented among all of the BNP systems. An important demonstration of CPMV-based vaccines and its potential to stimulate protective immunity was reported by Dalsgaard and coworkers [105] using the chimeric plant virus inserted with a short linear epitope derived from the amino-terminal region of VP2 of MEV. A single, subcutaneous injection of 1 mg of chimeric particles protected mink against challenge with MEV. In a following study, dogs immunized with ultraviolet (UV)-irradiated chimera elicited high titers of neutralizing antibodies and conferred resistance to canine parvovirus [175].

PVX, another plant-based antigen display vector, showed similar results in mice with the highly conserved ELDKWA epitope from HIV-1 gp41 expressed on the viral coat proteins [176]. The mice inoculated with the PVX-derived chimeric particles were able to elicit high levels of HIV-1 epitope-specific antibodies without adjuvants. Furthermore, the human immune response to chimeric viral particles was studied with severe combined immunodeficient mice reconstituted with human peripheral blood lymphocytes (hu-PBL-SCID). hu-PBL-SCID mice immunized with chimeric viral particle-pulsed autologous dendritic cells were able to mount a specific human primary antibody response against the gp41-derived epitope [176]. Remarkably, anti-HIV-1-neutralizing activity was present in the sera from both normal and hu-PBL-SCID mice. Similar vaccine studies with AlMV have also demonstrated that peptides containing antigenic determinants of rabies virus glycoprotein and nucleoprotein fused to the viral coat protein conferred immunity in mice against lethal challenge [177].

Chimeric TMV particles containing 10 or 15 amino acids from the spike protein of murine hepatitis virus (MHV) gave rise to intact chimeric viral particles with the MHV peptides displayed on the surface [116]. The study indicated that muscosal and parenteral immunization with the chimeric TMV particles protected the treated mice against lethal doses of MHV. However, displaying larger protein structures as genetic fusions to the capsid protein has not been possible on TMV. To address this issue, a reactive lysine was introduced near the amino-terminus of TMV CP, which was further modified with biotin [178]. The biotinylated end was then tagged with GFP–streptavidin or L2 protein of canine oral papillomavirus, resulting in TMV particles with GFP or L2 protein, respectively, decorated on the exterior. The L2 protein-coupled biotinylated-TMV was found to be more immunogenic in mice than uncoupled L2 protein fragments.

Chimeras expressing epitopes of a bacterial origin have also been shown to confer protective immunity. For example, a chimeric CPMV particle expressing amino acid sequences containing two epitopes from the outer membrane protein F (ompF) of *Pseudomonas aeruginosa* protected mice against challenge with *P. aeruginosa* in a model of chronic pulmonary infection [179, 180]. Likewise, a chimera plant virus expressing the D2 domain of the fibronectin-binding protein (FnBP) from *Staphylococcus aureus* has been shown to be able to protect rats against endocarditis [181]. Thus, plant virus-based chimeras carrying neutralizing epitopes can offer novel avenues for producing effective vaccines against various infectious viruses and, more generally, for the design of new vaccination strategies in humans. (See Refs. [20, 174] for more detailed reviews on plant virus-based vaccine development.)

13.5.2
Immune Modulation

In addition to the peptide displays, the BNPs can also be adapted to present multiple sugar residues on the exterior surface. The polyvalent scaffolds decorated with various carbohydrates have shown increased binding affinity and biological responses when compared with their monomeric constituents [182–184]. Similar to previous studies with polymers and other supports, the virus has been shown to accommodate multiple mannose residues via chemical coupling [80] and inhibit cell agglutination [51]. The virus–carbohydrate conjugate can further be designed to supplement immune responses or other biological processes.

The repetitive patterns on BNPs, while beneficial for antigen display in vaccine display, can become a major problem in adapting the BNPs for diagnostic and therapeutic applications. One modality has been to modify the particle surface with PEG polymers and other polymers to reduce the immunogenic response towards the particles [185]. In adenovirus, its bioavailability and pharmacokinetics have been investigated extensively with the intention of improving adenovirus-delivered gene therapeutics [44, 186]. To facilitate the use of other protein-based systems,

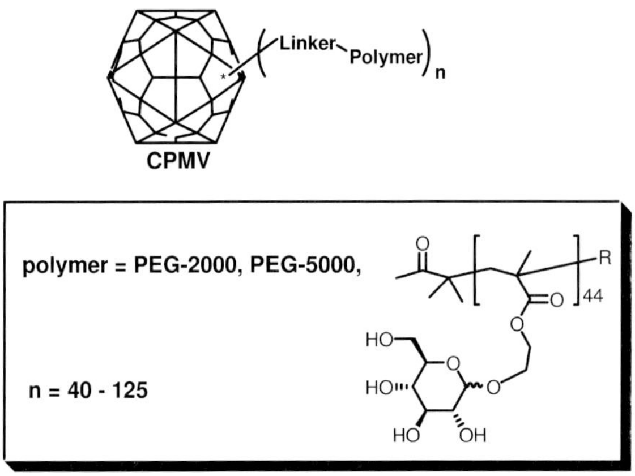

Figure 13.10. Schematic drawing of viral particle-modified polymer.

such as BNPs, Finn and his group studied the immune response towards viral particles modified with PEG and other polymers (Fig. 13.10) [49, 80]. The preliminary study was to assess the immunogenic response in mice towards PEG-modified CPMV. The levels of CPMV-specific antibodies in the mice treated with PEGylated CPMV were comparably similar to the levels in mice treated with unmodified CPMV, but the serum antibody level had drastically declined over the following 2 months in mice treated with modified CPMV compared with unmodified CPMV [49].

13.6 Future Directions

The major features of BNPs that were exploited for generating novel biotemplates in the nanometer range have been iterated throughout the chapter. In general, these protein structures naturally self-assemble to highly organized structures and many of the systems, either virus- or ferritin-based, demonstrate robust physical properties that can be exploited for variety purposes. The systems can be genetically engineered and chemically addressed to alter functionalities for future therapeutic applications. As platforms, the viruses provide a wide array of shapes such as rods and spheres, and vast ranges of sizes spanning from tens to hundreds of nanometers. Hsps and ferritin arrange as nanometer-sized materials with well-characterized hierarchical motifs as templates for mineralization. Several studies have demonstrated the feasibility of using various nanoparticles (BNPs, liposomal carriers, inorganic materials, etc.) tailored with ligands and small molecules to target different cell types for drug/gene delivery and cell imaging [56, 137, 151, 152, 164]. The nanosized probes can further be modified with chemical compounds, such as bioimaging agents (NIR fluorescent dyes, magnetic resonance imaging contrast agents) and drugs at high local concentrations to increase detection sensi-

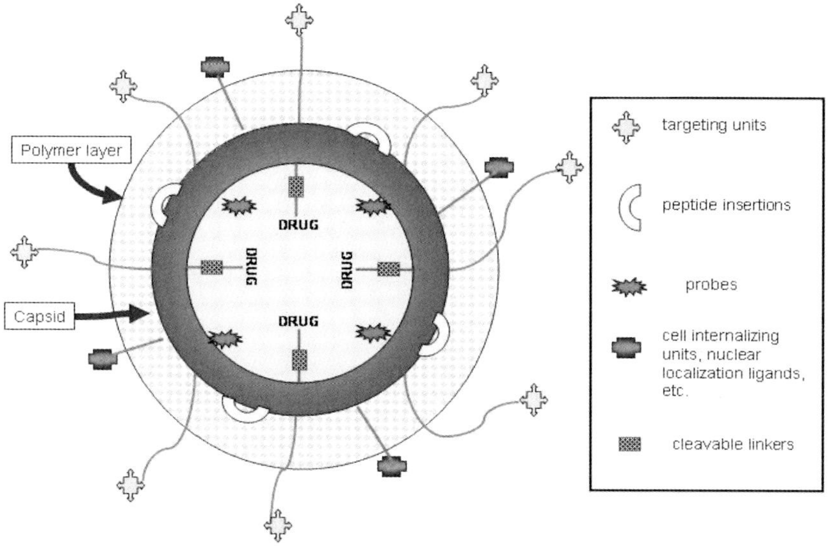

Figure 13.11. Multifunctional BNP hybrid.

tivity and efficacy for therapeutic applications [166, 187, 188]. Furthermore, the BNPs can be modified with polymers to boost the half-life of the biological system either by shielding the protein structures from enzymatic degradation or immune response. Ultimately, the combination of these multiple derivatizations on the nanoparticles could yield versatile units with specific cell targeting for drug/gene delivery, with simultaneous *in vivo* imaging for biomedical purposes (Fig. 13.11).

Acknowledgments

The authors are grateful of the Nanocenter of University of South Carolina, the USA Army–MURI program, DOD-DURIP, the W. M. Keck Foundation and the NSF-NER program.

References

1 C. M. Niemeyer, Nanoparticles, protein, and nucleic acids: biotechnology meets materials science. *Angew. Chem. Int. Ed.* **2001**, *40*, 4128–4158.
2 E. Dujardin, S. Mann, Bio-inspired materials chemistry. *Adv. Eng. Mater.* **2002**, *4*, 461–474.
3 N. C. Seeman, At the crossroads of chemistry, biology, and materials: structural dna nanotechnology. *Chem. Biol.* **2003**, *10*, 1151–1159.
4 W. M. Shih, J. D. Quispe, G. F. Joyce, A 1.7-kilobase single-stranded DNA that folds into a nanoscale octahedron. *Nature* **2004**, *427*, 618–621.
5 M. L. Flenniken, D. A. Willits, S. Brumfield, et al., The small heat

shock protein cage from *Methanococcus Jannaschii* is a versatile nanoscale platform for genetic and chemical modification. *Nano Lett.* **2003**, *3*, 1573–1576.

6 K. S. Raja, Q. Wang, Bionanoparticles and nanotechnology. *Encycl. Nanosci. Nanotechnol.* **2004**, *B*, 321–330.

7 N. Ban, A. McPherson, The structure of satellite panicum mosaic virus at 1.9 A resolution. *Nat. Struct. Biol.* **1995**, *2*, 882–890.

8 N. Nandhagopal, A. A. Simpson, J. R. Gurnon, et al., The structure and evolution of the major capsid protein of a large, lipid-containing DNA virus. *Proc. Natl Acad. Sci. USA* **2002**, *99*, 14758–14763.

9 W. J. McAleer, E. B. Buynak, R. Z. Maigetter, et al., Human hepatitis B vaccine from recombinant yeast. 1984. *Biotechnology* **1992**, *24*, 500–502.

10 D. M. Harper, E. L. Franco, C. Wheeler, et al., Efficacy of a bivalent L1 virus-like particle vaccine in prevention of infection with human papillomavirus types 16 and 18 in young women: a randomised controlled trial. *Lancet* **2004**, *364*, 1757–1765.

11 L. L. Villa, R. L. Costa, C. A. Petta, et al., Prophylactic quadrivalent human papillomavirus (types 6, 11, 16, and 18) L1 virus-like particle vaccine in young women: a randomised double-blind placebo-controlled multicentre phase II efficacy trial. *Lancet Oncol* **2005**, *6*, 271–278.

12 M. F. Bachmann, U. H. Rohrer, T. M. Kundig, et al., The influence of antigen organization on B cell responsiveness. *Science* **1993**, *262*, 1448–1451.

13 M. F. Bachmann, R. M. Zinkernagel, A. Oxenius, Immune responses in the absence of costimulation: viruses know the trick. *J. Immunol.* **1998**, *161*, 5791–5794.

14 K. K. W. Wong, T. Douglas, S. Gider, et al., Biomimetic synthesis and characterization of magnetic proteins (magnetoferritin). *Chem. Mater.* **1998**, *10*, 279–285.

15 T. Douglas, V. T. Stark, Nanophase cobalt oxyhydroxide mineral synthesized within the protein cage of ferritin. *Inorg. Chem.* **2000**, *39*, 1828–1830.

16 D. Ensign, M. Young, T. Douglas, Photocatalytic synthesis of copper colloids from Cu(II) by the ferrihydrite core of ferritin. *Inorg. Chem.* **2004**, *43*, 3441–3446.

17 C. Paavola, S. Chan, K. Mazzarella, et al., A versatile platform for nanotechnology based on circular permutation of a chaperonin protein. *Nanotechnology* **2006**, *17*, 1171–1176.

18 C. A. Kerfeld, M. R. Sawaya, S. Tanaka, et al., Protein structures forming the shell of primitive bacterial organelles. *Science* **2005**, *309*, 936–938.

19 G. P. Lomonossoff, J. E. Johnson, Use of macromolecular assemblies as expression systems for peptides and synthetic vaccines. *Curr. Opin. Struct. Biol.* **1996**, *6*, 176–182.

20 G. P. Lomonossoff, W. D. O. Hamilton, Cowpea mosaic virus-based vaccines. *Curr. Top. Microbiol. Immunol.* **1999**, *240*, 177–189.

21 L. Nieba, M. F. Bachmann, A new generation of vaccines. *Mod. Asp. Immunobiol.* **2000**, *1*, 36–39.

22 K. K. Hunt, S. A. Vorburger, Tech.Sight. Gene therapy. hurdles and hopes for cancer treatment. *Science* **2002**, *297*, 415–416.

23 D. Ferber, Gene therapy. Safer and virus-free? *Science* **2001**, *294*, 1638–1642.

24 T. Douglas, M. Young, Virus particles as templates for materials synthesis. *Adv. Mater.* **1999**, *11*, 679–681.

25 T. Douglas, M. Young, Host-guest encapsulation of materials by assembled virus protein cages. *Nature* **1998**, *393*, 152–155.

26 T. Douglas, E. Strable, D. Willits, et al., Protein engineering of a viral cage for constrained nanomaterials synthesis. *Adv. Mater.* **2002**, *14*, 405–418.

27 M. Allen, D. Willits, M. Young, et al., Constrained synthesis of cobalt

oxide nanomaterials in the 12-subunit protein cage from *Listeria* innocua. *Inorg. Chem.* **2003**, *42*, 6300–6305.
28 M. Allen, D. Willits, J. Mosolf, et al., Protein cage constrained synthesis of ferrimagnetic iron oxide nanoparticles. *Adv. Mater.* **2002**, *14*, 1562–1565.
29 C. E. Flynn, S.-W. Lee, B. R. Peelle, et al., Viruses as vehicles for growth, organization and assembly of materials. *Acta Mater.* **2003**, *51*, 5867–5880.
30 N. C. Seeman, A. M. Belcher, Emulating biology: building nanostructures from the bottom up. *Proc. Natl Acad. Sci. USA* **2002**, *99*, 6451–6455.
31 C. Mao, D. J. Solis, B. D. Reiss, et al., Virus-based toolkit for the directed synthesis of magnetic and semiconducting Nanowires. *Science* **2004**, *303*, 213–217.
32 C. Mao, C. E. Flynn, A. Hayhurst, et al., Viral assembly of oriented quantum dot nanowires. *Proc. Natl Acad. Sci. USA* **2003**, *100*, 6946–6951.
33 K. T. Nam, B. R. Peelle, S.-W. Lee, et al., Genetically driven assembly of nanorings based on the M13 virus. *Nano Lett.* **2004**, *4*, 23–27.
34 S.-W. Lee, A. M. Belcher, Virus-based fabrication of micro- and nanofibers using electrospinning. *Nano Lett.* **2004**, *4*, 387–390.
35 S.-W. Lee, B. M. Wood, A. M. Belcher, Chiral smectic C structures of virus-based films. *Langmuir* **2003**, *19*, 1592–1598.
36 S. W. Lee, C. Mao, C. E. Flynn, et al., Ordering of quantum dots using genetically engineered viruses. *Science* **2002**, *296*, 892–895.
37 S.-W. Lee, S. K. Lee, A. M. Belcher, Virus-based alignment of inorganic, organic, and biological nanosized materials. *Adv. Mater.* **2003**, *15*, 689–692.
38 C. E. Flynn, C. Mao, A. Hayhurst, et al., Synthesis and organization of nanoscale II–VI semiconductor materials using evolved peptide specificity and viral capsid assembly. *J. Mater. Chem.* **2003**, *13*, 2414–2421.
39 B. D. Reiss, C. Mao, D. J. Solis, et al., Biological routes to metal alloy ferromagnetic nanostructures. *Nano Lett.* **2004**, *4*, 1127–1132.
40 K. Wetz, R. R. Crichton, Chemical modification as a probe of the topography and reactivity of horse-spleen apoferritin. *Eur. J. Biochem.* **1976**, *61*, 545–550.
41 K. K. W. Wong, H. Colfen, N. T. Whilton, et al., Synthesis and characterization of hydrophobic ferritin proteins. *J. Inorg. Biochem.* **1999**, *76*, 187–195.
42 M. Li, K. K. W. Wong, S. Mann, Organization of inorganic nanoparticles using biotin-streptavidin connectors. *Chem. Mater.* **1999**, *11*, 23–26.
43 H. Romanczuk, C. E. Galer, J. Zabner, et al., Modification of an adenoviral vector with biologically selected peptides: a novel strategy for gene delivery to cells of choice. *Hum. Gene Ther.* **1999**, *10*, 2615–2626.
44 M. A. Croyle, N. Chirmule, Y. Zhang, et al., Pegylation of E1-deleted adenovirus vectors allows significant gene expression on readministration to liver. *Hum. Gene Ther.* **2002**, *13*, 1887–1900.
45 Q. Wang, K. S. Raja, K. D. Janda, et al., Blue fluorescent antibodies as reporters of steric accessibility in virus conjugates. *Bioconjug. Chem.* **2003**, *14*, 38–43.
46 Q. Wang, T. Lin, L. Tang, et al., Icosahedral virus particles as addressable nanoscale building blocks. *Angew. Chem. Int. Ed.* **2002**, *41*, 459–462.
47 Q. Wang, T. Lin, J. E. Johnson, et al., Natural supramolecular building blocks: cysteine-added mutants of cowpea mosaic virus. *Chem. Biol.* **2002**, *9*, 813–819.
48 Q. Wang, E. Kaltgrad, T. Lin, et al., Natural supramolecular building blocks: wild-type cowpea mosaic virus. *Chem. Biol.* **2002**, *9*, 805–811.
49 K. S. Raja, Q. Wang, M. J. Gonzalez, et al., Hybrid virus–polymer materials. 1. Synthesis and properties of peg-decorated cowpea mosaic virus. *Biomacromolecules* **2003**, *4*, 472–476.

50 A. Chatterji, L. L. Burns, S. S. Taylor, et al., Cowpea mosaic virus: from the presentation of antigenic peptides to the display of active biomaterials. *Intervirology* **2002**, *45*, 362–370.

51 K. S. Raja, Q. Wang, M. G. Finn, Icosahedral virus particles as polyvalent carbohydrate display platforms. *ChemBioChem* **2003**, *4*, 1348–1351.

52 E. Gillitzer, D. Willits, M. Young, et al., Chemical modification of a viral cage for multivalent presentation. *Chem. Commun.* **2002**, 2390–2391.

53 D. Taylor, Q. Wang, B. Bothner, et al., Correlation of chemical reactivity of nudaurelia capensis omega virus with a pH-induced conformational change. *Chem. Commun.* **2003**, 2770–2771.

54 T. L. Schlick, Z. Ding, E. W. Kovacs, et al., Dual-surface modification of the tobacco mosaic virus. *J. Am. Chem. Soc.* **2005**, *127*, 3718–3723.

55 H. N. Barnhill, V. S. Kotakadi, R. Ziessel, et al., Dual modification of turnip yellow mosaic virus: synthesis of a biotinylated luminescent nanoparticle. *ACS Meet. PMSE* **2006**, preprints.

56 H. N. Barnhill, W. Zhan, H. Tian, et al., Display of image contrast agents on bionanoparticles and their potential applications for *in vivo* imaging. *ACS Meet. PMSE* **2005**, *92*, 398.

57 J. M. Hooker, E. W. Kovacs, M. B. Francis, Interior surface modification of bacteriophage MS2. *J. Am. Chem. Soc.* **2004**, *126*, 3718–3719.

58 N. Maheshri, J. T. Koerber, B. K. Kaspar, et al., Directed evolution of adeno-associated virus yields enhanced gene delivery vectors. *Nat. Biotechnol.* **2006**, *24*, 198–204.

59 N. Muzyczka, K. H. Warrington, Jr., Custom adeno-associated virus capsids: the next generation of recombinant vectors with novel tropism. *Hum. Gene Ther.* **2005**, *16*, 408–416.

60 N. Krauzewicz, J. Stokrova, C. Jenkins, et al., Virus-like gene transfer into cells mediated by polyoma virus pseudocapsids. *Gene Ther.* **2000**, *7*, 2122–2131.

61 G. T. Hermanson, *Bioconjugate Techniques*. Academic Press, San Diego, **1996**.

62 S. Meunier, E. Strable, M. G. Finn, Crosslinking of and coupling to viral capsid proteins by tyrosine oxidation. *Chem. Biol.* **2004**, *11*, 319–326.

63 S. Sen Gupta, K. S. Raja, E. Kaltgrad, et al., Virus–glycopolymer conjugates by copper(I) catalysis of atom transfer radical polymerization and azide–alkyne cycloaddition. *Chem. Commun.* **2005**, 4315–4317.

64 M. L. Flenniken, L. O. Liepold, B. E. Crowley, et al., Selective attachment and release of a chemotherapeutic agent from the interior of a protein cage architecture. *Chem. Commun.* **2005**, 447–449.

65 C. Porta, V. E. Spall, T. Lin, et al., The development of cowpea mosaic virus as a potential source of novel vaccines. *Intervirology* **1996**, *39*, 79–84.

66 K. M. Taylor, T. Lin, C. Porta, et al., Influence of three-dimensional structure on the immunogenicity of a peptide expressed on the surface of a plant virus. *J. Mol. Recog.* **2000**, *13*, 71–82.

67 L. McLain, Z. Durrani, N. J. Dimmock, et al., A plant virus-HIV-1 chimera stimulates antibody that neutralizes HIV-1. *Vaccines 96: Mol. Approaches Control Infect. Dis.*, **1996**, pp. 311–316.

68 M. T. Klem, D. Willits, M. Young, et al., 2-D Array formation of genetically engineered viral cages on au surfaces and imaging by atomic force microscopy. *J. Am. Chem. Soc.* **2003**, *125*, 10806–10807.

69 K. K. W. Wong, N. T. Whilton, T. Douglas, et al., Hydrophobic proteins: synthesis and characterization of organic-soluble alkylated ferritins. *Chem. Commun.* **1998**, 1621–1622.

70 J. T. Russell, Y. Lin, A. Böker, et al., Self-assembly and cross-linking of bionanoparticles at liquid–liquid interfaces. *Angew. Chem. Int. Ed.* **2005**, *44*, 2420–2426.

71 Y. Lin, A. Boker, J. He, et al., Self-directed self-assembly of nanoparticle/copolymer mixtures. *Nature* **2005**, *434*, 55–59.

72 C. W. Tornoe, C. Christensen, M. Meldal, Peptidotriazoles on solid phase: [1,2,3]-triazoles by regiospecific copper(I)-catalyzed 1,3-dipolar cycloadditions of terminal alkynes to azides. *J. Org. Chem.* **2002**, *67*, 3057–3064.

73 V. V. Rostovtsev, L. G. Green, V. V. Fokin, et al., A stepwise Huisgen cycloaddition process: copper(I)-catalyzed regioselective "ligation" of azides and terminal alkynes. *Angew. Chem. Int. Ed.* **2002**, *41*, 2596–2599.

74 H. C. Kolb, M. G. Finn, K. B. Sharpless, Click chemistry: diverse chemical function from a few good reactions. *Angew. Chem. Int. Ed.* **2001**, *40*, 2004–2021.

75 A. J. Link, M. K. S. Vink, D. A. Tirrell, Presentation and detection of azide functionality in bacterial cell surface proteins. *J. Am. Chem. Soc.* **2004**, *126*, 10598–10602.

76 F. Perez-Balderas, M. Ortega-Munoz, J. Morales-Sanfrutos, et al., Multivalent neoglycoconjugates by regiospecific cycloaddition of alkynes and azides using organic-soluble copper catalysts. *Org. Lett.* **2003**, *5*, 1951–1954.

77 W. G. Lewis, F. G. Magallon, V. V. Fokin, et al., Discovery and characterization of catalysts for azide-alkyne cycloaddition by fluorescence quenching. *J. Am. Chem. Soc.* **2004**, *126*, 9152–9153.

78 Q. Wang, T. R. Chan, R. Hilgraf, et al., Bioconjugation by copper(I)-catalyzed azide–alkyne 3 + 2 cycloaddition. *J. Am. Chem. Soc.* **2003**, *125*, 3192–3193.

79 W. H. Zhan, H. N. Barnhill, K. Sivakumar, et al., Facile synthesis of new cyanine dyes for bioconjugation of bionanoparticles with "click" chemistry. *Tetrahedron Lett.* **2005**, *46*, 1691–1695.

80 S. Sen Gupta, J. Kuzelka, P. Singh, et al., Accelerated bioorthogonal conjugation: a practical method for the ligation of diverse functional molecules to a polyvalent virus scaffold. *Bioconjug. Chem.* **2005**, *16*, 1572–1579.

81 A. J. Link, D. A. Tirrell, Cell surface labeling of *Escherichia coli* via copper(I)-catalyzed 3 + 2 cycloaddition. *J. Am. Chem. Soc.* **2003**, *125*, 11164–11165.

82 A. Deiters, T. A. Cropp, M. Mukherji, et al., Adding amino acids with novel reactivity to the genetic code of *Saccharomyces cerevisiae*. *J. Am. Chem. Soc.* **2003**, *125*, 11782–11783.

83 A. Deiters, T. A. Cropp, D. Summerer, et al., Site-specific pegylation of proteins containing unnatural amino acids. *Bioorg. Med. Chem. Lett.* **2004**, *14*, 5743–5745.

84 F. Tian, M. L. Tsao, P. G. Schultz, A phage display system with unnatural amino acids. *J. Am. Chem. Soc.* **2004**, *126*, 15962–15963.

85 Z. Zhou, C. J. Fahrni, A fluorogenic probe for the copper(I)-catalyzed azide–alkyne ligation reaction: modulation of the fluorescence emission via (3)(N,Pi*)-(1)(Pi,Pi*) inversion. *J. Am. Chem. Soc.* **2004**, *126*, 8862–8863.

86 K. Sivakumar, F. Xie, B. Cash, et al., A fluorogenic 1,3-dipolar cycloaddition reaction of 3-azidocoumarins and acetylenes. *Org. Lett.* **2004**, *6*, 4603–4606.

87 S. D. Tilley, M. B. Francis, Tyrosine-selective protein alkylation using pi-allylpalladium complexes. *J. Am. Chem. Soc.* **2006**, *128*, 1080–1081.

88 N. S. Joshi, L. R. Whitaker, M. B. Francis, A three-component Mannich-type reaction for selective tyrosine bioconjugation. *J. Am. Chem. Soc.* **2004**, *126*, 15942–15943.

89 K. Uhde, R. Fischer, U. Commandeur, Expression of multiple foreign epitopes presented as synthetic antigens on the surface of potato virus X particles. *Arch. Virol.* **2005**, *150*, 327–340.

90 L. Liu, M. C. Canizares, W. Monger, et al., Cowpea mosaic virus-based systems for the production of antigens

and antibodies in plants. *Vaccine* **2005**, *23*, 1788–1792.

91 T. Yamada, M. Ueda, M. Seno, et al., Novel tissue and cell type-specific gene/drug delivery system using surface engineered hepatitis B virus nano-particles. *Curr. Drug Targets Infect. Disord.* **2004**, *4*, 163–167.

92 J. Xie, P. G. Schultz, Adding amino acids to the genetic repertoire. *Curr. Opin. Chem. Biol.* **2005**, *9*, 548–554.

93 A. Deiters, P. G. Schultz, In vivo incorporation of an alkyne into proteins in *Escherichia coli*. *Bioorg. Med. Chem. Lett.* **2005**, *15*, 1521–1524.

94 M. Bose, D. Groff, J. Xie, et al., The Incorporation of a photoisomerizable amino acid into proteins in *E. coli*. *J. Am. Chem. Soc.* **2006**, *128*, 388–389.

95 T. Hohsaka, Y. Ashizuka, H. Taira, et al., Incorporation of nonnatural amino acids into proteins by using various four-base codons in an *Escherichia coli in-vitro* translation system. *Biochemistry* **2001**, *40*, 11060–11064.

96 S. S. Cruz, S. Chapman, A. G. Roberts, et al., Assembly and movement of a plant virus carrying a green fluorescent protein overcoat. *Proc. Natl Acad. Sci. USA* **1996**, *93*, 6286–6290.

97 R. L. Toth, S. Chapman, F. Carr, et al., A novel strategy for the expression of foreign genes from plant virus vectors. *FEBS Lett.* **2001**, *489*, 215–219.

98 G. P. Lomonossoff, M. Shanks, C. L. Holness, et al., Comovirus capsid proteins: synthesis, structure, and evolutionary implications. *Proc. Phytochem. Soc. Eur.* **1991**, *32*, 76–91.

99 G. P. Lomonossoff, J. E. Johnson, The synthesis and structure of comovirus capsids. *Prog. Biophys. Mol. Biol.* **1991**, *55*, 107–137.

100 T. Lin, Z. Chen, R. Usha, et al., The refined crystal structure of cowpea mosaic virus at 2.8 Å resolution. *Virology* **1999**, *265*, 20–34.

101 L. Liu, G. Lomonossoff, Agro-infection as a rapid method for propagating cowpea mosaic virus-based constructs. *J. Virol. Methods* **2002**, *105*, 343–348.

102 D. J. Siler, J. Babcock, G. Bruening, Electrophoretic mobility and enhanced infectivity of a mutant of cowpea mosaic virus. *Virology* **1976**, *71*, 560–567.

103 C. Porta, V. E. Spall, K. C. Findlay, et al., Cowpea mosaic virus-based chimaeras. Effects of inserted peptides on the phenotype, host range, and transmissibility of the modified viruses. *Virology* **2003**, *310*, 50–63.

104 L. McLain, C. Porta, G. P. Lomonossoff, et al., Human immunodeficiency virus type 1-neutralizing antibodies raised to a glycoprotein 41 peptide expressed on the surface of a plant virus. *AIDS Res. Hum. Retroviruses* **1995**, *11*, 327–334.

105 K. Dalsgaard, A. Uttenthal, T. D. Jones, et al., plant-derived vaccine protects target animals against a viral disease. *Nat. Biotechnol.* **1997**, *15*, 248–252.

106 C. Porta, G. Wang, H. Cheng, et al., Direct imaging of interactions between an icosahedral virus and conjugate F(ab) fragments by cryoelectron microscopy and X-ray crystallography. *Virology* **1994**, *204*, 777–788.

107 I. W. Khor, T. Lin, J. P. Langedijk, et al., Novel strategy for inhibiting viral entry by use of a cellular receptor–plant virus chimera. *J. Virol.* **2002**, *76*, 4412–4419.

108 C. M. Hayden, A. M. Mackenzie, M. L. Skotnicki, et al., Turnip yellow mosaic virus isolates with experimentally produced recombinant virion proteins. *J. Gen. Virol.* **1998**, *79*, 395–403.

109 H. H. Bink, S. K. Roepan, C. W. Pleij, Two histidines of the coat protein of turnip yellow mosaic virus at the capsid interior are crucial for viability. *Proteins* **2004**, *55*, 236–244.

110 M. Leimkuhler, A. Goldbeck, M. D. Lechner, et al., The Formation of empty shells upon pressure induced decapsidation of turnip yellow mosaic virus. *Arch. Virol.* **2001**, *146*, 653–667.

111 M. Adrian, P. A. Timmins, J. Witz, In vitro decapsidation of turnip yellow mosaic virus investigated by cryo-

electron microscopy: a model for the decapsidation of a small isometric virus. *J. Gen. Virol.* **1992**, *73*, 2079–2083.

112 J. Haynes, J. Cunningham, A. von Seefried, et al., Development of a genetically-engineered, candidate polio vaccine employing the self-assembling properties of tobacco mosaic virus coat protein. *Biotechnology* **1986**, *4*, 637–641.

113 Y. Sugiyama, H. Hamamoto, S. Takemoto, et al., Systemic production of foreign peptides on the particle surface of tobacco mosaic virus. *FEBS Lett.* **1995**, *359*, 247–250.

114 H. Hamamoto, Y. Sugiyama, N. Nakagawa, et al., A new tobacco mosaic vector and its use for the systemic production of angiotensin-I-converting enzyme inhibitor in transgenic tobacco and tomato. *Biotechnology* **1993**, *11*, 930–932.

115 M. Bendahmane, M. Koo, E. Karrer, et al., Display of epitopes on the surface of tobacco mosaic virus: impact of charge and isoelectric point of the epitope on virus–host interactions. *J. Mol. Biol.* **1999**, *290*, 9–20.

116 M. Koo, M. Bendahmane, G. A. Lettieri, et al., Protective immunity against murine hepatitis virus (MHV) induced by intranasal or subcutaneous administration of hybrids of tobacco mosaic virus that carries an MHV epitope. *Proc. Natl Acad. Sci. USA* **1999**, *96*, 7774–7779.

117 L. Jiang, Q. Li, M. Li, et al., A modified TMV-based vector facilitates the expression of longer foreign epitopes in tobacco. *Vaccine* **2006**, *24*, 109–115.

118 L. A. Baratova, N. I. Grebenshchikov, E. N. Dobrov, et al., The organization of potato virus X coat proteins in virus particles studied by tritium planigraphy and model building. *Virology* **1992**, *188*, 175–180.

119 R. Koenig, L. Torrance, Antigenic analysis of potato virus X by means of monoclonal antibodies. *J. Gen. Virol.* **1986**, *67*, 2145–2151.

120 M. D. Ryan, A. M. King, G. P. Thomas, Cleavage of foot-and-mouth disease virus polyprotein is mediated by residues located within a 19 amino acid sequence. *J. Gen. Virol.* **1991**, *72*, 2727–2732.

121 L. Smolenska, I. M. Roberts, D. Learmonth, et al., Production of a functional single chain antibody attached to the surface of a plant virus. *FEBS Lett.* **1998**, *441*, 379–382.

122 M. Donini, C. Lico, S. Baschieri, et al., Production of an engineered killer peptide in *Nicotiana benthamiana* by using a potato virus X expression system. *Appl. Environ. Microbiol.* **2005**, *71*, 6360–6367.

123 N. D. Chasteen, P. M. Harrison, Mineralization in ferritin: an efficient means of iron storage. *J. Struct. Biol.* **1999**, *126*, 182–194.

124 R. M. Kramer, C. Li, D. C. Carter, et al., Engineered protein cages for nanomaterial synthesis. *J. Am. Chem. Soc.* **2004**, *126*, 13282–13286.

125 F. Uchiyama, Y. Tanaka, Y. Minari, et al., Designing scaffolds of peptides for phage display libraries. *J. Biosci. Bioeng.* **2005**, *99*, 448–456.

126 J. W. Kehoe, B. K. Kay, Filamentous phage display in the new millennium. *Chem. Rev.* **2005**, *105*, 4056–4072.

127 C. Gao, S. Mao, C. H. Lo, et al., Making artificial antibodies: a format for phage display of combinatorial heterodimeric arrays. *Proc. Natl Acad. Sci. USA* **1999**, *96*, 6025–6030.

128 A. B. Sanghvi, K. P. Miller, A. M. Belcher, et al., Biomaterials functionalization using a novel peptide that selectively binds to a conducting polymer. *Nat. Mater.* **2005**, *4*, 496–502.

129 O. J. Muller, F. Kaul, M. D. Weitzman, et al., Random peptide libraries displayed on adeno-associated virus to select for targeted gene therapy vectors. *Nat. Biotechnol.* **2003**, *21*, 1040–1046.

130 K. Ninomiya, T. Minohata, M. Nishimura, et al., In situ chemical aminoacylation with amino acid thioesters linked to a peptide nucleic acid. *J. Am. Chem. Soc.* **2004**, *126*, 15984–15989.

131 M. Sisido, K. Ninomiya, T. Ohtsuki, et al., Four-base codon/anticodon strategy and non-enzymatic aminoacylation for protein engineering with non-natural amino acids. *Methods* **2005**, *36*, 270–278.

132 T. Hohsaka, M. Fukushima, M. Sisido, Nonnatural mutagenesis in *E. coli* and rabbit reticulocyte lysates by using four-base codons. *Nucleic Acids Res. Suppl* **2002**, 201–202.

133 N. Muranaka, T. Hohsaka, M. Sisido, Four-base codon mediated mRNA display to construct peptide libraries that contain multiple nonnatural amino acids. *Nucleic Acids Res.* **2006**, *34*, e4.

134 H. Hamada, N. Kameshima, A. Szymanska, et al., Position-specific incorporation of a highly photodurable and blue-laser excitable fluorescent amino acid into proteins for fluorescence sensing. *Bioorg. Med. Chem.* **2005**, *13*, 3379–3384.

135 M. Manchester, J. E. Gairin, J. B. Patterson, et al., Measles virus recognizes its receptor, CD46, via two distinct binding domains within Scr1-2. *Virology* **1997**, *233*, 174–184.

136 M. Manchester, M. K. Liszewski, J. P. Atkinson, et al., Multiple isoforms of CD46 (membrane cofactor protein) serve as receptors for measles virus. *Proc. Natl Acad. Sci. USA* **1994**, *91*, 2161–2165.

137 R. Weissleder, K. Kelly, E. Sun, et al., Cell-specific targeting of nanoparticles by multivalent attachment of small molecules. *Nat. Biotechnol.* **2005**, *23*, 1418–1423.

138 A. E. Smith, H. Lilie, A. Helenius, Ganglioside-dependent cell attachment and endocytosis of murine polyomavirus-like particles. *FEBS Lett.* **2003**, *555*, 199–203.

139 Y. C. Shin, W. R. Folk, Formation of polyomavirus-like particles with different Vp1 molecules that bind the urokinase plasminogen activator receptor. *J. Virol.* **2003**, *77*, 11491–11498.

140 Z. Sandalon, A. Oppenheim, Self-assembly and protein–protein interactions between the SV40 capsid proteins produced in insect cells. *Virology* **1997**, *237*, 414–421.

141 D. Chang, C. Y. Fung, W. C. Ou, et al., Self-assembly of the JC virus major capsid protein, VP1, expressed in insect cells. *J. Gen. Virol.* **1997**, *78*, 1435–1439.

142 E. T. Gillock, S. Rottinghaus, D. Chang, et al., Polyomavirus major capsid protein VP1 is capable of packaging cellular DNA when expressed in the baculovirus system. *J. Virol.* **1997**, *71*, 2857–2865.

143 K. Sasnauskas, O. Buzaite, F. Vogel, et al., Yeast cells allow high-level expression and formation of polyomavirus-like particles. *Biol. Chem.* **1999**, *380*, 381–386.

144 U. Schmidt, J. Kenklies, R. Rudolph, et al., Site-specific fluorescence labeling of recombinant polyomavirus-like particles. *Biol. Chem.* **1999**, *380*, 397–401.

145 W. C. Ou, M. Wang, C. Y. Fung, et al., The major capsid protein, VP1, of human JC virus expressed in *Escherichia coli* is able to self-assemble into a capsid-like particle and deliver exogenous DNA into human kidney cells. *J. Gen. Virol.* **1999**, *80*, 39–46.

146 B. Tsai, J. M. Gilbert, T. Stehle, et al., Gangliosides are receptors for murine polyoma virus and SV40. *EMBO J.* **2003**, *22*, 4346–4355.

147 M. Caruso, L. Belloni, O. Sthandier, et al., Alpha4beta1 integrin acts as a cell receptor for murine polyomavirus at the post-attachment level. *J. Virol.* **2003**, *77*, 3913–3921.

148 M. Caruso, M. Cavaldesi, M. Gentile, et al., Role of sialic acid-containing molecules and the alpha4beta1 integrin receptor in the early steps of polyomavirus infection. *J. Gen. Virol.* **2003**, *84*, 2927–2936.

149 B. F. Sabath, E. O. Major, Traffic of JC virus from sites of initial infection to the brain: the path to progressive multifocal leukoencephalopathy. *J. Infect. Dis.* **2002**, *186*, S180–186.

150 M. Wang, T. H. Tsou, L. S. Chen, et al., Inhibition of simian virus 40 large tumor antigen expression in

human fetal glial cells by an antisense oligodeoxynucleotide delivered by the JC virus-like particle. *Hum. Gene Ther.* **2004**, *15*, 1077–1090.

151 D. Yu, C. Amano, T. Fukuda, et al., The specific delivery of proteins to human liver cells by engineered bio-nanocapsules. *FEBS J.* **2005**, *272*, 3651–3660.

152 T. Yamada, Y. Iwasaki, H. Tada, et al., Nanoparticles for the delivery of genes and drugs to human hepatocytes. *Nat. Biotechnol.* **2003**, *21*, 885–890.

153 M. L. Flenniken, D. A. Willits, A. L. Harmsen, et al., Melanoma and lymphocyte cell-specific targeting incorporated into a heat shock protein cage architecture. *Chem. Biol.* **2006**, *13*, 161–170.

154 S. Gleiter, H. Lilie, Coupling of antibodies via protein Z on modified polyoma virus-like particles. *Protein Sci.* **2001**, *10*, 434–444.

155 N. Krauzewicz, C. Cox, E. Soeda, et al., Sustained *ex vivo* and *in vivo* transfer of a reporter gene using polyoma virus pseudocapsids. *Gene Ther.* **2000**, *7*, 1094–1102.

156 A. Touze, L. Bousarghin, C. Ster, et al., Gene transfer using human polyomavirus BK virus-like particles expressed in insect cells. *J. Gen. Virol.* **2001**, *82*, 3005–3009.

157 S. Gleiter, H. Lilie, Cell-type specific targeting and gene expression using a variant of polyoma VP1 virus-like particles. *Biol. Chem.* **2003**, *384*, 247–255.

158 J. V. Osterman, A. Waddell, H. V. Aposhian, DNA and gene therapy: uncoating of polyoma pseudovirus in mouse embryo cells. *Proc. Natl Acad. Sci. USA* **1970**, *67*, 37–40.

159 C. Kimchi-Sarfaty, M. M. Gottesman, SV40 pseudovirions as highly efficient vectors for gene transfer and their potential application in cancer therapy. *Curr. Pharm. Biotechnol.* **2004**, *5*, 451–458.

160 C. Kimchi-Sarfaty, O. Ben-Nun-Shaul, D. Rund, et al., *In vitro*-packaged SV40 pseudovirions as highly efficient vectors for gene transfer. *Hum. Gene Ther.* **2002**, *13*, 299–310.

161 C. Kimchi-Sarfaty, M. Arora, Z. Sandalon, et al., High cloning capacity of *in vitro* packaged SV40 vectors with no SV40 virus sequences. *Hum. Gene Ther.* **2003**, *14*, 167–177.

162 C. Kimchi-Sarfaty, S. Brittain, S. Garfield, et al., Efficient delivery of RNA interference effectors via *in vitro*-packaged SV40 pseudovirions. *Hum. Gene Ther.* **2005**.

163 C. S. Rae, I. W. Khor, Q. Wang, et al., Systemic trafficking of plant virus nanoparticles in mice via the oral route. *Virology* **2005**, *343*, 224–235.

164 J. D. Lewis, G. Destito, A. Zijlstra, et al., Viral nanoparticles as tools for intravital vascular imaging. *Nat. Med.* **2006**, *12*, 354–360.

165 H. Ewers, A. E. Smith, I. F. Sbalzarini, et al., Single-particle tracking of murine polyoma virus-like particles on live cells and artificial membranes. *Proc. Natl Acad. Sci. USA* **2005**, *102*, 15110–15115.

166 C. Wu, H. Barnhill, X. Liang, et al., A new probe using hybrid virus-dye nanoparticles for near-infrared fluorescence tomography. *Optics Commun.* **2005**, *255*, 366–374.

167 I. L. Medintz, K. E. Sapsford, J. H. Konnert, et al., Decoration of discretely immobilized cowpea mosaic virus with luminescent quantum dots. *Langmuir* **2005**, *21*, 5501–5510.

168 A. Chatterji, W. F. Ochoa, T. Ueno, et al., A virus-based nanoblock with tunable electrostatic properties. *Nano Lett.* **2005**, *5*, 597–602.

169 N. G. Portney, K. Singh, S. Chaudhary, et al., Organic and inorganic nanoparticle hybrids. *Langmuir* **2005**, *21*, 2098–2103.

170 A. S. Blum, C. M. Soto, C. D. Wilson, et al., An engineered virus as a scaffold for three-dimensional self-assembly on the nanoscale. *Small* **2005**, *1*, 702–706.

171 G. R. Souza, D. R. Christianson, F. I. Staquicini, et al., Networks of gold nanoparticles and bacteriophage as biological sensors and cell-targeting agents. *Proc. Natl Acad. Sci. USA* **2006**, *103*, 1215–1220.

172 U. Schmidt, C. Gunther, R. Rudolph, et al., Protein and peptide delivery via engineered polyomavirus-like particles. *FASEB J.* **2001**, *15*, 1646–1648.

173 A. Abbing, U. K. Blaschke, S. Grein, et al., Efficient intracellular delivery of a protein and a low molecular weight substance via recombinant polyomavirus-like particles. *J. Biol. Chem.* **2004**, *279*, 27410–27421.

174 J. Johnson, T. Lin, G. Lomonossoff, Presentation of heterologous peptides on plant viruses: genetics, structure, and function. *Annu. Rev. Phytopathol.* **1997**, *35*, 67–86.

175 J. P. Langeveld, F. R. Brennan, J. L. Martinez-Torrecuadrada, et al., Inactivated recombinant plant virus protects dogs from a lethal challenge with canine parvovirus. *Vaccine* **2001**, *19*, 3661–3670.

176 C. Marusic, P. Rizza, L. Lattanzi, et al., Chimeric plant virus particles as immunogens for inducing murine and human immune responses against human immunodeficiency virus type 1. *J. Virol.* **2001**, *75*, 8434–8439.

177 V. Yusibov, D. C. Hooper, S. V. Spitsin, et al., Expression in plants and immunogenicity of plant virus-based experimental rabies vaccine. *Vaccine* **2002**, *20*, 3155–3164.

178 M. L. Smith, J. A. Lindbo, S. Dillard-Telm, et al., Modified tobacco mosaic virus particles as scaffolds for display of protein antigens for vaccine applications. *Virology* **2006**.

179 F. R. Brennan, L. B. Gilleland, J. Staczek, et al., A chimaeric plant virus vaccine protects mice against a bacterial infection. *Microbiology* **1999**, *145*, 2061–2067.

180 F. R. Brennan, T. D. Jones, L. B. Gilleland, et al., *Pseudomonas aeruginosa* outer-membrane protein F epitopes are highly immunogenic in mice when expressed on a plant virus. *Microbiology* **1999**, *145*, 211–220.

181 A. Rennermalm, Y. H. Li, L. Bohaufs, et al., Antibodies against a truncated *Staphylococcus aureus* fibronectin-binding protein protect against dissemination of infection in the Rat. *Vaccine* **2001**, *19*, 3376–3383.

182 J. J. Lundquist, E. J. Toone, The cluster glycoside effect. *Chem. Rev.* **2002**, *102*, 555–578.

183 J. J. Lundquist, S. D. Debenham, E. J. Toone, Multivalency effects in protein–carbohydrate interaction: the binding of the Shiga-like toxin 1 binding subunit to multivalent C-linked glycopeptides. *J. Org. Chem.* **2000**, *65*, 8245–8250.

184 J. E. Gestwicki, C. W. Cairo, L. E. Strong, et al., Influencing receptor–ligand binding mechanisms with multivalent ligand architecture. *J. Am. Chem. Soc.* **2002**, *124*, 14922–14933.

185 J. A. Harding, C. M. Engbers, M. S. Newman, et al., Immunogenicity and pharmacokinetic attributes of poly(ethylene glycol)-grafted immunoliposomes. *Biochim. Biophys. Acta* **1997**, *1327*, 181–192.

186 Z. L. Xu, H. Mizuguchi, F. Sakurai, et al., Approaches to improving the kinetics of adenovirus-delivered genes and gene products. *Adv. Drug Deliv. Rev.* **2005**, *57*, 781–802.

187 A. Dirksen, S. Langereis, B. F. de Waal, et al., A supramolecular approach to multivalent target-specific MRI contrast agents for angiogenesis. *Chem. Commun.* **2005**, 2811–2813.

188 H. Kobayashi, M. W. Brechbiel, Nano-sized MRI contrast agents with dendrimer cores. *Adv. Drug Deliv. Rev.* **2005**, *57*, 2271–2286.

14
Nanotechnology for Gene Therapy – HVJ-E Vector

Hironori Nakagami, Yasuhiko Tabata, and Yasufumi Kaneda

14.1
Introduction

Currently, more than 400 clinical protocols have been approved for human gene therapy. In 1995, the Orkin–Motulsky report indicated the importance of vector development in human gene therapy. Numerous vectors have been developed to date. In general, viral vectors are more effective for gene transfer; however, safety remains an issue [1]. In 1999, a young patient died following infusion of an adenoviral vector via the hepatic artery [2] and, in 2002, two patients with X-linked severe combined immunodeficiency treated with retroviral vector gene therapy developed leukemia-like symptoms, likely to have been induced by insertional mutagenesis of the retroviral DNA [3]. Hemophilia B gene therapy using the adeno-associated virus (AAV) vector looks promising [4], but several potential risks, such as germline transmission, remain. On the other hand, the safety of a nonviral vector has been evaluated, but inefficient gene transfection is a limitation of this vector system [5]. Therefore, the current consensus on vector development is that highly efficient and minimally invasive vectors are the most appropriate for human gene therapy. Before developing vector systems, we should analyze the biological barriers to gene transfer and create methods to overcome such difficulties.

All the current vector systems have their advantages and limitations [6]. Currently, there are several approaches to correct the limitations of each vector system. In adenovirus vector systems, one crucial improvement is reduced vector antigenicity and a helper-dependent or "gutless" vector in which most of the adenovirus genome is deleted has been developed [7]. However, the production of this "gutless" vector was much lower than that of the classical adenovirus vector. Another approach is to overcome the limitations of one vector system by drawing upon the strengths of another. Examples of chimeric vectors include the pseudo-type retrovirus vector in which the envelope component of the classical retrovirus vector is replaced with the vesicular stomatitis virus (VSV) G protein [8] and a new lentivirus vector containing human immunodeficiency virus (HIV) proteins with the pseudo-type retrovirus envelope-containing VSV G protein [9]. However, combinations of

Nanotechnologies for the Life Sciences Vol. 10
Nanomaterials for Medical Diagnosis and Therapy. Edited by Challa S. S. R. Kumar

ISBN: 978-3-527-31390-7

viral vector systems are thought to be of limited utility, because the components necessary for viral replication and packaging cannot be eliminated, and the constituent viruses may interfere with each other during vector production.

Limitations of vector systems are inevitable, and the introduction of foreign genes into cells is abnormal and is directed to disturb cellular function. Current gene therapy strategies mimic viral infection and cells are designed to resist the gene transfer. Cells have biological barriers that protect against invasion by foreign genes and inhibit expression of foreign gene products [5]. Protocols for *in vivo* gene transfection consist of several steps. The first step entails the approach of the vector to the target cell from the outside environment. The second is the introduction of the transgene into the cytoplasm. Third, the transgene must migrate to the nucleus. Finally, the transgene must be retained and stably expressed. Each of these steps has barriers. For example, serum proteins and immune cells can attack gene transfer vectors before they reach target cells, the cell membrane can prevent transfer of foreign genes to the cytoplasm, the nuclear envelope can restrict nuclear targeting of molecules, and expression of the transgene can be inhibited by degradation of the DNA or by transcriptional silencing. In a narrow sense, "gene transfer" means the introduction of a transgene into the cytoplasm, and it encompasses the first and second steps described above. However, it is pointless to only refer to the introduction of a transgene into the cell without considering the final step of gene expression. Thus, Section 14.2 highlights biological barriers from the first step (approach to the target cell) to the fourth step (effective expression of the transgene) and discusses potential solutions for each barrier with respect to future possibilities for gene transfer systems.

We have developed a unique vector, "HVJ-E (Hemagglutinating Virus of Japan-envelope)", that can rapidly transfer plasmid DNA, oligonucleotides and protein into cells by cell fusion. A detailed description is given in Section 14.3. However, this modality of targeting is still insufficient for rapid and specific accumulation of active vectors in target tissues. One solution is to engineer the surface proteins of viral vectors or to couple targeting ligands to viral as well as nonviral vectors, which might further improve tissue selectivity. Section 14.4 describes other candidates for nonviral vectors, such as cationized gelatin (CG) and magnetic nanoparticles. Finally, Section 14.5 discusses modification of the membrane surface of HVJ to achieve improvement as a future prospect. We modified HVJ-E conjugated with protamine sulfate (PS) and/or CG, which enhanced the transfection efficiency *in vitro* or *in vivo*. Moreover, we recently developed magnetic nanoparticle-conjugated HVJ-E. Importantly, the size and surface chemistry of magnetic particles could be tailored to meet specific demands of physical and biological characteristics. For example, coating with PS could be suitable for *in vitro*, but not *in vivo*, culture, whereas heparin sulfate was suitable for *in vivo* gene expression. Overall, CG or magnetic nanoparticles can enhance HVJ-E-based gene transfer by modification of the size or charge, which could potentially help to overcome fundamental limitations to gene therapy *in vivo*.

14.2 Biological Barriers to Gene Transfer

14.2.1 Reaching Target Cells

To achieve tissue-specific targeting, vector system development should be approached from at least three aspects: recognition by specific target tissues, avoidance of nonspecific uptake and resistance to degradation in the systemic circulation.

14.2.1.1 Recognition by Specific Target Tissues

Targeting vectors to specific tissues has been considered an ideal method for gene delivery. Ligand-specific delivery systems have been developed for tissue-specific targeting. In one experiment, asialoglycoprotein was conjugated with DNA–polylysine complexes [10]. Since asialoglycoprotein binds to receptors on hepatocytes, DNA can be delivered specifically to hepatocytes by receptor-mediated endocytosis using this complex [11]. Transferrin has also been used for receptor-mediated delivery of DNA to cancer cells, because cancer cells express high levels of the transferrin receptor [12]. These complexes worked well in cultured cells, but the efficiency of *in vivo* gene delivery was so good. Some viruses do, however, target specific tissues [13]. Epstein–Barr virus (EBV) primarily infects B lymphocytes, hepatitis virus B attacks hepatocytes, and HIV targets lymphocytes and macrophages. Currently, adenovirus-based gene delivery vectors are being used for many gene therapy applications because of the broad range of hosts [14]. Cellular tropism of the adenovirus vector in tissues is regulated by fiber proteins and, based on the tissue tropism of these viruses, targeting viral vectors can be developed [15–17].

14.2.1.2 Avoidance of Nonspecific Uptake

Colloidal particles with a diameter of more than 300 nm are trapped by reticuloendothelial system (RES) cells in the liver, spleen and lung [18]. HVJ-liposomes containing both hemagglutinin/neuraminidase (HN) protein and fusion (F) proteins target the liver, spleen and lung when the vector is injected into the saphenous vein of monkeys [19], probably because the phosphatidylserine residues [20] present on the envelope are recognized by the RES and the particle size is 470 nm in diameter. Some phospholipids such as phosphatidylserine are also recognized by the RES. The liposome–PS–plasmid DNA (LPD) vector targets the lung, kidney, heart, liver and spleen, with the highest level of gene expression in the lung [21, 22]. To avoid such nonspecific uptake, stealth liposomes have also been developed [23]. By selecting lipid components, the liposomes are retained in the systemic circulation much longer than other liposomes. Such stealth liposomes are used for drug delivery to tumor tissues [24]. In particular, liposomes conjugated with poly(ethylene glycol) (PEG) are also of the "stealth" type [25, 26]. Cationic lipid–

DNA complexes accumulate mostly into the lung, while "PEGylated" lipid–DNA complexes exhibit lower lung accumulation. The folate receptor is abundant in tumor tissues. When folate is conjugated with PEGylated lipid–DNA complexes, pulmonary accumulation of DNA is reduced and tumor-targeted DNA increases [27]. PEGylation of various types of vectors may regulate tissue-targeting when tissue-specific molecules are conjugated with the complex.

14.2.1.3 Resistance to Degradation in Systemic Circulation

In the human body, protective mechanisms against viral invasion exist. Anti-galactose antibodies present in human serum bind to retrovirus envelope proteins to induce complement-mediated lysis [28]. To avoid such lysis, a complement-resistant retrovirus has been developed [29]. Adenovirus is highly immunogenic and is attacked by the host immune system after repeated transfection [30]. As described above, to reduce immunogenicity, a "gutless" adenovirus vector has also been developed [7].

Another barrier to gene transfer is the penetration and distribution of vectors in tissues. To extrasavate from blood vessels to the target tissues and cells, vectors must penetrate endothelial cells. To induce gene expression in a large area of tissue, vectors must be spread diffusely throughout the entire area. Many viral vectors including adenovirus vector and AAV vector cannot penetrate endothelial cells when administered systemically [31]. Among the nonviral gene delivery systems, cationic liposomes are the most frequently used for gene transfer. When injected into the mouse tail vein, gene expression is detected primarily in the lung [32]. However, cationic liposomes cannot penetrate past the endothelial cells when injected into the vasculature [33]. In contrast, anionic liposomes are able to penetrate endothelial cells [34]. Moreover, anionic liposomes can distribute to broader areas in the target tissues than cationic liposomes. The mean size of liposomes is also important, because tissues are more permeable to smaller liposomes.

14.2.2 Crossing the Cell Membrane

After reaching the target cells, transgene DNA must cross the cell membrane, which is a very effective barrier that excludes foreign substances from cells. There are several ways to overcome this barrier. Although one is to facilitate DNA transfer by utilizing endocytosis or phagocytosis, in this process the foreign DNA must penetrate the membrane of the endosome or phagosome rapidly. Otherwise, the DNA will be degraded. Adenovirus can escape from the endosome by disrupting the endosomal membrane with penton fibers [35, 36]. This ability has been utilized to enhance the efficiency of gene transfer by transferrin/poly-L-lysine/DNA complexes [12]. Other viruses can fuse with the cell membrane to introduce their genomes into the cytoplasm. There are two different mechanisms of virus–cell fusion: pH-dependent and pH-independent. Influenza virus [37], Semliki forest virus (SFV) [38] and VSV [39] exhibit pH-dependent fusion, whereas HVJ (Sendai virus) [40] and retroviruses [41, 42] can fuse with the cell membrane at both acidic and neutral pH. Viral fusion proteins have been identified and synthetic vectors that express these viral fusion proteins can transfer foreign genes efficiently into the cytoplasm [43].

14.2.3 Nuclear Targeting

Transport of the foreign gene to the nucleus is required for gene expression in gene therapy. In nondividing cells especially, DNA is not transported efficiently to the nucleus where transcription occurs. However, it should be noted that naked plasmid DNA can be transported to the nucleus without breakdown of the nuclear envelope. The efficiency is generally 1–2% of the DNA in the cytoplasm [44]. Therefore, nuclear targeting increases gene expression, especially in tissues. Some viruses such as adenovirus, SV40, HIV and herpes virus are known to induce rapid migration of their genomes to the nucleus even in nondividing cells [43]. In SV40, viral capsid proteins contain nuclear localization sequences (NLSs) that trigger translocation of the virion to the nucleus and disassembly of the virion within the nucleus [44]. Although rapid nuclear transport also occurs with adenovirus, disassembly of the viral capsid occurs in the cytoplasm and the DNA-NLS-containing proteins are then sorted in the nucleus [45, 46]. In HIV, an integrase is required for nuclear migration of the viral genome [44]. However, the DNA–integrase complex, or preintegration complex, of oncoretroviruses such as Moloney leukemia virus cannot pass through the nuclear pores and, thus, transport of the transgene to the nucleus does not occur in nondividing cells in these retroviral systems [1]. In nonviral vector systems, nuclear transport of plasmid DNA occurs, but the efficiency is very low [5]. Enhancing nuclear migration of plasmid DNA is an important issue for increasing transgene expression. Complexes of plasmid DNA and nuclear proteins have been constructed to improve nuclear migration of DNA [47, 48]. It was recently reported that conjugation of the NLS peptide derived from SV40 with a luciferase gene fragment enhanced luciferase gene expression approximately 1000-fold compared with the luciferase gene without the NLS peptide [49]. The NLS peptide at either the 5′ or 3′ end of the DNA enhanced luciferase gene expression, but incorporation of the NLS at both ends was not effective. It is thought that positioning of the NLS at one end of the gene stimulates nuclear migration of the luciferase gene, whereas incorporation of the NLS at both ends ensnares the DNA at the nuclear envelope. However, it remains unknown whether NLS conjugation improves the nuclear migration of larger DNA molecules and if NLS conjugation improves the efficiency of translocation *in vivo*. This raises the question, does only a small fraction of all the plasmid DNA go to the nucleus? Recently, several papers have suggested that nuclear migration of plasmid DNA may be sequence dependent [50]. The SV40 enhancer sequence appears to facilitate nuclear migration of DNA by binding transcription factors [51] which are transported to the nucleus by the Ran/importin system.

RNA-based vectors have also been developed. Alphaviruses such as SFV and Sindvis virus are converted into gene expression recombinant RNA vectors [52,

53], which do not require the transport of DNA into the nucleus. In general, RNA vectors produce large amounts of proteins and this production inhibits host protein synthesis, inducing cell death (apoptosis) [54]. Thus, tight regulation of protein synthesis will be required for the use of gene therapy using RNA vector systems.

14.2.4 Regulation of Gene Expression

Effective expression of a transgene is also a major issue in gene therapy. We should view this step from at least two aspects. One is the stable retention of a transgene and the other is the regulation of transcription. The export of mRNA, translation and post-translational modification of polypeptides generally affect gene expression, but they are not specific for expression of a transgene. Therefore, this section focuses on the events occurring before mRNA production.

14.2.4.1 Stable Retention of Transgenes

There are two distinct approaches to this issue. One is the integration of the transgene into the host genome. Retroviruses can integrate into random sites of the host chromosomes, but integration occurs only in dividing cells [1]. HIV inserts its genome into the host chromosomes even in nondividing cells. A lentivirus vector system containing the recombinant HIV genome along with a therapeutic gene and the vesicular stomatitis virus G protein (VSVG) gene was used to generate long-term gene expression in mouse neurons [9]. The mechanism of insertion of the viral genome into host chromosomes has been investigated. However, reconstitution of the viral machinery that confers the ability of genome insertion to non-viral gene delivery systems has not yet been successful. In 1997, *sleeping beauty*, a fish transposon/transposase system, was developed [55]. This system inserts the neomycin-resistance gene into the HeLa cell genome with very high efficiency. Application of this system to gene transfer is currently under investigation. However, insertion of the transgene into the host genome occurs at random. Although AAV integrates specifically into the AAVS1 site of human chromosome 19 [56], the recombinant AAV vector is unable to do so because it does not express Rep 65 protein [57].

Another approach is the stable retention of an episomal piece of DNA. EBV has been analyzed thoroughly in terms of latent infection. The *cis*-acting oriP (the latent viral DNA replication origin) sequence and the *trans*-acting EBV nuclear antigen-1 (EBNA-1) gene are required for latent EBV infection, which is characterized by autonomous replication and nuclear retention of the EBV genome in host cells [58–60]. It has been reported that stable retention of the EBV genome is mediated by binding of the oriP sequence with the nuclear matrix. The EBV vector can transfer genes primarily to B lymphocytes, with minimal transfer to other somatic cells. To improve long-term transgene expression, an EBV replicon-based plasmid that contains oriP and EBNA-1 was constructed and transferred to various animal tissues using HVJ-liposomes. With the EBV replicon vector system, gene expression was sustained and enhanced both *in vitro* and *in vivo*, in several cell lines and mouse liver, respectively [61]. Without EBNA-1, transgene expression of an oriP-containing plasmid was diminished in mouse liver. However, by re-introducing EBNA-1 to the mouse liver, transgene expression was reactivated [62]. This indicates that EBNA-1 can restore gene expression of an episomal plasmid containing an oriP sequence within the nucleus. When the luciferase gene was introduced into a mouse melanoma cell line, with or without the EBV replicon components (oriP and EBNA-1), effective long-term gene expression was obtained in the plasmid containing the EBV replicon components. However, Southern blot analysis revealed that the copy number of the plasmid without the EBV components was much higher than that with the EBV replicon plasmid. This result suggests that effective gene expression by the EBV replicon plasmid results from transcriptional activation, and not from stable retention of the plasmid DNA. The regulation of transcription is further discussed below.

14.2.4.2 **Regulation of Transcription**

Silencing of transgene expression occurs in host cells, despite insertion of transgenes into the host genome [63]. Similar silencing has also been reported in certain viral infections. For example, retroviral gene expression was inhibited after retrovirus infection of mouse embryos [64, 65]. Although low or silenced transgene expression after transfection has been a major problem in human gene therapy [66], the mechanism(s) by which transgene expression is regulated have not yet been elucidated. Since it will be essential to control transgene expression in human gene therapy, basic research on transgene expression in human gene therapy should be pursued further.

Although transcription factors have been investigated extensively [67, 68], previous studies have not fully clarified the mechanism(s) of regulation of transcription in higher eukaryotes. Recent studies have shown that chromatin remodeling factors such as the switch/sucrose nonfermenting (SWI/SNF) family and the imitation switch (ISWI) family [69] are involved in regulation of transcription. It is thought that histone acetylase and deacetylase also regulate transcription by modifying chromatin [70, 71]. Acetylation and deacetylation of histones and other proteins associated with DNA have been shown to be important in the epigenetics of regulating gene expression [70–72]. Recently, amplification of transgene expression in animals treated with a novel histone deacetylase inhibitor was reported [73]. This amplification was more effective for transgene expression than for endogenous gene expression. These data suggest that transgene expression can be regulated by chromatin modifications, such as histone acetylation/deacetylation. Methylated DNA-binding protein MeCP2 is a component of the complex that contains histone deacetylase [74]. This suggests that DNA methylation status may dictate the state of histone acetylation/deacetylation in chromatin. To overcome the silencing of transgene expression and to sustain transgene expression, *cis*-elements such as "insulators" [75–77] that are not affected by chromatin modification may be applied for transgene expression in gene therapy.

Many significant barriers to gene transfer have been elucidated. If omnipotent vector systems are eventually developed, however, gene transfer may harm patients – this is far from therapeutic. An all-encompassing vector system may not be feasible and each vector system must be evaluated with respect to the target disease. In some diseases such as arteriosclerosis obliterans, transient gene expression would be sufficient to cure the disease and sustained gene expression would be detrimental. In other diseases such as SCID-X1 and hemophilia B, it may be necessary to induce transformation of only a small population of cells. Cancer gene therapy comprises more than 60% of current human gene therapy approaches and no remarkable successes have been reported in this area to date. When we consider why gene therapy is necessary for cancer treatment, the answer is that it should be used to inhibit tumor metastasis and suppress the recurrence of cancers. For these purposes, investigations on basic cancer cell biology and technological developments should be promoted much more than at present. The issues described in this chapter present a road map for future technological developments in cancer gene therapy. Thus, technology for gene therapy should be developed on the basis of analysis of the target tissues, target cells, cellular components and relevant molecules.

14.3
HVJ-E Vector

14.3.1
Development of HVJ-E Vector

HVJ is a mouse parainfluenza virus and is not a human pathogen. As molecules that enter the cell by phagocytosis or endocytosis often become degraded before reaching the cytoplasm, fusion-mediated delivery systems have been developed. A fusigenic viral liposome with a fusion proteins derived from HVJ was constructed [78]. HVJ fuses with the cell membrane at a neutral pH, and the HN protein and F protein of the virus contribute to cell fusion [79]. For fusion-mediated gene transfer, DNA-loaded liposomes were fused with ultraviolet (UV)-inactivated HVJ to form the fusigenic viral-liposome called the HVJ-liposome (Fig. 14.1).

Fusion-mediated delivery protected the molecules in the endosomes and lysosomes from degradation [80]. When fluorescein isothiocyanate (FITC)-tagged oligodeoxynucleotide (ODN) was introduced into vascular smooth muscle cells using HVJ-liposomes, fluorescence was detected in the nuclei 5 min after transfer and fluorescence was stable in the nucleus for at least 72 h. In contrast, fluorescence was observed in cellular components (most likely endosomes) and not in the nucleus when FITC-ODN was transferred directly in the absence of HVJ-liposomes and no fluorescence was detected 24 h after transfer. Using a fluorescence resonance energy transfer system, we demonstrated that more than 80% of oligonucleotides labeled with two different fluorescent dyes at the 5′ and 3′ ends were

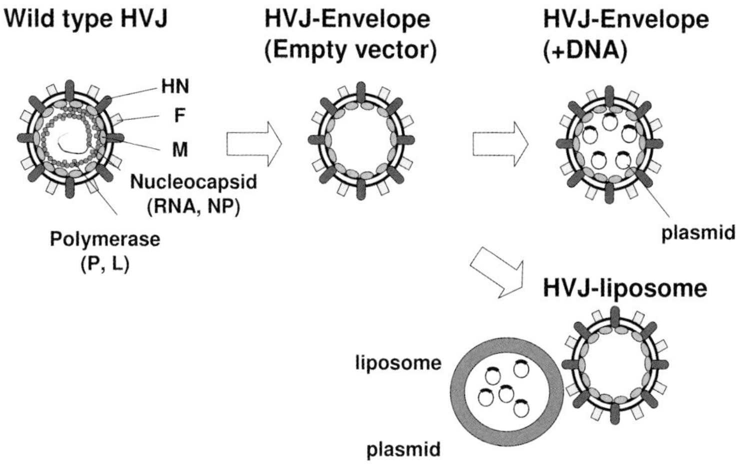

Figure 14.1. HVJ-E vector system. For constructing HVJ-E vector, plasmid DNA is mixed with inactivated HVJ particles, and the mixture is treated with mild detergent and centrifugation to incorporate DNA inside the particle. For constructing HVJ-liposome vector, plasmid DNA is incorporated in liposome and mixed with inactivated HVJ particles. HVJ can fuse with the cell membrane to directly transfer DNA into cells.

intact in the nucleus, while less than 30% of the oligonucleotides were intact when Lipofectin was used [81].

Another advantage of HVJ-liposomes is the ability to perform repeated injections. Gene transfer to rat liver cells was not inhibited by repeated injections. After repeated injections, the anti-HVJ antibodies generated in the rat were not sufficient to neutralize HVJ-liposomes. Cytotoxic T cells recognizing HVJ determinants were not detected in the rats transfected repeatedly with HVJ-liposomes [82].

A similar approach has been used to enhance the gene transfer efficiency of a receptor-mediated gene delivery system by combining fusion peptide derived from influenza virus hemagglutinin (HA) [83]. A tissue-specific gene delivery system has been developed by binding tissue-specific molecules to a poly-L-lysine/DNA complex [84]. Binding asialoglycoprotein and transferrin to a poly-L-lysine/DNA complex successfully targets DNA to hepatocytes and cancer cells, respectively [84, 85]. However, the limitation of this system is the degradation of the DNA in the lysosomes. To avoid such degradation, a fusion-mediated gene delivery system has been investigated using influenza fusion proteins. Influenza virus fuses with cell membranes at an acidic pH, and HA protein on the viral envelope is involved in the fusion between viral envelope and endosomal membrane. It has also been elucidated that a mutant N-terminal peptide of influenza HA subunit, HA-2, can fuse with cell membranes at neutral pH. The transferrin/poly-L-lysine/DNA complex bound with the HA-2 peptide increases gene transfer efficiency in cultured cancer cells more than 1000-fold compared with that in the absence of the peptide [83].

Reconstituted particles containing fusion proteins of HVJ have also been developed to promote fusion-mediated gene delivery [86, 87]. HVJ virion was completely lysed with detergent and the lysates were mixed with DNA solution. In some cases, several lipids were added to the mixture. By removing the detergent with dialysis or a column procedure, reconstituted HVJ particles containing DNA were constructed. Instead of the whole virion of HVJ, fusion proteins (F and HN) isolated from the virion were mixed with the lipid/DNA mixture in the presence or absence of detergent. Since F protein is recognized by the asialogycoprotein receptor on hepatocytes, reconstituted HVJ particles containing only F protein have been constructed to specifically target hepatocytes *in vivo* [88]. However, DNA trapping efficiency of the reconstituted particles was not so high. To improve the limitation, another approach was that liposomes containing fusion proteins of HVJ and DNA-loaded liposomes were prepared separately, and then both liposomes were fused together [89]. These reconstituted fusion liposomes were as effective as conventional HVJ-liposomes, which contain the fully intact HVJ virion, in terms of the delivery of FITC-ODN and the luciferase gene to cultured cells. The *LacZ* gene was also transferred directly to mouse skeletal muscle *in vivo* using these reconstituted fusion particles.

A more direct and practical approach is the conversion of a fusigenic virion to a nonviral gene delivery particle. Numerous viruses such as influenza, VSV and HVJ induce cell fusion. HVJ is the most abundantly produced in chick eggs. Therefore, we tried to construct an HVJ-E vector system by incorporating plasmid DNA into inactivated HVJ particle [90]. Our approach has been to use inactivated viral envelope in which the viral genome has been destroyed to develop highly efficient and minimally invasive vectors.

There are some drawbacks to HVJ-liposomes, although they have been widely used for gene transfer both *in vitro* and *in vivo*. One disadvantage of HVJ-liposomes is the complicated procedure used to isolate and produce both inactivated HVJ and DNA-loaded liposomes. Additionally, the fusion activity of the HVJ-liposomes decreases to approximately 2% of that of native HVJ because of the reduced density of fusion proteins on the surface of HVJ-liposomes. To simplify the vector system and to develop a more effective gene delivery system, we attempted to incorporate plasmid DNA into inactivated HVJ particles without using liposomes.

HVJ is a mouse parainfluenza virus and is not a human pathogen [79]. HVJ can fuse with cell membranes in both neutral and acidic conditions. Two distinct glycoproteins, HN and F, are required for cell fusion [79, 91]. HN is required for the binding of HVJ to cell surface sialic acid receptors and the subsequent degradation of the receptors by its sialidase activity. Then, F associates with lipids, such as cholesterol, in the cell membrane to induce cell fusion. The F glycoprotein is first synthesized as inactive F0 in cells infected with HVJ. F0 is then cleaved by host protease into the active F1 and F2 forms. F1 contains hydrophobic peptides with approximately 25 amino acids that induce cell fusion [91, 92]. F protein produced in chick eggs is converted to the active F1 form by the protease in chorioallantoic fluid, while the virus produced from cultured cells contains inactive F0 that needs to be cleaved by a protease to form active F1. Cells in the rodent airway contain enzymes to convert inactive F0 to active F1. Therefore, HVJ induces severe pneumonia in rodents but not in humans. Large amounts of viral proteins are produced in infected cells. Viral nucleocapsid protein induces cytotoxic T lymphocytes (CTLs) against infected cells [93]. However, nucleocapsid protein is indispensable for virus production. Therefore, to develop highly efficient and minimally invasive vectors based on HVJ, our approach has been to use inactivated viral envelope in which the viral genome has been destroyed.

For this purpose, we have converted HVJ to a nonviral vector containing therapeutic genes instead of the viral genome [90]. HVJ amplified in the chorioallantoic fluid of 10- to 14-day-old chick eggs was inactivated with β-propiolactone (0.0075–0.001%) [94] followed by UV irradiation (99 mJ cm^{-2}) [95]. Then, inactivated HVJ-E was purified by ion-exchange column chromatography and gel filtration (Nakajima and coworkers, unpublished method). With this inactivation procedure, virus replication was completely destroyed, but hemagglutinating activity was not affected. HVJ particles in the chorioallantoic fluid were very heterogeneous with a diameter ranging from 150 to 600 nm. More homogeneous HVJ-E was isolated with the improved purification method using the column procedure. The diameter of HVJ-E obtained from the column procedure was 280 nm and the ζ potential was approximately -5 mV.

Aliquots of the inactivated virus (3×10^{10} particles per 1.5-ml tube) were centrifuged (10 000 g, 5 min) and the viral pellet was mixed with exogenous plasmid DNA. Exogenous plasmid DNA was incorporated into inactivated HVJ by treatment with mild detergent and centrifugation. First, inactivated HVJ (3×10^{10}) particles were mixed with 0.24–0.80% Triton X-100 in the presence of plasmid DNA (200 μg) in less than 100 μl of Tris–EDTA buffer for 5 min on ice and the mixture was centrifuged at 10 000 g for 5 min to move the DNA into the HVJ particle. The DNA trapping efficiency of HVJ-E vector was approximately 15–20%. Without centrifugation, the DNA trapping efficiency was approximately 3%. Different detergents were available for the preparation of HVJ-E vector including NP-40, CHAPS, octylglucoside, sodium cholate and dodecyl maltoside, although the optimal concentration of detergent for preparation of HVJ-E vector is different. Without detergent treatment, DNA does not become incorporated into the viral particle. Electron microscopy confirms that DNA became incorporated into all of the particles of inactivated HVJ. The largest plasmid tested was 14 kb and its trapping efficiency was 18%.

The HVJ-E vector differs from the reconstituted HVJ particles that are prepared by reassembling lipids and fusion proteins after solubilization of the virus particle. To prepare HVJ-E vector, plasmid DNA is incorporated into inactivated HVJ particles by treatment with mild detergent. The virion is not destroyed, and not subjected to the dialysis, purification and addition of lipids or proteins that occurs during the preparation of reconstituted HVJ particles [86, 87, 89]. Protein analysis of HVJ-E vector using sodium dodecyl sulfate–polyacrylamide gel electrophoresis indicates that the composition of HVJ-E vector is very similar to that of native HVJ [90]. Most native HVJ proteins are retained in HVJ-E vector. Fusion proteins HN and F1 are retained, and the molar ratio of these proteins in HVJ-E vector was approximately 2:2.3, which is the same as the ratio in native HVJ [79]. This ratio of F and HN is very important for fusion activity. Therefore, the fusion activity of HVJ-E vector is as robust as wild-type HVJ. Electron microscopic observation confirmed that the fusion between HVJ-E vector and cell membrane occurs only 3–5 s after the attachment of the plasmid-containing HVJ-E vector to a cell surface.

In contrast to recombinant HVJ viral vector [96], the HVJ-E is a nonviral vector system that consists of an envelope derived from wild-type HVJ virus by inactivation and purification. Since the viral genome is inactivated in HVJ-E vector, the virus does not replicate and viral genes are not expressed in the cells that are transfected with HVJ-E vector. However, cells infected with recombinant HVJ viral vector produce viral proteins. The recombinant HVJ vector produces a large amount of therapeutic products, but it may cause cellular toxicity and be highly immunogenic, which make it less desirable for repeated administration.

For *in vitro* transfection, HVJ-E vector containing luciferase expression plasmid was mixed with PS and this mixture was added to culture cells. Protamine sulfate enhanced luciferase gene expression 10- to 50-fold in several cell lines and the optimum conditions for *in vitro* gene transfer have been previously summarized [90]. Small interfering RNA (siRNA) is an attractive and effective tool for suppressing target protein by specifically digesting its mRNA [97, 98]. siRNA is superior to antisense oligonucleotides and ribozyme in terms of efficiency and specificity [99, 100], but finding a suitable delivery system for siRNA has been problematic [101]. Drugs, synthetic oligonucleotides, proteins and peptides as well as siRNA can be incorporated into HVJ-E vector, and delivered into cells. The HVJ-E-mediated delivery efficiency of siRNA in cultured cells was 100%. Other researchers have also demonstrated that HVJ-E vector efficiently delivers siRNA to islet cell lines [102] and Jurkat cells [103].

HVJ-E vector system can be used for *in vivo* gene transfer. The HVJ-E vector has mediated gene transfer to a variety of tissues (lung, liver, uterus, eye, skin, muscle, brain and heart) in animals including mice, rats, rabbits and monkeys. In mouse liver, HVJ-E vector-mediated luciferase gene expression was 2 times higher than the expression mediated by HVJ-liposomes prepared from inactivated HVJ. In mouse skeletal muscle, consecutive injection of DNA-loaded HVJ-E vector did not inhibit gene transfection. In this experiment, empty HVJ-E vector was injected into mouse muscle tissue twice with a 2-week interval in one experimental group, while another group received saline injections. Two weeks later, HVJ-E vector-containing luciferase gene was intramuscularly injected in all mice. In the two groups, similar luciferase gene expression was observed. Thus, HVJ-E vector appears to be less immunogenic than other viral vector.

We reported the successful gene transfection into uterus and brains by HVJ-E vector [104, 105]. For the transfection into uterus, HVJ-E vector containing plasmid DNA was slowly injected into the uterine cavity and the cervix was clamped for 10 min. For the transfection into brain tissue, we intrathecally injected HVJ-E vector containing the *LacZ* gene into the cerebrospinal fluid (CSF). HVJ-envelop vector containing plasmid DNA was infused at the rate of 50 $\mu L\ min^{-1}$ after removing

100 μl of CSF. Then, the animals were placed head-down for 30 min. No behavioral changes, such as convulsions or abnormal movements, were observed. Cells that expressed β-galactosidase were present in the spiral ganglion cells (SGCs), cerebral cortex and medulla.

We also examined the transfection efficiency in the intravenous injection of HVJ-E vector. Luciferase gene-loaded HVJ-E vector (6×10^9 particles) was injected into the mouse tail vein and luciferase activity in several organs was measured 24 h after injection. Luciferase expression was detected in the spleen for at least 1 week. When HVJ-E vector containing FITC-ODNs was systemically injected, FITC-ODNs were observed in the marginal zone of the spleen. However, by intravenous injection of HVJ-E vector, coagulation functions in the mouse blood is transiently suppressed, but the functions are recovered at 24 h after the injection. It is probable that the hemagglutinating activity of HN protein will be necessary for systemic injection of HVJ-E vector to ensure the safety in gene therapy.

14.3.2 Approaches to Cancer Gene Therapy Utilizing HVJ-E Vector

14.3.2.1 Transfection of Dendritic Cells (DCs) with Melanoma-associated Antigen (MAA) using HVJ Envelope Vector for Immunotherapy of Melanoma

Our first approach for developing cancer gene therapy was to construct cancer vaccines using the HVJ-E vector system. Polyvalent tumor antigen vaccines have been evaluated to increase the repertoire of antitumor T cells [106]. In this study, we chose MAA genes, glycoprotein 100 (gp100) and tyrosine-related protein 2 (TRP2), and transfected DCs with these two genes to evaluate *ex vivo* vaccination for prophylactic and therapeutic melanoma treatment.

DCs are the most potent antigen-presenting cells. DCs are capable of highly effective presentation of antigens to naive T cells and they can initiate immune responses [107]. Several clinical studies have now been conducted in cancer patients with tumor-associated antigen (TAA)-loaded DCs [108, 109]. In several of these clinical studies the DCs were loaded by pulsing with protein antigens or with peptides derived from TAAs. Studies have demonstrated that *ex vivo* transfected DCs and adoptive therapy can be very effective in inducing antigen-specific immune responses. This type of strategy has been demonstrated in animals and pilot clinical studies for a variety of cancers [110, 111].

Transfected DCs with vectors expressing TAA genes have shown promising results. Studies have demonstrated that xenogeneic TAAs are very strong immunogens capable of cross-priming to host syngeneic TAAs. Human TRP2 and gp100 proteins have a high amino acid sequence homology to their mouse counterparts. We used xenogeneic TAAs for several reasons: to break self-antigen tolerance in the host, to induce strong antitumor immunity and to enhance individual TAA immunogenicity. The approach provides a large expression of TAAs and activates DC presentation. Therefore, highly efficient transfection system is absolutely necessary for efficient induction of tumor immunity. In recent studies, adenoviral vector was the original vector of choice for efficiently transfecting DCs [112, 113]. However, adenovirus has serious disadvantages as a vector for engineering DCs because of its high toxicity. Some studies have demonstrated that plasmid DNA in liposomes [114], vaccinia virus [115, 116] and retroviruses [117, 118] could be used to infect or transfect human DCs to present a variety of antigens. However, a highly efficient and minimally invasive vector system has not yet been achieved for transfection of DCs. To develop more efficient gene transfer to DCs that cause only minimal damage, we tested the potential of HVJ-E vector for transfection of DCs with two different TAA genes.

We used the luciferase gene to determine the optimal conditions for transfection of DCs. As previously reported, the optimum ratio of HVJ-E vector to cultured cells is 6×10^3 to 1.2×10^4 [90]. We identified 1.2×10^4 as the optimal ratio and determined the most effective transfection conditions. When DCs were incubated with HVJ-E vector containing the luciferase gene, luciferase gene expression was not significant. We attempted to increase the luciferase gene expression by centrifuging the mixture of DCs and HVJ-E vector. Centrifugation at 9000 *g* was much more effective for gene transfection than 3000 and 13 000 *g*. The viability of DCs after transfection was approximately 70%. The centrifugation time required for the most effective gene expression was 90 min. The highest luciferase gene expression was obtained in DCs that were centrifuged for 90 min at 9000 *g* and 37 °C. Six days after DCs were isolated was the best time to transfect the DCs for optimal luciferase gene expression. Thus, the optimal conditions for the most effective transfection of DCs were at 9000 *g* for 90 min at 37 °C in DCs cultured for 6 days after isolation from bone marrow. Under these optimal conditions, we assessed the expression of yellow fluorescent protein (YFP) expression to determine the transfected DCs population. Almost all DCs that were recognized with phycoerythrin (PE)-conjugated CD11c antibody expressed YFP, as determined by fluorescence microscopy. Flow cytometry analysis revealed that approximately 99% of DCs expressed YFP.

Surface markers of mature DCs were studied by flow cytometry analysis to confirm that differentiation was not inhibited by gene transfection using HVJ-E vector. The lipopolysaccharide (LPS)-induced expression of CD40, CD80, CD86 and HLA-DR was equivalent on nontransfected DCs and transfected DCs. The nonspecific phagocytotic activity of DCs (evaluated by uptake of FITC-labeled dextran) was suppressed in transfected DCs as well as in nontransfected DCs. Thus, gene transfer with HVJ-E vector did not inhibit LPS-induced maturation of DCs.

Next, we used HVJ-E vector to transfect the gp100 and TRP2 genes into DCs. The expression of each transfected antigen was detected by flow cytometry analysis of cells stained with antigen-specific antibody. On day 1, gp100 and TRP2 were detected in 36 and 63% of DCs, respectively. Approximately 80% of DCs expressed both antigens on day 7.

DCs transfected with either the gp100 or TRP2 gene or both genes after one day were injected intradermally into C57BL/6 mice. The delayed-type hypersensitivity (DTH) response was assessed in mice immunized with MAA-transfected DCs at 24, 48, and 72 h after TAA protein challenge. Significant cutaneous DTH was detected in mice immunized with MAA gene-transfected DCs compared to the control mice that were injected with DCs without MAA. The DTH response to gp100 was significant in the groups immunized with gp100-transfected DCs or gp100/TRP2-transfected DCs. The level of response was equivalent in the two groups. A similar response to TRP2 was obtained in the groups immunized with TRP2-transfected DCs or gp100/TRP2-transfected DCs.

We examined CTLs against BL6 tumor cells on day 7 after DC administration. TAA-specific CTLs were generated with variable response rates. Mice immunized with DCs expressing gp100 and TRP-2 had the highest level of CTL activity against ^{51}Cr – labeled BL6 target cells. Mice immunized with single TAA-transfected DCs generated significant CTL activity against BL6 cells when compared to the control groups that received HVJ-E vector containing pcDNA-3.1. However, these responses were lower than those generated by the cotransfer of gp100 and TRP2. Vaccination of DCs transfected with TAA genes induced TAA-specific cellular immunity consisting of CTL activity and DTH helper cell activity against melanoma cells.

We tested the effect of vaccination with MAA-transfected DCs on the inhibition of tumor growth in mice. No tumor growth was observed in mice immunized with gp100/TRP2 transfected DCs, although significant tumor masses were palpable in all control mice injected with DCs without TAA. Immunization with DCs transfected with single TAA gene was not effective, as small tumor masses were detected. However, the tumor growth rate was slower than that of the control group. In this prophylactic study, vaccination with DCs transfected with both gp100 and TRP2 was much more effective for inhibition of tumor growth than vaccination with DCs transfected with TRP2 alone.

To investigate the therapeutic effect of vaccination with TAA-transfected DCs, we vaccinated the mice with various DC vaccines 24 h after intravenous inoculation with 10^4 BL6 cells. All control mice injected with PBS-treated DCs and pcDNA3.1-transfected DCs died of lung metastasis in 45 and 62 days after inoculation, respectively. Vaccination with DCs that were transfected with a single TAA gene improved the survival. Vaccination with TRP2-transfected DCs was more effective than vaccination with gp100-transfected DCs. Vaccination with gp100/TRP2-transfected DCs significantly prolonged the survival rate. Eight of nine mice vaccinated with gp100/TRP2-transfected DCs survived more than 80 days after tumor inoculation. Vaccination with immature DCs that were not treated with LPS was not effective for improving survival and all of these mice died in 60 days (including the mice that received gp100/TRP2-transfected DCs).

14.3.2.2 **Fusion of DC Tumor Cells and Simultaneous Gene Transfer to the Hybrid Cells using HVJ-E for the Prevention and Treatment of Cancers**

TAAs have been identified in some cancers such as melanoma [119, 120]. However, TAAs in many cancers have not been identified. The identification of TAAs is required for the development of TAA-loaded DC vaccines.

To solve the problem, hybrid cell vaccines have been developed by fusing DCs with tumor cells [121, 122]. There is evidence that these DC–tumor fused cells possess the properties of both tumor cells containing known and unknown TAAs and

DCs with high levels of MHC class I and II molecules and costimulatory molecules for priming and activating naive $CD4^+$ and $CD8^+$ T cells. Therefore, even though tumor cells lose MHC class I molecules, TAAs can be presented on the surface of the fused cells by DC-derived MHC class I molecules. PEG and electroporation have been used to induce tumor cell–DC fusion. HVJ has been identified as a powerful fusogen. We stained mouse DCs with red fluorescent reagent. Mouse melanoma cells were stained green and irradiated with γ-rays. Both cells were mixed with inactivated HVJ. After 30 min, the fusion of DCs and tumor cells occurred with approximately 50% efficiency.

We used HVJ-E to generate powerful tumor–DC vaccines, because HVJ-E can induce tumor cell–DC fusion and simultaneously transfer DNA or proteins to activate the immune response. To confirm simultaneous fusion and gene transfer mediated by HVJ-E, DCs and tumor cells were mixed with HVJ-E containing the green fluorescent protein (GFP) gene. Fusion between DCs and irradiated-tumor cells was observed, and YFP expression was detected in fused cells as well as in DCs.

Using this system, we attempted to generate anti-tumor immunity using HVJ-E with or without the interleukin (IL)-12 gene. Ten days after the second immunization, spleen cells were isolated to assess cytolytic activity. The cytolytic activity of the effector cells obtained from the mice immunized with fused cells was significantly higher than that obtained from other vaccination protocols such as PBS, IL-12, "Mix" (mixture of DCs and tumor cells without fusion) and "Mix" plus IL-12. Higher cytolytic activity was observed in the mice that received fused cells plus IL-12 as compared with that in the mice that received fused cells alone.

First, we examined the effect of this hybrid cell vaccine on the prevention of tumor generation. After two vaccinations, melanoma cells or renal cancer cells were intradermally injected. The mice vaccinated with fused cells plus IL-12 had significantly increased survival; all of these mice were alive 60 days after tumor challenge in the B16BL6 tumor model. The survival rate was 20% in the mice vaccinated with fused cells without IL-12. All mice in the other groups died. The effect of fused cells and IL-12 on the enhancement of tumor-specific immunity in mice was also observed against renal cancer. Therefore, these findings indicate that immunization with fused cells plus IL-12 strongly induces T_h1 cytokines and activates tumor-specific CTLs, resulting in significant protection from melanoma, which has known TAAs or renal cancers which has unknown TAAs.

Next, we treated solid tumors by *in vivo* fusion and gene expression using HVJ-E vector. Mouse DCs and HVJ-E vector were injected into solid tumors. The effect of the transfer of a therapeutic gene by HVJ-E vector was also evaluated. To detect *in vivo* fusion of DCs with tumor cells, red-stained DCs were injected into melanoma masses expressing YFP with inactivated HVJ. Megakaryocytes, which indicate tumor cell–tumor cell fusion, were detected, as well as large orange-stained cells indicate DC–tumor cell fusion. However, the fusion efficiency *in vivo* was much less than that of *in vitro* cell fusion.

For therapeutic experiments, melanoma cells were intradermally injected. When the tumor diameter was greater than 5 mm, an injection of DCs and HVJ-E vector was administered. Spleen cells were isolated and assayed for antimelanoma CTL activity. No therapeutic genes were incorporated into HVJ-E vector. The coinjection of DCs and empty HVJ-E vector resulted in significant antimelanoma CTL activity. DCs or HVJ-E vector alone did not induce CTL activity. When tumor growth was observed, the coinjection of DCs and empty HVJ-E vector inhibited tumor growth, but the tumor volume still gradually increased. When DCs were coinjected with HVJ-E vector that contained the IL-12 gene, a greater inhibitory effect was obtained. The coinjection of DCs and HVJ-E vector effectively prolonged mouse survival. The most effective therapeutic effect was obtained when HVJ-E vector that contained IL-12 gene was coinjected with DCs into the tumor mass; approximately 60% of these mice survived 35 days after treatment.

Thus, we developed a novel cancer vaccine using HVJ-E-mediated DC–tumor cell fusion. The DC–tumor cell fusion was induced by HVJ-E vector at a high efficiency. Both known and unknown TAAs were presented on fused cells by MHC class I molecules from DCs. Furthermore, IL-12 gene transfer was achieved in the fused cells. The expression of IL-12 stimulates the maturation of naive T cells and promotes a T_h1 response [123]. It is believed that the presentation of TAAs and the promotion of a T_h1 response together induce an efficient antitumor CTL response.

The HVJ-E vector holds great promise for human gene therapy. We are improving the HVJ-E vector system so that it can be used in clinical trials. So far, the virus has been produced in chick eggs, but egg-derived HVJ is difficult to use for clinical trials. It has been very difficult to produce large amounts of the virus in cultured cells and the production in cultured cells are less than 2% of that in chick eggs. We recently developed the system in producing HVJ in human cells. We cloned HEK-293 cells that produce a high titer of HVJ after infection and determined the growth conditions for these cells in an animal product-free medium using a bioreactor. We are able to culture these cells in 10 L of serum-free medium at a density of more than 10^6 cells mL^{-1} and we can obtain HVJ at the efficiency of more than 3×10^9 particles mL^{-1}. The production in a 10-L culture is comparable to that in 500 chick eggs. A pilot plant to commercially produce clinical grade HVJ-E vector was established in a venture company named Genemidea (Japan; http//www.anges-mg.com/news/030324.htm). Genomidea created a working cell bank, master cell bank and master virus bank for producing clinical-grade HVJ for phase I and IIa trials. They also set up an apparatus to purify inactivated HVJ using two different column systems. The human cell-derived HVJ-E vector was more effective for gene transfection than the egg-derived HVJ-E vector. Human cell-derived HVJ-E vector is also available for drug delivery both *in vitro* and *in vivo*. This vector will be available for human gene therapy soon.

14.4 Biocompatible Polymer with HVJ-E

Recent advances in biotechnology have made it possible to produce various clinically useful DNA and proteins. While this technology has brought about the discovery and mass production of these bioactive macromolecules, several challenges need to be addressed with regard to their sustained delivery in a convenient, controlled manner and targeting formulations. It has been demonstrated that complexation with positively charged polymers enabled negatively charged DNA to have an enhanced stability and transfection efficiency to cells [124–126]. Recently, the use of biodegradable gelatin as a nonviral vector augmented adrenomedulin expression and thereby enhanced the therapeutic effects of adrenomedulin gene transfer which potentially induces angiogenesis [127]. They demonstrated that rhodamine isothiocyanate-labeled adrenomedulin DNA was incorporated into positively charged gelatin. In addition, intramuscular administration of adrenomedulin DNA–gelatin complexes strongly enhanced adrenomedulin production compared with that of naked adrenomedulin DNA. These results suggest that biodegradable gelatin may serve as a vector for gene transfer. In fact, adrenomedulin DNA–gelatin complexes induced more potent angiogenic effects in a rabbit model of hind limb ischemia than naked adrenomedulin DNA, as evidenced by significant increases in histological capillary density, calf blood pressure ratio, laser Doppler flow and muscle weight ratio, and a decrease in necrosis of lower hind limb and thigh muscles. These results suggest that the use of biodegradable gelatin as a nonviral vector augments adrenomedulin expression and enhances adrenomedulin-induced angiogenic effects. Adrenomedulin DNA–gelatin complexes were distributed mainly in connective tissues. They have recently demonstrated that gelatin–DNA complex is readily phagocytosed by macrophages, monocytes, endothelial progenitor cells, etc., resulting in gene expression within these phagocytes [128, 129]. These findings raise the possibility that adrenomedulin secreted from these cells acts on muscles in a paracrine fashion. Unlike adrenomedulin production in the naked adrenomedulin group, adrenomedulin overexpression in the adrenomedulin–gelatin group lasted for longer than 2 weeks. Thus, it is interesting to speculate that delaying gene degradation by gelatin may be responsible for the highly efficient gene transfer.

We succeeded in enhancing the transfection efficiency of HVJ-E by combining it with cationic polymers [130]. For cultured cells *in vitro*, the most efficient transfection was obtained by combining HVJ-E with both CG and PS. However, for *in vivo* transfection, CG–HVJ-E without PS resulted in the highest gene expression. These findings are consistent with our previous report indicating that the particle size of cationic liposomes may affect gene transfection efficiency [131]. By adding both PS and CG to HVJ-E, the size and charge of the resulting complex may have been the most suitable for *in vitro* transfection. PS and CG affected gene transfection efficiency in a variety of cell lines as well as in primary cells, although the efficiency was varied among cell types. The ratio of PS and CG used for these experiments was determined by gene transfection experiments with CT26 cells. Thus, gene expression in the other cell types may be enhanced when the conditions are optimized for each cell type.

We determined that cell fusion is the mechanism responsible for a PS–CG–HVJ-E-mediated gene transfer system. Although endocytosis appeared to be involved in gene transfection based on the wortmannin experiments, transfection was completely inhibited by antibody against the fusion protein of HVJ. Since the fusion activity of HVJ is pH independent, HVJ can fuse with the cell membrane both on the cell surface and in endocytotic vesicles. Even for the HVJ-E complex with PS and CG, the F protein of HVJ appeared to associate with the cell membrane, and fusion activity appeared to be necessary for gene transfection.

HVJ-E complexed with CG targeted the liver. With PS, gene expression in the liver after intravenous injection was lower than with CG–HVJ-E. We speculate that larger particles with positive charge are less mobile when intravenously administered. Comparison with PS–HVJ-E and PS–CG–HVJ-E suggests that CG–HVJ-E may have the appropriate size and potential for targeting the liver after intravenous injection. Our results suggest that the CG–HVJ-E vector may be effective and practical for the treatment of liver diseases, such as liver cirrhosis and hepatitis, when therapeutic genes encoding secreted proteins, such as human growth factor, soluble transforming growth factor-β receptor and decorin, are employed. An adverse effect of this treatment is that coagulation function is transiently decreased by CG–HVJ-E in mice, although it recovered in 1 day. This adverse effect is probably caused by HVJ hemagglutinating protein, which is necessary for binding with sialic acid, a virus receptor. When HVJ-E is complexed with CG, CG may perform the function of hemagglutinating protein and enhance the association with cell membranes. If HVJ-E without hemagglutinating protein is combined with CG, the complex may reduce adverse effects to a much lower level.

An additional advantage of CG is that it protects HVJ-E from degradation in fresh mouse serum. Although the *in vitro* transfection efficiency of HVJ-E was not inhibited by culture medium containing 10% FBS, the activity of HVJ-E was rapidly lost in the presence of fresh mouse serum. However, CG–HVJ-E was significantly stable in 50% fresh mouse serum. The high transfection activity of CG–HVJ-E after intravenous injection appears to be mediated by the stability of the vector in fresh serum. Liposomes composed of hydrogenated egg phosphatidylcholine and cholesterol activate the complement system in rats by interacting with IgG and IgM. Although it is unproven that HVJ is degraded by complement lysis in mouse serum, the interaction of serum proteins with HVJ-E may be involved in the loss of transfection activity of HVJ-E. Conjugation to CG appears to protect the surface molecules of HVJ-E from the detrimental effects of serum proteins.

The results of this study suggest that low-molecular-weight CG may be appropriate for complex formation with various envelope viruses, such as retrovirus, herpes virus and HIV, and that the CG-envelope virus vector may enhance transfection efficiency both *in vitro* and *in vivo*. This technology may lead to the achievement of an ideal vector system with high efficiency and minimal toxicity.

14.5
Magnetic Nanoparticles for Medicine

A novel transfection method, so called magnetofection, which comprises the association of vectors with superparamagnetic iron oxide nanoparticles and gene delivery under the application of a magnetic field, has been developed [132]. Using the method of magnetofection the efficiency of synthetic gene carriers has been enhanced up to several-hundred-fold. In particular, the duration of the transfection procedure has been reduced to minutes [132]. For magnetofection, gene carriers such as poly(ethylenimine) (PEI), which are associated with superparamagnetic iron oxide nanoparticles, are complexed with plasmid DNA (these complexes are called magnetofectins) and gene delivery is targeted by the application of a magnetic field. For an unrestricted use of magnetofection and its benefits it would be advantageous to gain more insights into the cellular uptake mechanism of the magnetofectins. For polyplexes an endocytic uptake mechanism, probably mediated by heparan sulfate proteoglycan receptors via endosomes, has been shown [133]. Due to its high buffering capacity, PEI is able to destabilize the endosomal membrane leading to the so-called endosomolysis. PEI apparently induces a massive proton accumulation in the endosomes followed by passive chloride influx leading to osmotic swelling of the endosomes and, finally, to its burst releasing the gene vectors into the cytoplasm as a prerequisite for the transport of DNA towards the nucleus. This effect is called the "proton sponge effect" [134–136]. In this context the question arises whether the PEI-based magnetofectins function in the same way as PEI gene vectors. In particular, we asked if the applied magnetic force result only in an increased accumulation of magnetofectins on the cell surface or if it is even able to pull them directly into the cells, circumventing endocytosis and leading to a different gene transfer mechanism as for PEI gene vectors.

Endocytosis is involved in various cellular processes like the transmission of neuronal, metabolic and proliferative signals, the uptake of many essential nutrients, and the ability of defense against invading microorganisms [137]. It is characterized by the formation of membrane vesicles at the plasma membrane. One distinguishes between clathrin-dependent and clathrin-independent endocytosis. The clathrin-dependent endocytosis is the best described so far. Here the vesicles (diameter of approximately 100 nm) are coated with clathrin [137, 138]. After internalization, the clathrin coat gets recycled and the vesicle fuses with an endosome where the sorting, mediated by microtubules, and the dissociation of potential receptors take place. This step is followed by degradation in lysosomes and further transport to the final destination [138]. Well-known examples for the clathrin-dependent uptake mechanism of receptor-bound ligands are transferrin and the low-density lipoprotein (LDL) [137]. The clathrin-independent pathways include phagocytosis, macropinocytosis, constitutive nonclathrin uptake and caveolae-mediated uptake [137]. Phagocytosis is generally restricted to macrophages, whereby macropinocytosis refers to the formation of large, irregular primary endocytic vesicles [138]. Clathrin-independent endocytosis in the absence of caveolae and caveolin is found and designated as constitutive nonclathrin uptake. The caveolae-mediated uptake is characterized by caveolae, which are omega-shaped, noncoated membrane invaginations (diameter 50–100 nm) present in many cell types, but especially abundant in endothelial cells [138]. Their structure is maintained by a family of cholesterol-binding proteins called caveolin. Besides caveolin, caveolae are enriched in cholesterol, sphingomyelin and glycosphingolipids [138]. There is some evidence for a potential role of caveolae in the internalization and intracellular delivery of gene-based therapeutics, as used for somatic gene transfer or single-stranded oligonucleotide technology [139].

We focused on magnetic nanoparticles, such as magnetite and maghemite, with an average size of from 20 to 50 nm, which can be positionally regulated by a magnetic force. Magnetic nanoparticles basically consist of oxidized iron, which is commonly used as a supplement for the treatment of anemia. We hypothesized that the association of magnetite and HVJ-E technology could allow the rapid attachment of HVJ-E and cells by application of a magnetic force, leading to enhanced transfection efficiency. Moreover, magnetic nanoparticles can be modified with several chemical compounds to allow modification of the charge, size and affinity. In addition, there is increasing interest in using magnetic resonance imaging (MRI) to monitor the *in vivo* behavior of proteins labeled with magnetic nanoparticles [140, 141]. Indeed, magnetic nanoparticles were recently used for gene transfection, because magnetic targeting exploits paramagnetic particles as drug carriers, guiding their accumulation in target tissues with strong local magnetic fields [142, 143].

To evaluate the HVJ-E vector system mixed with maghemite, we mixed several doses of maghemite with HVJ-E vector infusing luciferase plasmid. However, unexpectedly, we did not find any improvement in transfection efficiency. From these results, we speculated that there might be a close association, such as electrostatic interaction, between HVJ-E and maghemite. Since we have previously reported that PS, a low-molecular-weight naturally polycationic peptide (around 4000 Da), enhanced the transfection efficiency based on HVJ-E vector in an *in vitro* culture system, we coated the surface of maghemite with PS. After modification with PS, the ζ potential of maghemite was changed to 23.8 ± 1.8 from 17.5 ± 1.6 mV, which suggests that surface coating of maghemite enhanced its cationic charge. Interestingly, a mixture of PS-coated maghemite with HVJ-E vector significantly enhanced the transfection efficiency in a dose-dependent manner. Using the same system, high transfection efficiency into BHK cells was also achieved using the enhanced GFP (EGFP) gene or FITC-ODN. To confirm the interaction of magnetite and HVJ-E vector, we performed electron microscopy. PS-coated maghemite and HVJ-E vector co-existed even though a number of maghemite particles were aggregated around HVJ-E vector (Fig. 14.2).

To explore transfection *in vivo*, we further evaluated the maghemite-attached HVJ-E vector by direct injection into mouse liver. Unexpectedly, a mixture of maghemite surface-coated with PS did not enhance the transfection efficiency in the analysis of luciferase activity, differing from the *in vitro* system. Since cotreatment with heparin has been reported to enhance the transfection efficiency of HVJ-E vector in brain tissue, we next coated the surface of maghemite with heparin, which might antagonize the function of PS. The ζ potential of maghemite was changed to -10.1 ± 2.3 from 17.5 ± 1.6 mV, which suggests that the surface coating of maghemite was changed to a fairly negative net charge. A mixture of

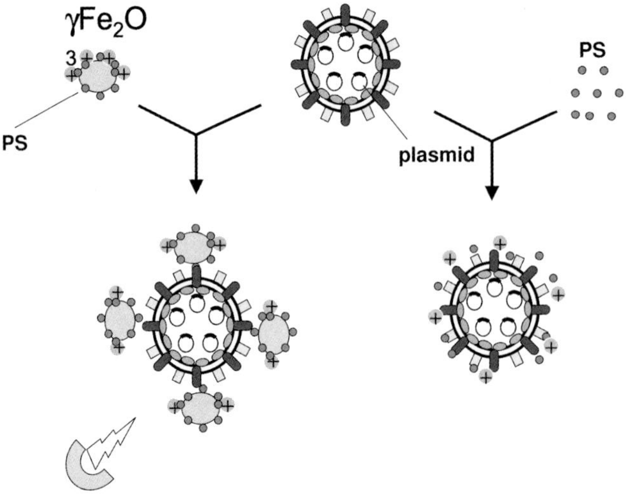

Figure 14.2. Modified HVJ-E vector. PS enhanced the transfection efficiency based on HVJ-E vector in an *in vitro* culture system. In addition, we coated the surface of magnetic nanoparticles with PS and further enhanced the transfection efficiency based on HVJ-E vector.

heparin-coated maghemite with HVJ-E vector significantly enhanced the transfection efficiency in the liver. These data suggest that suitable modifications for gene transfection differ between *in vitro* and *in vivo*. Analysis of EGFP expression in the liver by immunostaining, also confirmed marked expression obtained with heparin-coated maghemite with HVJ-E vector containing the EGFP gene as compared to PS-coated maghemite. For safety evaluation, the serum levels of alanine aminotransferase (ALT) and aspartate aminotransferase (AST) were not further elevated in the heparin-coated maghemite group compared to the control group. Furthermore, we tried to enhance the transfection efficiency under the influence of a magnetic field by placing a magnet on the surface of the liver. However, no obvious improvement in luciferase activity in the liver was observed. Probably, a stronger magnetic field or more accurate control of magnetite might be necessary to enhance it.

In the system of magnetofection, the gene carrier itself represents a hybrid system characterized by an iron oxide inner core and a coat consisting of the cationic PEI which might also assist the endosomal escape of a gene after transfection into cells. In contrast, in our system, transfection was mediated by a cell fusion process of HVJ-E vector, which did not require endosomal escape, are not by endocytosis. Thus, we selected PS as the coating material of maghemite in combination with the HVJ-E system, as PS is a low-molecular-weight polycationic peptide that has Food and Drug Administration approval as an antidote to heparin anticoagulation

[144, 145]. Since both the surface of HVJ-E and the cell membrane have a negative net charge, cationic charged PS-coated maghemite can be speculated to enhance the association of HVJ-E with the cell membrane. Thus, PS-coated maghemite would actively carry HVJ-E to cultured cells under a magnetic force.

However, in an *in vivo* system, heparin, but not PS, was suitable as the coating material in combination with HVJ-E vector, consistent with a previous *in vivo* report. Of special interest regarding this result was a previous report showing that coinfusion of trophic factors and heparin into the rat brain significantly enhanced the volume of distribution. Thus, we speculate that the distribution of these vectors may be a key to explaining this discrepancy between *in vitro* and *in vivo* gene transfer. In addition, no immunohistochemical data has been presented on potential toxic effects of heparin. The size and surface chemistry of magnetic particles could be tailored accordingly to meet specific demands of physical and biological characteristics.

Magnetically targeted drug delivery by particulate carriers to a localized disease site may be efficient as drugs and a very high concentrations of chemotherapeutic or radiological agent can be achieved near the target site, such as a tumor, without any toxic effects on normal surrounding tissue or the whole body. Magnetic carriers receive their magnetic responsiveness to a magnetic field from incorporated materials such as magnetite, iron, nickel, cobalt, neodymium–iron–boron or samarium–cobalt. As for biomedical applications, magnetic carriers must be water-based, biocompatible, nontoxic and nonimmunogenic. The first medical application directly applied magnetite or iron powder. The first clinical cancer therapy trial was performed in Germany for the treatment of advanced solid cancer in 14 patients using magnetic microspheres that were about 100 nm in diameter and filled with 4′-epidoxorubicin [146]. The phase I study clearly showed low toxicity of the method and accumulation of MMS in the target area. However, MRI measurements indicated that more than 50% of MMS ended up in the liver [147]. Conceptually, magnetic targeting is a very promising approach. However, there are a number of physical, magnetism-related properties which require careful attention. (i) More responsive magnetic materials with defined and homogenous material properties in a stable and defined oxidation state need to be synthesized. (ii) The size must be small enough that they do not clog the blood vessels through which they are guided to the target organ. (iii) Altering the surface of magnetite with appropriate molecules should be considered, to either increase or decrease the interaction of magnetite with tissues or organs. (iv) The magnetite size must be uniform enough to provide an equal probability of magnetic capture for each magnetite particle. (v) The fate of the particles in the body is an important consideration both for local and systemic short- and long-term toxicity. Thus, further improvements of this hybrid vector were required in future studies.

Overall, we have developed a novel hybrid vector of HVJ-E and magnetic nanoparticles with different surface modifications in an *in vitro* culture system as well as *in vivo*. Further modification of this system with MRI might provide new therapeutic potential to achieve tissue targeting.

Conclusion

If omnipotent vector systems are eventually developed, gene transfer may harm patients – this is far from therapeutic. An all-encompassing vector system may not be feasible and each vector system must be evaluated with respect to the target disease. In some diseases such as arteriosclerosis obliterans, transient gene expression would be sufficient to cure the disease and sustained gene expression would be detrimental. In other diseases, such as SCID-X1 and hemophilia B, it may be necessary to induce the transformation of only a small population of cells. Cancer gene therapy occupies more than 60% of current human gene therapy approaches and no remarkable successes have been reported in this area to date. When we consider why gene therapy is necessary for cancer treatment, the answer is that gene therapy should be used to inhibit tumor metastasis and suppress the recurrence of cancers. For these purposes, investigations in basic cancer cell biology and technological developments should be promoted much more than at present. The issues in this chapter present a road map for the future technological developments for gene therapy. Thus, technologies in gene therapy should be developed on the basis of analysis of the target tissues, target cells, cellular components and molecules which are relevant to the biology.

References

1 MULLIGAN, R. C., The basic science of gene therapy. *Science* **1993**, *260*, 926–932.
2 MARSHALL, E., Gene therapy death prompts review of adenovirus vector. *Science* **1999**, *286*, 2244–2245.
3 KAISER, J., Gene therapy. Seeking the cause of induced leukemias in X-SCID trial. *Science* **2003**, *299*, 495.
4 RAGNI, M. V., Safe passage: a plea for safety in hemophilia gene therapy. *Mol. Ther.* **2002**, *6*, 436–440.
5 LEDLEY, F. D., Nonviral gene therapy: the promise of genes as pharmaceutical products. *Hum. Gene Ther.* **1995**, *6*, 1129–1144.
6 KANEDA, Y., Gene therapy: a battle against biological barriers. *Curr. Mol. Med* **2001**, *1*, 493–499.
7 MORRAL, N., O'NEAL, W., RICE, K., LELAND, M., KAPLAN, J., PIEDRA, P. A., ZHOU, H., PARKS, R. J., VELJI, R., AGUILAR-CORDOVA, E., WADSWORTH, S., GRAHAM, F. L., KOCHANEK, S., CAREY, K. D., BEAUDET, A. L., Administration of helper-dependent adenoviral vectors and sequential delivery of different vector serotype for long-term liver-directed gene transfer in baboons. *Proc. Natl Acad. Sci. USA* **1999**, *96*, 12816–12821.
8 BURNS, J. C., FRIEDMANN, T., DRIEVER, W., BURRASCANO, M., YEE, J. K., Vesicular stomatitis virus G glycoprotein pseudotyped retroviral vectors: concentration to very high titer and efficient gene transfer into mammalian and nonmammalian cells. *Proc. Natl Acad. Sci. USA* **1993**, *90*, 8033–8037.
9 NALDINI, L., BLOMER, U., GALLAY, P., ORY, D., MULLIGAN, R., GAGE, F. H., VERMA, I. M., TRONO, D., *In vivo* gene delivery and stable transduction of nondividing cells by a lentiviral vector. *Science* **1996**, *272*, 263–267.
10 WU, G. Y., WU, C. H., Receptor-mediated *in vitro* gene transformation by a soluble DNA carrier system. *J. Biol. Chem.* **1987**, *262*, 4429–4432.

11 Wu, G. Y., Wu, C. H., Receptor-mediated gene delivery and expression *in vivo*. *J. Biol. Chem.* **1988**, *263*, 14621–14624.

12 Wagner, E., Zatloukal, K., Cotten, M., Kirlappos, H., Mechtler, K., Curiel, D. T., Birnstiel, M. L., Coupling of adenovirus to transferrin–polylysine/DNA complexes greatly enhances receptor-mediated gene delivery and expression of transfected genes. *Proc. Natl Acad. Sci. USA* **1992**, *89*, 6099–6103.

13 Flint, S. J., Enquist, L. W., Krug, R. M., Racaniello, V. R., Skalka, A. M. (Eds.). *Principles of Virology*. ASM Press, Washington, DC, **2000**.

14 Gall, J., Kass-Eisler, A., Leinwand, L., Falck-Pedersen, E., Adenovirus type 5 and 7 capsid chimera: fiber replacement alters receptor tropism without affecting primary immune neutralization epitopes. *J. Virol.* **1996**, *70*, 2116–2123.

15 Krasnykh, V. N., Mikheeva, G. V., Douglas, J. T., Curiel, D. T., Generation of recombinant adenovirus vectors with modified fibers for altering viral tropism. *J. Virol.* **1996**, *70*, 6839–6846.

16 Zabner, J., Chillon, M., Grunst, T., Moninger, T. O., Davidson, B. L., Gregory, R., Armentano, D., A chimeric type 2 adenovirus vector with a type 17 fiber enhances gene transfer to human airway epithelia. *J. Virol.* **1999**, *73*, 8689–8695.

17 Von Seggern, D. J., Huang, S., Fleck, S. K., Stevenson, S. C., Nemerow, G. R., Adenovirus vector pseudotyping in fiber-expressing cell lines: improved transduction of Epstein–Barr virus-transformed B cells. *J. Virol.* **2000**, *74*, 354–362.

18 Ikomi, F., Hanna, G. K., Schmid-Schonbein, G. W., Mechanism of colloidal particle uptake into the lymphatic system: basic study with percutaneous lymphography. *Radiology* **1995**, *196*, 107–113.

19 Tsuboniwa, N., Morishita, R., Hirano, T., Fujimoto, J., Furukawa, S., Kikumori, M., Okuyama, A., Kaneda, Y., Safety evaluation of Hemagglutinating Virus of Japan-artificial viral envelope liposomes in nonhuman primates. *Hum. Gene Ther.* **2001**, *12*, 469–487.

20 Allen, T. M., Williamson, P., Schlegel, R. A., Phosphatidylserine as a determinant of reticuloendothelial recognition of liposome models of the erythrocyte surface. *Proc. Natl Acad. Sci. USA* **1988**, *85*, 8067–8071.

21 Li, S., Huang, L., *In vivo* gene transfer via intravenous administration of cationic lipid–protamine–DNA (LPD) complexes. *Gene Ther.* **1997**, *4*, 891–900.

22 Li, S., Rizzo, M. A., Bhattacharya, S., Huang, L., Characterization of cationic lipid–protamine–DNA (LPD) complexes for intravenous gene delivery. *Gene Ther.* **1998**, *5*, 930–937.

23 Huang, S. K., Lee, K. D., Hong, K., Friend, D. S., Papahadjopoulos, D., Microscopic localization of sterically stabilized liposomes in colon carcinoma-bearing mice. *Cancer Res.* **1992**, *52*, 5135–5143.

24 Litzinger, D. C., Buiting, A. M., van Rooijen, N., Huang, L., Effect of liposome size on the circulation time and intraorgan distribution of amphipathic poly(ethylene glycol)-containing liposomes. *Biochim. Biophys. Acta* **1994**, *1190*, 99–107.

25 Blessing, T., Kursa, M., Holzhauser, R., Kircheis, R., Wagner, E., Different strategies for formation of pegylated EGF-conjugated PEI/DNA complexes for targeted gene delivery. *Bioconjug. Chem.* **2001**, *12*, 529–537.

26 Choi, Y. H., Liu, F., Choi, J. S., Kim, S. W., Park, J. S., Characterization of a targeted gene carrier, lactose-polyethylene glycol-grafted poly-L-lysine and its complex with plasmid DNA. *Hum. Gene Ther.* **1999**, *10*, 2657–2665.

27 Reddy, J. A., Abburi, C., Hofland, H., Howard, S. J., Vlahov, I., Wils, P., Leamon, C. P., Folate-targeted, cationic liposome-mediated gene transfer into disseminated peritoneal tumors. *Gene Ther.* **2002**, *9*, 1542–1550.

28 Pensiero, M. N., Wysocki, C. A., Nader, K., Kikuchi, G. E., Development of amphotropic murine retrovirus vectors resistant to inactivation by human serum. *Hum. Gene Ther.* **1996**, *7*, 1095–1101.

29 Oroszlan, S., Nowinski, R. C., Lysis of retroviruses with monoclonal antibodies against viral envelope proteins. *Virology* **1980**, *101*, 296–299.

30 Dickson, G., *Molecular and Cell Biology of Human Gene Therapeutics.* Chapman & Hall, London, **1995**.

31 Eslami, M. H., Gangadharan, S. P., Sui, X., Rhynhart, K. K., Snyder, R. O., Conte, M. S., Gene delivery to *in situ* veins: differential effects of adenovirus and adeno-associated viral vectors. *J. Vasc. Surg.* **2000**, *31*, 1149–1159.

32 Wheeler, C. J., Felgner, P. L., Tsai, Y. J., Marshall, J., Sukhu, L., Doh, S. G., Hartikka, J., Nietupski, J., Manthorpe, M., Nichols, M., Plewe, M., Liang, X., Norman, J., Smith, A., Cheng, S. H., A novel cationic lipid greatly enhances plasmid DNA delivery and expression in mouse lung. *Proc. Natl Acad. Sci. USA* **1996**, *93*, 11454–11459.

33 Sawa, Y., Suzuki, K., Bai, H. Z., Shirakura, R., Morishita, R., Kaneda, Y., Matsuda, H., Efficiency of *in vivo* gene transfection into transplanted rat heart by coronary infusion of HVJ liposome. *Circulation* **1995**, *92*, 479–482.

34 Yonemitsu, Y., Kaneda, Y., Morishita, R., Nakagawa, K., Nakashima, Y., Sueishi, K., Characterization of *in vivo* gene transfer into the arterial wall mediated by the Sendai virus (hemagglutinating virus of Japan) liposomes: an effective tool for the *in vivo* study of arterial diseases. *Lab. Invest.* **1996**, *75*, 313–323.

35 Seth, P., Mechanism of adenovirus-mediated endosome lysis: role of the intact adenovirus capsid structure. *Biochem. Biophys. Res. Commun.* **1994**, *205*, 1318–1324.

36 Greber, U. F., Webster, P., Weber, J., Helenius, A., The role of the adenovirus protease on virus entry into cells. *EMBO J.* **1996**, *15*, 1766–1777.

37 Maeda, T., Ohnishi, S., Activation of influenza virus by acidic media causes hemolysis and fusion of erythrocytes. *FEBS Lett.* **1980**, *122*, 283–287.

38 Marsh, M., Bolzau, E., Helenius, A., Penetration of Semliki Forest virus from acidic prelysosomal vacuoles. *Cell* **1983**, *32*, 931–940.

39 Blumenthal, R., Bali-Puri, A., Walter, A., Covell, D., Eidelman, O., pH-dependent fusion of vesicular stomatitis virus with Vero cells. Measurement by dequenching of octadecyl rhodamine fluorescence. *J. Biol. Chem.* **1987**, *262*, 13614–13619.

40 Okada, Y., Sendai virus-induced cell fusion. *Methods Enzymol.* **1993**, *221*, 18–41.

41 McClure, M. O., Sommerfelt, M. A., Marsh, M., Weiss, R. A., The pH independence of mammalian retrovirus infection. *J. Gen. Virol.* **1990**, *71*, 767–773.

42 McClure, M. O., Marsh, M., Weiss, R. A., Human immunodeficiency virus infection of CD4-bearing cells occurs by a pH-independent mechanism. *EMBO J.* **1988**, *7*, 513–518.

43 Wagner, E., Plank, C., Zatloukal, K., Cotten, M., Birnstiel, M. L., Influenza virus hemagglutinin HA-2 N-terminal fusogenic peptides augment gene transfer by transferrin–polylysine–DNA complexes: toward a synthetic virus-like gene-transfer vehicle. *Proc. Natl Acad. Sci. USA* **1992**, *89*, 7934–7938.

44 Izaurralde, E., Kann, M., Pante, N., Sodeik, B., Hohn, T., Viruses, microorganisms and scientists meet the nuclear pore. Leysin, VD, Switzerland, February 26–March 1, 1998. *EMBO J.* **1999**, *18*, 289–296.

45 Greber, U. F., Kasamatsu, H., Nuclear targeting of SV40 and adenovirus. *Trends Cell Biol.* **1996**, *6*, 189–195.

46 Greber, U. F., Suomalainen, M., Stidwill, R. P., Boucke, K., Ebersold, M. W., Helenius, A., The

role of the nuclear pore complex in adenovirus DNA entry. *EMBO J.* **1997**, *16*, 5998–6007.
47 Fritz, J. D., Herweijer, H., Zhang, G., Wolff, J. A., Gene transfer into mammalian cells using histone-condensed plasmid DNA. *Hum. Gene Ther.* **1996**, *7*, 1395–1404.
48 Sebestyen, M. G., Ludtke, J. J., Bassik, M. C., Zhang, G., Budker, V., Lukhtanov, E. A., Hagstrom, J. E., Wolff, J. A., DNA vector chemistry: the covalent attachment of signal peptides to plasmid DNA. *Nat. Biotechnol.* **1998**, *16*, 80–85.
49 Zanta, M. A., Belguise-Valladier, P., Behr, J. P., Gene delivery: a single nuclear localization signal peptide is sufficient to carry DNA to the cell nucleus. *Proc. Natl Acad. Sci. USA* **1999**, *96*, 91–96.
50 Dean, D. A., Import of plasmid DNA into the nucleus is sequence specific. *Exp. Cell Res.* **1997**, *230*, 293–302.
51 Wilson, G. L., Dean, B. S., Wang, G., Dean, D. A., Nuclear import of plasmid DNA in digitonin-permeabilized cells requires both cytoplasmic factors and specific DNA sequences. *J. Biol. Chem.* **1999**, *274*, 22025–22032.
52 Smerdou, C., Liljestrom, P., Alphavirus vectors: from protein production to gene therapy. *Gene Ther. Reg.* **2000**, *1*, 33–64.
53 Bredenbeek, P. J., Frolov, I., Rice, C. M., Schlesinger, S., Sindbis virus expression vectors: packaging of RNA replicons by using defective helper RNAs. *J. Virol.* **1993**, *67*, 6439–6446.
54 Liljeström, P., Garoff, H., A new generation of animal cell expression vectors based on the Semliki Forest virus replicon. *Biotechnology* **1991**, *9*, 1356–1361.
55 Ivics, Z., Hackett, P. B., Plasterk, R. H., Izsvak, Z., Molecular reconstruction of Sleeping Beauty, a Tc1-like transposon from fish, and its transposition in human cells. *Cell* **1997**, *91*, 501–510.
56 Summerford, C., Bartlett, J. S., Samulski, R. J., Adeno-associated viral vectors and successful gene therapy, the gap is closing. *Gene Ther. Reg.* **2000**, *1*, 9–32.
57 Rutledge, E. A., Russell, D. W., Adeno-associated virus vector integration junctions. *J. Virol.* **1997**, *71*, 8429–8436.
58 Lupton, S., Levine, A. J., Mapping genetic elements of Epstein–Barr virus that facilitate extrachromosomal persistence of Epstein–Barr virus-derived plasmids in human cells. *Mol. Cell. Biol.* **1985**, *5*, 2533–2542.
59 Yates, J. L., Warren, N., Sugden, B., Stable replication of plasmids derived from Epstein–Barr virus in various mammalian cells. *Nature* **1985**, *313*, 812–815.
60 Jankelevich, S., Kolman, J. L., Bodnar, J. W., Miller, G., A nuclear matrix attachment region organizes the Epstein–Barr viral plasmid in Raji cells into a single DNA domain. *EMBO J.* **1992**, *11*, 1165–1176.
61 Saeki, Y., Wataya-Kaneda, M., Tanaka, K., Kaneda, Y., Sustained transgene expression *in vitro* and *in vivo* using an Epstein–Barr virus replicon vector system combined with HVJ liposomes. *Gene Ther.* **1998**, *5*, 1031–1037.
62 Kaneda, Y., Saeki, Y., Nakabayashi, M., Zhou, W. Z., Kaneda, M. W., Morishita, R., Enhancement of transgene expression by cotransfection of oriP plasmid with EBNA-1 expression vector. *Hum. Gene Ther.* **2000**, *11*, 471–479.
63 Palmer, T. D., Rosman, G. J., Osborne, W. R., Miller, A. D., Genetically modified skin fibroblasts persist long after transplantation but gradually inactivate introduced genes. *Proc. Natl Acad. Sci. USA* **1991**, *88*, 1330–1334.
64 Harbers, K., Jahner, D., Jaenisch, R., Microinjection of cloned retroviral genomes into mouse zygotes: integration and expression in the animal. *Nature* **1981**, *293*, 540–542.
65 Jahner, D., Stuhlmann, H., Stewart, C. L., Harbers, K., Lohler, J., Simon, I., Jaenisch, R., *De novo* methylation and expression of retroviral genomes during mouse

embryogenesis. *Nature* **1982**, *298*, 623–628.

66 Grossman, M., Raper, S. E., Kozarsky, K., Stein, E. A., Engelhardt, J. F., Muller, D., Lupien, P. J., Wilson, J. M., Successful *ex vivo* gene therapy directed to liver in a patient with familial hypercholesterolaemia. *Nat. Genet* **1994**, *6*, 335–341.

67 Roeder, R. G., The role of general initiation factors in transcription by RNA polymerase II. *Trends Biochem. Sci.* **1996**, *21*, 327–335.

68 Tyler, J. K., Kadonaga, J. T., The "dark side" of chromatin remodeling: repressive effects on transcription. *Cell* **1999**, *99*, 443–446.

69 Luo, R. X., Dean, D. C., Chromatin remodeling and transcriptional regulation. *J. Natl. Cancer Inst.* **1999**, *91*, 1288–1294.

70 Kuo, M. H., Allis, C. D., Roles of histone acetyltransferases and deacetylases in gene regulation. *BioEssays* **1998**, *20*, 615–626.

71 Chen, W. Y., Bailey, E. C., McCune, S. L., Dong, J. Y., Townes, T. M., Reactivation of silenced, virally transduced genes by inhibitors of histone deacetylase. *Proc. Natl Acad. Sci. USA* **1997**, *94*, 5798–5803.

72 Dion, L. D., Goldsmith, K. T., Tang, D. C., Engler, J. A., Yoshida, M., Garver, R. I., Jr., Amplification of recombinant adenoviral transgene products occurs by inhibition of histone deacetylase. *Virology* **1997**, *231*, 201–209.

73 Yamano, T., Ura, K., Morishita, R., Nakajima, H., Monden, M., Kaneda, Y., Amplification of transgene expression *in vitro* and *in vivo* using a novel inhibitor of histone deacetylase. *Mol. Ther.* **2000**, *1*, 574–580.

74 Nan, X., Ng, H. H., Johnson, C. A., Laherty, C. D., Turner, B. M., Eisenman, R. N., Bird, A., Transcriptional repression by the methyl-CpG-binding protein MeCP2 involves a histone deacetylase complex. *Nature* **1998**, *393*, 386–389.

75 Wolffe, A. P., Transcriptional control: imprinting insulation. *Curr. Biol* **2000**, *10*, R463–465.

76 Steinwaerder, D. S., Lieber, A., Insulation from viral transcriptional regulatory elements improves inducible transgene expression from adenovirus vectors *in vitro* and *in vivo*. *Gene Ther.* **2000**, *7*, 556–567.

77 Muller, J., Transcriptional control: The benefits of selective insulation. *Curr. Biol* **2000**, *10*, R241–244.

78 Kaneda, Y., Saeki, Y., and Morishita, R., Gene therapy using HVJ-liposomes: the best of both worlds? *Mol. Med. Today* **1999**, *5*, 298–303.

79 Dzav, V., Mann, M. J., Morishita, R., Kaneda, Y., Fusigenic viral liposome for gene therapy in cardiovascular diseases. *Proc. Natl. Acad. Sci. USA* **1996**, *93*, 11421–11425.

80 Nakamura, N., Hart, D. A., Frank, C. B., Marchuk, L. L., Shrive, N. G., Ota, N., Taira, T., Yoshikawa, H., Kaneda, Y., Efficient transfer of intact pligonucleotides into the nucleus of ligament scar fibroblasts by HVJ-cationic liposomes is correlated with effective antisense gene inhibition. *J. Biochem.* **2001**, *129*, 755–759.

81 Hirano, T., Fujimoto, J., Ueki, T., Yamamoto, H., Iwasaki, T., Morishita, R., Kaneda, Y., Takahashi, H., Okamoto, E., Persistent gene expression in rat liver *in-vivo* by repetitive transfections using HVJ-liposome. *Gene Ther.* **1998**, *5*, 459–464.

82 Zenke, M., Steinlein, P., Wagner, E., Cotton, M., Beug, H., Birnstiel, M. L., Receptor-mediated endocytosis of transferrin–polycation conjugates: an efficient way to introduce DNA into hematopoietic cells. *Proc. Natl Acad. Sci. USA* **1990**, *87*, 3655–3659.

83 Bagai, S., Sarker, D. P., Targeted delivery of hygromycin B using reconstituted Sendai viral envelopes lacking hemagglutinin–neuraminidase. *FEBS Lett.* **1993**, *326*, 183–188.

84 Ramani, K., Bora, R. S., Kumar, M., Tyagi, S. K., Sarkar, D. P., Novel gene delivery to liver cells using engineered virosomes. *FEBS Lett.* **1997**, *404*, 164–168.

85 Ramani, K., Hassan, O., Venkaiah, B., Hasnain, S. E., Sarkar, D. P., Site-specific gene delivery *in vivo* through engineered Sendai virus envelopes. *Proc. Natl Acad. Sci. USA* **1998**, *95*, 11886–11890.

86 Suzuki, K., Nakashima, H., Sawa, Y., Morishita, R., Matsuda, H., Kaneda, Y., Reconstituted fusion liposomes for gene transfer *in vitro* and *in vivo*. *Gene Ther. Reg.* **2000**, *1*, 65–77.

87 Kaneda, Y., Nakajima, T., Nishikawa, T., Yamamoto, S., Ikegami, H., Suzuki, N., Nakamura, H., Morishira, R., Kotani, H., Hemagglutinating virus of Japan (HVJ) envelope vector as a versatile gene delivery system. *Mol. Ther.* **2002**, *6*, 219–226.

88 Yeagle, P. L., The fusion of Sendai virus. In *Viral Fusion Mechanisms*, Benty, J. (Ed.), CRC Press, London, **1993**, pp. 313–334.

89 Ghosh, J. K., Peisajovich, S. G., Shai, Y., Sendai virus internal fusion peptide: structural and functional characterization and a plausible mode of viral entry inhibition. *Biochemistry* **2000**, *39*, 1581–92.

90 Chen, Y., Webster, R. G., Woodland, D. L., Induction of $CD8^+$ T cell responses to dominant and subdominant epitopes and protective immunity to Sendai virus infection by DNA vaccination. *J. Immunol.* **1998**, *160*, 2425–2432.

91 Race, E., Stein, C. A., Wigg, M. D., Baksh, A., Addawe, M., Frezza, P., Oxford, J. S., A multistep procedure for the chemical inactivation of human immunodeficiency virus for use as an experimental vaccine. *Vaccine* **1995**, *13*, 1567–1575.

92 Kaneda, Y., In *Gene Therapy Protocol*, 2nd edn. (Morgan, J. R. (Ed.), Humana Press, Totowa, NJ, **2002**, pp. 63–72.

93 Yonemitsu, Y., Kitson, C., Ferrari, S., Farley, R., Griesenbach, U., Juda, D., Steel, R., Scheid, P., Zhu, J., Jeffery, P., Alton, E. F. W., Efficient gene transfer to airway epithelium using recombinant Sendai virus. *Nat. Biotechnol.* **2000**, *18*, 970–973.

94 Dorsett, Y., Tuschl, T., siRNAs: applications in functional genomics and potential as therapeutics. *Nat. Rev. Drug Discov.* **2004**, *3*, 318–329.

95 Tijsterman, M., Plasterk, R. H., Dicers at RISC; the mechanism of RNAi. *Cell* **2004**, *117*, 1–3.

96 Miyagishi, M., Hayashi, M., Taira, K., Comparison of the suppressive effects of antisense oligonucleotides and siRNAs directed against the same targets in mammalian cells. *Antisense Nucleic Acid Drug Dev.* **2003**, *13*, 1–7.

97 Yokota, T., Miyagishi, M., Hino, T., Matsumura, R., Tasinato, A., Urushitani, M., Rao, R. V., Takahashi, R., Bredesen, D. E., Taira, K., Mizusawa, H., siRNA-based inhibition specific for mutant SOD1 with single nucleotide alternation in familial ALS, compared with ribozyme and DNA enzyme. *Biochem. Biophys. Res. Commun.* **2004**, *314*, 283–291.

98 Sioud, M., Ribozyme- and siRNA-mediated mRNA degradation: a general introduction. *Methods Mol. Biol.* **2004**, *252*, 1–8.

99 Itoh, Y., Kawamata, Y., Harada, M., Kobayashi, M., Fujii, R., Fukusumi, S., Ogi, K., Hosoya, M., Tanaka, Y., Uejima, H., Tanaka, H., Maruyama, M., Satoh, R., Okubo, S., Kizawa, H., Komatsu, H., Matsumura, F., Noguchi, Y., Shinohara, T., Hinuma, S., Fujisawa, Y., Fujino, M., Free fatty acids regulate insulin secretion from pancreatic beta cells through GPR40. *Nature* **2003**, *422*, 173–176.

100 Ishii, T., Ohnuma, K., Murakami, A., Takasawa, N., Yamochi, T., Iwata, S., Uchiyama, M., Dang, N. H., Tanaka, H., Morimoto, C., SS-A/Ro52, an autoantigen involved in CD28-mediated IL-2 production. *J. Immunol.* **2003**, *170*, 3653–3661.

101 Nakamura, H., Kimura, T., Ikegami, H., Ogita, K., Kohyama, S., Shimoya, K., Tsujie, T., Koyama, M., Kaneda, Y., Murata, Y., Highly-efficient and minimally invasive *in vivo* gene transfer to the mouse uterus by Hemagglutinating Virus of Japan

(HVJ) envelope vector. *Mol. Hum. Reprod.* **2003**, *9*, 603–609.

102 Shimamura, M., Morishita, R., Endoh, M., Oshima, K., Aoki, M., Kurinami, H., Waguri, S., Uchiyama, Y., Ogihara, T., Kaneda, Y., Morishita, R., HVJ-envelope vector for gene transfer into central nervous system. *Biochem. Biophys. Res. Commun.* **2003**, *300*, 464–471.

103 Vilella, R., Benitez, D., Mila, J., Vilalta, A., Rull, R., Cuellar, F., Conill, C., Vidal-Sicart, S., Costa, J., Yachi, E., Palou, J., malvehy, J., Luig, S., marti, R., Mellado, B., Castel, T., Treatment of patients with progressive unresectable metastatic melanoma with a heterologous polyvalent melanoma whole cell vaccine. *Int. J. Cancer* **2003**, *106*, 626–631.

104 Figdor, C. G., de Vries, I. J., Lesterhuis, W. J., Melief, C. J., Dendritic cell immunotherapy: mapping the way. *Nat. Med.* **2004**, *10*, 475–480.

105 Nestle, F. O., Alijagic, S., Gilliet, M., Sun, Y., Grabbe, S., Dummer, R., Burg, G., Schadendorf, D., Vaccination of melanoma patients with peptide- or tumor lysate-pulsed dendritic cells. *Nat. Med.* **1998**, *4*, 328–332.

106 Thurner, B., Haendle, I., Roder, C., Dieckmann, D., Keikavoussi, P., Jonuleit, H., Bender, A., Maczek, C., Schreiner, D., von denDriesch, P., Brocker, E. B., Steinman, R. M., Enk, A., Kampgen, E., Schuler, G., Vaccination with mage-3A1 peptide-pulsed mature, monocyte-derived dendritic cells expands specific cytotoxic T cells and induces regression of some metastases in advanced stage IV melanoma. *J. Exp. Med.* **1999**, *190*, 1669–1678.

107 Gilboa, E., Nair, S. K., Lyerly, H. K., Immunotherapy of cancer with dendritic-cell-based vaccines. *Cancer Immunol. Immunother.* **1998**, *46*, 82–87.

108 Engleman, E. G., Dendritic cells: potential role in cancer therapy. *Cytotechnology* **1997**, *25*, 1–8.

109 Arthur, J. F., Butterfield, L. H., Roth, M. D., Bui, L. A., Kiertscher, S. M., Lau, R., Dubinett, S., Glaspy, J., McBride, W. H., Economous, J. S., A comparison of gene transfer methods in human dendritic cells. *Cancer Gene Ther.* **1997**, *4*, 17–25.

110 Kaplan, J. M., Yu, Q., Piraino, S. T., pennington, S. E., Shankara, S., Woodworth, L. A., Roberts, B. L., Induction of antitumor immunity with dendritic cells transduced with adenovirus vector-encoding endogenous tumor-associated antigens. *J. Immunol.* **1999**, *163*, 699–707.

111 Pecher, G., Spahn, G., Schirrmann, T., Kulbe, H., Ziegner, M., Schenk, J. A., Sandig, V., Mucin gene (MUC1) transfer into human dendritic cells by cationic liposomes and recombinant adenovirus. *Anticancer Res.* **2001**, *21*, 2591–2596.

112 Yang, S., Kittlesen, D., Slingluff, Jr., C. L., Vervaert, C. E., Seigler, H. F., Darrow, T. L., Dendritic cells infected with a vaccinia vector carrying the human gp100 gene simultaneously present multiple specificities and elicit high-affinity T cells reactive to multiple epitopes and restricted by HLA-A2 and -A3. *J. Immunol.* **2000**, *164*, 4204–4211.

113 Prabakaran, I., Menon, C., Xu, S., Gomez-Yafal, A., Czerniecki, B. J., Fraker, D. L., Mature $CD83^+$ dendritic cells infected with recombinant gp100 vaccinia virus stimulate potent antimelanoma T cells. *Ann. Surg. Oncol.* **2002**, *9*, 411–418.

114 Akiyama, Y., Maruyama, K., Watanabe, M., Yamauchi, K., Retroviral-mediated IL-12 gene transduction into human $CD34^+$ cell-derived dendritic cells. *Int. J. Oncol.* **2002**, *21*, 509–514.

115 Bello-Fernandez, C., Matyash, M., Strobl, H., Pickl, W. F., Majdic, O., Lyman, S. D., Knapp, W., Efficient retrovirus-mediated gene transfer of dendritic cells generated from $CD34^+$ cord blood cells under serum-free conditions. *Hum. Gene Ther.* **1997**, *8*, 1651–1658.

116 Boon, T., Cerottini, J. C., Van den Eynde, B., van der Bruggen, P., van Pel, A., Tumor antigens recognized by T lymphocytes. *Annu. Rev. Immunol.* **1994**, *12*, 337–365.

117 Kawakami, Y., Rosenberg, S. A., Human tumor antigens recognized by T-cells. *Immunol. Res.* **1997**, *16*, 313–339.

118 Gong, J., Chen, D., Kashiwaba, M., Kufe, D., Induction of antitumor activity by immunization with fusions of dendritic and carcinoma cells. *Nat. Med.* **1997**, *3*, 558–561.

119 Wang, J., Saffold, S., Cao, X., Krauss, J., Chen, W., Eliciting T cell immunity against poorly immunogenic tumors by immunization with dendritic cell–tumor fusion vaccines. *J. Immunol.* **1998**, *161*, 5516–5524.

120 Xu, S., Koski, G. K., Faries, M., Bedrosian, I., Mick, R., maeurer, M., Cheever, M. A., Cohen, P. A., Czerniecki, B. J., Rapid high efficiency sensitization of $CD8^+$ T cells to tumor antigens by dendritic cells leads to enhanced functional avidity and direct tumor recognition through an IL-12-dependent mechanism. *J. Immunol.* **2003**, *171*, 2251–2261.

121 Kabanov, A. V., Kabanov, V. A., DNA complexes with polycations for the delivery of genetic material into cells. *Bioconjug. Chem.* **1995**, *6*, 7–20.

122 Ledley, F. D., Nonviral gene therapy: the promise of genes as pharmaceutical products. *Hum. Gene Ther.* **1995**, *6*, 1129–1144.

123 Tomlinson, E., Rolland, A. P., Controllable gene therapy. Pharmaceutics of non-viral gene delivery systems. *J. Control. Release* **1996**, *39*, 357–372.

124 Tokunaga, N., Nagaya, N., Shirai, M., Tanaka, E., Ishibashi-Ueda, H., Harada-Shiba, M., Kanda, M., Ito, T., Shimizu, W., Tabata, Y., Uematsu, M., Nishigami, K., Sano, S., Kangawa, K., Mori, H., Adrenomedullin gene transfer induces therapeutic angiogenesis in a rabbit model of chronic hind limb ischemia: benefits of a novel nonviral vector, gelatin. *Circulation.* **2004**, *109*, 526–531.

125 Tabata, Y., Ikada, Y., Macrophage activation through phagocytosis of muramyl dipeptide encapsulated in gelatin microspheres. *J. Pharm. Pharmacol.* **1987**, *39*, 698–704.

126 Nagaya, N., Kangawa, K., Kanda, M., Uematsu, M., Horio, T., Fukuyama, N., Hino, J., Harada-Shiba, M., Okumura, H., Tabata, Y., Mochizuki, N., Chiba, Y., Nishioka, K., Miyatake, K., Asahara, T., Hara, H., Mori, H., Hybrid cell-gene therapy for pulmonary hypertension based on phagocytosing action of endothelial progenitor cells. *Circulation.* **2003**, *108*, 889–895.

127 Mima, H., Tomoshige, R., Kanamori, T., Tabata, Y., Yamamoto, S., Ito, S., Tamai, K., Kaneda, Y., Biocompatible polymer enhances the *in vitro* and *in vivo* transfection efficiency of HVJ envelope vector. *J. Gene Med.* **2005**, *7*, 888–897.

128 Saeki, Y., Matsumoto, N., Nakano, Y., Mori, M., Awai, K., Kaneda, Y., Development and characterization of cationic liposomes conjugated with HVJ (Sendai virus): reciprocal effect of cationic lipid for *in vitro* and *in vivo* gene transfer. *Hum. Gene Ther.* **1997**, *8*, 2133–2141.

129 Scherer, F., Anton, M., Schillinger, U., Henke, J., Bergemann, C., Krüger, A., Gänsbacher, B., Plank, C., Magnetofection: enhancing and targeting gene delivery by magnetic force *in vitro* and *in vivo*. *Gene Ther.* **2002**, *9*, 102–109.

130 Mislick, K. A., Baldeschwieler, J. D., Evidence for the role of proteoglycans in cation-mediated gene transfer. *Proc. Natl Acad. Sci. USA* **1996**, *93*, 12349–12354.

131 Boussif, O., Lezoualc'h, F., Zanta, M. A., Mergny, M. D., Scherman, D., Demeneix, B., Behr, J. P., A versatile vector for gene and oligonucleotide transfer into cells in culture and *in vivo*: polyethylenimine. *Proc. Natl Acad. Sci. USA* **1995**, *92*, 7297–7301.

132 Bieber, T., Meissner, W., Kostin, S., Niemann, A., Elsasser, H. P., Intracellular route and transcriptional competence of polyethylenimine–DNA complexes. *J. Control. Release* **2002**, *82*, 441–454.

133 Merdan, T., Kunath, K., Fischer, D., Kopecek, J., Kissel, T., Intracellular processing of poly(ethylene imine)/ribozyme complexes can be observed in living cells by using confocal laser scanning microscopy and inhibitor experiments. *Pharm. Res.* **2002**, *19*, 140–146.

134 Mellman, I., Endocytosis and molecular sorting. *Annu. Rev. Cell Dev. Biol.* **1996**, *12*, 575–625.

135 Nichols, B. J., Lippincott-Schwartz, J., Endocytosis without clathrin coats. *Trends Cell Biol.* **2001**, *11*, 406–412.

136 Gumbleton, M., Abulrob, A. G., Campbell, L., Caveolae: an alternative membrane transport compartment. *Pharm. Res.* **2000**, *17*, 1035–1048.

137 Arbab, A. S., Yocum, G. T., Kalish, H., Jordan, E. K., Anderson, S. A., Khakoo, A. Y., Read, E. J., Frank, J. A., Efficient magnetic cell labeling with protamine sulfate complexed to ferumoxides for cellular MRL. *Blood* **2004**, *104*, 1217–1223.

138 Bulte, J. W., Douglas, T., Witwer, B., Zhang, S. C., Strable, E., Lewis, B. K., Zywicke, H., Miller, B., van Gelderen, P., Moskowitz, B. M., Duncan, I. D., Frank, J. A., Magnetodendrimers allow endosomal magnetic labeling and *in vivo* tracking of stem cells. *Nat. Biotechnol.* **2001**, *19*, 1141–1147.

139 Scherer, F., Anton, M., Schillinger, U., Henke, J., Bergemann, C., Kruger, A., Gansbacher, B., Plank, C., Magnetofection: enhancing and targeting gene delivery by magnet force *in vitro* and *in vivo*. *Gene Ther.* **2002**, *9*, 102–109.

140 Huth, S., Lausier, J., Gersting, S. W., Rudolph, C., Plank, C., Welsch, U., Rosenecker, J., Insights into the mechanism of magnetofection using PEI-based magnetofections for gene transfer. *J. Gene Med.* **2004**, *6*, 923–936.

141 Bull, B. S., Huse, W. M., Brauer, F. S., Korpman, R. A., Heparin therapy during extracorporeal circulation. II. The use of a dose–response curve to individualize heparin and protamine dosage. *J. Thorac. Cardiovasc. Surg.* **1975**, *69*, 685–659.

142 Gervin, A. S., Complications of heparin therapy. *Surg. Gynecol. Obstet.* **1975**, *140*, 789–796.

143 Lubbe, A. S., Bergemann, C., Riess, H., Schriever, F., Reichardt, P., Possinger, K., Matthias, M., Dorken, B., Herrmann, F., Gurtler, R., Hohenberger, P., Haas, N., Sohr, R., Sander, B., Lemke, A. J., Ohlendorf, D., Huhnt, W., Huhn, D., Clinical experiences with magnetic drug targeting: a phase I study with 4′-epidoxorubicin in 14 patients with advanced solid tumors. *Cancer Res.* **1996**, *56*, 4686–4693.

144 Lubbe, A. S., Bergemann, C., Huhnt, W., Fricke, T., Riess, H., Brock, J. W., Huhn, D., Preclinical experiences with magnetic drug targeting: tolerance and efficacy. *Cancer Res.* **1996**, *56*, 4694–4701.

15
Nanotoxicology of Synthetic Gene Transfer Vectors: Poly(ethyleneimine)- and Polyfectin-mediated Membrane Damage and Apoptosis in Human Cell Lines

Seyed M. Moghimi

15.1
Introduction

Viral vectors are extremely efficient in transfecting cells; however, they can induce severe immunotoxicity and inflammatory responses, which restrain repeated administration [1]. The death of Jesse Gelsinger in September 1999 during an experimental adenoviral gene therapy trial conducted at the University of Pennsylvania is a grim reminder of these adverse effects. The autopsy findings confirmed that the adenoviral vector initiated an unusual and deadly immune system response that led to multiple organ failure and adult respiratory distress syndrome, and ultimately brain death. Another potential complication is insertional mutagenesis, which could pose additional risks in gene therapy programmes involving retroviruses, as evident from stem cell gene therapy trials for treatment of X-linked severe combined immunodeficiency disease at Necker Hospital, Paris, France [1–3]. Of 17 patients who participated in this programme, virtually all showed major improvement. However, three developed leukemia-like conditions; of these, one subsequently died. These issues, together with the limited loading capacity and difficulties in large-scale production of viral vectors, have generated a surge in design and engineering of synthetic cationic nonviral gene transfer systems. Examples include a plethora of cationic lipids (lipofectins) and polycations (polyfectins) such as poly(L-lysine) and poly(ethyleneimine) (PEI) in linear, branched and dendrimeric form, and variations thereof [poly(ethylene glycol)- and ligand-tagged] [4–6]. These materials can condense genetic materials into nanostructures readily amenable for transfection. PEIs have received considerable attention in gene transfer protocols as a result of excellent transfection efficiencies [4–6].

This chapter briefly reviews the structure and properties of PEI-based transfectants. PEI is also cytotoxic, but the molecular basis of its cytotoxicity is poorly understood and therefore not discussed in detail in previous reviews. The major part of this chapter critically examines recent breakthroughs in understanding of the molecular mechanisms of PEI-mediated cytotoxicity.

Nanotechnologies for the Life Sciences Vol. 10
Nanomaterials for Medical Diagnosis and Therapy. Edited by Challa S. S. R. Kumar

ISBN: 978-3-527-31390-7

15.2
PEI as a Nonviral Vector

15.2.1
Structure and Properties of PEI and PEI–DNA Complexes

PEI exists in both linear and branched form and is available in a broad range of molecular weights (from a few hundred Daltons to 1500 kDa). Ring-opening polymerization of 2-substituted 2-oxazoline leads to formation of poly(*N*-formalethylenimine), which is then hydrolyzed to yield linear PEI. In contrast, the branched form of PEI is produced by acid-catalyzed polymerization of aziridine.

PEI is capable of condensing DNA and RNA into stable toroidal and globular nanostructures mainly via electrostatic interactions, as supported by a range of biophysical characterization studies [7–10]. The physicochemical nature and stability of the PEI–DNA complex (polyplex) is dependent on a number of factors, including PEI type, molecular weight, charge density, ionic strength of the media, the tertiary structure of nucleic acids (e.g. linear versus supercoiled DNA), polymer:DNA ratio and even the sequence of component addition, and these are reviewed recently in detail by Neu and coworkers [6]. For example, low-molecular-weight PEIs (2 kDa and smaller) form larger polyplexes (greater than 500 nm) than their high-molecular-weight counterparts (less than 200 nm). Also, linear PEI possesses lower DNA condensation capacity when compared to a branched counterpart, which is attributed to its lower content in primary amines [6].

Polyplex formation not only protects DNA and RNA from degradation by nucleases, but also is a necessary prerequisite for the efficient delivery of nucleic acids into cells via endocytosis and macropinocytosis [10]. Following internalization, PEI can rapidly destabilize endosomal membrane following protonation. Indeed, every third atom of PEI is a nitrogen capable of protonation. PEI exhibits a very high buffering capacity above pH 7, which is attributed to the secondary amines in the structure, but additionally shows buffering capacity in the range of endosomal pH (pH 4–6). Thus, following internalization, PEI-based polyfectins act as proton sponges, buffering the low endosomal pH and inducing membrane rupture [11–14]. This releases PEI and PEI–DNA complexes into the cytoplasm.

15.2.2
Cytotoxicity

Various reports have indicated that PEI can induce cytotoxicity, often defined by assessing the *in vitro* metabolic activity of cells (e.g. MTT assay), but the mechanism(s) remain unclear [6, 15–17]. High-molecular-weight PEIs are more cytotoxic than their smaller counterparts and increasing the degree of branching induces more cytotoxic effects [15, 17]. The issue of PEI-induced cytotoxicity is particularly important in protocols that attempt to restore gene function, e.g. in metabolic disorders. PEI-induced cytotoxicity in normal and nontarget cells, particularly the type of cells that the cationic vectors will encounter when first administered to the patient, must also be considered. One of the most striking features of PEI polyplexes is the large amount of PEI that remains in the free form, which may induce cell dysfunction and explain the observed cytotoxicity [18]. However, the presence of free PEI is essential for modification and permeabilization of the endosomal membrane structure, thus affording polyplexes a mode of access into the cytoplasm [6, 18]. Indeed, partially purified PEI complexes were recently shown to induce less cytotoxicity, but this also led to a decrease in transfection efficiency [19]. The removal of excess PEI may also affect the stability of polyplexes, since complex formation is an equilibrium process [18].

In light of these observations and with the view that the intracellular levels of endogenous polyamines (e.g. spermine and spermidine) are tightly regulated by means of several homeostatic mechanisms, whereas their excessive cytoplasmic accumulation (e.g. resulting from insults to anionic cellular structures) transduces a death signal to mitochondria by an oxygen-independent mechanism [20, 21], we sought to investigate the effect of PEI and related polyfectins on human cell dysfunction and apoptosis. For the first time, we have identified PEI as an apoptotic agent [22, 23]. Our observations and findings may provide a likely explanation for previously reported transient gene expression associated with polyfectin vectors. A brief overview of our findings as well as recent breakthroughs in polycation-induced cytotoxicity mechanisms is therefore discussed.

15.3 PEI-mediated Cell Dysfunction and Apoptosis

15.3.1 PEI and PEI–DNA Complex Internalization

PEI and PEI–DNA complexes enter most cells presumably via binding to transmembrane heparan sulfate/chondroitin sulfate proteoglycans that belong to the syndecan family (e.g. syndecan-1 and -4) [24–27]. Cells, like fibroblasts, express glycosylphosphatidylinositol-anchored heparan sulfate proteoglycans (glypican) instead, which may also serve as a receptor for polyamine uptake [28].

Earlier, fluorescence-labeled studies have demonstrated that within 3 h of incubation with human cell lines, a significant fraction of PEI and PEI–DNA complexes appears in endosomes and endolysosomes [11]. Subsequent attempts with double fluorescence-labeled PEI–DNA complexes have shown disruption of some endosomes, beginning at 4 h postincubation, with evidence of some separation of DNA from PEI in cytosol [11]. Nuclear localization of PEI or PEI–DNA was relatively common by 3.5–4.5 h postincubation and the earliest localization of complexes within nuclei preceded the earliest observed transgene expression by 1 h [11]. The molecular basis of PEI–DNA complex localization to the nucleus still remains unclear, but such complexes may attract a lipophilic coating within cytosol, thus promoting fusion with the nuclear membrane. However, PEIs in the range of 5–25 kDa are most efficient in transfection experiments because of their small size (less than 200 nm) and relatively faster cytosolic movements [6].

15.3.2
Plasma Membrane Damage and Apoptosis

We have shown that exposure of three different primary human cell lines (hepatocytes, endothelial cells and lymphocytes) to branched (B)-PEI (25 kDa) or linear PEI (750 kDa) in both free form (10 and 30 μg mL^{-1}) as well as complexed with a mammalian DNA (regardless of PEI:DNA) causes considerable release of lactate dehydrogenase (LDH) within 1 h, followed by a time-dependent gradual rise in LDH release, thus confirming plasma membrane damage (Fig. 15.1A) [22]. Parallel to rapid LDH release, we also reported rapid (30–60 min) redistribution of phosphatidylserine (PS) from the inner plasma membrane to the outer cell surface with PEI concentrations of 20 μg mL^{-1} and above (Fig. 15.1B) [22]. PS redistribution was increased gradually with time. However, at lower PEI concentrations (e.g. 10 μg mL^{-1}) PS externalization was significant only after prolonged incubation periods (e.g. 24 h). PS translocation is a hallmark of apoptosis; caspase-3 in active form impairs the activity of aminophospholipid translocase, which leads to PS externalization [29, 30]. Early PS expression, however, was not inhibited in the pre-

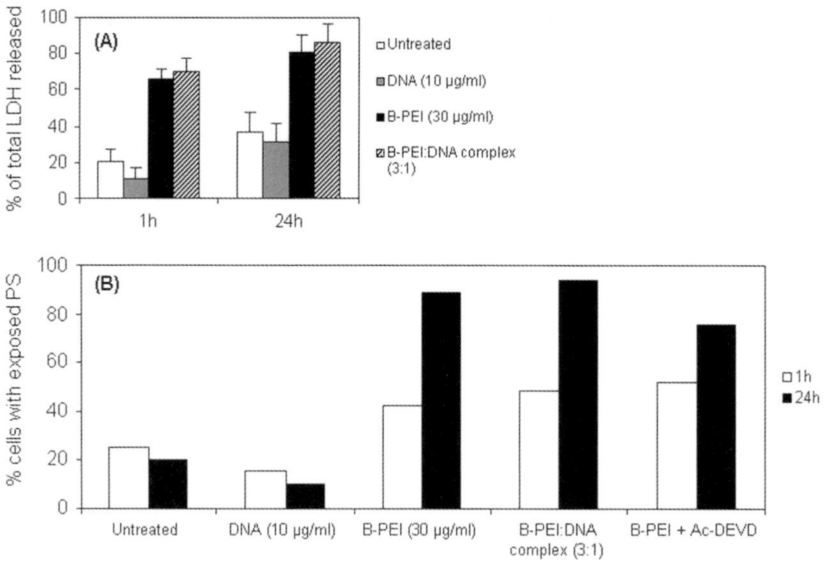

Figure 15.1. The effect of B-PEI in free form and DNA-complexed on Jurkat T cell plasma membrane integrity. The release of the cytoplasmic LDH from cells is shown in (A), whereas (B) demonstrates the extent of PS externalization from the inner to the outer cell surface. Detailed experimental procedures are outlined in reference [22].

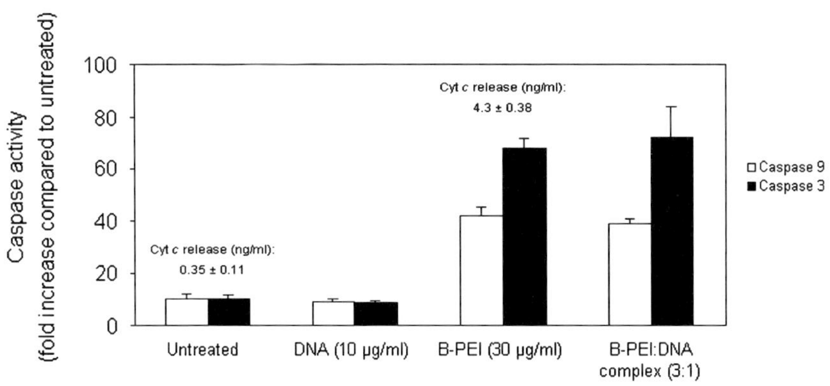

Figure 15.2. The effect of B-PEI in free form and DNA-complexed on caspase activation and cytochrome *c* release in Jurkat T cells.

sence of Ac-DEVD (a broad-spectrum caspase inhibitor) and therefore occurs independent of procaspase-3 cleavage. A substantial delay between PS exposure and activation of the executioner caspase-3 was also observed [22]. The activity of this protease was profound particularly at 24 h post-B-PEI/B-PEI–DNA treatment (Fig. 15.2) and could be inhibited by Ac-DEVD. Also, caspase-3 activation was detectable at 24 h post-treatment with lower concentrations of PEI and PEI–DNA complexes; this was in accord with PS expression in tandem with propidium iodide staining. Hence, both PEI types induce apoptosis, but early exposure of PS is presumably the result of plasma membrane destabilization during internalization processes, where PEI may crosslink syndecan molecules and/or induce syndecan clustering. Subsequently, syndecan/glypican clustering may mediate actin stress fiber formation and activate associated signaling pathways such as those of Src family of kinases, contractin, tubulin, microfilament-regulated processes and phosphatidylinositol 4,5-bisphosphate-dependent processes [27, 28, 31]. In certain cells these processes may initiate apoptosis via activation of protein kinases, depending on polycation type and architecture (discussed later). Dissociation of PEI–DNA complexes is also known to occur in the presence of negatively charged macromolecules [32]. It is likely that PEI may interact with actin and alter membrane integrity.

However, through which of the two primary caspase activation pathways, mitochondrially mediated and death receptor-mediated, do PEIs and PEI–DNA complexes induce apoptosis? Here, studies were restricted to PEI–DNA complexes that expressed positive ζ potential (PEI:DNA of 3:1), thus mimicking the established transfection protocols [6]. Stress-induced stimuli triggers mitochondrial permeabilization and causes the release of proapoptotic proteins such as cytochrome *c*, apoptosis-inducing factor (AIF), and Smac/DIABLO from mitochondrial intermembrane space [33, 35]. For example, cytochrome *c* release initiates apoptosis via the Apaf-1-containing apoptosome complex assembly. This results in subsequent cleavage of caspase-9, which, in turn, activates the executioner caspase-3 [33, 35]. On the other hand AIF, a 50-kDa protease, is capable of inducing DNA fragmentation and chromatin condensation directly [35]. PEI and PEI–DNA treatment in human cell lines was associated with substantial activation of both caspase-3 and -9; significant accumulation of cytochrome *c* in cytosol was also observed (Fig. 15.2) [22]. Since nuclear accumulation of PEI–DNA complexes was reported to occur within a few hours of transfection [11], PEI may also induce genotoxic stress via caspase-2 activation [36, 37]. Indeed, activated caspase-2 can directly permeabilize the outer mitochondrial membrane and stimulate the release of death-promoting proteins without the involvement of mitochondrial permeability transition [36, 37]. However, no evidence for caspase-2 activation even after prolonged periods following PEI and PEI–DNA complex treatment was reported [22, 38]. Also, the absence of caspase-8 activity further suggested that plasma membrane manipulation by PEI and PEI–DNA complexes has no effect on death receptor signaling, which could lead to activation of caspase-3 and -7 directly or indirectly via subsequent cleavage of the amino portion of cytosolic Bid. This would have generated truncated Bid, which, in turn, could activate proapoptotic Bax or Bak proteins to release cytochrome *c* from mitochondrial intermembrane space [35].

The loss of mitochondrial membrane potential (MMP) is also an early event in several types of apoptosis [39, 40]. In our hands, MMP in human cell lines was dramatically dropped in a time-dependent manner [22, 23] and was consistent with caspase activation (with peak activity at 24 h). MMP was determined by a specific cationic fluorescent probe, JC-1, which fluoresces differently in healthy and apoptotic cells (Fig. 15.3). JC-1 forms aggregates in healthy mitochondria with a high orange/red fluorescence, indicating a normal MMP, but following MMP loss these aggregates dissipate into the cytoplasm in the monomeric state, which is detectable with a concurrent gain in green fluorescence [22]. Therefore, these observations confirm that PEI and PEI–DNA complexes induce apoptosis via the mitochondrial pathway.

15.3.3
Effect of PEI on the Function of Isolated Mitochondria

To further understand the molecular basis of PEI-induced mitochondrially mediated apoptosis, attention was focused on studies with isolated mitochondria [22]. Here, PEI was able to release cytochrome *c* from the mitochondrial intermembrane space in a concentration-dependent manner. Indeed, cytochrome *c* release was detectable following treatment with both PEI types even at levels as low as 0.1 $\mu g\ mL^{-1}$. Interestingly, cytochrome *c* release was not associated with changes in mitochondrial volume (Fig. 15.4). This observation may indicate a minor role for permeability transition in the release of apoptogenic proteins from mitochondria. However, it should be emphasized that permeability transition is reversible; permeability transition may cause an individual mitochondrion to swell, releasing apoptogenic proteins, and then reverse and regenerate membrane potential [41]. Therefore, this route may still operate in intact cells.

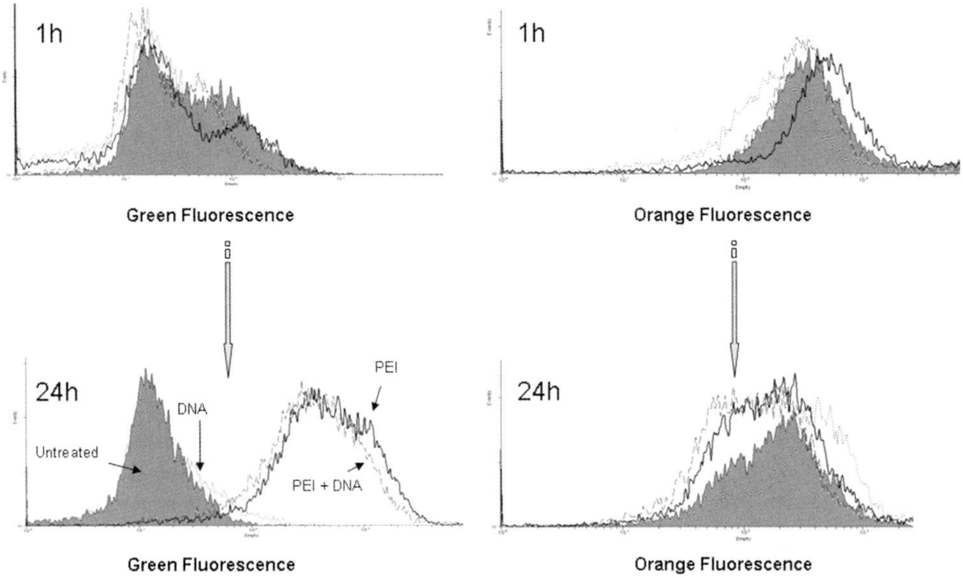

Figure 15.3. Time-dependent changes in MMP in Jurkat T cells by free (30 μg mL^{-1}) and DNA-complexed (PEI:DNA, weight ratio 3:1) branched PEI, as determined by specific MMP fluorescent probe JC-1. Detailed experimental procedures are outlined in Ref. [22].

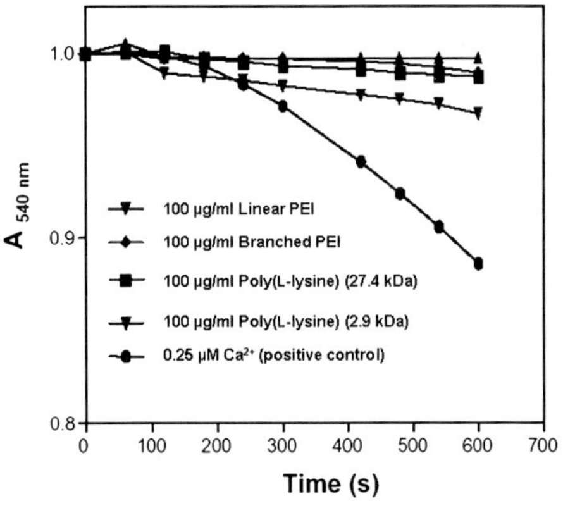

Figure 15.4. The effect of polycations on continuous swelling of isolated rat liver mitochondria, monitored as changes in A_{540} at room temperature. Detailed experimental procedures are outlined in Refs. [22, 50].

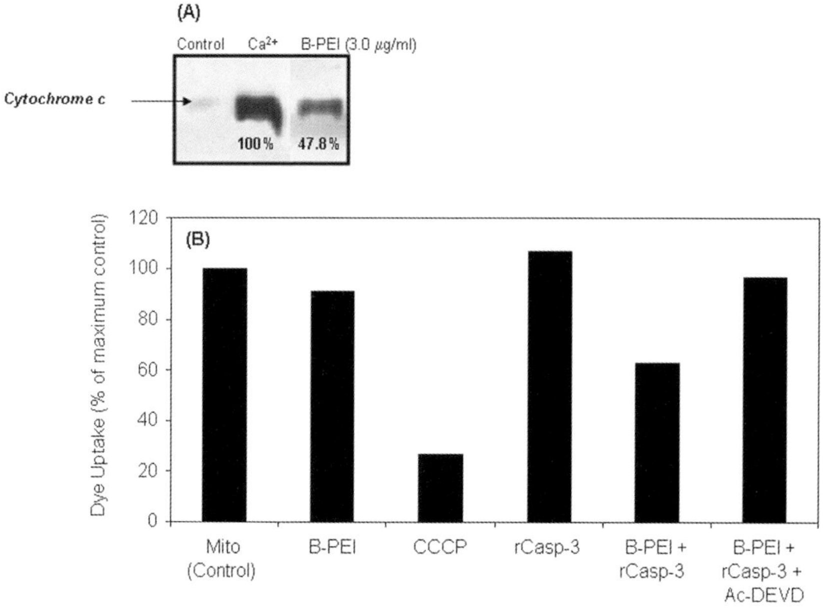

Figure 15.5. The effect of branched PEI on function of isolated rat liver mitochondria. (A) The effect of PEI on cytochrome *c* release (Western blot analysis). (B) The extent of $DiOC_6(3)$ uptake by isolated mitochondria at different treatment protocols. Following incubation with PEI and rCasp-3 (15 min), $DiOC_6(3)$ was added and the sample was incubated for a further 10 min at 22 °C. Samples were then diluted in the buffer, filtered and incubated for a further 10 min before flow cytometric analysis content of individual mitochondria.

Changes in the membrane potential of isolated mitochondria can be followed by measuring the uptake of the cationic lipophilic fluor $DiOC_6(3)$ (Fig. 15.5). This membrane potential-sensitive dye electrophoretically accumulates in the negatively charged matrix of healthy mitochondria. When mitochondrial depolarization occurs, accumulation of $DiOC_6(3)$ is reduced and can be followed by flow cytometry as a decrease in mitochondrial-associated green fluorescence. Interestingly, dye uptake remained unaltered in the presence of PEI (i.e. after cytochrome *c* release) when compared to healthy intact mitochondria (where no cytochrome *c* release is detectable) (Fig. 15.5). As a control experiment $DiOC_6(3)$ responded to acute changes in mitochondrial membrane potential induced by the protonophore carbonyl cyanide *p*-chlorophenylhydrazone (CCCP). Thus, cytochrome *c* release is independent of mitochondrial depolarization [22], but in intact cells PEI was capable of altering MMP. This discrepancy may indicate a role for activated caspases in altering MMP. Remarkably, the addition of an active recombinant human caspase 3 (rCasp-3) exerted no effect on dye accumulation in intact mitochondria, whereas in the presence of PEI dye uptake was reduced dramatically unless Ac-DEVD was present (Fig. 15.5). These experiments strongly support that PEI is capable of forming channels in the outer membrane large enough to allow the release of cytochrome *c*, presumably in a manner similar to proapoptotic peptides and oligomeric Bax [42, 43], without altering MMP. Thus, these observations are also in accord with the loss of MMP in intact cells following PEI or PEI–DNA uptake, which is believed to occur after cytochrome *c* release and presumably is mediated by activated caspases. Indeed, recently it was demonstrated that following cytochrome *c* release, activated caspases gain access to the intermembrane space of mitochondrion where they cleave the 75-kDa subunit of respiratory complex I, resulting in disruption of complex I activity, loss of MMP and production of reactive oxygen species [44].

15.3.4 Other Plausible Apoptotic Routes

Recently, a spatial and functional connection between Bax and the mitochondrial fission process was suggested [45, 46]. In normal interphase cells the mitochondria exists as a tubular network. During apoptosis, the mitochondrial network becomes fragmented and Bax colocalized with the fission- and fusion-related proteins (Drp1,

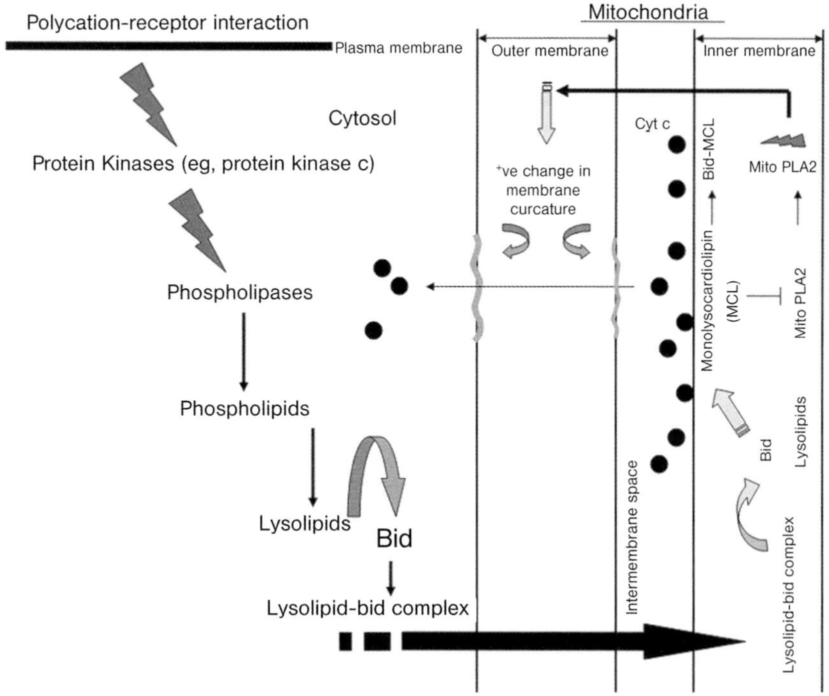

Figure 15.6. Schematic representation of possible polycation effect on protein kinase and phospholipase activation, and the role of full-length Bid in initiation of mitochondrially mediated apoptosis.

Mfn2) at fission sites in the outer mitochondrial membrane. Due to their polycationic nature and molecular architecture, PEI molecules could hypothetically promote mitochondrial fission, which may lead to destabilization of the outer mitochondrial membrane.

It can also be speculated that following binding to plasma membrane proteoglycans, such as syndecan or glypican, PEI and related polycations may initiate apoptosis via signaling and activation of protein kinases (Fig. 15.6). For example, poly(L-lysine)s and poly(arginine)s are known to stimulate a number of cellular kinases and protein phosphatases, particularly phospholipases, even at suboptimal cytotoxic concentrations [47]. For instance, poly(L-lysine) is capable of inducing phospholipase D activation in bovine pulmonary artery endothelial cells through the involvement of protein kinase C [47]. Phospholipase activation may lead towards insertion of lysolipids into the outer mitochondrial membrane via the recently identified lipid transfer capacity of full-length Bid [48]. Once bound to lysolipid, full-length Bid is suggested to transfer lysolipid to intracellular membranes rich in cardiolipin and monolysocardiolipin, towards which the protein has a "static" selectivity of binding, thereby altering cardiolipin homoeostasis [48]. Indeed, monolysocardiolipin is an inhibitor of mitochondrial phospholipase A2 [49] and thus tight binding of full-length Bid to monolysocardiolipin may lead to activation of this phospholipase. These modifications may induce a positive change in the outer mitochondrial membrane curvature leading to the release of apoptogenic factors, either directly or through other mediators.

15.4
Cell Damage and Apoptosis with Related Polycations and Cationic Lipids

Poly(L-lysine) are also used widely in DNA compaction and gene transfer protocols [4]. Recent observations from this laboratory have shown that poly(L-lysine)s are also capable of inducing mitochondrially mediated apoptosis in a wide range of human cell lines [50]. However, low- and high-molecular weight poly(L-lysine)s/poly(L-lysine)–DNA complexes had different effect on mitochondrial functions and initiated mitochondrially mediated apoptosis differently. For example, high-molecular-weight poly(L-lysine)s were not only capable of inducing cytochrome *c* release from isolated mitochondria, but were also able to dramatically alter mitochondrial respiration and membrane potential without swelling [50]. Interestingly, in intact cells inhibition of Bax channel-forming activity was shown to reduce the extent of cytochrome *c* release from mitochondria by half. In the case of low-molecular weight poly(L-lysine)s neither cytochrome *c* release nor changes in the function of isolated mitochondria was noticed, whereas in intact cells such treatments resulted in significant accumulation of cytochrome *c* in cytosol within 24 h with a concurrent MMP drop, and caspase-3 and -9 activation [50]. These observations may indicate a possible role for protein kinases and phospholipases in initiation of apoptosis by low-molecular weight poly(L-lysine)s, as discussed above (Fig. 15.6).

Poly[2-(dimethylamino)ethyl methacrylate] is another example of a cationic polymer that facilitates cell transfection. This polymer is also cytotoxic, but the mechanisms of its cytotoxicity is primarily due to necrotic cell death [51]. Nanoparticles made from poly(D,L-lactide-*co*-glycolide) have also been suggested for transfection studies; these particles can escape the endolysosomal compartment within minutes of internalization in intact form and reach the cytoplasm [52]. The mechanism of rapid escape is by selective reversal of the surface charge of nanoparticles from the anionic to the cationic state in endolysosomes, thus resulting in a local particle–membrane interaction with subsequent cytoplasmic release. However, degradation products arising from poly(L-lactic acid) particles also show cytotoxicity, and can induce apoptotic and necrotic cell death [53].

We have also proposed an apoptotic role for cationic surfactants and related structures (micelles), thus limiting the applicability of cationic drug carriers for intracellular drug release [54]. Cationic lipids have also been employed in gene transfer/therapy protocols [4], but recent studies have indicated that cationic lipids are also capable of inducing apoptosis [55]. For example, apoptosis in macrophage-like cell line RAW264.7 following treatment with stearylamine-incorporated liposomes was mediated by mitogen-activated protein kinase p38 and c-jun N-terminal kinase, and a caspase 8-dependent Bid cleavage pathway [55].

Furthermore, cDNA microarray expression profiling studies are beginning to reveal that the cationic delivery vehicle can adversely influence the desired effects of the delivered genetic agents [56], which is in agreement with the observation that polycations such as PEI and poly(L-lysine) in both free form and complexed with DNA can localize to the nucleus. Gene expression changes in a wide range of gene ontologies were recently demonstrated with PEI in both *in vitro* and *in vivo* studies [56]. Remarkably, both PEI concentration and architecture had a dramatic effect on non-target gene expression.

15.5 Conclusions and Future Outlook

Polycations such as PEI and poly(L-lysine) induce rapid perturbation of the plasma membrane (within 30–120 min of exposure) with characteristics resembling early necrotic-like changes, which is followed by activation of a "mitochondrially mediated" apoptotic programme at later stages (24 h), at least in human endothelial, lymphocyte and hepatic cell lines [22, 38, 50]. These findings are of relevance to transient gene expression following polycation-mediated DNA compaction and transfection both *in vitro* and *in vivo*. There are numerous developments with respect to the design and synthesis of "less cytotoxic" polycations [6, 57–59]. Cytotoxicity, however, is often assessed by the MTT assay, which is not indicative of apoptosis. Future cytotoxicity studies with newly designed cationic macromolecules and polyfectins should address and consider the time-dependent apoptotic processes, as apoptosis may compromise transcription and translation processes, and limit protein expression. Additionally, the process of apoptosis in intact cells is stochastic, with different cells entering apoptosis at different times. Furthermore, different cationic polymers may interact differently with mitochondria or the endoplasmic reticulum (leading to perturbation of intracellular calcium) and initiate apoptosis differently. The inherent heterogeneity of mitochondria that make up any particular population of these organelles should also be taken into the account.

Attempts in polycation-mediated gene transfer, however, could benefit through recent advances in high-throughput approaches to polymer design and screening [60]. Such approaches may enhance our understanding of the molecular basis of interaction between cationic polymers and intracellular membranes. An understanding of such events may eventually help to design novel and safer materials, particularly those that can provide duration period-specific gene expression in clinical scenarios.

References

1 Cavazzano-Calvo, M., Thrasher, A., Mavilio, F. The future of gene therapy, *Nature* **2004**, *427*, 779–781.

2 Gore, M. Gene therapy can cause leukemia: no shock, mild horror but a probe, *Gene Ther.* **2003**, *10*, 4–4.

3 Gansbacher, B. Report of a second serious adverse event in a clinical trial of gene therapy for X-linked severe combined immunodeficiency (X-SCID). Position of the European Society of Gene Therapy (ESGT), *J. Gene. Med.* **2003**, *5*, 261–262.

4 Schmidt-Wolf, G. D., Schmidt-Wolf, I. G. H. Non-viral and hybrid vectors in human gene therapy: an update, *Trend. Mol. Med.* **2003**, *9*, 67–72.

5 Kichler, A. Gene transfer with modified polyethylenimine, *J. Gene Med.* **2004**, *6*, S3–S10.

6 Neu, M., Fischer, D., Kissel, T. Recent advances in rational gene transfer vector design based on poly(ethyleneimine) and its derivatives, *J. Gene Med.* **2005**, *7*, 992–1009.

7 Tang, M. X., Szoka, F. C. The influence of polymer structure on the interaction of cationic polymers with DNA and morphology of the resulting complexes, *Gene Ther.* **1997**, *4*, 823–832.

8 Bloomfield, V. A., DNA condensation, *Curr. Opin. Struct. Biol.* **1996**, *6*, 334–341.

9 Bronich, T., Kabanov, A., Marky, L. A thermodynamic characterization of the interaction of a cationic copolymer with DNA, *J. Phys. Chem. B* **2001**, *105*, 6041–5050.

10 Oh, Y. K., Suh, D., Kim, J. M., Choi, H. G., Shin, K., Ko, J. J. Polyethylenimine-mediated cellular uptake, nucleus trafficking and expression of cytokine plasmid DNA, *Gene Ther.* **2002**, *9*, 1627–1632.

11 Godbey, W. T., Wu, K. K., Mikos, A. G. Tracking the intracellular path of poly(ethylenimine)/DNA complexes for gene delivery, *Proc. Natl Acad. Sci. USA* **1999**, *96*, 5177–5181.

12 Boussif, O., Lezoualc'h, F., Zanta, M. A., Mergny, M. D., Scherman, D., Demeneix, B., Behr, J.-P. A versatile vector for gene and oligonucleotide transfer into cells in culture and *in vivo*: polyethyleneimine, *Proc. Natl Acad. Sci. USA* **1995**, *92*, 7297–7301.

13 Clamme, J. P., Krishnamoorthy, G., Mély, Y. Intracellular dynamics of the gene delivery vehicle polyethylenimine during transfection: investigation by two-photon fluorescence correlation spectroscopy, *Biochim. Biophys. Acta Biomembr.* **2003**, *1617*, 52–61.

14 Forrest, M. L., Pack, D. W. On the kinetics of polyplex endocytic trafficking: Implications for gene delivery vector design, *Mol. Ther.* **2002**, *6*, 57–66.

15 Fischer, D., Bieber, T., Li, Y., Elasasser, H. P., Kissel, T. A novel non-viral vector for DNA delivery based on low molecular weight, branched polyethylenimine: effect of molecular weight on transfection efficiency and cytotoxicity, *Pharm. Res.* **1999**, *16*, 1273–1279.

16 Florea, B. I., Meaney, C., Junginger, H. E., Borchard, G. Transfection efficiency and toxicity of polyethylenimine in differentiated Calu-3 and nondifferentiated Cos-1 cell cultures, *AAPS PharmSci.* **2002**, *4*, article 12.

17 Fischer, D., von Harpe, A., Kunath, K., Petersen, H., Li, Y. X., Kissel, T. Copolymers of ethyeneimine and *N*-(2-hydroxyethyl)ethyleneimine as tools to study effects of polymer structure on physicochemical and biological properties of DNA complexes, *Bioconjug. Chem.* **2002**, *13*, 1124–1133.

18 Clamme, J. P., Azoulay, J., Mély, Y. Monitoring of the formation and dissociation of polyethylenimine/DNA complexes by two photon fluorescence spectroscopy, *Biophys. J.* **2003**, *84*, 1960–1968.

19 Boeckle, S., von Gersdorff, K., van der Piepen, S., Culmsee, C., Wangner, E., Ogris, M. Purification of polyethylenimine polyplexes highlights the role of free polycations in gene transfer, *J. Gene Med.* **2004**, *6*, 1102–1110.

20 Stefanelli, C., Bonavita, F., Stanic, I., Pignatti, C., Flamigni, F., Guarnieri, C., Caldarera, C. M. Spermine triggers the activation of caspase-3 in a cell-free model of apoptosis, *FEBS Lett.* **1999**, *451*, 95–98.

21 Stefanelli, C., Stanic, I., Zini, M., Bonavita, F., Flamigni, F., Zambonin, L., Landi, L., Pignatti, C., Guarnieri, C., Caldarera, C. M. Polyamines directly induce release of cytochrome c from heart mitochondria, *Biochem. J.* **2000**, *347*, 875–880.

22 Moghimi, S. M., Symonds, P., Murray, J. C., Hunter, A. C., Debska, G., Szewczyk, A. A two-stage poly(ethylenimine)-mediated cytotoxicity: implications for gene transfer/therapy, *Mol. Ther.* **2005**, *11*, 990–995.

23 Moghimi, S. M., Hunter, A. C., Murray, J. C. Nanomedicine: current status and future prospects, *FASEB J.* **2005**, *19*, 311–330.

24 Mislick, K. A., Baldeschwieler, J. D. Evidence for the role of proteoglycans in cation-mediated gene transfer. *Proc. Natl Acad. Sci. USA* **1996**, *93*, 12349–12354.

25 Mounkes, L. C., Zhong, W., Cipres-Palacin, Heath, T. D., Debs, R. J. Proteoglycans mediate cationic liposome–DNA complex-based gene delivery *in vitro* and *in vivo*, *J. Biol. Chem.* **1998**, *273*, 26164–26170.

26 Kopatz, I., Remy, J. S., Behr, J.-P. A model for non-viral gene delivery: through syndecan adhesion molecules and powered by actin, *J. Gene Med.* **2004**, *6*, 769–776.

27 Dull, R. O., Dinavahi, R., Schwartz, L., Humphries, D. E., Berry, D., Sasisekharan, R., Garcia, J. G. N. Lung endothelial heparan sulfate mediate cationic peptide-induced barrier dysfunction: a new role for the glycocalyx, *Am. J. Physiol. (Lung Cell. Mol. Physiol.)* **2003**, *285*, L986–L995.

28 Belting, M., Persson, S., Fransson, L.-A. Proteoglycan involvement in polyamine uptake, *Biochem. J.* **1999**, *338*, 317–323.

29 Martin, S. J., Finucane, D. M., Amarantemendes, G. P., O'Brien, G. A., Green, D. A. Phosphatidylserine externalization during CD95-induced apoptosis of cells and cytoplasts requires ICE/Ced-3 protease activity, *J. Biol. Chem.* **1996**, *271*, 28753–28756.

30 Mandal, D., Moitra, P. K., Saha, S., Basu, J. Caspase 3 regulates phosphatidylserine externalization and phagocytosis of oxidatively stressed erythrocytes, *FEBS Lett.* **2002**, *513*, 184–188.

31 Saoncella, S., Echtermeyer, F., Denhaz, F., Nowlen, J. K., Mosher, D. F., Robinson, S. D., Hynes, R., Goetinck, P. F. Syndecan-4 signals cooperatively with integrins in a Rho-dependent manner in the assembly of focal adhesions and actin stress fibers, *Proc. Natl Acad. Sci. USA* **1999**, *96*, 2805–2810.

32 Wong, G. C. L., Tang, J. X., Lin, A., Li, Y., Janmey, P. A., Safinya, C. R. Hierarchical self-assembly of F-actin and cationic lipid complexes: stacked three-layer tubule networks, *Science* **2000**, *288*, 2035–2039.

33 Newmeyer, D. D., Ferguson-Miller, S. Mitochondria: releasing power for life and unleashing the machineries of death, *Cell* **2003**, *112*, 481–490.

34 Kluck, R. M., Bossy-Wetzel, E., Green, D. R., Newmeyer, D. D. The release of cytochrome *c* from mitochondria: a primary site for Bcl-2 regulation of apoptosis, *Science* **1997**, *275*, 1132–1136.

35 Hengartner, M. O. The biochemistry of apoptosis, *Nature* **2000**, *407*, 770–776.

36 Robertson, J. D., Gogvadez, V., Kropotov, A., Vakifahmetoglu, H., Zhivotovsky, B., Orrenius, S. Processed caspase-2 can induce mitochondria-mediated apoptosis independently of its enzymatic activity, *EMBO Rep.* **2004**, *5*, 643–648.

37 Enoksson, M., Robertson, J. D., Gogvadez, V., Bu, P., Kropotov, A., Zhivotovsky, B. and Orrenius, S. Caspase-2 permeabilizes the outer mitochondrial membrane and disrupts the binding of cytochrome *c* to anionic phospholipids, *J. Biol. Chem.* **2004**, *279*, 49575–49578.

38 Moghimi, S. M., Symonds, P., Hunter, A. C., Murray, J. C. The molecular basis of immediate and delayed polycation/polyamine-induced cytotoxicity in gene transfer, *Toxicology* **2006**, *219*, 234–235.

39 Bortner, C. D., Cidlowski, J. A. Caspase independent/dependent regulation of K^+, cell shrinkage, and mitochondrial membrane potential during lymphocyte apoptosis, *J. Biol. Chem.* **1999**, *274*, 21953–21962.

40 Dinsdale, D., Zhuang, J., Cohen, G. M. Redistribution of cytochrome *c* precedes the caspase-dependent formation of ultra-condensed mitochondria, with a reduced inner membrane potential, in apoptotic monocytes, *Am. J. Pathol.* **1999**, *155*, 607–618.

41 Scarlett, J. L., Murphy, M. P. Release of apoptogenic proteins from the mitochondrial intermembrane space during the mitochondrial permeability transition, *FEBS Lett.* **1997**, *418*, 282–286.

42 Gogvadze, V., Robertson, J. D., Zhivotovsky, B., Orrenius, S. Cytochrome *c* release occurs via Ca^{2+}-dependent and Ca^{2+}-independent mechanisms that are regulated by Bax, *J. Biol. Chem.* **2001**, *276*, 19066–19071.

43 Letai, A., Bassik, M. C., Walensky, L. D., Sorcinelli, M. D., Weiler, S., Korsmeyer, S. J. Distinct BH3 domains either sensitize or activate mitochondrial apoptosis, serving as prototype cancer therapeutics, *Cancer Cell* **2002**, *2*, 183–192.

44 Ricci, J. E., Munoz-Pinedo, C., Fitzgerald, P., Bailly-Maitre, B., Perkins, G. A., Yadava, N., Scheffler, I. E., Ellisman, M. H., Green, D. R. Disruption of mitochondrial function during apoptosis is mediated by caspase cleavage of the p75 subunit of complex I of the electron transport chain, *Cell* **2004**, *117*, 773–786.

45 Frank, S., Gaume, B., Bergmann-Leitner, E. S., Leitner, W. W., Robert, E. G., Catez, F., Smith, C. L., Youle, R. J. The role of dynamin-related protein 1, a mediator of mitochondrial fission, in apoptosis, *Dev. Cell* **2001**, *1*, 515–525.

46 Karbowski, M., Lee, Y.-J., Gaume, B., Jeong, S.-Y., Frank, S., Nechushtan, A., Santel, A., Fuller, M., Smith, C. L., Youle, R. J. Spatial and temporal association of Bax with mitochondrial fission sites, Drp1, and Mfn2 during

apoptosis, *J. Biol. Chem.* **2002**, *159*, 931–938.

47 Vepa, S., Scribner, W. M., Natarajan, V. Activation of endothelial cell phospholipase D by polycations, *Am. J. Physiol. (Lung Cell. Mol. Physiol.)* **1997**, *272*, L608–L613.

48 Goonesinghe, A., Mundy, E. S., Smith, M., Khosravi-Far, R., Martinou, J. C., Espoti, M. D. Pro-apoptotic Bid induces membrane perturbation by inserting selected lysolipids into the bilayer, *Biochem. J.* **2005**, *387*, 109–118.

49 Reers, M., Pfeiffer, D. R. Inhibition of mitochondrial phospholipase A2 by mono- and dilysocardiolipin, *Biochemistry* **1987**, *26*, 8038–8041.

50 Symonds, P., Murray, J. C., Hunter, A. C., Debska, G., Szewczyk, A., Moghimi, S. M. Low and high molecular weight poly(L-lysine)s/poly(L-lysine)–DNA complexes initiate mitochondrial-mediated apoptosis differently, *FEBS Lett.* **2005**, *579*, 6191–6198.

51 Jones, R. A., Poniris, M. H., Wilson, M. R. pDMAEMA is internalised by endocytosis but does not physically disrupt endosomes, *J. Control. Release* **2004**, *96*, 379–391.

52 Panyam, J., Zhou, W. Z., Prabha, S., Sahoo, S. K., Labhasetwar, V. Rapid endo-lysosomal escape of poly(D,L-lactide-*co*-glycolide) nanoparticles: implications for drug and gene delivery, *FASEB J.* **2002**, *16*, 1217–1226.

53 Lam, K. H., Schakenraad, J. M., Esselbrugge, H., Feijen, J., Nieuwenhuis, P. The effect of phagocytosis of poly(L-lactic acid) fragments on cellular morphology and viability, *J. Biomed. Mat. Res.* **1993**, *27*, 1569–1577.

54 Moghimi, S. M., Hunter, A. C., Murray, J. C., Szewczyk, A. Cellular distribution of nonionic micelles, *Science* **2004**, *303*, 626–627.

55 Iwaoka, S., Nakamura, T., Takano, S., Tsuchiya, S., Aramaki, Y. Cationic liposomes induce apoptosis through p38 MAP kinase–caspase-8–bid pathway in macrophage-like RAW264.7 cells, *J. Leukoc. Biol.* **2006**, *79*, 184–191.

56 Hollins, J., Omidi, Y., Akhtar, S. Drug delivery system induced gene expression changes in cells *in vitro* and *in vivo*, *J. Pharm. Pharmacol. (Suppl.)* **2005**, *57*, S85.

57 Forrest, M. L., Koerber, J. T., Pack, D. W. A degradable polyethylenimine derivative with low toxicity for highly efficient gene delivery, *Bioconjug. Chem.* **2003**, *14*, 934–940.

58 Thomas, M., Lu, J. J., Ge, Q., Zhang, C., Chen, J., Klibanov, A. M. Full deacylation of polyethylenimine dramatically boosts its gene delivery efficiency and specificity to mouse lung, *Proc. Natl Acad. Sci. USA* **2005**, *102*, 5679–5684.

59 Yamashita, A., Choi, H. S., Ooya, T., Yui, N., Akita, H., Kogure, K., Harashima, H. Improved cell viability of linear polyethylenimine through γ-cyclodextrin inclusion for effective gene delivery, *ChemBioChem* **2006**, *7*, 297–302.

60 Anderson, D. G., Akinc, A., Hossain, N. and Langer, R. Structure/property studies of polymeric gene delivery using a library of poly(beta-amino esters), *Mol. Ther.* **2005**, *11*, 426–434.

16
Nanoparticles for the Treatment of Alzheimer's Disease: Theoretical Rationale, Present Status and Future Perspectives

Gang Liu, Ping Men, George Perry and Mark A. Smith

16.1
Introduction

Alzheimer's disease (AD) is the most common form of dementia among people over the age of 65 years, progressing slowly from mild forgetfulness to the need for total care [1]. This disease is a devastating neurodegenerative disorder with progressive and irreversible damage to thought, memory and language. In America alone, 360 000 new AD cases were identified in 2000, bringing the total to 4.5 million, and the affected population will continue to increase as the population ages [2, 3]. It is expected that the number of people with AD in the US and worldwide will be 14 and over 100 million, respectively, by 2050 if no effective prevention and treatment become available [4, 5]. As such, the disease poses a heavy economic and societal burden, with associated annual costs of care over US$100 billion [1]. In addition, AD places an incalculable emotional and physical drain on families and caretakers. The ravaging effects of the disease call for efforts to prevent, forestall and reverse the disease. Unfortunately, despite much interest, an explicative etiology or a viable cure is not available. The current Food and Drug Administration (FDA)-approved drugs, targeted towards managing cognitive symptoms such as changes in memory and perception, provide only partial benefit to select patients and fall tremendously short as adequate means of therapeutic management. In addition to donepezil (Aricept®), tacrine (Cognex®), rivastigmine (Exelon®) and galantamine (Reminyl®), memantine (Namenda®) has recently won FDA approval for the treatment of AD. Unlike the acetylcholinesterase inhibitors (Aricept, Exelon and Reminyl) and the cholinesterase inhibitor (Cognex), memantine blocks excess amounts of glutamate that can damage or kill nerve cells. This new drug is becoming the first-line choice for advanced stages of AD [6, 7]. In contrast, the earlier approved drugs mentioned above work in the early stages of AD by delaying the breakdown of acetylcholine, vital for nerve cell communication [8, 9]. Although treatment with these drugs provides symptomatic improvements or delays in the progression of cognitive, behavioral and functional deficits, this treatment does not stop or reverse the progression of AD.

There are many medications used to treat AD, including anti-inflammatory drugs [10–14], antioxidants and vitamins [15–24], hormones [25–30], calcium

Nanotechnologies for the Life Sciences Vol. 10
Nanomaterials for Medical Diagnosis and Therapy. Edited by Challa S. S. R. Kumar

ISBN: 978-3-527-31390-7

channel blockers [31, 32], angiotensin-converting enzyme (ACE) inhibitors [33], cholesterol-lowering statins [34–39], ethylenediaminetetraacetic acid (EDTA) and clioquinol [40–44], gabapentin, lamotrigine, prazosin and risperidone [15, 45–47], vaccines against amyloid-β (Aβ) [48–52], and even a drug (rosiglitazone) to treat insulin resistance [53, 54]. Antihypertensive medications or regular exercise are also suggested to reduce risk for AD and dementia among people aged 65 years and older [55–57]. Other medications and substances being investigated at the present time include cannabinoids, physostigmine, nerve growth factor, β-sheet breakers, valproate, huperzine and nicotine [58–65]. New studies on the regulation of Aβ protein precursor translation by Phenserine [66, 67], the regulation of Aβ by neprilysin [68], inhibition of the activity of amyloid precursor protein (APP) secretases [69–74] and CD45 [75] show promising progress toward the identification of new therapeutic agents. Other studies, such as targeting glycosaminoglycans or metalloprotein attenuating compounds, new chelation agents, tau phosphorylation inhibitors, NF-κB blocker, gene delivery and human embryonic stem cells are under investigation [51, 59, 76–95]. Unfortunately, none of the treatments or drugs currently available can prevent or cure AD. Indeed, it is likely that more than one type of drug will be required to control AD. A recent study shows that Aricept and Namenda work in tandem to ameliorate symptoms of AD [96]. These studies reveal the complexity of the disease, and indicate a great need for a better understanding of AD pathophysiology and for more effective therapeutic agents.

In addition to the complex mechanisms of AD development, another obstacle to a deeper understanding and better treatment of AD is the presence of the blood–brain barrier (BBB). Many drugs of interest cannot gain access to the brain by crossing the BBB. Its presence may also negatively affect drug efficacy and tolerance because a large dosage of drugs must be applied to achieve therapeutic effectiveness. Nanoparticulate drug delivery offers an opportunity to overcome this impediment. Accumulating studies provide evidence that this delivery method can improve drug targeting of the central nervous system and drug penetration of the BBB, thus reducing drug toxicity and improving therapeutic efficacy [97–105]. Although there are many promising studies regarding nanoparticle delivery of drugs across the BBB to treat central nervous system diseases, only a few address treatment of AD [106–110]. In this chapter, the rationale for nanoparticulate drug delivery in the treatment of AD is presented, the current studies of using this delivery systems for AD treatment are reviewed and brief perspectives on this new approach are outlined.

16.2 Rationales: The Ability of Nanoparticles to Cross the BBB – A Useful Tool to Deliver Drugs into the Brain

16.2.1 Physiological Functions of the BBB

The BBB, constituted by endothelial cells of the cerebral vasculature together with perivascular elements such as astrocytes, pericytes and basement membrane, strictly limits and specifically controls the passage of substances between the blood and the cerebral extracellular space [111, 112]. Brain blood vessel endothelial cells characteristically have tight continuous circumferential junctions between them, thus abolishing any aqueous paracellular pathways between the cells [113]. Due to the presence of the tight junctions and the lack of aqueous pathways between cells, polar solutes and lipid-insoluble substances are greatly restricted in movement across the cerebral endothelium [114]; however, noncharged, small, lipophilic molecules may cross the BBB through the endothelial membrane by passive diffusion. This pathway is closely checked by efflux pump systems, which include the multiple organic anion transporter (MOAT), P-glycoprotein (P-gp) and multidrug resistance-associated protein (MDR) [114]. As a result, even molecules with a favorable lipophilicity, which should enable them to cross the endothelial cells, may be rapidly pumped back to the blood stream. These efflux pump systems can also effectively prevent anions, amphipathic organic cations or neutral compounds from entering the central nervous system [114, 115]. As the BBB contains biochemical systems consisting of enzymes, many drugs and blood-borne substances are specifically metabolized before entering the brain [116]. In order to allow essential substances to enter the brain and metabolic waste to leave, the BBB provides specific routes such as receptor and transporter systems to accomplish this transport [114, 117, 118]. Substances that can be absorbed or eliminated by the brain using these carrier-mediated transporter systems include amino acids, hexoses, monocarbonic substances, lipoproteins, insulin and purine compounds [99, 100]. Nanoparticulate drug delivery systems may utilize the low-density lipoprotein (LDL) receptor and the transferrin transcytosis systems to transport drugs into the brain [117, 118]. These transport pathways at the BBB are depicted in Fig. 16.1 [119].

16.2.2
Strategies for Drug BBB Penetration

Although the BBB's existence is absolutely necessary to isolate the central nervous system, with broad consequences for physiology, biology, pharmacology and pathology (most of which remain to be fully elucidated), the BBB represents an insurmountable difficulty for brain uptake of many therapeutic agents. These agents include some antibiotics, antineoplastic drugs and central nervous system-active therapeutics, especially neuropeptides [99, 100]. To overcome this obstacle, various strategies have been developed, which include osmotic opening of the brain endothelial cell tight junctions [120], prodrug preparation [121, 122], and utilization of carrier-mediated transporter systems such as antibodies [123–125], carbohydrate conjugation [126–129], viral and nonviral gene delivery vectors [130–132], peptide vectors [133, 134], liposomes [135–137], micelles [138, 139], and nanoparticles [100, 102, 103, 140–142]. While these studies have shown promise, most of these methods have been of limited use [133, 140]. For example, use of osmotic pressure to open tight junctions is a very invasive procedure and the opened junctions enable the passage of unwanted molecules. Prodrugs designed with higher lipophilicity and/or the ability to circumvent the efflux pump systems may enable them

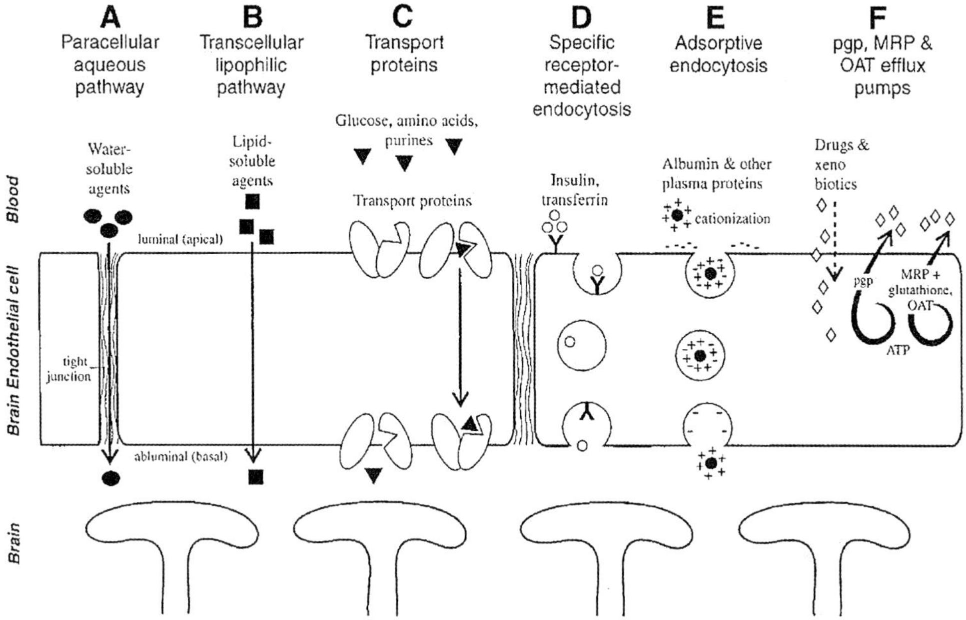

Figure 16.1. Physiological functions of the BBB (with permission after Ref. [119], see original article for full details).

more effectively to penetrate the BBB and transport into the brain, but this approach is not often possible [99]. It is common to use viral vectors for transfecting the expression of specific protein, but this drug delivery method shows certain disadvantages such as safety of both vector and expressed transgene, and stability and regulation of transgene expression [130]. Drugs conjugated to a natural protein molecule as carrier, so called vector-mediated drug delivery utilizing chimerical peptide technology, have shown effectiveness in brain delivery; however, the amount of transported drugs is limited because the maximal ratio of drug to carrier protein is usually about 1:1 [142]. Carbohydrate drug delivery, using sugar-mediated transporters in the BBB, may only work for drugs with small molecular sizes. On the other hand, colloidal drug delivery systems including liposomes, micelles and polymeric nanoparticles have become an important tool to transport drugs into the brain [100, 102, 103, 105, 124, 140]. Compared with other colloidal systems, the polymeric nanoparticle delivery system in particular has the advantage of easier preparation and higher stability in biological fluids [141, 143]. Controlled and sustained drug release is an added virtue of the nanoparticulate drug delivery systems [104, 141]. However, passive targeting of nanoparticles, which refers to the natural distribution of a drug delivery system in organs containing sessile actively phagocytosing cells such as liver and spleen, has to be solved, especially with parenteral administration [143–147]. This passive uptake represents a major problem for nanoparticle targeting to other parts of the body including the brain. Fortunately, studies have demonstrated that, by modification of the properties of nanoparticulate drug delivery systems, they can actively target specific organs or cells [141]. These modifications can be approached through various means that include (i) surfactant or macromolecule coating to alter system surface properties, (ii) conjugating specific antibodies to the system surface, (iii) changing the particle size and/or electric charge on the surface, and (iv) incorporating magnetite particles into the system and using a magnetic field for targeting. These techniques open the door for nanoparticulate drug targeting development and provide many possibilities to optimize particle-targeting delivery.

16.2.3
Preparation of Polymeric Nanoparticulate Drug Delivery Systems

Drugs delivered by polymeric nanoparticles can be dissolved, entrapped or encapsulated in the nanoparticles, forming a solid solution or dispersion. Also, the drugs can be adsorbed onto the particle surface or chemically attached (Fig. 16.2) [99, 100, 104]. Nanoparticles of 10–1000 nm, composed of either natural or synthetic macromolecules as therapeutic adjuvants and/or drug carriers, have potential for pharmaceutical and medical uses [99, 100, 141]. With respect to drug delivery to the brain, nanoparticles that are too small in size may result in reduced brain uptake due to rapid dissolution in the blood [101, 141]. Also, at smaller sizes it becomes difficult to obtain a monodispersed particle population [104]. On the other hand, larger size particles may suffer an increase in uptake by the mononuclear phagocytic system before reaching the brain, and increase the risk of blood capillary blockade and embolism, especially with intravenous administration [101, 148–150]. Nanoparticles in the region of 200 nm have, with surface modification, the ability to deliver drugs such as central nervous system-active substances and anticancer agents across the BBB, as shown by therapeutic efficacy [98, 100, 102, 141, 142, 151, 152].

Nanospheres (Fig. 16.2A), generally defined as a dense polymeric matrix in which drugs are dispersed, can be prepared via an emulsion and/or dispersion po-

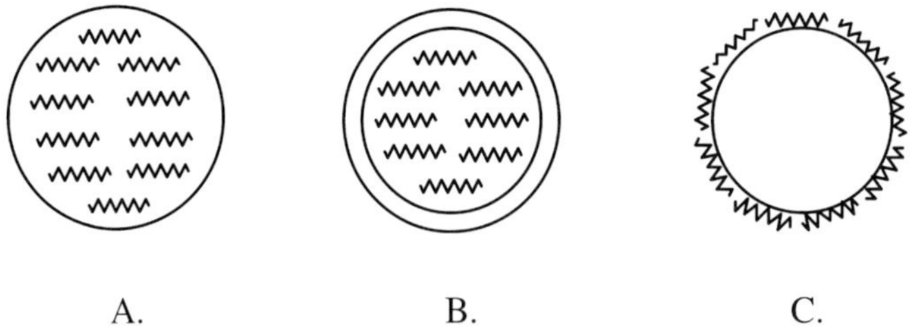

Figure 16.2. Different types of nanoparticulate drug delivery systems such as: (A) nanosphere with drug incorporated in polymeric matrix, (B) nanocapsule with drug surrounded by a thin polymeric envelope and (C) drug absorbed or chemically attached on the polymeric nanoparticle surface.

lymerization of monomers, depending on the nature of the polymers used [103, 110, 153] or by preformed polymers [103]. For example, poly(alkylcyanoacrylate) nanospheres, which are rapidly biodegradable and widely used for *in vivo* studies of drug delivery to the brain, are obtained by the emulsion polymerization process. In this method, droplets of water-insoluble monomers are emulsified in aqueous solution and stabilized by surfactants. The anionic polymerization reaction is initiated by the water itself and started in micelles after diffusion of monomers through the aqueous phase. Polymeric chains continue growing until prohibited by free-radical termination, then aggregate into fine particles. To incorporate them into nanospheres, drugs can be dissolved in the polymerization medium either before the monomer introduction or after its polymerization [104]. Using the solution-emulsification technique, nanosphere drug delivery systems can be obtained from preformed, well-defined macromolecules. This approach can avoid some potential problems associated with polymerization of monomers such as residual monomer and drug interaction and inactivation [104]. An example of this method is briefly described here. Polyester is dissolved in chloroform and this solution is mixed with an aqueous phase to form a uniform oil/water emulsion [154, 155]. Continuous emulsification under mixing is necessary to prevent organic droplet coalescence and to allow spontaneous solvent evaporation and particle formation [104]. To obtain particles with sizes less than 1 μm, ultrafine emulsification must be performed and microfluidization was recently used for this purpose [156]. An improved method based on desolvation has been developed, in which macromolecules can be precipitated from solution following the introduction of a third component or a nonsolvent miscible with the solution. Many nanoparticulate drug delivery systems are prepared using this technique or its modifications, as reviewed in [104].

Nanocapsules (Fig. 16.2B) are characterized by the presence of a liquid core surrounded by a thin polymeric shell. Interfacial deposition and emulsification diffusion are the two main approaches for nanocapsule preparation. The interfacial deposition procedure involves mixing a water-miscible organic phase containing oil (with or without lipophilic surfactant) with an aqueous solution containing hydrophilic surfactants. This approach can also use either preformed polymers or monomers that polymerize at the oil/water interface [104, 157, 158]; preformed macromolecules should first be dissolved in the organic phase (or in a phase that can dissolve them). After mixing the organic and aqueous phases, the macromolecules diffuse with the organic solvent and are stranded at the oil/water interface. If monomers are used, e.g. alkylcyanoacrylates, they are dissolved in ethanol and oil, then dispersed in water containing surfactants. Polymerization in the oil phase is initiated at the interface, resulting in the formation of nanocapsules [104]. The emulsification diffusion technique provides a simple approach to produce nanocapsules. It also has several advantages including a large choice, small solvent quantities, and controlled size and shell thickness [104]. Using this method, nanocapsules with an inner aqueous core can be prepared [159]. Emulsification diffusion is based on the initial formation of an oil/water emulsion, which contains a polymer, a drug and oil in the organic solvent, in an aqueous solution of a stabilizing agent. Then, displacement of the organic solvent into the external phase is conducted by adding excess water [104, 160]. It is worth noting that nanocapsules have higher drug-loading capacity and lower polymeric content than nanospheres.

Drugs can also be adsorbed onto the surface of preformed nanoparticles (Fig. 16.2C) by mixing the particles with the drugs in solutions. The absorptive capacity is dependent on several factors such as the polymer, the drug and the medium pH [141, 161]. In some cases, chemical binding of drugs to nanoparticle surface (Fig. 16.2C) may be necessary as described later in our studies. The covalent bonds can be formed through chemical reactions between functional groups present in the drugs and the particles [141, 162]. Apart from polymeric nanoparticulate drug delivery, drug nanocrystals (nanosuspensions), lipid–drug conjugate nanoparticles and lipid nanoparticles are also widely used and take advantage of high drug-loading capacity. Their features, including preparation and medical application, are reviewed in Refs. [101, 102].

The nanoparticle sizes and their distribution can be evaluated by elastic light scattering. This can also be done using scanning or transmission electron microscopy (SEM, TEM), which may provide information about nanoparticle structure [103, 104, 141]. Measurement of the ζ potential is often made to characterize the nanoparticle surface properties such as electrical surface potential, drug location and particle stability [103, 104, 141]. Some more commonly performed characterizations such as drug loading and releasing capacities are summarized in Refs. [103, 141].

16.2.4
Possible Mechanisms by which Nanoparticles Cross the BBB

There is a little doubt that nanoparticles conjugated with antibody against transferrin receptor (TfR) or ligands such as thiamine are transported across the BBB by utilizing TfR or thiamine-mediated transport systems, respectively [123, 142, 148, 163]. However, the mechanisms by which nonantibody or non-ligand-coated nanoparticles deliver drugs into the brain are not fully understood. Surface coating of nanoparticles, e.g. using poly(ethylene glycol) (PEG) [164–166] and some poloxamers [100, 167, 168], and especially with polysorbates [151, 152, 169, 170] and apolipoprotein E and/or B (ApoE and/or B) [100, 167, 171], plays a critical role in nanoparticle-mediated drug transport across the BBB. The coating with these materials apparently alters the natural blood opsonization process of the nanoparticles, thus reducing macrophage recognition in the liver and spleen. This effect consequently increases the nanoparticle blood half-life and extravasation to non-reticuloendothelial systems including the brain [142].

To further elucidate the role of coating, patterns of human plasma protein absorption on the nanoparticle surface have been examined after incubation of nanoparticles in the plasma. Analyses were performed by separating the nanoparticles and releasing the absorbed plasma proteins followed by two-dimensional polyacrylamide gel electrophoresis (2-D PAGE). These analyses showed that polysorbate-coated nanoparticles preferentially absorb ApoE on their surface. In contrast, no such adsorption was found after incubation of noncoated nanoparticles or nanoparticles coated with many other surfactants [100, 167, 168]. Moreover, in *in vivo* studies on central nervous diseases, only drugs delivered via polysorbate or ApoE (and/or B) coated nanoparticles have therapeutic effectiveness and ApoE-deficient animals exhibit a reduced therapeutic response compared to controls [172]. These findings strongly indicate the involvement of ApoE and B in nanoparticle-mediated drug transport across the BBB and the surfactant on the particle surface may serve as an anchor for ApoE [171]. It is well known that ApoE plays a key role in the transport of LDLs into the brain, and the LDL receptor exists on the BBB [118, 173–177]. Also, lipoprotein particles containing ApoE and ApoA-I are found in human cerebrospinal fluid [178]. After the polysorbate coated nanoparticles absorb ApoE from blood plasma, it is very possible that nanoparticles mimic LDL particles and interact with the LDL receptor. Thus, brain capillary endothelial cells take up the nanoparticles by receptor-mediated endocytic processes [99]. Endocytosis of nanoparticles coated with polysorbate has been demonstrated in both *in vitro* and *in vivo* studies [169, 171, 172, 179, 180]. Significant and rapid uptake of polysorbate-coated nanoparticles by endothelial cells is found at an incubation temperature of 37 °C, whereas only minimal uptake is observed for noncoated nanoparticles [169, 172]. Further evidence shows that uptake is inhibited at lower temperatures (4 °C) or by cytochalasin B (a potent phagocytic uptake inhibitor) pretreatment [169, 172].

After nanoparticle endocytotic uptake, the nanoparticles may be transcytosed through the brain blood vessel endothelial cells since LDL transcytosis across the BBB has been demonstrated [118]. It is also possible that the drug is released from the nanoparticle in the endothelial cells and diffuses into the brain [99]. Several other mechanisms involved in nanoparticle-mediated drug transport across the BBB have been suggested [99]. For example, opening of the tight junctions between the brain endothelial cells by nanoparticles could occur, and the drug could then penetrate through the opened junctions either with the particles and/or in free form. Studies show that inulin spaces, an indicator of the tight junction opening, are increased only by 10 and 99% after 10 and 45 min, respectively, in rats treated with polysorbate-coated nanoparticles. In contrast, the increase of these spaces is 1000–2000% by osmotic methods [180–184]. These studies indicate that the coated nanoparticles increase the volume available to the intravascular inulin; however, they do not disrupt the BBB significantly. The slight opening of the tight junctions caused by the particles may result from folding-up of the cell membrane accompanied by endocytotic events or from an increase in fluid-phase endocytosis of inulin associated with the internalization of the nanoparticles [99]. It is known that some surfactants such as polysorbate show the ability to inhibit P-gp present in the brain endothelial cells and responsible for the multidrug resistance [185–187]. This inhibition of the efflux pump by surfactant could be responsible for nanoparticle-mediated drug delivery into the brain [99]. It may be significant that nanoparticle brain penetration increases when brain pathologies such as cancer [188, 189] and allergic encephalomyelitis [164] occur. The potential toxicity of the polysorbate-coated nanoparticle to the brain endothelial cell has also been suggested to facilitate particulate drug delivery across the BBB [170]. In fact, many studies show that there are no significant signs of toxicity associated with this process [99, 190, 191]. However, it should be mentioned that nanoparticle surface charges may affect BBB function and studies show that cationic nanoparticles pose a toxic effect on the BBB, while the neutral or anionic nanoparticles at low concentrations do not disrupt BBB integrity [192]. Lipid coating may prevent the toxic effect of the ionically charged particles to the endothelial cell and enable the particles to cross the endothelial cell layer via transcytosis with no or little degradation [99, 193].

The preparation of the drug–nanoparticle system is relatively easy and in general the system is very stable. It is also important that there is a large variety of ways to improve the bioavailability and specific targeting of the particulate drug delivery systems and to minimize the toxicity of the systems. Based on the nanoparticle-mediated transport technology, a novel approach was recently developed in our laboratories [109]. This approach allows the nanoparticles not only to deliver metal chelation agents into the brain for the treatment of AD and other metal-mediated neurodegenerative diseases, but also to bring the toxic metals out of the brain, thus increasing therapeutic efficacy and limiting metal-chelate toxicity. This principle may be useful for other biomedical applications in the delivery of drugs to disease targets and/or depletion of toxicants using nanoparticle transport technology.

16.3
Status: Nanoparticle Targeting Transport of Therapeutic Agents for Potential Treatment of AD

The technology of nanoparticulate drug delivery has been developed for many years, and has been demonstrated not only to improve drug safety and efficacy, but also to lead to new therapeutic agents. However, its application in the treatment of AD has only appeared recently in very limited studies, due perhaps to the complexity of the disease pathogenesis and to an incomplete understanding of the mechanisms by which nanoparticles deliver drugs across the BBB. A lack of collaboration between scientists in differing, but relevant, disciplines may also impede application. In order to understand how to advance nanoparticle application, a review of recent developments in nanoparticulate drug delivery for AD treatment is now presented.

16.3.1
Nanoparticle Targeting of Aβ to Deliver Potentially Therapeutic Agents

Senile plaques in the brain, composed mainly of insoluble deposits of Aβ peptide with 39–43 amino acids, are a major hallmark of AD [69]. Studies, albeit controversial studies, show that the accumulation of Aβ derived from APP by proteolytic cleavage are neurotoxic and believed to be responsible for the neurodegeneration observed in AD [194, 195]. Therefore, preventing and reversing the Aβ accumulation is an important pharmacological target in AD treatment and several potential therapeutics such as β-sheet breakers [196, 197], regulators of APP translation [66, 198–200], inhibitors of APP secretases [69–74], vaccines against Aβ [48] and metal chelators [42, 76–78] have been developed and tested. As many potential drugs are electrically charged hydrophilic and/or large size molecules, a lack of ability to enter the brain may hamper their treatment efficacy. Although nanoparticles serving as a vehicle can provide a valuable approach to carry many otherwise impermeable drugs across the BBB, the tissue distribution of nanoparticles and drug release are not fully elucidated. However, a recent study showed that the nanoparticles as well as delivered drugs are present predominantly in microglia and also in neurons [106], where the Aβ accumulation may occur and cause neurotoxicity [69, 194, 195, 201].

In this study, core–shell latex particles containing Thioflavin-(TfT) as a marker for fibrillar Aβ were synthesized by aqueous polymerization of butylcyanoacrylate and seeded onto polystyrene cores filled with TfT, then collected by ultrafiltration. The cores were prepared using emulsion polymerization of styrene in aqueous ethanol solution containing TfT and purified by dialysis against deionized water [202]. The formed core–shell nanoparticles are reported to be sphere-shaped with a diameter of about 90 nm, as demonstrated by SEM and TEM (Fig. 16.3A and B). The nanoparticles were injected into the hippocampus (AP $= -1.7$ mm, L $= 1$ mm and DV $= 2$ mm, relative to bregma) of C57B6 mice after anesthesia. Three days postinjection, the animals were transcardially perfused with 4% paraformaldehyde and 0.5% glutaraldehyde in 0.1 M phosphate buffer (pH 7.4). The brains were then fixed in 4% paraformaldehyde overnight and coronal vibratome 50-μm sections of the dentate gyrus were cut. Using the oxygen-enriched photoconversion method [203], the TfT was photoconverted into an electron-dense material to localize the TfT-containing nanoparticles in the brain. After washing, osmication and dehydration, the brain tissue blocks were embedded in Ducurpan and semithin or ultrathin sections were prepared. Aggregated nanoparticles were detected in dentate granule cells and vacuolated cytoplasm in the vicinity of nanoparticle aggregates using light microscopy (Fig. 16.3C). Using TEM, this study also found clustered nanoparticles in microglia (Fig. 16.3D) and in neurons (Fig. 16.3E and F). Moreover, vacuolated inclusions and amorphous structures with moderated electron density were found in both cell types. The core–shell structure of the nanoparticles and the TfT delivered from the nanoparticles were further confirmed by TEM at higher power (Fig. 16.3F).

This study indicates that nanoparticles and the nanoparticle-delivered drugs may target Aβ in the brain, and provides strong evidence to further support the possibility of nanoparticle drug delivery for AD treatment with increased efficacy and lowered toxicity.

16.3.2
Nanoparticulate Antioxidant Delivery to Increase Efficacy against Aβ-mediated Oxidative Stress

One of the neurotoxic effects of Aβ is to induce lipid peroxidation [204–207] that can lead to the formation of cytosolic free radicals and reactive oxygen species

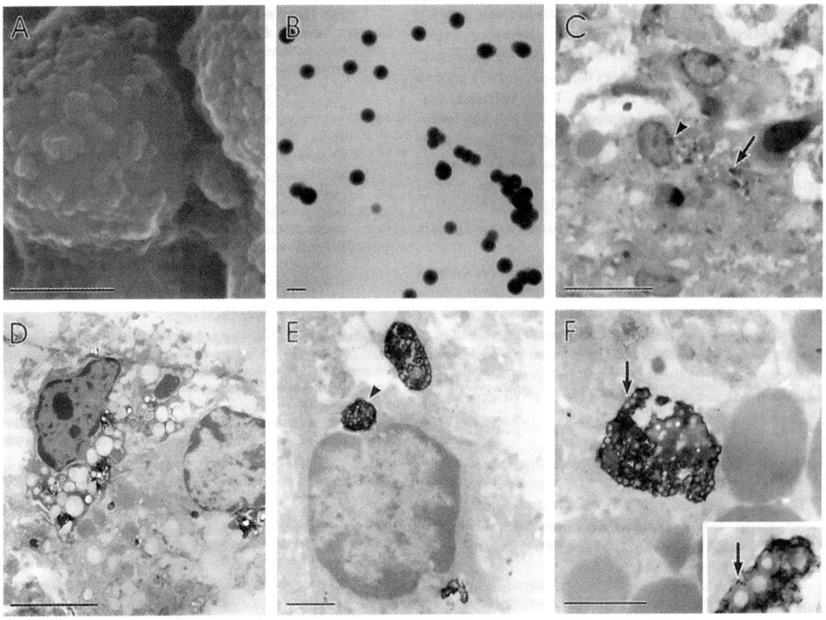

Figure 16.3. (A) The TfT-containing latex nanoparticles with a diameter of about 90 nm (SEM analysis). (B) Image of the nanoparticles on a Pioloform-coated slot grid (TEM analysis). (C) Light microscopic analysis of a section from fixed and plastic-embedded mouse dentate gyrus after 3-day intrahippocampal injection of nanoparticles and following photoconversion of TfT. Arrows and arrowheads indicate representative adducts of photoconversion. (D–F) TEM analyses of cells in the dentate gyrus after 3-day TfT particle injection and photoconversion. (D) Analyses show clusters of aggregated particles incorporated in microglia (left) and in a granular cell (right). The vacuolar inclusions and amorphous structures with moderate electron density are found in both cells. (E) Photoconverted, aggregated latices are located in the cytoplasm of a granule cell and an arrowhead marks the same cluster in (C). (F) High magnification of intraneuronal particle clusters. Photoconverted electron-dense materials surround the most core–shell-type microspheres (arrows), indicating TfT delivered by the nanoparticles. Scale bar: 1 μm for A, E and F; 0.1 μm for B; 20 μm for C; 5 μm for D. (With permission after Ref. [106].)

(ROS) [208]. Free radicals and ROS are highly active and can cause oxidative damage to all classes of biomolecules found *in vivo*, which include cellular lipids, nucleic acids, proteins and carbohydrates [209, 210]. This is believed to be a key factor in AD development [211, 212]. With aging, the endogenous antioxidant systems may gradually lose their ability to provide adequate neuroprotection and fail to compensate for the increased ROS formation [213]. Thus, antioxidant intake may provide protective effects against oxidative neurodegeneration [214, 215]; however, as discussed before, one impediment to the success of AD antioxidant therapy is the BBB that may limit appropriate antioxidant concentrations within the brain, thus diminishing its efficacy. Reduced efficacy may also result from the inability of antioxidants to reach specific targets. It is known that vitamin E, a lipophilic antioxidant, shows mixed results in the treatment of AD [19, 216–218]. Furthermore, although vitamin E is capable of preventing $A\beta$-induced ROS in cultured cells, the cells have to be treated with vitamin E before $A\beta$ exposure, or treated simultaneously with vitamin E and $A\beta$. In contrast, antioxidants that can enter the cytosolic compartment of these cells give neuroprotection even if applied after $A\beta$ exposure [219–221]. This limitation is suggested to be a consequence of the lipophilic nature of vitamin E. The lipophilicity of vitamin E reduces its access to the hydrophilic cytosolic compartment, thus minimizing its ability to quench cytosolic ROS, as well as ROS produced from antecedent membrane oxidative damage [208]. It is possible that nanoparticle-mediated drug delivery cannot only send antioxidants into the brain more effectively, but also facilitate targeting specific locations, hence increasing their antioxidative effects.

A recent study [108] showed that vitamin E encapsulated in nanoparticles possesses an improved ability to quench $A\beta$-induced ROS even if applied about 1 h after $A\beta$ exposure; in contrast, nonencapsulated vitamin E does not have such a capability. This study indicates that although vitamin E can protect against $A\beta$-mediated ROS, it lacks the ability to access the secondary ROS, which radiates into the cytosolic compartment following prior $A\beta$ exposure, due to the lipophilicity of vitamin E [205–208, 213, 221].

In this study, nanoparticles containing vitamin E were prepared by mixing PEG 1500 decanyl polymer and vitamin E in chloroform solution. After removal of the solution, the mixture of PEG polymer and vitamin E was redissolved into water to induce self-assembly by vortexing. Resultant vitamin E-containing nanoparticles were purified by dialysis against water to remove unencapsulated vitamin E [222]. To examine the antioxidative efficacy of vitamin E encapsulated in PEG polymer nanoparticles, SH-SY-5Y human neuroblastoma cells were used. The cells were cultured in DMEM with 10% fetal calf serum and differentiated for 7 days with 10 μM retinoic acid. Cell cultures were exposed to $A\beta$ (25–35) for 2 h. Vitamin E and vitamin E encapsulated in nanoparticles were added to additional cultures either simultaneously with, or 1 h following, the addition of $A\beta$. To monitor the intracellular peroxide concentrations as an index of ROS, 2′7′-dichlorofluorescein diacetate was added to cultures for 20 min and then cultures visualized under fluorescein UV optics. The results indicate that vitamin E prevents an increase in ROS induced in differentiated neuroblastoma cells following $A\beta$ treatment only if applied prior to or simultaneously with $A\beta$ (Fig. 16.4). In contrast, vitamin E encapsulated in nanoparticles can prevent ROS even 1 h after $A\beta$ exposure. The protective effectiveness was same as application of an equivalent concentration of nonencapsulated vitamin E simultaneously with $A\beta$ exposure (Fig. 16.4). Nanoparticles without encapsulated vitamin E do not have neuroprotective ability. This result that the nanoparticles can deliver vitamin E into cytosol, thus increasing vitamin E antioxidative capability to quench cytosolic ROS, indicates that nanoparticle-mediated delivery may serve as a valuable tool for targeted transportation of antioxidants or other therapeutic agents for the treatment of AD. However, this result needs to be confirmed using normal neuro-cells and *in vivo* studies.

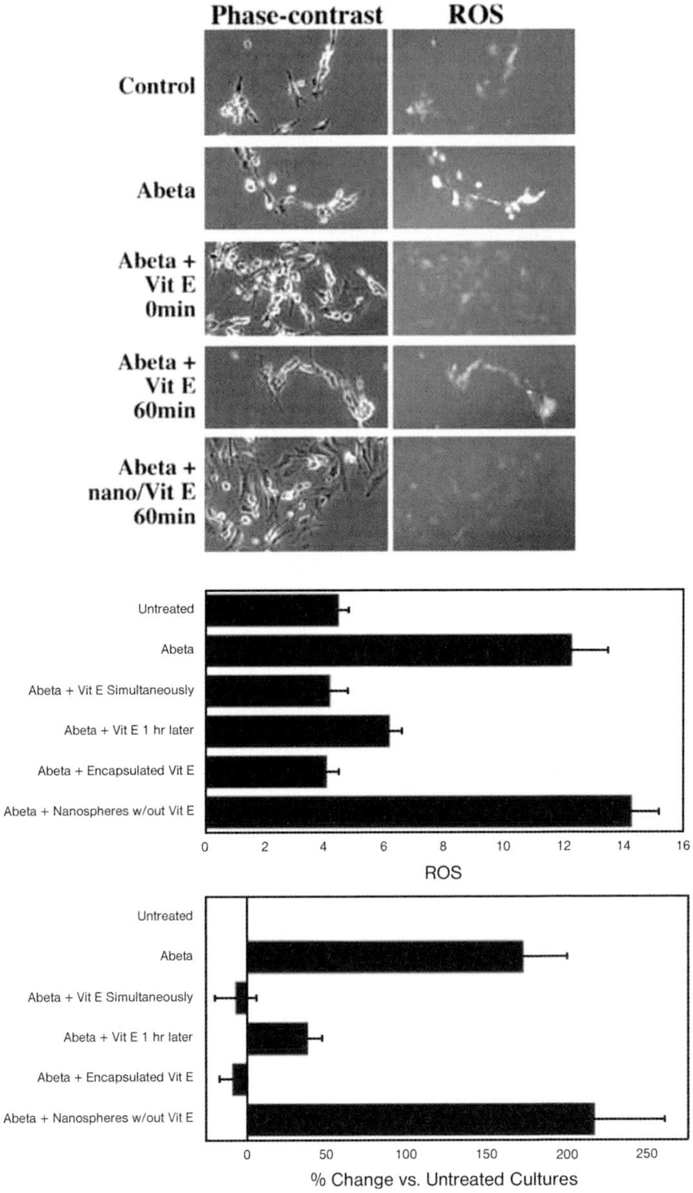

Figure 16.4. Nanoparticulate drug delivery improves the efficacy of delayed application of vitamin E against Aβ-induced ROS. Panels present phase-contrast and fluorescent images of SH-SY-5Y neuroblastoma cells examined for ROS before (control) or 1 h following addition of Aβ with or without vitamin E or nanoparticulated vitamin E at the indicated intervals. Note the increase in ROS following addition of Aβ. Note that this increase is prevented by simultaneous, but not delayed, addition of vitamin E, yet is prevented by delayed addition of nanoparticulated vitamin E. The accompanying graphs present the mean 2′7′-dichlorofluorescein diacetate (DCF-DA) fluorescent intensity ± standard deviation of at least 50 cells. Values are also presented in the percent change in fluorescent intensity for each condition versus untreated controls (the mean intensity for controls are defined as 1). (With permission after Ref. [108].)

16.3.3 Nanoparticle Delivery of Copper Chelator for Preventing and Reversing Aβ Deposition

Copper and zinc are essential in the body, but their excess is toxic. Accumulation of these metals in the central nervous system is believed to contribute to the oxidative stress and inflammation associated with AD [223–225]. Studies reveal that Aβ has the ability to bind copper and zinc with high affinity, and that these metals may, in turn, mediate the Aβ deposition in AD [226–233]. The evidence showing the association of these metals with Aβ deposition is that simple coincubation of Aβ from postmortem AD brain tissue with copper and/or zinc chelators results in resoluble aqueous Aβ [234]. This association is also demonstrated by other findings from both animal experimental studies and human clinical trails [42, 43, 77, 80, 235]. Severe changes in some metal distributions are found in the brain of AD patients compared with healthy controls [225]. Concentrations of copper and zinc are significantly elevated in amyloid plaques and neuropil regions in the brains of AD patients (about 400 μM for copper and 1 mM for zinc) compared to the healthy brains (70 μM for copper and 350 μM for zinc) [226, 236]. Treatment of APP transgenic mice (an AD mouse model) with the copper and zinc chelator, clioquinol, was shown to reverse Aβ deposition [237], leading to a near halving of Aβ deposition in the animal brain, compared with sham-treated controls [77]. The reduction of Aβ deposition was accompanied by a significant improvement in behavior and general health parameters. Clinical studies also demonstrate that AD patients treated with clioquinol show significantly slowed cognitive deterioration and lowered plasma Aβ levels [42, 43]. There were no indications of toxicity associated with chelation treatment for either experimental or clinical studies. These results suggest a potential approach that can prevent and treat AD by targeting the interaction of copper and zinc with Aβ using chelation agents. However, an implication of clioquinol toxicity in an epidemic of subacute myelo-optic neuropathy in Japan has forced withdrawal of the drug from the market. For neuro-chelation therapy, the BBB represents a major hurdle for most available chelation therapeutics [109, 238]. To gain a deeper understanding of the roles of metals in AD development and to make progress in AD chelation therapy, there is a great need to develop more effective and safer chelation agents. Nanoparticle-mediated drug transport as an alternative means of drug delivery to the brain may provide an opportunity for such development [109, 110].

A recent study showed that D-penicillamine, a specific copper chelator for Wilson's disease (copper overload), can be successfully conjugated to nanoparticles through covalent bonding [107]. The nanoparticles have a long circulating ability in the blood and have been shown to be taken up by the brain *in situ* and *in vivo* without significant changes in BBB integrity or permeability [107, 147, 239, 240]. The nanoparticles containing 1,2-dioleoyl-*sn*-glycero-3-phosphoethanolamine-*N*-[4-(*p*-maleimidophenyl)butyramide] (MPB-PE) or 1,2-dioleoyl-*sn*-glycero-3-phosphoethanolamine-*N*-[3-(2-pyridyldithio)propionate] (PDP-PE) were synthesized by warming microemulsion precursors composed of emulsifying wax and surfactants such as Brij 78 or Tween 80 [107, 241]. These core components of the nanoparticles are considered nontoxic and nonirritant materials [107, 241]. This study shows that the stability of these nanoparticles is greatly affected by the final concentration of surfactants, and the use of 4–6 mM of Brij and 2 mg mL^{-1} of emulsifying wax can form the most-stable particles. A further increase in Brij concentration leads to the formation of less-stable nanoparticles. This study provides a simple preparation method for stable nanoparticles that can anchor chelation agents with them. In the preparation procedure, emulsifying wax was first melted and then stirred at 50–55 °C after adding deionized and filtered water in order to form a homogenous milky slurry. The surfactant was then added with continuously stirring. After microemulsions were formed, the mixture was cooled to room temperature to produce nanoparticles. The formed particles were characterized using a Coulter N4 Plus Sub-micron Particle Sizer. To provide functional sites on the nanoparticles for covalent conjugation with the sulfhydryl group in D-penicillamine, various amounts of MPB-PE or PDP-PE were incorporated into the particles by adding different concentrations of MPB-PE or PDP-PE in chloroform. The solvent was removed by evaporation before adding the emulsifying wax. The diameter of the formed nanoparticles was less than 100 nm with a narrow size range. Size is influenced by the MPB-PE or PDP-PE concentration, although not significantly [107]; however, if the concentration of MPB-PE or PDP-PE reaches 15% w/w, the microemulsion cannot be formed and the size of the resulting particles is relatively large. This study suggests that the hydrophilic heads of MPB or PDP are exposed on the nanoparticle surface while the lipophilic dioleoyl groups in both MPB-PE and PDP-PE insert into the lipophilic core of nanoparticles [107, 241, 242]. This molecular orientation, leaving the functional groups on the nanoparticle surface, is favorable for chelator conjugation. D-Penicillamine contains a sulfhydryl group and can either react with MPB-PE or PDP-PE to form thioether or disulfide bonds, respectively, which link the chelator and nanoparticles [243–245] (Scheme 16.1). The reactions were conducted at room temperature in approximately neutral aqueous solution (pH 6.5 for MPB-PE containing particles; pH 8.0 for PDP-PE containing particles). Nitrogen gas was used to prevent atmospheric oxygen from disturbing the conjugation reaction. The chelator-conjugated nanoparticles were purified by gel permeation chromatography using a Sephadex G75 column. The short-term stability of the chelator-nanoparticles containing PDP-PE was tested by particle size measured at intervals. The stability of the particles to salt or serum was also examined: D-penicillamine-conjugated nanoparticles are stable at 37 °C for 30 min in several different biologically compatible media such as saline, 10 mM phosphate-buffered saline solution (PBS), 10% lactose and 10% fetal bovine serum in saline. The linkage of disulfide bonds between D-penicillamine and PDP-PE incorporated into particles is also quite stable in PBS at pH 6, 7 and 8. Both D-penicillamine conjugated PDP-PE nanoparticles and MPB-PE nanoparticles are stable when treated with simulated serum, thus being suitable for chelator delivery *in vivo*. D-penicillamine conjugated MPB-PE nanoparticles are more stable than D-penicillamine–PDP-PE conjugated ones because of the formation of a more stable thioether linkage of D-penicillamine–MPB compared to the less stable disulfide link between D-penicillamine and PDP [245].

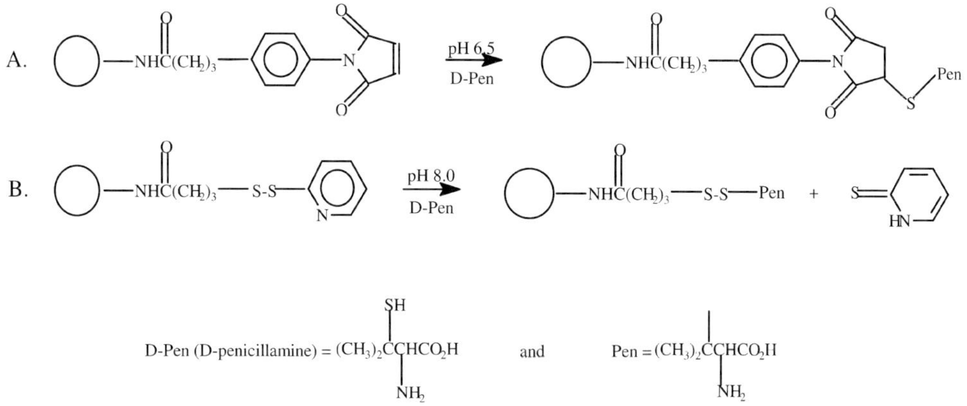

Scheme 16.1. Conjugation reactions of D-penicillamine to (A) MPB– and (B) PDP–nanoparticles. (Minor modification from Ref. [107].)

It should be mentioned that linkages using the sulfhydryl group of D-penicillamine totally deprive its copper binding activity. This, however, may provide a targeting chelation approach by which D-penicillamine can chelate copper within the brain only if it is released from nanoparticles, thus minimizing chelator toxicity in other places. To restore the chelation activity of D-penicillamine, it was proposed that the release could take place when the D-penicillamine conjugated nanoparticles react with reducing agents such as glutathione under normal physiological conditions. In cells, glutathione is the most concentrated nonprotein thiol and its concentration is about 1–6 mM [107, 246]. In order to test this hypothesis, a reducing agent, dithiothreitol (DTT) was used to incubate with the D-penicillamine-conjugated nanoparticles. After a 1-h incubation at 37 °C in water at pH 6.7, D-penicillamine was partially released from PDP-PE-containing particles by DTT, indicating cleavage of the disulfide bond between D-penicillamine and PDP. Although this result indicates the possibility of D-penicillamine release from nanoparticles by reducing agents, further studies are warranted such as increasing the releasing efficacy in both *in vitro* and *in vivo* investigations. As Aβ is known to bind metals with high affinity and its aggregates are associated with copper, the ability of D-penicillamine, D-penicillamine–nanoparticles and D-penicillamine released from nanoparticles to reverse copper-mediated Aβ aggregates were evaluated in this study. The Aβ deposition is obtained from incubation of Aβ(1–42) with cupric chloride in Tris buffer (pH 7.4) for 1 h at 37 °C and then incubated with those chelation agents for a further 1 h at 37 °C. To determine the redissolved copper Aβ aggregates in the soluble fraction, the samples were centrifuged (10 000 g for 20 min) and the supernatants were analyzed for protein concentrations using the Pierce method [107]. In order to release D-penicillamine from nanoparticles, the chelator-conjugated PDP-PE-containing particles were incubated in basic aqueous solution (0.1 M, sodium hydroxide) at 45 °C for 1 h. Under these conditions, the

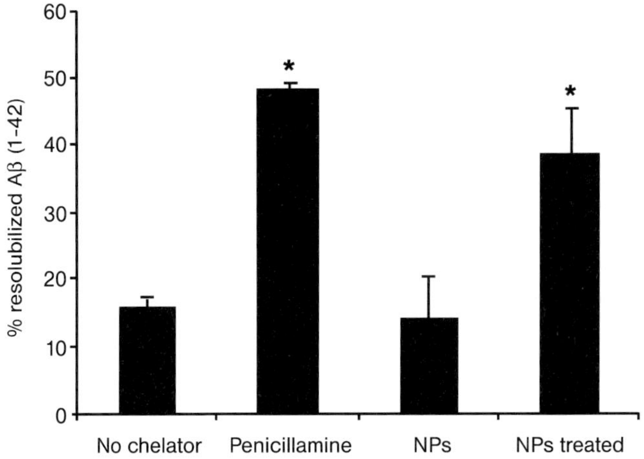

Figure 16.5. Experiments of Cu-Aβ(1–42) aggregate resolubilization. The treatments are control (no chelator), D-penicillamine, D-penicillamine conjugated to PDP-NPs (NPs) and D-penicillamine conjugated to PDP-NPs (NPs) after being treated in 0.1 N NaOH at 45 °C for 1 h (NPs treated). An asterisk indicates that the values for D-penicillamine and treated NPs are not different from each other, but are significantly higher than that of no chelator and NPs. (With permission after Ref. [107].)

disulfide bond of D-penicillamine–particle linkage is more labile [243, 247]. Results show that the D-penicillamine conjugated to nanoparticles can no longer resolubilize the insoluble Aβ aggregates mediated by copper while the free D-penicillamine does. D-Penicillamine released from nanoparticles restores its ability to effectively resolubilize the copper–Aβ aggregates (Fig. 16.5).

This study provides a method to prepare D-penicillamine-conjugated nanoparticles that may have the ability to cross the BBB without adverse effects on cerebral perfusion, BBB integrity and permeability [107, 239, 240]. This study also shows that the nanoparticle-delivered chelator may be released after targeting and resolubilize metal-mediated Aβ deposition, thus being able to prevent and treat AD. D-Penicillamine is used to treat Wilson's disease, wherein copper is accumulated initially in the liver and eventually in other organs including the brain [248]. D-Penicillamine can conveniently be administered orally and its effect on urinary copper excretion is dramatic [249]. However, development of D-penicillamine intolerance is frequently seen among patients and the ability of D-penicillamine to cross the BBB is not clear [107, 250, 251]. Thus, nanoparticle D-penicillamine delivery may increase the brain targeting of D-penicillamine and reduce its intolerance. Although more *in vivo* studies are needed and this chelation may be imperfect due to the possible accumulation of the chelator–metal complexes in the brain, this study provides evidence to support nanoparticle drug delivery as a potential approach for AD management.

16.3.4
Nanoparticle Transport of Iron Chelators and Metal Chelator Complexes Into and Out of the Brain, Respectively

16.3.4.1 Increased Levels of Various Metals in the Brain of AD Patients

It is already known from the above that copper and zinc play an important role in the accumulation of Aβ deposits, which in the form of preamyloid lesions and neuritic plaques, are one of the key neuropathological features of AD [107, 195]. Other metal ions are also known to be toxic and may be potential risk factors for AD. For example, excess iron in the body is extremely dangerous even though it is an essential nutrient for virtually all mammalian cells. Studies demonstrate that in individuals with primary or secondary iron overload disease, extreme iron accumulation in organs is recognized as a contributor to the manifestation of other diseases, including cardiac, hepatic, endocrine and bone disorders as well as cancer [252–254]. Even moderate elevations of iron in the body, which may be associated with age, is believed to play a significant role in causing diseases such as atherosclerosis, cancer, diabetes, dementia and osteoporosis [210, 255–260]. The toxic effects of excess iron and copper result largely from their ability to catalyze free radical generation through the Fenton reaction or Haber–Weiss reaction [209]. Iron also plays a key role in the regulation of cellular functions such as respiration, oxygen transport, DNA synthesis, nitric oxide formation and other redox reactions [209]. Therefore, iron levels in particular biological compartments have a close association with various disease processes. Although the etiology of AD is not well understood, accumulating evidence supports the hypothesis that oxidative stress generated by various mechanisms may be among the major risk factors that initiate and promote neurodegeneration [16, 211, 261–263]. Compared with other tissues, the central nervous system may be particularly susceptible to oxidative damage [264, 265]. Since iron and copper catalyze oxidation reactions, the likelihood that an oxidation reaction will take place is probably increased by regional concentrations of these metals [209, 223]. Substantial studies show that the metabolism of iron is involved in AD and that the concentration of iron, like copper, in the brain of AD patients is elevated [224, 266–270]. The iron levels in neuropil of human brain are 39 $\mu g\ g^{-1}$ for AD patients and 19 $\mu g\ g^{-1}$ for controls determined by microparticle-induced X-ray emission [236, 271–273]. Studies also demonstrate that iron can induce Aβ aggregation at acidic pH [232], a pathological value found in inflammatory disorders. Another metal ion, aluminum, has also received attention in AD [274], although its role in AD development has not yet been convincingly demonstrated. Nonetheless, aluminum is found in high concentrations in both senile plaques and intra-neuronal fibrillar tangles in the brains of subjects with AD, which suggests that this metal may be involved in the etiopathology of AD [224, 269, 275, 276]. Aluminum, unlike iron and copper, is unable to participate in redox cycles of electron transfer reactions due to a fixed oxidation state of 3+ in biological systems, but growing evidence suggests that it can act synergistically with iron to increase free radical damage [264, 277]. A recent study shows that accumulated aluminum in the central nervous system modulates Aβ formation and deposition [278]. As mentioned early, evidence already shows that copper [211, 236, 279–283] and zinc [229, 236, 269, 284, 285] are implicated in the development of AD. In the AD brain, the concentration of copper is elevated in the rim of senile plaques and the concentration of zinc is significantly elevated in senile plaques. Taken together, these studies indicate that the environmental conditions in AD, exacerbated by imbalances in several metals, have the potential of catalyzing and stimulating free radical formation [109], and of facilitating Aβ aggregation and deposition [286], thus enhancing neurodegeneration.

Simultaneously elevated levels of multiple metals promoting oxidative damage to the brain present a complex system of pathophysiology that is not yet fully understood. Despite this complexity, metal dysregulation may in fact be the Achilles' heel of AD, opening a door for chelation therapy. A chelator, regardless of synthetic or natural origin, may have high affinity for one metal ion, but it can also undesirably chelate other metals in the body leading to serious side-effects. The affinity for multiple metals such as aluminum, copper, iron and zinc may pose useful rather than detrimental effects since various metals are implicated as oxidative instigators. Perhaps this is why desferrioxamine (DFO), a specific iron chelator also with high affinities for aluminum, copper and zinc, has demonstrated some therapeutic benefits for patients with AD. Thus, simultaneous chelation of several excess metals in the AD brain may provide a novel approach for safe and effective treatment of AD.

16.3.4.2 **Problems with Iron Chelators for Simultaneous Removal of Multimetal Ions for Treatment of AD**

Iron chelation therapy shows potential as an alternative treatment for AD by simultaneously chelating multiple excess metals. However, this promising approach is hindered by chelator toxicity and/or poor bioavailability, especially BBB impenetrability. A few clinically available iron chelators also negatively affect the development of iron chelation therapy for this disease.

DFO and deferasirox (ICL670, Exjade®) are the only iron chelation drugs approved by the FDA for iron overload disease (Fig. 16.6). Their therapy can promote iron excretion, and has led to great improvements in the quality and duration of life of patients who suffer from β-thalassemia and other refractory anemias [287,

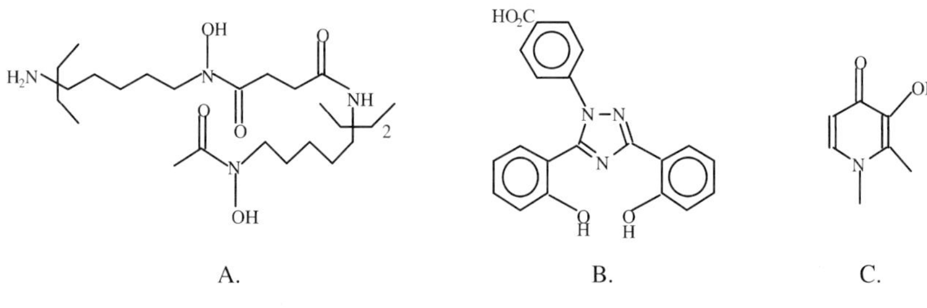

Figure 16.6. Chemical structures of (A) DFO, (B) ICL670 and (C) L1.

288]. Although there are no reports yet on deferasirox for potential treatment of AD, DFO is found to significantly slow the progression of AD in one clinical trial [289]. In this study, only the chelation of aluminum was examined, but it is possible that the therapeutic effect may also have been due to removal of iron since DFO preferably chelates iron forming 1:1 complex (DFO, a hexadentete chelator) [290, 291]. DFO also has an appreciable affinity for copper and zinc [290, 292]. The affinity constants of DFO for Fe(III), Al(III), Cu(II), and Zn(II) are 30.6, 22.0, 14.1 and 11.1 (log K), respectively [293]. In this particular clinical study, copper and zinc were not monitored. Thus, it is unclear if the DFO treatment simultaneously removes these metals and/or whether such a removal plays a role in slowing the clinical progression of AD. However, 2 years after the initial publication, a verbal report at the International Conference on Alzheimer's Disease (Padua, Italy, 1992) provides evidence that iron and zinc concentrations are decreased in a postmortem analysis for DFO-treated patients [271, 290]. This clinical study, in addition to the follow-up report, provides strong evidence that multiple metal accumulations in the brain may be key contributors to AD development and simultaneous removal of them mitigates disease progression. Aside from effective chelation of several metals, DFO also inhibits nigrostriatal degeneration induced by 6-hydroxydopamine [294]. Unfortunately, DFO has serious side-effects including neurotoxicity and neurological changes [223, 274, 295–300]. Furthermore, DFO is poorly absorbed by the gastrointestinal tract and rapidly degrades after administration [301]. Therefore, it requires long subcutaneous administration to yield significant iron excretion [287, 291, 302]. Moreover, some studies show DFO does not easily penetrate the BBB due to its hydrophilic nature [303], although this point remains open to debate [304]. Indeed, some penetration may occur due to a compromised BBB via lesion sites [303]. Nonetheless, the neurotoxicity and difficulty of administration and delivery present serious hindrances to the use of DFO for AD treatment.

Another iron chelator, L1 (deferiprone or 1,2-dimethyl-3-hydroxyl-4-pyridinone), is a bidentate chelator and approved in Europe, but not in the US, for iron or aluminum overload diseases [305–307] (Fig. 16.6). It chelates iron and aluminum with very high stability constants of $\log \beta = 37$ and 32, respectively. Since it can also chelate copper and zinc with appreciable efficiencies ($\log \beta = 19.6$ for copper and 13.5 for zinc), L1 is capable of simultaneously chelating these metal ions. L1 virtually lacks affinity for calcium or magnesium; therefore, unlike many other chelators, L1 has no toxic effects due to chelation of these essential metals [307]. L1 also has high oral activity and BBB penetration because of its lipophilicity and relatively small molecular size. However, its use is limited because of serious side-effects [308, 309]. Moreover, studies show that L1 lacks the ability to remove iron from the brain [304] probably due to strong hydrophilicity of the iron–L1 complex. Additionally, there is no carrier-mediated transport system available to remove the complex from the brain. Other L1 derivatives with higher lipophilicity also have the ability to cross the BBB and complex iron in the brain, but they also possess considerable neurotoxicity [295, 298, 308]. Deferasirox is a tridentate iron chelator with oral bioavailability, which is currently approved by FDA for treatment of transfusional iron overload in thalassemia. However, its long-term profiles are not yet available [288]. Furthermore, its lipophilic nature like L1 may raise questions concerning potential toxicity in AD treatment.

Thus, the use of the currently available iron chelators to simultaneously remove several excess metals in the brain of AD is limited because of their toxicity and/or poor transference across the BBB. Most bi- or tridentate iron chelators with small molecular weight and high lipophilicity have the ability to penetrate the BBB, but show toxicity [310]. On the other hand, hexadentate iron chelators are considered better candidates for chelation therapy than bi- and tridentate ones because of their lower toxicity before and after chelation [310], but they have difficulty penetrating the BBB [122, 304, 310] due to their hydrophilicity and relative high molecular weight. One strategy to increase the BBB penetration is by enhancing the lipophilicity and lowering the molecular weight of the iron chelators, but this is believed to increase toxicity [311]. In addition, the increase in lipophilicity of iron chelators will decrease the solubility in aqueous solution with probable a decrease in bioavailability [309]. Also, it is possible that some lipophilic chelators which normally should cross the brain endothelial cells are rapidly pumped back into the blood stream by extremely effective efflux pumps, as mentioned before [99]. Many promising attempts have been made to develop iron chelators with oral activity (membrane penetration) and low toxicity for the treatment of iron overload disease [312–347]. This leads to the hope, that if successful, some iron chelators may also be suitable for simultaneous chelation of several excess metal ions for AD treatment.

Some existing USP drugs such as clioquinol (iodochlorohydroxyquin) that possess chelation properties and BBB penetration ability have shown therapeutic benefits in AD [42, 43]. Clioquinol is an antibiotic agent and chelator with high affinity for zinc and copper, and less for calcium and manganese [77]. As mentioned before, oral administration of clioquinol in APP transgenic mice with advanced Aβ deposition leads to a significant reduction of Aβ deposition in the mouse brain compared to nontreated animals. This reduction of Aβ deposition is reported to be associated with copper and zinc chelation by clioquinol [77]. In clinical studies with clioquinol, the clinical rate of cognitive decline is slowed in a subset of AD patients compared with controls [42, 43]. Interestingly, the zinc concentration in plasma of AD patients treated with clioquinol was significantly higher than that of controls although no parallel change in plasma copper concentration has been indicated [43]. However, further investigation with this new approach is hindered by clioquinol toxicity. It should also be mentioned that this type of chelator generally may have a low affinity for iron and would be toxic at doses needed for sufficient iron removal [293]. EDTA has also shown some clinical improvements in the patients with dementia, including AD, in a small clinical trial and a large retrospective study [40, 41].

Currently, chelators with a hydroxyquinoline backbone or with high lipophilicity show BBB permeability and neuroprotective potential in experimental studies [78–80]. However, the toxicity of these chelators related to their lipophilicity has not been studied. Other therapeutic approaches are being explored to overcome the impediment of the BBB. For example, a prochelator has been designed for the purpose of easily entering the BBB. The functional groups of the prochelator are then activated by enzymatic or nonenzymatic reactions after they have entered the target organ [121]. Another example is to use simple inorganic silicate that can form very stable complexes with many metals and probably has the ability to enter the BBB [348]. A newly developed copper chelator (tetrathiomolybdate) for Wilson's disease is also suggested as a potential treatment for AD [85, 349]. Iron chelators designed with near-optimal lipophilic/hydrophilic balance of the free chelator and iron complex for the purpose of passage into and out of the cell have been synthesized and studied [309]. However, no clear-cut clinical evidence for a beneficial effect of these chelators in AD has been demonstrated and new approaches are necessary.

16.3.4.3 Nanoparticle Transport Technology to Improve Chelation Therapy for AD

The use of nanoparticles to transfer chelators represents an exciting therapeutic option that may prove safer and more effective for chelation therapy. There are four advantages to this particle chelator delivery approach: (i) the chelators need not be lipophilic to cross the BBB, (ii) the lipophilic character of the chelators no longer contributes to potential toxicity and (iii) hydrophilic hexadentate iron chelators with large molecular weights may be used, as previously demonstrated with nanoparticle technology [152, 350, 351]. Finally, the most important advantage is that the chelator conjugated to nanoparticles has the potential to leave the brain after complexing metals, thus further improving chelation safety and efficacy.

For metal chelation to be effective, the chelators must be capable of leaving the brain with the corresponding complexed metal ions. Many chelators are unable to prevent iron from catalyzing free radical formation via Fenton or Haber–Weiss reaction even though the chelators can complex iron tightly [352]. Thus, the metal–chelator complexes in the brain may still catalyze free radical formation, with possible new adverse effects on the brain. In fact, there is no systematic solution for this problem and finding the solution remains a big challenge in chelation therapy for AD as well as other neurodegenerative diseases associated with metal toxicity. If the nanoparticles are not biodegradable within the brain and can mimic lipoprotein particles by preferentially absorbing ApoA-I, known to facilitate the removal of particles from the brain [99, 353], the same carrier mediated transport systems of LDL will be able to carry the metal-complex nanoparticles out of the brain. This is in contrast to lipophilic chelators that can enter the brain, but when complexed with metals, are unable to cross the BBB due to a change in their lipophilicity. For example, the distribution coefficient (DC) of free L1 determined in *n*-octanol/Tris–HCl buffer system is 0.24, but when complexed with iron is down to about 0.001 [354]. Therefore, although L1 can reportedly penetrate the BBB, it fails to remove iron from the brain [304]. Obviously, the use of nanoparticles may provide a novel approach to transport of metal–chelator complexes out of the brain. The use of nanoparticles conjugated with chelators to mimic lipoprotein particles and transfer iron chelators into and out of the brain through selected apolipoprotein absorption not only provides a useful means of improving the efficacy and minimizing the toxicity of chelation therapy, but also provides insights into the mechanisms of AD development. This novel approach can also open a new area for nanoparticle technology to clean unwanted substances from diseased sites.

16.3.4.4 Experimental Descriptions

To conjugate nanoparticles covalently, iron chelators must have a functional group to react with an active moiety on the particle surface. The functional group introduced into the iron chelators should not possess adverse effects on the chelator–metal binding. Synthetic methods to produce a series of iron chelators with such functional side-chains have been developed [126, 127, 355]. The metal binding properties of these chelators and some biological properties such as the *in vitro* ability to remove iron from tissue sections of AD brains and from ferritin (an important protein for iron storage) have been examined [126, 355]. Some of these chelators can remove iron from ferritin and are capable of depleting iron from tissue sections of the AD brain more effectively than DFO. Methods for conjugation of various iron chelators to nanoparticles have also been developed. The particles can be made of biocompatible synthetic or natural macromolecules [99, 100, 356] with functional groups such as amino and carboxyl groups on their surface for covalent bonding with chelators [162, 243]. After conjugation, the amounts of chelator that conjugate to the particles and the ability of the chelator–particle systems to bind iron are determined. Interestingly, some bidentate iron chelators converted to hexadentate chelators after conjugation to particles because the particles provided backbone linkages. This phenomenon greatly improved the metal binding stability and lowered toxicity associated with metal–chelator complexes. The human plasma protein absorption patterns on iron chelator particle systems are examined using 2-D PAGE technology [99, 357]. These studies show that the protein absorption pattern on the iron chelator particle systems is totally different from that of the human plasma proteins. Through changing the system surface properties, such as chelators and surfactants, the chelator–particle systems can preferentially absorb ApoE. With the same kind of changes, it is also found that the chelator–particle systems after binding metals can preferentially absorb ApoA-I. Such preferential absorptions allow the systems to mimic the ApoE or ApoA-I nanoparticles and to cross the BBB through LDL transport mechanisms [350, 353]. Uniform coating of the systems with ApoE, B or A-I can also be achieved by overcoating of these apolipoproteins, which may enable the systems to cross the BBB with high efficiency [171]. These studies indicate that iron chelator–nanoparticle systems have the potential to enter the brain and bring excess metals out of the brain, thus effectively preventing metal-associated oxidative damage. The results also show the potential to obtain chelator–nanoparticle systems with optimal surface properties via changing chelators, linkages, coating materials and nanoparticles with different surfaces. These findings are promising and suggest that this novel method of chelation may prove useful in the treatment of AD. More studies are warranted to demonstrate the chelation efficacy of the chelator–nanoparticle systems, to evaluate the system toxicity and to optimize their capability to cross the BBB. Some experiments are briefly described as follows.

16.3.4.4.1 **Synthesis of Iron Chelators with Functional Groups for Nanoparticle Conjugation** Iron chelators containing active functional groups have been synthesized. The preparation procedures are simple and product yields are good. The synthetic chelators have been characterized using standard methods such as

^{1}H-nuclear magnetic resonance (NMR), mass spectrometry (MS), ultraviolet (UV)-vis and elemental analysis. Their preparations are briefly given below.

2-Methyl-*N*-(2′-aminoethyl or 3′-aminopropyl)-3-hydroxyl-4-pyridinone (MAEHP and MAPHP) The chelators were synthesized using a modified procedure as previously described (Scheme 16.2) [358, 359]. In brief, 3-hydroxyl-2-methyl-4-pyranone and benzyl chloride were mixed in a solution of water and methanol in the presence of NaOH. The mixture was refluxed for several hours with magnetic stirring. After removing methanol under vacuum, water was added and the 3-benzyloxy-2-methyl-4-pyranone was extracted with methylene chloride. The methylene chloride solution was then washed with 5% NaOH aqueous solution followed by water and dried over $MgSO_4$. The product was obtained after evaporation of the solvent under vacuum and then reacted with 1,2-diaminoethane or 1,3-diaminopropane in aqueous ethanol solution at room temperature. After 1 week, solvents and residual diamines were evaporated under vacuum and the residue was dissolved in chloroform, washed with water and dried with Na_2SO_4. After removing solvent, methanol was added and the pH is adjusted to 1 with HCl. 1-(2′-Aminoethyl)-3-benzyloxy-2-methyl-4-pyridinone or 1-(3′-aminopropyl)-3-benzyloxy-2-methyl-4-pyridinone was precipitated as dihydrochloride salt and collected by filtration. The pure products were obtained by recrystallization from methanol and ether, and further reacted with BBr_3 (1.0 M CH_2Cl_2 solution) in CH_2Cl_2. The mixture was stirred overnight at room temperature under a nitrogen atmosphere. Water was added and stirring was continued for an additional 4 h. The aqueous phase containing the MAEHP or MAPHP was separated and evaporated under vacuum. The crude MAEHP or MAPHP was purified through recrystallization from an ethanol/ether solution.

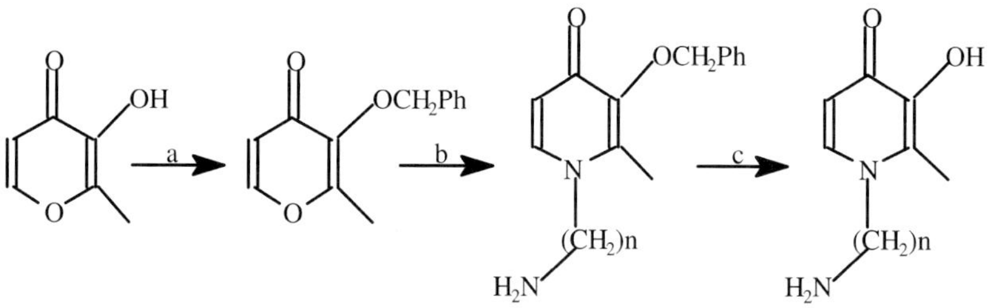

Scheme 16.2. (a) Benzylchloride/NaOH. (b) $NH_2(CH_2)_nNH_2$, $n = 2, 3$. (c) BBr_3 in CH_2Cl_2 at 4 °C or hydrogenation with H_2/Pt on active carbon. (With permission after [359].)

2-Methyl (or ethyl)-*N*-(2′-hydroxyethoxy)methyl-3-hydroxyl-4-pyridinone (MHEMHP or EHEMHP) The chelators were synthesized using established methods (Scheme 16.3) [355, 360]. Briefly, 3-benzyloxyl-2-alkyl-4-pyridinone was synthesized as reported in reference [358] with a minor modification. First, to protect the 3-hydroxyl group, 2-alkyl-3-hydroxyl-4-pyranone with benzyl chloride was refluxed under alka-

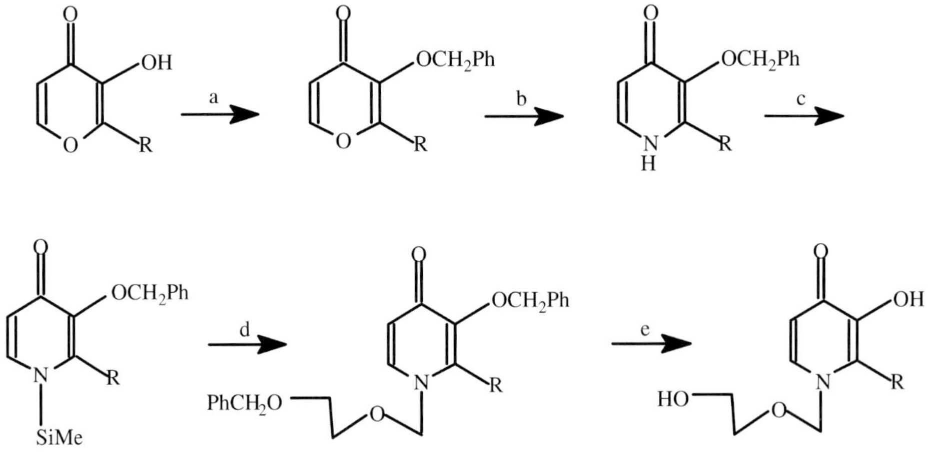

Scheme 16.3. R = Me and Et. (a) $PhCH_2Cl$/NaOH/refluxing/6 h. (b) NH_4OH/room temperature/48 h. (c) Hexamethyldisilazane, chlorotri-methylsilane. (d) Benzyloxyethoxy-methylchloride, trimethylsilyl trifluoro-methanesulfonate in 1,2-dichloroethane. (e) H_2, Pd/C, AcOH in 95% EtOH. (With permission after [355].)

line conditions, as described above. Then, the ring oxygen of 3-benzyloxyl-2-alkyl-4-pyranone was replaced by a nitrogen atom via a substitution reaction with aqueous ammonia at room temperature for 48 h. The 3-benzyloxyl-2-alkyl-4-pyridinone was silylated in hexamethyldisilazane under refluxing and nitrogen gas for 2 h. After evaporation of the solvent under vacuum, the residue was redissolved in 1,2-dichloroethane and then benzyloxyethoxymethylchloride that could be replaced by (2-acetoxyethoxy)methyl bromide [361] was added in the presence of a catalytic amount of trimethylsilyl trifluoromethanesulfonate ($SnCl_4$ could also be used as catalyst in the alkylation reaction, but might result in separation difficulties and low yields) [362]. The resulting mixture was stirred at room temperature for 4 h and then treated with an aqueous solution saturated with sodium bicarbonate. After removing the aqueous phase, the organic phase was dried with sodium sulfate and the solvent evaporated under vacuum. Both of the protection groups were removed simultaneously by hydrogenation with H_2/Pt on activated carbon in acidic aqueous ethanol at room temperature for 24 h or by BBr_3 in CH_2Cl_2 at 4 °C [306, 363, 364]. The chelators were obtained in pure form after recrystallization from a 1:1 solution of CH_3Cl:MeOH. To evaluate whether the linked (2′-hydroxyethoxy)methyl moiety affected the geometry of the iron binding site in the chelators, molecular and crystal structures of EHEMHP were determined by X-ray crystallographic analysis. A piece of colorless crystal (0.33 mm × 0.33 mm × 0.11 mm) formed in methanol/ethyl acetate solution was used for X-ray measurement with an Enraf-Nonius CAD-4 diffractometer equipped with a graphite monochromator of MoK_α (0.71073 Å) [355]. An Oak Ridge Thermal Ellipsoid Plot (ORTEP) stereoview of the EHEMHP molecular structure is depicted in Fig. 16.7.

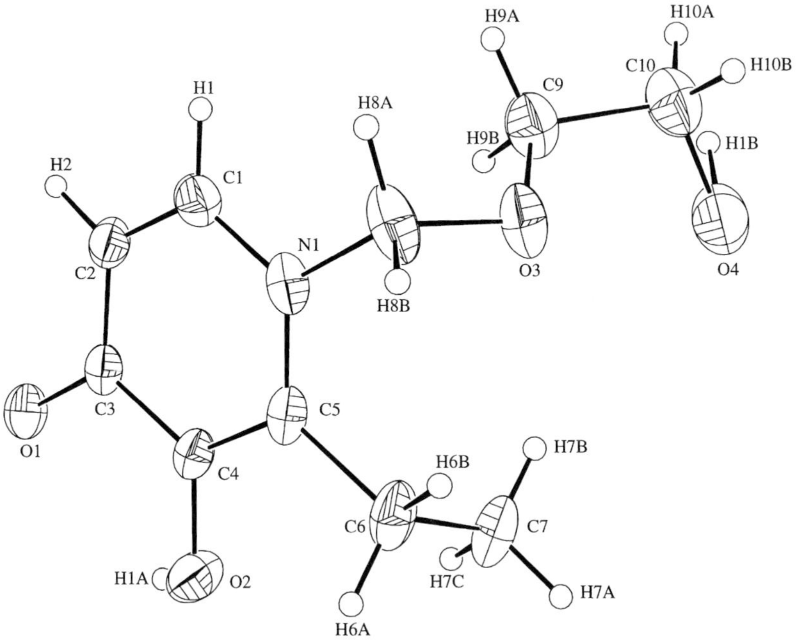

Figure 16.7. ORTEP stereoview of chelator EHEMHP. (With permission after Ref. [355].)

2-Methyl-3-hydroxy-1-(β-D-ribofuranosyl or ribopyranosyl)-4-pyridinone (MHRFP or MHRPP) The synthesis of these chelators was similar to that of MHEMHP and EHEMHP above using a modified Hilbert–Johnson reaction (Scheme 16.4) [127, 360, 365]. In brief, after silylation the silylated 3-benzyloxyl-2-methyl-4-pyridinone

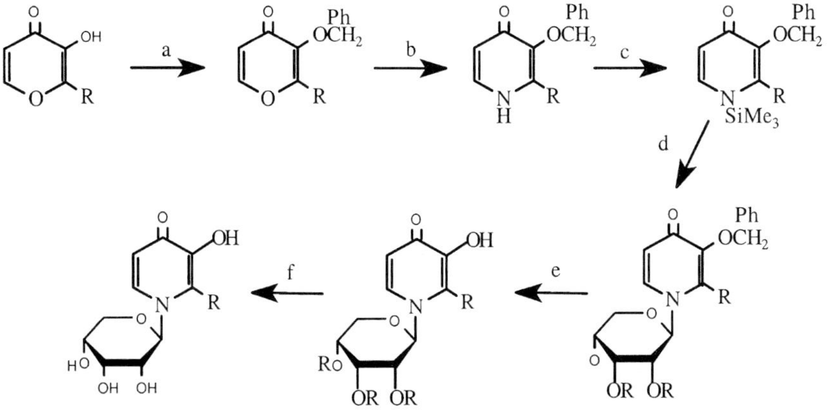

Scheme 16.4. R = Me. (a) $PhCH_3Cl/NaOH/$refluxing/6 h. (b) NH_4OH/room temperature/24 h. (c) $Me_3SiCl/Me_3SiNHSiMe_3$. (d) A prototype, 1,2,3,4-tetra-*O*-acetyl-β-D-ribopyranose/trimethylsilyltrifluoromethanesulfonate. (e) H_2, Pd/C in aqueous methanol with acetic acid. (f) NH_3-MeOH solution. (With permission after [127].)

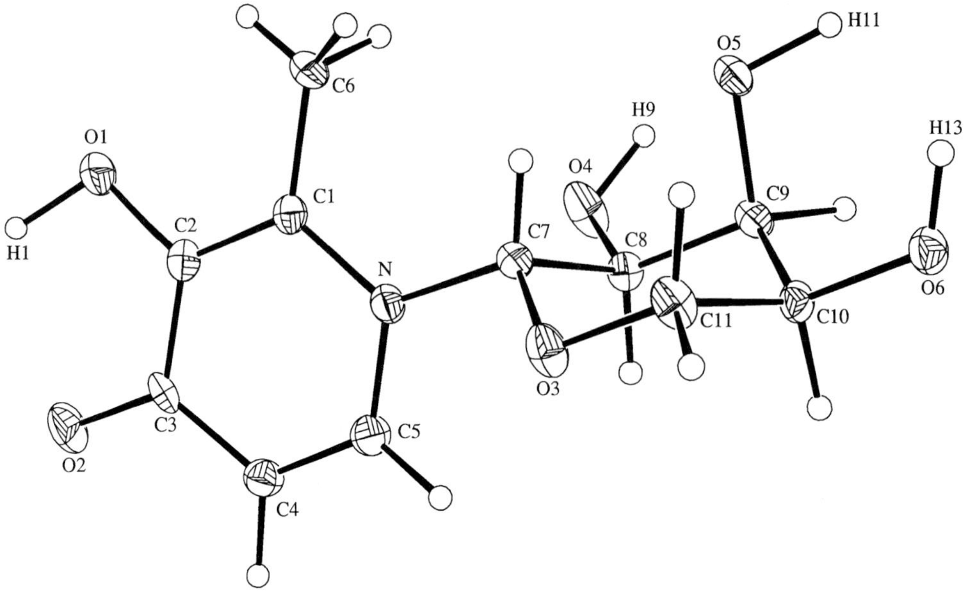

Figure 16.8. The molecular structure of chelator MHRPP. (With permission after Ref. [126].)

was alkylated by β-D-ribofuranosyl or ribopyranosyl groups. The benzyl protection group on the pyridinone was first removed by hydrogenation under H_2/Pt on activated carbon in acidic aqueous methanol [306, 363, 364]. Then, the hydroxyl groups of the sugar moiety were deprotected by basic hydrolysis in an NH_3/methanol medium overnight at room temperature. The chelators were obtained in pure form after recrystallization from a 1:1 solution of CH_3Cl:MeOH. Molecular and crystal structures of MHRPP were determined using X-ray crystallographic analysis to further evaluate the effects of the linked sugar moiety on the iron binding geometry in the chelators. An ORTEP stereoview of the molecular structure of MHRPP is depicted in Fig. 16.8.

16.3.4.4.2 **Ability of the Chelators to Complex Iron**

Reaction of Chelators with Iron Ions in Buffer Solution The reaction between iron and chelators was indicated by a color change of buffer solutions (Tris buffer, 25 mM, pH 7.5, 22 °C) containing chelators following ferric iron [$Fe(NO_3)_3$] addition to the solution. The chelators and iron formed purple complexes with the chelator:iron stoichiometry of 3:1 [126, 355]. The typical visible absorption λ_{max} for free chelators and chelator–iron complexes was about 280 and over 450 nm, respectively (shown in Fig. 16.9). The stoichiometry was determined spectrophotometrically by titration of chelators in Tris buffer with freshly prepared iron solution

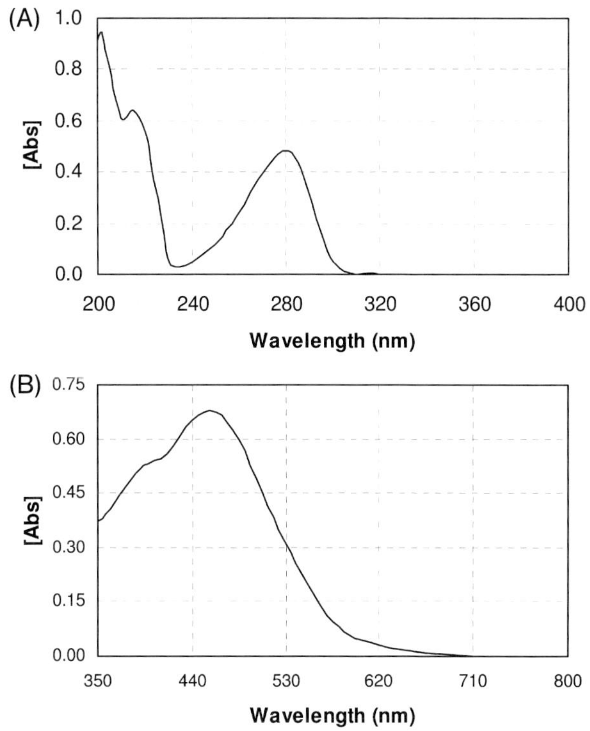

Figure 16.9. A. The UV-vis absorption of free MAPHP ($\lambda_{max} = 281$ nm, $\varepsilon = 1.43 \times 10^4$ Mcm^{-1}) and B. The absorption of iron–MAPHP complexes ($\lambda_{max} = 455$ nm, $\varepsilon = 3.02 \times 10^3$ Mcm^{-1}).

at room temperature. The iron solution was added gradually and the change in absorbance of the chelator–iron complexes was monitored by UV-vis spectrophotometery after the chelation reaction reaches equilibrium. Typical titration curves using MHEMHP and EHEMHP are presented in Fig. 16.10 and the endpoints of the titration indicate the formation of chelator:iron (3:1) complexes [355].

Iron Mobilization by Chelators from Ferritin The removal of iron from ferritin was studied by incubation of horse spleen ferritin with chelators in Tris buffer (25 mM, pH 7.5). Each chelator was mixed with the ferritin and incubated at 37 °C. The changes in absorbance of the iron–chelator complexes were measured spectrophotometrically at different time intervals. The concentrations of iron–chelator complexes were estimated from ε_{max} values at the wavelength of λ_{max} of the complexes [126, 355]. The kinetics of the iron release was investigated for periods up to 72 h. Figure 16.11 shows the iron removal from ferritin by MHEMHP and EHEMHP as a prototype compared with DFO.

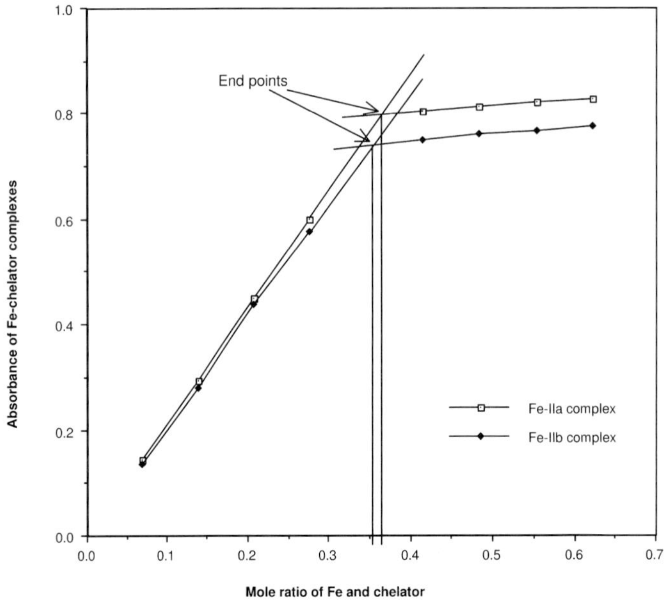

Figure 16.10. Titration of MHEMHP (IIa) and EHEMHP (IIb) with iron. (With permission after [355].)

Iron Mobilization by Chelators from AD Brain Sections *In Vitro* The ability of chelators to remove iron from brain sections was examined using a histochemical method [366]. Briefly, hippocampal tissues were collected from Alzheimer's disease patients, then fixed in methacarn (methanol:chloroform:acetic acid 6:3:1) overnight at 4 °C. After fixation, the tissues were placed in 50% ethanol, dehydrated in ascending concentrations of ethanol and embedded in paraffin. Six 6-μm sections of the tissues were cut and then mounted on silane-coated slides (Sigma). The sections were deparaffinized with two changes of xylene (10 min each) and rehydrated through graded ethanol/TBS (50 mM Tris, 150 mM NaCl, pH 7.6). Then, 40 μL of each chelator in PBS at various concentrations were applied to each section and incubated over night at 37 °C. The sections were rinsed thoroughly with TBS. After a 2-h incubation at 37 °C in 7% potassium ferrocyanide in aqueous hydrochloric acid (3%), the sections were rinsed with Tris buffer and subsequently incubated in 0.75 mg mL^{-1} 3,3′-diaminobenzidine and 0.015% H_2O_2 for 5–10 min. Finally, sections were dehydrated through graded ethanol and cover slip.

16.3.4.4.3 **Conjugation of MAPHP and DFO with Nanosphere or Microsphere Particles** A variety of covalent bonds such as amido, amino, ether and thioether can easily be formed for conjugation of chelators and particles, depending on the existing functional groups located on chelator side-chains and on the surface of

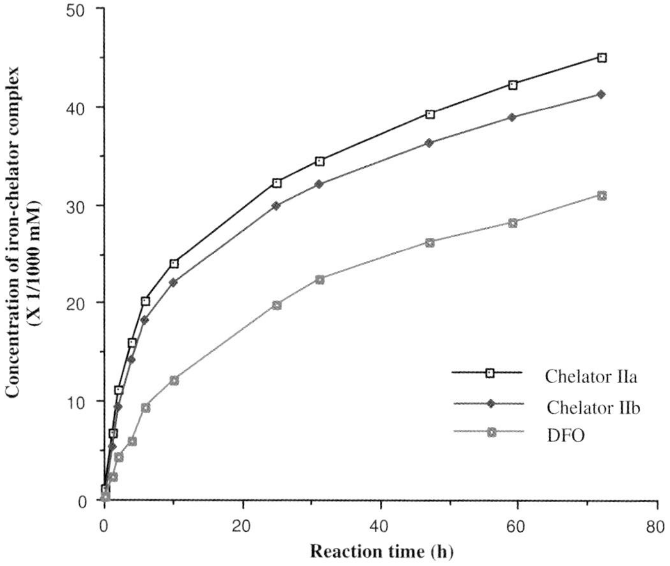

Figure 16.11. Removal of iron from ferritin by the chelators of MHEMHP (IIa), EHEMHP (IIb) and DFO. (With permission after [355].)

particles [162, 243]. Here, a simple method of particle–chelator conjugation by forming an amido bond is presented as a prototype. Monodispersed polystyrene particles with carboxyl groups on the surface were used to conjugate MAPHP or DFO, each of which contained a free primary amino group available for the conjugation. The preparation of the chelator–particle conjugates is presented in Scheme 16.5. The carboxylic acid functional groups on the particle surface were preactivated by *N*-cyclohexyl-*N*′-(2-morpholinoethyl)carbodiimide methyl-*p*-toluensulfonate (CMC) and conjugated with MAPHP or DFO as described in Refs. [162, 243, 367]. The carboxylated particles were resuspended through pipetting and vortexing, and then the particles were immediately transferred into a microcentrifuge tube and the supernatant removed by centrifugation. The particles were suspended in 0.01 M NaOH solution, mixed well and the process was repeated. The particles were washed twice with 0.1 M of 2-(*N*-morpholino)ethane sulfonic acid (MES) buffer (pH 5.0) and once with cold Milli-Q water. Carboxyl groups on the particles were activated by adding cold Milli-Q water containing CMC (0.01 M) and incubating for 10 min at 4 °C with slow tilt rotation. After removal of the supernatant, CMC solution was added again along with MES buffer (0.3 M, pH 5.0). The mixture was vortexed and incubated as described above for 30 min. The particles with activated carboxyl groups were washed twice with cold 0.1 M MES as quickly as possible and resuspended in MES buffer (0.1 M, pH 5.0) containing excess MAPHP or DFO (0.01 M). The mixture was vortexed, followed by incubation

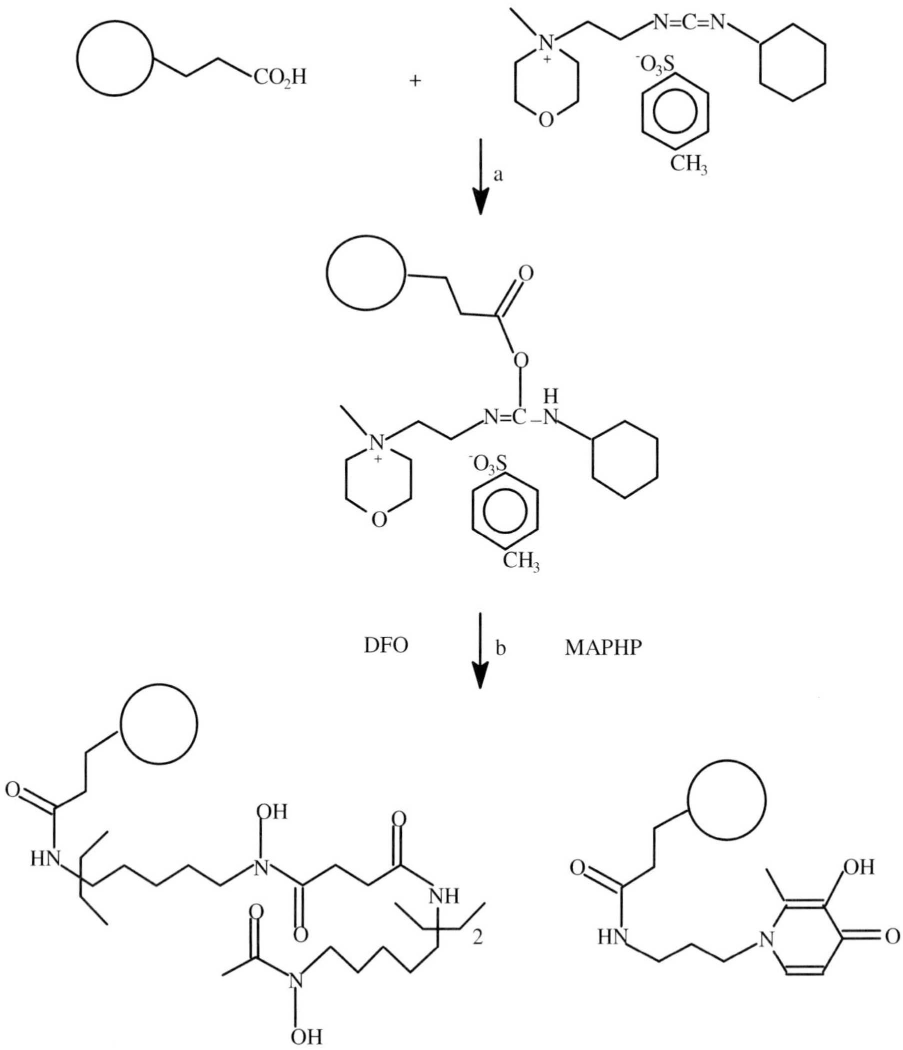

Scheme 16.5. Conjugation of MAPHP and DFO to particles. (a) Reaction of CMC with carboxylic acid on particle surface in MES at room temperature for 30 min and (b) reactions of the activated carboxyl groups with excess chelators in MES for 30 min at room temperature.

for 30 min at room temperature with tilt rotation. The particles conjugated with chelators were washed with 0.1 M MES buffer twice and PBS (pH 7.4) twice and stored in PBS at 4 °C. The yield of conjugation was determined by measurements of the free chelator concentrations in the solutions before and after conjugation using high-performance liquid chromatography (HPLC) or UV-vis spectrometry at the wavelength of maximum absorption [162]. The concentration and size distribution of the chelator–particle systems could be determined using a Beckman Coulter Multisizer II in a counting cuvette containing Isoton II diluent or using a Coulter N4 Plus Sub-micron Particle Sizer.

16.3.4.4.4 **Reaction of MAPHP– or DFO–Particle Systems with Ferric Iron** An aliquot of freshly prepared ferric iron solution [$Fe(NO_3)_3$, 0.002 M] in MES buffer (0.01 M, pH 5.0) was added to MES (0.01 M, pH 5.0) solution containing suspended MAPHP–particles or plain particles as a control. The mixture was rotated at room temperature for 4 h. The iron–chelator–particle systems and supernatant were separated by centrifugation. The systems were thoroughly washed with MES buffer 5 times to remove noncomplexed iron ions. After combining the supernatants, excess MAPHP in MES buffer (0.01 M) was added to complex the iron ions that did not react with the chelator–particle systems. The visible absorbance of the iron–MAPHP complex was measured using UV-vis spectrophotometry at a maximum wavelength of 455 nm ($\varepsilon = 3.02 \times 10^3$) after the chelating reaction reached equilibrium. A standard curve for iron concentration was obtained by measuring several solutions of iron–MAPHP complex with known iron concentrations. The identical procedure was applied in the investigation of the reaction of DFO–particle systems with ferric iron.

16.3.4.4.5 **Protein Absorption Patterns of Chelator–Particle Systems and Chelator–Particle Systems with Iron** The protein absorption patterns of chelator–particle systems and chelator–particle systems with iron, which were obtained by reaction of ferric iron with chelator–particle systems, were evaluated using 2-D PAGE analyses. In brief, the chelator–particle systems, overcoated with Polysorbate 80 at room temperature, and the chelator–particle system with iron (100 μL of each system, 2.5% w/v in PBS buffer) were incubated separately in 1 mL of citrated human plasma (Sigma) for 5 min at 37 °C [357]. After separation by centrifugation and washing 4 times with Milli-Q water, the adsorbed proteins were eluted from the particle surface with a protein-solubilizing solution [5% sodium dodecyl sulfate (SDS), 5% dithioerythritol, 10% glycerol and 60 mM Tris, pH 6.8] [357] and analyzed by 2-D PAGE. In the first dimension, isoelectric focusing (IEF), the proteins were separated only according to their isoelectric points (pI). The IEF was carried out in glass tubes of inner diameter 2.0 mm using 2.0% pH 3.5–10 ampholines for 9600 Vh. In the second dimension, SDS–polyacrylamide gel electrophoresis (PAGE), the separation was based on molecular weight. Each tube was equilibrated for 10 min in buffer (2.3% SDS, 50 mM dithioerythritol, 10% glycerol and 62.5 mM Tris, pH 6.8) and sealed to the top of a stacking gel that was on top of a 10% acrylamide slab gel (145 mm × 145 mm × 0.75 mm). SDS slab gel electrophoresis was performed for about 4 h at 12.5 mA per gel. After SDS–PAGE, the gels were dried between sheets of cellophane and silver-stained [357].

16.3.4.5 Results and Discussion

16.3.4.5.1 Preparation of Iron Chelators with Functional Groups for Particle Conjugation In order for chelators to conjugate with nanoparticles, the chelators must have a functional group to allow formation of a covalent bond between the two. As described above, several methods have been successfully developed to modify L1 by adding various side-chains that contain functional groups. The synthetic approaches are simple and the reaction yields in general are very high. In L1 (Fig. 16.6), the methyl group on the nitrogen atom at position 1 can be very easily replaced through various reactions, which provide many possibilities to obtain new chelators with functional groups. Also, the replacement has little effect on the geometry of metal-binding sites. Therefore, it is expected that the high binding affinity of L1 to iron as well as aluminum, copper and zinc will remain after its modification, enabling the new chelators to simultaneously complex multiple metals. The geometry of the metal-binding site in the modified chelators has been examined by X-ray crystallographic analysis. The analysis shows that the C3–O2, C2–O1 and C2–C3 bond distances of the metal binding site in MHRPP are 1.269(6), 1.361 and 1.428(7) Å, respectively (Fig. 16.8) [126]. These data compare well with the corresponding bond lengths of 1.271, 1.364 and 1.438 Å in L1 (Fig. 16.6) [368]. The unchanged geometry of the metal-binding site indicates that the affinity for iron as well as other metals is not affected [126, 355, 368, 369]. In EHEMHP, the C3–O1, C4–O2 and C3–C4 bond distances of iron binding site are 1.302(3), 1.350(3) and 1.418(4) Å, respectively (Fig. 16.7). The bond lengths of C4–O2 and C3–C4 are similar to that of L1, but the C3–O1 carbonyl bond distance is about 0.031 Å longer. These phenomena are explained by the increased electron donor effect of the ethyl group in EHEMHP compared with that of the methyl group in L1 on the 2 position of the pyridinone ring. Since the carbonyl group on the pyridinone ring is an electron draw group, the greater the electron density on the pyridinone ring donated by alkyl groups (ethtyl > methyl), the longer the carbonyl bond length should be. Interestingly, the carbonyl bond distance of EHEMHP is close to that of the iron–L1 complex [370]. In the complex, the corresponding carbonyl bond length is 1.299(8) Å. The C4–O2 and C3–C4 bond lengths in EHEMHP also compare very well with the corresponding bond lengths of 1.342(7) and 1.408(7) Å in iron–L1 complex [370]. These observations indicate that the replacement of the 2-hydroxyethoxymethyl group has no negative effect on iron binding and that the iron-binding site of EHEMHP may be more favorable for iron chelation than L1 because of the preorganizated effect [371].

16.3.4.5.2 Examination of Modified Chelators Complexing to Iron The ability of the modified chelators to complex metals was examined by titration of the chelators with iron in Tris buffer solution. The chelators react with iron forming purple complexes which have the chelator:iron stoichiometry of 3:1. The titration result also reveals that the functional groups in the side-chains are not involved in iron complexation under physiological conditions. This is important, because it ensures that the use of the functional groups in chelator side-chains for conjugation with nanoparticles will not affect the chelator–metal binding ability.

To further examine the ability of the chelators to complex metals, the reaction of chelators with ferritin was evaluated. This protein is important for iron storage and in brain tissue most of nonheme iron is in the form of ferritin [266, 372]. Evidence shows that iron metabolism is altered in the brain of AD patients, with alterations including chelatable iron, ferritin and transferrin [267, 268, 275, 373]. The *in vitro* extraction of iron from the ferritin core by chelators is a convenient measurement of the potential efficacy of *in vivo* removal of iron from iron-overloaded organs [374]. All of the modified chelators can mobilize iron from ferritin in a slow reaction, which is monitored by the increase in absorbance of the iron–chelator complexes using a spectrophotometric method [126, 355, 374]. The formation of iron–chelator complexes in all the reactions indicated a common kinetic mobilization pattern that is characterized by initial rapid iron removal, followed by a slower iron removal rate. The end of the reaction as judged from stable absorbance. The modified chelators were more effective than DFO in mobilizing iron from ferritin at physiological pH. The initial rate of removal was faster with the modified chelators than with DFO, while the rate after 24 h was about the same, which can be seen in Fig. 16.11.

In vitro tests of iron removal from AD brain sections with various iron chelators were also performed and examinations of the sections using differential interference microscopy demonstrated that iron chelators have the ability to strip iron from the brain tissues. Results showed that the iron removal efficacy depends on the chelator chemical structures and concentrations used. For example, both MAEHP and MHEMHP had better ability to remove iron from AD brain sections, compared with DFO and MHRPP, at concentrations of 0.01 M (Tab. 16.1). The histochemical evaluation of iron in an AD brain section treated with MAEHP is presented in Fig. 16.12, showing remarkably less staining for iron compared with an untreated control. Importantly, this finding provides further support for the possible mechanism of metal-associated oxidative damage in AD development, by show-

Tab. 16.1. Iron evaluation by histochemical staining in AD brain sections after being treated with various iron chelators.

	0.1 M	**0.01 M**
Untreated	positive	positive
DFO	negative	very positive
MHRPP	few positive blood vessels	very positive
MHEMHP	negative	weakly positive
MAEHP	negative	weakly positive

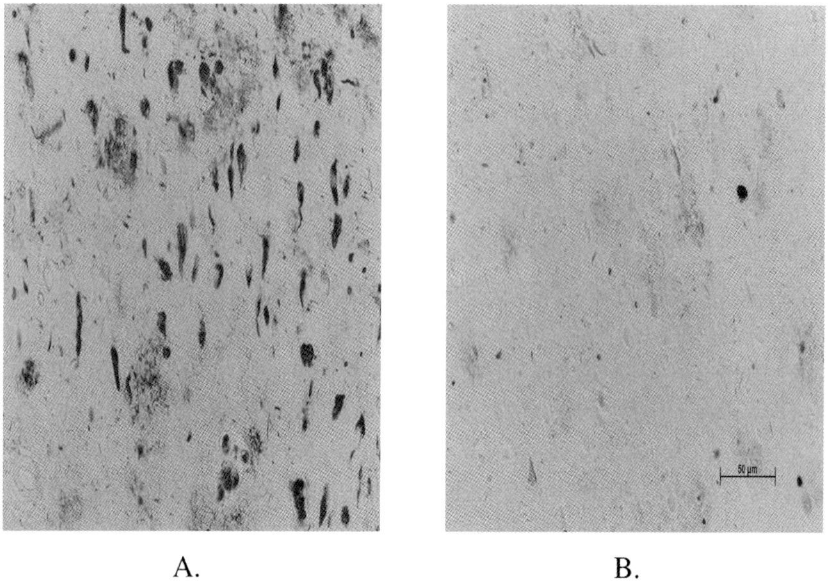

Figure 16.12. Lesion-associated chelatable iron in AD brain sections was depleted with iron chelator, which was evaluated by histochemistry. (A) Control and (B) MAEHP-treated section (with permission after [375]).

ing the existence of chelatable iron in the AD brain. The chelatable iron is believed to be one of the culprits that catalyze free radical formation, causing oxidative damage to all types of biomolecules [209]. Furthermore, this result indicates the potential of chelation therapy of AD by depletion of excess metals, hence preventing metal-mediated neuro-oxidative damage. These results are consistent with early reports that chelation treatment can affect iron accumulations that are closely associated with the places of senile plaques and neurofibrillary tangles in cases of AD [366]. This iron specifically localized to the lesions of AD could participate in *in situ* oxidation and catalyze an H_2O_2-dependent oxidation [366]. Our current study also identifies a useful tool to screen potential chelators which have suitable ability to mobilize iron from the AD brain *in vitro*. This method provides important information for selecting optimal chelators to use for conjugation with nanoparticles in our studies.

As discussed previously, currently available iron chelators used in chelation therapy are problematic due to both toxicity and/or poor bioavailability. It is difficult to develop iron chelators with an optimal balance of bioavailability and low toxicity by adjusting chelator size and lipophilicity. Therefore, other strategies have been explored in order to develop therapeutic iron chelators with suitable bioavailability as well as tolerable levels of toxicity. Relevant to particulate drug delivery, attempts to improve the pharmacological properties of current clinical iron chelators include covalently conjugating DFO to dextran and hydroxyethyl-starch [376–378] or conjugating DFO to large agarosepolyacrolein microsphere beads [379]. Results from these studies are consistent with our studies that the conjugation does not appear to affect the normal high iron-binding affinity of DFO. Also, improved bioavailability and/or stability of DFO as well as decreased toxicity are observed. Formulations of DFO with *n*-decanesulfonate or poly(fumaric anhydride-*co*-sebacic anhydride) produced particles with increased efficiency in chelation treatment by slowing down the release of DFO from the particles [380, 381]. In addition, microencapsulated formulations of L1 with Eudragit RS, RL and L90, and cellulose acetate phthalate have been developed to further improve its bioavailability [382]. Despite all of these improvements, there still is a tremendous need to develop iron chelators with specific organ-targeting ability. Optimal organ-targeting may in itself further improve bioavailability of chelators and limit toxicity. In addition to the primary purpose of correcting primary and secondary iron overload, this particular approach may also make it possible for chelation therapy to prevent and treat other diseases especially neurodegenerative disorders associated with excess metals.

16.3.4.5.3 **Chelator–Particle Conjugation, Metal Complexation and Potential BBB Penetration** Nanoparticulate drug delivery provides an opportunity for drugs to penetrate the BBB. The nanoparticle drug system also possesses the advantage of easy preparation and high stability. To explore the possibility of nanoparticle–chelator transport for AD treatment, practical methods for chelator conjugation with nanoparticles were investigated. Here, the reaction of MAPHP or DFO, each containing one primary amino group, with polystyrene nano/microparticles with a surface carboxylic acid moiety is presented as a prototypic conjugation. As mentioned before, it also is possible to synthesize iron chelators containing different functional groups that readily react to the nanoparticle surface active sites without any adverse effects on the chelator metal binding.

Carboxylic acid functional groups on the surface of the particles used here allowed the particles to conjugate with chelators by forming covalent amido bonds. Prior to conjugation, the carboxylic acid groups were activated using carbodiimide in MES buffer at an acidic pH value to form an active intermediate ester. To remove excess carbodiimide, the particles were rapidly washed with cool Mill-Q water since the ester is unstable and undergoes hydrolysis. An alternative method, such as adding a water-soluble *N*-hydroxyl compound like sulfo-*N*-hydroxysuccinimide (NHS), could increase the coupling yield since NHS is known to form a more stable intermediate ester by replacing the oacylisourea intermediate formed by carbodiimide. The NHS-formed ester is less susceptible to hydrolysis but still highly reactive toward amino groups [383, 384]. The primary amino group in the chelators reacts with active ester intermediates derived from carboxyl groups on the particle surface, consequently forming covalent amido bond linkages in good quality yields (over 70%). Coupling yields were determined by (i) measuring the free chelator concentration in solution before and after conjugation, using HPLC or UV-vis spectrophotometery readings, and (ii) calculating the difference between the two concentrations to indicate the amounts of the chelators conjugated to particles. After the conjugation reaction, the particle size distribution was

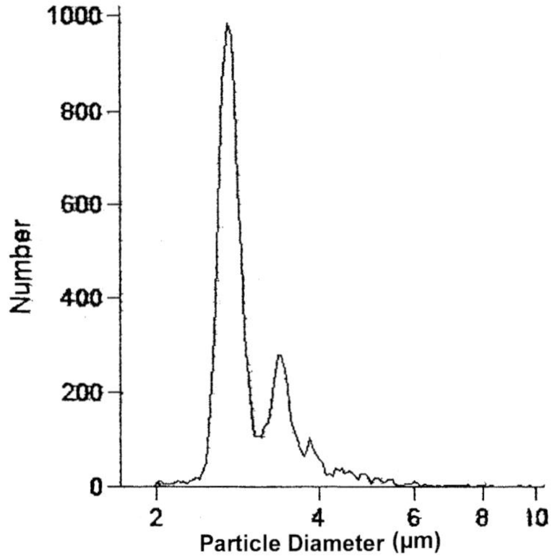

Figure 16.13. Particle size distributions measured by Multizer analyzer II. There is no distribution change between particles conjugated with MAPHP and particles without conjugation.

measured and compared with the distribution prior to conjugation. A distribution change was not observed, which indicated that there was no particle clumping (Fig. 16.13). A useful protocol for particle conjugation with various molecules can be found in Ref. [162].

With rapid development of nanoparticle technology in biomedical applications, most processes for preparing various nanoparticles with different sizes and properties have become routine and standard, and many of these nanoparticles are even commercially available. The technologies to make the nanoparticles virtually monodispersed, with a narrow diameter deviation, spherical shape and constant surface area, has really advanced the development of nanoparticulate drug delivery. Also, it has become easier to obtain suitable nanoparticles with various functional groups on their surface for the purpose of covalent bond conjugation by utilizing simple chemical reactions, as demonstrated by our studies.

To test whether chelators retain their ability to complex metals after conjugation with nanoparticles, the chelator–nanoparticle systems were incubated with a $Fe(NO_3)_3$ solution. After the reaction was complete, the $Fe(NO_3)_3$ solution was removed and noncomplexed iron was determined by adding MAPHP and measuring the iron–MAPHP complexes using UV-vis spectroscopy. Results indicated that about two MAPHP molecules conjugated to particles complexed with every iron atom. As each MAPHP can provide only two oxygen donors to chelate iron, two more iron-binding sites are needed to form a highly stable iron complex with an octahedral coordination sphere. According to our earlier studies [385], the oxygen atoms in amido groups may be involved in chelating iron; thus, two oxygen donors

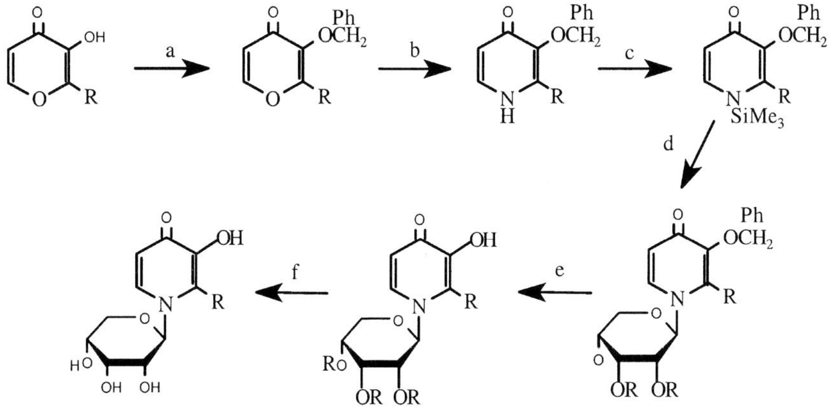

Figure 16.14. Four oxygen donors from two MAPHPs and two oxygen donors from amido groups constructing a hexadentate chelator through particle surface as the backbones.

from two amido groups and four oxygen donors from two MAPHPs may assemble into a hexadentate chelator, using particle surface linkages as the backbone (Fig. 16.14). This is significant, as hexadentate iron chelators possess many advantages including kinetic stability, concentration independence of iron affinity and low toxicity [310]. In addition, attempts to convert bi- or tridentate iron chelators into hexadentate chelators with various backbones suffer mainly from decreased bioavailability and the risk of potential toxicity. By contrast, the use of nano/microparticles to convert bi- or tridentate chelators to hexadentate chelators may circumvent these problems due to the particle targeting ability. In this manner, many bidentate or tridentate iron chelators, even with intolerable toxicity, can be modified by conjugation with nano/microparticles, since the toxic character of the free chelators may be diminished after particle conjugation. Our results also revealed that DFO still retains the 1:1 complex ratio with iron – an indication that conjugation with particles does not affect its iron binding ability. It is also worth mentioning that the bioavailability of some hexadentate iron chelators with high molecular weights and hydrophilicity can be improved after forming the chelator–particle delivery systems [386].

In order to demonstrate the possibility that chelator–nanoparticle systems enter the brain and that the chelator–nanoparticle systems leave the brain after chelation with metals, the protein absorption patterns of MAPHP–particle system and iron–MAPHP–particle system were evaluated; 2-D PAGE analyses were used to conduct this evaluation after incubation of the systems with human plasma. The 2-D PAGE images are presented in Fig. 16.15 and show that the protein patterns on the systems are totally different from that of the human plasma protein (Fig. 16.15a).

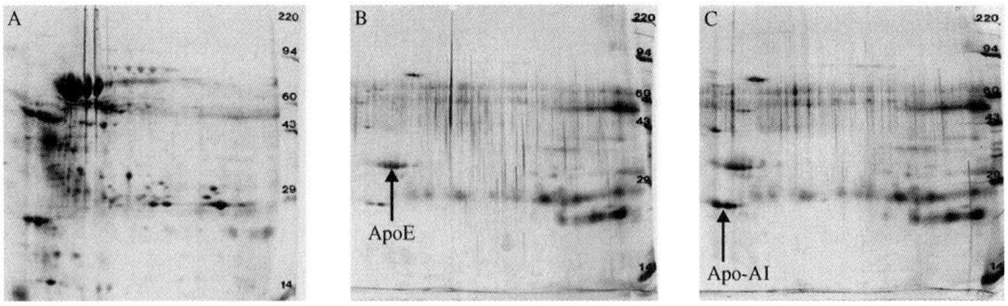

Figure 16.15. Images of plasma protein patterns examined by 2-D PAGE. (A) Plasma, (B) nanoparticle–chelator systems coated with Polysorbate 80 and (C) nanoparticle–chelator systems complexed with iron (with permission after [375]).

Through changing the surface properties of MAPHP–particle system by coating surfactants such as Polysorbate 80, the system preferentially absorbed ApoE (Fig. 16.15b). On the other hand, after complexing of MAPHP–particle system with iron, the iron–MAPHP–particle system possessed the absorption preference for ApoA-I (Fig. 16.15c). Such preferential protein absorptions may allow the MAPHP–particle system and iron–MAPHP–particle system to mimic the ApoE and A-I nanoparticle, respectively, and therefore to enter brain without metal chelation and leave the brain with complexed metals via LDL transport mechanisms.

Simultaneous chelation of iron and other metals such as aluminum, copper and zinc may provide a useful therapeutic option for AD treatment. The use of nanoparticles to transport iron chelators into and out of the brain could lead to a safer and more effective chelation therapy for AD by means of decreasing the multiple metal load in neuro-tissue, and thereby staving off the harmful effects of oxidative damage and its sequelae. Iron chelators with functional groups can be synthesized and the functional groups can be used for conjugation with nanoparticles. The conjugation of such chelators to nanoparticles does not alter the chelator metal-binding ability and, in some cases, the conjugation even improves the chelation coordination property. The nanoparticles can be made of biocompatible synthetic or natural macromolecules with functional groups on their surface for conjugation with chelators. The macromolecules can be non- or controlled biodegradable for specific purposes. Changing nanoparticle surface properties can optimize the preferential protein absorption, thus improving the ability of the particle to cross the BBB. Many approaches to adjust particle surface properties can be used, such as coating with different surfactants or proteins, conjugating with different chelators or with various linkers and using antibodies to increase lipoprotein preferential absorption. Further studies with the chelator–nanoparticle system may provide more insights into the mechanisms of AD pathophysiology, and may show the possibility of prevention and treatment for other iron-mediated neurodegenerative diseases such as Friedrich ataxia, Huntington's disease, Parkinson's disease and Hallervorden–Spatz Syndrome. More studies are needed to demonstrate the protective efficacy of the chelator–nanoparticle systems, to evaluate their toxicity and to optimize their capability to cross the BBB. Our studies may also open the door for the use of a nanoparticle-mediated transport to facilitate extraction of toxins from defective places in the body for disease prevention and treatment.

16.4 Perspectives

Nanoparticulate drug delivery for AD prevention and treatment shows great potential; however, it is still at a very early stage of development. In order to advance this technology for AD application, knowledge is urgently needed in several basic research areas. For example, there is no study on the *in vivo* treatment of AD using nanoparticulate drug delivery technology. With the AD animal models available, the efficacy of nanoparticulate agents delivered to the brain that may offer therapeutic effects on AD based on a current understanding of AD pathogenesis should be evaluated. This will not only provide insights into the mechanisms of AD development, but also lead to more effective and safer therapeutics for the disease. It also is necessary to fully study whether the nanoparticulate drug systems possess adverse effects on the BBB and brain as well as other parts of the body, at tissue, cell and molecular levels. Additionally, the pharmacology and pharmacokinetics of the systems need to be examined, which will ensure the further development of the nanoparticulate drug systems for clinical use. Furthermore, it is suggested that the nanoparticle surface, and perhaps also the particle components, can be used to manipulate particle uptake into the brain via the LDL receptor, because nanoparticles preferentially absorb ApoE and/or B in blood, and thereby mimic these protein particles. However, the exact mechanisms are not fully understood, and thorough studies could provide valuable information that will help improve the ability of nanoparticulate drug systems to cross the BBB. Moreover, studies on improving drug-loading capacity in nanoparticulate drug systems, which should not affect the ability of these systems to enter the brain, must be carried out in order to reach sufficient drug level in the AD brain. In this regard, drug nanosuspensions have the advantage that no polymeric materials are required as carriers. Lipid nanoparticulate drug systems also show promise; both need to be investigated. Finally, because of the highly interdisciplinary nature of developing the technology of nanoparticulate drug delivery for AD treatment, it is necessary to bring together chemists, bioengineers and life scientists in order to accomplish this task.

Specifically, it would be useful to focus on nanoparticle chelation agents as a possible drug for AD treatment, because metal-mediated toxicity is believed to be an important contributor to AD development and chelation therapy shows some benefits to AD patients. In addition to nanoparticle delivery of drugs into the brain, which has seen achieved in some cases, the ability of nanoparticles to bring chelator–metal complexes out of the AD brain needs to be demonstrated *in vivo*. Effects of the nanoparticulate chelator system on metal biokinetics and excretion should be studied, which will provide important information about chelation efficacy and toxicity.

Further studies should utilize the nanoparticulate drug delivery systems, one of the few valuable tools to deliver drugs into the brain, to transport available therapeutics to prevent or treat AD in clinical studies. This approach may significantly improve the efficacy of these therapeutic agents and minimize systemic side-effects or make it possible for some potential therapeutics such as nerve growth factors, non-brain-distributing ACE inhibitors and hydrophilic chelators with large molecular size to enter the brain for AD treatment. The use of this technology will also facilitate the development of other promising treatments such as antibody, gene and stem cell therapies. Simultaneous multidrug delivery can also be achieved through nanoparticle technology, which may provide better therapeutic efficacy. Biocompatible or biodegradable polymers to serve as carriers in nanoparticulate drug systems are now being developed, as are potential AD therapeutics. Coupling these studies may result in more rapid identification of more effective and safer drugs for the treatment of AD. As many nanoparticulate drug delivery systems are designed for intravenous administration, the possibility of oral administration as well as transdermal, ocular, nasal and inhalation routes should be investigated. The development of these patient-administrable nanoparticulate drug delivery systems would greatly facilitate the care of AD patients and benefit patients over extended time periods of therapy.

It is worth noting that an outstanding feature of nanoparticulate drug delivery technology is its simplicity of preparation, optimization and application. For example, the nanoparticles used for chelator transport can be made of synthetic or natural macromolecules with functional groups such as amino and carboxyl moieties on their surface for covalently bonding with chelators. Changing the chelators, linkages, surfactants and the nanoparticle surface can result in nanoparticulate chelator systems with desirable surface properties, which enable the systems to cross the BBB. Also, directly coating the chelator–nanoparticle with apolipoproteins or their antibodies may facilitate high-efficiency penetration of the BBB. In addition to nanoparticle delivery of drugs, nanoparticle conjugation with drugs or prodrugs can also offer the possibility of developing new therapeutics that not only possess specific organ targeting, but also have improved therapeutic efficacy and minimized toxicity for AD treatment. It is also possible that nanoparticles can serve as vehicles to bring toxic materials out of the brain, which will be a huge advance in nanoparticle technology for disease prevention and treatment.

The fundamentals of nanoparticulate drug delivery into the brain indicate the possibility of transporting therapeutic agents across the BBB for treatment of AD. Current investigations provide evidence to support this possibility and show promise. Further studies are needed to demonstrate therapeutic efficacy and tolerance. Enthusiasm for nanoparticle transport of drugs for AD treatment is high because this approach will not only provide more insights into the mechanisms of AD development, but also will lead to safer and more effective therapies for the disease. This approach can also be used for prevention and treatment other neurological diseases as well as for disease diagnosis.

Acknowledgments

We are grateful for the financial support by the National Institutes of Health. We would also like to thank Drs. Mark Smith and Peggy Harris of the Case Western Reserve University for their histochemical analysis of AD brain tissues. Finally, we would want to thank all the various publishers for their kind permission to reproduce figures and schemes used in this chapter.

References

1 Smith MA. Alzheimer disease. *Int. Rev. Neurobiol. 42*, **1998**, 1–54.

2 Brookmeyer R, Gray S, Kawas C. Projections of Alzheimer's disease in the United States and the public health impact of delaying disease onset. *Am. J. Public Health 88*, **1998**, 1337–42.

3 Hebert LE, Scherr PA, Bienias JL, Bennett DA, Evans DA. Alzheimer's disease in the US population: prevalence estimates using the 2000 census. *Arch. Neurol. 60*, **2003**, 1119–22.

4 Hebert LE, Beckett LA, Scherr PA, Evans DA. Annual incidence of Alzheimer's disease in the United States projected to the years 2000 through 2050. *Alzheimer Dis. Assoc. Disord. 15*, **2001**, 169–73.

5 Scorer CA. Preclinical and clinical challenges in the development of disease-modifying therapies for Alzheimer's disease. *Drug Discov. Today 6*, **2001**, 1207–19.

6 Marder K, Memantine approved to treat moderate to severe Alzheimer's disease. *Curr. Neurol. Neurosci. Rep. 4*, **2004**, 349–50.

7 Sonkusare SK, Ramarao CLKP. Dementia of Alzheimer's disease and other neurodegenerative disorder – memantine, a new hope. *Pharmac. Res. 51*, **2005**, 1–17.

8 Coyle J, Kershaw P. Galantamine. A cholinesterase inhibitor that allosterically modulates nicotinic receptors: effects on the course of Alzheimer's disease. *Biol. Psychiatry 49*, **2001**, 289–99.

9 Farlow MR. Pharmacokinctic profilcs of current therapies for Alzheimer's disease: implications for switching to galantamine. *Clin. Ther. 23 (Suppl. A)*, **2001**, A13–24.

10 Szekely CA, Thorne JE, Zandi PP, Ek M, Messias E, Breitner JC, Goodman SN. Nonsteroidal anti-inflammatory drugs for the prevention of Alzheimer's disease: a systematic review. *Neuroepidemiology 23*, **2004**, 159–69.

11 Weggen S, Eriksen JL, Das P, Sagi SA, Wang R, Pietrzik CU, Findlay KA, Smith TE, Murphy MP, Bulter T, Kang DE, Marquez-Sterling N, Golde TE, Koo EH. A subset of NSAIDs lower amyloidogenic Abeta42 independently of cyclo-oxygenase activity. *Nature 414*, **2001**, 212–6.

12 McAdam BF, Catella-Lawson F, Mardini IA, Kapoor S, Lawson JA, FitzGerald GA. Systemic biosynthesis of prostacyclin by cyclooxygenase (COX)-2: the human pharmacology of a selective inhibitor of COX-2. *Proc. Natl Acad. Sci. USA 96*, **1999**, 272–7.

13 Montine TJ, Sidell KR, Crews BC, Markesbery WR, Marnett LJ, Roberts LJ. 2nd, Morrow JD. Elevated CSF prostaglandin E_2 levels in patients with probable AD. *Neurology 53*, **1999**, 1495–8.

14 Zandi PP, Anthony JC, Hayden KM, Mehta K, Mayer L, Breitner JC. Cache County Study Investigators. Reduced incidence of AD with NSAID but not H2 receptor antagonists: the

Cache County Study. *Neurology 59*, **2002**, 880–6.

15 Prevention of Alzheimer's Disease by Vitamin E and Selenium (PREADVISE). http://www.nia.nih.gov/HealthInformation/ClinicalTrials.htm.

16 Prasad KN, Hovland AR, Cole WC, Prasad KC, Nahreini P, Edwards-Prasad J, Andreatta CP. Multiple antioxidants in the prevention and treatment of Alzheimer disease: analysis of biologic rationale. *Clin. Neuropharmacol. 23*, **2000**, 2–13.

17 Casadesus G, Zhu X, Atwood CS, Webber KM, Perry G, Bowen RL, Smith MA. Beyond estrogen: targeting gonadotropin hormones in the treatment of Alzheimer's disease. *Curr. Drugs, Targets CNS Neurol. Disord. 3*, **2004**, 281–5.

18 Webber KM, Bowen R, Casadesus G, Perry G, Atwood CS, Smith MA. Gonadotropins and Alzheimer's disease: the link between estrogen replacement therapy and neuroprotection. *Acta Neurobiol. Exp. (Wars) 64*, **2004**, 113–8.

19 Zandi PP, Anthony JC, Khachaturian AS, Stone SV, Gustafson D, Tschanz JT, Norton MC, Welsh-Bohmer KA, Breitner JC; Cache County Study Group. Reduced risk of Alzheimer disease in users of antioxidant vitamin supplements: the Cache County Study. *Arch. Neurol. 61*, **2004**, 82–8.

20 Suh YH, Checler F. Amyloid precursor protein, presenilins, and alpha-synuclein: molecular pathogenesis and pharmacological applications in Alzheimer's disease. *Pharmacol. Rev. 54*, **2002**, 469–525.

21 Corrada M, Kawas CH, Hallfrisch J, Muller D, Brookmeyer R. Reduced risk of Alzheimer's disease with high folate intake: The Baltimore Longitudinal Study of Aging. *Alzheimer's & Dementia 1*, **2005**, 11–8.

22 Sano M, Ernesto C, Thomas RG, Klauber MR, Schafer K, Grundman M, Woodbury P, Growdon J, Cotman CW, Pfeiffer E, Schneider LS, Thal LJ. A controlled trial of selegiline, alpha-tocopherol, or both as treatment for Alzheimer's disease. The Alzheimer's Disease Cooperative Study. *N. Engl J. Med. 336*, **1997**, 1216–22.

23 Morris MC, Evans DA, Bienias JL, Tangney CC, Bennett DA, Wilson RS, Aggarwal N, Schneider J. Consumption of fish and $n-3$ fatty acids and risk of incident Alzheimer disease. *Arch. Neurol. 60*, **2003**, 940–6.

24 Morris MC, Evans DA, Bienias JL, Tangney CC, Hebert LE, Scherr PA, Schneider JA. Dietary folate and vitamin B12 intake and cognitive decline among community-dwelling older persons. *Arch. Neurol. 62*, **2005**, 641–5.

25 Cholerton B, Gleason CE, Baker LD, Asthana S. Estrogen and Alzheimer's disease: the story so far. *Drugs Aging 19*, **2002**, 405–27.

26 Sherwin BB. Estrogen and cognitive aging in women. *Trends Pharmacol. Sci. 23*, **2002**, 527–34.

27 Mulnard RA, Corrada MM, Kawas CH. Estrogen replacement therapy, Alzheimer's disease, and mild cognitive impairment. *Curr. Neurol. Neurosci. Rep. 4*, **2004**, 368–73.

28 Rosin RA, Raskind MA. Gonadotrophin-releasing hormone agonist treatment of aggression in Alzheimer's disease: a case report. *Int. Psychogeriatr. 17*, **2005**, 313–8.

29 Rasgon NL, Small GW, Siddarth P, Miller K, Ercoli LM, Bookheimer SY, Lavretsky H, Huang SC, Barrio JR, Phelps ME. Estrogen use and brain metabolic change in older adults. A preliminary report. *Psychiatry Res. 107*, **2001**, 11–8.

30 Dunkin J, Rasgon N, Wagner-Steh K, David S, Altshuler L, Rapkin A. Reproductive events modify the effects of estrogen replacement therapy on cognition in healthy postmenopausal women. *Psychoneuroendocrinology 30*, **2005**, 284–96.

31 Yasar S, Corrada M, Brookmeyer R, Kawas C. Calcium channel blockers and risk of AD: the Baltimore Longitudinal Study of Aging. *Neurobiol. Aging 26*, **2005**, 157–63.

32 Ohrui T, Matsui T, Yamaya M, Tomita N, Sato-Nakagawa T, Maruyama M, Niwa K, Arai H, Sasaki H. ACE inhibitors and incidence of Alzheimer disease in Japan. *J. Am. Geriatr. Soc. 52*, **2004**, 649–50.

33 Ohrui T, Tomita N, Sato-Nakagawa T, Matsui T, Maruyama M, Niwa K, Arai H, Sasaki H. Effects of brain-penetrating ACE inhibitors on Alzheimer disease progression. *Neurology 63*, **2004**, 1324–5.

34 Zamrini E, McGwin G, Roseman JM. Association between statin use and Alzheimer's disease. *Neuroepidemiology 23*, **2004**, 94–8.

35 Kojro E, Gimpl G, Lammich S, Marz W, Fahrenholz F. Low cholesterol stimulates the non-amyloidogenic pathway by its effect on alpha-secretase ADAM 10. *Proc. Natl Acad. Sci. USA 98*, **2001**, 5815–20.

36 Simons M, Keller P, De Strooper B, Beyreuther K, Dotti CG, Simons K. Cholesterol depletion inhibits the generation of beta-amyloid in hippocampal neurons. *Proc. Natl Acad. Sci. USA 95*, **1998**, 6460–4.

37 Simons M, Schwarzler F, Lutjohann D, von Bergmann K, Beyreuther K, Dichgans J, Wormstall H, Hartmann T, Schulz JB. Treatment with simvastatin in normocholesterolemic patients with Alzheimer's disease: A 26-week randomized, placebo-controlled, double-blind trial. *Ann. Neurol. 52*, **2002**, 346–50.

38 Fassbender K, Simons M, Bergmann C, Stroick M, Lutjohann D, Keller P, Runz H, Kuhl S, Bertsch T, von Bergmann K, Hennerici M, Beyreuther K, Hartmann T. Simvastatin strongly reduces levels of Alzheimer's disease beta-amyloid peptides Abeta 42 and Abeta 40 *in vitro* and *in vivo*. *Proc. Natl Acad. Sci. USA 98*, **2001**, 5856–61.

39 Kwak B, Mulhaupt F, Myit S, Mach F. Statin as a newly recognized type of immunomodulator. *Nat. Med. 6*, **2000**, 1399–402.

40 Casdorph HR. EDTA chelation therapy: efficacy in brain disorders. In *A Textbook on DETA Chelation Therapy*, 2nd edn, Cranton EM (Ed.). Hampton Roads Publishing, Charlottesville, VA, **2001**, pp. 142–63.

41 Olszewer E, Carter JP. EDTA chelation therapy: a retrospective study of 2870 patients. In *A Textbook on DETA Chelation Therapy*, 2nd edn, Cranton EM (Ed.). Hampton Roads Publishing, Charlottesville, VA, **2001**, pp. 210–24.

42 Regland B, Lehmann W, Abedini I, Blennow K, Jonsson M, Karlsson I, Sjogren M, Wallin A, Xilinas M, Gottfries CG. Treatment of Alzheimer's disease with clioquinol. *Dement. Geriatr. Cogn. Disord. 12*, **2001**, 408–14.

43 Ritchie CW, Bush AI, Mackinnon A, Macfarlane S, Mastwyk M, MacGregor L, Kiers L, Cherny R, Li QX, Tammer A, Carrington D, Mavros C, Volitakis I, Xilinas M, Ames D, Davis S, Beyreuther K, Tanzi RE, Masters CL. Metal–protein attenuation with iodochlorhydroxyquin (clioquinol) targeting Abeta amyloid deposition and toxicity in Alzheimer disease: a pilot phase 2 clinical trial. *Arch. Neurol. 60*, **2003**, 1685–91.

44 Ibach B, Haen E, Marienhagen J, Hajak G. Clioquinol treatment in familiar early onset of Alzheimer's disease: a case report. *Pharmacopsychiatry 38*, **2005**, 178–9.

45 Raudino F, Mascalzi MG, Zagami A. Gabapentin and behavioral disorders in severe Alzheimer disease. *J. Clin. Psychopharmacol. 24*, **2004**, 459–60.

46 De Leon OA. Treatment of psychotic symptoms with lamotrigine in Alzheimer disease. *J. Clin. Psychopharmacol. 24*, **2004**, 232–3.

47 Mintzer J, Greenspan A, Caers I, Van Hove I, Kushner S, Weiner M, Gharabawi G, Schneider LS. Risperidone in the treatment of psychosis of Alzheimer disease: results from a prospective clinical trial. *Am. J. Geriatr. Psychiatry 14*, **2006**, 280–91.

48 Nash JM. Alzheimer's disease. New insights into its cause lead to new drug strategies. *Time 157*, **2001**, 80–1, 85.
49 Dominguez DI, De Strooper B. Novel therapeutic strategies provide the real test for the amyloid hypothesis of Alzheimer's disease. *Trends Pharmacol. Sci. 23*, **2002**, 324–30.
50 Schenk D. Amyloid-beta immunotherapy for Alzheimer's disease: the end of the beginning. *Nat. Rev. Neurosci. 3*, **2002**, 824–8.
51 Hirschfield GM, Hawkins PN. Amyloidosis: new strategies for treatment. *Int. J. Biochem. Cell Biol. 35*, **2003**, 1608–13.
52 McGeer PL, McGeer E. Is there a future for vaccination as a treatment for Alzheimer's disease? *Neurobiol. Aging 24*, **2003**, 391–5.
53 Schmitt B, Bernhardt T, Moeller HJ, Heuser I, Frolich L. Combination therapy in Alzheimer's disease: a review of current evidence. *CNS Drugs 18*, **2004**, 827–44.
54 Risner ME, Saunders AM, Altman JF, Ormandy GC, Craft S, Foley IM, Zvartau-Hind ME, Hosford DA, Roses AD. Efficacy of rosiglitazone in a genetically defined population with mild-to-moderate Alzheimer's disease. *Pharmacogenomics J 6*, **2006**, 246–54.
55 Larson EB, Wang L, Bowen JD, McCormick WC, Teri L, Crane P, Kukull W. Exercise is associated with reduced risk for incident dementia among persons 65 years of age and older. *Ann. Intern. Med. 144*, **2006**, 73–81.
56 Khachaturian AS, Zandi PP, Lyketsos CG, Hayden KM, Skoog I, Norton MC, Tschanz JT, Mayer LS, Welsh-Bohmer KA, Breitner JCS; for the Cache County Study Group. Antihypertensive medication use and incident Alzheimer disease: The Cache County Study. *Arch. Neurol. 63*, **2006**, 686–92.
57 Hendrie HC, Albert MS, Butters MA, Gao S, Knopman DS, Launer LJ, Yaffe K, Cuthbert BN, Edwards E, Wagster MV. The NIH cognitive and emotional health project: Report of the critical evaluation study committee. *Alzheimer's & Dementia 2*, **2006**, 12–32.
58 Ramirez BG, Blazquez C, Gomez del Pulgar T, Guzman M, de Ceballos ML. Prevention of Alzheimer's disease pathology by cannabinoids: neuroprotection mediated by blockade of microglial activation. *J. Neurosci. 25*, **2005**, 1904–13.
59 National Institute on Aging/National Institutes of Health, Progress Report on Alzheimer's Disease, 2000. http://www.alzheimers.org/prog00.htm.
60 Smith DE, Roberts J, Gage FH, Tuszynski MH. Age-associated neuronal atrophy occurs in the primate brain and is reversible by growth factor gene therapy. *Proc. Natl Acad. Sci. USA 96*, **1999**, 10893–8.
61 Kordower JH, Isacson O, Emerich DF. Cellular delivery of trophic factors for the treatment of Huntington's disease: is neuroprotection possible? *Exp. Neurol. 159*, **1999**, 4–20.
62 Bachurin SO. Medicinal chemistry approaches for the treatment and prevention of Alzheimer's disease. *Med. Res. Rev. 23*, **2003**, 48–88.
63 Tariot PN, Loy R, Ryan JM, Porsteinsson A, Ismail S. Mood stabilizers in Alzheimer's disease: symptomatic and neuroprotective rationales. *Adv. Drug Deliv. Rev. 54*, **2002**, 1567–77.
64 Bai DL, Tang XC, He XC, Huperzine A, a potential therapeutic agent for treatment of Alzheimer's disease. *Curr. Med. Chem. 7*, **2000**, 355–74.
65 Newhouse PA, Potter A, Singh A. Effects of nicotinic stimulation on cognitive performance. *Curr. Opin. Pharmacol. 4*, **2004**, 36–46.
66 Shaw KT, Utsuki T, Rogers J, Yu QS, Sambamurti K, Brossi A, Ge YW, Lahiri DK, Greig NH. Phenserine regulates translation of beta-amyloid precursor protein mRNA by a putative interleukin-1 responsive element, a target for drug development. *Proc. Natl Acad. Sci. USA 98*, **2001**, 7605–10.

67 Witt A, Macdonald N, Kirkpatrick P. Memantine hydrochloride. *Nat. Rev. Drug Discov. 3*, **2004**, 109–10.
68 Iwata N, Tsubuki S, Takaki Y, Shirotani K, Lu B, Gerard NP, Gerard C, Hama E, Lee HJ, Saido TC. Metabolic regulation of brain Abeta by neprilysin. *Science 292*, **2001**, 1550–2.
69 Selkoe DJ. Alzheimer's disease: genes, proteins and therapy. *Phys. Rev. 81*, **2001**, 741–66.
70 Cai H, Wang Y, McCarthy D, Wen H, Borchelt DR, Price DL, Wong PC. BACE1 is the major beta-secretase for generation of Abeta peptides by neurons. *Nat. Neurosci. 4*, **2001**, 233–4.
71 Doerfler P, Shearman MS, Perlmutter RM. Presenilin-dependent gamma-secretase activity modulates thymocyte development. *Proc. Natl Acad. Sci. USA 98*, **2001**, 9312–7.
72 Cumming JN, Iserloh U, Kennedy ME. Design and development of BACE-1 inhibitors. *Curr. Opin. Drug Discov. Dev. 7*, **2004**, 536–56.
73 Thompson LA, Bronson JJ, Zusi FC. Progress in the discovery of BACE inhibitors. *Curr. Pharm. Des. 11*, **2005**, 3383–404.
74 Steiner H. Uncovering gamma-secretase. *Curr. Alzheimer Res. 1*, **2004**, 175–81.
75 Penninger JM, Irie-Sasaki J, Sasaki T, Oliveira-dos-Santos AJ. CD45: new jobs for an old acquaintance. *Nat. Immunol. 2*, **2001**, 389–96.
76 Treiber C, Simons A, Strauss M, Hafner M, Cappai R, Bayer R, Multhaup G. Clioquinol mediates copper uptake and counteracts copper efflux activities of the amyloid precursor protein of Alzheimer's disease. *J. Biol. Chem. 279*, **2004**, 51958–64.
77 Cherny RA, Atwood CS, Xilinas ME, Gray DN, Jones WD, McLean CA, Barnham KJ, Volitakis I, Fraser FW, Kim Y, Huang X, Goldstein LE, Moir RD, Lim JT, Beyreuther K, Zheng H, Tanzi RE, Masters CL, Bush AI. Treatment with a copper–zinc chelator markedly and rapidly inhibits beta-amyloid accumulation in Alzheimer's disease transgenic mice. *Neuron 30*, **2001**, 665–76.
78 Shachar DB, Kahana N, Kampel V, Warshawsky A, Youdim MB. Neuroprotection by a novel brain permeable iron chelator, VK-28, against 6-hydroxydopamine lesion in rats. *Neuropharmacology 46*, **2004**, 254–63.
79 Youdim MBH, Stephenson G, Shachar DB. Ironing iron out in Parkinson's disease and other neurodegenerative disease with iron chelators. A lesson form 6-hydroxydopamine and iron chelators, desferal and VK-28. *Ann. NY Acad. Sci. 1012*, **2004**, 306–25.
80 Lee JY, Friedman JE, Angel I, Kozak A, Koh JY. The lipophilic metal chelator DP-109 reduces amyloid pathology in brains of human beta-amyloid precursor protein transgenic mice. *Neurobiol. Aging 25*, **2004**, 1315–21.
81 Reznichenko L, Amit T, Zheng H, Avramovich-Tirosh Y, Youdim MB, Weinreb O, Mandel S. Reduction of iron-regulated amyloid precursor protein and beta-amyloid peptide by (−)-epigallocatechin-3-gallate in cell cultures: implications for iron chelation in Alzheimer's disease. *J. Neurochem. 97*, **2006**, 527–36.
82 Zheng H, Weiner LM, Bar-Am. O, Epsztejn S, Cabantchik ZI, Warshawsky A, Youdim MB, Fridkin M. Design, synthesis, and evaluation of novel bifunctional iron-chelators as potential agents for neuroprotection in Alzheimer's, Parkinson's, and other neurodegenerative diseases. *Bioorg. Med. Chem. 13*, **2005**, 773–83.
83 Richardson DR. Novel chelators for central nervous system disorders that involve alterations in the metabolism of iron and other metal ions. *Ann. NY Acad. Sci. 1012*, **2004**, 326–41.
84 Shin RW, Kruck TP, Murayama H, Kitamoto T. A novel trivalent cation chelator Feralex dissociates binding

of aluminum and iron associated with hyperphosphorylated tau of Alzheimer's disease. *Brain Res. 961*, **2003**, 139–46.
85 Venti A, Giordano T, Eder P, Bush AI, Lahiri DK, Greig NH, Rogers JT. The integrated role of desferrioxamine and phenserine targeted to an iron-responsive element in the APP-mRNA 5′-untranslated region. *Ann. NY Acad. Sci. 1035*, **2004**, 34–48.
86 Wolozin B, Brown III J, Theisler C, Silberman S. The cellular biochemistry of cholesterol and statins: insights into the pathophysiology and therapy of Alzheimer's disease. *CNS Drug Rev. 10*, **2004**, 127–46.
87 Bartzokis G, Tishler TA, Shin IS, Lu PH, Cummings JL. Brain ferritin iron as a risk factor for age at onset in neurodegenerative diseases. *Ann. NY Acad. Sci. 1012*, **2004**, 224–36.
88 Brown M. Gene therapy success for Alzheimer's? *Drug Discov. Today 8*, **2003**, 474–5.
89 Clausen T, Bullock R. Medical treatment and neuroprotection in traumatic brain injury. *Curr. Pharm. Des. 7*, **2001**, 1517–32.
90 Helmuth L. New therapies. New Alzheimer's treatments that may ease the mind. *Science 297*, **2002**, 1260–2.
91 Scarpini E, Scheltens P, Feldman H. Treatment of Alzheimer's disease: current status and new perspectives. *Lancet Neurol. 2*, **2003**, 539–47.
92 Mandelkow E. Alzheimer's disease The tangled tale of tau. *Nature 402*, **1999**, 588–9.
93 Ahn JS, Radhakrishnan ML, Mapli M, Choi S, Tidor B, Cuny GD, Musacchio A, Yrh L-A, Kosik KS. Defining Cdk5 ligand chemical space with small molecule inhibitors of tau phosphorylation. *Chem. Biol. 12*, **2005**, 811–23.
94 Sung S, Yang H, Uryu K, Lee EB, Zhao L, Shinenman D, Trojanowski JQ, Lee VM, Pratico D. Modulation of nuclear factor-kappa B activity by indomethacin influences A beta levels but not A beta precursor protein metabolism in a model of Alzheimer's disease. *Am. J. Pathol. 165*, **2004**, 2197–206.
95 Hong CS, Goins WF, Goss JR, Burton EA, Glorioso JC. Herpes simplex virus RNAi and neprilysin gene transfer vectors reduce accumulation of Alzheimer's disease-related amyloid-beta peptide *in vivo*. *Gene Ther. 13*, **2006**, 1068–79.
96 Tariot PN, Farlow MR, Grossberg GT, Graham SM, McDonald S, Gergel I. Memantine treatment in patients with moderate to severe Alzheimer disease already receiving donepezil: a randomized controlled trial. *J. Am. Med. Ass. 291*, **2004**, 317–24.
97 Ravi Kumar MN. Nano and microparticles as controlled drug delivery devices. *J. Pharm. Pharm. Sci. 3*, **2000**, 234–58.
98 Gutman R, Peacock G, Lu D. Targeted drug delivery for brain cancer treament. *J. Control. Release 65*, **2000**, 31–41.
99 Kreuter J. Nanoparticulate systems for brain delivery of drugs. *Adv. Drug Deliv. Rev. 47*, **2001**, 65–81.
100 Kreuter J. Influence of the surface properties on nanoparticle-mediated transport of drugs to the brain. *J. Nanosci. Nanotechnol. 4*, **2004**, 484–8.
101 Muller RH, Jacobs C, Kayser O. Nanosuspensions as particulate drug formulations in therapy. Rationale for development and what we can expect for the future. *Adv. Drug Deliv. Rev. 47*, **2001**, 3–19.
102 Muller RH, Keck CM. Drug delivery to the brain-realization by novel drug carriers. *J. Nanosci. Nanotechnol. 4*, **2004**, 471 –83.
103 Couvreur P, Couarraze G, Devissaguet JP, Puisieux F. Nanoparticles: preparation and characterization. In *Microencapsulation: Methods and Industrial Applications*, Benita S (Ed.). Marcel Dekker, New York, **1996**, pp. 183–211.
104 Barratt G, Couarraze G, Couvreur P, Dubernet C, Fattal E, Gref R, Labarre D, Legrand P, Ponchel G, Vauthier C. Polymeric Micro- and nanoparticles as drug carriers. In

Polymeric Biomaterials, 2nd edn, Dumitriu S (Ed.). Marcel Dekker, New York, **2002**, pp. 753–81.

105 Muldoon LL, Tratnyek PG, Jacobs PM, Doolittle ND, Christoforidis GA, Frank JA, Lindau M, Lockman PR, Manninger SP, Qiang Y, Spence AM, Stupp SI, Zhang M, Neuwelt EA. Imaging and nanomedicine for diagnosis and therapy in the central nervous system: report of the eleventh annual blood–brain barrier disruption consortium meeting. *Am. J. Neuroradiol. 27*, **2006**, 715–21.

106 Hartig W, Paulke BR, Varga C, Seeger J, Harkany T, Kacza J. Electron microscopic analysis of nanoparticles delivering thioflavin-T after intrahippocampal injection in mouse: implications for targeting beta-amyloid in Alzheimer's disease. *Neurosci. Lett. 338*, **2003**, 174–6.

107 Cui Z, Lockman PR, Atwood CS, Hsu CH, Gupte A, Allen DD, Mumper RJ. Novel D-penicillamine carrying nanoparticles for metal chelation therapy in Alzheimer's and other CNS diseases. *Eur. J. Pharm. Biopharm. 59*, **2005**, 263–72.

108 Shea TB, Ortiz D, Nicolosi RJ, Kumar R, Watterson AC. Nanosphere-mediated delivery of vitamin E increases its efficacy against oxidative stress resulting from exposure to amyloid beta. *J. Alzheimer's Dis. 7*, **2005**, 297–301.

109 Liu G, Garrett MR, Men P, Zhu X, Perry G, Smith MA. Nanoparticle and other metal chelation therapeutics in Alzheimer disease. *Biochem. Biophys. Acta 1741*, **2005**, 246–52.

110 Roney C, Kulkarni P, Arora V, Antich P, Bonte F, Wu A, Mallikarjuana NN, Manohar S, Liang HF, Kulkarni AR, Sung HW, Sairam M, Aminabhavi TM. Targeted nanoparticles for drug delivery through the blood–brain barrier for Alzheimer's disease. *J. Control. Release 108*, **2005**, 193–214.

111 Couraud PO, Scherman D. Preface. In *Biology and Physiology of the Blood–Brain Barrier. Transport, Cellular Interactions, and Brain Pathologies*, Couraud PO, Scherman D (Eds.). Plenum Press, New York, **1996**, p. vii.

112 Ballabh P, Braun A, Nedergaard M. An overview, structure, regulation and clinical implication. *Neurobiol. Dis. 16*, **2004**, 1–13.

113 Brightman M. Ultrastructure of the brain endothelium. In *Physiology and pharmacology Of The Blood–Brain Barrier. Handbook of Experimental Pharmacology*, Bradbury MWB (Ed.). Springer, Berlin, **1992**, vol. 103, pp. 1–22.

114 Begley D. The blood–brain barrier: principles for targeting peptides and drugs to the central nervous system. *J. Pharm. Pharmacol. 48*, **1996**, 136–46.

115 Habgood MD, Liu ZD, Dehkordi LS, Khodr HH, Abbott J, Hider RC. Investigation into the correlation between the structure of hydroxy-pyridinones and blood–brain barrier permeability. *Biochem. Pharmacol. 57*, **1999**, 1305–10.

116 Minn A, El-Bacha RDS, Bayol-Denizot C, Lagrange P, Suleman FG. Drug metabolism in the brain: benefits and risks. In *The Blood–Brain Barrier and Drug Delivery to the CNS*, Begley DJ, Bradbury MW, Kreuter J (Eds). Marcel Dekker, New York, **2000**, pp. 145–70.

117 Rapoport SI. Modulation of the blood–brain barrier perability. *J. Drug Target. 3*, **1996**, 417–25.

118 Dehouck B, Fenart L, Dehouck M-P, Pierce A, Torpier G, Cecchelli R. A new function for the LDL receptor: transcytosis of LDL across the blood–brain barrier. *J. Cell Biol. 138*, **1997**, 877–89.

119 Neuwelt EA. Mechanisms of disease: the blood-brain barrier. *Neurosurgery. 54*, **2004**, 131–40.

120 Gummerloch MK, Neuwalt EA. Drug entry into the brain and its pharmacologic manipulation. In *Physiology and pharmacology Of The Blood–Brain Barrier. Handbook of Experimental Pharmacology*, Bradbury MWB (Ed.). Springer, Berlin, **1992**, vol. 103, pp. 525–42.

121 Galey JB, Dumats J, Beck I, Fernandez B, Hocquaux M. *N,N'*-bis-dibenzyl ethylenediaminediacetic acid (DBED): a site-specific hydroxyl radical scavenger acting as an "oxidative stress activatable" iron chelator *in vitro*. *Free Radic. Res. 22,* **1995**, 67–86.
122 Gassen M, Youdim MB. The potential role of iron chelators in the treatment of Parkinson's disease and related neurological disorders. *Pharmacol. Toxicol. 80,* **1997**, 159–66.
123 Pardridge WM, Buciak JL, Friden PM. Selective transport of an anti-transferrin receptor antibody through the blood–brain barrier *in vivo*. *J. Pharmacol. Exp. Ther. 259,* **1991**, 66–70.
124 Pardridge WM. *Brain Drug Targeting.* Cambridge University Press, Cambridge, **2001**.
125 Pardridge WM. Drug and gene targeting to the brain with molecular Trojan horses. *Nat. Rev. Drug Discov. 1,* **2002**, 131–9.
126 Liu G, Bruenger FW, Miller SC, Arif AM. Molecular structure and biological and pharmacological properties of 3-hydroxy-2-methyl-1-(β-D-ribofuranosyl or pyranosyl)-4-pyridinone: potential iron overload drugs for oral administration. *Bioorg. Med. Chem. Lett. 8,* **1998**, 3077–80.
127 Liu G, Bruenger FW, Barrios AM, Miller SC. Synthesis of 2-alkyl-3-hydroxy-4-pyridinone-ribonucleosides. Potential oral iron chelators. *Nucleosides Nucleotides 14,* **1995**, 1091–104.
128 Fokt I, Conrad CA, Madden T, Yung AW, Lang FF, Thapar N, Priebe W. The discovery and development of blood–brain barrier (BBB) penetrating anthracyclines for the treatment of brain tumors. Presented at *AACR–NCI–EORTC International Conference on Molecular Targets and Cancer Therapeutics: Discovery, Biology, and Clinical Application.* Philadelphia, PA, 2005, meeting abstract A199.
129 Fokt I, Grynkiewicz G, Skibicki P, Przewloka T, Priebe W. New strategies towards synthesis of doxorubicin analogs. *Polish J. Chem. 79,* **2005**, 349–59.
130 Cristiano RJ, Xu B, Nguyen D, Schumacher G, Kataoka M, Spitz FR, Roth JA. Viral and nonviral gene delivery vectors for cancer gene therapy. *Cancer Detect. Prev. 22,* **1998**, 445–54.
131 Isacson O, Breakefield XO. Benefits and risks of hosting animal cells in the human brain. *Nat. Med. 3,* **1997**, 964–9.
132 Schumacher JM, Isacson O. *Neuron*al xenotransplantation in Parkinson's disease. *Nat. Med. 3,* **1997**, 474–5.
133 Temsamani J, Rousselle C, Rees AR, Scherrmann JM. Vector-mediated drug delivery to the brain. *Expert Opin. Biol. Ther. 1,* **2001**, 773–82.
134 Temsamani J, Bonnafous C, Rousselle C, Fraisse Y, Clair P, Granier LA, Rees AR, Kaczorek M, Scherrmann JM. Improved brain uptake and pharmacological activity profile of morphine-6-glucuronide using a peptide vector-mediated strategy. *J. Pharmacol. Exp. Ther. 313,* **2005**, 712–9.
135 Zhou X, Huang L. Targeted delivery of DANN by liposomes and polymers. *J. Control. Release 19,* **1992**, 269–74.
136 Chen D, Lee KH. Biodistribution of calcitonin encapsulated in liposomes in mice with particular reference to the central nervous system. *Biochem. Biophys. Acta, 1158,* **1993**, 244–50.
137 Huwyler J, Wu D, Pardridge WM. Brain drug delivery of small molecules using immunoliposomes. *Proc. Natl Acad. Sci. USA 93,* **1996**, 14164–9.
138 Kataoka K, Harada A, Nagasaki Y. Block copolymer micelles for drug delivery: design, characterization and biological significant. *Adv. Drug Deliv. Rev. 47,* **2001**, 113–31.
139 Allen C, Maysinger D, Eisenberg A. Nano-engineering block copolymer aggregates for drug delivery. *Colloids Surf. B 16,* **1999**, 3–27.
140 Maysinger D, Savic R, Tam J, Allen C, Eisenberg A. Recent Developments in drug to the nervous system.

In *Polymeric Biomaterials*, 2nd edn, Dumitriu S (Ed.). Marcel Dekker, New York, **2002**, pp 1083–99.
141 Kreuter J. Nanoparticles. In *Encyclopedia of Pharmaceutical Technology*, Swarbrick J, Boylan JC (Eds.). Dekker, New York, **1994**, vol. 10, pp. 165–90.
142 Aktas Y, Yemisci M, Andrieux K, Gursoy RN, Alonso MJ, Fernandez-Megia E, Novoa-Carballal R, Quinoa E, Riguera R, Sargon MF, Celik HH, Demir AS, Hincal AA, Dalkara T, Capan Y, Couvreur P. Development and brain delivery of chitosan–PEG nanoparticles functionalized with the monoclonal antibody OX26. *Bioconjug. Chem. 16*, **2005**, 1503–11.
143 Troester SD, Mueller U, Kreuter J. Modification of the body distribution of poly(methylmethacrylate) nanoparticles in rats by coating with surfactants. *Int. J. Pharm. 61*, **1990**, 85–100.
144 Juhlin L. Retention of particles by the reticuloendothelial system. *Acta Physiol. Scand. 48*, **1960**, 78–87.
145 Kreuter J, Taeuber U, Illi V. Distribution and elimination of poly(methyl-2-^{14}C-methacrylate) nanoparticle radioactivity after injection in rats and mice. *J. Pharm. Sci. 68*, **1979**, 1443–7.
146 Lenaerts V, Nagelkerke JF, Van Berkel TJC, Couvreur P, Grislain L, Roland M, Speiser P. *In vivo* uptake and cellular distribution of biodegradable polymeric nano-particles. In *Sinusoidal Liver Cells*, Knook DL, Wisse E (Eds.). Elsevier, Amsterdam, **1982**, pp. 343–52.
147 Reszka R, Beck P, Fichtner I, Hentschel M, Richter J, Kreuter J. Body distribution of free, liposomal and nanoparticle-associated mitoxantrone in B16-melanoma-bearing mice. *J. Pharmacol. Exp. Ther. 280*, **1997**, 232–7.
148 Lockman PR, Oyewumi MO, Koziara J, Roder KE, Mumper RJ, Allen DD. Brain uptake of thiamine-coated nanoparticles. *J. Control. Release 93*, **2003**, 271–82.
149 Craft TKS, Mahoney JH, Courtney DeVries A, Sarter M. Microsphere embolism-induced cortical cholinergic deafferentation and impairments in attentional performance. *Eur. J. Neurosci. 21*, **2005**, 3117–32.
150 Sekiguchi M, Takagi K, Takagi N, Date I, Takeo S, Tanaka O, Yamato I, Kobashikawa S, Torigoe K, Nowakowski RS. Time course and sequence of pathological changes in the cerebellum of microsphere-embolized rats. *Exp. Neurol. 191*, **2005**, 266–75.
151 Gulyaev AE, Gelperina SE, Skidan IN, Antropov AS, Kivman GY, Kreuter J. Significant transport of doxorubicin into the brain with polysorbate 80-coated nanoparticles. *Pharm. Res. 16*, **1999**, 1564–9.
152 Schroeder U, Sommerfeld P, Ulrich S, Sabel BA. Nanoparticle technology for delivery of drugs across the blood–brain barrier. *J. Pharm. Sci. 87*, **1998**, 1305–7.
153 Gubha S, Mandal B. Dispersion polymerization of acrylamide. *J. Colloid Interface Sci. 271*, **2004**, 55–9.
154 Gurny R, Peppas N, Harrington DD, Banks GS. Development of biodegradable and injectable lattices for controlled release of potent drugs. *Drug Dev. Ind. Pharm. 7*, **1981**, 1–25.
155 Krause HJ, Schwartz A, Rohdewald P. Polylactic acid nanoparticles, a colloidal drug delivery system for lipophilic drugs. *Int. J. Pharm. 27*, **1985**, 145–55.
156 Verracchia T, Spenlehauer G, Bazile DV, Murry-Brelier A, Archimbaud Y, Veillard M. Non-stealth (poly(lactic acid/albumin) and stealth (poly(lactic acid–poly-ethylene glycol)) nanoparticles as injectable drug carriers. *J. Control. Release 36*, **1995**, 49–61.
157 Fessi H, Puisieux F, Devissaguet JP, Ammoury N, Benita S. Nanocapsule formation by interfacial deposition following solvent displacement. *Int. J. Pharm. 55*, **1989**, R1–4.
158 Al Khouri N, Fessi H, Roblot-Treupel L, Devissaguet JP, Puisieux F. An original procedure for pre-

paring nanocapsules of polyalkylcyanoacrylates for interfacial polymerization. *Pharm. Acta Helv. 61*, **1986**, 274–81.

159 Vranckx H, De Moutier M, De Leers M. Pharmaceutical compositions containing nanocapsules. *US Patent 5,500,224*, **1996**.

160 Ravi Kumar MN, Bakowsky U, Lehr CM. Preparation and characterization of cationic PLGA nanospheres as DNA carriers. *Biomaterials 25*, **2004**, 1771–7.

161 Illum L, Khan MA, Mak E, Davis SS. Evaluation of carrier capacity and release characteristics for poly (butyl 2-cyanoacry-late)nanoparticles. *Int. J. Pharm. 30*, **1986**, 17–28.

162 Bangs Laboratories. *TechNote 201: Working with Microspheres*. Bangs Laboratories, Fishers, IN, **1999**.

163 Jefferies WA, Brandon MR, Hunt SV, Williams AF, Gatter KC, Mason DY. Transferrin receptor on endothelium of brain capillaries. *Nature 312*, **1984**, 162–3.

164 Calvo P, Gouritin B, Villarroya H, Eclancher F, Giannavola C, Klein C, Andreux JP, Couvreur P. Quantification and localization of PEGylated polycyanoacrylate nanoparticles in brain and spinal cord during experimental allergic encephalomyelitis in the rat. *Eur. J. Neurosci. 15*, **2002**, 1317–26.

165 Calvo P, Gouritin B, Chacun H, Desmaele D, D'Angelo J, Noel JP, Georgin D, Fattal E, Andreux JP, Couvreur P. Long-circulating PEGylated polycyanoacrylate nanoparticles as new drug carrier for brain delivery. *Pharm. Res. 18*, **2001**, 1157–66.

166 Peracchia MT, Vauthier C, Desmaele D, Gulik A, Dedieu JC, Demoy M, D'Angelo J, Couvreur P. Pegylated nanoparticles from a novel methoxypolyethylene glycol cyanoacrylate–hexadecyl cyanoacrylate amphiphilic copolymer. *Pharm. Res. 15*, **1998**, 550–6.

167 Lueck M. Plasmaproteinadsorption als moeglicher Schluesselfaktor fuer eine kontrollierte Arzneistoffapplikation mit partikulaeren Traegern. *PhD Thesis*. Freie Universitaet, Berlin, **1997**, pp. 14–24 and 137–54.

168 Kreuter J, Petrov VE, Kharkevich DA, Alyautdin RN. Influence of the type of surfactant on the analgesic effects induced by the peptide dalargin after its delivery across the blood-brain barrier using surfactant-coated nanoparticles. *J. Control. Release 49*, **1997**, 81–7.

169 Ramge P, Unger RE, Oltrogge JB, Zenker D, Begley D, Kreuter J, Von Briesen H. Polysorbate-80 coating enhances uptake of polybutylcyanoacrylate (PBCA)-nanoparticles by human and bovine primary brain capillary endothelial cells. *Eur. J. Neurosci. 12*, **2000**, 1931–40.

170 Olivier JC, Fenart L, Chauvet R, Pariat C, Cecchelli R, Couet W. Indirect evidence that drug brain targeting using polysorbate 80-coated polybutylcyanoacrylate nanoparticles is related to toxicity. *Pharm. Res. 16*, **1999**, 1836–42.

171 Kreuter J, Shamenkov D, Petrov V, Ramge P, Cychutek K, Koch-Brandt C, Alyautdin R. Apolipoprotein-mediated transport of nanoparticle-bound drugs across the blood–brain barrier. *J. Drug Target. 10*, **2002**, 317–25.

172 Ramge P. *Untersuchungen zur Ueberwindung der Blut-Hirn-Schranke mit Hilfe von Nanopartikeln*. Shaker Verlag, Aachen, **1998**, pp. 99–110 and 123–39.

173 Meresse S, Delbart C, Fruchart JC, Cecchelli R. Low-density lipoprotein receptor on endothelium of brain capillaries. *J. Neurochem. 53*, **1989**, 340–5.

174 de Vries HE, Kuiper J, de Boer AG, van Berkel TJ, Breimer DD. Characterization of the scavenger receptor on bovine cerebral endothelial cells *in vitro*. *J. Neurochem. 61*, **1993**, 1813–21.

175 Dehouck B, Dehouck MP, Fruchart JC, Cecchelli R. Upregulation of the low density lipoprotein receptor at the blood–brain barrier: intercommunications between

brain capillary endothelial cells and astrocytes. *J. Cell Biol.* *126*, **1994**, 465–73.

176 Lucarelli M, Gennarelli M, Cardelli P, Novelli G, Scarpa S, Dallapiccola B, Strom R. Expression of receptors for native and chemically modified low-density lipoproteins in brain microvessels. *FEBS Lett.* *401*, **1997**, 53–8.

177 Cecchelli R, Fenart L, Decamps L, Torpier G, Dehouck MP. Receptor-mediated transcytosis of blood-borne molecules through blood–brain barrier endothelial cells: drug targeting by endogenous transport routes. *Proc Int. Symp. Control. Release Bioact. Mater.* *24*, **1997**, 221–2.

178 Pitas RE, Boyles JK, Lee DH, Foss D, Maley RW. Astrocytes synthesize apolipoprotein E and metabolize apolipoprotein E-containing lipoproteins. *Biochem. Biophys. Acta* *917*, **1987**, 148–61.

179 Kreuter J, Alyautdin RN, Kharkevich DA, Ivanov AA. Passage of peptides through the blood–brain barrier with colloidal polymer particles (nanoparticles). *Brain Res.* *674*, **1995**, 171–4.

180 Alyaudtin RN, Reichel A, Lobenberg R, Ramge P, Kreuter J, Begley DJ. Interaction of poly-(butylcyanoacrylate) nanoparticles with the blood–brain barrier *in vivo* and *in vitro*. *J. Drug Target.* *9*, **2001**, 209–21.

181 Fenstermacher JD, Patlak CS, The exchange of materials between cerebrospinal fluid and brain. In *Fluid Environment of the Brain*, Cserr HF, Fenstermacher JD, Fencl V (Eds.). Academic Press, New York, **1975**, pp. 201–14.

182 Kessler JA, Fenstermacher JD, Owens ES. Spinal subarachnoid perfusion of rhesus monkeys, *Am. J. Physiol.* *230*, **1976**, 614–8.

183 Cremer JE, Seville MP. Regional blood low, blood volume, and haematocrit values the adult rat, *J. Cereb. Blood Flow Metab.* *3*, **1983**, 254–6.

184 Fenstermacher JD, Gross P, Sposito N, Acuff V, Pettersen S, Gruber K. Structural and functional variations in capillary systems within the brain. *Ann. NY Acad. Sci.* *529*, **1988**, 21–30.

185 Woodcock DM, Linsenmeyer ME, Chojnowski G, Kriegler AB, Nink V, Webster LK, Sawyer WH. Reversal of multidrug resistance by surfactants. *Br. J. Cancer* *66*, **1992**, 62–8.

186 Nerurkar MM, Burton PS, Borchardt RT. The use of surfactants to enhance the permeability of peptides through Caco-2 cells by inhibition of an apically polarized efflux system. *Pharm. Res.* *13*, **1996**, 528–34.

187 Cordon-Cardo C, O'Brien JP, Casals D, Rittman-Grauer L, Biedler JL, Melamed MR, Bertino JR. Multidrug-resistance gene (P-glycoprotein) is expressed by endothelial cells at blood–brain barrier sites. *Proc. Natl Acad. Sci. USA* *86*, **1989**, 695–8.

188 Brigger I, Morizet J, Aubert G, Chacun H, Terrier-Lacombe MJ, Couvreur P, Vassal G., Poly(ethylene glycol)-coated hexadecylcyanoacrylate nanospheres display a combined effect for brain tumor targeting. *J. Pharmacol. Exp. Ther.* *303*, **2002**, 928–36.

189 Pulfer SK, Gallo JM. Enhanced brain tumor selectivity of cationic magnetic polysaccharide microspheres. *J. Drug Target.* *6*, **1998**, 215–27.

190 Kreuter J, Ramge P, Petrov V, Hamm S, Gelperina SE, Engelhardt B, Alyautdin R, von Briesen H, Begley DJ. Direct evidence that polysorbate-80-coated poly(butylcyanoacrylate) nanoparticles deliver drugs to the CNS via specific mechanisms requiring prior binding of drug to the nanoparticles. *Pharm. Res.* *20*, **2003**, 409–16.

191 Gelperina SE, Khalansky AS, Skidan IN, Smirnova ZS, Bobruskin AI, Severin SE, Turowski B, Zanella FE, Kreuter J. Toxicological studies of doxorubicin bound to polysorbate 80-coated poly(butyl cyanoacrylate) nanoparticles in healthy rats and rats with intracranial glioblastoma. *Toxicol. Lett.* *126*, **2002**, 131–41.

192 Lockman PR, Koziara JM, Mumper RJ, Allen DD. Nanoparticle surface charges alter blood–brain barrier integrity and permeability. *J. Drug Target.* *12*, **2004**, 635–41.

193 Fenart L, Casanova A, Dehouck B, Duhem C, Slupek S, Cecchelli R, Betbeder D. Evaluation of effect of charge and lipid coating on ability of 60-nm nanoparticles to cross an *in vitro* model of the blood–brain barrier. *J. Pharmacol. Exp. Ther.* *291*, **1999**, 1017–22.

194 Klein WI, Krafft GA, Finch CE. Targeting small Ab oligomers: the solution to an Alzheimer's disease conundrum? *Trends Neurosci.* *24*, **2001**, 219–24.

195 Ghiso J, Frangione B. Amyloidosis and Alzheimer's disease. *Adv. Drug Deliv. Rev.* *54*, **2002**, 1539–51.

196 Permanne B, Adessi C, Fraga S, Frossard MJ, Saborio GP, Soto C. Are beta-sheet breaker peptides dissolving the therapeutic problem of Alzheimer's disease? *J. Neural. Transm. Suppl.* *62*, **2002**, 293–301.

197 Permanne B, Adessi C, Saborio GP, Fraga S, Frossard MJ, Van Dorpe J, Dewachter I, Banks WA, Van Leuven F, Soto C. Reduction of amyloid load and cerebral damage in a transgenic mouse model of Alzheimer's disease by treatment with a beta-sheet breaker peptide. *FASEB J.* *16*, **2002**, 860–2.

198 Lleo A, Berezovska O, Growdon JH, Hyman BT. Clinical, pathological, and biochemical spectrum of Alzheimer disease associated with PS-1 mutations. *Am. J. Geriatr. Psychiatry* *12*, **2004**, 146–56.

199 Rogers JT, Randall JD, Eder PS, Huang X, Bush AI, Tanzi RE, Venti A, Payton SM, Giordano T, Nagano S, Cahill CM, Moir R, Lahiri DK, Greig N, Sarang SS, Gullans SR. Alzheimer's disease drug discovery targeted to the APP mRNA 5′-untranslated region. *J. Mol. Neurosci.* *19*, **2002**, 77–82.

200 Rogers JT, Randall JD, Cahill CM, Eder PS, Huang X, Gunshin H, Leiter L, McPhee J, Sarang SS, Utsuki T, Greig NH, Lahiri DK, Tanzi RE, Bush AI, Giordano T, Gullans SR. An iron-responsive element type II in the 5′-untranslated region of the Alzheimer's amyloid precursor protein transcript. *J. Biol. Chem.* *277*, **2002**, 45518–28.

201 Marchesi VT. An alternative interpretation of the amyloid Abeta hypothesis with regard to the pathogenesis of Alzheimer's disease. *Proc. Natl Acad. Sci. USA* *102*, **2005**, 9093–8.

202 Paulke B-R, Moeglich P-M, Knippel E, Budde A, Nitzsche R, Mueller RH. Electrophoretic 3D-mobility profiles of latex particles with different surface groups. *Langmuir* *11*, **1995**, 70–4.

203 Kacza J, Hartig W, Seeger J. Oxygen-enriched photoconversion of fluorescent dyes by means of a closed conversion chamber. *J. Neurosci. Methods* *71*, **1997**, 225–32.

204 Koppal T, Drake J, Butterfield DA. *In vivo* modulation of rodent glutathione and its role in peroxynitrite-induced neocortical synaptosomal membrane protein damage. *Biochim. Biophys. Acta* *1453*, **1999**, 407–11.

205 Butterfield DA, Koppal T, Subramaniam R, Yatin S. Vitamin E as an antioxidant/free radical scavenger against amyloid beta-peptide-induced oxidative stress in neocortical synaptosomal membranes and hippocampal neurons in culture: insights into Alzheimer's disease. *Rev. Neurosci.* *10*, **1999**, 141–9.

206 Butterfield DA, Howard B, Yatin S, Koppal T, Drake J, Hensley K, Aksenov M, Aksenova M, Subramaniam R, Varadarajan S, Harris-White ME, Pedigo NW Jr, Carney JM. Elevated oxidative stress in models of normal brain aging and Alzheimer's disease. *Life Sci.* *65*, **1999**, 1883–92.

207 Butterfield DA, Yatin SM, Varadarajan S, Koppal T. Amyloid beta-peptide-associated free radical oxidative stress, neurotoxicity, and

Alzheimer's disease. *Methods Enzymol. 309*, **1999**, 746–68.

208 Subramaniam R, Koppal T, Green M, Yatin S, Jordan B, Drake J, Butterfield DA. The free radical antioxidant vitamin E protects cortical synaptosomal membranes from amyloid beta-peptide(25–35) toxicity but not from hydroxynonenal toxicity: relevance to the free radical hypothesis of Alzheimer's disease. *Neurochem. Res. 23*, **1998**, 1403–10.

209 Halliwell B, Gutteridge JMC. *Free Radicals in Biology and Medicine*, 3rd edn. Oxford University Press, New York, **1999**.

210 Liu G, Men P, Kenner GH, Miller SC. Age-associated iron accumulation in bone: Implications for post-menopausal osteoporosis and a new target for prevention and treatment by chelation. *BioMetals 19*, **2006**, 245–51.

211 Markesbery WR, Carney JM. Oxidative alternations in Alzheimer's disease. *Brain Pathol. 9*, **1999**, 133–46.

212 Zhu X, Raina AK, Lee HG, Casadesus G, Smith MA, Perry G. Oxidative stress signaling in Alzheimer's disease. *Brain Res. 1000*, **2004**, 32–9.

213 Rottkamp CA, Nunomura A, Raina AK, Sayre LM, Perry G, Smith MA. Oxidative stress, antioxidants, and Alzheimer disease. *Alzheimer Dis. Assoc. Disord. 14*, **2000**, S62–66.

214 Polidori MC, Mattioli P, Aldred S, Cecchetti R, Stahl W, Griffiths H, Senin U, Sies H, Mecocci P. Plasma antioxidant status, immunoglobulin G oxidation and lipid peroxidation in demented patients: relevance to Alzheimer disease and vascular dementia. *Dement. Geriatr. Cogn. Disord. 18*, **2004**, 265–70.

215 Anlasik T, Sies H, Griffiths HR, Mecocci P, Stahl W, Polidori MC. Dietary habits are major determinants of the plasma antioxidant status in healthy elderly subjects. *Br. J. Nutr. 94*, **2005**, 639–42.

216 Berman K, Brodaty H. Tocopherol (vitamin E) in Alzheimer's disease and other neurodegenerative disorders. *CNS Drugs 18*, **2004**, 807–25.

217 Growdon JH. Incorporating biomarkers into clinical drug trials in Alzheimer's disease. *J. Alzheimer's Dis. 3*, **2001**, 287–92.

218 Vina J, Lloret A, Orti R, Alonso D. Molecular bases of the treatment of Alzheimer's disease with antioxidants: prevention of oxidative stress. *Mol. Aspects Med. 25*, **2004**, 117–23.

219 Dhitavat S, Rivera ER, Rogers E, Shea TB. Differential efficacy of lipophilic and cytosolic antioxidants on generation of reactive oxygen species by amyloid-beta. *J. Alzheimer's Dis. 3*, **2001**, 525–9.

220 Ekinci FJ, Linsley MD, Shea TB. Beta-amyloid-induced calcium influx induces apoptosis in culture by oxidative stress rather than tau phosphorylation. *Brain Res. Mol. Brain Res. 76*, **2000**, 389–95.

221 Ekinci FJ, Malik KU, Shea TB. Activation of the L voltage-sensitive calcium channel by mitogen-activated protein (MAP) kinase following exposure of neuronal cells to beta-amyloid. MAP kinase mediates beta-amyloid-induced neurodegeneration. *J. Biol. Chem. 274*, **1999**, 30322–7.

222 Kumar R, Chen MH, Parmar VS, Samuelson LA, Kumar J, Nicolosi R, Yoganathan S, Watterson AC. Supramolecular assemblies based on copolymers of PEG600 and functionalized aromatic diesters for drug delivery applications. *J. Am. Chem. Soc. 126*, **2004**, 10640–4.

223 Olanow CW. An introduction to the free radical hypothesis in Parkinson's disease. *Ann. Neurol. 32*, **1992**, S2–9.

224 Markesbery WR, Ehmann WD. Oxidative stress in Alzheimer disease. In *Alzheimer Disease*, Terry RD, Katzman R, Bick KL, Sisodia SS (Eds.). Lippincott Williams & Wilkins, Philadelphia, PA, **1999**, pp. 401–14.

225 Ehmann WD, Markesberg WR, Alauddin M, Hossain TI, Brubaker EH. Brain trace elements in Alzheimer's disease. *Neurotoxicology 7*, **1986**, 195–206.

226 Huang X, Atwood CS, Moir RD, Hartshorn MA, Vonsattel JP,

Tanzi RE, Bush AI. Zinc-induced Alzheimer's Abeta1–40 aggregation is mediated by conformational factors. *J. Biol. Chem. 272*, **1997**, 26464–70.

227 Atwood CS, Perry G, Zeng H, Kato Y, Jones WD, Ling KQ, Huang X, Moir RD, Wang D, Sayre LM, Smith MA, Chen SG, Bush AI. Copper mediates dityrosine cross-linking of Alzheimer's amyloid-beta. *Biochemistry 43*, **2004**, 560–8.

228 Atwood CS, Scarpa RC, Huang X, Moir RD, Jones WD, Fairlie DP, Tanzi RE, Bush AI. Characterization of copper interactions with Alzheimer amyloid beta peptides: identification of an attomolar-affinity copper binding site on amyloid beta1–42. *J. Neurochem. 75*, **2000**, 1219–33.

229 Bush AI, Pettingell WH, Multhaup G, d Paradis M, Vonsattel JP, Gusella JF, Beyreuther K, Masters CL, Tanzi RE. Rapid induction of Alzheimer A beta amyloid formation by zinc. *Science 265*, **1994**, 1464–7.

230 Bush AI, Masters CL, Tanzi RE. Copper, beta-amyloid, and Alzheimer's disease: tapping a sensitive connection. *Proc. Natl Acad. Sci. USA 100*, **2003**, 11193–4.

231 Jobling MF, Huang X, Stewart LR, Barnham KJ, Curtain C, Volitakis I, Perugini M, White AR, Cherny RA, Masters CL, Barrow CJ, Collins SJ, Bush AI, Cappai R. Copper and zinc binding modulates the aggregation and neurotoxic properties of the prion peptide PrP106–126. *Biochemistry 40*, **2001**, 8073–84.

232 Cherny RA, Legg JT, McLean CA, Fairlie DP, Huang X, Atwood CS, Beyreuther K, Tanzi RE, Masters CL, Bush AI. Aqueous dissolution of Alzheimer's disease Abeta amyloid deposits by biometal depletion. *J. Biol. Chem. 274*, **1999**, 23223–8.

233 Loske C, Gerdemann A, Schepl W, Wycislo M, Schinzel R, Palm D, Riederer P, Munch G. Transition metal-mediated glycoxidation accelerates cross-linking of beta-amyloid peptide. *Eur. J. Biochem. 267*, **2000**, 4171–8.

234 Cherny RA, Barnham KJ, Lynch T, Volitakis I, Li QX, McLean CA, Multhaup G, Beyreuther K, Tanzi RE, Masters CL, Bush AI. Chelation and intercalation: complementary properties in a compound for the treatment of Alzheimer's disease. *J. Struct. Biol. 130*, **2000**, 209–16.

235 Lynch T, Cherny RA, Bush AI. Oxidative processes in Alzheimer's disease: the role of abeta-metal interactions. *Exp. Gerontol. 35*, **2000**, 445–51.

236 Lovell MA, Robertson JD, Teesdale WJ, Campbell JL, Markesbery WR. Copper, iron and zinc in Alzheimer's disease senile plaques, *J. Neurol. Sci. 158*, **1998**, 47–52.

237 Padmanabhan G, Becue I, Smith JA. Clioquinol. In *Analytical Profiles of Drug Substances*, Florey K (Ed.). Academic Press, New York, **1989**, pp 57–90.

238 Andersen O. Chemical and biological considerations in the treatment of metal intoxications by chelating agents. *Mini-Rev. Med. Chem. 4*, **2004**, 11–21.

239 Lockman PR, Koziara J, Roder KE, Paulson J, Abbruscato TJ, Mumper RJ, Allen DD. *In-vivo* and *in-vitro* assessment of baseline blood–brain barrier parameters in the presence of novel nanoparticle. *Pharm. Res. 20*, **2003**, 705–13.

240 Koziara JM, Lockman PR, Allen DD, Mumper RJ. *In-situ* blood–brain barrier of nanoparticles. *Pharm. Res. 20*, **2003**, 1772–8.

241 Cui Z, Mumper RJ. Plasmid DNA-entrapped nanoparticles engineered from microemulsion precursors: *in-vitro* and *in-vivo* evaluation. *Bioconjug. Chem. 13*, **2002**, 1319–27.

242 Oyewumi MO, Mumper RJ. Influence of formulation parameters on gadolinium entrapment and tumor cell uptake using folate-coated nanoparticles. *Int. J. Pharm. 251*, **2003**, 85–97.

243 Wong SS. *Chemistry of Protein Conjugation and Cross-Linking.* CRC Press, Bioca Raton, FL, **1991**.

244 Martin FJ, Papahadjopoulos D. Irreversible coupling of immuno-

globulin fragments to preformed vesicles. *J. Biol. Chem. 257*, **1982**, 286–8.

245 Martin FJ, Hubbell WL, Papahadjopoulos D. Immunospecific targeting of liposomes to cells: a novel and efficient method for covalent attachment of Fab' fragments via disulfide bonds. *Biochemistry 20*, **1981**, 4229–38.

246 Kato N, Nakamura M, Uchiyama T. ^{1}H NMR studies of the reactions of copper(I) and copper(II) with D-penicillamine and glutathione. *J. Inorg. Biochem. 75*, **1999**, 117–21.

247 Danehy JP, Hunter WE. The alkaline decomposition of organic disulfides. II. Alternative pathways as determined by structure. *J. Org. Chem. 32*, **1967**, 2047–53.

248 Subramanian ZF, Vanek ZF. Diagnosis and treatment of Wilson's disease. *Curr. Neurol. Neurosci. Rep. 2*, **2002**, 317–23.

249 Walshe JM. Penicillamine, a new oral therapy for Wilson's disease. *Am. J. Med. 21*, **1956**, 487–95.

250 Walshe JM. Copper chelation in patients with Wilson's disease. A comparison of penicillamine and triethylene tetramine dihydrochloride. *Q. J. Med. 42*, **1973**, 441–52.

251 Walshe JM. Treatment of Wilson's disease with trientine (triethylene teramine) dihydrochloride. *Lancet i*, **1982**, 643–7.

252 Powell LW, Jazwinska E, Halliday JW. Primary iron overload. In *Iron Metabolism in Health and Disease*, Brock JH, Halliday JW, Pippard MJ, Powell LW (Eds.). Saunders, London, **1994**, pp. 227–270.

253 Pippard MJ. Secondary iron overload. In *Iron Metabolism in Health and Disease*, Brock JH, Halliday JW, Pippard MJ, Powell LW (Eds.). Saunders, London, **1994**, pp. 271–309.

254 Crichton RR. *Inorganic Biochemistry of Iron Metabolism from Molecular Mechanis to Clinical Consequences*, 2nd edn. Wiley, Chichester, **2001**.

255 Sullivan JL. Iron and the sex difference in heart disease risk. *Lancet 1*, **1981**, 1293–4.

256 Stadler N, Lindner RA, Davies MJ. Direct detection and quantification of transition metal ions in human atherosclerotic plaques: evidence for the presence of elevated levels of iron and copper. *Arterioscler. Thromb. Vasc. Biol. 24*, **2004**, 949–54.

257 Stevens RG, Jones DY, Micozzi MS, Taylor PR. Body iron stores and the risk of cancer. *N. Engl J. Med. 319*, **1988**, 1047–52.

258 Woo J, Mak YT, Law LK, Swaminathan R. Plasma ferritin in an elderly population living in the community. *J. Med. 20*, **1989**, 123–34.

259 Moirand R, Mortaji AM, Loreal O, Paillard F, Brissot P, Deugnier Y. A new syndrome of liver iron overload with normal transferrin saturation. *Lancet 349*, **1997**, 95–7.

260 Rouault TA. Iron on the brain. *Nat. Genet. 28*, **2001**, 299–300.

261 Lovell MA, Ehmann WD, Butler SM, Markesbery WR. Elevated thiobarbituric acid-reactive substances and antioxidant enzyme activity in the brain in Alzheimer's disease. *Neurology 45*, **1995**, 1594–601.

262 Perry G, Castellani RJ, Hirai K, Smith MA. Reactive oxygen species mediate cellular damage in Alzheimer disease. *J. Alzheimer's Dis. 1*, **1998**, 45–55.

263 Casadesus G, Smith MA, Zhu X, Aliev G, Cash AD, Honda K, Petersen RB, Perry G. Alzheimer disease: evidence for a central pathogenic role of iron-mediated reactive oxygen species. *J. Alzheimer's Dis. 6*, **2004**, 165–9.

264 Gutteridge JM. Hydroxyl radicals, iron, oxidative stress, and neurodegeneration. *Ann. NY Acad. Sci. 738*, **1994**, 201–13.

265 Evans PH. Free radicals in brain metabolism and pathology. *Br. Med. Bull. 49*, **1993**, 577–87.

266 Connor JR, Menzies SL, St Martin SM, Mufson EJ. Cellular distribution of transferrin, ferritin, and iron in normal and aged human brains. *J. Neurosci. Res. 27*, **1990**, 595–611.

267 Connor JR, Snyder BS, Beard JL, Fine RE, Mufson EJ. Regional

distribution of iron and iron-regulatory proteins in the brain in aging and Alzheimer's disease. *J. Neurosci. Res. 31*, **1992**, 327–35.

268 Connor JR, Menzies SL, St Martin SM, Mufson EJ. A histochemical study of iron, transferrin, and ferritin in Alzheimer's diseased brains. *J. Neurosci. Res. 31*, **1992**, 75–83.

269 Christen Y. Oxidative stress and Alzheimer disease. *Am. J. Clin. Nutr. 71*, **2000**, 621S–9S.

270 Collingwood JF, Mikhaylova A, Davidson M, Batich C, Streit WJ, Terry J, Dobson J. In situ characterization and mapping of iron compounds in Alzheimer's disease tissue. *J. Alzheimer's Dis. 7*, **2005**, 267–72.

271 Finefrock AE, Bush AI, Doraiswamy PM. Current status of metals as therapeutic targets in Alzheimer's disease. *J. Am. Geriatr. Soc. 51*, **2003**, 1143–8.

272 Suh SW, Jensen KB, Jensen MS, Silva DS, Kesslak PJ, Danscher G, Frederickson CJ. Histochemically-reactive zinc in amyloid plaques, angiopathy, and degenerating neurons of Alzheimer's diseased brains. *Brain Res. 852*, **2000**, 274–8.

273 Lee JY, Mook-Jung I, Koh JY. Histochemically reactive zinc in plaques of the Swedish mutant B-amyloid precursor protein transgenic mice. *J. Neurosci. 19*, **1999**, RC10.1–5.

274 McLachlan DR, Kruck TP, Lukiw WJ, Krishnan SS. Would decreased aluminum ingestion reduce the incidence of Alzheimer's disease? *Can. Med. Ass. J. 145*, **1991**, 793–804.

275 Good PF, Perl DP, Bierer LM, Schmeidler J. Selective accumulation of aluminum and iron in the neurofibrillary tangles of Alzheimer's disease: a laser microprobe (LAMMA) study. *Ann. Neurol. 31*, **1992**, 286–92.

276 Kong S, Liochev S, Fridovich I. Aluminum(III) facilitates the oxidation of NADH by the superoxide anion. *Free Radic. Biol. Med. 13*, **1992**, 79–81.

277 Bondy SC, Guo-Ross SX, Truong AT. Promotion of transition metal-induced reactive oxygen species formation by beta-amyloid. *Brain Res. 799*, **1998**, 91–6.

278 Pratico D, Clark CM, Liun F, Rokach J, Lee VY, Trojanowski JQ. Increase of brain oxidative stress in mild cognitive impairment: a possible predictor of Alzheimer disease. *Arch. Neurol. 59*, **2002**, 972–976.

279 Kennard ML, Feldman H, Yamada T, Jefferies WA. Serum levels of the iron binding protein p97 are elevated in Alzheimer's disease. *Nat. Med. 2*, **1996**, 1230–5.

280 Jefferies WA, Food MR, Gabathuler R, Rothenberger S, Yamada T, Yasuhara O, McGeer PL. Reactive microglia specifically associated with amyloid plaques in Alzheimer's disease brain tissue express melanotransferrin. *Brain Res. 712*, **1996**, 122–6.

281 Multhaup G, Schlicksupp A, Hesse L, Beher D, Ruppert T, Masters CL, Beyreuther K. The amyloid precursor protein of Alzheimer's disease in the reduction of copper(II) to copper(I). *Science 271*, **1996**, 1406–9.

282 Sayre LM, Perry G, Smith MA. Redox metals and neurodegenerative disease. *Curr. Opin. Chem. Biol. 3*, **1999**, 220–5.

283 Linder MC, Hazegh-Azam M. Copper biochemistry and molecular biology. *Am. J. Clin. Nutr. 63*, **1996**, 797S–811S.

284 Hensley K, Carney JM, Mattson MP, Aksenova M, Harris M, Wu JF, Floyd RA, Butterfield DA. A model for beta-amyloid aggregation and neurotoxicity based on free radical generation by the peptide: relevance to Alzheimer disease. *Proc. Natl Acad. Sci. USA 91*, **1994**, 3270–4.

285 Butterfield DA. beta-Amyloid-associated free radical oxidative stress and neurotoxicity: implications for Alzheimer's disease. *Chem. Res. Toxicol. 10*, **1997**, 495–506.

286 House E, Collingwood J, Khan A, Korchazkina O, Berthon G, Exley C. Aluminium, iron, zinc and copper influence the *in vitro* formation of amyloid fibrils of Abeta42 in a manner which may have consequences

for metal chelation therapy in Alzheimer's disease. *J. Alzheimer's Dis. 6*, **2004**, 291–301.
287 Hershko C. Iron chelators for thalassaemia. *Br. J. Haematol. 101*, **1998**, 399–406.
288 Neufeld EJ. Oral chelators deferasirox and deferiprone for transfusional iron overload in Thalassemia major: new data, new questions. Blood *107*, **2006**, 3436–41.
289 McLachlan DR, Dalton AJ, Kruck TP, Bell MY, Smith WL, Kalow W, Andrews DF. Intramuscular desferrioxamine in patients with Alzheimer's disease. *Lancet, 337*, **1991**, 1304–8.
290 Cuajungco MP, Faget KY, Huang X, Tanzi RE, Bush AI. Metal chelation as a potential therapy for Alzheimer's disease. *Ann. NY Acad. Sci. 920*, **2000**, 292–304.
291 Richardson DR, Ponka P. Development of iron chelators to treat iron overload disease and their use as experimental tools to probe intracellular iron metabolism. *Am. J. Hematol. 58*, **1998**, 299–305.
292 Keberle H. The biochemistry of desferrioxamine and its relation to iron metabolism. *Ann. NY Acad. Sci. 119*, **1964**, 758–68.
293 Hider RC, Hall AD. Clinically useful chelators of tripositive elements. *Prog. Med. Chem. 28*, **1991**, 41–173.
294 Ben-Shachar D, Riederer P, Youdim MB. Iron–melanin interaction and lipid peroxidation: implications for Parkinson's disease. *J. Neurochem. 57*, **1991**, 1609–14.
295 Floor E. Iron as a vulnerability factor in nigrostriatal degeneration in aging and Parkinson's disease. *Cell Mol. Biol. 46*, **2000**, 709–20.
296 Blake DR, Winyard P, Lunec J, Williams A, Good PA, Crewes SJ, Gutteridge JM, Rowley D, Halliwell B, Cornish A, Hider RC. Cerebral and ocular toxicity induced by desferrioxamine. *Q. J. Med. 56*, **1985**, 345–55.
297 Kruck TP, Fisher EA, McLachlan DR. A predictor for side-effects in patients with Alzheimer's disease treated with deferoxamine mesylate. *Clin. Pharmacol. Ther. 53*, **1993**, 30–7.
298 Struck M, Waldmeier P, Berdoukas V. The treatment of iron overload – psychiatric implication. In *Iron in Central Nervous System Disorders*, Riederer P, Youdim MBH (Eds.). Springer Verlag, Wien, **1993**, pp. 189–96.
299 Klaasen CD. Heavy metals and heavy-metal antagonists. In *Goodman and Gilman's The Pharmacological Basis of Therapeutics*, Hardman JG, Limbird LE, Molinoff PB, Ruddon RW, Gilman AG (Eds.). McGraw-Hill, New York, **1996**, pp. 1649–71.
300 Jenner P, Olanow CW. Understanding cell death in Parkinson's disease. *Ann. Neurol. 44*, **1998**, S72–S84.
301 May PM, Bulman RA. The present status of chelating agents in medicine. *Prog. Med. Chem. 20*, **1983**, 225–336.
302 Olivieri NF, Brittenham GM. Iron-chelating therapy and the treatment of thalassemia. *Blood 89*, **1997**, 739–61.
303 Lynch SG, Fonseca T, Levine SM. A multiple course trial of desferrioxamine in chronic progressive multiple sclerosis. *Cell Mol. Biol. 46*, **2000**, 865–9.
304 Crowe A, Morgan EH. Effects of chelators on iron uptake and release by the brain in the rat. *Neurochem. Res. 19*, **1994**, 71–6.
305 Kontoghiorghes GJ. New concepts of iron and aluminium chelation therapy with oral L1 (deferiprone) and other chelators. A review. *Analyst 120*, **1995**, 845–51.
306 Nelson WO, Timothy B, Karpishin TB, Retting SJ, Orvig C. Aluminum and gallium compounds of 3-hydroxy-4-pyridinones: synthesis, characterization, and crystallography of biologically active complexes with unusual hydrogen bonding. *Inorg. Chem. 27*, **1988**, 1045–51.
307 Hoffbrand AV. Oral iron chelation. *Semin. Hematol. 33*, **1996**, 1–8.
308 Ward RJ, Dexter D, Florence A, Aouad F, Hider R, Jenner P, Crichton RR. Brain iron in the ferrocene-loaded rat: its chelation and

influence on dopamine metabolism. *Biochem. Pharmacol. 49*, **1995**, 1821–6.

309 Richardson DR. The therapeutic potential of iron chelators. *Expert Opin. Invest. Drugs 8*, **1999**, 2141–58.

310 Hider RC, Porter JB, Singh S. The design of therapeutically useful iron chelators. In *The Development of Iron Chelators for Clinical Use*. Bergeron RJ, Brittenham GM (Eds.). CRC, Boca Raton, FL, **1994**, pp. 353–71.

311 Porter JB, Morgan J, Hoyes KP, Burke LC, Huehns ER, Hider RC. Relative oral efficacy and acute toxicity of hydroxypyridin-4-one iron chelators in mice. *Blood 76*, **1990**, 2389–96.

312 Raymond KN, Xu J. Siderophore-based hydroxypyridonate sequestering agents. In *The Development of Iron Chelators for Clinical Use*, Bergeron RJ, Brittenham GM (Eds.). CRC Press, Boca Raton, FL, **1994**, pp. 354–71.

313 Zhou T, Liu ZD, Neubert H, Kong XL, Ma YM, Hider RC. High affinity iron(III) scavenging by a novel hexadentate 3-hydroxypyridin-4-one-based dendrimer: synthesis and characterization. *Bioorg. Med. Chem. Lett. 15*, **2005**, 5007–11.

314 Hider RC, Choudhury R, Rai BL, Dehkordi LS, Singh S. Design of orally active iron chelators. *Acta Haematol. 95*, **1996**, 6–12.

315 Martell AE, Motekaitis RJ, Sun Y, Ma R, Welch MJ, Pajeau T. New chelating-agents suitable for the treatment of iron overload. *Inorg. Chim. Acta 291*, **1999**, 238–46.

316 Caravan P, Orvig C. Tripodal aminophenolate ligand complexes of aluminum(III), gallium(III), and indium(III) in water. *Inorg. Chem. 36*, **1997**, 237–48.

317 Faller B, Spanka C, Sergejew T, Tschinke V. Improving the oral bioavailability of the iron chelator HBED by breaking the symmetry of the intramolecular H-bond network. *J. Med. Chem. 43*, **2000**, 1467–75.

318 Richardson DR, Ponka P. Pyridoxal isonicotinoyl hydrazone and its analogs: potential orally effective iron-chelating agents for the treatment of iron overload disease. *J. Lab. Clin. Med. 131*, **1998**, 306–15.

319 Richardson DR. Friedreich's ataxia: iron chelators that target the mitochondrion as a therapeutic strategy? *Expert Opin. Invest. Drugs 12*, **2003**, 235–45.

320 Galanello R, Piga A, Alberti D, Rouan MC, Bigler H, Sechaud R. Safety, tolerability, and pharmacokinetics of ICL670, a new orally active iron-chelating agent in patients with transfusion-dependent iron overload due to beta-thalassemia. *J. Clin. Pharmacol. 43*, **2003**, 565–572.

321 Donovan JM, Plone M, Dagher R, Bree M, Marquis J. Preclinical and clinical development of deferitrin, a novel, orally available iron chelator. *Ann. NY Acad. Sci. 1054*, **2005**, 492–4.

322 Sterba M, Simunek T, Mazurova Y, Adamcova M, Popelova O, Kaplanova J, Ponka P, Gersl V. Safety and tolerability of repeated administration of pyridoxal 2-chlorobenzoyl hydrazone in rabbits. *Hum. Exp. Toxicol. 24*, **2005**, 581–9.

323 Lovejoy DB, Kalinowski D, Bernhardt PV, Richardson DR. PCTH: a novel orally active chelator for the treatment of iron overload disease. *Hemoglobin 30*, **2006**, 93–104.

324 Kontoghiorghes GJ, Eracleous E, Economides C, Kolnagou A. Advances in iron overload therapies. prospects for effective use of deferiprone (L1), deferoxamine, the new experimental chelators ICL670, GT56-252, L1NA11 and their combinations. *Curr. Med. Chem. 12*, **2005**, 2663–81.

325 Bergeron RJ, Bharti N, Wiegand J, McManis JS, Yao H, Prokai L. Polyamine-vectored iron chelators: the role of charge. *J. Med. Chem. 48*, **2005**, 4120–37.

326 Fisher AE, Naughton DP. Metal ion chelating peptides with superoxide dismutase activity. *Biomed. Pharmacother. 59*, **2005**, 158–62.

327 Apostol M, Baret P, Serratrice G, Desbrieres J, Putaux JL, Stebe MJ, Expert D, Pierre JL. Self-assembly of an amphiphilic iron(III) chelator:

mimicking iron acquisition in marine bacteria. *Angew. Chem. Int. Ed. 44*, **2005**, 2580–2.

328 Novakovic J, Tesoro A, Thiessen JJ, Spino M. Metabolic and pharmacokinetic evaluation of a novel 3-hydroxypyridinone iron chelator, CP502, in the rat. *Eur. J. Drug Metab. Pharmacokinet. 29*, **2004**, 221–4.

329 Hochhauser E, Ben-Ari Z, Pappo O, Chepurko Y, Vidne BA. TPEN attenuates hepatic apoptotic ischemia/reperfusion injury and remote early cardiac dysfunction. *Apoptosis 10*, **2005**, 53–62.

330 Lebedev AV, Ivanova MV, Levitsky DO. Echinochrome, a naturally occurring iron chelator and free radical scavenger in artificial and natural membrane systems. *Life Sci. 76*, **2005**, 863–75.

331 Chong HS, Torti SV, Ma R, Torti FM, Brechbiel MW. Synthesis and potent antitumor activities of novel 1,3,5-*cis,cis*-triaminocyclohexane *N*-pyridyl derivatives. *J. Med. Chem. 47*, **2004**, 5230–4.

332 Hodges YK, Antholine WE, Horwitz LD. Effect on ribonucleotide reductase of novel lipophilic iron chelators: the desferri-exochelins. *Biochem. Biophys. Res. Commun. 315*, **2004**, 595–8.

333 Lewis JA, Puerta DT, Cohen SM. Metal complexes of the *trans*-influencing ligand thiomaltol. *Inorg. Chem. 42*, **2003**, 7455–9.

334 Halper SR, Cohen SM. Synthesis, structure, and spectroscopy of phenylacetylenylene rods incorporating meso-substituted dipyrrin ligands. *Chemistry 9*, **2003**, 4661–9.

335 Brandon MS, Paszczynski AJ, Korus R, Crawford RL. The determination of the stability constant for the iron(II) complex of the biochelator pyridine-2,6-bis(monothiocarboxylic acid). *Biodegradation 14*, **2003**, 73–82.

336 Laden K, Zaklad H, Simhon ED, Klein JY, Cyjon RL, Winchell HS. *N,N′,N″*-tris(dihydroxyphosphorylmethyl)-1,4,7-triazacyclononane (Deofix) – a high-affinity, high-specificity chelator for first transition series metal cations with significant deodorant, anti-microbial, and antioxidant activity. *J. Cosmet. Sci. 54*, **2003**, 251–61.

337 Persson HL, Yu Z, Tirosh O, Eaton JW, Brunk UT. Prevention of oxidant-induced cell death by lysosomotropic iron chelators. *Free Radic. Biol. Med. 34*, **2003**, 1295–305.

338 Dhungana S, Heggemann S, Gebhardt P, Mollmann U, Crumbliss AL. Fe(III) coordination properties of a new saccharide-based exocyclic trihydroxamate analogue of ferrichrome. *Inorg. Chem. 42*, **2003**, 42–50.

339 Ferrali M, Bambagioni S, Ceccanti A, Donati D, Giorgi G, Fontani M, Laschi F, Zanello P, Casolaro M, Pietrangelo A. Design, synthesis, and physicochemical and biological characterization of a new iron chelator of the family of hydroxychromenes. *J. Med. Chem. 45*, **2002**, 5776–85.

340 Kicic A, Chua AC, Baker E. The desferrithiocin (DFT) class of iron chelators: potential as antineoplastic agents. *Anticancer Drug Des. 16*, **2001**, 195–207.

341 Royt PW, Honeychuck RV, Ravich V, Ponnaluri P, Pannell LK, Buyer JS, Chandhoke V, Stalick WM, DeSesso LC, Donohue S, Ghei R, Relyea JD, Ruiz R. 4-hydroxy-2-nonylquinoline: a novel iron chelator isolated from a bacterial cell membrane. *Bioorg. Chem. 29*, **2001**, 387–97.

342 Dhungana S, Heggemann S, Heinisch L, Mollmann U, Boukhalfa H, Crumbliss AL. Fe(III) coordination properties of two new saccharide-based enterobactin analogues: methyl 2,3,4-tris-*O*-[*N*-[2,3-di(hydroxy)benzoyl-glycyl]-aminopropyl]-alpha-D-glucopyranoside and methyl 2,3,4-tris-*O*-[N-[2,3-di-(hydroxy)-benzoyl]-aminopropyl]-alpha-D-glucopyranoside. *Inorg. Chem. 40*, **2001**, 7079–86.

343 Samuni AM, Krishna MC, DeGraff W, Russo A, Planalp RP, Brechbiel MW, Mitchell JB. Mechanisms underlying the cytotoxic effects of Tachpyr – a novel metal chelator.

Biochim. Biophys. Acta 1571, **2002**, 211–8.

344 Ferrali M, Donati D, Bambagioni S, Fontani M, Giorgi G, Pietrangelo A. 3-Hydroxy-(4H)-benzopyran-4-ones as potential iron chelating agents *in vivo*. *Bioorg. Med. Chem. 9*, **2001**, 3041–7.

345 Naughton DP, Grootveld M. EDTA bis-(ethyl phenylalaninate): a novel transition metal-ion chelating hydroxyl radical scavenger with a potential anti-inflammatory role. *Bioorg. Med. Chem. Lett. 11*, **2001**, 2573–5.

346 Borsari M, Gabbi C, Ghelfi F, Grandi R, Saladini M, Severi S, Borella F. Silybin, a new iron-chelating agent. *J. Inorg. Biochem. 85*, **2001**, 123–9.

347 Galey JB, Destree O, Dumats J, Genard S, Tachon P. Protection against oxidative damage by iron chelators: effect of lipophilic analogues and prodrugs of *N,N'*-bis(3,4,5-trimethoxybenzyl)ethylenediamine-*N,N'*-diacetic acid (OR10141). *J. Med. Chem. 43*, **2000**, 1418–21.

348 Fasman GD, Moore CD. The solubilization of model Alzheimer tangles: reversing the beta-sheet conformation induced by aluminum with silicates. *Proc. Natl Acad. Sci. USA 91*, **1994**, 11232–5.

349 Brewer GJ. Neurologically presenting Wilson's disease: epidemiology, pathophysiology and treatment. *CNS Drugs 19*, **2005**, 185–92.

350 Alyautdin RN, Tezikov EB, Ramge P, Kharkevich DA, Begley DJ, Kreuter J. Significant entry of tubocurarine into the brain of rats by adsorption to polysorbate 80-coated polybutylcyanoacrylate nanoparticles: an in situ brain perfusion study. *J. Microencapsul. 15*, **1998**, 67–74.

351 Alyautdin RN, Petrov VE, Langer K, Berthold A, Kharkevich DA, Kreuter J. Delivery of loperamide across the blood–brain barrier with polysorbate 80-coated polybutylcyanoacrylate nanoparticles. *Pharm. Res. 14*, **1997**, 325–8.

352 Luo Y, Han Z, Chin SM, Linn S. Three chemically distinct types of oxidants formed by iron-mediated Fenton reactions in the presence of DNA. *Proc. Natl Acad. Sci. USA 91*, **1994**, 12438–42.

353 Davson H, Segal MB. *Physiology of the CSF and Blood–Brain Barriers*. CRC Press, Boca Raton, FL, **1996**.

354 Porter JB, Gyparaki M, Burke LC, Huehns ER, Sarpong P, Saez V, Hider RC. Iron mobilization from hepatocyte monolayer cultures by chelators: the importance of membrane permeability and the iron-binding constant. *Blood 72*, **1988**, 1497–503.

355 Liu G, Men P, Kenner GH, Miller SC, Bruenger FW. Acyclonucleoside iron chelators of 1-(2-hydroxyethoxy)-methyl-2-alkyl-3-hydroxy-4-pyridinones: potential oral iron chelation therapeutics. *Nucleosides Nucleotides Nucleic Acids 23*, **2004**, 599–611.

356 Brem H, Walter KA, Tamargo RJ, Olivi A, Langer R. Drug delivery to the brain. In *Polymeric Site-Specific Pharmacotherapy*, Domb AJ (Ed.). Wiley, New York. **1994**, pp. 117–39.

357 Blunk T, Hochstrasser DF, Sanchez JC, Muller BW, Muller RH. Colloidal carriers for intravenous drug targeting: plasma protein adsorption patterns on surface-modified latex particles evaluated by two-dimensional polyacrylamide gel electrophoresis. *Electrophoresis 14*, **1993**, 1382–7.

358 Dobbin PS, Hider RC, Hall AD, Taylor PD, Sarpong P, Porter JB, Xiao G, van der Helm D. Synthesis, physicochemical properties, and biological evaluation of *N*-substituted 2-alkyl-3-hydroxy-4(1H)-pyridinones: orally active iron chelators with clinical potential. *J. Med. Chem. 36*, **1993**, 2448–58.

359 Liu G, Miller SC, Bruenger FW. Synthesis of lipophilic 3-hydroxy-2-methyl-4-pyridinone derivatives. *Synth. Commun. 25*, **1995**, 3247–53.

360 Liu G, Miller SC, Bruenger FW. Efficient synthesis of *N*-[2-hydroxyethoxy)methyl]-2-alkyl-3-hydroxy-4-pyridinone by a modified

Hilbert–Johnson reaction. *Synthetic Commun.* *26*, **1996**, 2681–6.
361 Robins MJ, Hatfield PW. Nucleic acid related compounds. 37. Convenient and high-yield synthesis of *N*-[(2-hydroxyethoxy)methyl] heterocycles as "acyclic nucleoside" analogues. *Can J. Chem.* *60*, **1982**, 547–53.
362 Schaeffer HJ, Gurwara S, Vince R, Bittner S. Novel substrate of adenosine deaminase. *J. Med. Chem.* *14*, **1971**, 367–9.
363 Streater M, Taylor PD, Hider RC, Porter J. Novel 3-hydroxy-2(1H)-pyridinones. Synthesis, iron(III)-chelating properties, and biological activity. *J. Med. Chem.* *33*, **1990**, 1749–55.
364 Harris RLN. Potential wool growth inhibitors. Improved synthesis of mimosine and related 4(1H)-pyridones. *Aust. J. Chem.* *29*, **1976**, 1329–34.
365 Niedballa U, Vorbrueggen H. A general synthesis of pyrimidine nucleosides. *Angew Chem. Int. Ed.* *9*, **1970**, 461–2.
366 Smith MA, Harris PL, Sayre LM, Perry G. Iron accumulation in Alzheimer's disease is a source of redox-generated free radicals. *Proc. Natl Acad. Sci. USA* *94*, **1997**, 9866–8.
367 Arano Y, Matsushima H, Tagawa M, Koizumi M, Endo K, Konishi J, Yokoyama A. A novel bifunctional metabolizable linker for the conjugation of antibodies with radionuclides. *Bioconjug. Chem.* *2*, **1991**, 71–6.
368 Hider RC, Taylor PD, Walkinshaw M, Wang JL, van der Helm D. Crystal structure of 3-hydroxy-1,2-dimethyl-pyridin-4(1H)-one: an iron (III) chelator study. *J. Chem. Res. Synop.* *10*, **1990**, 316–7.
369 Nelson WO, Karpishin TB, Retting SJ, Orvig C. Physical and structural studies of *N*-substituted-3-hydroxy-2-methyl-4(1H)-pyridinones. *Can. J. Chem.* *66*, **1988**, 123–31.
370 Charalambous J, Dodd A, McPartlin M, Matondo SOC, Pathirana ND, Powell HR. Synthesis and X-ray crystal structure of tris(1,2-dimethyl-3-hydroxypyrid-4-onato)iron(III). *Polyhedron* *7*, **1988**, 2235–7.
371 Xiao GY, van der Helm D, Hider RC, Rai BL. Molecular modeling studies of a ferric hexadentate 3-hydroxy-2(1*H*)-pyridinone complex and an analogue by molecular mechanics, molecular dynamics, and free energy perturbation simulations. *J. Phys. Chem.* *100*, **1996**, 2345–52.
372 Kaneko Y, Kitamato T, Tateishi J, Yamaguchi K. Ferritin immunohistochemistry as a marker for microglia. *Acta Neuropathol.* *79*, **1989**, 129–36.
373 Thompson CM, Markesbery WR, Ehmann WD, Mao YX, Vance DE. Regional brain trace-element studies in Alzheimer's disease. *Neurotoxicology* *9*, **1988**, 1–7.
374 Kontoghiorghes GJ. Iron mobilization from ferritin using α-oxohydroxy heteroaromatic chelators. *Biochem. J.* *233*, **1986**, 299–302.
375 Liu G, Men P, Harris PL, Rolston RK, Perry G, Smith MA. Nanoparticle iron chelators: a new therapeutic approach in Alzheimer disease and other neurologic disorders associated with trace metal imbalance. *Neurosci Lett.* *406*, **2006**, 189–93.
376 Hallaway PE, Eaton JW, Panter SS, Hedlund BE. Modulation of deferoxamine toxicity and clearance by covalent attachment to biocompatible polymers. *Proc. Natl Acad. Sci. USA* *86*, **1989**, 108–12.
377 Panter SS, Braughler JM, Hall ED. Dextran-coupled deferoxamine improves outcome in a murine model of head injury. *J. Neurotrauma* *9*, **1992**, 47–53.
378 Drugas GT, Paidas CN, Yahanda AM, Ferguson D, Clemens MG. Conjugated desferoxamine attenuates hepatic microvascular injury following ischemia/reperfusion. *Circ. Shock* *34*, **1991**, 278–83.
379 Horowitz D, Margel S, Shimoni T. Iron detoxification by haemoperfusion through deferoxamine-conjugated agarose-polyacrolein microsphere beads. *Biomaterials* *6*, **1985**, 9–16.

380 Golenser J, Domb A, Teomim D, Tsafack A, Nisim O, Ponka P, Eling W, Cabantchik ZI. The treatment of animal models of malaria with iron chelators by use of a novel polymeric device for slow drug release. *J. Pharmacol. Exp. Ther. 281*, **1997**, 1127–35.

381 Lowther N, Sparks K, Nicklin J, Jin Y. A novel depot preparation of desferrioxamine-B: development of formulation principles. *Drug Dev. Ind. Pharm. 25*, **1999**, 1157–66.

382 Venkataram S, Khohlokwane M. Microencapsulation of an iron chelator for sustained release and crystal habit modification. *J. Microencapsul. 13*, **1996**, 519–25.

383 Anjaneyulu PS, Staros JV. Reactions of *N*-hydroxysulfosuccinimide active esters. *Int. J. Pept. Protein Res. 30*, **1987**, 117–24.

384 Staros JV, Wright RW, Swingle DM. Enhancement by *N*-hydroxysulfosuccinimide of water-soluble carbodiimide-mediated coupling reactions. *Anal. Biochem. 156*, **1986**, 220–2.

385 Shi Y, Eyring EM, van Eldik R, Liu G, Bruenger FW, Miller SC. Kinetics and mechanisms of Fe(III) complexation by lipophilic 3-hydroxy-2methyl-1(γ-stearoamidopropyl)-4-pyridinone (HMSP). *J. Bioinorg. Chem. 2*, **1997**, 728–43.

386 Michaelis M, Langer K, Arnold S, Doerr HW, Kreuter J, Cinatl Jr J. Pharmacological activity of DTPA linked to protein-based drug carrier systems. *Biochem. Biophys. Res. Commun. 323*, **2004**, 1236–40.

Index

Nanotechnologies for the Life Sciences Vol. 10
Nanomaterials for Medical Diagnosis and Therapy. Edited by Challa S. S. R. Kumar

ISBN: 978-3-527-31390-7

d

o

Related Titles

Kumar, C. S. S. R., Hormes, J., Leuschner, C. (eds.)

Nanofabrication Towards Biomedical Applications

Techniques, Tools, Applications, and Impact

442 pages with 161 figures and 19 tables
2005. Hardcover
ISBN-13: 978-3-527-31115-6
ISBN-10: 3-527-31115-7

Schleef, M. (ed.)

DNA-Pharmaceuticals

Formulation and Delivery in Gene Therapy, DNA Vaccination and Immunotherapy

275 pages with 37 figures and 11 tables
2005. Hardcover
ISBN-13: 978-3-527-31187-3
ISBN-10: 3-527-31187-4

Prendergast, G. C. (ed.)

Molecular Cancer Therapeutics

Strategies for Drug Discovery and Development

approx. 368 pages
2004. Hardcover
ISBN-13: 978-0-471-43202-9
ISBN-10: 0-471-43202-4

Seifert, R., Wieland, T. (eds.)

G Protein-coupled Receptors as Drug Targets

Analysis of Activation and Constitutive Activity

304 pages
2005. Hardcover
ISBN-13: 978-3-527-30819-4
ISBN-10: 3-527-30819-9

Goodsell, D. S.

Bionanotechnology

Lessons from Nature

338 pages
2004. Hardcover
ISBN-13: 978-0-471-41719-4
ISBN-10: 0-471-41719-X